FIRST AID FOR THE®
BASIC SCIENCES

Organ Systems

Third Edition

SENIOR EDITORS

TAO LE, MD, MHS
Associate Clinical Professor
Chief, Section of Allergy and Immunology
Department of Medicine
University of Louisville School of Medicine

WILLIAM L. HWANG, MD, PhD
Resident, Harvard Radiation Oncology Program
Massachusetts General Hospital
Brigham & Women's Hospital

EDITORS

VINAYAK MURALIDHAR, MD, MSc
Resident, Harvard Radiation Oncology Program
Massachusetts General Hospital
Brigham & Women's Hospital

JARED A. WHITE, MD
Resident, Department of Surgery
Division of Plastic and Reconstructive Surgery
University of Florida College of Medicine

M. SCOTT MOORE, DO
Clinical Research Fellow
Affiliated Laboratories

Mc
Graw
Hill
Education

New York / Chicago / San Francisco / Athens / London / Madrid / Mexico City
Milan / New Delhi / Singapore / Sydney / Toronto

NOTICE

Medicine is an ever-changing science. As new research and clinical experience broaden our knowledge, changes in treatment and drug therapy are required. The authors and the publisher of this work have checked with sources believed to be reliable in their efforts to provide information that is complete and generally in accord with the standards accepted at the time of publication. However, in view of the possibility of human error or changes in medical sciences, neither the authors nor the publisher nor any other party who has been involved in the preparation or publication of this work warrants that the information contained herein is in every respect accurate or complete, and they disclaim all responsibility for any errors or omissions or for the results obtained from use of the information contained in this work. Readers are encouraged to confirm the information contained herein with other sources. For example and in particular, readers are advised to check the product information sheet included in the package of each drug they plan to administer to be certain that the information contained in this work is accurate and that changes have not been made in the recommended dose or in the contraindications for administration. This recommendation is of particular importance in connection with new or infrequently used drugs.

Disclosure: The opinions or assertions contained herein are the private views of the authors and are not to be construed as official or as reflecting the views of the Department of Defense, the United States Military, or the Department of Health and Human Services.

The editor was Christina M. Thomas.
The production supervisor was Jeffrey Herzich.
Project management was provided by Rainbow Graphics.

Library of Congress Cataloging-in-Publication Data
Le, Tao.
 First aid for the basic sciences. Organ systems / Tao Le.
  p. ; cm.
 Organ systems
 Third edition. | New York : McGraw-Hill Education, [2017] | Includes index.
 LCCN 2016017904 | ISBN 9781259587030 (paperback : alk. paper) | ISBN 1259587037
 (paperback : alk. paper)
 1. MESH: Internal Medicine | Outlines.
 LCC R834.5 | NLM WB 18.2 | DDC 616.0076--dc23 LC record available at https://lccn.loc.gov/2016017904

DEDICATION

To the contributors to this and future editions, who took time to share their knowledge,
insight, and humor for the benefit of students and physicians everywhere.

and

To our families, friends, and loved ones, who supported us
in the task of writing this book.

Contents

Contributing Authors vi
Faculty Reviewers vii
Preface ix
How to Use This Book x
Acknowledgments xi
How to Contribute xiii

CHAPTER 1. Cardiovascular 1
Embryology 2
Anatomy 9
Physiology 14
Pathology 52
Imaging/Diagnostic Tests 90
Pharmacology 91

CHAPTER 2. Endocrine 107
Hypothalamus and Pituitary 108
Thyroid and Parathyroid 126
Adrenal Gland 147
Pancreas 158

CHAPTER 3. Gastrointestinal 171
Embryology 172
Anatomy 178
Physiology 192
Pathology 210
Pharmacology 258

CHAPTER 4. Hematology and Oncology 265
Embryology 266
Anatomy 267
Pathology 272
Pharmacology 310

CHAPTER 5. Musculoskeletal, Skin, and Connective Tissue 323
Embryology 324
Anatomy 335
Physiology 354
Pathology 362
Pharmacology 402

CHAPTER 6. Neurology and Special Senses ... 411
Embryology, Anatomy, and Physiology 412
Histology 464
Pathology 468
Pharmacology 507

CHAPTER 7. Psychiatry 533
Basic Definitions and Concepts 534
Pathology 539

CHAPTER 8. Renal 583
Embryology 584
Anatomy 587
Histology 590
Physiology 594
Pathology 623
Pharmacology 655

CHAPTER 9. Reproductive 661
Embryology 662
Anatomy 674
Physiology 681
Pathology—Genetic Diseases 700
Pathology—Female 703
Pathology—Male 733
Pharmacology 741

CHAPTER 10. Respiratory 747
Embryology 748
Anatomy 753
Histology 758
Physiology 761
Pathology 779
Pharmacology 818

Image Acknowledgments 825
Index 841
About the Editors 896

CONTRIBUTING AUTHORS

Haripriya S. Ayyala, MD
Resident, Department of Surgery
Rutgers New Jersey Medical School

James E. Bates, MD
Resident, Department of Radiation Oncology
University of Florida, College of Medicine

Deep Bhatt, MD
University of Iowa Carver College of Medicine
Class of 2016

Aaron J. Cohen
Harvard Medical School
Class of 2017

Eric Dowling, MD
University of North Dakota School of Medicine & Health
    Sciences
Class of 2016

Rachelle Dugue, PhD
SUNY Downstate Medical Center
Class of 2018

Reed Gilbow, MD
Resident, Department of Otolaryngology–Head and Neck Surgery
University of Virginia School of Medicine

Thomas P. Howard
Harvard Medical School
Class of 2020

Toufic R. Jildeh, MD
Resident, Department of Orthopaedic Surgery
Henry Ford Hospital

Zachary Johnson, MD
Resident, Department of Neurological Surgery
University of Texas Southwestern Medical Center

James J. Jones Jr., MD
Resident, Transitional Year Department
San Antonio Military Medical Center

James Murchison, MD
Texas Tech University Health Sciences Center School of
    Medicine
Class of 2016

Michael Oh, MD
Resident, Department of Medicine
McGaw Medical Center of Northwestern University

Brent Pickrell, MD
Resident, Plastic & Reconstructive Surgery
Harvard Medical School

Jasmine Rana
Harvard Medical School
Class of 2017

Heather Schopper
University of Iowa Carver College of Medicine
Class of 2017

Harrison To, MD
Resident, Department of Anesthesiology
University of California, San Diego

Elisa Walsh
Harvard Medical School
Class of 2017

Benjamin Weisenthal, MD
Resident, Department of Orthopaedic Surgery and
    Rehabilitation
Vanderbilt University Medical Center

Wenhui Zhou
Tufts University School of Medicine
Class of 2019

Andrew Zureick
University of Michigan Medical School
Class of 2018

FACULTY REVIEWERS

Zafia Anklesaria, MD
Fellow, Division of Pulmonary and Critical Care Medicine
Department of Medicine
David Geffen School of Medicine at UCLA

Mary Beth Babos, PharmD
Associate Professor of Pharmacotherapy
DeBusk College of Osteopathic Medicine
Lincoln Memorial University

Brooks D. Cash, MD
Professor of Medicine, Division of Gastroenterology
University of South Alabama School of Medicine

Ammar Chaudhry, MD
Neuroradiologist, Department of Radiology
Johns Hopkins Medical Institute

Jaimini Chauhan, MD
Physician, Geriatric Psychiatry and Adult Psychiatry
Lincoln Medical and Mental Health Center
Weill Cornell Medical College

Jeffrey J. Gold, MD, PhD
Associate Professor, Department of Neurology
University of California, San Diego School of Medicine

Nancy Hsu, MD
Fellow, Pulmonary and Critical Care Medicine
David Geffen School of Medicine at UCLA

Peter Marks, MD, PhD
Center for Biologics Evaluation and Research
U.S. Food and Drug Administration

Kathryn Melamed, MD
Fellow, Pulmonary and Critical Care Medicine
David Geffen School of Medicine at UCLA

Jeannine Rahimian, MD, MBA
Associate Professor, Obstetrics and Gynecology
David Geffen School of Medicine at UCLA

Soroush Rais-Bahrami, MD
Assistant Professor, Urology and Radiology
The University of Alabama at Birmingham School of Medicine

Melanie Schorr, MD
Assistant in Medicine, Department of Medicine
Massachusetts General Hospital

Prashant Vaishnava, MD
Assistant Professor, Department of Medicine
Mount Sinai Hospital and Icahn School of Medicine

Tisha Wang, MD
Associate Clinical Professor, Division of Pulmonary and Critical
  Care Medicine
Department of Medicine
David Geffen School of Medicine at UCLA

Adam Weinstein, MD
Assistant Professor, Pediatric Nephrology
Geisel School of Medicine at Dartmouth

Preface

With this third edition of *First Aid for the Basic Sciences: Organ Systems*, we continue our commitment to providing students with the most useful and up-to-date preparation guides for the USMLE Step 1. For the past year, a team of authors and editors have worked to update and further improve this third edition. This edition represents a major revision in many ways.

- Every page has been carefully reviewed and updated to reflect the most high-yield material for the Step 1 exam.
- New high-yield figures, tables, and mnemonics have been incorporated.
- Margin elements, including flashcards, have been added to assist in optimizing the studying process.
- Hundreds of user comments and suggestions have been incorporated.
- Emphasis is on deeper understanding and integration of critical concepts.

This book would not have been possible without the help of the hundreds of students and faculty members who contributed their feedback and suggestions. We invite students and faculty to please share their thoughts and ideas to help us improve *First Aid for the Basic Sciences: Organ Systems*. (See How to Contribute, p. xiii.)

Louisville   Tao Le
Boston   William Hwang

How to Use This Book

Both this text and its companion, *First Aid for the Basic Sciences: General Principles*, are designed to fill the need for a high-quality, in-depth, conceptually driven study guide for the USMLE Step 1. They can be used either alone or in conjunction with the original *First Aid for the USMLE Step 1*. In this way, students can tailor their own studying experience, calling on either series, according to their mastery of each subject.

Medical students who have used the previous editions of this guide have given us feedback on how best to make use of the book.

- **It is recommended that you begin using this book as early as possible** when learning the basic medical sciences. We advise that you use this book as a companion to your preclinical medical school courses to provide a guide for the concepts that are most important for the USMLE Step 1.
- As you study each discipline, **use the corresponding section in *First Aid for the Basic Sciences: Organ Systems*** to consolidate the material, deepen your understanding, or clarify concepts.
- As you approach the test, use both *First Aid for the Basic Sciences: General Principles* and *First Aid for the Basic Sciences: Organ Systems* to review challenging concepts.
- Use the margin elements (ie, Flash Forward, Flash Back, Key Fact, Clinical Correlation, Mnemonic, Flash Cards) to test yourself throughout your studies.

To **broaden** your learning strategy, you can **integrate** your *First Aid for the Basic Sciences: Organ Systems* study with *First Aid for the USMLE Step 1*, *First Aid Cases for the USMLE Step 1*, and *First Aid Q&A for the USMLE Step 1* on a chapter-by-chapter basis.

Acknowledgments

This has been a collaborative project from the start. We gratefully acknowledge the thoughtful comments and advice of the residents, international medical graduates, medical students, and faculty who have supported the editors and authors in the development of *First Aid for the Basic Sciences: Organ Systems*.

For support and encouragement throughout the process, we are grateful to Thao Pham. Thanks to Louise Petersen for organizing and supporting the project.

Furthermore, we wish to give credit to our amazing editors and authors, who worked tirelessly on the manuscript. We never cease to be amazed by their dedication, thoughtfulness, and creativity.

Thanks to our publisher, McGraw-Hill Education, for their assistance and guidance. For outstanding editorial work, we thank Isabel Nogueira, Emma Underdown, and Catherine Johnson. Thank you to our USMLE-Rx/ScholarRx team of editors, Virginia Abbott, Allison Battista, Linda Geisler, Ruth Kaufman, and Hannah Warnshuis. A special thanks to Rainbow Graphics, especially David Hommel, for remarkable production work.

We are also very grateful to Dr. Artemisa Gogollari and our medical illustrator, Hans Neuhart, for their creative work on the new illustrations. We also acknowledge, with thanks, Dr. Herman Singh Bagga, Dr. John Breinholt, and Dr. Howard M. Steinman for their review of the new illustrations. Thanks also to the faculty at Uniformed Services University of the Health Sciences for use of their images and Dr. Richard Usatine for his outstanding dermatologic and clinical image contributions.

For contributions and corrections, we thank Patrick Achkar, Tareq Al Saadi, Ashley Aluko, Nicholas Alvey, Joseph Anaya, M. Anna, Christie Atchison, Nicholas Austin, Maria Bakkal, Konstantinos Belogiannis, Rayyan Bhuiyan, Luigi Bonini, Wynne Callon, Anup Chalise, Alex Chan, Christopher Chan, Vincent Chan, Shengchieh Chang, Bridget Chen, Emanuela Cimpeanu, Dave Comstock, Steven Core, Malcolm Debaun, Douglas Dembinski, Nolan Derr, Baljinder Dhillon, Keith Do, Devin Dunatov, Mohamed Ebrahim, Alejandra Ellison-Barnes, Matt Fishman, Maikel Ragaei Ramzi Gerges, Gregory Giles, Hillary Glick, Richard Godby, Carma Goldstein, Jan Andre Grauman, Joshua Gross, Priscilla Haakenson, Jessie Hanna, John Haydek, Jennifer Hou, Jennifer Hsu, David Hung, Mohammad Ismail, Victoria Jang, Caroline Jones, Kamran Karim, Ari Kassardjian, Raphael Keegan, Richard Kozinski, Joe Lai, Michael Larkin, Jesse Lee, Nicholas Linkous, Huy Ly, James Malcolm, Deborah Marshall, Lucas Mihalovich, Jan Neander, Paul Nicholson, Lola Ogunsuyi, Mario Weert Pande, Aaron Parzuchowski, Jay Patel, Toral Patel, Yelyzaveta Plechysta, Stephanie Pollard, Nathan Potter, Jennifer Pruitt, Chayawut Punsriwong, Pim Puttawibul, Ryan Qasawa, Peter Francis Raguindin, Eric Raynal, Thea Recai, Amanda Ries, Syed Rizvi, John Roberts, Paul Rutkowski, Tor Sauter, Jeffrey Savin, James Seymour, Christienne Shams, Joshua Siewert, Racquel Skold, Justin Smith, Peter Soh, Allison Sweeney, Jacob Szafranski, John Thomas, Akesh Thomas, David Tobin, Judy Trieu, Chris Tufts, Michael Turgeon, Itzel Vazquez, Grace Wang, Lily Wang, Joseph Wilson, Teepawat Witeerungrot, Matthew Wolcott, Alisa Yamasaki, Raymond Yeow, Carl Youssef, and Parvin Zafarani.

Louisville	Tao Le
Boston	William Hwang

How to Contribute

To continue to produce a high-yield review source for the USMLE Step 1, you are invited to submit any suggestions or corrections. We also offer paid internships in medical education and publishing ranging from three months to one year (see below for details). Please send us your suggestions for:

- New facts, mnemonics, diagrams, and illustrations
- High-yield topics that may reappear on future Step 1 examinations
- Corrections and other suggestions

For each new entry incorporated into the next edition, you will receive up to a $20 **Amazon.com gift card** as well as personal acknowledgment in the next edition. Significant contributions will be compensated at the discretion of the authors. Also let us know about material in this edition that you feel is low yield and should be deleted.

All submissions including potential errata should ideally be supported with hyperlinks to a dynamically updated Web resource such as UpToDate, AccessMedicine, or ClinicalKey.

We welcome potential errata on grammar and style if the change improves readability. Please note that *First Aid* style is somewhat unique; for example, we have fully adopted the AMA *Manual of Style* recommendations on eponyms ("We recommend that the possessive form be omitted in eponymous terms") and on abbreviations (no periods with eg, ie, etc).

The preferred way to submit new entries, clarifications, mnemonics, or potential corrections with a valid, authoritative reference is via our website: **www.firstaidteam. com.**

Alternatively, you can email us at: **firstaidteam@yahoo.com.**

NOTE TO CONTRIBUTORS

All contributions become property of the authors and are subject to editing and reviewing. Please verify all data and spellings carefully. Contributions should be supported by at least two high-quality references. In the event that similar or duplicate entries are received, only the first complete entry received with valid, authoritative references will be credited. Please follow the style, punctuation, and format of this edition as much as possible.

AUTHOR OPPORTUNITIES

The *First Aid* author team is pleased to offer part-time and full-time paid internships in medical education and publishing to motivated medical students and physicians. Internships range from a few months (eg, a summer) up to a full year. Participants will have an opportunity to author, edit, and earn academic credit on a wide variety of projects, including the popular *First Aid* series.

English writing/editing experience, familiarity with Microsoft Word, and Internet access are required. For more information, email us at **firstaidteam@yahoo.com** with a résumé and summary of your interest or sample work.

CHAPTER 1

Cardiovascular

EMBRYOLOGY   2
  Development of the Heart   2
  Summary of Congenital Heart Lesions   4
  Congenital Cardiac Defect Associations   7
  Fetal-Postnatal Derivatives   8
  Fetal Erythropoiesis   8
  Fetal Circulation   8

ANATOMY   9
  Surfaces and Borders of the Heart   9
  Relationships of the Heart and Great Vessels   10
  Heart Valves and Sites of Auscultation   10
  Layers of the Heart   10
  Coronary Artery Anatomy   12
  Conduction System   13

PHYSIOLOGY   14
  Cardiac Electrophysiology   14
  Cardiac Muscle and Contraction   20
  Cardiac Output   23
  Pressure-Volume Loops   26
  Cardiac and Vascular Function Curves   27
  The Cardiac Cycle   29
  Hemodynamics and Peripheral Vascular Circulation   32
  Measurement and Regulation of Arterial Pressure   35
  Electrocardiography   40
  Arrhythmias   46

PATHOLOGY   52
  Hypertension   52
  Arteriosclerosis   54
  Myocarditis   57

Endocarditis   58
Rheumatic Fever   60
Cardiomyopathies   61
Congestive Heart Failure   63
Aneurysms   66
Heart Murmurs   67
Cardiac Tumors   73
Venous Disease   73
Emboli   76
Shock   77
Pericardial Disease   78
Peripheral Vascular Disease   81
Ischemic Heart Disease   86
Coronary Steal Phenomenon   86
Myocardial Infarction   87
Chronic Ischemic Heart Disease   89

IMAGING/DIAGNOSTIC TESTS   90
  Radiography   90
  Echocardiography   90
  Cardiac Catheterization   90
  Nuclear Imaging   90
  Stress Testing   90
  Pericardiocentesis   91

PHARMACOLOGY   91
  Antihypertensive Agents   91
  Antianginal Therapy   100
  Drugs Used in Heart Failure   101
  Antiarrhythmics   103
  Lipid-Lowering Agents   103

Embryology

DEVELOPMENT OF THE HEART

Embryonic Heart Structures and Adult Derivatives

By the third week of development, the rapidly growing embryo can no longer rely on simple diffusion from the placenta for its metabolic and oxygen requirements. It is no surprise, then, that the heart is the first functioning organ in vertebrate embryos, and a primitive heart begins to beat by week 4 of development (Table 1-1).

Development and Looping of Heart Tube

A primitive heart tube develops from mesodermal cells at the cranial end of the embryo during gastrulation. The steps of looping are as follows:

1. Primitive heart chambers lined with endothelial cells form along the cranial-caudal axis of the heart tube.
2. Rapid elongation of the heart tube occurs in a confined space (the pericardial cavity), requiring that it bend into a U-shaped loop that places the primitive atrium behind the more-prominent primitive ventricle. Note that in the early stages, the primitive atrium is connected to the ventricle via a common **atrioventricular (AV) canal.**

Formation of Septa

Heart septa divide the atrioventricular canal, atrium, ventricle, and aortiocopulmonary (ventricular outflow) tract into discrete chambers. Septa form between the fourth and sixth weeks of development from inward growth of the innermost (endocardial) cardiac surface. Although all septation events occur simultaneously, for clarity, these steps are detailed individually for each structure below.

Atrioventricular Canal Septum

The common AV canal is split into two canals by **endocardial cushions,** which are endocardial inward growths that fuse together from the anterior and posterior canal walls.

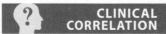

CLINICAL CORRELATION

Defects in **dynein** (protein in cilia involved in L/R asymmetry) or cardiac looping can lead to **dextrocardia,** a condition in which the heart lies on the right side of the thorax. It often accompanies Kartagener syndrome, an autosomal recessive genetic disorder that results in dysfunctional cilia in the reproductive and genitourinary tracts as well.

CLINICAL CORRELATION

Patent foramen ovale (PFO) results from failure of the septum primum and septum secundum to fuse after birth. Because no atrial septal tissue is absent, it is not a true atrial septal defect (ASD). It is usually asymptomatic if left atrial pressure exceeds right atrial pressure, which forces the septum primum—although not fused—to stay closed up against the septum secundum.

TABLE 1-1.   Embryonic Heart Structures and Adult Derivatives

EMBRYONIC STRUCTURE	ADULT STRUCTURE
Truncus arteriosus	Ascending aorta and pulmonary trunk
Bulbus cordis	Smooth parts (outflow tract) of left and right ventricles
Primitive ventricle	Trabeculated parts of left and right ventricles
Primitive atrium	Trabeculated parts of left and right atria
Left horn of sinus venosus (SV)	Coronary sinus (largest venous drainage of heart)
Right horn of SV	Smooth part of right atrium
Right common cardinal vein and right anterior cardinal vein	Superior vena cava
Vitelline veins	Portal system

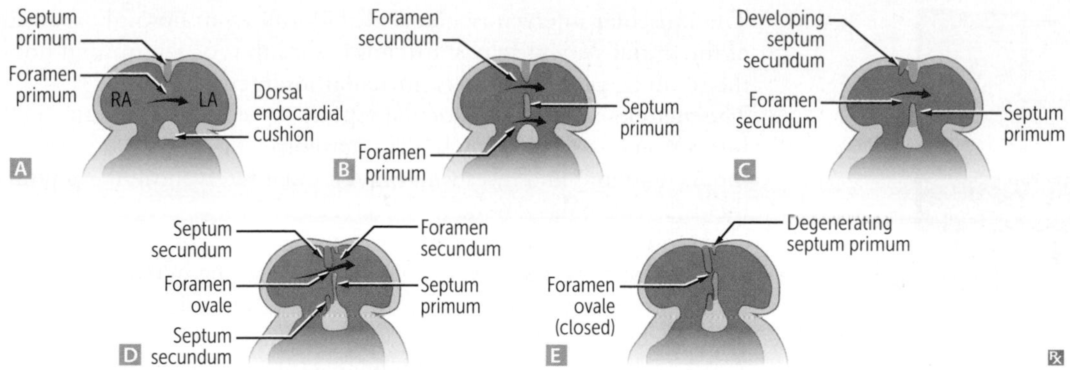

Septum primum — Foramen primum — RA → LA — Dorsal endocardial cushion

A

Foramen secundum — Septum primum — Foramen primum

B

Developing septum secundum — Foramen secundum — Septum primum

C

Septum secundum — Foramen ovale — Septum secundum — Foramen secundum — Septum primum

D

Degenerating septum primum — Foramen ovale (closed)

E

FIGURE 1-1. **Embryologic development of the atrial septum.**

Abnormal fusion of endocardial cushions can lead to **endocardial cushion defects**, which are a broad class of congenital heart defects with abnormal septation of the atria, ventricle, and/or AV canal.

Atrial Septum

The atrial septum is responsible for the initial division of the primitive atrium into the left and right atria. The steps of development are as follows:

1. The **septum primum** begins to grow toward the atrioventricular (AV) cushions (Figure 1-1A). The orifice (ie, ostium) between the leading edge of the septum primum and the AV cushions is termed the **ostium primum** (aka foramen primum). The ostium primum is obliterated when the septum primum reaches the AV septum.
2. The **ostium secundum** (aka foramen secundum) is formed as tissue degenerates in the superior septum primum (Figure 1-1B).
3. The **septum secundum** forms alongside the right edge of the septum primum (Figure 1-1C).
4. The septum secundum contains the **foramen ovale**, which allows blood to be shunted from the right atrium (RA) to the left atrium (LA) during fetal life (Figure 1-1D). The septum primum to the left of the septum secundum helps act as a one-way valve for right-to-left flow. After birth, the increase in pressure in the LA causes the septum primum to close and fuse against the septum secundum, forming the mature interatrial septum (Figure 1-1E).

An **atrial septal defect (ASD)** is an opening in the atrial septum, allowing blood to flow between the atria (Figure 1-2). The **most common form is the ostium secundum type** located in the region of the foramen ovale, which is due to excessive resorption of the septum primum or inadequate formation of the septum secundum. Patients are typically asymptomatic until adulthood, but the clinical course depends on the size of the defect.

Classic signs of ASD include the following:

- **Wide, fixed splitting of S$_2$:** Normal splitting occurs because of increased right ventricle preload during inspiration that delays closure of pulmonary valve. In ASD, the right ventricle is always preload overloaded from the left-to-right shunt, and thus there is no increase in splitting during inspiration.
- **Pulmonic flow murmur** due to increased flow across the pulmonary valve heard best in the second intercostal space along the left sternal border.

Interventricular Septum

The interventricular septum consists of two parts: the **muscular** portion and the **membranous** portion.

CLINICAL CORRELATION

Due to left-to-right shunting in ASD, right atrial and ventricle enlargement occurs. On ECG, this results in tall P waves (best seen in leads II and V$_1$/V$_2$), which reflect atrial enlargement, and signs of RVH (eg, QRS right axis deviation).

CLINICAL CORRELATION

A failure of the septum primum to fuse with the endocardial cushions can lead to an **ostium primum** ASD at the inferior part of the atrial septum. This type of endocardial cushion defect is associated with trisomy 21.

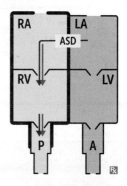

FIGURE 1-2. **Atrial septal defect (ASD).** In ASD, there is a left-to-right shunt between the atria. The right atrium (RA), right ventricle (RV), and pulmonary artery (P) become enlarged (indicated by bolded borders of heart chambers) owing to the influx of additional blood via the ASD left-to-right shunt. A, aorta; LA, left atrium; LV, left ventricle.

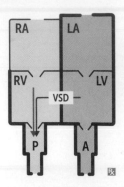

FIGURE 1-3. Ventricular septal defect (VSD). In VSD, there is a left-to-right shunt between the ventricles. The left atrium (LA) and left ventricle (LV) become enlarged (indicated by bolded borders of heart chambers) as a result of blood flow through this left-to-right shunt into the pulmonary artery and back into the left atrium and ventricle. Right ventricle (RV) and right atrium (RA) enlargement may also be present. Over time, Eisenmenger syndrome can occur as a result of the VSD. A, aorta; P, pulmonary artery.

MNEMONIC

The 5 T's of early cyanosis (right-to-left shunts):

1. **T**runcus arteriosus (1 vessel)
2. **T**ransposition (2 switched vessels)
3. **T**ricuspid atresia (3 = tri)
4. **T**etralogy of Fallot (4 = tetra)
5. **T**APVR (5 letters in the name)

CLINICAL CORRELATION

Persistent truncus arteriosis is often associated with **DiGeorge syndrome.**

MNEMONIC

Tetralogy of Fallot—

PROVe

Pulmonic stenosis
RV hypertrophy
Overriding aorta
VSD

- The **muscular** interventricular **septum** forms as an upward expansion of the base of the primitive ventricle. It extends toward the AV septum but does not reach it; the resulting gap is the **interventricular foramen.**
- The **membranous** interventricular **septum** is created by the fusion of the aorticopulmonary septum with the muscular intraventricular septum. It grows downward from the AV cushions and fuses with the muscular interventricular septum, obliterating the interventricular foramen.

Ventricular septal defect (VSD), an abnormal opening in the interventricular septum, is **the most common congenital heart malformation** (Figure 1-3). The most common location is in the membranous interventricular septum, resulting from incomplete fusion of the AV cushions with aorticopulmonary septum. Clinical manifestations of a VSD vary depending on the size of the defect. Fifty percent of small VSDs undergo complete or sufficient partial closure by age 2 and do not require intervention. Larger VSDs result in left-to-right shunting of blood, and, as a result, may present with late cyanosis.

- A classic symptom is **easy fatigability.**
- Cardiac auscultation reveals a **harsh holosystolic murmur** heard best at the left lower sternal border.

Aorticopulmonary Septum

The **aorticopulmonary (AP) septum** is derived from **neural crest cells** that migrate into the primitive ventricular outflow tract. It is responsible for separating the **truncus arteriosus** into the aorta and pulmonary artery. As the septum descends, it **spirals 180 degrees** so that the aorta becomes the left ventricular outflow tract and the pulmonary trunk becomes the right ventricular outflow tract. Failure of spiraling leads to congenital malformations that involve **right-to-left shunting and early cyanosis in the newborn period.**

- **Persistent truncus arteriosus** results from abnormal migration of neural crest cells and subsequent **failure of formation of the AP septum.** Therefore, separation of the left ventricular and right ventricular outflow tracts never occurs. The aorta and pulmonary trunk form a common tract leaving the ventricles, which allows mixing of oxygenated and deoxygenated blood.
- **Transposition of the great vessels** occurs when the AP septum fails to spiral 180 degrees. The left ventricle (LV) is connected to the pulmonary trunk, and the right ventricle (RV) is connected to the aorta (Figure 1-4). This condition results in a complete **right-to-left shunt** and **early cyanosis.**
- **Tetralogy of Fallot** is caused by **anterior displacement of the AP septum.** The four abnormalities are overriding aorta, pulmonic stenosis, RV hypertrophy, and VSD (Figure 1-5). The primary defect is termed an "**overriding aorta,**" because the misplaced aorta partially obstructs the right ventricular outflow tract, leading to **right ventricular outflow obstruction (pulmonic stenosis).** Pulmonic stenosis leads to increased pressures in the RV and subsequent **right ventricular hypertrophy.** The **membranous VSD** results from a failure of fusion between the AP septum and the muscular portion of the intraventricular septum (IVS). **Right-to-left shunting** results in **early cyanosis.**

SUMMARY OF CONGENITAL HEART LESIONS

Congenital heart lesions are classified as **cyanotic** or **noncyanotic** based on the appearance of the infant at birth. **Cyanosis** is the purple-blue skin and mucous membrane discoloration due to an increased level of deoxyhemoglobin from decreased oxygen levels in systemic circulation.

Cyanotic Congenital Heart Lesions

Cyanosis is caused by lesions that lead to **right-to-left shunting** of blood, in which blood coming from the right ventricle bypasses lungs to various degrees before entering systemic circulation.

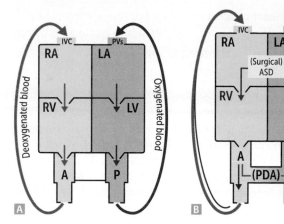

FIGURE 1-4.   **Transposition of the great vessels.** Developmental defect in which the left ventricle connects to the pulmonary artery and the right ventricle connects to the aorta, resulting in two closed circuits. **A** Without a patent ductus arteriosus (PDA) and atrial septal defect (ASD), a closed circuit results that is incompatible with life. **B** With a PDA and ASD, a left-to-right shunt is created at the atrial level, and systemic circulation can receive oxygenated blood. Note: For infants awaiting more definitive surgical repair, prostaglandin E_1 (PGE) can be administered to maintain a PDA and an ASD can be surgically created. A, aorta; IVC, inferior vena cava; LA, left atrium; LV, left ventricle; P, pulmonary artery; PVs, pulmonary veins; RA, right atrium; RV, right ventricle.

These lesions can be remembered as the 5 Ts:

1. Tetralogy of Fallot (most common cause of early cyanosis)
2. Transposition of the great vessels
3. Truncus arteriosus
4. Total anomalous pulmonary venous return
5. Tricuspid atresia (Figure 1-6)

Squatting increases left-sided pressure or systemic vascular resistance (SVR) by compression of femoral arteries; this can make SVR higher than PVR (pulmonary vascular resistance, or right-sided pressure) and thus may decrease right-to-left shunting and allow more blood to pass through the pulmonary circulation before entering the systemic circulation, alleviating symptoms of cyanosis.

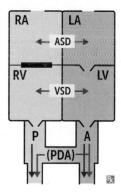

FIGURE 1-6.   **Tricuspid atresia.** Failure of the tricuspid valve to develop, preventing blood from flowing from the right atrium (RA) into the right ventricle (RV). In order for oxygenated blood to reach the body, an atrial septal defect (ASD) and ventricular septal defect (VSD) must simultaneously be present in order for blood from the RA to reach the RV and flow to the lungs to be oxygenated. A patent ductus arteriosus (PDA) can be maintained via the administration of prostaglandin E_2 (PGE_2) to permit blood flow from an ASD into the pulmonary artery (P), thereby allowing blood from the RA to flow into the P for oxygenation.

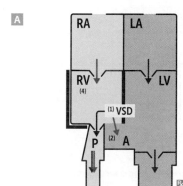

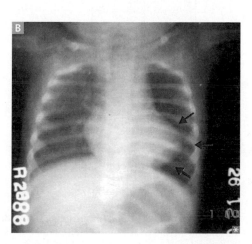

FIGURE 1-5.   **Tetralogy of Fallot.** **A** Four concurrent defects: (1) Ventricular septal defect (VSD), (2) an overriding aorta, causing (3) right ventricular outflow obstruction (pulmonic stenosis) and subsequent (4) right ventricular hypertrophy. The extent of R-L shunting is determined by the degree of pulmonic stenosis present. **B** As seen on x-ray, the heart appears boot-shaped (arrows). (A, aorta; LA, left atrium; LV, left ventricle; P, pulmonary artery; RA, right atrium; RV, right ventricle.)

Acyanotic Congenital Heart Lesions

Defects that do not produce early cyanosis at birth are termed **acyanotic** lesions and can be due to **stenotic lesions** or **left-to-right shunts**.

Stenotic Lesions

Coarctation of the Aorta

Coarctation of the aorta is aortic narrowing that typically occurs proximal to the ductus arteriosus (can be termed "preductal" or "postductal" based on location of the stenosis in relation to the ductus arteriosus), resulting in increased LV afterload. Coarctation can be symptomatic early (infantile form) or later in life (adult form), depending on severity of stenosis and if there is a patent ductus arteriosus (PDA) at birth:

- **Infantile form:** Aortic narrowing proximal to a PDA, which can lead to cyanosis of the lower half of the body due to right-to-left shunting via the PDA to vessels below the aortic arch. Note that the upper half of the body is supplied by branches of the aortic arch, which are unaffected by the distal right-to-left shunt (Figure 1-7A).

- **Adult form:** Aortic narrowing distal to the aortic arch without PDA (Figure 1-7B). Presents later in life, with hypertension in upper extremities (supplied by the branches of the aortic arch) and hypotension in lower extremities from decreased blood flow across the coarctation and absence of PDA. As a result, collateral circulation usually develops to route blood from the aorta to the lower extremities (from the proximal aorta via the subclavian artery, to the internal thoracic artery, to the superior epigastric artery, to the inferior epigastric artery, to the external iliac artery). Increased blood flow to the intercostal arteries causes them to dilate and eventually erode into ribs. This process results in the characteristic "rib notching" associated with coarctation of the aorta.

Congenital Aortic Stenosis

Congenital aortic stenosis is caused most often by abnormal development of the aortic valve that results in stenosis in the neonate. Bicuspid valves generally do not cause any obstruction at birth, but are more susceptible to calcification and fibrosis than normal tricuspid valves and often result in early-adulthood aortic stenosis.

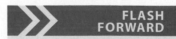

FLASH FORWARD

Indomethacin, a nonsteroidal anti-inflammatory drug (NSAID), is used to close a patent ductus arteriosus (PDA). Exogenous administration of prostaglandins (PGE$_2$) is used to keep a PDA open.

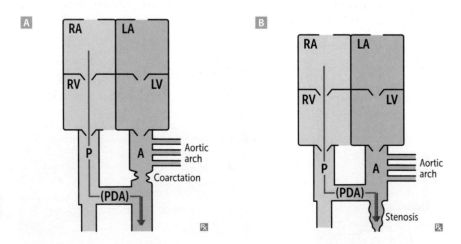

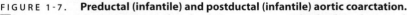

FIGURE 1-7. **Preductal (infantile) and postductal (infantile) aortic coarctation.**
A Narrowing of the aorta proximal to the ductus arteriosus. This leads to decreased blood flow distal to the coarctation, and a right-to-left shunt if the patent ductus arteriosus (PDA) is kept open (can lead to cyanosis of the lower half of the body). **B** Narrowing of the aorta distal to the ductus arteriosus. This leads to decreased blood flow to the lower body. A, aorta; LA, left atrium; LV, left ventricle; P, pulmonary artery; RA, right atrium; RV, right ventricle.

Left-to-Right Shunts

Ventricular Septal Defect

VSD is one of the most common congenital cardiac abnormalities; see earlier VSD discussion.

Atrial Septal Defect

An atrial septal defect has a loud S_1 and a wide, fixed split S_2; see earlier ASD discussion.

Patent Ductus Arteriosus

Within hours after birth, the increased oxygenation of blood and decreased circulation of prostaglandins through the ductus arteriosus mediate closure of the ductus. When this does not occur, a **patent ductus arteriosus** (PDA) can persist, leaving a connection between the left pulmonary artery and aortic arch (Figure 1-8). Because the left heart has higher pressures than right heart at birth, a left-to-right shunt develops, with blood flowing from the aorta into the pulmonary artery. It is most common in premature infants who are hypoxic. It does not result in early cyanosis, because there is no right-to-left shunting.

- Results in a continuous "machine-like" murmur because blood is flowing throughout systole and diastole from aorta into pulmonary artery.
- Administration of prostaglandin inhibitors (eg, indomethacin, nonsteroidal anti-inflammatory drugs [NSAIDs]) enhances closure of the PDA.

If these left-to-right shunts do not close, and high blood flow continues through the pulmonary circulation, the pulmonary arterial system becomes hypertrophic and even fibrotic, resulting in pulmonary hypertension. Increased right-sided pressure leads to right ventricular hypertrophy. When the right-sided pressure becomes higher than left-sided pressure, the shunt reverses and becomes right-to-left. This shunt reversal is termed **Eisenmenger syndrome** and causes **late cyanosis** in early adulthood from shunting of deoxygenated blood into systemic circulation.

CONGENITAL CARDIAC DEFECT ASSOCIATIONS

Certain disorders are associated with particular congenital cardiac malformations (Table 1-2).

TABLE 1-2. Disorders and Associated Cardiac Defects

DISORDER	CARDIAC DEFECT
22q11 Deletions	Truncus arteriosus, tetralogy of Fallot
Down syndrome	VSD, ASD, AV septal defect (endocardial cushion defect)
Turner syndrome	Coarctation of the aorta, bicuspid aortic valve, aortic dissection in adulthood
Offspring of a diabetic mother	Most commonly, transposition of the great vessels, VSD, and aortic stenosis
Congenital rubella	Septal defects, PDA, pulmonary artery stenosis
Marfan syndrome	Aortic insufficiency (due to aortic root dilation), mitral valve prolapse, aortic aneurysm/dissection

ASD, atrial septal defect; AV, atrioventricular; PDA, patent ductus arteriosus; VSD, ventricular septal defect.

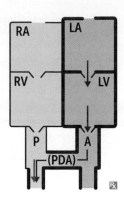

FIGURE 1-8. Patent ductus arteriosus (PDA). In PDA, a left-to-right shunt is present between the aorta (A) and pulmonary artery (P) due to the persistence of prostaglandins, a decrease of which normally triggers the closure of the PDA shortly after birth. A persistent PDA results in a continuous, machine-like murmur throughout systole and diastole. The left atrium (LA), left ventricle (LV), P and A become enlarged as a result of increased blood return to the left side of the heart. RA, right atrium; RV, right ventricle.

KEY FACT

Enlargement of the LA, a characteristic finding in mitral valve (MV) insufficiency, may cause dysphagia due to impingement on the esophagus.

CLINICAL CORRELATION

The use of certain drugs during pregnancy (lithium, benzodiazepines) has been associated with a rare congenital defect called Ebstein anomaly, in which tricuspid valve leaflets are located deep in the right ventricle. If there is an associated ASD, build-up of blood in the right atrium secondary to poor tricuspid valve function can lead to right-to-left shunting and cyanosis.

QUESTION

A 30-year-old magician swallows an open safety pin as part of his show. Which chamber of the heart is most likely to be punctured?

FETAL-POSTNATAL DERIVATIVES

Some important fetal structures and their postnatal counterparts follow:

- AllaNtois → urachus—**mediaN** umbilical ligament (Note: urachus is part of allantoic duct between bladder and umbilicus.)
- Ductus arteriosus → ligamentum arteriosum
- Ductus venosus → ligamentum venosum
- Foramen ovale → fossa ovalis
- Notochord → nucleus pulposus
- UmbiLical arteries → **mediaL** umbilical ligaments
- Umbilical vein → ligamentum teres hepatis (Note: contained in falciform ligament.)

FETAL ERYTHROPOIESIS

Organ Involvement

Fetal erythrocytes are produced in different locations throughout the life of the fetus.

- **Y**olk sac (3–8 weeks) during organogenesis
- **L**iver (7 weeks–birth)
- **S**pleen (9–28 weeks)
- **B**one marrow (22 weeks–adult axial skeleton [pelvis, ribs, sternum, vertebrae] and long bones' proximal epiphyses)

Hemoglobin

Fetal hemoglobin consists of two alpha subunits and two gamma subunits (α_2 and γ_2). Because fetal hemoglobin has a higher affinity for oxygen due to its lower affinity for 2,3-bisphosphoglycerate (2,3-BPG) than does adult hemoglobin, the transfer of oxygen across the placenta from maternal to fetal circulation is ensured.

After birth, there is a gradual decrease in red cell production, caused by increased oxygenation of systemic circulation, and a switch from fetal to adult hemoglobin (consists of two alpha and two beta subunits). This results in a physiologic anemia that nadirs around 4–8 weeks of life before a new steady-state production of adult hemoglobin is established.

FETAL CIRCULATION

The fetal circulation is designed to meet the needs of the growing fetus without utilizing the oxygenating capacity of the lungs, which are filled with amniotic fluid in utero. To accomplish this, oxygenated blood from the mother travels from the placenta via the **umbilical vein** to the fetal systemic circulation, and deoxygenated blood from the fetus travels back to the placenta via the **umbilical arteries** (Figure 1-9). There are three important shunts in the fetal circulation:

1. Blood entering the fetus through the umbilical vein is conducted via the **ductus venosus** into the IVC, bypassing hepatic circulation.
2. Most of the highly oxygenated blood reaching the heart via the IVC is directed through the **foramen ovale** and pumped into the aorta to supply the head and body.
3. Deoxygenated blood from the SVC passes through the right atrium → right ventricle → main pulmonary artery → **patent ductus arteriosus (PDA)** → descending aorta. This shunt via the PDA can occur because of the high fetal pulmonary artery resistance (due in part to low fetal oxygen tension and high concentration of circulating vasodilators like nitric oxide and prostaglandins).

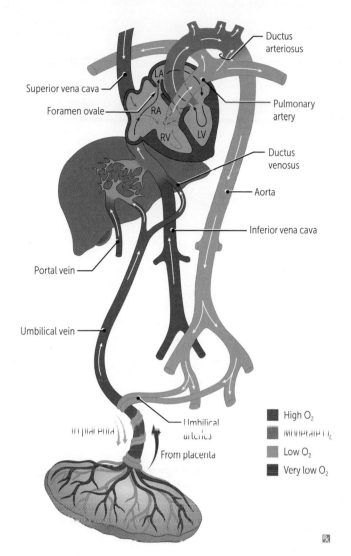

Ductus arteriosus

Superior vena cava

Foramen ovale

LA

RA

RV LV

Pulmonary artery

Ductus venosus

Aorta

Inferior vena cava

Portal vein

Umbilical vein

To placenta

Umbilical arteries

From placenta

 High O_2
Moderate O_2
Low O_2
Very low O_2

FIGURE 1-9. Fetal circulation. Most of the oxygenated blood reaching the heart via the umbilical vein (O_2 saturation ~ 80%) and inferior vena cava is diverted through the foramen ovale into the left atrium and pumped out into aortic arch vessels to the head, neck, and upper extremities (O_2 saturation ~ 60%), while deoxygenated blood returned via the superior vena cava is mostly pumped through the pulmonary artery and ductus arteriosus to the feet and the umbilical arteries.

After birth, as the neonate begins to breathe, the pulmonary arterial resistance decreases due to increased oxygen tension and decreased circulating vasodilators. For the first time, pressures in the left heart exceed pressures in the right heart. The increase in left atrial pressure forces the septum primum against the septum secundum, closing the foramen ovale (now called **fossa ovalis**). Closure of the ductus arteriosus and ductus venosus is mediated by falling levels of prostaglandins due to increased oxygen content in the circulation.

Anatomy

SURFACES AND BORDERS OF THE HEART

- The **anterior (sternal) surface** is formed by the RV (Figure 1-10A).
- The **posterior surface** is formed by the LA and is in close proximity to the esophagus.
- The **right border** is formed by the right atrium.

KEY FACT

In cardiomegaly the apex is shifted laterally; therefore the point of maximal impulse (PMI) is palpated more lateral than the midclavicular line.

QUESTION

An 18-year-old man is stabbed with a knife just to the right of the sternum between the fourth and fifth ribs. Which cardiac structure is penetrated by the knife?

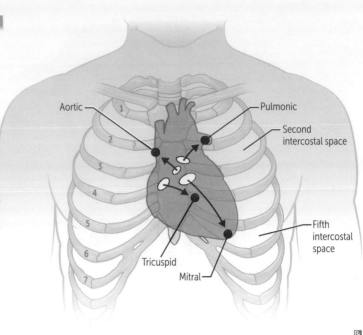

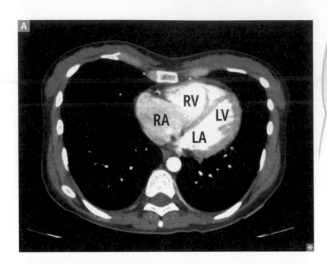

FIGURE 1-10.   Anatomic relationships of the heart. A Axial CT of the heart. B Anatomic relationship of valves in the heart. LA, left atrium; LV, left ventricle; RA, right atrium; RV, right ventricle.

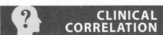

CLINICAL CORRELATION

Aortic stenosis (AS) and hypertrophic obstructive cardiomyopathy (HOCM) both produce **systolic crescendo-decrescendo murmurs.** In AS, the murmur is best heard in the right upper sternal border and radiates to the carotids and/or cardiac apex. In HOCM, the murmur does not typically radiate and is best heard at the left sternal border; it also increases in intensity with Valsalva (AS murmur decreases in intensity with Valsalva).

CLINICAL CORRELATION

Mitral regurgitation (MR) causes a **holosystolic blowing murmur,** heard best at the cardiac apex. It can sometimes be confused with tricuspid regurgitation; however, the murmur of tricuspid regurgitation becomes louder with inspiration.

 ANSWER

The right atrium forms the right border of the heart. Note that the right ventricle forms the anterior portion of the heart to the left of the sternum.

- The **left border** is formed by the LA and LV.
- The **apex** is formed by the LV.

RELATIONSHIPS OF THE HEART AND GREAT VESSELS

- The **right border** is formed by the right atrium and is located between the third and sixth ribs along the right sternal border.
- The **left border** is formed by the left ventricle and is located between the third and sixth ribs between the midclavicular line and left sternal border.
- The apex is located at the fifth intercostal space, midclavicular line. The point of maximal impulse (PMI) is normally palpated here.
- The **aortic arch** is located at the level of the sternal notch, corresponding to vertebral level T2.
- The **superior vena cava (SVC)** enters the RA at the level of the third rib.

HEART VALVES AND SITES OF AUSCULTATION

The four heart valves are the **aortic, pulmonic, mitral,** and **tricuspid valves** (Table 1-3). It is important to understand how valve movement relates to the cardiac cycle (discussed in The Cardiac Cycle).

Many cardiac diseases and valvular lesions result in abnormal heart sounds. Abnormal heart sounds are due to aberrant blood flow; therefore, the site of auscultation of a particular valve is downstream to the direction of flow through that valve (Figure 1-10B).

LAYERS OF THE HEART

The heart is composed of three layers: **endocardium, myocardium,** and **pericardium** (Figure 1-11).

TABLE 1-3. **Characteristics of Heart Valves**

VALVE	LOCATION	STRUCTURE	SITE OF AUSCULTATION	PHASE WHEN VALVE IS OPEN
Aortic	Between LV and aorta	Semilunar (3 cusps)	Right second IS at the SB	Systole
Pulmonic	Between RV and pulmonary trunk	Semilunar (3 cusps)	Left second IS at the SB	Systole
Mitral	Between LA and LV	Bicuspid	Left fifth IS at the midclavicular line	Diastole
Tricuspid	Between RA and RV	Tricuspid	Left fifth IS at the SB	Diastole

IS, intercostal space; LA, left atrium; LV, left ventricle; RA, right atrium; RV, right ventricle; SB, sternal border.

Endocardium

The endocardium is the innermost layer and contacts the blood in the heart chambers. It is composed of simple squamous epithelium (endothelium) and underlying connective tissue.

Myocardium

The myocardium is the middle and thickest layer composed of myocytes, the contractile cells responsible for pumping blood through the heart.

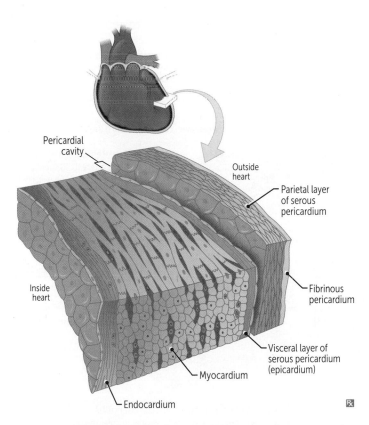

FIGURE 1-11. **Layers of the heart.** The three layers are epicardium, myocardium, and endocardium. The pericardial space is lined by a visceral and parietal layer of pericardium that encloses a thin layer of serous fluid.

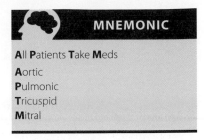

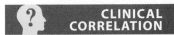

CLINICAL CORRELATION

Cardiac tamponade is the compression of the heart by fluid (ie, blood) in the pericardial sac, leading to decreased cardiac output (CO). Classic signs are distended neck veins, hypotension, and muffled heart sounds (Beck triad). Treatment is pericardiocentesis.

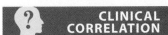

CLINICAL CORRELATION

Hypertrophy of the myocardium occurs in hypertrophic obstructive cardiomyopathy (HOCM) and can result in sudden death due to ventricular arrythmias from poorly functional myocytes.

QUESTION

Which heart vessel carries the most deoxygenated blood?

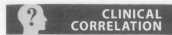

Pericardium

The pericardium is composed of two layers: the outer **fibrous pericardium** and the inner **serous pericardium**. It covers the heart and proximal portion of the great vessels.

- **Fibrous pericardium** is the tough connective tissue that tethers the heart in place via its connections to the sternum anteriorly and the central tendon of the diaphragm inferiorly.
- **Serous pericardium** comprises two layers: the parietal layer and the visceral layer.
    - The parietal layer is continuous with the internal aspect of the fibrous pericardium.
    - The visceral layer, also known as the **epicardium**, is the thin innermost layer of the pericardium. This layer contains the major branches of the coronary arteries.

CORONARY ARTERY ANATOMY

Major Branches

The coronary arteries arise from the proximal portion of the aorta (the aorta's first branches) as the **right coronary artery (RCA)** and the **left coronary artery (LCA)** (Figure 1-12). These vessels lie just deep to the epicardium on the surface of the heart.

The heart receives a dual blood supply: The **epicardium** and **myocardium** are supplied by the **coronary arteries** and their branches, whereas the **endocardium** receives O₂ and nutrients from distal branches of the coronary arteries and has direct contact with blood inside the heart chambers.

When flow through a coronary artery is compromised, the subendocardial tissue is most vulnerable to ischemic injury because it lies in the zone farthest from either blood supply.

Flow through the coronary arteries occurs mainly during diastole. The contraction of the myocardium during systole increases external pressure on the vessels and inhibits blood flow through them.

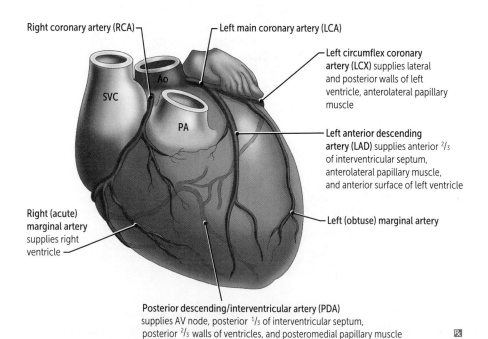

FIGURE 1-12. **Coronary artery circulation.** Ao, aorta; PA, pulmonary artery; SVC, superior vena cava.

Major branches of the LCA are the **left anterior descending artery (LAD)** and **left circumflex artery.**

Major branches of the RCA are the **marginal artery** and the **posterior descending artery.**

Dominant Circulation

The coronary artery that supplies the posterior descending artery (PDA) is considered the dominant artery of the heart.

- Right-dominant circulation = 85% (PDA arises from RCA.)
- Left-dominant circulation = 8% (PDA arises from left circumflex coronary artery [LCX].)
- Co-dominant circulation = 7% (PDA arises from RCA and LCX.)

Acute Coronary Syndrome

Acute coronary syndrome (ACS) describes a spectrum of serious clinical diagnoses (unstable angina, non-ST elevation myocardial infarction [NSTEMI], and ST-elevation myocardial infarction [STEMI]) that affect individuals with coronary artery disease. The most common cause of ACS is occlusion due to thrombus from an atherosclerotic plaque (Figure 1-13).

The coronary artery **most commonly occluded** (40–50%) is the **LAD,** followed by the RCA, and then the left circumflex. STEMI results in characteristic ECG changes demonstrated in Figure 1-14 and Table 1-4.

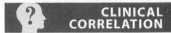

CONDUCTION SYSTEM

The cardiac conduction system is responsible for distributing electrical impulses throughout the heart so that the atria and ventricles function in concert as an effective pump. The sequence of electrical activation in the heart is outlined below and in Figure 1-15:

1. **Sinoatrial (SA) node:** Called the **native pacemaker** of the heart, the SA node is where the electrical impulse is initiated. It is located at the junction of RA and SVC and contains specialized myocytes that have the ability to depolarize spontaneously **(automaticity)** at a regular rate of 60–100 beats per minute at rest.
2. The electrical impulse from the SA node travels through both atria (right → left) until it eventually reaches the **AV node.**

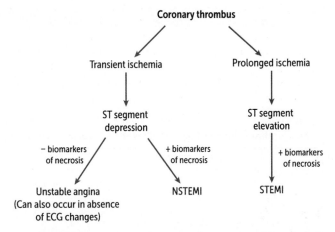

FIGURE 1-13. Spectrum of acute coronary syndrome. A coronary thrombus, depending on how occlusive it is and/or how much ischemia it causes, can lead to unstable angina, non-ST elevation myocardial infarction (NSTEMI), or ST-elevation myocardial infarction (STEMI), which are distinguished by ECG findings (ST segment elevation/depression) and biomarkers of necrosis (eg, troponins).

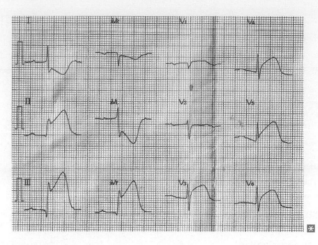

FIGURE 1-14. **ECG findings in myocardial infarction.** ST-segment elevation in the inferior (II, III, and aVF) and anterior (V_3–V_6) leads.

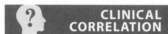

Conduction block is a type of arrhythmia that occurs when there is cellular damage to conducting cells, outlined in Figure 1-15. Complete AV block, for example, can lead to no conduction between atria and ventricles, often requiring a pacemaker.

3. **Atrioventricular (AV) node:** Located in the posteroinferior part of the interatrial septum near the coronary sinus, the AV node delays conduction from the atria to the ventricles (100 msec delay) to allow time for the atria to depolarize and fully empty their contents into the ventricles before ventricular contraction.
4. After a brief delay in the AV node, the electrical impulse spreads through the ventricular conduction system, which contains specialized myocytes from below the AV node to walls of both ventricles: **Bundle of His** → divides into the **right and left bundle branches** along the interventricular septum (note that the **left bundle branch** splits into the **left anterior** and **left posterior fascicles**) → bundles and fascicles terminate in specialized conducting fibers termed **Purkinje fibers** in the walls of both ventricles to distribute the electrical impulse to allow for full ventricular contraction.

Physiology

The cardiovascular (CV) system, which can be modeled as a pump (heart) and a set of tubes (blood vessels), distributes O_2, nutrients, and other substances to the tissues while removing metabolic by-products from the tissues.

CARDIAC ELECTROPHYSIOLOGY

To generate an electrical signal that can regularly contract the atria and ventricles, the heart contains two populations of cells: **conducting** and **contractile cells.** Conducting (nodal) myocytes form the specialized conduction pathway of the heart (SA node, AV node, bundle of His, bundle branches, Purkinje fibers). They have the ability to

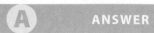

RCA. ST elevation in inferior leads (II, III, and aVF). Recall that RCA perfuses the AV node. Ischemia of the AV node can cause nodal dysfunction and result in bradycardia and various degrees of heart block.

TABLE 1-4. **ECG Findings With ST Segment Elevation Myocardial Infarction (STEMI)**

AREA OF INFARCT	CORONARY ARTERY INVOLVED	LEADS WITH ST ELEVATION
Inferior wall (RV)	RCA	II, III, aVF
Anterior wall (may include septum)	LAD	V_2, V_3
Lateral wall (LV)	Left circumflex	I, aVL, V_5, V_6

aVF, augmented voltage foot; aVL, augmented voltage left arm; LAD, left anterior descending; LV, left ventricle; RCA, right coronary artery; RV, right ventricle.

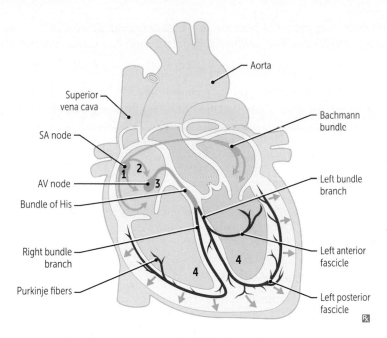

FIGURE 1-15. **Anatomy of the conduction system in the heart.**

spontaneously generate action potentials (APs). APs travel along the normal conduction pathway (Figure 1-15) to stimulate surrounding contractile myocytes via electrical gap junctions to contract and generate enough force to pump blood into the circulation.

Resting Membrane Potential

By convention, the resting membrane potential of a cell is measured in mV relative to the extracellular space. Excitable cells, like cardiac myocytes, neurons, and skeletal myocytes, have resting membrane potentials between −70 and −90 mV. The membrane potential (Vm) in all cells can be explained by:

- The relative conductance of the cell membrane for certain ions (eg, K+, Na+, Ca2+). This determines which ion's equilibrium potential predominates. The membrane potential at any point in the AP is determined by the relative contribution of different ion conductances.
- The relative intracellular and extracellular concentrations of these ions.

At rest, the membrane conductance is higher for K+ than it is for the other major ions (Na+ or Ca2+). This explains why the resting membrane potential is close to the equilibrium potential for K+ (a function of the intracellular ($[K^+]_i$) and extracellular ($[K^+]_e$) potassium concentration gradient). Since $[K^+]_i \gg [K^+]_e$, K+ diffuses out of the cell and down its concentration gradient, causing the V_m to become more negative (losing positive charge to the outside). At a certain membrane potential, the net force driving K+ along its electrochemical gradient equals the net concentration gradient driving ions across the membrane. This potential at which there is no net movement of ions across the membrane is the **equilibrium (or Nernst) potential (E_K)** and can be calculated:

$$E_K = \frac{-61}{z} \log \frac{[K^+]_i}{[K^+]_e}$$

(z = 1 because K+ is monovalent)

If [K+]e = 4 mEq/L and [K+]i = 120 mEq/L, the membrane potential for K+ = 91 mV, which closely approximates the resting membrane potential for a ventricular contractile myocyte (−90 mV). Notably, conducting myocytes (eg, SA and AV node) have a

KEY FACT

Membrane conductance describes the cell membrane's permeability to a particular ion. It is a function of whether the ion channels specific to a particular ion are open. Because an action potential triggers voltage-gated channels to open and close, ion conductance varies throughout an action potential.

KEY FACT

Inward current positive charge (eg, Ca2+, K+, Na+) enters cell → depolarizes V_m (makes less negative).
Outward current positive charge (eg, K+) leaves cell → hyperpolarizes V_m (makes more negative).

less-negative resting potential because of a higher conductance to Ca^{2+} and Na^+ at less-negative voltages due to spontaneous depolarization (see Cardiac Action Potentials below).

In contrast to K^+, since the $[Na^+]$ is higher in the extracellular space, Na^+ tends to enter the cell and make the membrane potential more positive. The Na^+-K^+-ATPase pump maintains the ionic gradient across the cell membrane by pumping 3 Na^+ out for every 2 K^+ pumped in. This maintains the resting Na^+ and K^+ intracellular and extracellular concentration gradients (Figure 1-16).

Cardiac Action Potentials

Cardiac myocytes produce two types of action potentials (APs): fast response and slow response (Figure 1-17). These APs, which measure the electrical potential of the cell over time, differ in their shape and conduction velocity (Table 1-5).

Fast-Response (Ventricular) Action Potential

Fast-response APs occur in the atrial and ventricular myocytes, the bundle of His, and Purkinje fibers.

- Phase 0: Rapid upstroke and depolarization. Voltage-gated Na^+ channels open.
- Phase 1: Initial repolarization. Inactivation of voltage-gated Na^+ channels. Voltage-gated K^+ channels begin to open.
- Phase 2: Plateau. Ca^{2+} influx through voltage-gated **L-type** Ca^{2+} channels balances K^+ efflux. Ca^{2+} influx triggers Ca^{2+} release of intracellular Ca^{2+} from sarcoplasmic reticulum and myocyte contraction.
- Phase 3: Repolarization. Massive K^+ efflux due to opening of voltage-gated slow K^+ channels and closure of voltage-gated Ca^{2+} channels (via calcium-dependent inactivation).
- Phase 4: Resting potential. High K^+ permeability through K^+ channels.

Slow-Response (Pacemaker) Action Potential

Slow-response APs occur in the SA and AV nodes.

- Phase 0: Upstroke (less rapid and steep than fast-response AP) and depolarization. Opening of voltage-gated **T-type** Ca^{2+} channels. A greater proportion of fast voltage-gated Na^+ channels are inactivated in pacemaker cells (they have a less negative resting membrane voltage than ventricular myocytes). In the AV node, this results in a slow conduction velocity to prolong transmission from atria to ventricles.
- Phase 1: Not present.
- Phase 2: Not present (no plateau).

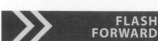

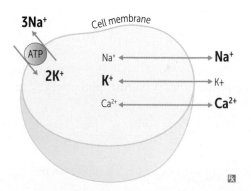

FIGURE 1-16.   Intracellular and extracellular concentrations of Ca^{2+}, Na^+, and K^+ in mEq/L. The ATP-powered Na^+/K^+ pump maintains the baseline membrane potential, which is largely determined by $[K^+]$.

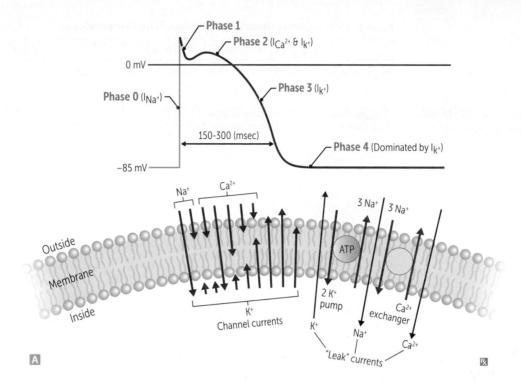

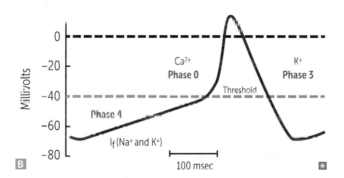

FIGURE 1-17. **Fast response** **and slow response** B **cardiac action potentials.** I_X denotes the current (ie, flow of charge) of the specified ion (x) through the ion channel in the direction noted. Note that for the fast response action potential, the AP duration (150–300 msec) varies by location of conducting pathways (Purkinje fibers > ventricle > atria).

- Phase 3: Repolarization. Inactivation of the voltage-gated Ca^{2+} channels and increased K^+ conductance causes K^+ efflux.
- Phase 4: Slow diastolic depolarization. Membrane potential spontaneously depolarizes as Na^+ conductance increases through **I(f) "funny" Na^+ channels.** Accounts for the automaticity of the SA and AV nodes.

Cardiac Pacemakers

Myocytes in the SA node, AV node, bundle of His, and Purkinje system all have the capacity to act as pacemakers of the heart, and each has different intrinsic firing rates (**automaticity**):

- SA node: 60–100 bpm
- AV node and proximal bundle of His: 50–60 bpm
- Purkinje cells: 30–40 bpm

The myocytes with the fastest intrinsic firing rates (ie, SA node) are the **native pacemakers** of the heart because they **overdrive suppress** the **latent pacemakers** (ie, AV node,

> **KEY FACT**
>
> "Funny" Na^+ channels are funny because, unlike fast-acting voltage-gated Na^+ channels activated by depolarization, funny Na^+ channels are activated by **hyperpolarization.**

TABLE 1-5. **Comparison of Slow and Fast Action Potentials**

	SLOW PACEMAKER ACTION POTENTIAL	FAST ACTION POTENTIAL
Length of AP	150 ms (SA, atria), 250–300 ms (AV, ventricular)	100 ms
Conduction velocity	0.01–0.10 m/sec	0.3–3.0 m/sec
Tissues involved	SA and AV nodes	Atria, ventricles, bundle of His, Purkinje fibers
Phases	0. Increased $I_{Ca^{2+}}$	0. Increased I_{Na^+}
	1. Increased I_{K^+}	1. Decreased I_{Na^+}, increased I_{K^+}
	4. Increased $I_{f(Na^+)}$	2. Increased $I_{Ca^{2+}}$, increased I_{K^+}
		3. Decreased $I_{Ca^{2+}}$, increased I_{K^+}
Targeting antiarrhythmics	Class II β-blockers (phase 4), class IV Ca channel blockers (phase 0)	Class Ia, Ib, Ic (phase 0), class III (phase 3)

AP, action potential; AV, atrioventricular; SA, sinoatrial.

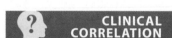

Electrolyte changes can also affect the shape of APs. **Calcium gluconate,** for example, is often administered to counteract the effects of hyperkalemia. Persistent hyperkalemia causes depolarization of the membrane potential and inactivates Na+ channels, ultimately decreasing membrane excitability and predisposing to life-threatening arrhythmias. Calcium reverses this effect and restores membrane potential by a mechanism that is not fully understood.

bundle of His, Purkinje system) to maintain a regular rate and rhythm. If the SA node fails to fire, the next fastest pacemaker cells (ie, AV node) will take over, and if the AV node fails to fire, the next fastest pacemaker cells (bundle of His and Purkinje cells) will take over.

Although pacemaker cells have automaticity, autonomic nervous system input (along with drugs that mimic their effects) can affect the heart rate (HR). Table 1-6 highlights the effect of sympathetic and parasympathetic stimulation on portions of the pacemaker action potential to increase and decrease heart rate, respectively.

Conduction Velocity

Conduction velocity (m/sec) is the speed at which APs travel through the myocardium. The speed depends on the size of inward current during the AP upstroke (phase 0); the

TABLE 1-6. **Effect of Autonomic Nervous System and Drugs on Pacemaker Action Potentials**

STIMULATION	EFFECT ON HEART RATE	EFFECT ON RESTING MEMBRANE POTENTIAL	EFFECT ON SLOPE OF PHASE 4 DEPOLARIZATION	EFFECT ON THRESHOLD POTENTIAL
↑ Acetylcholine (parasympathetic ANS) ↑ Adenosine ↑ β-blockers	↓	More negative	Decreased (due to ↓ I_f)	More positive
↑ Catecholamines (sympathetic ANS, caffeine, cocaine)	↑	More positive	Increased (due to ↑ I_f)	More negative

ANS, autonomic nervous system; HR, heart rate.

larger the inward current, the faster the electrical impulse can spread to neighboring myocytes via gap junctions. A point that often causes confusion: AP duration (from depolarization to repolarization) does not impact conduction velocity, because conduction velocity measures how fast APs spread **between** cells (a function of inward current). Conduction velocity is fastest in the Purkinje system (2–4 m/sec) and slowest in the AV node (0.01–0.05 m/sec). A slower conduction velocity in the AV node means that the excitation of the ventricles is delayed. The AV nodal delay enables the atria to empty fully into the ventricles prior to depolarization of the ventricles, thus improving ventricular filling and increasing cardiac output in a given beat. Fast conduction velocity in the Purkinje fibers ensures uniform and efficient ventricular contraction to maintain cardiac output.

Refractory Period

The duration of cardiac myocyte APs (150–300 msec) is longer than the duration of neuron and skeletal myocyte APs (1–2 msec). Since duration of an AP is directly proportional to duration of its **refractory period,** it follows that cardiac myocytes have long refractory periods to ensure the heart has enough time to fill during diastole and to prevent tetany.

The underlying basis of the refractory period is **closure of Na⁺ channel inactivation gates** (Figure 1-18). Depolarization activates Na⁺ channel gates to open and simultaneously initiates Na⁺ channel inactivation gates to close (at a slower rate), which results in termination of the upstroke (phase 0). Na⁺ channel inactivation gates progressively reopen during repolarization, resulting in three degrees of excitability during the refractory period (Figure 1-19):

- **Absolute:** Begins at phase 0 (upstroke) to the end of phase 2 (plateau). "Absolutely" no AP can be generated, regardless of amount of inward current, because nearly all Na⁺ inactivation gates are closed.
- **Effective:** Begins at phase 0 (upstroke) to the beginning of phase 3 (start of repolarization). An "effective" AP (ie, an AP that can conduct to neighboring cells) cannot be generated because not enough Na⁺ inactivation gates have yet recovered.
- **Relative:** Begins at end of absolute refractory period to approximately end of phase 3 (repolarization). Because more Na⁺ inactivation channels recover during this period, a "relatively" larger-than-normal stimulus is able to generate a second AP.

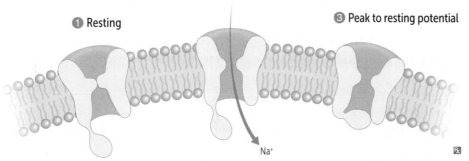

② Threshold to peak potential

① Resting

③ Peak to resting potential

Na⁺

FIGURE 1-18. **Voltage-gated inactivation and activation gates.** (1) At rest, the sodium activation gate is closed and sodium inactivation gate is open. (2) Depolarization causes the voltage-gated sodium activation gate to open. (3) As depolarization causes the cell to reach its maximum cell potential, it triggers the voltage-gated sodium inactivation gate to close, making the cell refractory to additional depolarizing stimuli. The inactivation gate reopens during repolarization as the cell returns to its resting membrane potential (1).

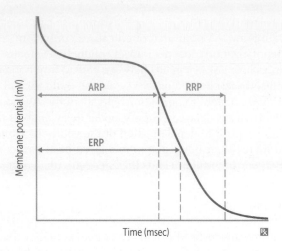

FIGURE 1-19.   Absolute (ARP), effective (ERP), and relative (RRP) refractory periods in the ventricle. Sodium inactivation gates reopen with increasing time of phase 3 (repolarization), resulting in these three degrees of excitability. Note that ARP and ERP both start at phase 0 and RRP starts at the end of ARP.

CARDIAC MUSCLE AND CONTRACTION

Contraction of the cardiac muscle cell is initiated by the AP signal acting on intracellular organelles to evoke the generation of tension and shortening of the cell. These APs are profoundly different from those of skeletal muscle cells. Cardiac and skeletal muscles differ physiologically (Table 1-7).

Excitation-Contraction Coupling

Excitation-contraction coupling occurs for all excitable cells and refers to the ability of an AP to cause contractile force in the cell. Ca^{2+} facilitates generation of contractile force in all three types of muscle in the body (skeletal, cardiac, smooth muscle), but the path that causes APs to generate intracellular Ca^{2+} varies for different cell types.

In contrast to skeletal myocytes, for example, cardiac myocytes use Ca^{2+} influx through **L-type Ca^+ channels** during phase 2 of the AP to directly trigger more Ca^{2+} release from intracellular stores (**Ca^{2+}-induced Ca^{2+} release**). Skeletal myocytes lack Ca^{2+} influx during the AP (no phase 2) and thus mechanically couple voltage-gated chan-

TABLE 1-7.   Characteristics of Cardiac and Skeletal Myocytes

MEMBRANE CHARACTERISTIC	CARDIAC MYOCYTES	SKELETAL MYOCYTES
Duration of AP	150–300 msec	1–2 msec
Plateau (phase 2 of AP) of non-pacemaker cells	Present (Ca^{2+} ions involved in cell depolarization)	Absent (no Ca^{2+} involved in cell depolarization)
Automaticity	Present in conducting cells	Absent
Gap junctions	Present	Absent
Mitochondria	↑↑↑	↑
Generation of contractile force	Increase in the individual fiber contractility	Increase in number of skeletal muscle fibers activated

AP, action potential.

nels activated by the AP to release Ca^{2+} inside the cell. The downstream mechanism of Ca^{2+}-generating contractile force is similar for skeletal and cardiac myocytes.

Excitation-contraction coupling depends on several structures in the cardiac myocyte (see Figure 1-20) that coordinate the contraction response to the cardiac AP:

- **Sarcomere:** Smallest contractile unit of cardiac muscle. Note that each cardiac myocyte contains multiple **myofibrils** that are composed of repeating sarcomere units. Each sarcomere unit is composed of thick (myosin) and thin (actin, tropomyosin, troponin) fibrous proteins that slide against each other, facilitating muscular contraction and relaxation. When viewed under a microscope, these filaments form dark and light bands that have been given different names (Figure 1-20):
    - I band: Contains actin. Shortens with contraction.
    - A band: Contains myosin. Length unchanged with contraction.
    - H band: Contains myosin. Shortens with contraction.
    - Z line: Marks borders of the sarcomere. Z lines come closer together with contraction.
    - M line: Marks the center of the sarcomere and midpoint of the thick filaments. Location unchanged with contraction.
- **T tubules:** Parts of the cell membrane that invaginate at the Z lines. They carry APs into the cell interior.
- **Sarcoplasmic reticulum:** Intracellular site of storage and release of Ca^{2+}, which facilitates Ca^{2+}-induced Ca^{2+} release.
- **Intercalated disks:** Located at the ends of cells (not shown in Figure 1-20). Mediate adhesion between cells.
- **Gap junctions:** Occur at the intercalated disks. Provide a path of low resistance for APs to rapidly spread between cells.

Myocardial Contraction and Relaxation

The cardiac myocyte translates the electrical signal (AP) into a physical response (contraction) through the following steps: Extracellular Ca^{2+} enters myocardial cell → Ca^{2+} induces intracellular Ca^{2+} release → myocardial contraction, and finally myocardial relaxation.

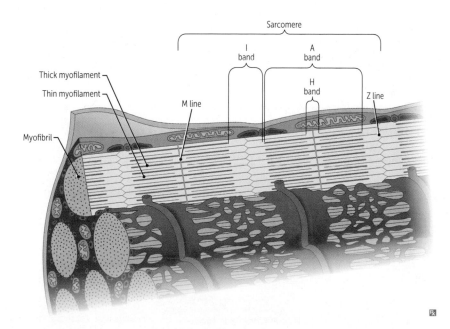

FIGURE 1-20. Schematic of the smallest contractile unit of a myocyte, the sarcomere.
Labelled bands correspond to segments of thick (myosin) and thin (actin) filaments.

KEY FACT

During contraction, the H, I, and Z bands shorten. Only the A band stays constant throughout the cycle.

MNEMONIC

HIZ shrinkage. **A** band is **A**lways the same length.

- **Influx of extracellular Ca^{2+} into myocardial cells:** Action potential spreads along the cell membrane into the T tubules. During the plateau (phase 2) of the AP, extracellular Ca^{2+} enters the cell through voltage-gated Ca^{2+} (**L-type Ca^{2+}**) channels.

- **Ca^{2+}-induced Ca^{2+} release:** The influx of extracellular Ca^{2+} is not sufficient to induce muscle contraction. Therefore, extracellular Ca^{2+} binds to **ryanodine receptors** on the sarcoplasmic reticulum (SR), inducing a conformational change that releases Ca^{2+} from the SR.

- **Myocardial contraction:** Ca^{2+} release from the SR increases intracellular $[Ca^{2+}]$ to cause sarcomere contraction according to the following steps (Figure 1-21):

  1. Released Ca^{2+} binds to **troponin C,** causing a conformational change that moves **tropomyosin** (normally blocks interaction between myosin and actin) away from the myosin-binding groove on actin filaments. Energy released from the hydrolysis of ATP → ADP + PO_4^{3-} is used to "cock" the myosin head into a high-energy state that can bind newly exposed actin filaments.

  2. The high-energy-state myosin binds to actin on the myosin-binding groove.

  3. The high-energy-state myosin uses its energy to undergo a "power stroke," in which it pulls the actin filaments attached to Z lines on either side of the M line toward the M line → sarcomere shortens → muscular contraction.

  4. Myosin will continue to stay bound to actin in its so-called "rigor conformation" until a new molecule of ATP attaches to the myosin head to facilitate detachment of myosin from actin.

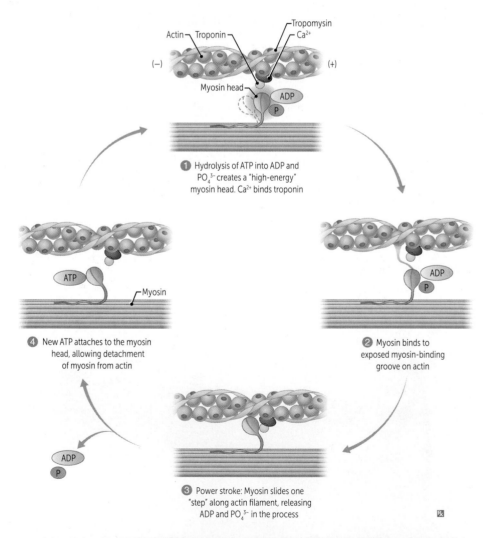

FIGURE 1-21. One cycle of skeletal muscle contraction at the level of the sarcomere. In the presence of Ca^{2+}, myosin moves along actin filaments via a "power stroke," fueled by the hydrolysis of ATP. ADP, adenosine diphosphate; ATP, adenosine triphosphate.

These steps continue in a cycle when calcium is present. Each round of the cycle produces an additional "step" of myosin along actin, ultimately producing sufficient contractile force.

- **Myocardial relaxation:** Occurs when Ca^{2+} is pumped back into the SR via a Ca^{2+}-ATPase (SERCA) and expelled into the extracellular space with the help of a Ca^{2+}/Na^+ pump (see Figure 1-17A). This reduces intracellular $[Ca^{2+}]$ and removes Ca^{2+} from troponin, which terminates contraction of the sarcomere.

CARDIAC OUTPUT

The volume of blood pumped per minute from either ventricle, which should be equal in the absence of pathology, is known as **cardiac output (CO).** Normal resting CO is 4–8 L/min and can increase five- to sixfold during exercise. CO can be calculated using SV and HR ($CO = SV \times HR$) or measured using Fick's O_2 method.

Fick's Cardiac Output

Cardiac output is indirectly measured by measuring O_2 consumption. Based on conservation of mass, the amount of O_2 delivered to the body (product of CO and the difference in pulmonary artery and vein $[O_2]$) must equal O_2 consumed. The O_2 consumption for a 70-kg man is 250 mL/min, and the $[O_2]$ in the pulmonary vein can be measured from a peripheral artery (no significant utilization of O_2 by tissues at this point), and the $[O_2]$ in the pulmonary artery can be measured from the pulmonary artery or right ventricle.

$$O_2 \text{ delivered} - O_2 \text{ removed} = O_2 \text{ consumed}$$
$$CO \times ([O_2]pv - [O_2]pa) = O_2 \text{ consumed}$$
$$\text{Fick } CO = O_2 \text{ consumed}/([O_2]pv - [O_2]pa)$$

where

CO = cardiac output (L/min)
O_2 consumed = O_2 used by body (mL O_2/min) = 250 mL/min in a 70-kg man
$[O_2]pa$ = O_2 in pulmonary artery (mL O_2/L blood)
$[O_2]pv$ = O_2 in pulmonary vein (mL O_2/L blood)

Stroke Volume

Stroke volume is the difference between end-diastolic volume and end-systolic volume, or the volume of blood ejected by the LV during a heartbeat. It varies directly as a function of contractility and preload and varies inversely with afterload. SV increases with increased preload, decreased afterload, or increased contractility. Other variables that affect SV and contractility are summarized in Table 1-8.

Ejection Fraction

The ejection fraction (EF) is the fraction of blood received by the LV (end-diastolic volume) that is ejected (SV) and directly reflects the state of contractility of the heart. A larger percentage of LV blood volume ejected (larger EF) reflects an increased contractile state.

$$EF = \frac{\text{stroke volume}}{\text{end-diastolic volume}} \times 100 \text{ (normal)} = 55\text{–}75\%$$

$$SV = \frac{CO}{HR} = EDV - ESV$$

KEY FACT

Mean systemic pressure is increased by:
- Increased blood volume
- Decreased venous compliance (blood shifted from veins to arteries)
- Exercise (sympathetic stimulation)

KEY FACT

Factors that increase O_2 consumption:
- Increased afterload
- Increased contractility
- Increased HR
- Increased size of heart (increases radius → increases tension via LaPlace's law)

MNEMONIC

SV CAP

Stroke **V**olume affected by:
Contractility
Afterload
Preload

KEY FACT

EF ↓ in systolic HF.
EF normal in diastolic HF.

TABLE 1-8.   Factors Affecting Contractility

CONTRACTILITY AND STROKE VOLUME ↑ "POSITIVE INOTROPIC EFFECT"	CONTRACTILITY AND STROKE VOLUME ↓ "NEGATIVE INOTROPIC EFFECT"
↑ **HR** (Ca^{2+} clearance is less efficient during shorter relaxation times → ↑ intracellular $[Ca^{2+}]$)	↓ **HR** (Ca^{2+} clearance is more efficient during longer relaxation times → ↓ intracellular $[Ca^{2+}]$)
Sympathetic stimulation (↑ catecholamines → stimulation of β_1 receptors → ↑ intracellular $[Ca^{2+}]$ and ↑ activity of SR Ca^{2+} ATPase)	**Parasympathetic stimulation** (↑ ACh → stimulation of muscarinic receptors → ↓ intracellular $[Ca^{2+}]$)
Digitalis (inhibition of myocardial cell membrane $Na^+/K^+/ATPase$ → ↑ intracellular $[Na^+]$ → decreased $[Na^+]$ gradient across cell membrane → less intracellular Ca^{2+} removed by Na^+/Ca^{2+} exchanger → ↑ intracellular $[Ca^{2+}]$)	β_1-blockade (↓ cAMP) HF with systolic dysfunction Acidosis Hypoxia/hypercapnia (↓ Po_2/↑ Pco_2) Non-dihydropyridine Ca^{2+} channel blockers

Determinants of Cardiac Output

Cardiac output is influenced by three major parameters affecting the left ventricle: **afterload, preload, and contractility.** As shown in Figure 1-22, these three parameters directly affect SV, which is a major determinant of CO in addition to HR.

Afterload

Afterload is the load that myocytes must contract against to generate CO. Afterload is more formally defined as **wall stress (σ)** on the LV during contraction (systole). Wall stress reflects the tensile force ("tension") per unit area the heart must generate during systole to eject blood across the aortic valve—it reflects the "load" the myocytes are contracting against. Laplace's law applied to the ventricle illustrates two key principles:

1. Wall stress **increases** with increased ventricular pressure (eg, hypertension) and increased ventricular radius (eg, dilated cardiomyopathy).
2. Wall stress **decreases** with increased ventricular thickness (eg, concentric hypertrophy of myocytes → more sarcomeres added in parallel per myocyte → reduced wall stress "felt" by each myocyte).

$$\sigma = \frac{P \times r}{2h}$$

where P is ventricular pressure, r is ventricular chamber radius, and h is ventricular wall thickness.

KEY FACT

In the absence of valvular pathology (eg, aortic stenosis), LV afterload during systole is proportional to systemic blood pressure (BP). In the RV, afterload (absent valvular pathology like pulmonic stenosis) is proportional to pulmonary artery pressure.

CLINICAL CORRELATION

LV compensates for ↑ afterload by thickening (hypertrophy) in order to ↓ wall tension.

FLASH FORWARD

- Vasodilators (eg, hydralazine) → ↓ afterload
- ACE inhibitors and ARBs → ↓ preload and afterload
- Chronic hypertension → ↑ afterload → LV hypertrophy (compensatory)

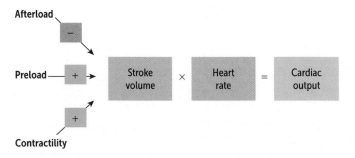

FIGURE 1-22.   The determinants of cardiac output are stroke volume (SV) and heart rate. SV is directly proportional to contractility and preload and indirectly proportional to afterload.

Preload

The amount of "stretch" felt by the filled LV at the end of relaxation (diastole) before contraction (systole). In other words, it is the "wall stress" at the end of diastole (vs afterload, which is the wall stress during systole). Measurements of pressure or volume at end diastole are thus often used as proxies for preload: LV end-diastolic volume (LVEDV) and LV end-diastolic pressure (LVEDP).

Length-Tension Relationship and Contractility (Inotropy)

Two mechanisms can influence force generation in cardiac muscle:

- Change in muscle fiber length
- Change in **contractility** or **inotropy** (independent of fiber length)

The first mechanism, involving change in muscle fiber length, is known as the **length-tension relationship** for myocytes. Derived from experimental observations, it reveals that sarcomere length impacts the force of contraction (Figure 1-23). At the optimal length, there is maximal actin-myosin overlap, which results in the maximum systolic contraction. Sarcomere length is directly related to **preload** (how "stretched out" ventricle is at end diastole).

Contractility describes the amount of force generated by cardiac myocytes, **independent** of the intrinsic length-tension relationship for myocytes. Specifically, it describes how external factors, such as drugs (eg, calcium channel blockers [CCBs], β-blockers, digoxin), cell mediators (eg, catecholamines, intracellular [Ca^{2+}]), and pathologies (eg, CHF, hypoxia, acidosis) can influence contraction of the heart. Because increased contractile force of the heart → increased SV at a given LVEDV, the ejection fraction (= SV/LVEDV) can be a useful proxy in measuring how contractility ("inotropic state") of the heart changes with different interventions. Normal EF = 55–75%. Table 1-8 highlights important factors that affect contractility.

Frank-Starling Relationship

The greater the venous return, the greater the CO. In steady-state, the Frank-Starling principle ensures that venous return equals CO. It is one of the fundamental principles in cardiac physiology and is simply the **length-tension relationship** applied to ventricles. Since the "length" of a ventricle is proportional to **preload** (**LVEDV** or **LVEDP**) just before contraction, and the "tension" generated is proportional to measurable proxies of pressure generated in the LV (**CO** or **SV**), a curve with these axes (similar to the one drawn in Figure 1-23, notably without the descending limb) is often drawn to illustrate the Frank-Starling "curve" (Figure 1-24).

KEY FACT

Preload is affected by ventricular **compliance** (ie, how "stiff" the ventricle is; more compliant → less ΔP for a given ΔV):

- ↓ compliance (eg, ventricular hypertrophy, diastolic heart failure) → ↓ **LVEDV** at a given EDP
- ↑ compliance (eg, dilated cardiomyopathy) → ↑ **LVEDV** at a given EDP

KEY FACT

↓ **venous return** (eg, hemorrhage, vasodilation) → ↓ **preload**
↑ **venous return** (eg, administration of IV fluids, vasoconstriction) → ↑ **preload**

KEY FACT

Agents that ↑ contractility are referred to as positive inotropes. Agents that ↓ contractility are referred to as negative inotropes.

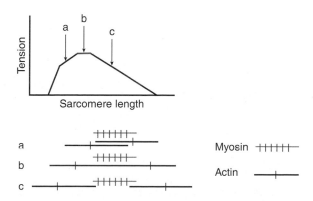

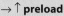

FIGURE 1-23. **Effect of sarcomere length on the force of contraction.** There is an ideal length that maximizes the overlap between actin and myosin (b) and maximizes tension generated. If the sarcomere is too short (a) or too long (c), the myosin and actin cannot interact optimally to produce maximal tension.

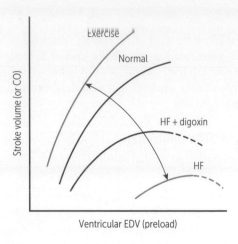

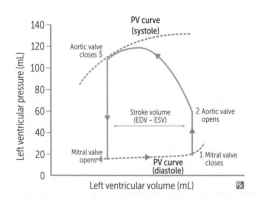

FIGURE 1-24. **Frank-Starling curve.** CO, cardiac output; EDV, end-diastolic volume; HF, heart failure.

The "normal" curve in Figure 1-24 illustrates that up to a certain point, force of systolic contraction (**SV** or **CO**) is directly proportional to the length of the cardiac muscle (**preload**). This rule holds up to a certain threshold preload. The heart at its strongest and contracting most vigorously can handle only so much venous return before it becomes overstretched. At a preload beyond this threshold value, actin-myosin overlap is no longer optimal, as cross-bridges cannot form. As a result, contractility decreases as preload continues to increase, resulting in the descending limb (not shown in Figure 1-24) of the Frank-Starling curve at excessively high preloads. Other curves in Figure 1-24 illustrate how the Frank-Starling curve shifts up or down with factors that increase and decrease contractility, respectively (Table 1-8). Specifically, at a given preload, **positive inotropic agents** increase ventricular function (↑ SV or CO), and **negative inotropic agents** decrease it.

PRESSURE-VOLUME LOOPS

Pressure-volume (PV) loops describe the relationship between LV volume and pressure during one full cardiac cycle, including contraction (systole) and relaxation (diastole) (Figure 1-25). PV loops are constructed in part by combining a pseudo–Frank-Starling curve (pressure-volume relationship in LV during systole) with another curve called the **compliance curve** (pressure-volume relationship in LV during diastole). The left ventricle PV loop for one full cardiac cycle has four main phases (contraction, ejection, relaxation, and filling), detailed below:

> **KEY FACT**
>
> Increased venous return → increased cardiac output.

> **KEY FACT**
>
> **Ventricular diastole** begins with aortic valve closure and lasts through the mitral valve closure, whereas **ventricular systole** is defined as the part of the cardiac cycle from mitral valve closure to aortic valve closure.

FIGURE 1-25. **Left ventricular pressure-volume loop with overlayed systolic (top) and diastolic (bottom) PV curves.** Note that the systolic PV curve is the principle behind the Frank-Starling curve. The diastolic PV curve is also referred to as the "compliance curve" for the ventricle during diastole. Increase in preload, for example, moves the PV loop "up" the compliance curve.

1 → 2: Isovolumetric Contraction (Systole)

Period between mitral valve (MV) closure, marking the end of diastole, and aortic valve (AoV) opening. Since the MV and AoV are closed, the LV is a closed chamber and contracts under a constant (isovolumetric) volume. No blood is ejected from the LV in this phase. The ventricular pressure continues to rise until LV pressure > aortic pressure.

2 → 3: Ventricular Ejection (Systole)

Eventually LV pressure > aortic pressure and AoV opens. Contraction of LV continues, allowing ejection of blood from the LV into the aorta. Volume ejected from the LV in this phase is the SV (width of the PV loop). When aortic pressure > LV pressure, AoV closes. Note that the maximum pressure generated during systole can be graphed directly on the pseudo–Frank-Starling curve.

3 → 4: Isovolumetric Relaxation (Diastole)

Period between AoV closing, marking the end of systole, and MV opening. Once again, the LV is a closed chamber and relaxes under a constant (isovolumetric) volume. No blood is ejected from the LV in this phase. The ventricular pressure continues to drop until LA pressure > LV pressure.

4 → 1: Ventricular Filling (Diastole)

When LA pressure > LV pressure, the MV opens. Blood moves from the LA (receiving venous return throughout cardiac cycle) into the LV. **Rapid filling** occurs just after MV opening caused by atrial contraction, followed by **slow filling** just before MV closing.

Variables That Affect PV Loops

PV loops are useful for visualizing changes in preload, afterload, or contractility. Increases or decreases in these parameters alter the shape of the PV loop; the effect of increasing these parameters on PV loops is highlighted in Figure 1-26.

CARDIAC AND VASCULAR FUNCTION CURVES

The cardiac and vascular function curves illustrate how CO and venous return change with respect to RA pressure or end-diastolic volume (EDV). It is important to understand that each curve goes in opposite directions (Figure 1-27) because, because each answers a different question:

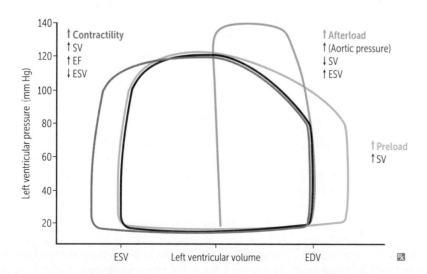

FIGURE 1-26. Effect of increased contractility, afterload, and preload on the pressure-volume loop. EDV, end-diastolic volume; EF, ejection fraction; ESV, end-systolic volume; SV, stroke volume.

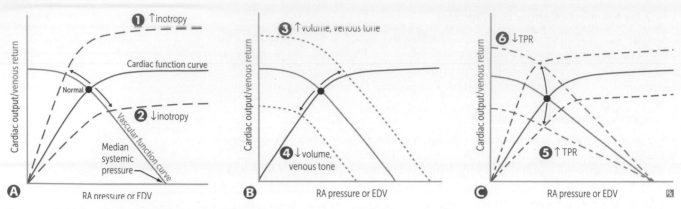

Intersection of curves = operating point of heart (ie, venous return and CO are equal).

GRAPH	EXAMPLES
A Inotropy	**❶** Catecholamines, digoxin ⊕
	❷ Uncompensated HF, narcotic overdose, sympathetic inhibition ⊖
B Venous return	**❸** Fluid infusion, sympathetic activity ⊕
	❹ Acute hemorrhage, spinal anesthesia ⊖
C Total peripheral resistance	**❺** Vasopressors ⊕
	❻ Exercise, AV shunt ⊖

Changes often occur in tandem, and may be reinforcing (eg, exercise ↑ inotropy and ↓ TPR to maximize CO) or compensatory (eg, HF ↓ inotropy → fluid retention to ↑ preload to maintain CO).

FIGURE 1-27.   Cardiac (red) and vascular (blue) function curves. Changes in inotropy, venous return, and total peripheral resistance often occur in tandem. CO, cardiac output; EDV, end-diastolic volume; HF, heart failure; RA, right atrium; SVR, systemic vascular resistance.

- **Cardiac function curve:** How does preload (RA pressure or EDV) affect CO? This should sound familiar; it is the Frank-Starling relationship! As preload increases, up to a certain point, CO also increases.

- **Vascular function curve:** How does preload (RA pressure or EDV) affect venous return? Venous return is blood returning from systemic circulation to the right heart, and is influenced by RA pressure and preload (EDV). Venous return increases with decreasing RA pressure and EDV, because the pressure gradient from the systemic veins to the right atrium increases. The flat portion of the vascular curve corresponds to negative RA pressures. At negative pressures, veins collapse, preventing an increase in venous return to the heart (maximum venous return).

Figure 1-27 shows how several factors (eg, inotropic agents, changes in circulating volume, and changes in total peripheral resistance) alter the shape of the curves. Parameters that can be measured on the combined cardiac-vascular function curves include:

- **Steady-state CO and venous return:** Intersection of the cardiac and vascular function curves (panels A, B, and C) represents the new "steady-state" CO and venous return for a given set of parameters. Note in panel A, for example, how inotropic agents shift the cardiac function curve up or down (analogous to Figure 1-24), moving the point of intersection up or down, respectively. Increased contractility, for example, results in increased CO that shifts the cardiac function curve upward; vascular function curve does not change because venous return is not affected by changes in contractility. Note, however, that the new point of intersection is at a decreased RA pressure/EDV, which reflects the fact that ejection fraction increases (ie, more blood is ejected per beat) with increasing contractility.

■ **Mean systemic pressure:** The pressure throughout the circulatory system if the heart stopped beating (ie, venous pressure = arterial pressure). If systemic pressure is equal everywhere, there is no gradient for any venous return to the heart, which corresponds to the **x-intercept of the vascular function curve** (= zero venous return). Increase in blood volume (eg, transfusion) or vasoconstriction (eg, sympathetic activation) results in an increase in the x-intercept/mean systemic pressure (Figure 1-27, panel B). Notably, the cardiac function curve is unchanged by change in blood volume, but the point of intersection is altered (often described as moving "up" or "down" the Frank-Starling curve with increasing or decreasing blood volume, respectively).

■ **Systemic vascular resistance (SVR):** Changes in SVR affect both function curves (Figure 1-27, panel C). Increase in SVR secondary to arteriolar vasoconstriction (because arterioles are the major determinant of SVR) results in increased afterload that causes decreased CO (shifts cardiac function curve down). Increased SVR also results in less venous return for a given RA pressure due to vasoconstriction (rotates the vascular function curve counterclockwise). Note that the vascular function curve rotates up or down with changes in SVR, but the x-intercept is unchanged if mean systemic pressure is fixed.

A summary of parameters that alter cardiac and vascular function curves is provided in Table 1-9.

> **? CLINICAL CORRELATION**
>
> Venodilators (eg, nitroglycerin) increase the **compliance** of veins, allowing them to hold more blood. Thus, less blood will be stored in "stiffer" arteries → decrease in mean systemic pressure.

THE CARDIAC CYCLE

The heart as a "pump" is more accurately described as two pumps in series (left and right sides of the heart). The right side (RA and RV) pumps deoxygenated blood into the lungs, and the left side (LA and LV) pumps oxygenated blood from the lungs to systemic circulation. The Frank-Starling principle ensures that the right and left "pumps" work in concert so that an increase in venous return leads to an increase in CO. For blood to move simultaneously and efficiently through the right and left sides of the heart, it relies on coordinated electrical conduction pathways to ensure well-timed ventricular contraction bilaterally.

The Wiggers diagram (named after a cardiac physiologist) is used to illustrate valvular and electrical events in one full cardiac cycle with accompanying pressure and volume changes (Figure 1-28). For clarity, the Wiggers diagram is shown only for the left side of the heart (similar events are occurring on the right side of the heart at a lower pressure).

The Wiggers diagram is divided into seven phases (divided by vertical lines) that are best studied left to right with the valvular and electrical events that occur in each phase. Recall that PV loops divide the cardiac cycle into four phases: (1) isovolumetric contraction, (2) ventricular ejection, (3) isovolumetric relaxation, and (4) LV filling. The Wiggers diagram includes each of these phases, including subdivisions of some, accounting for the seven phases (labeled at the top of Figure 1-28).

TABLE 1-9.   **Parameters That Alter Cardiac and Vascular Function Curves**

	POSITIVE INOTROPES	NEGATIVE INOTROPES	↑ BLOOD VOLUME	↓ BLOOD VOLUME	↑ SVR	↓ SVR
Cardiac Function Curve	↑ shift	↓ shift	No change	No change	↓ shift	↑ shift
Vascular Function Curve	No change	No change	↑ shift	↓ shift	Counterclockwise rotation	Clockwise rotation

SVR, systemic vascular resistance.

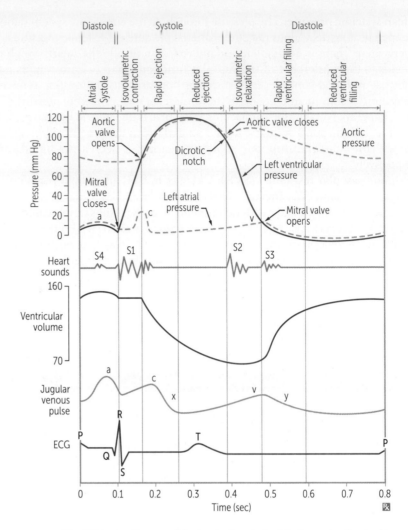

FIGURE 1-28. **The Wiggers diagram.** Mechanical and electrical events of a single cardiac cycle.

Pressure Tracings During the Cardiac Cycle

Pressure Changes in Diastole and Systole

Ventricular diastole begins with AoV closure (S_2) and lasts through the MV closure (S_1), whereas **ventricular systole** is defined as the part of the cardiac cycle from MV closure (S_1) to AoV closure (S_2) (Figure 1-28).

Pressure Changes in Left Ventricular Pressure, Aortic Pressure, and Jugular Venous Pressure

 CLINICAL CORRELATION

Atrial fibrillation can cause loss of the "atrial kick" → decreased CO.

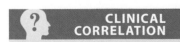 **KEY FACT**

- Heart valves OPEN when pressure upstream > pressure downstream.
- Heart valves CLOSE when pressure downstream > pressure upstream.

- **LV pressure:** The LV pressure curve is a function of changes in ventricular volume/pressure changes during diastole and systole.
  - Diastole: AoV closure marks the beginning of diastole. The LV relaxes and the pressure inside decreases. MV opens when LA pressure is higher than LV pressure. Blood enters the LV from the LA passively along a favorable pressure gradient. At the end of diastole, during atrial systole, the atrium contracts and actively fills the LV ("atrial kick"). When LV pressure exceeds LA pressure, the MV closes, marking the end of diastole and beginning of systole.
  - Systole: MV closure marks the beginning of systole. The LV contracts and LV pressure rapidly rises during isovolumetric contraction. When LV pressure is higher than aortic pressure, the AoV opens. As blood rushes out of the LV into the aorta, LV pressure drops. The AoV closes when aortic pressure exceeds LV pressure, marking the end of systole and beginning of diastole.

- **Aortic pressure:** The aortic pressure curve reflects pressure/volume changes in the aorta during diastole and systole.
  - Diastole: Aortic pressure is higher than LV pressure during diastole (ventricular filling); thus the AoV remains closed. Normal diastolic pressure in adults is 80–90 mm Hg.
  - Systole: LV pressure exceeds AoV during systole; thus the AoV is open. Pressure in the aorta increases as the stroke volume is ejected, but begins to decrease as ejection rate slows. Normal systolic pressure in adults is 120–140 mm Hg.
- **Jugular venous pulses:** Provides another complementary pressure tracing to follow mechanical (as opposed to valvular) events of systole and diastole; mirrors left atrial pressure (LAP) since the LA is continuous with jugular vein via the SVC; consists of *a*, *c*, and *v* waves, and *y* descent (see Figure 1-28).
  a wave: **A**trial contraction
  c wave: RV **c**ontraction (tricuspid valve bulging into the RA)
  v wave: Increased RA pressure due to filling against closed tricuspid valve
  y descent: Corresponds to rate of atrial emptying as the tricuspid valve opens

Pressures in the various heart chambers are measured by doing a right-heart catheterization, which involves placing a pulmonary artery catheter (sometimes referred to as a Swan-Ganz catheter) into the SVC → right atrium → right ventricle → pulmonary artery (Figure 1-29). This allows right-sided pressures and waveforms to be obtained. When the catheter is "wedged" in a pulmonary branch, it forms a closed chamber that is continuous with the left atrium and allows measurement of a pulmonary capillary wedge pressure (PCWP) that is a good approximation of LAP.

Heart Sounds

The state of valve closure, ventricular filling, or pathology can be extrapolated from four heart sounds (Table 1-10). The relative timing of the four heart sounds in relation to the cardiac cycle is shown in Figure 1-30.

S₁ and S₂, Splitting

S_1 and S_2 are due to valve closures. S_1 is due to closure of the mitral and tricuspid valves; S_2 is due to closure of the aortic and pulmonic valves. S_1 is usually auscultated as a single sound. S_2, which is really composed of two sounds closely linked in time

KEY FACT

The slope of the *y* descent in the JVP waveform decreases in tamponade (ie, RA empties more slowly) and increases in constrictive pericarditis (ie, RA empties more quickly, filling ends more abruptly).

CLINICAL CORRELATION

Jugular venous distention (JVD) is common in right heart failure (RHF) due to elevated right atrial pressure.

MNEMONIC

Nickel, dime, quarter rule for heart pressures:
RA ~ 5 mm Hg (nickel)
LA ~ 10 mm Hg (dime)
RV ~ 25 mm Hg (quarter)
LV ~ 120 mm Hg (systemic BP)

CLINICAL CORRELATION

PCWP can be used to distinguish between isolated left heart failure (LHF) and right heart failure (RHF):
- LHF → ↑ LAP → ↑ PCWP
- Isolated RHF → normal LAP → normal PCWP

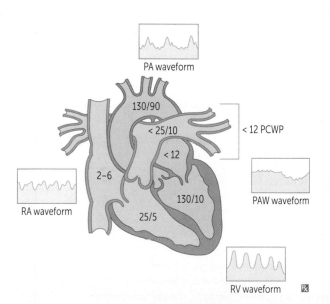

FIGURE 1-29. **Normal pressures in the heart in millimeters of mercury (mm Hg).** Superior vena cava, 5; right atrium, 2–6; right ventricle, 25/5; left atrium, < 12; left ventricle, 130/10; aorta, 130/90. PA, pulmonary artery; PAW, pulmonary artery wedge; PCWP, pulmonary capillary wedge pressure; RA, right atrial; RV, right ventricular.

TABLE 1-10. **Heart Sounds and Significance**

SOUND	SIGNIFICANCE
S_1	MV and tricuspid valve closure; the MV closes before the tricuspid, so S_1 may be split (but usually not discernible).
S_2	Aortic and pulmonary valve closure; the AoV (A_2) closes before the pulmonic valve (P_2); inspiration causes increased physiological splitting of S_2.
S_3	Ventricular gallop. Occurs right after S_2 in early diastole due to turbulent blood flow. Normal in children, young adults, and pregnancy. In older adults (age > 40), is associated with states of volume overload (heart failure, high-output heart failure).
S_4	Atrial gallop. Occurs right before S_1 in late diastole, when the atrium contracts ("atrial kick") against a stiff ventricle. Associated with ventricular hypertrophy and acute myocardial infarction. May be a feature of hypertension (secondary to ventricular hypertrophy). Abnormal in children.

AoV, aortic valve; MV, mitral valve.

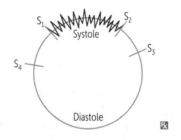

FIGURE 1-30. **Relative timing of the four heart sounds (S_1-S_4) in one full cardiac cycle.**

(AoV closure, A_2, and pulmonic valve closure, P_2), exhibits a normal splitting during inspiration. Examples of normal and pathological splitting are in Table 1-11.

HEMODYNAMICS AND PERIPHERAL VASCULAR CIRCULATION

Physical factors such as blood flow, velocity, resistance, and capacitance govern blood flow within the circulatory system. The components of blood and the circulatory system (ie, types of vasculature) are reviewed briefly.

Blood

Normal adult blood composition is illustrated in Figure 1-31. Note that serum = plasma – clotting factors (eg, fibrinogen).

TABLE 1-11. **Splitting**

TYPE OF SPLITTING	PATHOPHYSIOLOGY	ILLUSTRATION OF SPLITTING
Normal	Inspiration → drop in intrathoracic pressure → ↑ venous return → ↑ RV filling → ↑ RV stroke volume → ↑ RV ejection time → delayed closure of pulmonic valve. ↓ pulmonary impedance (↑ capacity of the pulmonary circulation) also occurs during inspiration, which contributes to delayed closure of pulmonic valve.	E / I : S1, A2 P2 — Normal delay
Wide	Seen in conditions that delay RV emptying (eg, pulmonic stenosis, right bundle branch block). Delay in RV emptying causes delayed pulmonic sound (especially on inspiration). An exaggeration of normal splitting.	E / I : S1, A2 P2 — Abnormal delay
Fixed	Heard in ASD. ASD → left-to-right shunt → ↑ RA and RV volumes → ↑ flow through pulmonic valve such that, regardless of breath, pulmonic closure is greatly delayed.	E / I : S1, A2 P2 (=)
Paradoxical	Heard in conditions that delay aortic valve closure (eg, aortic stenosis, left bundle branch block). Normal order of valve closure is reversed so that P_2 sound occurs before delayed A_2 sound. Therefore on inspiration, P_2 closes later and moves closer to A_2, thereby "paradoxically" eliminating the split (usually heard in expiration).	E / I : S1, P2 A2

E = Expiration
I = Inspiration

Modified with permission from Le T, et al. *First Aid for the USMLE Step 1: 2017.* New York: McGraw-Hill Education, 2017.

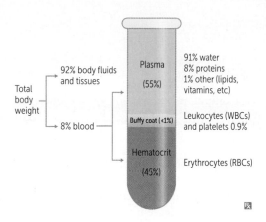

FIGURE 1-31. **Composition of blood post-centrifugation in average adult.** Note that a "normal" hematocrit can vary depending on age and gender.

Components of the Vasculature

The vasculature includes arteries, arterioles, capillaries, venules, and veins, each of which has different composition and function (Table 1-12).

Hemodynamic Parameters

Velocity of Blood Flow

$$v = Q/A$$

where

v is velocity (cm/min)
Q is blood flow (mL/min)
A is cross-sectional area (cm^2)

Velocity is directly proportional to blood flow (↑ blood flow → ↑ velocity), and inversely proportional to area (ie, blood flow velocity is greater in the aorta [smaller cross-sectional area] than in the capillaries [larger **total** cross-sectional area]).

> **KEY FACT**
>
> **Arterioles:** Site of highest resistance in the CV system
> **Capillaries:** Largest total cross-sectional and surface area (remember, this facilitates gas and nutrient exchange!)
> **Veins:** Site of highest capacitance (or compliance) in the CV system

TABLE 1-12. **Function and Composition of the Vasculature**

	COMPOSITION	PRESSURE	FUNCTION
Artery	Thick-walled with elastic tissue, smooth muscle	High	Delivers oxygenated blood to tissues
Arteriole	Smooth muscle with innervation from autonomic nerve fibers	High	Smallest branch of an artery; dilates or constricts in response to neurohormonal stimuli and thus is major determinant of systemic vascular resistance
Capillary	Single layer of endothelial cells, thin-walled	Low	Exchanges nutrients, water, and gases with surrounding tissues
Venule	Thin-walled	Low	Formed from merging capillaries; site of margination, adhesion, and transmigration of inflammatory cells into surrounding tissue
Vein	Thin-walled, highly compliant	Low	The largest vein, the vena cava, returns blood to the heart

Blood Flow

$$Q = \Delta P / R$$

Relationship is analogous to Ohm's law ($I = V/R$), where

Q (blood flow or cardiac output, mL/min)	$\leftrightarrow$	I (current)
ΔP (pressure gradient, mm Hg)	$\leftrightarrow$	V (voltage)
R (resistance, mm Hg/mL/min)	$\leftrightarrow$	R

Blood flow (Q) is directly proportional to pressure gradient (ΔP) and inversely proportional to resistance (R). Blood flows from high (aorta) to low (vena cava) pressure. Various hormones and drugs can cause **vasoconstriction** (increase in R) or **vasodilation** (decrease in R) to decrease and increase blood flow, respectively.

Resistance (r)

$$\text{Resistance} = \frac{\text{driving pressure }(\Delta P)}{\text{flow }(Q)} = \frac{8\eta(\text{viscosity}) \times \text{length}}{\pi r^4} \text{ (Poiseuille's law)}$$

Resistance is inversely proportional to the fourth power of the blood vessel radius, so increasing the radius by 2 times decreases the resistance by a factor of $2^4 = 16$! Resistances in parallel or series can be calculated with the following equations:

- In **parallel** (eg, systemic circulation in which each organ is supplied by an artery that branches off the aorta)

$$1/R_{\text{total}} = 1/R_a + 1/R_b + \ldots + 1/R_n$$

- In **series** (eg, the arrangement of blood vessels in a given organ; the incoming large artery becomes arterioles, capillaries, and veins that are arranged in series)

$$R_{\text{total}} = R_{\text{artery}} + R_{\text{capillaries}} + R_{\text{veins}}$$

- The same volume of blood flows through each set of vessels (ie, blood flow through the largest artery is the same as through all the capillaries).

Arterioles are the site of greatest resistance, and they are responsible for the largest drop in arterial pressure.

Capacitance (Compliance)

$$C = \Delta V / \Delta P$$

where

C is capacitance (mL/mm Hg)
V is volume (mL)
P is pressure (mm Hg)

Capacitance (or compliance) describes how distensible a blood vessel is and is inversely related to elastance. Since veins are more compliant than arteries, more blood is stored in veins than in arteries. With aging, vessels stiffen and become less compliant.

Laminar Versus Turbulent Flow

Laminar flow is streamlined (ie, travels in a straight line). Turbulent flow is not and causes audible vibrations (bruits). Turbulent flow is more likely in states with the following:

- Decreased blood viscosity (eg, anemia)
- Increased blood velocity (eg, narrower vessel, increased CO)

? CLINICAL CORRELATION

Organ removal (eg, nephrectomy) → ↑ total peripheral resistance and ↓ flow (cardiac output).

KEY FACT

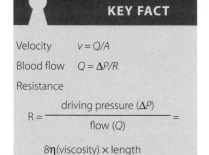

Velocity $v = Q/A$

Blood flow $Q = \Delta P/R$

Resistance

$$R = \frac{\text{driving pressure }(\Delta P)}{\text{flow }(Q)} =$$

$$\frac{8\eta(\text{viscosity}) \times \text{length}}{\pi r^4}$$

(Poiseuille's law)

Capacitance (or compliance) $C = \Delta V/\Delta P$

Capillary Fluid Exchange

Fluid movement is determined by osmotic and hydrostatic pressures in the capillary and interstitial spaces, which are known as Starling forces (Figure 1-32). These include:

- P_c = Capillary hydrostatic pressure: Tends to push fluid out of the capillary
- P_i = Interstitial hydrostatic pressure: Tends to push fluid into the capillary
- π_c = Capillary oncotic pressure: Tends to pull fluid into the capillary
- π_i = Interstitial oncotic pressure: Tends to pull fluid out of the capillary

Net Filtration Pressure

The net filtration pressure (P_{net}) is the sum of the Starling forces. $P_{net} > 0$ favors net filtration into the interstitial space. $P_{net} < 0$ favors net absorption into the capillary. Under normal circumstances, $P_{net} > 0$ entering the capillary (arteriolar end) to promote filtration into the interstitial space and $P_{net} < 0$ leaving the capillary (venular end) to reabsorb filtered blood and ensure no significant intravascular volume loss.

$$P_{net} = [(P_c - P_i) - (\pi_c - \pi_i)]$$

FLASH FORWARD

The determinants of glomerular filtration rate (GFR) of the kidney are also dictated by Starling forces, in which the Bowman capsule is analogous to the interstitial space.

Net Fluid Flow

The net fluid flow (J_v, mL/min) is determined by P_{net} and K_f, the filtration constant (capillary permeability). This relationship is known as the **Starling equation.** A positive J_v means net fluid movement out of the capillary (filtration).

$$J_v = K_f \times P_{net} = K_f[(P_c - P_i) - (\pi_c - \pi_i)]$$

Lymphatics

Lymph from the right side of the upper body empties into the right lymphatic duct. All other lymph from the rest of the body empties via the **thoracic duct** (at the junction of the left subclavian vein and left internal jugular vein) into the venous system. Lymph has a similar composition as the surrounding interstitial fluid.

Edema

Changes in Starling forces and capillary permeability (K_f) can result in edematous states by increasing the net fluid flow (J_v) (Table 1-13). If changes in Starling forces predominantly cause edema, it is classified as **transudative.** If changes in capillary permeability (K_f) largely cause edema, it is classified as **exudative** (Table 1-14).

MEASUREMENT AND REGULATION OF ARTERIAL PRESSURE

Mean arterial pressure (MAP) is determined by CO, systemic vascular resistance (SVR), and central venous pressure (CVP), according to Ohm's law applied for blood flow:

$$\Delta P = Q \times R$$
$$MAP - CVP = CO \times SVR$$
$$MAP = (CO \times SVR) + CVP$$

Because CVP is usually ~ 0 mm Hg, this is simplified to:

$$MAP = CO \times SVR$$

Accordingly, **changes in CO or SVR affect MAP** (Figure 1-33). In simple terms, there are three determinants of blood pressure: (1) how well the "pump" works (CO), (2) how much blood there is (intravascular volume regulated by kidney, which indirectly impacts CO), and (3) SVR (arteriolar dilation or constriction).

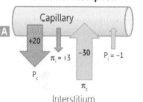

Net pressure = −31 + 23 = −8 mm Hg
Favors **net absorption**

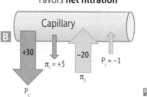

Net pressure = −21 + 33 = +12 mm Hg
Favors **net filtration**

FIGURE 1-32. Starling forces that favor net absorption A and net filtration B across a capillary. Numbers represent hypothetical magnitudes of Starling forces in mm Hg. By convention, negative pressures favor net absorption into the capillary while positive pressures favor net filtration out of the capillary. It is the sum of Starling forces that determines if there is net filtration (eg, arteriole end of capillary) or net absorption (eg, venule end of capillary).

TABLE 1-13.   Causes and Examples of Edema

CAUSE	EXAMPLES
↑ P_c	↑ venous pressure secondary to: ■ CHF (eg, pulmonary edema) ■ Venous obstruction (eg, deep venous thrombosis) ■ Cirrhosis (eg, portal hypertension) ■ Standing, which causes edema in the dependent limbs
↓ π_c	↓ plasma protein concentration (primarily of albumin) secondary to: ■ ↓ Synthesis (liver disease) ■ ↓ Intake (protein malnutrition) ■ ↑ Excretion (nephrotic syndrome)
↑ K_f	Burns Inflammation (eg, histamine, bradykinin) secondary to: ■ Allergic reactions ■ Sepsis ■ Acute respiratory distress syndrome
↑ interstitial pressure	Lymphatic obstruction secondary to: ■ Post-mastectomy ■ Malignancy ■ Congenital lymphedema ■ Filariasis

Due to changes in aortic pressure during diastole and systole, the arterial pressure correspondingly varies in a pulsatile pattern during the cardiac cycle. It is assessed by measuring systolic pressure and diastolic pressure; both values are used to calculate MAP and pulse pressure (Figure 1-34).

- **Systolic pressure:** Highest arterial pressure of the cardiac cycle. Measured after the heart contracts and blood has been ejected into the arterial system. In older patients, it is increased due to age-related stiffening of large arteries. In younger patients, it is increased due to increased SV. Decreases with dehydration, β-blockers, diuretics, and blood loss.
- **Diastolic pressure:** Lowest arterial pressure of the cardiac cycle. Corresponds to the time when the heart is relaxed and blood is returning to the heart via the venous

TABLE 1-14.   Types of Edema

	TRANSUDATE	EXUDATE
Mechanism	↑ capillary pressure (P_c) or ↓ oncotic pressure (π_c)	More permeable vessels (↑ K_f). Due to inflammation, etc
	Fluid from the vessel is either pushed out or leaves based on differences in osmotic pressure	The vessel becomes leakier; therefore both protein and fluid leave
Composition of fluid	Protein-poor Hypocellular Specific gravity < 1.012	Protein-rich Cellular Specific gravity > 1.020
Examples	■ Pulmonary edema from CHF (↑ pulmonary venous pressure) ■ Lower extremity edema from CHF (↑ plasma volume) ■ Ascites (↑ portal pressure and ↓ oncotic pressure)	■ Malignant pleural effusion ■ Parapneumonic pleural effusion

CHF, congestive heart failure.

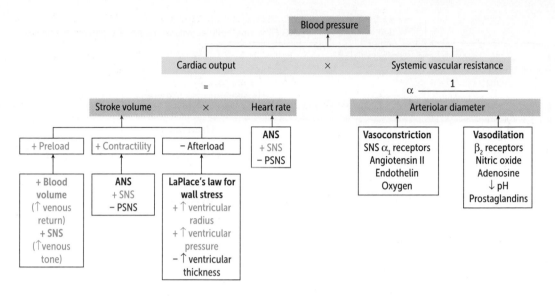

FIGURE 1-33. **Determinants of blood pressure.** Blood pressure = stroke volume × heart rate. Note systemic vascular resistance is **inversely** proportional to arteriolar diameter. ANS, autonomic nervous system; PSNS, parasympathetic nervous systems; SNS, sympathetic nervous system.

system. Decreases with aortic stiffening (decreased compliance), which results in less blood volume in the aorta at the onset of diastole.

- **Pulse pressure:** Difference between systolic and diastolic pressure; depends mainly on SV. Decreased aortic compliance secondary to aging (think stiffer pipes) increases the pulse pressure since systolic pressure increases and diastolic pressure decreases.

$$\textbf{MAP} = \text{diastolic pressure} + {}^1/_3 \times (\text{pulse pressure})$$
$$\textbf{Pulse pressure} = \text{systolic pressure} - \text{diastolic pressure}$$

Regulation of Mean Arterial Pressure

Changes in MAP are detected by either baroreceptors or the kidney as decreased extracellular circulating volume (ECV) (Figure 1-35). In the carotid sinus and aortic arch, decreased baroreceptor firing is centrally processed and relayed to the autonomic nervous system (ANS). In the kidney, decreased ECV and activation of the sympathetic nervous system (via B_1 receptors on the juxtaglomerular apparatus) activate the renin-

CLINICAL CORRELATION

Aortic regurgitation characteristically presents with increased pulse pressure due to (1) regurgitation of blood into the LV (decreases diastolic pressure) and (2) increased stroke volume from chronic regurgitation (increases systolic pressure).

KEY FACT

Diastolic pressure impacts MAP more than does systolic pressure, because diastole is longer than systole.

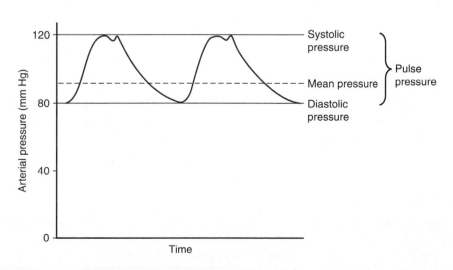

FIGURE 1-34. **Arterial pressure during the cardiac cycle.**

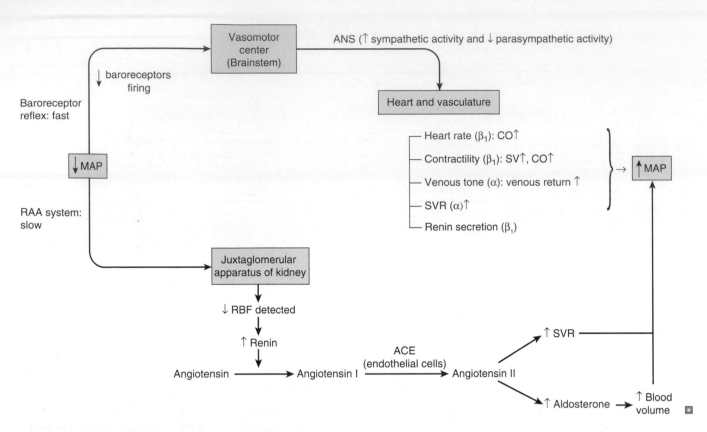

FIGURE 1-35. **Control of mean arterial pressure (MAP).** ANS, autonomic nervous system; CO, cardiac output; RAA, renin–angiotensin–aldosterone; RBF, renal blood flow; SV, stroke volume; SVR, systemic vascular resistance.

angiotensin-aldoesterone system (RAAS). The baroreceptor reflex is neurally controlled and has a fast (minute-to-minute) response, whereas the RAAS is hormonally controlled with a slower regulation response.

Mechanisms other than the fast baroreceptor reflex and slower RAAS to regulate arterial pressure are based on P_{CO_2}, P_{O_2}, blood volume, and atrial pressure (Table 1-15).

TABLE 1-15. **Other Mechanisms That Regulate Arterial Pressure**

TRIGGER	RESPONSE
↑ P_{CO_2} in brain tissue (cerebral ischemia)	↑ sympathetic outflow to heart and blood vessels.
↓ P_{O_2} detected by chemoreceptors in carotid and aortic bodies	Vasoconstriction to increase systemic vascular resistance (SVR) and arterial pressure.
↓ blood volume of at least 10% (eg, hemorrhage)	Release of vasopressin (ADH) leads to vasoconstriction, which increases SVR and water reabsorption.
↑ atrial pressure	Release of atrial natriuretic peptide (ANP) to relax vascular smooth muscle to reduce SVR and increase natriuresis to reduce blood volume.
↑ ventricular pressure	Release of B-type natriuretic peptide (BNP), which has similar actions as ANP. Of note, however, BNP is generally elevated during the stretch of diseased myocytes (eg, CHF exacerbation, MI).

ADH, antidiuretic hormone; CHF, congestive heart failure; MI, myocardial infarction.

Baroreceptor Reflex: Short-Term Regulation of Blood Pressure

Stretch receptors located within the walls of the carotid sinus and aortic arch respond to changes in BP. Carotid sinus baroreceptors are tonically active, so increased activity indicates an increase in BP, and decreased firing indicates decreased BP. Changes in firing rate at the carotid sinus (transmitted by CN IX) and at the aortic arch (transmitted by CN X) are relayed to the solitary nucleus of the brain stem and elicit an ANS response.

For example, decreased firing secondary to perceived drop in BP leads to decreased parasympathetic and increased sympathetic outflow to the heart, leading to increased HR, contractility, SV, and vasoconstriction of arterioles and veins. Accordingly, increased baroreceptor firing leads to increased parasympathetic and decreased sympathetic outflow, leading to decreased HR, contractility, and SV, and vasodilation of arterioles and veins.

Maneuvers that affect baroreceptor reflex:

- Increased sympathetic nervous system (SNS) output, decreased parasympathetic nervous system (PNS) output: leads to increase in blood pressure.
  - Carotid occlusion, cutting afferents, orthostasis/lying to standing, and fluid loss.
- Increased PNS output, decreased SNS output: leads to a dramatic decrease in blood pressure.
  - Carotid massage, volume loading, and weightlessness.

Autonomic Nervous System

Table 1-16 summarizes effects of parasympathetic and sympathetic nervous stimulation on the main determinants of arterial blood pressure (CO = HR × SV and SVR). Of note, the effect of ANS on HR is often referred to as "chronotropic effect." Parasympathetic stimulation causes negative chronotropic effects, and sympathetic stimulation causes positive chronotropic effects.

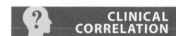

CLINICAL CORRELATION

Angiotensin-converting enzyme (ACE) inhibitors and angiotensin II receptor blockers (ARBs) impede the RAAS pathway and thus are commonly used in the management of hypertension.

Renin-Angiotensin-Aldosterone System: Long-Term Regulation of Blood Pressure

Decreased BP activates the RAAS. Renin is secreted from specialized smooth muscle cells in the kidney called **juxtaglomerular cells** (JG cells) in response to three triggers:

1. ↓ perfusion pressure (detected by stretch receptors in JG cells of the nephron)
2. ↓ Na^+ in distal tubule (detected by specialized cells in the macula densa of the nephron)
3. ↑ sympathetic stimulation (detected by β_1 receptors on JG cells)

Renin cleaves angiotensinogen (produced in the liver) to angiotensin I. Angiotensin converting enzyme (ACE), secreted by endothelial cells, then converts angiotensin I

TABLE 1-16. Autonomic Effects on the Heart and Blood Vessels

	SYMPATHETIC		PARASYMPATHETIC	
	ACTION	RECEPTOR	ACTION	RECEPTOR
Heart rate	↑	β_1	↓	M_2
Contractility	↑	β_1	↓	M_2
Vascular smooth muscle tone	Constriction[a]	α_1	Dilation	M_3

[a]Vascular smooth muscle in skeletal muscle also contains β_2 receptors, which cause vascular smooth muscle dilation.

to angiotension II (AII), a peptide hormone that increases SVR/intravascular volume to ↑ BP by two main mechanisms:

- Vasconstriction (via AII receptors on vascular smooth muscle)
- Release of aldosterone (via AII receptor on adrenal cortex) → acts on mineralocorticoid receptors in nephron to reabsorb Na^+/H_2O

AII also has direct effects on various organs to maintain increase in BP:

- Heart (↑ contractility and ventricular hypertrophy)
- Kidney (directly increases Na^+ reabsorption)
- Posterior pituitary (stimulates antidiuretic hormone [ADH] secretion)

Autoregulation

Each organ has a different mechanism to **autoregulate** or maintain constant blood flow over a wide range of perfusion pressures. Recall Ohm's law applied to blood flow:

$$Q = \Delta P/R$$

If perfusion pressure (ΔP) of an organ decreases, autoregulation in blood vessels attempts to decrease resistance (R) to maintain blood flow (Q). Autoregulation is particularly important in maintaining blood flow to highly metabolic organs like the brain, heart, and kidney. For example, in hemorrhage, autoregulation ensures preferential vasodilation of cerebral and coronary vascular beds despite vasoconstriction mediated by the SNS via the baroreceptor reflex. Autoregulation also allows maintenance of blood flow to organs, despite a chronic decrease in perfusion pressure (eg, due to progressive atherosclerosis) by vasodilation of arterioles downstream of narrowed arteries.

Myogenic, endothelial, and metabolic mechanisms contribute to autoregulation independent of neural and hormonal input. Myogenic behavior is the intrinsic ability of vascular smooth muscle to constrict and dilate in response to an acute increase and decrease in pressure, respectively, to maintain blood flow. Endothelial cells can also release vasodilators (nitric oxide, prostacyclin) and vasoconstrictors (endothelin). Inflammation and ischemia can alter the normal balance of vasodilators and vasoconstrictors (eg, acute MI, atherosclerosis), thereby affecting vascular tone. Finally, metabolic needs also influence blood flow. For example, except for the pulmonary vasculature, in which hypoxia induces vasoconstriction, hypoxia causes vasodilation in all other organs to increase delivery of blood/O_2 to starved tissues. Metabolites that play important roles in vasodilating specific organ beds in response to metabolic needs are listed in Table 1-17.

ELECTROCARDIOGRAPHY

Electrocardiograms (ECGs) provide important information about cardiac structure and function by measuring the electrical impulse flowing through the heart.

TABLE 1-17.   Autoregulation in Various Organs

ORGAN (% CARDIAC OUTPUT RECEIVED)	MAJOR VASODILATOR(S)
Coronaries in the heart (5)	Adenosine
Skeletal muscle (20)	Lactic acid, K^+
Brain (15)	CO_2 (pH)

KEY FACT

Circulation through organs:
Liver: Largest proportion of systemic cardiac output
Kidney: Highest blood flow per gram of tissue
Heart: Largest arteriovenous O_2 difference; ↑ O_2 demand met by ↑ coronary blood flow.

Electrocardiogram Leads

In a conventional 12-lead ECG, there are 12 electrical axes or leads (six on the frontal plane and six on the transverse/horizontal plane) that are formed by electrodes placed on the chest wall and extremities. The electrical axes the leads form are shown in Figure 1-36.

Imagine 12 leads taking "snapshots" from different angles of the heart's net electrical activity. The net electrical activity (measured in volts on the ECG's y axis) is essentially an average of all of the tiny electrical vectors flowing through the heart at any given time point. The net "electrical vector" is directed toward the heart's apex for most of its journey from the atria to ventricles; it ultimately swings to the thicker left posterior aspect of the heart, which contains a high density of myocytes and thus more conduction pathways.

> **KEY FACT**
>
> Locations and corresponding leads:
> Inferior = II, III, aVF
> Septal = V_1, V_2
> Lateral = I, V_5, V_6, aVL

Electrocardiogram Waveforms

Important waveforms (P wave, QRS complex, and T wave) of the ECG are illustrated in Figure 1-37. Each waveform corresponds to a specific part of the action potential in one cardiac cycle:

- Atrial depolarization → P wave
- Ventricular depolarization → QRS complex
- Ventricular repolarization → T wave

Note: Atrial repolarization is masked by the QRS complex.

> **KEY FACT**
>
> A tiny positive deflection following the T wave, called a U wave, is rarely seen and is associated with bradycardia and hypokalemia.

Waveforms, as described below, reflect the net depolarization and repolarization vectors of action potentials spreading through the heart.

There are four golden rules of ECGs:

1. Depolarization toward a (+) pole of a lead produces an upward deflection on ECG.
2. Depolarization toward a (−) pole of a lead produces a downward deflection on ECG.

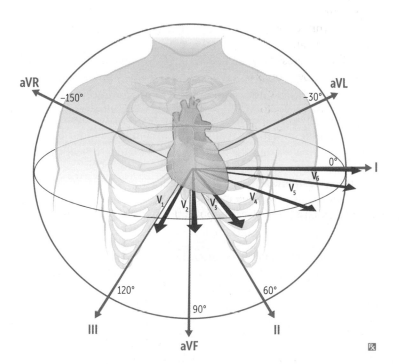

FIGURE 1-36. **Electrical axes of the heart.** Six limb leads (blue) and six precordial leads (red) create electrical axes in the frontal and transverse planes, respectively. By convention, the arrowhead is (+) pole of the lead with (−) pole of the same lead being directly opposite the arrowhead in the same plane.

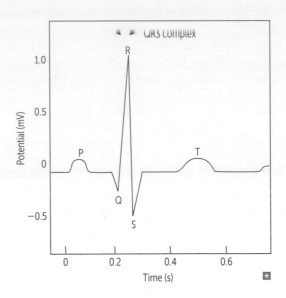

FIGURE 1-37. **Waveforms.** P wave, QRS complex, and T wave in one cardiac cycle.

3. The magnitude of deflection (up or down) is proportional to how parallel the net electrical vector is to the lead measuring it.
4. A net electrical vector records zero magnitude in any lead perpendicular to it.

With these golden rules in mind, it is possible to understand why the waveforms look slightly different in magnitude and direction in each of 12 ECG leads. During interpretation of an ECG, different leads provide useful information depending on the clinical question (eg, determining location of MI, assessing for LV and RV hypertrophy, calculating mean QRS axis).

Electrocardiogram Interpretation

ECGs should be interpreted using a systematic sequence of steps each time. Note the x-axis of an ECG strip is time (1 small box = 0.04 sec), and the y-axis of an ECG strip measures electrical potential (1 small box = 1 mV). Recall that deflections on the ECG strip are measuring the net electrical vector of the heart at a given time during the cardiac cycle. Below is a straightforward method to use for interpreting ECGs.

- **Heart rhythm:** Rhythm describes where the heart beat originates and how it is conducted (often described as "regular" or "irregular"). Under physiologic conditions, rhythm originates from the SA node and is regular. So-called "sinus rhythm" is present if
  - Every P wave is followed by a QRS complex.
  - Every QRS complex is preceded by P wave.
  - P wave is upright in leads I, II, and III.
  - PR interval > 0.12 sec (three small boxes).

  If the above criteria are not met, an arrhythmia is present (discussed in the Arrhythmia section). Note that an arrhythmia may still be present even if the criteria for sinus rhythm are met, because the defect may still be in the conduction of the electrical impulse (eg, bundle branch blocks, first-degree AV block); therefore, to detect an arrhythmia, it is important to assess ALL the waveforms and segments (below).

- **Heart Rate:** Normal rate is 60–100 bpm (bradycardia < 60 bpm, tachycardia > 100 bpm)
  - Because ECG speed is 25 mm/sec (1 mm = 1 small box), the heart rate can be calculated by counting the number of boxes between two QRS complexes (also known as the R-R distance):

$$\text{Heart rate} = \frac{25 \text{ mm/sec} \times 60 \text{ sec/min}}{\text{Number of mm between beats}}$$
$$\text{(bpm)}$$

$$\text{Heart rate} = \frac{1{,}500}{\text{Number of small boxes between two consecutive beats}}$$
$$\text{(bpm)}$$

- If the beat is irregular, calculate HR:

$$\text{HR} = \# \text{ of QRS complexes in 6 seconds} \times 10$$

- **Intervals (PR, QRS, QT):** Intervals include a wave (P, QRS, or T) and a portion of the ECG baseline. Clinically important intervals, their normal width (measured in seconds), and their relationship to the cardiac conduction pathway are detailed in Table 1-18.
- **Mean QRS axis:** Measures the direction of the net electrical vector generated during ventricular depolarization in the frontal plane (Figure 1-38). The normal path of

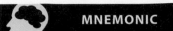

MNEMONIC

Drug-induced long QT (**ABCDE**):
Anti**A**rrhythmics (class IA, III)
Anti**B**iotics (eg, macrolides)
Anti"**C**"cychotics (eg, haloperidol)
Anti**D**epressants (eg, TCAs)
Anti**E**metics (eg, ondansetron)

KEY FACT

↑ HR leads to ↓ PR interval and ↓ QT interval.

TABLE 1-18.   **Electrocardiographic Intervals**

INTERVAL		NORMAL RANGE	PART OF THE CARDIAC CYCLE	EXAMPLE OF ARRHYTHMIAS WITH ABNORMAL INTERVALS
PR		0.12–0.20 sec (3–5 small boxes)	Corresponds to time it takes for the electrical impulse to travel from SA node, through AV node, to the start of ventricular depolarization	First-degree AV heart block: sinus rhythm and PR interval > 0.20
QRS		≤ 0.10 sec (≤ 2.5 small boxes)	Corresponds to ventricular depolarization	QRS complexes > 0.10 sec may reflect delayed conduction **within** (eg, bundle branch block) or **outside** of the specialized conduction pathway of the heart (eg, ventricular tachycardia)
QT		Heart rate 60–100 bpm: QT ≤ half the distance between two consecutive QRS complexes (R-R distance) Heart rate < 60 or > 100 bpm: Use the corrected QT: = QT/√(R-R) ≤ 0.44 seconds	Corresponds to mechanical contraction of the ventricles	Long QT syndrome can be inherited or acquired (eg, from QT-prolonging medications) and predisposes to a form of ventricular tachycardia called torsade de pointes

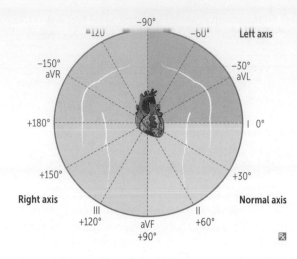

FIGURE 1-38. **Calculation of the QRS axis.** Mean QRS axis is determined by which quadrant the net electrical vector falls in, as determined by the direction of the QRS complex in leads I and aVF.

conduction creates a net electrical vector in the direction of the cardiac apex (0 to 90 degrees). An abnormal axis may indicate a fascicular block and/or ventricular hypertrophy. Estimation of mean QRS axis is determined by the direction of the QRS complex in leads I and aVF (some texts suggest using leads I and II), as described in Table 1-19, which correlates with a net electrical vector in a normal, left-deviated, or right-deviated quadrant on the electrical axes (Figure 1-38).

■ **P-wave abnormalities:** Increased height and/or splitting of the P wave in leads II (most parallel to net electrical vector of atrial depolarization) or V_1 can be useful for detecting right or left atrial enlargement, which can accompany conditions like systolic heart failure and/or any valvular defects (eg, mitral stenosis) that cause elevated atrial pressures.

■ **QRS abnormalities:** The amplitude and width of the QRS complex is useful for noting hypertrophy and bundle branch blocks, respectively.

   ■ **Left (LV) or right (RV) ventricular hypertrophy:** Increased muscle mass leads to increased "signal" of the electrical activity of the heart. Using this principle and knowing that QRS axis shifts may accompany hypertrophy, criteria have been proposed to diagnose RV and LV hypertrophy (Table 1-20).

   ■ **Bundle branch block (BBB):** Damage anywhere along the left or right bundle branch (Figure 1-15) can cause a BBB. Central to diagnosing a left or right BBB is detecting a wide QRS complex, resulting from asymmetric, slower cell-to-cell conduction in the part of the ventricle that is "blocked" from the normal pathway of faster Purkinje fiber conduction. By definition, a "complete block" has a QRS width higher than 0.12 sec (3 small boxes), and an "incomplete block" has a QRS width between 0.10 and 0.12 sec (2.5–3.0 small boxes). Notably, if only the

TABLE 1-19. **Mean QRS axis.**

DIRECTION OF QRS COMPLEX IN LEAD I	DIRECTION OF QRS COMPLEX IN LEAD aVF	MEAN QRS AXIS
↑	↑	Normal
↑	↓	Left-deviated (eg, left anterior fascicular block, LV hypertrophy)
↓	↑	Right-deviated (eg, RV hypertrophy, RV strain from acute pulmonary embolism, left posterior fascicular block)

LV, left ventricular; RV, right ventricular.

TABLE 1-20.   Left Ventricular (LV) and Right Ventricular (RV) Hypertrophy Criteria

	CRITERIA
LV hypertrophy[1]	▪ S in V_1 + R in V_5 or $V_6 \geq 35$ mm OR ▪ R in aVL > 11 mm OR ▪ R in lead I > 15 mm
RV hypertrophy	▪ R > S in lead V_1 ▪ Right axis deviation

[1]Many criteria proposed for LV Hypertrophy. Listed are three criteria commonly used.

anterior or posterior fascicle of the left bundle branch is blocked (a hemiblock), QRS width is typically normal (only part of LV activation is compromised), but mean QRS axis deviation, as described above, may occur. Finally, because BBB results in an altered sequence of ventricular depolarization, leads V_1 (anterior) and V_6 (posterior) are useful for detecting additional changing waveforms associated with left and right BBBs (Table 1-21).

▪ **Signs of Acute Coronary Syndrome (ACS):** The earliest ECG changes in ACS (eg, unstable angina, NSTEMI, STEMI) are in the ST segment, because depolarization is more susceptible to ischemic injury than repolarization. Ischemia inhibits the ATP Na/K pumps, making the resting membrane potential of injured myocytes more positive than healthy myocytes. One accepted theory to explain ST changes in ACS is as follows: The difference in membrane potential between healthy and injured myocytes forms a voltage gradient that leads to a "current of injury" detected in leads adjacent to the area of injury during repolarization (ST segment).

  ▪ In subendocardial ischemia, the net vector of ST "injury current" goes toward the endocardium → ST depression (from perspective of leads on the chest wall).

  ▪ In transmural ischemia, the net vector of ST "injury current" goes toward the epicardium → ST elevation (from perspective of leads on the chest wall).

Notably, these findings must be in multiple leads in the same anatomic site (Table 1-4) to be diagnostic of an infarction. Not all ST changes are due to ischemic injury. If there are no accompanying T- and/or Q-wave changes (T-wave inversion and prominent Q waves may develop hours to days after infarction), and the ST changes do not fall within an anatomic region supplied by the coronary arteries, consider other common causes of ST elevation and depression:

ST depression:
  ▪ Hypertrophy
  ▪ Drugs (eg, digoxin)
  ▪ Hypokalemia
ST elevation:
  ▪ Pericarditis
  ▪ Hyperkalemia
  ▪ Brugada syndrome

TABLE 1-21.   Abnormal Waveforms in Leads V_1 and V_6 Typically Seen on ECG for Right and Left BBBs in Addition to Widened QRS Complex

	V_1	V_6
Right BBB	RSR' complex ("bunny ears")	Prominent S wave
Left BBB	Prominent S wave (no R wave)	Wide and notched R wave

BBBs, bundle branch blocks.

ARRHYTHMIAS

Arrhythmias are abnormalities of electrical rhythm that result from abnormal impulse formation, impulse conduction, or both. Clinically, it is important to:

- Identify common arrhythmias and their clinical presentations
- Understand underlying pathophysiology
- Determine if/what treatment is necessary

It is useful to organize clinically common and important arrhythmias into **bradyarrhythmias** (heart rate < 60 bpm) and **tachyarrhythmias** (heart rate > 100 bpm). Within this framework, arrhythmias can be further subdivided based on their etiology within or outside of the heart's conduction system (ie, SA node, AV node, atria, or ventricles); refer to Figure 1-39. Please note that BBBs, a type of arrhythmia described in the Electrocardiography section, are not included in this scheme because they often *coexist* with normal sinus rhythm.

Bradyarrhythmias

Arrhythmias with HR < 60 bpm. Classified by location of arrhythmia origin (SA or AV node).

SA Node: Sinus Bradycardia

IDENTIFICATION AND CLINICAL PRESENTATION: Usually asymptomatic and physiologic in many people during rest or in athletes with increased vagal tone; sinus bradycardia is slowing of sinus rhythm normally generated at the SA node. Look for normal P waves and QRS complexes on ECG with a rate < 60 bpm.

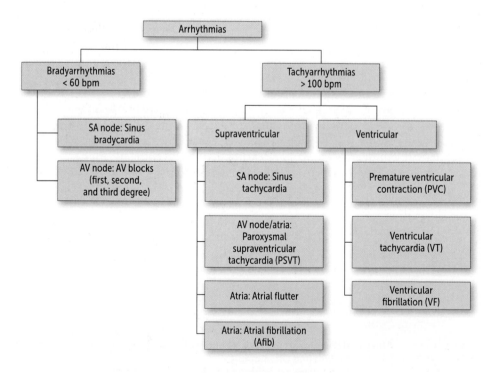

FIGURE 1-39. Clinically common and important arrhythmias. Organized scheme of arrhythmias by rate (bradyarrhythmias or tachyarrhythmias) and location (eg, SA node, AV node, atria, and ventricle).

PATHOPHYSIOLOGY: Secondary to **decreased automaticity** at the SA node, which can be physiologic and/or desired (eg, increased parasympathetic tone during sleep and rest, use of β-blockers and nondihydropyridine CCBs) or pathologic (eg, hypothyroidism, cardiomyopathy, aging, and ischemic heart disease).

TREATMENT: If asymptomatic, no treatment is required. If bradycardia causes symptoms of hypoperfusion (eg, syncope, altered mental status), treat with anticholinergics (eg, atropine). Pacemaker if condition is chronic.

AV Node: Conduction Blocks

A delay or failure in conduction through the AV node can result in three types (or degrees) of AV block based on ECG findings. The three degrees of AV block are described below.

First-Degree AV Block

IDENTIFICATION AND CLINICAL PRESENTATION: First-degree AV block is present if PR interval, which represents delay between atrial and ventricular depolarization mediated by the AV node, is prolonged more than 0.2 sec or 5 small boxes on ECG. Note the preservation of one P wave for every QRS complex in Figure 1-40 (1:1 P-to-QRS relationship). Asymptomatic.

PATHOPHYSIOLOGY: Delayed conduction through the AV node can be due to a reversible transient cause (eg, vagal tone, transient ischemia, β-blockers, nondihydropyridine CCBs, antiarrhythmics, Lyme disease) or permanent structural cause (eg, MI, infiltrative conditions like amyloidosis and sarcoidosis, and degeneration of the AV node conduction pathways with aging).

TREATMENT: Because first-degree AV block is generally asymptomatic, it does not require treatment. However, it may indicate underlying disease in the AV node that can progress to higher degrees of AV block or become a symptomatic bradyarrhythmia with additional reversible or structural superimposing influences discussed above.

Second-Degree AV Block

IDENTIFICATION AND CLINICAL PRESENTATION: Intermittent failure of AV conduction that results in a P wave not followed by QRS complex *with* (**Mobitz type I**) or *without* (**Mobitz type II**) preceding gradual lengthening of the PR interval.

- **Mobitz Type I (Wenckebach):** Look for progressive lengthening of PR interval on ECG until a beat is "dropped" (Figure 1-41A). Usually asymptomatic and rarely progresses to third-degree AV block.
- **Mobitz Type II (Hay):** Look for sudden, unpredictable dropped beat (P wave not followed by QRS) on ECG that is not preceded by PR interval lengthening as in type I (Figure 1-41B). It is often described using the ratio of P waves to QRS complexes. If the block persists for two or more beats (ie, a P-to-QRS ratio ≥ 2:1), it is considered a **high-grade** AV block. QRS interval may be normal or widened. Usually without symptoms, but may progress to third-degree AV block without warning.

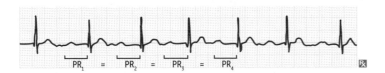

FIGURE 1-40. ECG tracing of first-degree AV block.

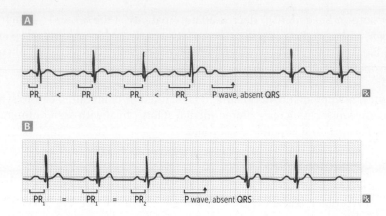

FIGURE 1-41.   **ECG tracing of second-degree AV block.** A Mobitz type I and B Mobitz type II.

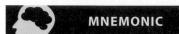
PATHOPHYSIOLOGY: Unlike Mobitz type II, Mobitz type I block is usually due to **delayed AV node conduction** from physiologic (eg, vagal tone, sleep, athletes) or pathologic (eg, MI, ischemia of AV node) etiologies. A Mobitz type II block is usually due to a block **distal** to the AV node in the ventricular conduction system, which is why it may have wide QRS complexes, as might be encountered in BBBs. Mobitz type II is due most often to pathologic degeneration of ventricular conduction system from MI or aging.

TREATMENT: Treat Mobitz type II block (even if asymptomatic) with a pacemaker, because it can progress at any moment to third-degree AV block!

Third-Degree (Complete) AV Block

IDENTIFICATION AND CLINICAL PRESENTATION: "Complete" failure of impulse to be conducted from the atria to ventricles, resulting in **AV dissociation** (ie, the atria and ventricles beat independently of each other), as shown in Figure 1-42. Ventricles are depolarized by latent pacemakers in the AV node (normal QRS width) or ventricular conduction pathway (wide QRS width). On ECG, look for P waves and QRS complexes with no relationship; atrial rate is faster than the ventricular rate. A slower ventricular rate may cause symptoms of hypoperfusion (eg, syncope and altered mental status) from impaired CO.

PATHOPHYSIOLOGY: Most common causes in adults include MI and age-related damage to the conduction pathways. Rarely, may also be due to infectious (eg, Lyme disease) and autoimmune (eg, congenital complete heart block in infants of mothers with SLE; hypothyroidism can cause acquired AV block) causes. Hyperkalemia can also reduce myocyte excitability (depolarizes membrane potential, more Na^+ channels inactivated) → AV block.

TREATMENT: Identify reversible causes (eg, ischemia, hyperkalemia, hypothyroidism). Pacemaker required to alleviate hypoperfusion symptoms and prevent degeneration of

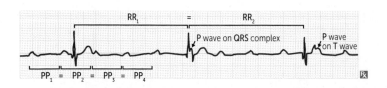

FIGURE 1-42.   **ECG tracing of third-degree (complete) AV block.** AV dissociation is evident by the fact that P waves and QRS complexes are both present, but are "beating" independently of one another. Note that the atrial rate (PP/time) is faster than ventricular rate (RR/time).

AV block into ventricular fibrillation. Avoid administering any AV nodal blocking agents (eg, β-blockers, nondihydropyridine CCBs, adenosine, digoxin).

Tachyarrhythmias

Tachyarrhythmias are arrhythmias with HR higher than 100 bpm. Classified into arrhythmias that originate above the ventricle (supraventricular) or below the ventricle (ventricular).

Supraventricular

Supraventricular tachyarrhythmias are arrhythmias that originate above the ventricles and therefore have normal-width ("narrow") QRS complexes. They are further subdivided by location of arrhythmia origin (SA node or atria). The supraventricular arrhythmias listed below all have regular rhythms except for atrial fibrillation (AF; irregularly irregular rhythm).

SA Node: Sinus Tachycardia

IDENTIFICATION AND CLINICAL PRESENTATION: Sinus tachycardia is characterized by faster sinus rhythm generated at the SA node. Look for normal P waves and QRS complexes on ECG with a rate higher than 100 bpm. Patients may report heart palpitations.

PATHOPHYSIOLOGY: Secondary to **increased automaticity** at the SA node, which can be physiologic (eg, response to emotional stimuli, exercise) or pathologic (eg, hypoxemia, fever, hyperthyroidism, side effect of β-agonist drugs).

TREATMENT: Treat underlying cause of pathologic sinus tachycardia (eg, replenish volume in hypovolemic patient, reduce fever, administer drugs to decrease thyroxine synthesis).

AV Node (Most of the Time): Paroxysmal Supraventricular Tachycardia

IDENTIFICATION AND CLINICAL PRESENTATION: As the name implies, **paroxysmal** SVT is characterized by bouts of supraventricular tachycardia (140–250 bpm). The most common type of PSVT is **atrioventricular nodal re-entrant tachycardia (AVNRT)**, which involves a re-entrant pathway in the AV node. Patients may report palpitations with/without precipitants (eg, stress, caffeine, alcohol). On ECG, retrograde P waves (via a reentry circuit) may be inverted or hidden.

PATHOPHYSIOLOGY: AVNRT is caused by a re-entry circuit in the AV node. It may occur in young (otherwise healthy) adults who have a "slow" and "fast" pathway in the AV node. In this scenario, a premature beat from the atrium may travel down the slow **or** fast pathway (but not both pathways, because they have different refractory periods). Distally, the transmitted impulse may travel in a retrograde fashion through the pathway that was initially refractory (repolarized by the time the impulse travels distally), which can then travel back through the atrium and establish a re-entrant pathway.

TREATMENT: Most AVNRTs in young, healthy adults are terminated by vagal maneuvers (eg, carotid massage, Valsalva), which slow conduction in the AV node. If that is not successful, IV adenosine (also slows AV node conduction) is a rapid therapy. For more long-term control, pharmacologic options include AV nodal blockers (eg, β-blockers, nondihydropyridine CCBs), ablation, and class IA or IC antiarrhythmics.

Atria: Atrial Flutter

IDENTIFICATION AND CLINICAL PRESENTATION: Characterized on ECG by regular, rapid atrial rhythm (250–350 bpm). Look for a rapid succession of identical and back-to-back atrial depolarization waves ("P waves") that give a "sawtooth" appearance to the baseline on ECG, as shown in Figure 1-44. Because not all atrial impulses are transmitted to ventricles owing to the longer refractory period of the AV node, the ventricular rate

KEY FACT

Latent pacemakers maintain the heart rate when SA node conduction is impaired. A **junctional escape rhythm** originates from the AV node or proximal bundle of His (40–60 bpm). A **ventricular escape rhythm** (30–40 bpm) may originate anywhere distal to the bundle of His, including ventricular myocytes outside the specialized conduction pathway.

KEY FACT

Narrow QRS complexes (≤ 0.10 sec or 2.5 small boxes) originate at or above the AV node (ie, **supraventricular**). Broad QRS complexes (> 0.10 sec) may originate below the AV node (ie, **ventricular**) and reflect slow conduction outside the specialized conduction pathways, or they may originate above the AV node and be delayed due to electrolyte abnormalities (eg, hyperkalemia), ventricular conduction blocks (eg, BBBs), or drug effects (eg, sodium-channel blockers).

CLINICAL CORRELATION

Wolff-Parkinson-White syndrome occurs in individuals with an accessory pathway ("bundle of Kent") between the atria and ventricles. As in AVNRT, this creates a "fast" (bundle of Kent) and "slow" (AV node) pathway between atrium and ventricle, predisposing to a re-entry circuit and SVT. Characterized by a delta wave on ECG (Figure 1-43), which reflects earlier ventricular depolarization.

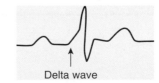

Delta wave

FIGURE 1-43. **Characteristic delta wave seen in Wolff-Parkinson-White syndrome.**

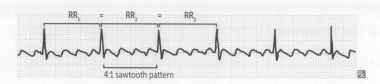

FIGURE 1-44.   ECG tracing of atrial flutter with a 4:1 AV block (only every fourth atrial beat is transmitted across AV node). Note the sawtooth baseline pattern, formed by the back-to-back identical P waves.

is slower than the atrial rate. For example, if there is a "4:1" conduction block at AV node, and the atrial rate is 300 bpm, ventricular rate will be 300/4 = 75 bpm. Patients may report sensations of regular palpitations; usually well-tolerated if ventricular rate is < 100 bpm.

PATHOPHYSIOLOGY: Most often in patients with existing heart disease, it is caused by a re-entry over a fixed circuit in the atrial cardiac tissue (ie, the repeated depolarization occurs in the same re-entry pathway beat-to-beat, producing the identical back-to-back atrial depolarization waves).

TREATMENT: Vagal maneuvers (eg, carotid sinus massage) can temporarily decrease ventricular rate by increasing refractory period at the AV node. More definitive therapy may include restoration of sinus rhythm with cardioversion, AV-blocking drugs to slow the ventricular rate (eg, β-blockers, nondihydropyridine CCBs), ablation, and class IA, IC, or III antiarrhythmics (often for chronic prevention).

Atria: Atrial Fibrillation

IDENTIFICATION AND CLINICAL PRESENTATION: Characterized by rapid atrial rhythm (350–600 bpm) that is "irregularly irregular," which refers to the fact that atrial depolarizations are irregular in no particular pattern. This chaotic depolarization creates an erratic baseline with no discernable P waves (Figure 1-45). Degree of symptoms (eg, palpitations, syncope from impaired CO) largely depends on the ventricular rate, which on average is between 140 and 160 bpm owing to some degree of physiologic AV nodal rate control. A "pulse deficit" may occur since not all ventricular beats are conducted effectively to produce a peripheral pulse.

PATHOPHYSIOLOGY: Often associated with right or left atrial enlargement (eg, from mitral stenosis, hypertension, congestive heart failure [CHF]), which makes the formation of multiple re-entry circuits more likely → irregular atrial depolarization. Excessive alcohol intake and thyrotoxicosis are also associated with development of atrial fibrillation.

TREATMENT: Life-threatening side effects of atrial fibrillation include (1) impaired CO due to rapid ventricular rate and (2) formation of thrombi due to relative stasis in atria without an organized firing pattern. Thus, treatment targets (1) rate control and (2) anticoagulation to reduce formation of thrombi that could otherwise potentially embolize to the systemic circulation from the left atrium.

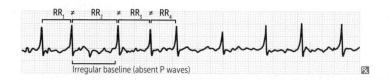

FIGURE 1-45.   ECG tracing of atrial fibrillation. Note irregularly irregular rhythm characterized by unequal RR distances between beats and a chaotic baseline.

Ventricular

Ventricular tachyarrhythmias are arrhythmias that originate in the ventricles in which the generated depolarization travels outside of the His-Purkinje conduction pathway, leading to wide QRS complexes. These tend to be more life-threatening arrhythmias than supraventricular tachycardias.

Premature Ventricular Contraction

IDENTIFICATION AND CLINICAL PRESENTATION: Premature ventricular contractions (PVCs) are often asymptomatic and can occur in otherwise healthy adults or those with structural heart disease. On ECG, they appear as a premature widened QRS complexes with no association to any prior P wave. Some patients report palpitations or feeling a "skipped beat."

PATHOPHYSIOLOGY: In healthy adults, isolated PVCs usually arise from ectopic foci in the ventricle (often without known underlying cause). In patients with heart disease, re-entry and digoxin toxicity can be other precipitants.

TREATMENT: PVCs alone are not life threatening and do not increase the risk of fatal arrhythmias in individuals without underlying heart disease, so reassurance is often provided. Avoidance of PVC triggers that increase automaticity of ectopic foci (eg, caffeine) and electrolyte repletion may be helpful.

Ventricular Tachycardia

IDENTIFICATION AND CLINICAL PRESENTATION: Ventricular tachycardia (VT) is defined as a series of at least three or more consecutive PVCs. On ECG, VT is characterized by (and distinguished from most supraventricular tachycardias) a wide-QRS complex tachycardia at a regular and rapid rate (usually 100–200 bpm). There is an arbitrary classification of VT:

- **Sustained VT:** Rhythm persists > 30 seconds, causes symptoms (eg, syncope from impaired CO), or requires pharmacologic therapy.
- **Nonsustained VT:** Rhythm self-terminates and does not meet criteria above.

PATHOPHYSIOLOGY: Monomorphic VT (identical QRS complexes) is usually caused by a single ectopic focus or re-entry in a diseased heart. **Polymorphic VT** (nonidentical QRS complexes) can be caused by multiple ectopic foci (eg, precipitated by ischemia after MI) or re-entry. **Torsade de pointes** is one type of polymorphic VT (QRS amplitude and axis change cyclically) that often occurs in patients with abnormal repolarization due to a prolonged QT interval (eg, from long QT syndrome, electrolyte abnormalities).

TREATMENT: Because sustained VT can degenerate into ventricular fibrillation (and sudden cardiac arrest), it requires immediate termination. Electrical cardioversion is first line for hemodynamically unstable monomorphic VT; if patient is hemodynamically stable, IV amiodarone and lidocaine are antiarrhythmic options. IV magnesium is often given for torsade de pointes if hypomagnesemia is a suspected cause. ICD placement and/or long-term pharmacologic therapy is often considered for patients with underlying heart disease, because recurrent VT is not uncommon in these patients.

Ventricular Fibrillation

IDENTIFICATION AND CLINICAL PRESENTATION: On ECG, ventricular fibrillation (VF) is characterized by rapid, irregular ventricular depolarizations that make individual waveforms indiscernible (Figure 1-46). The patient may report syncope, chest pain, shortness of breath (due to impaired CO secondary to uncoordinated ventricular contraction; imagine a quivering ventricle without coordinated contraction) and may, depending on the severity and prolongation, be unconscious and/or hemodynamically unstable.

KEY FACT

Escape rhythms are late and slower relative to the base conduction rate. **Ectopic rhythms** are premature and faster relative to the base conduction rate.

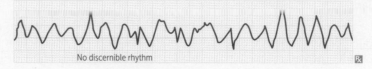

No discernible rhythm

FIGURE 1-46. **ECG tracing of ventricular fibrillation.** Note the erratic baseline with no discernible P waves.

PATHOPHYSIOLOGY: Most often, VF develops from untreated sustained VT in patients with underlying heart disease. In a minority of cases, idiopathic VF can develop (ie, there is no underlying heart disease or other known cause).

TREATMENT: Because VF impairs CO, this is a fatal arrhythmia unless treated with quick cardiac defibrillation. Underlying precipitants (eg, electrolyte abnormalities, hypoxia) should be addressed once sinus rhythm is established. Most individuals who survive VT receive an ICD to prevent future occurrences.

Pathology

HYPERTENSION

Hypertension affects more than 30% of US individuals over age 20 and is a major risk factor for several cardiovascular diseases. It is defined as persistent systolic pressure > 140 mm Hg and/or diastolic pressure > 90 mm Hg. Risk factors include advanced age, obesity, diabetes, physical inactivity, excess salt or alcohol consumption, family history, smoking, oral contraceptive use, and race (black > white > Asian). Hypertension has several stages (Table 1-22).

Primary hypertension is the most common type of hypertension, comprising 95% of cases. By definition, there is no single identifiable cause. However, it tends to be familial and likely represents an intersection of genetics with other factors, such as excessive salt intake and increased adrenergic tone. Prevalence increases with age, and individuals with relatively higher BPs at a young age are at increased risk of developing essential hypertension.

The long-term consequences of hypertension include the following:

- **Cardiac:**
  - Coronary artery disease (CAD)
  - Left ventricular hypertrophy (LVH)
  - Heart failure
  - Atrial fibrillation

TABLE 1-22. **Stages of Hypertension**

	SYSTOLIC (MM HG)	DIASTOLIC (MM HG)
Normal	< 120	*and* < 80
Prehypertension	120–139	*or* 80–89
Stage 1	140–159	*or* 90–99
Stage 2	≥ 160	*or* ≥ 100

KEY FACT

Cardioversion, a therapy option for terminating most arrhythmias, is a **synchronized** administration of shock during the R wave or QRS complex. **Defibrillation** is **nonsynchronized** administration of shock during the cardiac cycle and is indicated for VF (no prominent R or QRS complex).

KEY FACT

The most common risk factor for atrial fibrillation in the United States is hypertension.

CLINICAL CORRELATION

If a patient's BP is 118/93 mm Hg, then the patient is considered to have stage 1 hypertension. Remember, it is the highest level of either systolic **or** diastolic.

CLINICAL CORRELATION

For each 20-mm Hg ↑ in systolic or 10-mm Hg ↑ in diastolic pressure above 115/75 mm Hg, the CV disease risk doubles.

KEY FACT

Thiazide diuretics are usually the initial drug of choice for treatment of primary hypertension.

- **Large arterial:**
  - Aortic dissection
  - Aortic aneurysm
- **Neurologic:** Stroke
- **Renal:** Chronic kidney disease
- **Ophthalmologic:** Retinopathy

Primary (Essential) Hypertension

DIAGNOSIS

BP of > 140/90 mm Hg, confirmed on at least **two** separate occasions, or a single reading of > 170/110 mm Hg. Since primary hypertension is a diagnosis of exclusion, secondary hypertension must be ruled out.

TREATMENT

Initial treatment is aimed at **therapeutic lifestyle modifications,** such as weight loss, increased exercise, decreased sodium and alcohol intake, and smoking cessation.

Medical therapy involves the use of diuretics, β-adrenergic antagonists, angiotensin-converting enzyme (ACE) inhibitors, angiotensin receptor blockers (ARBs), calcium channel blockers, or α-adrenergic antagonists.

Secondary Hypertension

Secondary hypertension is increased systemic arterial pressure as a result of other identifiable conditions. Features of secondary hypertension may include onset of hypertension at ages < 20 or > 50 years old, BP > 180/110 mm Hg, abdominal bruits, and/or a **family history** of renal disease or **uncontrolled hypertension** despite maximal doses of three antihypertensive agents. Causes include:

- **Renal:**
  - **Renal artery stenosis:** Causes include atherosclerosis (older patients and usually bilateral) and **fibromuscular dysplasia** (young women, "beaded appearance" on arteriogram).
  - **Renal parenchymal disease:** Treat with ACE inhibitors, which slow progression.
- **Drug-induced:**
  - Oral contraceptives
  - Glucocorticoids
  - Phenylephrine
  - NSAIDs (preferentially constrict the afferent arteriole).
- **Endocrine:**
  - **Pheochromocytoma:** Adrenal tumor secreting catecholamines. Manifests with **triad** of **hypertension, diaphoresis,** and **tachycardia.**
  - **Primary aldosteronism (Conn syndrome):** Aldosterone-producing tumor causes **triad** of **hypertension, hypokalemia,** and **metabolic alkalosis.**
  - Hyperthyroidism (→ increased β-adrenergic receptors).
  - Cushing syndrome (→ excess cortisol → upregulates α₁-receptors on arterioles → ↑ sensitivity to norepinephrine and epinephrine).
- **Vascular:**
  - **Coarctation of the aorta:** Constriction of the aortic segment usually distal to the left subclavian artery. Leads to high BP in upper extremities, low BP in lower extremities. Differential cyanosis is seen in the infantile form of the disease if a patent ductus arteriosus is present.
  - **Fibromuscular dysplasia:** A disease resulting in narrowing of small and medium-sized arteries (primarily renal arteries), leading to hypertension. Often diagnosed in young women who present with headaches and uncontrollable hypertension.

CLINICAL CORRELATION

ACE inhibitors have been proven to lower mortality and morbidity in diabetic hypertensives. They decrease renal hypertension by decreasing vasoconstriction of the efferent arteriole. This lowers intraglomerular pressure and helps prevent proteinuria.

CLINICAL CORRELATION

In a patient with severe, ongoing, drug-resistant hypertension, suspect unilateral renal artery stenosis. On gross pathology, the kidney will appear shrunken. Biopsy will show crowding with tubulointerstitial atrophy, fibrosis, and focal inflammation.

CLINICAL CORRELATION

Percutaneous transluminal angioplasty (PTA) with or without stenting is the best treatment in fibromuscular dysplasia. Conversely, renal artery stenosis due to arteriosclerosis is generally managed with statins, antiplatelet agents, and antihypertensives.

CLINICAL CORRELATION

To distinguish primary hyperaldosteronism from conditions causing renin excess, the recommended screening tool is the aldosterone-to-renin ratio (ARR). An ARR > 20:1 is highly predictive of primary hyperaldosteronism.

QUESTION

A 26-year-old woman arrives at her primary care provider for follow-up of persistent hypertension. She is now on three antihypertensive agents. However, she reports continued malaise as well as severe, generalized headaches. Her BP is 160/90 mm Hg. What is the most likely diagnosis?

PRESENTATION

Patients are usually asymptomatic but can present with signs and symptoms of end-organ damage, such as chest pain, peripheral edema, vision changes, and claudication. Additionally, the following may be found on physical exam and routine lab work:

- **Cardiac:** S_4 due to atrial contraction against a stiff LV secondary to increased afterload from hypertension.
- **Renal:** Microalbuminuria, proteinuria.
- **Vascular:** Carotid bruits, hyaline arteriosclerosis, abdominal bruits.
- **Ophthalmologic:** Loss of venous pulsations, arteriovenous nicking, hemorrhages, and papilledema.

DIAGNOSIS

A thorough history and physical exam are necessary to detect clinical features of secondary hypertension. Specific diagnostic tests can also be very helpful.

- **Pheochromocytoma:** Symptoms of sweating and palpitations; increased urinary **catecholamines, metanephrines, and vanillylmandelic acid (VMA).**
- **Renal artery stenosis:** Auscultation of abdominal bruits on physical exam; increased plasma renin levels.
- **Hyperthyroidism:** Symptoms of **heat intolerance,** weight loss, weakness, and fatigue; decreased thyroid-stimulating hormone (TSH).
- **Coarctation of the aorta:** Absent or decreased femoral pulses on physical exam.

TREATMENT

Treatment varies depending on the underlying cause. Nonpharmacologic treatment includes weight loss, sodium restriction, smoking cessation, exercise, and reduction in alcohol intake. Pharmacologic treatments for hypertension include ACE inhibitors, ARBs, diuretics, vasodilators, calcium channel blockers, and α- and β-blockers.

Malignant Hypertension

Malignant hypertension is a severe, **rapid increase** in BP, usually > 240/120 mm Hg, associated with **organ damage.** Clinically it is characterized by chest pain, dyspnea, angina, and headache with papilledema, evidence of LV hypertrophy, and retinal hemorrhages on physical examination. End-organ damage can manifest as pulmonary edema, azotemia ("flea-bitten kidneys"), retinal hemorrhages, encephalopathy, seizures, and coma.

ARTERIOSCLEROSIS

Arteriosclerosis comprises a group of diseases that involve arterial wall thickening and loss of elasticity. They are divided into three categories (Table 1-23).

Arteriolosclerosis

Affects the **intima** of small arterioles and arteries and is most often seen in the elderly and in patients with diabetes, metabolic syndrome, or hypertension.

Microscopically there are two types of arteriolosclerosis:

- **Hyaline arteriolosclerosis:** In patients with diabetes, it results from advanced glycosylation end products deposited in the basement membrane of vessels. In patients with essential hypertension, it results from proteins forced into the vascular wall due to increased arterial blood pressure (Figure 1-48A).

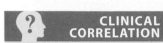

CLINICAL CORRELATION

Hypertensive urgency: BP > 180/120 mm Hg with no end-organ damage

Hypertensive emergency: BP > 180/120 mm Hg with end-organ damage

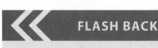

FLASH BACK

Metabolic syndrome is a group of risk factors in a single individual that increases risk for CV disease. These include insulin resistance, hypertension, abdominal obesity, dyslipidemia, and prothrombotic states.

ANSWER

In a young woman with headaches and uncontrollable hypertension, suspect **fibromuscular dysplasia** (Figure 1-47), which causes narrowing of the small and medium-sized arteries (primarily renal arteries).

TABLE 1-23. **Features of Arteriosclerosis**

	ARTERIOLOSCLEROSIS	MÖNCKEBERG	ATHEROSCLEROSIS
Artery size	Small	Medium	Medium to large
Affected layer	Intima	Media	Intima
Distinguishing feature	Onion skinning	Calcification	Foam cells
Risk factors	↑ Age, DM, metabolic syndrome, HTN	↑ Age, DM, CKD, SLE, ↑ vitamin D	↑ Age, DM, metabolic syndrome, HTN, obesity, smoking, sedentary lifestyle, OCP use, male gender, family history, homocystinuria
Prognosis	Progressive vessel obstruction	Benign	Progressive vessel obstruction

CKD, chronic kidney disease; DM, diabetes mellitus; HTN, hypertension; OCP, oral contraceptive pill; SLE, systemic lupus erythematosus.

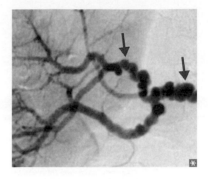

FIGURE 1-47. **Fibromuscular dysplasia.** "String of beads" appearance (arrows) of the renal artery in fibromuscular dysplasia.

■ **Hyperplastic arteriolosclerosis:** Seen in **malignant hypertension,** it is visualized as an increase in smooth muscle proliferation and basement membrane duplication, leading to "**onion skinning**" (concentric wall thickening). Effects are especially prevalent in the renal arterioles (Figure 1-48B), which can lead to nephrosclerosis.

Mönckeberg Arteriosclerosis

Uncommon. A benign medial calcification of the elastic lamina not involving the intima, leading to vascular stiffening without obstruction. It tends to affect medium-sized arteries in the radial, ulnar, tibial, uterine, or femoral arteries in the elderly. It has a "pipestem" appearance on x-ray (Figure 1-48C). It is generally asymptomatic and benign.

Atherosclerosis

Atherosclerosis is caused by the deposition of cholesterol plaques in the intima of medium and large arteries. The arteries most often affected by atherosclerosis, listed from

FLASH FORWARD

In the kidney, hyaline arteriosclerosis is termed *benign* nephrosclerosis, and hyperplastic arteriosclerosis is termed *malignant nephrosclerosis.*

MNEMONIC

Mönckeberg is **M**edial calcification of the **M**edium-sized arteries.

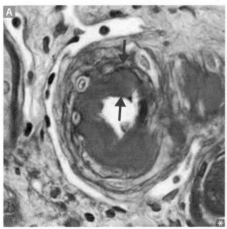
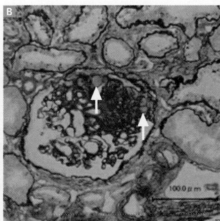
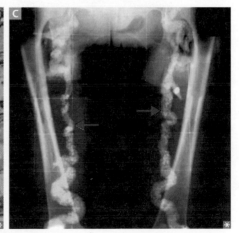

FIGURE 1-48. **Features of arteriosclerosis.** A Hyaline arteriolosclerosis with thickened vessel walls; B Segmental glomerulosclerosis in perihilar lesion. This glomerulus contains perihilar hyalinosis (arrowheads); C Mönckeberg arteriosclerosis with "pipestem" appearance on x-ray.

most to least likely, are abdominal aorta > coronary artery > popliteal artery > internal carotid artery > circle of Willis. The common carotid arteries are often spared. The risk factors for atherosclerosis are divided into modifiable and nonmodifiable categories:

- **Modifiable:** Hyperlipidemia, hypertension, smoking, diabetes, obesity, sedentary lifestyle, oral contraceptive use
- **Nonmodifiable:** Age, gender (men and postmenopausal women), homocystinuria, family history

PATHOGENESIS

The pathogenesis of atherosclerosis is explained in Figure 1-49.

HISTOPATHOLOGY

- **Fatty streaks** are flat and yellow and contain foam cells (lipid-laden macrophages), which can be visualized on histopathology.
- **Fibrous plaques** are elevated white plaques that contain a necrotic core of cholesterol, lipids, foam cells, and debris surrounded by a fibrous cap of collagen, smooth muscle, and lymphocytes (Figure 1-50).

COMPLICATIONS

The complications of atherosclerosis can be severe. Plaque rupture and subsequent thrombosis can lead to unstable angina, myocardial infarction (MI), stroke or transient ischemic attacks, and proximal renal thrombosis leading to activation of the renin-angiotensin-aldosterone system and hypertension. Chronic atherosclerosis can lead to ischemia in

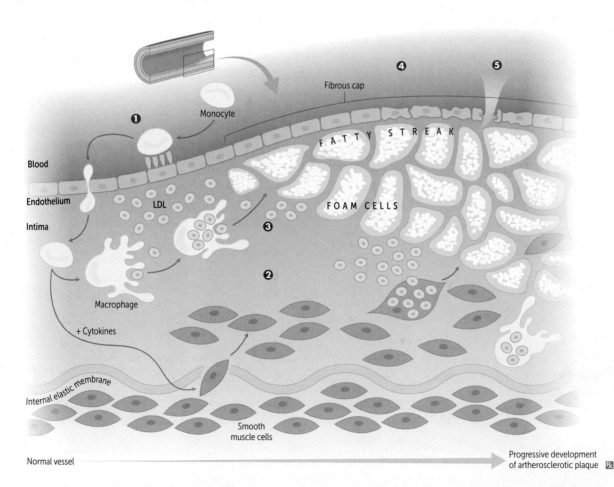

FIGURE 1-49. Pathogenesis of atherosclerosis. ❶ Endothelial cell injury causes monocyte emigration into intima. **❷** Activated macrophages release cytokines causing smooth muscle cells to migrate into intima. **❸** Macrophages form foam cells into a fatty streak, and a fibrous cap develops. **❹** As intimal muscle cells become senescent and die, fibrous matrix degrades. **❺** Fibrous cap (plaque) calcifies and ulcerates, causing vessel thrombosis.

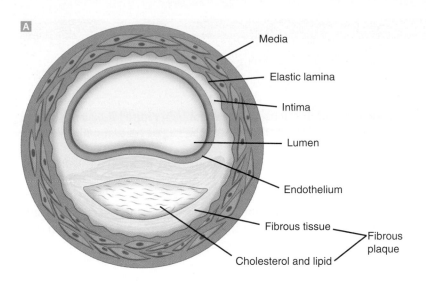

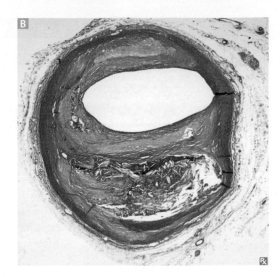

FIGURE 1-50. **Fibrous plaque.** **A** Schematic of fibrous plaque. **B** Histopathology demonstrating an atherosclerotic plaque within the left anterior descending coronary artery. The plaque is narrowing the lumen to approximately 25% of its normal area.

distal regions, manifesting as renal artery ischemia, peripheral vascular occlusive disease, impotence, and claudication. Finally, artery wall degeneration can predispose to aneurysm formation.

MYOCARDITIS

Myocarditis is inflammation of the heart muscle due to various causes, including infections, toxins, autoimmune diseases, and drug reactions. The most common cause of myocarditis in developed countries is a **viral infection** caused by coxsackie B virus, rubella virus, and cytomegalovirus; however, the most common cause worldwide is **Chagas disease** (caused by *Trypanosoma cruzi*).

Bacteria such as *Staphylococcus aureus, Corynebacterium diphtheriae,* and *Haemophilus influenzae* can also cause myocarditis. For patients with HIV, myocarditis may result from toxoplasmosis or Kaposi sarcoma metastases. Other causes of myocarditis include Lyme disease, acute renal failure, rheumatic fever, lupus, and drugs such as doxorubicin.

PRESENTATION

Patients may present with symptoms of congestive heart failure (CHF) including **chest pain,** peripheral edema, and dyspnea, **palpitations** from arrhythmias, and viral sequelae including **fever,** diarrhea, and fatigue. On physical exam, patients may demonstrate a muffled S_1, an S_3, and/or mitral regurgitation (MR) murmur.

DIAGNOSIS

ECG shows **diffuse T wave inversions** and **ST segment elevations,** which can mimic an MI or pericarditis. Cardiac biopsy is the gold standard, demonstrating edematous myocardial interstitium with lymphocytic infiltrate. Creatine kinase–myocardial bound fraction (CK-MB) and troponin may also be elevated.

TREATMENT

Supportive therapy for acute heart failure with diuretics, ACE inhibitors, or nitrates is often necessary. Viral myocarditis requires symptomatic treatment, including NSAIDs for inflammation and diuretics for ventricular failure. Bacterial myocarditis requires antibiotics.

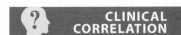

CLINICAL CORRELATION

Cellular infiltrates in myocarditis:
Neutrophilic → bacterial myocarditis
Mononuclear → viral myocarditis

KEY FACT

Bacterial myocarditis is rare in patients who are immunocompetent.

FLASH BACK

Virulence factors of **S aureus** include **protein A** to inhibit phagocytic engulfment and **catalase** (breaks down H_2O_2, which is important in O_2-dependent killing) to enhance survival in phagocytes.

ENDOCARDITIS

Endocarditis is an inflammation of the lining of the heart and heart valves.

Infective Endocarditis

Heart valves are avascular, and thus leukocytes cannot be recruited if bacteria adhere to the valves. Endocarditis can be acute (days) or subacute (weeks to months).

Acute infective endocarditis tends to affect **normal heart valves** and is most often associated with *S aureus*, which is extremely virulent. IV drug users are particularly at risk.

Subacute infective endocarditis usually colonizes a **previously damaged or abnormally developed valve** in the setting of bacteremia from oral surgery or poor dentition. It is most commonly associated with *Streptococcus viridans* (Table 1-24).

PRESENTATION

Patients with infective endocarditis classically present with fevers, chills, weight loss, systemic emboli, petechiae, **Janeway lesions** (small, painless erythematous lesions on the palms and soles), **Osler nodes** (painful raised lesions on the finger and toe pads), **splinter hemorrhages** (linear streaks under the fingernails and toenails), **Roth spots** (round white spots on the retina surrounded by hemorrhage), and **valvular involvement** (mitral > aortic > tricuspid) (Figure 1-51).

DIAGNOSIS

The Duke criteria for infective endocarditis include positive serial blood cultures, prior infective endocarditis, IV drug use, fever, vascular or immune phenomena, and valvular lesions on echocardiography.

TREATMENT

Intravenous antibiotics targeted to the specific organism. For acute endocarditis, start antibiotics empirically—nafcillin and gentamicin provide good coverage. For subacute endocarditis, obtain blood cultures before starting antibiotics. Choices include ampicillin + gentamicin for native valves, and vancomycin, gentamicin, and rifampin for prosthetic valves.

TABLE 1-24.   **Bacterial Causes of Endocarditis**

RISK FACTOR/PRESENTING FACTOR	BACTERIA TO CONSIDER
Prosthetic device	*Staphylococcus epidermidis*
Colon cancer	*Streptococcus bovis*
Dental procedure	Viridans group streptococci
GI surgery	*Enterococcus*
Total parenteral nutrition	Fungal
Alcoholics or the homeless	*Bartonella henselae*
Fastidious and culture negative	HACEK organisms

HACEK, *Haemophilus, Actinobacillus, Cardiobacterium, Eikenella,* and *Kingella*.

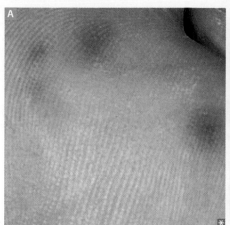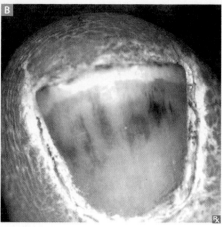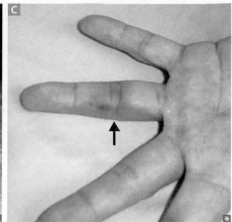

FIGURE 1-51. **Classic signs of endocarditis.** A Janeway lesions; B splinter hemorrhages; and C Osler nodes.

COMPLICATIONS

- Chordae rupture, leading to mitral or tricuspid regurgitation.
- Septic emboli:
  - Right-sided emboli enter pulmonary circulation and cause lung abscess.
  - Left-sided emboli enter systemic circulation and can injure highly perfused organs such as the kidney, brain, and spleen.
- Glomerulonephritis.
- Suppurative pericarditis.

Marantic Endocarditis

Nonbacterial endocarditis (also known as nonbacterial thrombotic endocarditis [NBTE]) occurs when small, sterile fibrin vegetations deposit on the heart valves of people with debilitating disease. This can occur as a **paraneoplastic syndrome** of mucin-secreting tumors (usually of the colon or pancreas) in which mucin deposition on heart valves creates a nidus for platelet aggregation and infection. NBTE may also be caused by a hypercoagulable state and lupus. A major complication is a sterile embolus, leading to cerebral infarct. The prognosis is generally poor.

Libman-Sacks Endocarditis

Libman-Sacks endocarditis (LSE) is a sequela of systemic lupus erythematosus (SLE) wherein autoantibodies target and damage the heart valves. Sterile vegetations (composed of fibrin, neutrophils, lymphocytes, and histiocytes) form on **both sides of the heart valves.** Often the patient is asymptomatic, but the condition can be picked up by the presence of a heart murmur, which usually affects the mitral valve and presents as a holosystolic "blowing" murmur.

Carcinoid Syndrome

Carcinoid tumors synthesize and secrete high levels of serotonin (5-HT). Increased serotonin leads to systemic vasodilation as well as thickening, contraction, and decreased mobility of right-sided heart valves. This results in reduced preload and end-diastolic volume. The left side of the heart is protected by serotonin inactivation by monoamine oxidase in the lungs. The difference between **carcinoid syndrome** and **carcinoid tumors** is as follows:

- **Carcinoid syndrome** is only seen in 5% of carcinoid tumors, which most commonly affect the terminal ileum or appendix. Usually, the tumors are too small to be symptomatic. However, if the tumor is large enough to overwhelm the liver's metabolic capacity, or if it metastasizes to the liver, then serotonin can escape

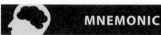

MNEMONIC

Bacteria **FROM JANE:**
Fever
Roth spots
Osler nodes
Murmur
Janeway lesions
A
Nailbed hemorrhage
Emboli

CLINICAL CORRELATION

Carcinoid syndrome can lead to **pellagra** (niacin deficiency syndrome) because tryptophan is the common precursor for niacin and serotonin synthesis. Increased serotonin synthesis from the tumor → ↓ niacin synthesis.

QUESTION

A 25-year-old woman arrives at her annual primary care appointment. At her last appointment, she was noted to have hypertension with a blood pressure of 138/87 mm Hg. Today, her blood pressure is 135/86 mm Hg. She follows a low-sodium diet and exercises regularly. Her only medication is an oral contraceptive pill (OCP). What is the next best step?

MNEMONIC

Sydenham chorea
Transient migratory arthritis
Rheumatic subcutaneous nodules
Erythema marginatum
Pancarditis

 MNEMONIC

JONES PEACE
Major criteria:

Joints: migratory arthritis
Carditis: new-**O**nset murmur
Nodules, subcutaneous: extensor
    surfaces
Erythema marginatum`
Sydenham chorea
Minor criteria:

PR interval, prolonged
ESR elevated
Arthralgias
CRP elevated
Elevated temperature (fever)

 CLINICAL CORRELATION

Evidence of streptococcal infection:
■ Antistreptolysin O (ASO) titers
■ Positive throat culture for
    streptococci group A

 ANSWER

Discontinue the OCP, a common cause of secondary hypertension in an otherwise healthy individual, and recommend an alternative method of birth control. At next follow-up, remeasure blood pressure. If it has not improved, consider other causes of hypertension.

hepatic degradation and enter systemic circulation. Systemic symptoms include abdominal pain, flushing, secretory diarrhea, and bronchoconstriction leading to wheezing in addition to the valvular pathology.

DIAGNOSIS

Elevated levels of **5-hydroxindoleacetic acid (5-HIAA)**, a serotonin metabolite, are detected in the urine. CT, MRI, and indium-111 pentetreotide scan can also be used to locate the carcinoid tumor.

TREATMENT

The first-line treatment is surgery to remove the tumor. In patients in whom surgery is not an option, a somatostatin analog, **octreotide,** can decrease serotonin secretion from the tumor.

RHEUMATIC FEVER

Rheumatic fever is a multisystem inflammatory disease that may occur following pharyngeal infection with **group A β-hemolytic streptococci.** It usually affects children aged 5–10 years. It has been postulated that the streptococcal antigens elicit production of antibodies that cross-react with cardiac antigens.

Classically, patients complain of a pharyngeal infection 1–4 weeks prior and present with classic symptoms that are collectively referred to as the **Jones criteria** (Table 1-25).

Acute Rheumatic Heart Disease

The most serious complication of rheumatic fever. It affects all 3 layers of the heart and can be divided into:

■ **Fibrinous pericarditis:** Presents with friction rub and chest pain.
■ **Myocarditis:** focal interstitial myocardial inflammation in which collagen and fibrinoid material form nodules (**Aschoff bodies**) and are surrounded by macrophages (**Anitschkow cells**), lymphocytes, plasma cells, and multinucleated giant cells (**Aschoff cells**) (Figure 1-52).
■ **Endocarditis:** The valve leaflets become red and swollen, and small verrucae (rubbery fibrin vegetations) form along the lines of closure. Eventually the valves become fibrotic, thickened, and calcified. Valvular disease can lead to either insufficiency

TABLE 1-25. **Jones Criteria**

MAJOR CRITERIA	MINOR CRITERIA
Migratory polyarthritis	Arthralgia (most common)
Carditis	Fever
Subcutaneous nodules	High ESR/CRP
Erythema marginatum	Long PR interval
Sydenham chorea	High WBC count

Diagnosis is confirmed in the presence of **two major criteria,** *or* **one major and two minor criteria,** in addition to evidence of streptococcal infection including **rising ASO or DNAse titers.**

CRP, C-reactive protein; ESR, erythrocyte sedimentation rate; WBC, white blood cell.

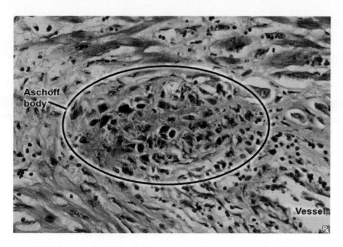

FIGURE 1-52.   **Aschoff body in fibrous tissue next to myocardial vessel.**

or stenosis. The mitral and aortic valves are most often affected since the left heart sees the highest pressure gradients.

Chronic Rheumatic Heart Disease

Mitral and aortic valvular fibrosis causes valve thickening and calcifications, fusion of commissures ("fish-mouth" appearance), and short, thick chordae tendineae. The chronic form can lead to **mitral stenosis (MS),** MR, aortic regurgitation, and CHF. It can also predispose to infectious endocarditis.

DIAGNOSIS

Diagnosis is usually made through clinical suspicion and fulfillment of the Jones criteria (Table 1-25) including evidence of prior streptococcal infection. Positive antibody titers against streptococci can verify a prior infection. Echocardiography can aid in diagnosing cardiac complications.

TREATMENT

Antibiotic therapy for rheumatic heart disease targets group A streptococci with **high-dose penicillin.** Additionally, symptomatic treatment is often employed. Steroids and salicylates aid in reducing pain and inflammation, whereas digitalis may reduce symptoms of heart failure. Haloperidol is the treatment of choice for Sydenham chorea, if present.

CARDIOMYOPATHIES

Cardiomyopathy refers to a spectrum of diseases that affect the myocardium and lead to cardiac dysfunction (summarized in Table 1-26).

Dilated Cardiomyopathy

Dilated cardiomyopathy represents approximately 90% of nonischemic cardiomyopathies. Echocardiography often reveals four-chamber enlargement.

Causes include: idiopathic, alcohol abuse, wet beriberi (thiamine deficiency), coxsackie B virus myocarditis, chronic cocaine use, Chagas disease, doxorubicin toxicity, hemochromatosis, HIV, Lyme disease, sarcoidosis, hypothyroidism, acromegaly, and peripartum cardiomyopathy.

FLASH FORWARD

Mitral stenosis causes increased left atrial pressure, which reflects back into the pulmonary system to produce pulmonary hypertension and hemoptysis. Eventually, elevated pulmonary pressures lead to right ventricular hypertrophy and then to RHF.

KEY FACT

Aschoff bodies contain both Aschoff cells and Anitschkow cells.

KEY FACT

Myocarditis leading to cardiac failure is a cause of death in acute rheumatic fever.

CLINICAL CORRELATION

Complications of dilated cardiomyopathy include cardiac arrhythmias, mural thrombi, CHF, bundle-branch blocks, and death.

QUESTION

A 32-year-old man arrives in the emergency department with fevers greater than 101°F, chills, and general malaise. On history, he denies illicit drug use but has been a known IV drug user. On examination, he is found to have a new murmur and splinter hemorrhages on his nail beds. What are the next best steps?

TABLE 1-26. Nonischemic Cardiomyopathies

	DILATED	HYPERTROPHIC	RESTRICTIVE
Cause	Idiopathic, ethanol abuse, coxsackie B virus infection, cocaine abuse, Chagas disease, peripartum	Autosomal dominant	Senile/primary amyloidosis, sarcoidosis, Loeffler ("eosinophilic") endomyocarditis
Clinical presentation	↓ EF, fatigue, cardiomegaly, dyspnea	Dyspnea, angina, S_4, syncope	Peripheral edema, dyspnea, ascites, JVD
Special notes	Most common form on chest film: balloon heart	Young athlete with echocardiogram showing asymmetric LVH preferentially involving the septum	

EF, ejection fraction; JVD, jugular venous distention; LVH, left ventricular hypertrophy.

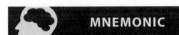
PRESENTATION

Can manifest as right or left heart failure. Signs and symptoms can include decreased ejection fraction (EF), jugular venous distention (JVD), edema, orthopnea, hepatomegaly, cardiomegaly, arrhythmias, the presence of S_3 heart sound, or a systolic regurgitant murmur.

DIAGNOSIS

Radiography shows an enlarged cardiac silhouette with pulmonary congestion. **Echocardiography** is the key diagnostic study and shows a dilated LV with a decreased EF (Figure 1-53A). In dilated cardiomyopathy due to coxsackie B virus myocarditis, pathology may demonstrate a lymphocytic infiltrate with myocyte necrosis.

TREATMENT

Dilated cardiomyopathy treatment is centered around improving symptoms of CHF: Digitalis, β-blockers, ACE inhibitors, ARBs, diuretics, or vasodilators. Patients are also treated with sodium restriction. If ejection fraction < 35% despite optimal medical therapy, consider ICD placement to control arrhythmias or even heart transplantation.

Hypertrophic Cardiomyopathy

Hypertrophic cardiomyopathy (HCM) leads to marked ventricular hypertrophy. Sixty percent to 70% of cases are familial, inherited in an autosomal dominant fashion and commonly associated with a β-myosin heavy-chain mutation. It may also be associated with Friedrich ataxia. Asymmetric septal hypertrophy causes a decrease in LV compliance and diastolic dysfunction. Blood flows at an increased velocity over the hypertrophied septum, which creates negative pressure, drawing the anterior mitral leaflet into the outflow tract (Venturi effect). This causes subaortic obstruction to outflow, leading to syncope during exercise. It can also lead to sudden cardiac death in young athletes due to ventricular arrhythmias.

PRESENTATION

Patients may present with **syncope, dyspnea,** and **chest pain brought on by exercise** and **relieved by rest.** On physical exam, patients may demonstrate an **S_4 cardiac gallop** (due to an atrial kick into a noncompliant ventricle), a **harsh systolic crescendo-decrescendo murmur** best appreciated at the left-upper sternal border, and the systolic murmur of

mitral valve regurgitation. Patients may also demonstrate pulsus bisferiens (a biphasic pulse), consisting of two strong systolic pulse peaks.

DIAGNOSIS

Imaging reveals **cardiomegaly** (secondary to aberrant, disorganized fibers in the myocardium) and a **dilated left atrium. Echocardiography** is normally used for diagnosis and shows asymmetrical left ventricular hypertrophy (LVH) preferentially involving the septum, MR, and diastolic dysfunction. Biopsy shows myofibrillar disarray and fibrosis (Figure 1-53B).

TREATMENT

The goal is to **maintain ventricular filling** in order to prevent obstruction. β-Blockers and calcium channel blockers are often used to slow the heart rate (HR) and increase diastolic filling time, as well as decrease myocardial O_2 consumption. Implantable cardioverter defibrillators (ICDs) are often implanted in high-risk patients to prevent sudden cardiac death. Patients with HCM are also advised to cease high-intensity athletics.

Restrictive Cardiomyopathy

Restrictive cardiomyopathy is the least common type of cardiomyopathy, and is caused by diseases that infiltrate the myocardium to impede diastolic filling of the heart. Major causes include sarcoidosis, amyloidosis, postradiation fibrosis, endocardial fibroelastosis (thick fibroelastic tissue in endocardium of young children), Löeffler syndrome (endomyocardial fibrosis with a prominent eosinophilic infiltrate), glycogen storage disorders (Pompe disease), inborn errors of metabolism (Gaucher and Fabry diseases), and hemochromatosis (dilated cardiomyopathy can also occur).

PRESENTATION

Dyspnea, weakness, exercise intolerance, peripheral edema, ascites, JVD, S_4 gallop, **pulsus paradoxus**, CHF, and arrhythmias from conduction defects.

DIAGNOSIS

Radiography shows mild cardiomegaly. In cases of amyloidosis, ECG shows **low voltage** despite thick myocardium.

TREATMENT

There is no effective therapy except to treat the underlying disease. In severe cases, heart transplantation may be necessary.

CONGESTIVE HEART FAILURE

Congestive heart failure (CHF) is defined as the inability of the heart to generate sufficient cardiac output to meet the metabolic demands of the body. It is a syndrome or diagnosis, not a specific disease. Heart failure can be the final manifestation of most cardiac disease, from hypertension to cardiomyopathy. The incidence in the United States is increasing due to the growth of the aging population and prolonged survival after cardiac insults. CHF is usually attributed to left heart failure; however, left and right heart failure often occur concurrently (in fact, the most common cause of right-sided HF is left-sided HF).

Left-Sided Heart Failure

Left-sided HF may be divided into two categories (Figures 1-54 and 1-55):

Heart failure with reduced ejection fraction: Heart failure occurring due to impaired ventricular emptying because of (1) impaired contractility and/or (2) increased after-

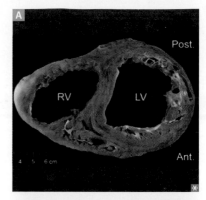

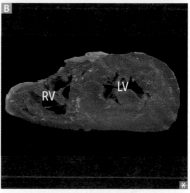

FIGURE 1-53. **Cardiomyopathies.** **A** Dilated cardiomyopathy. Note enlarged cavities and thinned walls of both ventricles. **B** Hypertrophic cardiomyopathy. Note concentric hypertrophy of left ventricle.

KEY FACT

Any maneuver that ↓ end-diastolic volume, such as Valsalva maneuver or exercise, ↑ the murmur's intensity in both mitral valve prolapse (MVP) and hypertrophic cardiomyopathy because the ↓ volume leads to a ↓ chamber size and ↑ obstruction.

KEY FACT

Primary amyloidosis is a disorder in which amyloid light-chain protein fibers are deposited in tissues and organs, impeding their function. It is diagnosed by apple-green birefringence on Congo red staining.

KEY FACT

An S_3 **heart sound** is caused by vibration and turbulence as blood fills a ventricle that already has excess fluid due to systolic dysfunction.

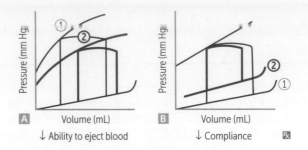

FIGURE 1-54. **Systolic and diastolic dysfunction.** [A] Systolic failure: downward + rightward shift of end-systolic pressure-volume relation (ESPVR) → ↓ SV, ↓ EF, ↑ LVEDV, ↑ LVEDP (preload). [B] Diastolic failure: upward shift of passive diastolic pressure-volume curve → ↑ LVEDP, ↓ LVEDV, preserved EF.

load. This results in a reduced ejection fraction and increased left ventricular ESV. While this in turn increases EDV and EDP, leading to increased stroke volume via the Frank-Starling mechanism, it is not enough to overcome the original deficit, and **EF remains lower than normal.**

Heart failure with preserved ejection fraction: Heart failure occurring due to reduced compliance resulting from (1) impaired diastolic relaxation and/or (2) impaired ventricular filling. This causes the ventricular pressure to increase, further decreasing EDV. EF is preserved due to preserved systolic function.

PRESENTATION

Left-sided pump dysfunction leads to pulmonary congestion and low perfusion. Patients typically present with orthopnea (shortness of breath when supine), dyspnea on exertion, paroxysmal nocturnal dyspnea (PND; breathless awakening from sleep), and fatigue. Physical examination may demonstrate rales, JVD, and pitting edema. Patients may also have S_3 or S_4 heart sounds.

Microscopically, intra-alveolar hemosiderin-laden macrophages (heart failure cells), alveolar edema, and cardiac myocyte hypertrophy are seen. Complications include pulmonary congestion, cardiogenic shock, and hyperaldosteronism secondary to RAAS activation upon reduced blood flow to kidneys.

TREATMENT

Acute treatment involves relieving dyspnea and congestion with O_2, diuretics, nitrates, and morphine. Long-term management includes counteracting rise in hormone levels

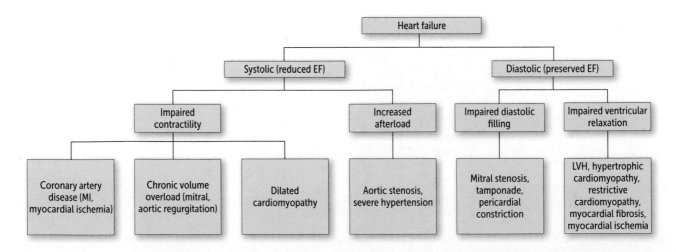

FIGURE 1-55. **Causes of left-sided heart failure.** EF, ejection fraction; LVH, left ventricular hypertrophy; MI, myocardial infarction.

with β-blockers, ACE inhibitors, and ARBs. **ACE inhibitors** lead to decreased afterload, resulting in reduced aldosterone-mediated salt and water retention, and have been proven to reduce mortality in CHF patients. **Diuretics** are also a mainstay in preventing volume overload. **β-Blockers** lead to augmented cardiac output, stabilized hemodynamics, and improved survival. **Digoxin** and other inotropes may be helpful in systolic failure due to improved contractility, but do not aid in diastolic heart failure because they do not improve ventricular relaxation properties. In general, systolic heart failure is more responsive to these agents, whereas diastolic heart failure is best treated by reversing the underlying cause.

Of these agents, select β-blockers, ACE inhibitors/ARBs, and mineralocorticoid antagonists all reduce mortality in patients with heart failure with reduced ejection fraction.

Right-Sided Heart Failure

The most common cause of right-sided heart failure is left-sided heart failure. Other causes include **cor pulmonale,** right-sided heart failure secondary to pulmonary hypertension, and pulmonary or tricuspid valve disease.

PRESENTATION

Right-sided pump failure leads to systemic congestion. Patients may present with splenomegaly, hepatomegaly ("nutmeg" liver), peripheral edema, and jugular venous distention due to fluid backup from the right heart. Renal hypoxia further exacerbates fluid retention caused by right-sided pump failure, due to RAAS activation for perceived low-volume status. This leads to severe pitting edema (beginning in the ankles), pleural effusions, and ascites (Figures 1-56 and 1-57). Cirrhosis may occur in long-standing congestion.

TREATMENT

Treatment for right-sided heart failure entails ACE inhibitors, which decrease afterload and prevent aldosterone mediated salt and water retention. ACE inhibitors have been shown to **decrease mortality** rates in CHF patients, but should be used cautiously, because patients with stiff LVs are very preload dependent.

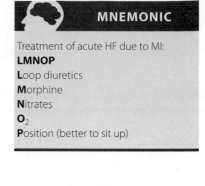

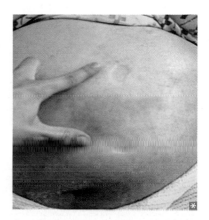

FIGURE 1-56. **Pitting edema above the umbilicus.**

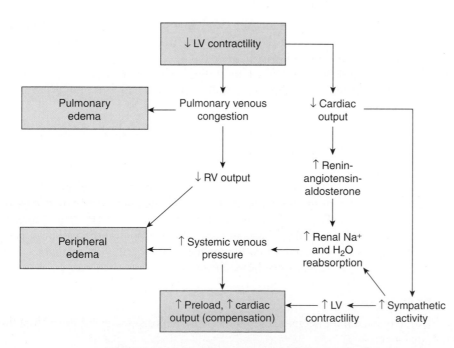

FIGURE 1-57. **Pathophysiology of congestive heart failure.** LV, left ventricular; RV, right ventricular.

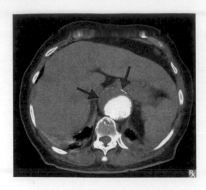

FIGURE 1-58. Abdominal aortic aneurysm. CT showing large suprarenal aneurysm with eccentric mural thrombus (arrows).

KEY FACT

The Law of Laplace states that:

$$\text{Wall stress} = \frac{(\text{Pressure} \times \text{radius})}{(2 \times \text{wall thickness})}$$

In an aneurysm, the radius of the vessel is steadily increasing. Eventually, the stress increases to the point of aortic rupture.

ANEURYSMS

Aneurysms are congenital or acquired **abnormal dilatations** of either an artery or vein due to weakness of the vessel wall. There are many types of aneurysms (discussed as follows). Complications of aneurysms include thrombus formation, erosion into nearby structures, and rupture leading to hypotension, shock, or death.

Abdominal Aortic Aneurysm

Abdominal aortic aneurysm (AAA) is the most common form of aneurysm. Typically affects male smokers > 50 years old with **atherosclerosis** and occurs between the renal arteries and the aortic bifurcation at the L4 level. Classically manifests as a palpable pulsating abdominal mass (Figure 1-58). AAAs can become large and may result in rupture (with subsequent loss of massive amounts of blood into the peritoneal cavity), obstruction or compression of other structures, or release of emboli (resulting in stroke or MI). Abdominal ultrasound screening is recommended for past or active male smokers between 65 and 75 years old.

Thoracic Aortic Aneurysms

Atherosclerotic Aneurysms

Caused by atheroma formation leading to weakening of the media. Usually due to atherosclerotic disease or coronary artery disease (CAD) and associated with **hypertension** and smoking.

Syphilitic Aneurysms

Syphilis is a sexually transmitted disease (STD) that has primary, secondary, and tertiary stages. Tertiary syphilis damages the **vasa vasorum** of the aorta with consequent atrophy of vessel wall and dilatation of the aorta and valve ring, leading to aneurysm formation. Calcification of the aortic root and ascending aortic arch may be seen, causing a "tree bark" appearance of the aorta. Involvement of the aortic valve can lead to aortic insufficiency.

Connective Tissue Disorder Aneurysms

Connective tissue disorder aneurysms are caused by several inherited and acquired disorders and characterized by weakening of connective tissue. The major structural protein molecules, **collagen** and **elastin,** are often affected. The aortic wall, which is exposed to significant shear stress while transporting high-pressure blood, is particularly vulnerable. The intrinsic weakening of the wall of the aorta can thus progress to aneurysm and, eventually, dissection.

Miscellaneous Aneurysms

Berry Aneurysms

These are small, congenital, saccular lesions seen most often in the **circle of Willis.** Although not present at birth, these lesions develop at congenital sites of medial weakness at the **bifurcations of cerebral arteries** (posterior cerebral artery [PCA] and anterior cerebral artery [ACA], especially). They are associated with polycystic kidney disease, and rupture can lead to subarachnoid hemorrhage. A patient with a subarachnoid hemorrhage presents with "the worst headache of my life."

Mycotic Aneurysms

Usually due to bacterial infection (most often salmonellosis) involving the wall of the abdominal aorta.

Microaneurysms

These are small aneurysms usually seen in diabetes and hypertension.

Aortic Dissection

Luminal blood dissects the medial layers through a longitudinal intimal tear, forming a **false lumen** (Figure 1-59). This can be limited to the ascending aorta, propagate from the ascending aorta, or propagate from the descending aorta. From this point, it can progress to pericardial tamponade, aortic rupture, and death (Figure 1-60).

Often, dissection results from cystic medial necrosis, in which elastic tissue and muscle within the tunica media have degenerated. Predisposing factors include **hypertension,** bicuspid aortic valve, and **inherited connective tissue disorders,** such as Marfan syndrome and Ehlers-Danlos syndrome.

Patients can present with a tearing chest pain of sudden onset, radiating to the back. They may or may not have markedly unequal blood pressures in each arm, which indicates involvement of the subclavian artery. X-ray of the chest will show mediastinal widening.

Treatment depends on the location of the dissection. Stanford Type A dissections (proximal) involve the ascending aorta and are managed surgically (due to potential involvement of the aortic valve). Stanford Type B dissections (distal) involve the descending aorta and can be managed medically with β-blockers, then vasodilators.

Arteriovenous Fistula

This is an abnormal communication between an artery and a vein, usually secondary to trauma. The diversion of blood can result in **ischemic changes,** increased venous pressure causing **aneurysm** formation, and hypervolemia leading to **high-output cardiac failure** associated with a palpable thrill on physical examination (increased venous return → increased preload → increased cardiac output → eventual HF).

HEART MURMURS

Normally, blood travels through the cardiovascular system with laminar flow, which is silent. However, hemodynamic or structural changes may disturb laminar flow and produce **turbulent flow,** creating an audible murmur. Mechanisms for murmur generation include (1) increased blood flow, (2) flow into a dilated chamber, (3) regurgita-

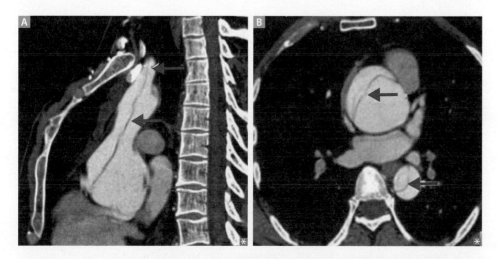

FIGURE 1-59.   Aortic dissection. CT shows intraluminal tear (arrows) forming a flap separating true and false lumen, involving the ascending and descending aorta.

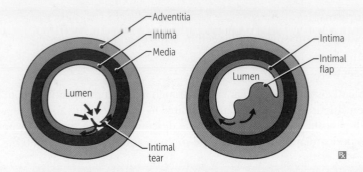

FIGURE 1-60. **Progression of arterial dissection.**

tion through an incompetent valve, (4) blood forced through an obstruction, and (5) abnormal shunting between chambers. In general (although not always), the **intensity** correlates with the amount of turbulent blood flow.

Murmurs can be classified according to several different characteristics (Table 1-27):

- **Timing:** Systolic (between S_1 and S_2), diastolic (between S_2 and S_1), and continuous.
- **Intensity:** Quantified by a grading system.
- **Location:** Area of highest intensity (Figure 1-10).
- **Pitch:** Frequency of the murmur (low or high).
- **Shape:** How the murmur changes in intensity from onset to completion.
- **Radiation:** Transmission of primary murmur to other areas.
- **Maneuver response:** Change of the murmur with certain actions, such as Valsalva and standing.

Systolic Murmurs

Mitral Regurgitation

Insufficiency of the mitral valve allows for backflow of blood from the LV into the LA. Consequences include (1) **increased LA pressure and volume,** (2) **increased LV volume** due to receiving the additional regurgitated volume during diastole, and (3) **reduction of forward flow.** In acute MR, the LA is very stiff; thus pressure increases substantially with regurgitation. This can result in rapid pulmonary edema. In chronic MR, the LA dilates via eccentric hypertrophy due to volume overload and develops increased compliance such that LA pressure (and thus backflow into the pulmonary system) decreases. However, this also leads to reduced forward CO.

Acute causes of MR include **papillary muscle rupture,** endocarditis, or ruptured chordae tendineae. Chronic causes include **rheumatic heart disease,** ischemic cardiomyopathy, dilated cardiomyopathy, hypertrophic cardiomyopathy, mitral valve prolapse,

> **CLINICAL CORRELATION**
>
> The murmur of **mitral valve prolapse** (MVP), often seen in patients with Marfan syndrome and in young women, is exaggerated by the Valsalva maneuver.

TABLE 1-27. **Classification of Murmurs**

	SYSTOLIC		DIASTOLIC		CONTINUOUS
EJECTION	HOLOSYSTOLIC	LATE SYSTOLIC	EARLY	LATE	
Aortic stenosis	MR	MVP	Aortic regurgitation	Mitral stenosis	PDA
Pulmonic stenosis	Tricuspid regurgitation	HCM	Pulmonic regurgitation	Tricuspid stenosis	VSD

HCM, hypertrophic cardiomyopathy; MR, mitral regurgitation; MVP, mitral valve prolapse; PDA, patent ductus arteriosus; VSD, ventricular septal defect.

endocardial fibroelastosis, or endocarditis (Table 1-28). Mitral valve prolapse is the most common cause of MR in the developed world.

PRESENTATION

Clinically, patients with acute MR tend to present with symptoms of **pulmonary edema.** Patients with chronic MR may present with symptoms of **low cardiac output** (fatigue, weakness), **pulmonary congestion** (dyspnea, orthopnea, PND), and even **RHF** (peripheral edema, ascites) in severe cases.

On physical examination, an S_3 and a **holosystolic,** high-pitched, blowing murmur are heard best at the apex, radiating toward the left axilla. The murmur is holosystolic since LV pressure is always greater than LA pressure in systole. The increased flow in the LA can lead to increased LA pressure and **pulmonary edema**.

DIAGNOSIS

ECG changes include LV hypertrophy and LA enlargement. Echocardiography shows a **regurgitant mitral valve** +/– underlying pathology (such as vegetations of endocarditis or MVP) as well as **LA and LV enlargement.** X-ray of the chest may show pulmonary edema. Pulmonary capillary wedge pressure tracings will show a prominent **v wave,** indicative of increased LA pressure (Figure 1-61).

TREATMENT

The goal is to increase forward flow, reduce regurgitation, and decrease pulmonary venous hypertension. Medications include diuretics (relief of pulmonary edema), vasodilators (reduced resistance to forward flow), and digitalis (increased cardiac output). MV repair or replacement is usually required for symptomatic severe MR.

Aortic Stenosis

In **aortic stenosis** (AS), blood cannot flow past the aortic valve during systole. Initially, the LV compensates with **concentric hypertrophy,** allowing generation of pressures high enough to crack open the stenosed valve and maintain normal CO. However, over time, this compensatory measure fails, resulting in decreased CO.

The most common cause is **age-related thickening and calcification** of the valves. However, it may also occur in younger patients (younger than 65 years) with a history of **rheumatic heart disease or bicuspid aortic valve** (the bicuspid valve is anatomically more susceptible to earlier calcification than the normal tricuspid valve).

PRESENTATION

- Patients with advanced AS may present with the "SAD" triad:
  - Syncope: Hypertrophied LV cannot significantly increase cardiac output during exercise due to fixed obstruction → decreased cerebral perfusion → loss of consciousness

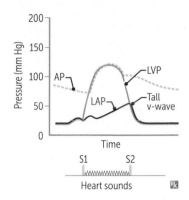

FIGURE 1-61.   Mitral regurgitation. AP, aortic pressure; LAP, left atrial pressure; LVP, left ventricular pressure.

KEY FACT

An S_3 occurs in early diastole and implies volume overload in older adults. It can be normal in children and young adults.

CLINICAL CORRELATION

Tricuspid regurgitation is a blowing holosystolic murmur heard at the left lower sternal border that increases with inspiration due to the increase in venous return to the right side of the heart.

KEY FACT

Coronary perfusion pressure = aortic diastolic pressure – LV end-diastolic pressure (LVEDP)

TABLE 1-28.   Acute vs Chronic Mitral Regurgitation

	ACUTE MITRAL REGURGITATION	CHRONIC MITRAL REGURGITATION
LA end-diastolic pressure	↑↑	Normal
LA compliance	Normal	↑
LV size	Normal	↑ (eccentric hypertrophy)
Cardiac output	Normal	↓
Pulmonary congestion	+	–

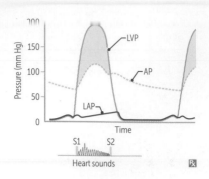

FIGURE 1-62. Aortic stenosis.
Pressure tracing demonstrating LVP > AP during ejection. Notice the crescendo-decrescendo pattern that is due to blood being forced through the narrowed aortic valve. AP, aortic pressure; LAP, left atrial pressure; LVP, left ventricular pressure.

? CLINICAL CORRELATION

Pulmonic stenosis (often congenital; also caused by carcinoid syndrome and rheumatic fever) is also a systolic ejection murmur that can radiate to the neck or shoulder and is loudest in the left upper sternal border.

« FLASH BACK

A single ventricular chamber is divided into two chambers by a **muscular** and **membranous** interventricular septum. Most VSDs are in the membraneous (upper) septum owing to failure of septal fusion with AV endocardial cushions.

KEY FACT

Left-to-right shunting can lead to increased pulmonary and right atrial pressure; if these pressures eventually become greater than the left-sided pressures, the shunt will reverse and become right-to-left. This is called **Eisenmenger syndrome.**

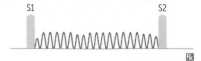

FIGURE 1-63. Ventricular septal defect.

- Angina: Imbalance between myocardial oxygen demand (LVH, increased wall stress) and oxygen supply (reduced cardiac output, coronary perfusion pressure).
- Dyspnea: Increased LV pressure → increased LA pressure → pulmonary congestion → symptoms of CHF
- Note that the order in which these symptoms appear is different from the mnemonic: (angina → syncope → dyspnea).
- **Crescendo-decrescendo systolic ejection murmur** that begins shortly after the S_1 heart sound. Murmur intensifies (crescendo) after AoV opens due to the large pressure gradient between LV and aorta. The murmur subsides (decrescendo) during late systole as the pressure gradient decreases with ejection of blood into the aorta. The high-frequency murmur is best heard in the right upper sternal border and usually radiates to the carotids (in the direction of turbulent blood flow) (Figure 1-62).
- Weak and delayed pulse at the carotid artery due to stenosis (**pulsus parvus et tardus**).

DIAGNOSIS

ECG shows a stenosed valve and LVH.

TREATMENT

Surgical correction or balloon valvuloplasty.

Ventricular Septal Defect

Ventricular septal defect (VSD) is a developmental defect in the interventricular septum that allows the two ventricles to communicate.

PRESENTATION

A defect in this septum leads to **left-to-right shunting** of blood, which may result in increased pulmonary blood flow and pulmonary artery pressure. Infants with this congenital defect may present with a harsh systolic murmur, fatigue with feeding, poor growth, and respiratory infections.

DIAGNOSIS

The VSD murmur is a **harsh, nonradiating holosystolic murmur** best heard over the left sternal border at the third and fourth intercostal spaces. The smaller the VSD, the more turbulent the flow through it, resulting in a louder murmur over the entire precordium. Extremely large VSDs may be entirely silent (Figure 1-63).

TREATMENT

May resolve spontaneously before age 2, but otherwise treated with surgery.

Mitral Valve Prolapse

Mitral valve prolapse (MVP) is a common syndrome that affects up to 7% of women aged 14–30 years. Often called floppy valve disease, it occurs when the MV leaflets do not close properly and billow into the LA during ventricular systole. It can be an autosomal dominant disorder or acquired as part of a connective tissue disorder. The normal collagen and elastin are replaced by myxomatous connective tissue. Connective tissue disorders such as Marfan syndrome, SLE, the mucopolysaccharidoses, and Ehlers-Danlos syndrome can manifest with MVP.

PRESENTATION

Usually **asymptomatic;** however, it can cause chest pain, palpitations, labored breathing, or fatigue. The murmur heard in MVP is a **late systolic murmur preceded by a midsystolic click** that corresponds to the tensing of the mitral leaflet/chordae tendineae as they are forced into the LA. The murmur corresponds to the regurgitation of blood from the LV into the LA (Figure 1-64).

Valsalva maneuver decreases preload, and squatting increases preload. Any maneuver that decreases the volume of the LV, such as Valsalva or standing, allows the prolapse to occur sooner, causing an increase in the intensity of the murmur. Squatting, which increases venous return, increases ventricular volume, helping to maintain tension on the chordae tendineae and allowing the valve to stay shut longer, thus causing a decrease in the intensity of the murmur.

DIAGNOSIS

Doppler echocardiography can show systolic displacement of the mitral leaflets.

TREATMENT

β-Blockers for chest pain or arrhythmias. Surgical treatment is rare. Endocarditis prophylaxis is no longer indicated.

Diastolic Murmurs

Aortic Valve Regurgitation

In **aortic regurgitation** (AR), blood backflows from the aorta into the LV during diastole. Thus, the LV must eject the regurgitant volume in addition to usual filling from the LA. In **acute AR,** the LV is relatively noncompliant; thus pressure rises dramatically with increased volume, with transmission into the LA and pulmonary circulation leading to congestive symptoms. In **chronic AR,** the LV and LA enlarge via **eccentric hypertrophy** to accommodate the increased volume without increase in pressure. LV systolic pressure increases while aortic diastolic pressure decreases, leading to a **widened pulse pressure** and reduced coronary perfusion pressure.

Causes include rheumatic heart disease, infectious endocarditis, aortic dissection, hypertension, syphilis, or Marfan syndrome.

PRESENTATION

Patients typically present with:

- Dyspnea on exertion.
- **Angina** due to shorter diastole and decreased coronary artery filling.
- Fatigue.
- Wide pulse pressures.
- S_3 and a **high-pitched, "blowing" early diastolic decrescendo murmur** (due to a decreasing pressure gradient from the aorta to LV during diastole) heard best at the second right intercostal space (Figure 1-65).
- **Austin Flint murmur,** a mid-diastolic, low-pitched rumbling that occurs when the regurgitated blood hits the MV leaflet in diastole, preventing an opening snap (differentiating AR from MS).

DIAGNOSIS

Echocardiography demonstrates a dilated LV and aorta and aortic regurgitant flow. Regurgitation can cause a "pseudovalve" or "bird's-nest deformity" on the ventricular septum on pathologic examination.

TREATMENT

The goal is **afterload reduction** with ACE inhibitors and vasodilators. Diuretics and digitalis are also used. Valve replacement can help if EF decreases or symptoms develop.

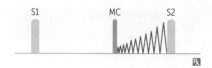

FIGURE 1-64. Mitral valve prolapse. Notice the midsystolic click that precedes the systolic murmur.

 CLINICAL CORRELATION

MVP and hypertrophic cardiomyopathy are the only two murmurs with this paradoxic relationship. All other murmurs increase in intensity with increased preload (squatting) and decrease in intensity with decreased preload (Valsalva).

KEY FACT

In both AR and MR, the extent of regurgitation relies on
- Size of regurgitant lesion
- Pressure gradient across valve during diastole
- Duration of diastole

 CLINICAL CORRELATION

Grading system for systolic murmurs:
I: Barely audible
II: Faint but audible
III: Easily heard
IV: Easily heard and associated with palpable thrill
V: Easily heard with stethoscope barely touching chest
VI: Easily heard without stethoscope touching chest

 CLINICAL CORRELATION

Several key physical examination findings are seen in aortic regurgitation:
- Corrigan (water-hammer) pulse: Marked distention and collapse
- de Musset sign: Head-bobbing with systole
- Quincke sign: Capillary pulsations visible in nail beds
- Bisferiens pulse: Double systolic impulse in carotid or brachial artery
Note: All related to widened pulse pressure.

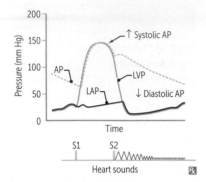

FIGURE 1-65. Aortic regurgitation. Pressure tracing demonstrates increased aortic systolic pressure, decreased aortic diastolic pressure, and increased LA/LV pressure. The murmur caused by aortic regurgitation has a decrescendo shape because there is a rapid diastolic relaxation of the left ventricle, and therefore a rapid pressure gradient is generated between the high-pressure aorta and the low-pressure ventricle. An Austin Flint murmur, however, has a crescendo-decrescendo pattern.

Mitral Stenosis

In **mitral stenosis,** there is obstruction to blood flow across the mitral valve from the LA to LV. This impedes LA emptying and thus increases LA pressure. This transmits into the pulmonary circulation, resulting in high pulmonary venous and capillary pressures. This can lead to **pulmonary edema** and even rupture of bronchial veins, leading to **hemoptysis.** Chronic MS can lead to reactive pulmonary hypertension and thus RHF. Chronically elevated LA pressure also leads to LA dilation, which can predispose to **atrial fibrillation** due to disruption of the conducting system.

The most common cause is **rheumatic heart disease,** producing commissural fusion ("fish mouth" valve). Less common causes include calcification in elderly patients, congenital stenosis, and endocarditis with large vegetations.

PRESENTATION

Clinically, patients may present with dyspnea, fatigue, orthopnea, paroxysmal nocturnal dyspnea, and, in severe cases, signs of RHF. Presentations may also include atrial fibrillation (due to enlarged LA), thromboembolism (from LA stasis), infective endocarditis, and hemoptysis.

The characteristic murmur of MS is best heard at the apex and includes the **high-pitched opening snap after S_2, followed by a decrescendo "diastolic rumble"** with accentuation at the end of the diastole (Figure 1-66).

DIAGNOSIS

Echocardiography shows thick MV leaflets and LA enlargement. ECG shows P mitrale (an **M**-shaped P wave) due to an enlarged atrium (Figure 1-67).

TREATMENT

Mainstays include diuretics and a salt-restricted diet to minimize symptoms of vascular congestion. Do not use inotropes because the ventricle has not failed. Treatment may also include **warfarin** to prevent thromboembolism and β-blockers to reduce heart rate and thus improve diastolic LV filling. Mechanical options include percutaneous balloon mitral valvoplasty (cracking open the stenosis), open mitral commissurotomy (cutting open the stenosis), and mitral valve replacement.

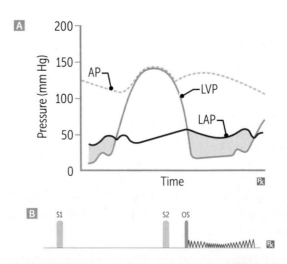

FIGURE 1-66. Mitral stenosis pressure tracing and murmur. **A** This figure illustrates the difference in pressure between the left atrium and the left ventricle. Also evident is the increase in pressure at the end of diastole, due to LA contraction. This is why there is a decrescendo-crescendo murmur associated with mitral stenosis. **B** Mitral stenosis murmur.

Continuous Murmur

Patent Ductus Arteriosus

Patent ductus arteriosus (PDA) is a congenital disorder with persistent communication between the aorta and the pulmonary artery via a patent ductus arteriosus.

PRESENTATION

CHF and late cyanosis are often seen. Because the aortic pressure is always greater than pulmonary artery pressure in both diastole and systole, the **machinery-like murmur** is heard throughout the cardiac cycle at the left infraclavicular area (Figure 1-68).

DIAGNOSIS

Doppler echocardiography.

TREATMENT

Indomethacin (an NSAID) is often used to close the PDA.

CARDIAC TUMORS

Primary cardiac tumors are very rare (more rare than secondary tumors) and include **myxomas** and **rhabdomyomas**. Most cardiac tumors are **metastatic** from bronchogenic carcinoma, malignant melanoma, malignant lymphoma, and carcinoma of the pancreas and esophagus.

Cardiac Myxoma

The most common primary cardiac tumor in the **adult**. They are benign and found in the **LA** in 90% of adults. They arise from endocardial mesenchymal cells, which proliferate and protrude into cardiac chambers (often pedunculated). On microscopy, myxoma cells, endothelial cells, and smooth muscle cells are found in a mucopolysaccharide background. They may cause tumor emboli or **ball-valve** obstruction and syncopal episodes as they act on the MV (Figure 1-69). On physical examination, they may produce a diastolic "plop" sound.

Cardiac Rhabdomyoma

The most common primary cardiac tumor in **children**. They usually arise within the myocardium and are associated with **tuberous sclerosis.**

VENOUS DISEASE

Varicose Veins

Varicose veins are tortuous, dilated, superficial vessels that normally involve the lower extremities. More common in women, they are thought to result from increased intraluminal pressure from incompetent venous valves, intrinsic weakness of the vessel wall, or congenital defects of the valves that impair forward flow to the heart.

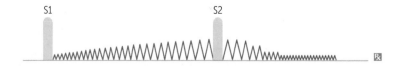

FIGURE 1-68. **Patent ductus arteriosus murmur.**

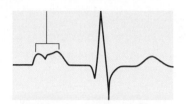

FIGURE 1-67. **P mitrale.** Note the M-shaped P wave (bracket) due to an enlarged left atrium that is often seen in mitral stenosis.

CLINICAL CORRELATION

In patients with a PDA, think about **congenital rubella and prematurity.** A common complication is infective endarteritis.

FLASH BACK

PDA closure is usually mediated by a decrease in circulating prostaglandins (PGs) at birth. Administering an NSAID (eg, indomethacin) decreases cyclooxygenase-mediated production of PG, facilitating PDA closure.

FLASH BACK

Tuberous sclerosis is an autosomal dominant disorder manifesting with hamartomas (benign tumor-like growths) affecting several organ systems, with cortical tubers, hypopigmented "ash leaf" skin lesions, facial angiofibromas (adenoma sebaceum), renal angiomyolipomas, and cardiac rhabdomyomas.

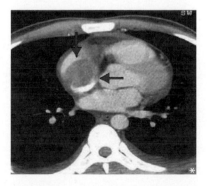

FIGURE 1-69. Cardiac myxoma. CT image showing cardiac myxoma in the right atrium (arrows).

PRESENTATION

Patients have a history of pregnancy, prolonged standing, or obesity. Many people seek treatment for cosmetic reasons; however, symptoms can also include a dull aching pressure after long periods of standing, swelling and skin ulceration from valvular dysfunction, and thrombosis and hematoma from stasis of blood.

TREATMENT

Treatment includes elevation of the legs, compression stockings to offset the increased venous hydrostatic pressure, and IV sclerosing agents. Surgical therapies such as vein stripping, ligation, and cryotherapy are generally used only in patients with symptomatic recurrent thrombosis or ulcers.

Deep Venous Thrombosis

Blood clots most often occur in the **calf veins,** although they can also affect the popliteal, femoral, or iliac veins. Risk factors are summarized in **Virchow triad:** Stasis of blood flow, vascular endothelium damage, and hypercoagulability (Table 1-29).

PRESENTATION

Patients can be asymptomatic or present with calf or thigh discomfort, unilateral leg swelling, edema, erythema, and warmth or tenderness on palpation over the vein. Homans sign—dorsiflexion of the foot producing calf pain—is often used as a test but is unreliable.

TABLE 1-29. **Virchow Triad**

SIGN OR SYMPTOM	EXAMPLES	PATHOGENESIS
Stasis/turbulence of blood flow	▪ Immobilization (cast applied for bone fracture may cover damaged vessels as well) ▪ Inactivity (postsurgery, long plane or car rides) ▪ Hyperviscosity (polycythemia vera) ▪ Turbulence (aneurysms) particularly common at the carotid bifurcation ▪ Deep sea diving (compression of legs and stasis)	Disruption of laminar flow → increased platelet-endothelium contact → coagulation factor excess→ thrombosis

Endothelial damage	▪ Trauma
	▪ IV catheters
	▪ Atherosclerosis
		Endothelial damage
		    → exposed collagen
		    → increased vWF binding
		    → initiation of clotting cascade
		Endothelial damage
		    → prevention of antithrombotic secretion

Hypercoagulable state	▪ Clotting disorders (antithrombin III deficiency, antiphospholipid antibodies) ▪ High-estrogen states (pregnancy, oral contraceptives) ▪ Smoking ▪ Neoplasm (direct secretion of coagulation factors from necrotic tumor cells)	Excess of procoagulants → thrombosis

vWF, von Willebrand factor.

KEY FACT

The most common place for a DVT to develop is in the calves; however, it may also form in the deep veins of the thigh or even the upper extremities.

DIAGNOSIS

Usually made through clinical judgment and laboratory testing. An increased D-dimer (fibrin degradation product) is sensitive but not specific. Lower extremity **venous duplex ultrasonography** uses Doppler ultrasound to assess blood flow within the vein. This test is both sensitive and specific. The gold standard is angiography, but it is invasive so is not generally used to make a clinical diagnosis.

TREATMENT

The main objective is to prevent complications such as **pulmonary embolism (PE)** and postthrombotic syndrome (chronic venous insufficiency syndrome). Elevation of the extremity helps reduce edema, and anticoagulation with heparin is started to prevent thrombus enlargement. For patients who cannot comply with anticoagulation or have medical conditions preventing anticoagulation, an intravascular filter is placed in the inferior vena cava (IVC) to prevent emboli from traveling from the extremity to the lungs.

Migratory Thrombophlebitis (Trousseau Syndrome)

Hypercoagulability secondary to malignancy resulting in venous thromboses appearing at one site, disappearing, and then reappearing in other veins. Occurs as a paraneoplastic syndrome (lung, pancreas, and colon cancer).

Superior Vena Cava Syndrome

Caused by neoplasms (bronchogenic carcinoma and mediastinal lymphomas) compressing or invading the superior vena cava (SVC), leading to impaired drainage of the vessels above the level of the blockage. Symptoms include dyspnea, face and neck edema, and dilation of head, neck, and arm veins, as well as collaterals on the chest wall (Figure 1-70). Often accompanied by respiratory distress (pulmonary venous compression).

Inferior Vena Cava Syndrome

Obstruction of the IVC manifests with edema in the legs, distention of the superficial veins of the lower abdomen, and, if renal veins are involved, massive proteinuria. Caused by neoplasms (liver and kidney cancers) or thrombi that compress or occlude the IVC.

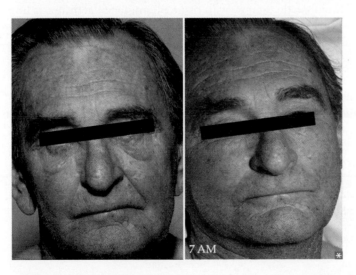

FIGURE 1-70. Superior vena cava syndrome. In image on the right, note facial edema, ruddy features, and development of swollen collateral veins.

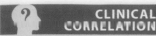

EMBOLI

An **embolus** is any mass (solid, liquid, or gaseous) that travels through the bloodstream and becomes trapped within the arterial vasculature. Thromboembolism refers to the trapping of fragmented thrombi in various parts of human vasculature. Thrombi are the most common types of emboli; however, other forms such as fat emboli and gas emboli also occur (Table 1-30).

Pulmonary Emboli

Pulmonary emboli usually arise from a DVT that has fragmented, with small portions traveling through the IVC and into branches of the pulmonary artery. This creates a ventilation-perfusion mismatch ($\dot{V}/\dot{Q}$ mismatch) leading to increased dead space, which means there is no perfusion with preserved ventilation. This causes hypoxemia with respiratory alkalosis.

PRESENTATION

Often clinically silent, this diagnosis is frequently missed in the hospital setting. Patients can present with tachycardia, tachypnea, dyspnea, hemoptysis, cough, and/or chest pain.

DIAGNOSIS

Once clinically suspected, the diagnostic test of choice is spiral CT angiography, provided there is no contraindication (Figure 1-71). A $\dot{V}/\dot{Q}$ **scan** can be used instead if the patient has renal insufficiency and cannot receive contrast. This will reveal a ventilation-perfusion mismatch. Other tests include pulmonary angiogram, Doppler ultrasound, and increased D-dimer. Arterial blood gas testing will show reduced PaO_2 and $PaCO_2$ as well as a respiratory alkalosis secondary to hyperventilation.

TREATMENT

Options include anticoagulation therapy with heparin and oral anticoagulants such as warfarin, or IVC filter placement to prevent future emboli. Heparin binds to the enzyme inhibitor antithrombin III (AT), causing a conformational change that results in its activation through an increase in the flexibility of its reactive site loop. The activated AT then inactivates thrombin and other proteases involved in blood clotting, most notably factor Xa. Thrombolytic therapy with tissue plasminogen activator is limited to those with a pulmonary embolism that causes hemodynamic compromise. However, there is an increased risk of bleeding and stroke with thrombolytics.

PROGNOSIS

The majority of patients, if receiving the correct diagnosis, have no sequelae. Obstruction of the pulmonary artery can lead to a hemorrhagic pulmonary infarction in which the

TABLE 1-30. Types of Embolism

CLASS	SOURCE
Thromboembolism (blood clot)	Arterial thrombosis
Cholesterol embolism	Atherosclerotic plaque inside vessel
Fat embolism	Bone fracture
Air embolism	IV, procedures with open vasculature, lung trauma
Septic embolism (bacteria)	Infection
Amniotic fluid embolism	Via placental bed of uterus

patient presents with shortness of breath, hemoptysis, and pleuritic chest pain. Sudden death occurs in cases of a **saddle embolus,** an embolus located at the bifurcation of the main pulmonary artery, and a minority of patients with recurrent pulmonary emboli can develop chronic pulmonary hypertension.

Arterial Emboli

An **arterial embolus** usually arises from a mural thrombus in the left atrium.

Arterial thromboemboli often cause infarction involving the brain (branches of the carotid artery), kidney (branches of the renal artery), and the intestine (branches of the mesenteric artery). Other sites affected can include the spleen and lower extremities.

Paradoxical Emboli

Paradoxical emboli are venous emboli that cross over from the right side of the heart to the left side and access the systemic circulation. Most common coexisting defects are ASDs or a patent foramen ovale (PFO).

Fat Emboli

Bone marrow particles and fatty tissue travel to the lungs, brain, and kidney following severe long-bone fractures (occurs 24–48 hours post trauma). Patients present with **petechiae, neurologic abnormalities,** and **pulmonary distress.**

Gas Emboli

Caused by the introduction of air into the circulation. This is often seen in deep-sea divers who ascend from depth too rapidly. Nitrogen bubbles precipitate and block circulation, causing musculoskeletal pain also known as **"the bends."**

Amniotic Fluid Emboli

A complication of labor in which amniotic fluid leaks into the maternal circulation, most commonly after trauma or placenta abruptio. Complications include disseminated intravascular coagulation (80%) and **death** (20–90%).

SHOCK

Shock is a state of generalized hypoperfusion of tissues and cells in which O_2 delivery cannot meet O_2 demand. Initially the injury is reversible; however, as the hypoperfusion continues, the injuries become permanent and lead to multiple organ dysfunction syndrome (MODS). MODS can follow any type of shock and frequently involves the lung, kidney, heart, and liver (Table 1-31).

Presentation

Patients usually present with tachycardia, oliguria, hypotension, weak pulses, mental status changes, and cool extremities.

Stages of Shock

- **Compensation:** Reflex mechanisms maintain perfusion of vital organs. These mechanisms include increased HR, increased peripheral resistance, release of catecholamines, and activation of the RAAS.
- **Decompensation:** After greater than 15–20% of blood volume is lost, reflex mechanisms can no longer compensate, leading to tissue hypoperfusion, reversible tissue injury, and metabolic imbalance (eg, metabolic acidosis and renal insufficiency).
- **Irreversible injury:** End-organ damage and failure ultimately leading to death.

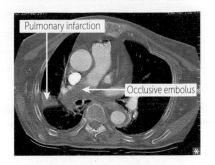

FIGURE 1-71. Pulmonary thromboembolism. Spiral CT showing pulmonary thromboembolism.

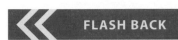

FLASH BACK

Three congenital heart defects that do not cause early cyanosis:
AS**D**
VS**D**
PD**A**

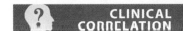

CLINICAL CORRELATION

Arterial embolism to an extremity → remember the 5 Ps
Pain
Pulselessness
Pallor
Paresthesias
Paralysis

TABLE 1-31.   Types of Shock

	CAUSED BY	PATHOPHYSIOLOGY	SKIN	CVP (PRELOAD)	CO	SVR (AFTERLOAD)	TREATMENT
Hypovolemic	Hemorrhage, dehydration, burns	Low circulating blood volume	Cold, clammy	↓↓	↓	↑	IV fluids
Cardiogenic	Acute MI, HF, valvular dysfunction, arrhythmia	Pump failure (often LV)	Cold, clammy	↑	↓↓	↑	Inotropes, diuresis
Obstructive	Cardiac tamponade, PE	Physical obstruction of great vessels	Cold, clammy	↑	↓↓	↑	Relieve obstruction
Distributive	Sepsis, CNS injury, anaphylaxis	▪ Septic → endotoxin release → NO release → peripheral vasodilation ▪ CNS trauma (ie, neurogenic shock) → loss of sympathetic drive → peripheral vasodilation ▪ Anaphylaxis → histamine release → peripheral vasodilation	Warm, dry	↓	↑	↓↓	Pressors, IV fluids

↓↓, primary insult. CVP, central venous pressure; HF, heart failure; MI, myocardial infarction; PE, pulmonary embolism; SVR, systemic vascular resistance.

Systemic inflammatory response syndrome (≥ 2: fever/hypothermia, tachycardia, tachypnea, leukocytosis/leukopenia). First sign of shock is tachycardia. Multiple organ dysfunction syndrome (MODS) is the end result of shock.

KEY FACT

Left anterior descending (LAD) infarction can cause left bundle-branch block (LBBB), anterior wall rupture, and mural thrombi. Right coronary artery (RCA) infarction can cause LV papillary rupture, posterior flail leaflet, and MR.

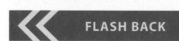

FLASH BACK

CO = HR × SV
SVR = (MAP − CVP) / CO

Pathology

- Kidney: Acute tubular necrosis, oliguria.
- Intestines: Mucosal ischemic necrosis and patchy hemorrhages, sepsis.
- Brain: Necrosis.
- Liver: Centrilobular necrosis ("shock liver").
- Adrenal: Waterhouse-Friderichsen syndrome with acute hemorrhagic infarction and adrenal insufficiency.

PERICARDIAL DISEASE

The **pericardium** is a double-layered sac that surrounds the heart, with the visceral pericardium lining the heart and the parietal pericardium on the outside. In between the two layers is pericardial fluid that helps to decrease friction.

Pericardial Effusion

Increased fluid accumulation sometimes occurs in the pericardial space. The volume of fluid, the rate of increase, and pericardial compliance all factor into the clinical symptoms of effusion. It can be acute or chronic (Table 1-32).

PRESENTATION

Usually asymptomatic, clinical features can include soft heart sounds, dullness over the posterior left lung and left-sided chest ache, or compressive symptoms such as dysphagia (compression of the esophagus), hoarseness, or dyspnea.

TABLE 1-32.   Acute Versus Chronic Pericardial Effusion

	ACUTE	CHRONIC
Cause	Pericarditis, cardiac surgery, uremia, and collagen vascular disease	TB, cancer (lung, breast, or bone), SLE, HIV
Presentation	Chest pain, pericardial friction rub, pericardiocentesis reveals **small amounts** of fluid	With or without symptoms, **large amounts** of fluid on pericardiocentesis, symptom relief may or may not be seen after fluid is drained

HIV, human immunodeficiency virus; SLE, systemic lupus erythematosus; TB, tuberculosis.

DIAGNOSIS

Echocardiography can quantify the volume of fluid in the pericardial sac. ECG shows low voltages, and an increased cardiac silhouette is seen on chest radiograph.

TREATMENT

Involves treatment of the underlying disorder or pericardiocentesis.

Cardiac Tamponade

Cardiac tamponade is a pericardial effusion with enough fluid and pressure to compress the heart chambers, leading to impaired cardiac filling. The most common causes include neoplasms; postviral; uremia; and hemorrhage from trauma, ruptured LV following LAD MI, active tuberculosis, or dissecting aortic aneurysm.

PRESENTATION

Principal features include systemic venous congestion exhibited by JVD, peripheral edema and hepatomegaly, pulmonary venous congestion demonstrated by crackles (rales) on exam, and decreased cardiac output evidenced by hypotension and tachycardia. Other features include elevated diastolic intracardiac pressure, decreased heart sounds, and **pulsus paradoxus.**

Normally with inspiration the intrathoracic pressure becomes more negative, leading to increased venous return and increased filling of the right heart. This leads to intraventricular septal bulging into the LV, causing decreased cardiac output and BP. Any disease that causes high negative intrathoracic pressures (eg, status asthmaticus) or impaired right ventricular filling (eg, restrictive cardiomyopathy) or outflow will exaggerate this mechanism, causing a > 10-mm Hg decline in systolic BP upon inspiration **(pulsus paradoxus).**

DIAGNOSIS

Echocardiography can help evaluate for pericardial effusion. In tamponade, there is collapse of the RA and RV during diastole. Definitive diagnosis is by cardiac catheterization, which shows **diastolic pressure equalization in all four chambers.** ECG shows low voltage because the surrounding fluid attenuates the signal. **Electrical alternans** may also be seen, which will manifest as beat-to-beat variation of the QRS complex amplitude with or without a wandering ECG baseline. This occurs because the heart moves more freely in the enlarged pericardial sac and thus alters its position relative to the recording electrodes.

KEY FACT

The Beck triad of cardiac tamponade includes:
- Muffled heart sounds
- Elevated jugular venous pressure (JVP)
- Low systolic blood pressure

KEY FACT

Pulsus paradoxus is defined by a fall in blood pressure (>10 mm Hg) during inspiration. In healthy individuals, inspiration leads to negative intrathoracic pressure relative to atmospheric pressure, which increases venous return to the right heart but also expands pulmonary vasculature. Overall, this causes blood to pool in the lungs and decreases flow to the left heart, which leads to reduced stroke volume and thus a small decrease in systolic blood pressure (<10 mm Hg). In pericardial tamponade, diastolic dysfunction leads to reduced LV filling and thus exaggerates this reduced stroke volume during inspiration. This leads to a systolic blood pressure drop >10 mm Hg.

FLASH BACK

Subxiphoid pericardiocentesis requires the needle to pass through the skin, superficial and deep fascia, pectoralis major muscle, external intercostal membrane, internal intercostal membrane, transversus thoracis muscle, fibrous pericardium, and the parietal layer of the serous pericardium.

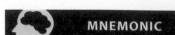

MNEMONIC

Causes of pericarditis—
CARDIAC RIND

Collagen vascular disease
Aortic aneurysm
Radiation
Drugs (hydralazine)
Infections
Acute renal failure
Cardiac Infarction
Rheumatic fever
Injury
Neoplasms
Dressler syndrome

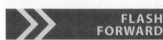

FLASH FORWARD

Dressler syndrome is a delayed pericarditis (believed to be autoimmune reaction against cardiac antigens formed in inflammation during MI) that develops 2–10 weeks after an MI.

TREATMENT

Removal of fluid through pericardiocentesis. The two locations for pericardiocentesis are in between the fifth and sixth intercostal space along the left sternal border or an infrasternal approach starting just inferior to the xiphoid process.

Acute Pericarditis

Inflammation of the Pericardium

There are four subtypes of pericarditis: serous, fibrinous, suppurative (productive of pus), and hemorrhagic (Table 1-33). These may resolve or lead to scarring and chronic adhesive or chronic constrictive pericarditis. The most common cause is idiopathic, often presumed secondary to occult viral infection.

PRESENTATION

Patients present with retrosternal chest pain (worse on inspiration or coughing; relief while sitting or leaning forward), fever, hypotension, JVD, **pericardial friction rub,** and distant heart sounds.

DIAGNOSIS

Clinical suspicion with the presence of pleuritic and positional pain with a friction rub; ECG with diffuse ST segment elevation and PR depression are often seen (Figure 1-72).

TREATMENT

Treat the underlying cause, including NSAIDs for pain in viral pericarditis or Dressler syndrome.

Chronic Constrictive Pericarditis

Gradual resorption of acute pericarditis can lead to fusion of the pericardial layers and scar formation with possible calcifications leading to a stiff pericardium (see Table 1-32). This results in inhibition of diastolic filling, and signs similar to those of CHF may become evident. The most common cause worldwide is TB; however, it may also be secondary to pyogenic organisms or *Staphylococcus* spp leading to obliteration of the pericardial cavity.

PRESENTATION

Patients tend to develop symptoms over months to years. Reduced CO leads to fatigue, hypotension, and reflex tachycardia. Elevated systemic venous pressures lead to JVD, peripheral edema, and hepatomegaly with ascites. **Kussmaul sign,** or failure of the

TABLE 1-33.   Types of Pericarditis

DISEASE	EXUDATE	ASSOCIATIONS
Serous	Protein-rich, straw-colored, few inflammatory cells	Associated with SLE, rheumatic fever, uremia, and viral infection (coxsackie B)
Fibrinous	Fibrin-rich with plasma proteins	Associated with MI (Dressler syndrome), uremia, or rheumatic fever; can lead to scar formation and diastolic filling defects
Suppurative	Cloudy fluid with many inflammatory cells	Caused by bacterial infection leading to erythematous serosal surfaces
Hemorrhagic	Bloody and inflammatory fluid	Due to tumor invasion or TB

MI, myocardial infarction; SLE, systemic lupus erythematosus; TB, tuberculosis.

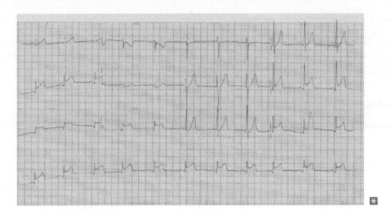

FIGURE 1-72. **ECG findings in acute pericarditis.** Notice the diffuse concave upward ST segment elevation.

jugular veins to collapse during inspiration, is also seen. Heart sounds are distant, and a pericardial "knock"—an early apical diastolic sound representing the sudden cessation of ventricular filling due to the stiffened pericardium—may be heard.

DIAGNOSIS

Chest radiograph may show an enlarged cardiac silhouette, and CT or MRI may show pericardial thickening. Confirmation is by cardiac catheterization showing increased diastolic pressures. A prominent *y* descent is visible in the atrial pressure curve.

TREATMENT

Effective treatment requires removal of the pericardium (pericardiectomy).

PERIPHERAL VASCULAR DISEASE

Large-Vessel Vasculitis

Temporal (Giant Cell) Arteritis

Temporal arteritis, also known as giant-cell arteritis (GCA), affects **medium** to **large** arteries, particularly the carotid and aortic branches. It is characterized by nodular inflammation, intimal fibrosis, and granulomas containing multinucleated giant cells. It most often affects woman more than 50 years old.

PRESENTATION

Often affects the temporal artery. Symptoms include unilateral headache, sudden-onset vision loss, facial pain, and jaw claudication. Palpation of the artery may reveal absence of pulse. Ophthalmic artery involvement can lead to **blindness.**

Patients can also have polymyalgia rheumatica, characterized by severe stiffness and aches in the axial skeleton (neck, shoulder girdle, and pelvic girdle).

DIAGNOSIS

Definitive diagnosis is by biopsy of the affected vessel, usually the temporal artery, showing granulomatous inflammation. Elevated erythrocyte sedimentation rate (ESR) and CRP levels are also seen due to inflammation.

TREATMENT

After confirming elevated ESR, it is essential to administer **high-dose, systemic corticosteroids** to prevent permanent loss of vision. The biopsy may be performed afterwards.

MNEMONIC

Konstrictive pericarditis presents with **K**ussmaul sign and a pericardial **K**nock.

KEY FACT

In usual physiology, inspiration leads to negative intrathoracic pressure that enhances right heart filling. In constrictive pericarditis, the rigid pericardium prevents right heart filling, leading blood to accumulate in the jugular veins during inspiration. This produces **Kussmaul sign,** a paradoxical distention of the jugular veins during inspiration.

Takayasu Arteritis

Takayasu arteritis, also known as "pulseless disease," is an inflammation of elastic arteries—most commonly affecting the **aorta** and **its upper branching vessels.** It often occurs in Asian woman younger than 40 years old.

PRESENTATION

Loss of the carotid, ulnar, and radial pulse leads to the distinctive "pulseless disease" designation. Inflammation of the affected vessels can lead to myocardial ischemia, hypertension, and visual defects. Systemic inflammatory effects such as fever, night sweats, arthralgia, and weight loss are also seen.

DIAGNOSIS

Angiography will demonstrate narrowing of the aortic arch and proximal great vessels due to granulomatous inflammation. Elevated ESR.

TREATMENT

Steroids and cytotoxic drugs are used to reduce inflammation.

Medium-Vessel Vasculitis

Polyarteritis Nodosa

Polyarteritis nodosa (PAN) is a necrotizing, immune complex–mediated inflammation of **small** to **medium** arteries, frequently involving destruction of the media and internal elastic lamina. It most commonly affects middle-aged to older men, peaking at 50 years of age. It is common in patients with **hepatitis B** infection ($\leq 30\%$ are infected).

PRESENTATION

Symptoms are either inflammatory in nature (eg, fever and musculoskeletal pain) or due to decreased organ blood flow (eg, headache, abdominal pain, and hypertension). Ischemia of vessels can lead to distal disruption including **ischemic heart disease, arthritis,** and **renal lesions** (multiple organ involvement). Neurologic dysfunction can occur as **mononeuritis multiplex** (a motor peripheral neuropathy affecting at least two unrelated nerve regions), as well as cutaneous symptoms (palpable purpura, livedo reticularis, subcutaneous nodules). There is **no lung involvement.**

DIAGNOSIS

Definitive diagnosis is by biopsy of the affected vessels (transmural inflammation of the arterial wall and fibrinoid necrosis is present). Necrosis is accompanied by a prominent polymorphonuclear infiltrate. Antineutrophil cytoplasmic antibodies (ANCA) are highly suggestive of microscopic polyarteritis nodosa. Arteriogram will show innumerable renal microaneurysms and spasms.

TREATMENT

Immunosuppressants (eg, cyclophosphamide), prednisone.

Kawasaki Disease

A mucocutaneous disease characterized by acute necrotizing inflammation of the small, medium, and larger arteries. It is often found in children younger than 4 years. The most serious sequelae include coronary vessel involvement, leading to aneurysms.

PRESENTATION

Symptoms include:

- Fever present for at least 5 days
- Cervical lymphadenitis

FLASH BACK

Cytoplasmic antineutrophil cytoplasmic antibody (c-ANCA) is often associated with change to granulomatosis with polyangiitis (GPA).
Perinuclear antineutrophil cytoplasmic antibody (p-ANCA) is often seen in Churg-Strauss syndrome, microscopic polyangiitis, and primary sclerosing cholangitis.

KEY FACT

The triad of granulomatosis with polyangiitis is (1) focal necrotizing vasculitis, (2) necrotizing granulomas of the lungs and upper airway, and (3) necrotizing glomerulonephritis.

- Bilateral conjunctival injection
- Red, fissured lips
- Oral erythema ("strawberry tongue")
- Diffuse maculopapular erythematous rash
- Desquamation of the hands and feet

DIAGNOSIS

Diagnosis is made clinically; coronary angiogram is performed to diagnose coronary artery aneurysms.

TREATMENT

Aspirin and IV immunoglobin aid as anti-inflammatory agents. Long-term treatment in those with CAD includes aspirin and antiplatelet therapy. Anticoagulation is used in those with coronary aneurysms.

Thromboangiitis Obliterans

Also known as Buerger disease, thromboangiitis obliterans is a full-thickness, segmental, thrombosing inflammation of the distal extremity medium-sized arteries, veins, and nerves. It is strongly associated with **young men** who are **heavy smokers.**

PRESENTATION

Triad of distal arterial occlusion, Raynaud phenomenon, and migrating superficial vein thrombophlebitis. Intermittent claudication may lead to gangrene and/or auto-amputation of digits.

DIAGNOSIS

Arteriography may show distal stenotic corkscrew vessels. Definitive diagnosis involves tissue biopsy.

TREATMENT

Smoking cessation.

Small-Vessel Vasculitis

Granulomatosis with Polyangiitis

Granulomatosis with polyangiitis (GPA) is characterized by necrotizing, granulamatous inflammation affecting **small vessels** in the renal system and respiratory tract. It is defined by a triad of:

- Focal necrotizing vasculitis
- Necrotizing granulomas in the lungs and upper airways
- Necrotizing glomerulonephritis

PRESENTATION

- Renal: Hematuria, red cell casts in the urine.
- Lower respiratory tract: Hemoptysis, cough, dyspnea.
- Upper respiratory tract: Nasal septum perforation, chronic sinusitis, otitis media, mastoiditis.
- Skin: Purpura.

DIAGNOSIS

Ninety percent of patients are c-ANCA/PR3-ANCA positive, and definitive diagnosis is made through biopsy showing necrosis and granuloma formation. Chest radiography shows nodular densities. Hematuria/red cell casts also aid in diagnosis.

KEY FACT

Raynaud phenomenon occurs when cold or stress exposure induces vasoconstriction of the digital arteries, causing the fingers/toes to turn white or blue. Primary Raynaud phenomenon (Raynaud disease) occurs in the absence of an underlying cause and is usually found in women, whereas secondary Raynaud phenomenon is usually found in men with a secondary systemic disorder.

MNEMONIC

Patients with Kawasaki disease **CRASH** and **BURN.**
They have 4/5 of the following:
Conjunctivitis (with sparing of the limbus)
Rash (truncal)
Adenopathy (unilateral and cervical)
Strawberry tongue (+/- dry, cracked lips)
Hands and feet (edema followed by desquamation)
PLUS
BURN = fever of at least 5 days

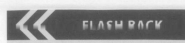

FLASH BACK

The main side effect of
Cyclophosphamide is **C**ystitis. **Mesna**
is used to prevent cyclophosphamide-
induced cystitis by binding to the
metabolite acrolein in the bladder.

TREATMENT

Cyclophosphamide and corticosteroids.

Churg-Strauss Syndrome

Churg-Strauss syndrome is a granulomatous, necrotizing vasculitis affecting **small to medium**-sized arteries. It is characterized by the presence of **eosinophilia.**

PRESENTATION

The presentation may involve many systems and includes:

- Upper respiratory tract: Sinusitis, allergic rhinitis
- Lower respiratory tract: Asthma, cough
- Musculoskeletal: Arthralgias
- Dermatologic: Palpable purpura
- Neurologic: Peripheral neuropathy (ie, foot drop)
- Gastrointestinal: Melena, colitis

Cardiac and renal manifestations (pauci-immune glomerulonephritis) may also be seen.

DIAGNOSIS

Criteria include asthma, peripheral eosinophilia (increased IgE), paranasal sinusitis, pulmonary infiltrates, histologic proof of vasculitis, and polyneuropathy. Often p-ANCA-positive (70%).

TREATMENT

Supportive therapy and glucocorticoids.

Microscopic Polyangitis

A necrotizing vasculitis most commonly involving **small vessels** of the lungs, kidneys, and skin. Characterized by pauci-immune glomerulonephritis and palpable purpura.

PRESENTATION

Similar to GPA but lacking nasopharyngeal involvement.

DIAGNOSIS

Positive for p-ANCA/MPO-ANCA. No granulomas will be seen on biopsy.

TREATMENT

Cyclophosphamide and corticosteroids.

Henoch-Schönlein Purpura

Henoch-Schönlein Purpura (HSP) is the most common childhood systemic vasculitis, with inflammation secondary to **IgA complex deposition** affecting **small vessels.** It often follows an upper respiratory infection in children.

PRESENTATION

The classic triad involves:

- Palpable purpura on the buttocks and legs
- Polyarthralgias
- Colicky abdominal pain

Edema, hematuria (due to IgA nephropathy), hypertension, and melena may also be seen.

DIAGNOSIS

The diagnosis is made clinically, since laboratory tests are often normal.

TREATMENT

Supportive therapy with analgesics is often employed. If renal involvement is found, children must be followed long-term for development of chronic kidney disease (CKD) and/or hypertension. Therapy may sometimes include corticosteroids.

Cryoglobulinemic Vasculitis

Cryoglobulinemic vasculitis is a small-vessel disease in which serum proteins precipitate out in the cold.

DIAGNOSIS

Often due to hepatitis C infection, it is diagnosed with purpura, low complement, and immune deposits in vascular walls.

TREATMENT

Treatment involves plasmapheresis and hepatitis C treatment (interferon-α and ribavirin).

ISCHEMIC HEART DISEASE

Ischemic heart disease (IHD) occurs when myocardial oxygen demand exceeds oxygen supply. While this often involves an interruption of arterial blood flow to the heart, as with atherosclerotic narrowing of the coronary arteries, it may also be a consequence of profound anemia (low oxygen-carrying capacity). Risk factors include hypertension, family history, smoking, hypercholesterolemia (LDL > 160 mg/dL or HDL < 35 mg/dL), diabetes mellitus, age (male > 45 years old or female > 55 years old/postmenopausal), and tobacco use. IHD can present as angina pectoris or MI.

Angina Pectoris

Episodic chest pain caused by a disparity between cardiac perfusion and cardiac demand, leading to transient hypoxia of the myocardium. No necrosis occurs.

PRESENTATION

Typically manifests as **retrosternal chest pain or pressure** that can radiate to the neck, jaw, or left arm, and lasts anywhere from 15 seconds to 15 minutes. Patients are often diaphoretic and nauseated. Symptoms are very similar to those of MI, but the ECG does not show any acute changes. Precipitating factors include cold, food, and stress, whereas relieving factors include rest and nitroglycerin. There are three types: stable angina, unstable angina, and Prinzmetal angina.

- **Stable angina:** The most common form in which pain is **induced by exertion** (usually the same amount of exertion causes pain); the pain is **relieved by rest** or nitroglycerin. Pain is thought to be due to **stenosis** of the atherosclerotic coronary arteries, which can no longer supply enough O_2 to meet the increased demands of the heart during exertion. If pain occurs with exertion, the coronaries are generally > 70% stenotic.
- **Unstable angina:** Pain at **rest** or with increasing frequency, intensity, and duration of pain during activity. Thought to be induced by a ruptured atherosclerotic plaque that leads to thrombosis and embolization. Unstable angina is more likely to lead to **MI** than is stable angina. ECG may show ST segment depressions and T-wave inversions, but never ST segment elevations. Cardiac biomarkers will be **normal.** If pain occurs at rest, the arteries are > 90% stenotic. Treatment involves aspirin, nitrates, β-blockers, and statins for lipid management. Heparin or glycoprotein IIb/IIIa inhibitors are also used. Patients are often sent for coronary angiography.

DIAGNOSIS

The diagnosis is made clinically, since laboratory tests are often normal.

TREATMENT

Supportive therapy with analgesics is often employed. If renal involvement is found, children must be followed long-term for development of chronic kidney disease (CKD) and/or hypertension. Therapy may sometimes include corticosteroids.

Cryoglobulinemic Vasculitis

Cryoglobulinemic vasculitis is a small-vessel disease in which serum proteins precipitate out in the cold.

DIAGNOSIS

Often due to hepatitis C infection, it is diagnosed with purpura, low complement, and immune deposits in vascular walls.

TREATMENT

Treatment involves plasmapheresis and hepatitis C treatment (interferon-α and ribavirin).

KEY FACT

Platelet counts are often normal or elevated in HSP, whereas they are decreased in idiopathic thrombocytopenic purpura (ITP).

ISCHEMIC HEART DISEASE

Ischemic heart disease (IHD) occurs when myocardial oxygen demand exceeds oxygen supply. While this often involves an interruption of arterial blood flow to the heart, as with atherosclerotic narrowing of the coronary arteries, it may also be a consequence of profound anemia (low oxygen carrying capacity). Risk factors include hypertension, family history, smoking, hypercholesterolemia (LDL > 160 mg/dL or HDL < 35 mg/dL), diabetes mellitus, age (male > 45 years old or female > 55 years old/postmenopausal), and tobacco use. IHD can present as angina pectoris or MI.

Angina Pectoris

Episodic chest pain caused by a disparity between cardiac perfusion and cardiac demand, leading to transient hypoxia of the myocardium. No necrosis occurs.

PRESENTATION

Typically manifests as **retrosternal chest pain or pressure** that can radiate to the neck, jaw, or left arm, and lasts anywhere from 15 seconds to 15 minutes. Patients are often diaphoretic and nauseated. Symptoms are very similar to those of MI, but the ECG does not show any acute changes. Precipitating factors include cold, food, and stress, whereas relieving factors include rest and nitroglycerin. There are three types: stable angina, unstable angina, and Prinzmetal angina.

- **Stable angina:** The most common form in which pain is **induced by exertion** (usually the same amount of exertion causes pain); the pain is **relieved by rest** or nitroglycerin. Pain is thought to be due to **stenosis** of the atherosclerotic coronary arteries, which can no longer supply enough O_2 to meet the increased demands of the heart during exertion. If pain occurs with exertion, the coronaries are generally > 70% stenotic.
- **Unstable angina:** Pain at **rest** or with increasing frequency, intensity, and duration of pain during activity. Thought to be induced by a ruptured atherosclerotic plaque that leads to thrombosis and embolization. Unstable angina is more likely to lead to **MI** than is stable angina. ECG may show ST segment depressions and T-wave inversions, but never ST segment elevations. Cardiac biomarkers will be **normal.** If pain occurs at rest, the arteries are > 90% stenotic. Treatment involves aspirin, nitrates, β-blockers, and statins for lipid management. Heparin or glycoprotein IIb/IIIa inhibitors are also used. Patients are often sent for coronary angiography.

KEY FACT

Transmural ischemia = ST elevation Subendocardial/partial thickness ischemia = ST depression

■ **Prinzmetal angina:** Also called variant angina, it presents as **intermittent chest pain at rest** that is not related to activity, stress, or BP. Known triggers include tobacco, cocaine, and triptans, but the cause is often unknown. Often occurs during the night. It is thought to be due to **coronary artery vasospasm.** ECG may demonstrate transient ST segment elevations. Cardiac catheterization may not demonstrate atherosclerosis, and spasm can be precipitated with ergonovine. Definitive diagnosis involves exaggerated spasm of coronary arteries after injection with provocative agents, such as ergonovine, during coronary angiography. Treatment includes calcium channel blockers and nitrates.

DIAGNOSIS

Multiple diagnostic modalities are available. ECG may show prior MI or signs of ischemia. Stress testing via exercise or medication (traditionally vasodilators such as dipyramidole or adenosine, or positive chronotropic agents such as dobutamine) may reveal inducible ischemia visible by echocardiogram or myocardial perfusion imaging. Finally, cardiac catheterization can directly visualize coronary obstruction.

TREATMENT

Modification of risk factors through smoking cessation, diet control, active lifestyle, weight loss, and treatment of diseases such as hypertension, hyperlipidemia, and diabetes is always helpful. Medical therapy for stable angina is shown in Table 1-34.

Surgical therapy includes **coronary artery bypass graft (CABG),** which replaces diseased vessels with healthy veins and arteries from other parts of the body, and **percutaneous transluminal coronary angioplasty,** which uses a balloon threaded from a peripheral artery to inflate the stenosed area. In both cases, stents (bare metal or drug-eluting) are often placed to ensure the vessel remains patent.

CORONARY STEAL PHENOMENON

In CAD, the vessel distal to the stenosis will be maximally dilated at baseline to allow for adequate tissue perfusion. Therefore, administration of a vasodilator such as dipyramidole will dilate normal vessels but cannot further dilate the stenosed vessels. This leads to shunting of blood toward well-perfused areas, leading to reduced flow to poststenotic regions. This principle is useful for pharmacologic stress testing.

TABLE 1-34. Drug Treatment for Stable Angina Pectoris

DRUG	REASON FOR USE	SIDE EFFECTS
Nitrates	Venous dilation to ↓ preload (main effect), arteriolar dilatation to ↓ afterload, and coronary artery dilatation to ↑ O_2 supply	Orthostatic hypotension, reflex tachycardia, blushing, headache
β-Blockers	↓ Sympathetic drive will ↓ myocardial O_2 demand and improve survival	Bronchoconstriction, insomnia, depression, GI disturbances
Calcium channel blockers	↓ Preload and afterload	Hypotension, reflex tachycardia, flushing, headache

MYOCARDIAL INFARCTION

MI is due to myocardial necrosis secondary to inadequate cardiac tissue perfusion, most often secondary to acute rupture of a coronary artery atherosclerotic plaque. This leads to microscopic changes in the heart and release of myocardial enzymes into the bloodstream (Table 1-35). Risk factors include increasing age, hypercoagulable states, vasculitis, and those that predispose to atherosclerosis.

PRESENTATION

Patients describe prolonged (> 30–45 minutes) crushing chest pain similar to angina, but **not relieved by nitroglycerin,** as well as nausea, vomiting, sweating, shortness of breath, and weakness. There are two patterns of myocardial involvement: nontransmural and transmural.

- **Non-ST-elevation myocardial infarct (NSTEMI):** This is an MI that is limited to the inner one-half to one-third of the LV wall. Coronary artery atherosclerosis results in decreased coronary blood flow and loss of perfusion to the wall. **ST-segment depression** is seen on ECG.
- **ST-elevation myocardial infarct (STEMI):** This occurs following atherosclerotic plaque rupture and thrombosis leading to complete vessel occlusion (no blood flow!). Necrosis of the entire myocardial wall is seen. ECG is characterized by **ST-segment elevation** (Figure 1-73). Q waves may develop hours after and persist long after MI.

Coronary artery thrombosis most commonly affects LAD > RCA > left circumflex coronary artery.

DIAGNOSIS

ST segment elevation is seen in transmural infarcts. ECG changes in contiguous leads corresponding to geographic location of MI (Table 1-36 and Figure 1-73) include:

- Tall peaked T waves starting immediately and lasting up to several minutes
- ST segment elevation starting shortly after MI, due to injured myocytes
- Prolonged Q waves starting 1–4 days after MI, due to coagulative necrosis
- T wave inversion starting within 1 day, signifying ischemia at the periphery of the infarct
- New left-bundle branch block, poor R wave progression

KEY FACT

Cocaine can cause MI by precipitating coronary vasospasm and thrombosis.

KEY FACT

NSTEMI and unstable angina (UA) are similar entities along the acute coronary syndrome (ACS) spectrum. Distinguished by absence (UA) or presence (NSTEMI) of cardiac enzymes. Management is often very similar.

KEY FACT

Red infarcts occur in tissues with collateral circulation, such as the lungs or intestines.
Pale infarcts occur in solid tissues with a single blood source, such as brain, heart, and kidney.

TABLE 1-35. **Gross and Microscopic Changes to the Heart in Myocardial Infarction**

TIME	CELLULAR EVENTS	INFILTRATE
0–4 hr	None	None
4–24 hr	Early coagulative necrosis with edema, hemorrhage, and "wavy fibers" If reperfusion occurs → contraction bands (due to free radical damage)	Neutrophils
1–3 days	Extensive coagulative necrosis and acute inflammation	Neutrophils
3–14 days	Continued inflammation, granulation tissue at margins	Macrophages
2 wk onwards	Contracted scar complete	None

Modified with permission from Le T, et al. *First Aid for the USMLE Step 1: 2017.* New York: McGraw-Hill Education, 2017.

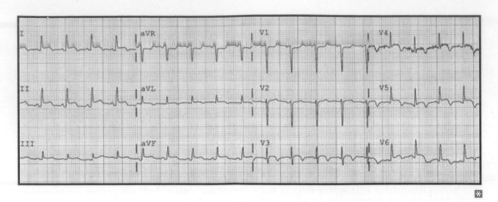

FIGURE 1-73. **ECG finding in ST elevation myocardial infarction.** Notice the ST-segment elevation present in leads I, II, III, AVL, AVF, V$_3$–V$_6$ and T-wave inversion from V$_3$ to V$_6$ and in AVL. Note the absence of Q waves.

Echocardiogram can show ventricular wall hypokinesia or akinesia.

Cardiac enzymes are widely used for diagnosis (Figure 1-74).

- **Troponin** starts to elevate 4–6 hours after the pain starts and lasts 7–10 days. It is more specific than CK-MB.
- **CK-MB** is an enzyme predominantly found in the myocardium, but may also be released from skeletal muscle. Elevation starts 6–12 hours after the pain begins, peaks within 24 hours, and returns to baseline within 48 hours. It is the test of choice in the first 24 hours post-MI because if it disappears and a second spike occurs, this signals another MI is occurring (troponin would be elevated the entire time).

Prognosis

Fatality is common in the period immediately after an MI. Causes include the following:

- **0–3 days post-MI:**
  - Cardiac arrhythmias.
  - Sudden cardiac death.
  - Acute post-infarction fibrinous pericarditis (listen for friction rub).

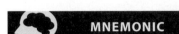

MNEMONIC

To remember the time course of CK-MB, note that it peaks at 24 hrs and disappears by 48 hrs (same # of characters as CK-MB):

- CK-MB
- 24-48

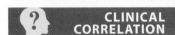

CLINICAL CORRELATION

At 7–10 days there is an increased chance of ventricular aneurysms or rupture of the papillary muscle due to the central softening.

TABLE 1-36. **Electrocardiographic Localization of Infarct in ST-Elevation Myocardial Infarction**

INFARCT LOCATION	LEADS WITH ST ELEVATIONS OR Q WAVES
Anteroseptal (LAD)	V$_1$–V$_2$
Anteroapical (distal LAD)	V$_3$–V$_4$
Anterolateral (LAD or LCX)	V$_5$–V$_6$
Lateral (LCX)	I, a**V**L
In**F**erior (RCA)	II, III, a**V**F
Posterior (PDA)	V$_7$–V$_9$, ST depression in V$_1$–V$_3$ with tall R waves

Modified with permission from Le T, et al. *First Aid for the USMLE Step 1: 2017.* New York: McGraw-Hill Education, 2017.

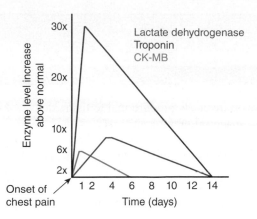

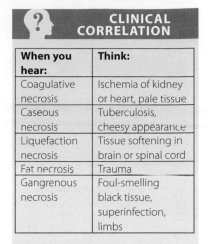

When you hear:	Think:
Coagulative necrosis	Ischemia of kidney or heart, pale tissue
Caseous necrosis	Tuberculosis, cheesy appearance
Liquefaction necrosis	Tissue softening in brain or spinal cord
Fat necrosis	Trauma
Gangrenous necrosis	Foul-smelling black tissue, superinfection, limbs

FIGURE 1-74. **Cardiac enzyme changes with myocardial infarction.** CK-MB, creatine kinase-myocardial bound fraction.

- Cardiogenic shock.
- **3–14 days post-MI:**
  - Ventricular free wall rupture resulting in cardiac tamponade (LAD).
  - Papillary muscle rupture resulting in acute mitral regurgitation (RCA).
  - Interventricular septum rupture resulting in VSD.
  - Ventricular pseudoaneurysm resulting in reduced CO, arrhythmia, and risk of embolus from mural thrombus.
- **2 weeks to months post-MI:**
  - True ventricular aneurysm resulting in dyskinesia, associated with fibrosis.
  - Dressler syndrome or autoimmune fibrinous pericarditis.

Additionally, patients may suffer from nonfatal arrhythmias, heart block, and CHF after an MI. Of note, diabetics and elderly patients with reduced sensory input secondary to neuropathy may have silent MIs and must be carefully monitored.

TREATMENT

Unstable angina/NSTEMI:

- Acute treatment: **M**orphine, **O**xygen, **N**itroglycerin, **A**spirin (MONA).
- Anticoagulation (ie, heparin).
- Antiplatelet therapy (ie, aspirin and one among clopidogrel, prasugrel and ticagrelor) decreases post-MI mortality. These agents are mandatory following intracoronary stenting.
- β-blockers have been shown to decrease mortality rates post-MI.
- ACE inhibitors.
- Statins.
- Nitrates for symptom relief (no benefit for mortality).
- Morphine for symptom relief.

STEMI:

- In addition to the therapies listed above, reperfusion therapy via percutaneous coronary intervention is preferred over fibrinolysis with tPA or streptokinase.

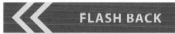

FLASH BACK

Pericarditis presents with a friction rub on auscultation.

CHRONIC ISCHEMIC HEART DISEASE

Ischemic heart damage causes CHF that can lead to chronic ischemic heart disease (CIHD). Often found in the elderly, infarction leads to cardiac hypertrophy and decompensation. Typically, the patient has no history of angina.

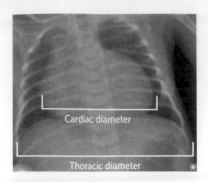

FIGURE 1-75.   Cardiomegaly.
Note that the cardiac silhouette occupies > 50% of the width of the thorax.

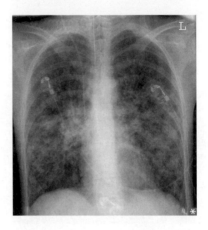

FIGURE 1-76.   Pulmonary edema.
Note increased interstitial markings.

Imaging/Diagnostic Tests

RADIOGRAPHY

- X-ray penetration is inversely proportional to tissue density. Less X-ray absorption leads to a darker image. Therefore, air is seen as black, while bone or metal is seen as white. Soft tissue is not well visualized on X-ray.
- Posteroanterior view describes the direction of the beam: The X-rays are transmitted from behind the patient onto a film placed anterior to the patient's chest.
- The normal cardiac silhouette occupies ≤ 50% of the width of the thorax in an adult. Cardiomegaly is apparent when the silhouette occupies > 50% of the width of the thorax (Figure 1-75).
- Increased pulmonary vasculature can be a sign of heart failure (Figure 1-76).
- It is imperative to be able to visualize both heart borders, as pneumonia can blur the border lines.

ECHOCARDIOGRAPHY

- A safe, noninvasive imaging modality using ultrasound.
- Can be used with Doppler to help evaluate blood flow, direction, turbulence, and estimation of pressure gradients across valves.
- Can be transthoracic or transesophageal (better sensitivity, but more invasive).
- Used to evaluate pericardial fluid, ventricular function, valvular abnormalities, pericardial disease, cardiomyopathies, or CAD.

CARDIAC CATHETERIZATION

- Used to measure the pressures within each heart chamber as well as to perform contrast angiography to assess vascular structure.
- Right-sided pressures are normally measured by inserting a catheter through the femoral or jugular vein, whereas left-sided pressures are measured by inserting a catheter through the radial or femoral artery.

See Figure 1-29 for a diagram of normal pressures of the cardiac chambers and great vessels on catheterization.

NUCLEAR IMAGING

- Used to evaluate myocardial perfusion and viability.
- Uses ^{99m}technetium (Tc)-labeled compounds or thallium-201.

STRESS TESTING

- Can employ **exercise** or **drugs** (exercise preferred).
- In a nuclear stress test, a patient is asked to exercise to maximum level and then a radioactive isotope (thallium or technetium) is injected into the bloodstream. The isotope enters the coronary arteries that supply the myocardium. Any area that does not receive adequate blood flow receives fewer isotopes, which is evident on the images. Stress images are compared with resting images.
- If a patient is unable to exercise, **dipyridamole** or **adenosine** is given to increase cardiac blood flow. As partially occluded arteries are already maximally dilated to preserve adequate blood flow, they are unable to dilate further and thus receive less blood flow than neighboring vessels. This is the phenomenon of "coronary

steal," which can reproduce symptoms of cardiac ischemia. **Dobutamine** is given to increase inotropy.

■ Abnormal results can signify CAD. The test can also be used for prognosis of patients post-MI and to determine the causes of chest pain in low-risk patients.

■ Absolute contraindications to stress testing include **acute MI within 2 days,** severe aortic stenosis, acute myocarditis/pericarditis, acute pulmonary embolus, acute aortic dissection, **decompensated heart failure, hemodynamically unstable arrhythmias,** and **pulmonary embolism.**

PERICARDIOCENTESIS

■ More than 20–30 mL of fluid accumulation in the pericardial sac is usually abnormal. A change in the cardiac silhouette is seen when > 250 mL of fluid accumulates.

■ Indications include pericardial tamponade, symptomatic pericardial effusion, pericardial biopsy, and purulent pericarditis.

■ **Parasternal pericardiocentesis** (the more common procedure) requires the needle to pass through the skin, superficial and deep fascia, pectoralis major muscle, external intercostal membrane, internal intercostal membrane, transversus thoracis muscle, fibrous pericardium, and finally the parietal layer of the serous pericardium.

■ **Subcostal pericardiocentesis** requires the needle to pass through skin, superficial fascia, deep fascia, outer layer of the rectus sheath, rectus abdominis muscle, posterior layer of the rectus sheath, fibers of the diaphragm at its attachment to the costal margin, endothoracic fascia of the diaphragm, fibrous pericardium, and finally the serous parietal pericardium.

Pharmacology

ANTIHYPERTENSIVE AGENTS

Hypertension is a common and serious disease with many sequelae, including MI, stroke, systemic vascular disease, and renal disease. See Figure 1-77 for an overview of the major classes of antihypertensive agents.

Diuretics

Diuretics act on the kidney with the primary purpose of reducing blood volume by increasing the rate of urine excretion. Reduction of blood volume leads to a decrease in BP. There are several types of diuretics, and they can be divided into separate classes based on their mechanism and site of action. Figure 1-78 serves as a review of the major diuretics and their mechanism of action in the kidney.

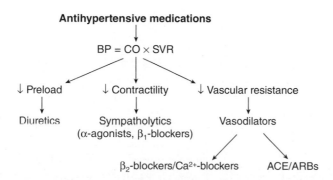

FIGURE 1-77. Overview of major classes of antihypertensive agents. ACE, angiotensin-converting enzyme; ARB, angiotensin receptor blocker; BP, blood pressure; CO, cardiac output; SVR, systemic vascular resistance.

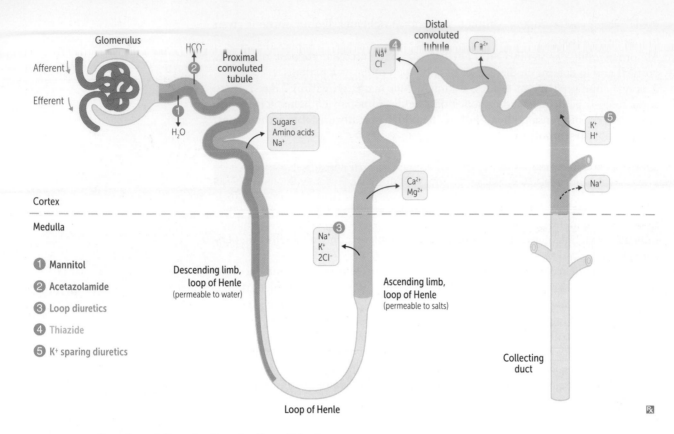

Afferent

Efferent

Glomerulus

Proximal convoluted tubule

HCO_3^-

H_2O

Sugars
Amino acids
Na^+

Cortex

Medulla

1 Mannitol

2 Acetazolamide

3 Loop diuretics

4 Thiazide

5 K^+ sparing diuretics

Descending limb, loop of Henle
(permeable to water)

Distal convoluted tubule

Na^+
Cl^-

Ca^{2+}

K^+
H^+

Na^+

Ca^{2+}
Mg^{2+}

Na^+
K^+
$2Cl^-$

Ascending limb, loop of Henle
(permeable to salts)

Collecting duct

Loop of Henle

FIGURE 1-78. **Overview of sites of action of various diuretics.**

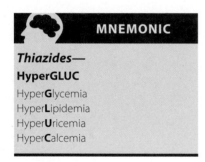

Thiazide Diuretics (eg, Hydrochlorothiazide, Metolazone)

MECHANISM. Inhibit Na^+-Cl^- symporter, thereby blocking Na^+ and Cl^- reabsorption in the distal convoluted tubule. NaCl is excreted along with water into the urine. They also increase Ca^{2+} reabsorption.

SITE OF ACTION. Early distal convoluted tubule (Figure 1-79).

USES. Often first line for moderate/mild hypertension; mild CHF, nephrogenic diabetes insipidus, nephrolithiasis secondary to idiopathic hypercalciuria.

SIDE EFFECTS. Hyperglycemia, hyperlipidemia, hyperuricemia, **hypercalcemia**, sulfa allergy (hydrochlorothiazide), hypokalemia.

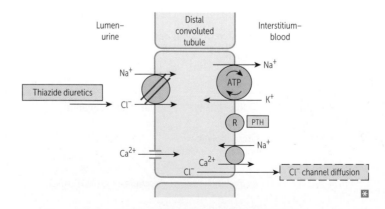

Lumen–urine

Distal convoluted tubule

Interstitium–blood

Thiazide diuretics

Na^+

Cl^-

ATP

Na^+

K^+

R PTH

Na^+

Ca^{2+}

Ca^{2+}

Cl^-

Cl^- channel diffusion

FIGURE 1-79. **Ion physiology at the distal convoluted tubule.**

Loop Diuretics (eg, Furosemide, Ethacrynic Acid, Bumetanide)

MECHANISM. Inhibit Na^+-K^+-$2Cl^-$ channel in the thick ascending limb of the loop of Henle. By preventing Na^+ and K^+ reabsorption into the renal medulla, they abolish the hypertonicity of the medulla (so urine cannot be concentrated in the collecting ducts). This results in marked diuresis. They also **increase Ca^{2+} excretion** because they reduce the lumen positive potential in the loop of Henle.

SITE OF ACTION. Thick ascending limb of loop of Henle (Figure 1-80).

USES. The **most efficacious diuretics,** used for edema (CHF, cirrhosis, nephrotic syndrome, and pulmonary edema), moderate to severe hypertension, hypercalcemia, and hyperkalemia.

SIDE EFFECTS. Ototoxicity (especially in combination with aminoglycoside), **hypokalemia,** hypercalciuria, hypocalcemia, dehydration, allergy to sulfa (furosemide, not ethacrynic acid), nephritis, gout.

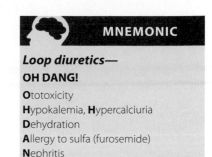

Potassium-Sparing Diuretics (eg, Spirinolactone, Triamterene, Amiloride, and Eplerenone)

MECHANISM

- **Spironolactone and eplerenone: Competitive antagonists at the aldosterone receptor** in the collecting tubule (indirectly inhibit Na^+ reabsorption).
- **Triamterene and amiloride:** Directly block Na^+ channels in the collecting tubule.

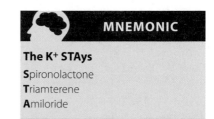

Reasons for the K-sparing properties of this class:

- Less K^+ secretion occurs due to inhibition of Na^+ reabsorption in the distal tubule (Na^+ reabsorption and K^+ secretion are coupled in this segment of the nephron).
- Because they are not active in the proximal portions of the tubules, these agents do not greatly increase tubular flow (high flow rates through the tubules increase secretion of K^+).

SITE OF ACTION. Collecting tubule and collecting duct (Figure 1-81).

USES. Primarily used in combination with more efficacious diuretics (eg, loop diuretics) to **prevent associated K^+ wasting.** Spironolactone has been proven to increase survival in patients with CHF. Also used to treat ascites in patients with cirrhosis. The antiandrogen effect of K^+-sparing diuretics (mainly spironolactone) is useful for treating hirsutism in polycystic ovarian syndrome (PCOS).

SIDE EFFECTS. Hyperkalemia; spironolactone causes gynecomastia.

ELECTROLYTE CHANGES ASSOCIATED WITH DIURETIC USE. All diuretics affect the reabsorption and/or secretion of various electrolytes in the kidney, so electrolyte abnormalities may

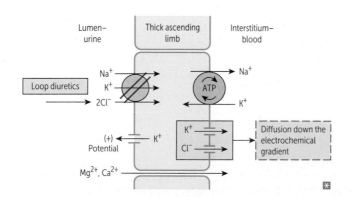

FIGURE 1-80. **Ion physiology at the loop of Henle.**

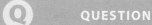

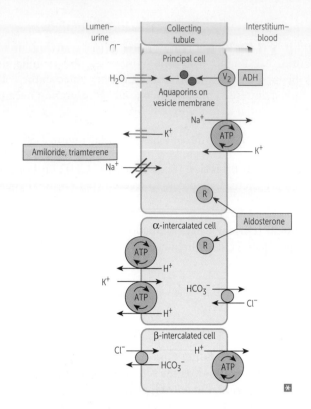

FIGURE 1-81. **Ion physiology at the collecting tubule and collecting duct.**

accompany the use of these drugs. See Table 1-37 for a review of some alterations in electrolytes in the urine and blood for various diuretics.

Osmotic Diuretics (eg, Mannitol)

MECHANISM. Increase kidney tubular fluid osmolarity. The drug is filtered through the glomerulus into the kidney tubule, where it pulls water from the interstitial space into the tubules via osmosis. This process results in **more water excreted** into the urine and less water reabsorbed into the circulation.

SITE OF ACTION. In the kidney at the **proximal tubule** (site of major water reabsorption) (Figure 1-82).

USES. Rarely used for hypertension. More commonly used for patients with increased intracranial pressure (ICP) or increased intraocular pressure (IOP).

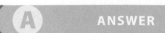

ANSWER

The patient likely developed hypokalemia as a side effect of the loop diuretic. You could change to a K+-sparing diuretic, such as spironolactone.

TABLE 1-37. **Electrolyte Changes with Various Diuretics**

DRUG	URINE NACL	URINE K+	URINE CA+	URINE HCO_3^-	BLOOD PH
Osmotic diuretics	↑↑	↑	↑	↑	NC
Carbonic anhydrase inhibitors	↑	↑↑	NC	↑↑	↓
Loop diuretics	↑↑↑	↑↑	↑↑	NC	↑
Thiazide diuretics	↑	↑↑	↓	NC	↑
Potassium-sparing diuretics	↑	↓	NC	NC	↓

NC, no change.

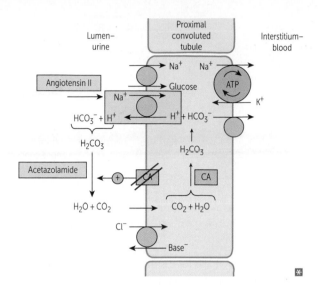

FIGURE 1-82. **Ion physiology at the proximal convoluted tubule.** CA, carbonic anhydrase.

SIDE EFFECTS. Can cause major problems if the drug cannot be filtered through the glomerulus (eg, in anuria). In this situation, the drug remains in the circulation and pulls water from the interstitial tissues into the blood. This results in increased blood volume (the exact opposite of its intended effect), leading to peripheral and/or pulmonary edema.

Carbonic Anhydrase Inhibitors (eg, Acetazolamide)

MECHANISM. Inhibits carbonic anhydrase, thereby preventing the conversion of bicarbonate (HCO_3^-) into CO_2, at the brush border of the proximal tubule. This inhibition results in **excretion of HCO_3^- along with water** into the urine.

SITE OF ACTION. In the kidney at the **proximal convoluted tubule** (see Figure 1-82).

USES. Rarely used for hypertension. More commonly used for patients with metabolic alkalosis, altitude sickness, glaucoma, or intracranial hypertension (eg, due to pseudotumor cerebri).

SIDE EFFECTS. Metabolic acidosis due to increased excretion of HCO_3^-. The loss of this major source of alkalinity causes a rise in urinary pH and a drop in blood pH. In addition, acetazolamide contains a sulfa group, which causes allergic reactions in some patients.

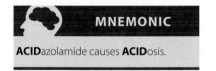

MNEMONIC

ACIDazolamide causes **ACID**osis.

Sympatholytics

Function of Sympathetic Receptors

Sympatholytic, or sympathoplegic, drugs reduce the effects of the sympathetic nervous system (SNS) on the CV system (Figure 1-83). Recall that arterial BP = cardiac output × systemic vascular resistance (SVR). Cardiac output is the product of HR and SV.

Since multiple factors contribute to BP control, pharmacologic agents that target different parameters can be used to decrease BP.

Sympathetic activity increases BP by increasing all of the following:

- HR
- Cardiac contractility
- Venous return to the heart (preload)
- SVR (or afterload)
- Renin production in the juxtaglomerular cells of the kidney

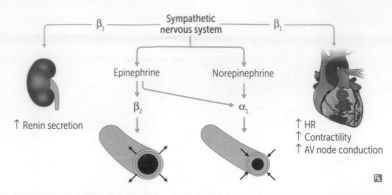

FIGURE 1-83. **End-organ effects of sympathetic nervous system activity relating to blood pressure control.** AV, atrioventricular; HR, heart rate.

Drugs that inhibit sympathetic activity reduce some or all of these parameters and thus lower BP. (Review the major functions of the sympathetic receptor subtypes in Table 1-38.)

β-Adrenergic Receptor Antagonists (β-Blockers; eg, Propranolol, Atenolol, Metoprolol, Esmolol, Carvedilol)

MECHANISM

- Nonselective β-receptor (β$_1$ and β$_2$) antagonists (propanol, nadolol, pindolol, timolol):
  - Reduce HR by blocking β$_1$ effects.
  - Reduce contractility by blocking β$_1$ effects.
  - Inhibit renin production by blocking β$_1$ effects.
  - More side effects because of their action on β$_2$-receptors (see Side Effects section).
- Selective β$_1$-receptor antagonists (atenolol, metoprolol, esmolol, acebutalol, betaxolol):
  - Same as above due to β$_1$-blockade
  - Fewer side effects
- Mixed α- and β-receptor antagonists (carvedilol, labetalol):
  - Same as above due to β$_1$-blockade
  - Plus decreased SVR due to α-blockade

SITE OF ACTION. β$_1$-Receptors on heart and kidney, β$_2$-receptors on arterioles.

USES. Hypertension, angina, patients with previous MI, CHF. Esmolol is an ultra-short-acting agent used in acute hypertensive emergencies.

SIDE EFFECTS

- **Bradycardia:** Important to remember when checking vital signs on patients who are taking β-blockers.

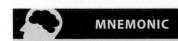

MNEMONIC

Drugs with β-blocking action end in **-OLOL.**

Drugs with both α- and β-blocking action end in either **-ILOL** or **-ALOL.**

TABLE 1-38. **Function of Sympathetic Receptors Within the Cardiovascular System**

RECEPTOR	MAJOR EFFECTS ON CV SYSTEM
α$_1$	Vasoconstriction
α$_2$	- Central receptors: ↓ sympathetic outflow - Peripheral receptors: arterial vasodilation
β$_1$	↑ Heart rate, ↑ cardiac contractility, ↑ renin release
β$_2$	Vasodilation

- **Bronchoconstriction** and asthma exacerbation (especially nonselective agents with β_2 antagonism).
- Blunted response to hypoglycemia. May be especially **dangerous in diabetics** on insulin therapy. Hypoglycemic episodes are marked by pallor, trembling, diaphoresis, and tachycardia (all mediated by increased β-receptor activity). With β-blockade, these important clues of hypoglycemia may be absent.
- **Other:** Impotence, CNS adverse effects. Avoid in cocaine users owing to unopposed α-agonist activity.

α-Adrenergic Receptor Antagonists (α-Blockers; eg, Prazosin, Doxazosin, Terazosin)

MECHANISM. Selective α_1-receptor antagonists; α_1-blockade decreases SVR by preventing arteriolar vasoconstriction. The result is decreased BP.

SITE OF ACTION. Primarily α_1-receptors on arterioles. Of note, also blocks α_1-receptors at the bladder sphincter (see later discussion for clinical uses).

USES. Mild to moderate hypertension. Most common use of α_1-blockers is to treat urinary hesitancy for patients with prostatic hypertrophy (by preventing bladder sphincter contraction).

SIDE EFFECTS. First-dose hypotension, reflex tachycardia, secondary Na^+ retention in kidney (use in combination with diuretic), orthostatic hypotension. Be careful when combining with another vasodilator (eg, nitrates, sildenafil).

Centrally Acting Sympatholytics (eg, Methyldopa, Clonidine)

MECHANISM. Selective α_2 agonists. By activating α_2 receptors in the brain stem, these agents reduce central sympathetic outflow. The result is decreased cardiac output and SVR.

SITE OF ACTION. Brain stem.

USES. Rarely used for hypertension due to poor side effect profile, but methyldopa is traditionally considered the drug of choice for hypertension in pregnant patients.

SIDE EFFECTS

- Methyldopa: Sedation, **positive Coombs test** in 10% of patients (reversible upon discontinuation of drug).
- Clonidine: Sedation, dry mouth, **severe rebound hypertension** with abrupt discontinuation (should not be used in patients who may have difficulty obtaining/taking medication as directed).

Calcium Channel Blockers and Other Vasodilators

Vasodilators **decrease SVR** by relaxing smooth muscle in arteriole walls through a number of different mechanisms. The result is the same, however—by increasing arteriolar diameter, SVR (also known as afterload) is reduced, which also reduces BP (remember, BP = cardiac output × SVR).

Calcium Channel Blockers (eg, Nifedipine, Amlodipine, Verapamil, Diltiazem)

MECHANISM. Block L-type Ca^{2+} channels, inhibiting entry of Ca^{2+} into arteriolar smooth muscle; this action results in arteriole dilation and reduced SVR.

SITE OF ACTION

- **Vasoselective agents** work predominantly at the arteriolar smooth muscle. The most commonly used class is the **dihydropyridines** (including nifedipine and amlodipine).
- **Nonselective agents** act equally on the heart and the arterioles. Their vasodilating action is not as potent as that of the dihydropyridines, but they also reduce cardiac contractility. Examples are **verapamil** and **diltiazem**.

KEY FACT

β_2-receptors in the lung mediate bronchodilation. β_2-Blockade can impair breathing in patients with asthma or chronic obstructive pulmonary disease (COPD), so avoid nonspecific β-blocker use in these patients.

MNEMONIC

α-Blockers end in **-OSIN.**

KEY FACT

Methyldopa is the drug of choice to lower BP in pregnant patients.

KEY FACT

Dihydropyridines are more active at the arterioles than the heart. Their names end in **-PINE.**

USES. Mild to moderate hypertension. Angina (especially Prinzmetal), Raynaud phenomenon, rate control in atrial fibrillation/flutter.

SIDE EFFECTS. Constipation, bradycardia, AV block, peripheral edema (especially dihydropyridines), gingival hyperplasia.

Nitric Oxide Releasers (eg, Nitroprusside)

MECHANISM. Spontaneously releases nitric oxide, via an increase in cGMP, causing relaxation of both arterial and venous smooth muscle. This action results in rapid reduction of SVR and BP.

SITE OF ACTION. Arteriolar > venule smooth muscle.

USES. Hypertensive emergencies (given in IV form).

SIDE EFFECTS. By-products of metabolism include cyanide and thiocyanate, which can be harmful to patients with poor renal function (antidote is sodium thiosulfate). Other side effects include excessive hypotension and reflex tachycardia.

Hydralazine

MECHANISM. Exact mechanism unknown. Vasodilator of arterioles more than veins.

SITE OF ACTION. Arteriolar smooth muscle.

USES. Severe hypertension.

SIDE EFFECTS. May cause **drug-induced lupus;** reflex tachycardia, and sodium retention (therefore, it is given in combination with a β-blocker and a diuretic).

Minoxidil

MECHANISM. Opens K^+ channels, causing hyperpolarization of smooth muscle cells and arteriolar dilation.

SITE OF ACTION. Arteriolar smooth muscle.

USES. Mild to moderate hypertension and baldness (see following section).

SIDE EFFECTS. Hirsutism, or excessive hairiness (minoxidil is the main ingredient in Rogaine, which is used for the treatment of alopecia, or hair loss); also reflex tachycardia and sodium retention (also given in combination with a β-blocker and a diuretic).

Fenoldopam

MECHANISM. Selective dopaminergic D_1 receptor agonist leading to vasodilation, improved renal perfusion, decreased BP, and increased natriuresis.

SITE OF ACTION. D_1 receptors of arteries, arterioles, and kidney.

USES. Hypertensive emergencies (IV).

Angiotensin Inhibitors

The RAAS plays an intricate role in BP regulation. Two classes of drugs are used to alter this system and thereby reduce BP. Both classes reduce the action of angiotensin II, which is a molecule that increases SVR by directly causing vasoconstriction. Angiotensin II also increases Na^+ and water reabsorption in the kidney (via aldosterone). The RAAS is shown in Figure 1-84.

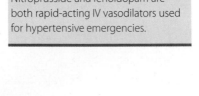
KEY FACT

Nitroprusside and fenoldopam are both rapid-acting IV vasodilators used for hypertensive emergencies.

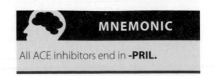
MNEMONIC

All ACE inhibitors end in **-PRIL.**

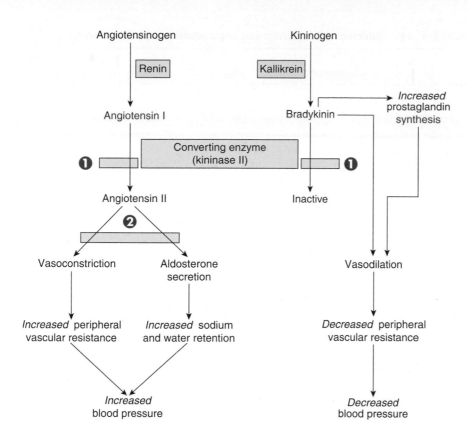

FIGURE 1-84. **Renin angiotensin aldosterone pathway and sites of action of ACE inhibitors and angiotensin receptor blockers.** ❶, ACE inhibitors; ❷, angiotensin receptor blockers.

Angiotensin-Converting Enzyme (ACE) Inhibitors (eg, Captopril, Lisinopril, Enalapril)

MECHANISM. These drugs **block ACEs,** thus preventing conversion of angiotensin I to angiotensin II. They also inhibit degradation of bradykinin (an intrinsic vasodilator). This action results in **decreased SVR and decreased Na⁺ and water reabsorption (via reduced aldosterone).**

SITE OF ACTION. The active site of the enzyme (found on the endothelial membrane and in plasma).

USES. Mild to moderate hypertension, heart failure, diabetic renal disease (usually first-line treatment for diabetics with hypertension).

SIDE EFFECTS. Cough (due to increased release of bradykinin), **hyperkalemia,** angioedema, proteinuria, taste changes, hypotension, fetal renal problems, rash. Contraindicated in patients with bilateral renal artery stenosis.

Angiotensin II Receptor Antagonists (Also Called Angiotensin Receptor Blockers [ARBs]; eg, Losartan, Valsartan)

MECHANISM. Blockade of angiotensin II receptors, producing similar downstream effects as ACE inhibitors (namely, decreased SVR).

SITE OF ACTION. Heart, kidney, adrenal cortex.

USES. Mainly used in patients who cannot tolerate ACE inhibitors.

SIDE EFFECTS. Less cough than ACE inhibitors, fetal renal damage.

ACE inhibitors and ARBs affect levels of various products within the RAAS (see Figure 1-84 and Table 1-39).

KEY FACT

Angiotensin II is an enzyme responsible for aldosterone synthesis in the adrenal cortex and is also a direct vasoconstrictor.

MNEMONIC

CAPTOPRIL

Cough
Angioedema
Proteinuria
Taste changes
Hyp**O**tension
Pregnancy problems
Rash
Increased renin
Lower angiotensin II

MNEMONIC

All ARBs end in **-ARTAN.**

TABLE 1-39. Effects of ACE Inhibitors and Angiotensin Receptor Blockers

	ACE INHIBITORS	ARBS	ALISKIREN/DIRECT RENIN INHIBITOR
Renin	↑	↑	↓
AT I	↓	↑	↓
AT II	↓	↑	↓
Aldosterone	↓	↓	↓
Bradykinin	↑	no change	no change

Aliskiren

MECHANISM

Directly binds and inhibits renin, thus preventing cleavage of angiotensinogen to angiotensin I; as a result, there is a decrease in angiotensin II.

USES

Essential hypertension.

SIDE EFFECTS

Angioedema, hyperkalemia, hypotension.

ANTIANGINAL THERAPY

Angina is chest pain resulting from myocardial ischemia. Ischemia occurs when the demand of the heart exceeds that supplied by the coronary arteries. Therefore, **reducing O_2 demand of the heart is the goal of treatment** so that supply is greater than demand. Some of the important factors that contribute to O_2 demand include **preload, afterload, HR,** and **cardiac contractility.** The major agents used to alter these parameters are nitrates, β-blockers, and calcium channel blockers. After reviewing the drugs, see Table 1-40 for a recap on how the drugs affect myocardial O_2 demand.

TABLE 1-40. Antianginal Therapy

COMPONENT	NITRATES	β-BLOCKERS	NITRATES + β-BLOCKERS
End-diastolic volume	↓	No effect or ↑	No effect or ↓
Blood pressure	↓	↓	↓
Contractility	No effect	↓	Little/no effect
Heart rate	↑ (reflex response)	↓	No effect or ↓
Ejection time	↓	↑	Little/no effect
MVO$_2$	↓	↓	↓↓

MVO$_2$, myocardial oxygen consumption.

Reproduced with permission from Le T, et al. *First Aid for the USMLE Step 1 2017*. New York, NY: McGraw-Hill Education; 2017.

Types of Angina

There are three major forms of angina:

- **Stable (effort) angina:** Due to fixed narrowing of coronary arteries.
    - Occurs with increased activity.
    - Is relieved by rest and nitroglycerin.
- **Unstable angina/NSTEMI:** Due to **acute formation of thrombus** on atherosclerotic plaque.
    - Occurs at rest or with progressively decreasing levels of activity.
    - Is not relieved by rest but may be relieved by nitroglycerin.
    - More likely to progress to MI.
- **Variant (Prinzmetal) angina:** Due to **coronary artery vasospasm.**

Nitrates (eg, Nitroglycerin, Isosorbide Dinitrate, Isosorbide Mononitrate)

MECHANISM. Vasodilates via release of nitric oxide; major effect is preload reduction (veins dilate, blood pools in veins, and venous return to the heart decreases), resulting in decreased O_2 demand. May cause some afterload reduction also.

USES. Stable angina, unstable angina, and variant angina.

SIDE EFFECTS. Tachycardia, orthostatic hypotension, headache.

β-Blockers (eg, Metoprolol, Atenolol, Propranolol)

MECHANISM. Reduce O_2 demand by reducing HR and cardiac contractility.

USES. Stable angina, **not variant (Prinzmetal) angina** (because β blockade can disrupt the balance of α and β effects and worsen vasospasms). Headache prophylaxis and essential tremor.

SIDE EFFECTS. Bradycardia, AV block. Contraindicated in asthma and COPD patients (only beta-blockers selective for β_2-receptors, such as atenolol and metoprolol, can be used).

Calcium Channel Blockers (eg, Verapamil, Diltiazem, Nifedipine)

MECHANISM. Decrease O_2 demand:

- Verapamil, diltiazem: Decrease HR and contractility (like β-blockers).
- Nifedipine: Decreases afterload via vasodilation.

USES. Stable angina and variant (Prinzmetal) angina (calcium channel blockers are the drugs of choice).

SIDE EFFECTS. Nifedipine may cause reflex tachycardia (increased O_2 demand); verapamil and diltiazem can cause constipation, bradycardia, and AV block. Verapamil has negative inotropic effects and can cause signs of heart failure.

DRUGS USED IN HEART FAILURE

Heart failure is defined as cardiac output insufficient for the **O_2 demands of the body.** It can be thought of as a chronic disease with intermittent acute exacerbations. Heart failure is characterized by poor cardiac output, and the response is to increase SNS tone and increase retention of sodium and water. Decreased cardiac output could be due to poor contractility (systolic heart failure) or impaired ventricular relaxation and filling (diastolic heart failure).

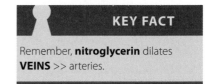

KEY FACT

Remember, **nitroglycerin** dilates **VEINS** >> arteries.

KEY FACT

Calcium channel blockers are the drugs of choice for variant (Prinzmetal) angina.

QUESTION

A 27-year-old, otherwise healthy woman complains of intermittent chest pain at rest that typically occurs in clusters. What is the most likely diagnosis and what class of medication can be used to improve her symptoms?

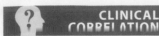

The goals of long-term therapy are to prevent cardiac remodeling and improve mortality. Other drugs are used to increase cardiac output and improve symptoms. Several drugs used in heart failure have been discussed previously. These include diuretics (eg, furosemide, spironolactone), β-blockers (eg, metoprolol, carvedilol), ACE inhibitors (eg, captopril), ARBs (eg, losartan), and vasodilators (eg, nitroprusside, nitroglycerin). Long-term use of β-blockers, ACE inhbitors/ARBs, and the combination of isosorbide dinitrate/hydralazine has been shown to improve mortality in systolic heart failure. In addition, spironolactone has been shown to prolong lifespan in patients with severe systolic heart failure. Review these drugs in the previous sections and study Table 1-41 for their benefits in heart failure. Other drugs used to treat heart failure include agents that directly increase cardiac output, such as β-agonists, cardiac glycosides, and phosphodiesterase inhibitors. In addition, diuretics (usually loop diuretics) are used for symptomatic treatment of fluid overload.

β-Agonists (eg, Dobutamine)

MECHANISM

Selective β_1-agonist; this action increases HR and cardiac contractility, leading to an increase in cardiac output.

SITE OF ACTION

Primarily the heart.

USES

Acute exacerbations of heart failure (given IV and has a very short half-life). Does not improve overall mortality.

TABLE 1-41.   Drugs Used in the Treatment of Heart Failure

DRUG CLASS	EXAMPLES	BENEFITS IN HEART FAILURE
Diuretics	Furosemide, spironolactone	Reduced sodium/water retention → reduced preload and afterload; spironolactone prevents detrimental effects of aldosterone (myocardial fibrosis).
β-Blockers	Metoprolol, carvedilol	Reduced sympathetic tone → reduced afterload. Improves mortality.
ACE inhibitors/ARBs	Captopril, losartan	Reduced sympathetic tone, reduced aldosterone → reduced afterload. Improves mortality by preventing negative remodeling.
Vasodilators	Nitroglycerin, nitroprusside	Vasodilation → reduced preload and reduced afterload.
Cardiac glycosides	Digoxin	Increased cardiac contractility → increased cardiac output. Does not improve mortality.
β_1-Agonists	Dobutamine	Increased cardiac contractility → increased cardiac output.
Phosphodiesterase inhibitors	Milrinone, inamrinone	Increased cardiac contractility → increased cardiac output. Used only to treat acute heart failure, not chronic heart failure.

SIDE EFFECTS

Angina (due to increased myocardial O_2 demand), tachycardia, arrhythmias.

Cardiac Glycosides (eg, Digoxin)

MECHANISM

Blocks Na^+-K^+ ATPase, resulting in increased intracellular Na^+. The high levels of intracellular Na^+ reduce the activity of the Na^+-Ca^{2+} exchanger and more Ca^{2+} remains intracellular. This high level of intracellular Ca^{2+} **improves cardiac contractility** (leading to higher cardiac output). Digoxin also has some parasympathetic activity and **decreases AV nodal conduction velocity** (increased filling).

SITE OF ACTION

Membrane of cardiac myocytes.

USES

Chronic heart failure, also atrial fibrillation.

SIDE EFFECTS

Arrhythmias, blurry yellow vision, nausea, vomiting, AV block. Toxicities are highly **increased with hypokalemia** (important because many patients taking digoxin also take furosemide, a major cause of hypokalemia).

Phosphodiesterase Inhibitors (eg, Inamrinone, Milrinone)

MECHANISM

Block the action of phosphodiesterase, leading to increased levels of cAMP and increased Ca^{2+} flow into the cardiac myocyte. The result is increased cardiac contractility and cardiac output. Also cause some vasodilation.

USES

Acute exacerbations of heart failure.

SIDE EFFECTS

Arrhythmias.

ANTIARRHYTHMICS

Pharmacotherapy of arrhythmias is very complex (Table 1-42).

LIPID-LOWERING AGENTS

Hyperlipidemia refers to increases in blood levels of lipoproteins or triglycerides or both. It is a major risk factor for CV diseases such as angina, MI, and stroke. Several pharmacologic agents are used to treat hyperlipidemia, and it is important to understand the key differences between the major classes of lipid-lowering agents (Table 1-43 and Figure 1-85).

MNEMONIC

To remember class III medications, think of **AIDS** (**A**miodarone, **I**butilide, **D**ofetilide, **S**otalol).

CLINICAL CORRELATION

In patients with hemodynamically unstable **supraventricular tachycardias** (SVTs), use electric cardioversion. For stable SVTs, consider rate control strategy with class II or class IV antiarrythmics.

CLINICAL CORRELATION

For patients on amiodarone, remember to monitor thyroid, liver, and pulmonary function.

KEY FACT

Common action potential (AP) changes associated with antiarrhythmics:
- Increased QT interval: class IA, class III
- Increased PR interval: class II, class IV
- Increased AP: class IA, class III
- Decreased AP: class IB
- No change in AP: class IC

TABLE 1-42. **Overview of Drugs Used to Treat Arrhythmias**

CLASS	EXAMPLE(S)	MECHANISM	CLINICAL USE	SIDE EFFECTS
I (Na+ channel blockers)				
IA	Quinidine, procainamide, disopyramide	Decrease ventricular conduction (increased QRS interval on ECG); prolong ventricular action potential **(increased QT interval on ECG)**	Atrial and ventricular arrhythmias	Quinidine: cinchonism (headache, tinnitus) and **torsades de pointes (due to increased QT interval);** procainamide: **drug-induced lupus**
IB	Lidocaine	Slow conduction and increased threshold for firing of abnormal cells	Acute ventricular arrhythmias, post-MI arrhythmias	CV and CNS depression with overdose
IC	Flecainide, propafenone	Decrease ventricular conduction (increased QRS interval on ECG)	Ventricular arrhythmias	Can cause arrhythmias, contraindicated in patients with structural heart disease or a previous MI
II (β-Blockers)	Esmolol (IV, rapid acting), metoprolol, propranolol	Decrease AV nodal conduction (increased PR interval on ECG)	Ventricular and supraventricular arrhythmias	Bradycardia, AV block
III (K+ channel blockers)	Amiodarone, sotalol	Prolong ventricular action potential **(increased QT interval on ECG)**	Treatment and prevention of ventricular arrhythmias	Amiodarone: pulmonary fibrosis, hepatotoxicity, thyroid disease
IV (Ca2+ channel blockers)	Verapamil, diltiazem	Decrease AV nodal conduction	Supraventricular arrhythmias	Constipation, bradycardia, AV block
Other	Adenosine	Decrease AV nodal conduction	Supraventricular arrhythmias	Flushing, hypotension, chest pain
	Magnesium (Mg2+)	Unknown	Torsades de pointes	Respiratory depression

AV, atrioventricular; CNS, central nervous system; CV, cardiovascular; MI, myocardial infarction.

TABLE 1-43.   Commonly Used Lipid-Lowering Agents

DRUG CLASS	EXAMPLE(S)	MECHANISM	LDL	HDL	TGS	SIDE EFFECTS
HMG-CoA reductase inhibitors ("statins")	Lovastatin, pravastatin, simvastatin, atorvastatin	Inhibit rate-determining step in cholesterol synthesis, leading to increased synthesis of LDL receptors. First-line agent for hypercholesterolemia.	↓↓↓	↑	↓	Increased LFTs, myositis
Bile acid resins	Cholestyramine, colestipol	Bind bile salts in the intestine thus preventing their reabsorption (along with cholesterol) in the intestine.	↓↓	–	↑	Bad taste, bloating, constipation, impaired absorption of fat-soluble vitamins, cholesterol gallstones
Cholesterol absorption inhibitors	Ezetimibe	Block absorption of cholesterol in the small intestine.	↓↓	–	–	Rarely increased LFTs. Diarrhea
Fibrates	Gemfibrozil, fenofibrate, clofibrate	Increase synthesis of lipoprotein lipase via activation of peroxisome proliferator-activated receptor-α (PPAR-α).	↓	↑	↓↓↓	Myositis, increased LFTs, cholesterol gallstones
Other	Niacin (nicotinic acid, vitamin B_3)	Decreases formation and secretion of VLDL resulting in less formation of LDL.	↓↓	↑↑	↓	Flushed face (can be prevented by aspirin through prostaglandin-mediated effect)

HMG-CoA, 3-hydroxy-3-methylglutaryl coenzyme A; LDL, low-density lipoprotein; LFTs, liver function tests; VLDL, very low-density lipoprotein.

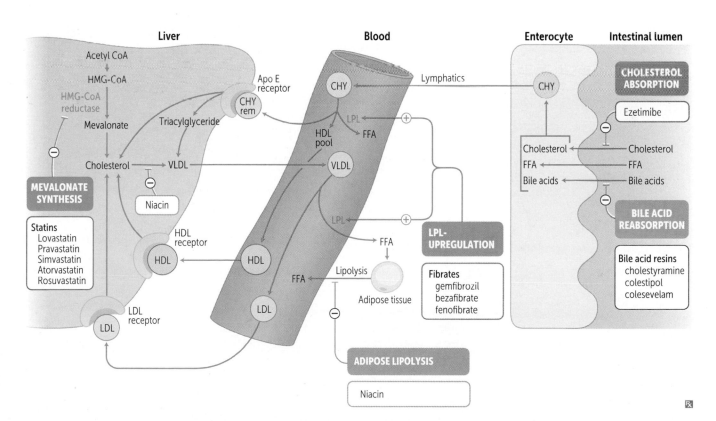

FIGURE 1-85. Overview of mechanisms of various lipid-lowering agents. CHY-rem, chylomicron remnant; FFA, free fatty acid; HDL, high-density lipoprotein; HMG-CoA, 3-hydroxy-3-methylglutaryl coenzyme A; LDL, low-density lipoprotein; VLDL, very low-density lipoprotein.

NOTES

CHAPTER 2

Endocrine

HYPOTHALAMUS AND PITUITARY 108
Hormone Basics 108
Hypothalamic-Pituitary Axis 112
Anterior Pituitary Disease 119
Posterior Pituitary Disease 122
Pituitary/Hypothalamic Pharmacology 124

THYROID AND PARATHYROID 126
Thyroid 126
Disorders of the Thyroid 131
Drugs for Hypothyroidism 135
Antithyroid Drugs 136
Parathyroid Gland 137
Calcium and Phosphate Homeostasis 139
Calcium Disorders 144
Calcium Drugs 146

ADRENAL GLAND 147
Anatomy 147

Embryology 147
Histology 148
Steroid Hormone Synthesis 149
Glucocorticoids 150
Mineralocorticoids 152
Adrenal Androgens 153
Disorders of the Adrenal Gland 153

PANCREAS 158
Anatomy 158
Embryology 159
Histology 159
Insulin 159
Glucagon 161
Somatostatin 162
Disorders of the Endocrine Pancreas 162
Tumors of Islet Cells 165
Diabetes Drugs 166
Oral Hypoglycemic Drugs 167

Hypothalamus and Pituitary

HORMONE BASICS

The endocrine system maintains many complex communication systems between cells, tissues, and organ systems. These interactions take place locally or at a distance and are mediated by peptides, amines, and steroids called hormones.

Site of Action

Endocrine signals can be characterized by the relationship between the site of secretion and the relative location of target receptors:

- **Autocrine secretion:** Released signal affects the cell from which it was secreted (eg, upon antigen binding, T cells release factors to stimulate their own proliferation).
- **Paracrine secretion:** Released signal acts on neighboring cells that have the appropriate receptors (eg, when exposed to an allergen, mast cells release histamine, which acts on vascular smooth muscle to induce vasodilation).
- **Endocrine secretion:** Released signal enters the **bloodstream** and acts on distant receptors (eg, follicle-stimulating hormone [FSH] is secreted from the anterior pituitary and acts on granulosa cells of the ovary).
- **Exocrine secretion:** Released signal enters a **duct** and acts on epithelial surface of the skin/gut (eg, pancreas releases amylase into the duodenum).
- **Multifunctional signals:** Signals can produce different effects depending on the mode of action and the target tissue. For example, testosterone released by Leydig cells in the testes acts on muscles to stimulate growth (endocrine) but also acts on seminiferous tubules, along with FSH, to promote spermatogenesis (paracrine).

KEY FACT

The pancreas has both endocrine and exocrine functions. The endocrine pancreas regulates glucose metabolism, while the exocrine pancreas facilitates the chemical digestion of food.

Types of Hormones by Mechanism of Action

Hormones fall into three classes of molecules: peptides, steroids, and amines. (Table 2-1).

- **Peptides and proteins:** Preprohormone typically synthesized by rough endoplasmic reticulum (RER) → signal peptide cleavage in RER produces prohormone.
  - Transport within the Golgi apparatus results in further processing and final active hormone structure.

TABLE 2-1.   Peptide, Steroid, and Amine Hormones

	PEPTIDE/PROTEIN HORMONES	STEROID	AMINES
Precursors	Amino acids	Cholesterol	Tyrosine
Site of synthesis	Rough ER	Smooth ER	Cytosol, colloid
Storage	Yes (stored in vesicles)	No (produced on demand)	Yes (stored in vesicles, colloid)
Carrier proteins	No (majority soluble in blood)	Yes (bound to carrier proteins)	Yes (only for thyroid hormone)
Location of receptors	Target cell membrane	Intracytoplasmic, transported into nucleus	Target cell membrane, nucleus (thyroid hormone)
Signal propagation	Via second messengers	Via new gene transcription	Via second messengers or gene expression
Kinetics	Fast acting +/− long-term actions	Slow-acting	Fast acting +/− long-term actions
Examples	ACTH, LH, insulin	Estrogen, testosterone	Epinephrine, norepinephrine, thyroid hormone

ACTH, adrenocorticotropic hormone; ER, endoplasmic reticulum; LH, luteinizing hormone.

- Stored in secretory vesicles and released via exocytosis into the bloodstream (water-soluble).
- Act on cell surface receptors and second-messenger systems of target tissues (fast-acting effects).
- **Steroids:** Synthesized from cholesterol on demand (not stored) → lipid solubility, which allows for rapid diffusion across membrane.
  - Transported in blood bound to plasma carrier proteins due to limited solubility.
  - Diffuse across target cell membrane and bind to intracytoplasmic protein receptors.
  - Resultant steroid hormone–receptor complex enters nucleus and activates transcription of specific genes for new protein synthesis (slow-acting effects).
- **Amines:** Synthesized from tyrosine precursors. Examples of amine hormones include thyroid hormone, epinephrine, and norepinephrine. Epinephrine and norepinephrine are synthesized, stored, released, and act on targets in a manner similar to peptide hormones. Thyroid hormone exhibits aspects of both peptide and steroid hormones.

Plasma Transport of Lipid-Soluble Hormones

Most steroid hormones (and thyroid hormones) are hydrophobic. Plasma proteins bind to these hormones to enable them to circulate in the bloodstream. These carrier proteins, produced by the liver, may either be nonspecific or specialized for a given hormone.

Example: Corticosteroid-binding globulin has a greater affinity for cortisol and aldosterone than for other steroid hormones. Conversely, albumin is relatively nonspecific, binding a variety of steroid hormones with equal affinity (Table 2-2).

Carrier proteins allow for another level of control within the signaling network, as hormone-protein complexes are unable to diffuse across membranes and activate target cells. Instead, free and bound forms of hormone exist in equilibrium. Only free hormone is biologically active. Therefore, the amount of free hormone in plasma determines how much hormone is available to target tissues.

Peptide Hormones: Second-Messenger Pathways

Peptide/protein hormones stimulate membrane-bound receptors on target cells, generating conformational changes in the receptors. The intracellular propagation of the signal proceeds via the action of second messengers (Table 2-3, Figure 2-1). The major second-messenger systems include:

- **Adenylate cyclase mechanism:** Hormone binds G protein-coupled receptor (GPCR) → activated G protein (G_s) stimulates adenylate cyclase (AC).

> **KEY FACT**
>
> In men, increased sex hormone-binding globulin (SHBG) → decreased free testosterone → increased risk of unopposed estrogen activity → gynecomastia. In women, decreased SHBG → increased free testosterone → hirsutism.

TABLE 2-2. Hormone Transport Proteins

CARRIER PROTEIN	HORMONE TRANSPORTED	SERUM CONCENTRATIONS
Corticosteroid-binding globulin (CBG)	Cortisol, aldosterone	↓ in cirrhosis, nephrotic syndrome, hyperthyroidism, and protein malnutrition
Sex hormone–binding globulin (SHBG)	Estrogen, testosterone	↑ by estrogen, OCPs, and exogenous thyroid hormone
Thyroxine-binding globulin (TBG)	Thyroxine (T_4), triiodothyronine (T_3)	↑ by estrogen, pregnancy, and OCPs
Serum albumin	Nonspecific steroid transporter, T_4, and T_3	↓ in cirrhosis, nephrotic syndrome, and protein malnutrition

OCPs, oral contraceptive pills.

TABLE 2-3.   Hormone Signal Propagation Mechanisms

cAMP	cGMP	INOSITOL TRIPHOSPHATE	INTRACELLULAR RECEPTOR	INTRINSIC TYROSINE KINASE	RECEPTOR-ASSOCIATED TYROSINE KINASE
FSH	ANP	**G**nRH	**V**itamin D	Insulin	**P**rolactin
LH	BNP	**O**xytocin	**E**strogen	IGF-1	**I**mmunomodulators (eg, cytokines, IL-2, IL-6, IFN)
ACTH	NO	**A**DH (V$_1$ receptor)	**T**estosterone	FGF	**G**H
TSH		**T**RH	**T**$_3$/T$_4$	PDGF	**G**-CSF
CRH		**H**istamine (H$_1$)	**C**ortisol	EGF	**E**rythropoietin
hCG		**A**ngiotensin II	**A**ldosterone		**T**hrombopoietin
ADH (V$_2$ receptor)		**G**astrin	**P**rogesterone		
MSH					
PTH					
Calcitonin					
GHRH					
Glucagon					
"FLAT CHAMP"	Think vasodilators	**"GOAT HAG"**	**"VETTT CAP"**	Think growth factors	**"PIGGIET"**

ACTH, adrenocorticotropic hormone; ADH, antidiuretic hormone; ANP, atrial natriuretic peptide; BNP, brain natriuretic peptide; cAMP, cyclic adenosine monophosphate; cGMP, cyclic guanosine monophosphate; CRH, corticotropin-releasing hormone; EGF, epidermal growth factor; FGF, fibroblast growth factor; FSH, follicle-stimulating hormone; GH, growth hormone; GHRH, growth hormone-releasing hormone; G-CSF, granulocyte colony-stimulating factor; GnRH, gonadotropin-releasing hormone; hCG, human chorionic gonadotropin; IGF-1, insulin-like growth factor 1; IFN, interferon; IL, interleukin; LH, luteinizing hormone; MSH, melanocyte-stimulating hormone; NO, nitric oxide; PDGF, platelet-derived growth factor; PTH, parathyroid hormone; T$_3$, triiodothyronine; T$_4$, thyroxine; TRH, thyrotropin-releasing hormone; TSH, thyroid-stimulating hormone.

- AC catalyzes formation of cAMP.
- cAMP activates protein kinase A (PKA).
- PKA exerts downstream effects via phosphorylation of other proteins.
- Other hormones inhibit adenylate cyclase through a separate GPCR, using an inhibitory G protein (G$_i$).
- cAMP is inactivated by the enzyme phosphodiesterase (PDE).
- **Inositol triphosphate (IP$_3$) mechanism:** Hormone binds GPCR → activated G protein (G$_q$) stimulates phospholipase C.
  - Phospholipase C cleaves phosphatidylinositol 4,5-bisphosphate (PIP$_2$), a membrane lipid, producing IP$_3$ and diacylglycerol (DAG).
  - IP$_3$ opens calcium channels in endoplasmic reticulum, releasing calcium into cytoplasm.
  - DAG and calcium facilitate activation of protein kinase C (PKC).
  - PKC exerts downstream effects via phosphorylation of other proteins.
- **Receptor tyrosine kinase (RTK) mechanism:** Hormone binds two adjacent cell membrane receptors → activated receptor dimer with tyrosine kinase activity.
  - Intracytoplasmic ends cross-phosphorylate each other as well as other proteins.
  - Many of these other proteins are also tyrosine kinases, which continue to phosphorylate other proteins and transcription factors.
- **Janus kinase/signal transducer and activator (JAK/STAT) mechanism:** Hormone binds two identical cell membrane receptors → activated JAKs on cytoplasmic ends.
  - JAKs phosphorylate tyrosine residues on receptors.

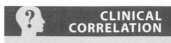

CLINICAL CORRELATION

Janus kinase (JAK) inhibitors, approved for a variety of autoimmune diseases, can exert anti-inflammatory effects by preventing signal propagation of a number of cytokines.

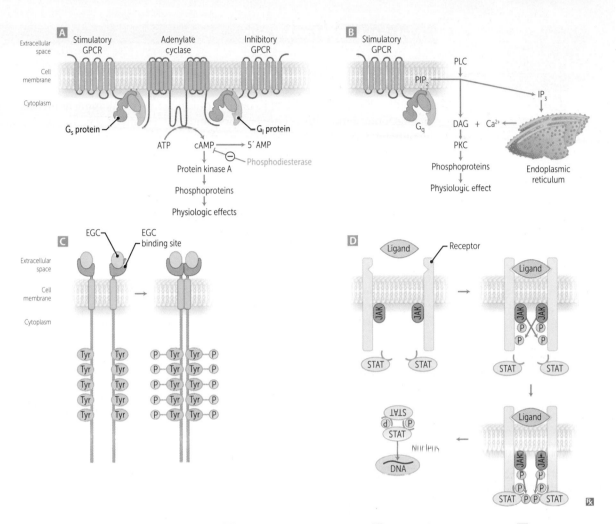

FIGURE 2-1.   Signal propagation mechanisms. A Adenylate cyclase pathway. B Phospholipase C pathway. C Receptor tyrosine kinase pathway. D JAK/STAT pathway. CaBP, calcium-binding protein; DAG, diacylglycerol; EGC, (–)-epigallocatechin; ER, endoplasmic reticulum; G_s, G_i and G_q, G protein; IP_3, inositol 1,4,5-triphosphate; JAK/STAT, Janus kinase/signal transducer and activator; P, phosphate; PDE, PiP_2, phosphatidylinositol 4,5 bisphosphate; PKC, protein kinase C; PLC, phospholipase C; Tyr, tyrosine.

- JAKs then recruit and phosphorylate STATs.
- Activated STATs dimerize and translocate to nucleus to modify gene expression.

Regulatory Control

- **Receptor up- and downregulation:** Target cells can upregulate/downregulate the number of receptors or receptor affinity for their ligands (eg, insulin receptors are internalized and degraded after sustained stimulation).
- **Negative feedback:** A hormone (or product of hormone signaling) acts upstream along its endocrine axis to increase or decrease its release toward the normal range (eg, thyroid hormone inhibits the release of thyroid-stimulating hormone [TSH]).
- **Positive feedback:** Instead of maintaining homeostasis, a hormone can perpetuate an increase or decrease of its own release away from the normal range via reinforcement along its endocrine axis (eg, during childbirth, pressure receptors in the cervix stimulate oxytocin release, which then induces uterine contractions that increase pressure).
  - Feedback can occur via alterations in gene transcription, posttranslational processing, or hormone release.
  - Hormones may exhibit both positive and negative feedback controls (eg, estrogen inhibits luteinizing hormone [LH] release during the follicular phase of the menstrual cycle [negative feedback] but at midcycle promotes the LH surge and ovulation [positive feedback]).

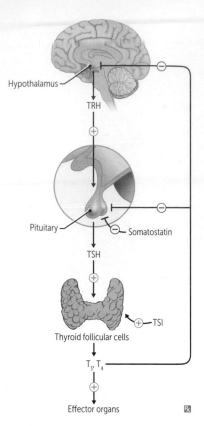

FIGURE 2-2. Hypothalamic-pituitary-thyroid axis. The final hormone produced often feeds back to inhibit the production of upstream hormones in order to maintain homeostasis. TRH, thyrotropin-releasing hormone; TSH, thyroid-stimulating hormone; TSI, thyroid-stimulating immunoglobulin.

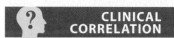

CLINICAL CORRELATION

Empty sella syndrome (ESS): In primary ESS, increased pressure in the sella turcica flattens the pituitary along the walls of the cavity. Secondary ESS is the regression of the pituitary secondary to injury or radiation. Both give the impression of an empty sella on imaging. This syndrome occasionally results in endocrine dysfunction.

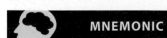

MNEMONIC

Anterior pituitary hormones—

FLAT PiG
FSH
LH
ACTH
TSH
PRL
GH

HYPOTHALAMIC-PITUITARY AXIS

Hypothalamus

The hypothalamus is located below the thalamus and above the pituitary gland (which sits in the sella turcica). Each of its nuclei contributes to maintaining homeostasis: water balance, body temperature, hunger, thirst, and even emotions. The hypothalamus links the nervous system to the endocrine system, primarily through the pituitary gland (Figure 2-2). It does so by regulating the timing and amount of pituitary hormones secreted.

The hypothalamus exerts direct control over anterior pituitary hormone secretion via releasing/inhibiting factors (Table 2-4). These factors are synthesized by neural cell bodies in the hypothalamus, stored in granules at axon terminals, and released into the hypothalamo-hypophyseal circulation.

Pituitary

The pituitary, or hypophysis, is composed of two embryologically and morphologically distinct glands (anterior and posterior) connected to the hypothalamus by the pituitary stalk. The gland rests in a bony cavity at the base of the skull called the sella turcica (Figure 2-3).

Anterior Pituitary (Adenohypophysis)

The anterior pituitary forms from the embryonic invagination of pharyngeal epithelium (**oral ectoderm**) called the pouch of Rathke. It is composed of five different hormone-producing cell populations, all of which are regulated by hypothalamic releasing and inhibiting hormones. The neurons that secrete these releasing hormones converge in the median eminence of the hypothalamus and act on the anterior pituitary via the hypophyseal circulation (a portal system).

Posterior Pituitary (Neurohypophysis)

The posterior pituitary forms from **neuroectoderm** derived from the hypothalamus. During development, it fuses with the pouch of Rathke. The posterior pituitary, composed of neural tissue, releases hormones in response to neurotransmission (not circulating hormones).

Anterior Pituitary Cell Types and Regulation

The adenohypophysis is composed of five major cell types, each of which produces one or more peptide hormones (Table 2-5).

Cell populations of the anterior pituitary can be further generalized according to reactions to histochemical stains. Periodic acid-Schiff (PAS) stain identifies three groups: Acidophils (stain orange), basophils (stain purple), and chromophobes (no stain reaction).

- **Acidophils:** Somatotropes (growth hormone [GH]), lactotropes (prolactin)
- **Basophils:** Gonadotropes (FSH, LH), corticotropes (adrenocorticotropic hormone [ACTH]), thyrotropes (TSH) ("**B-FLAT**")
- **Chromophobes:** "Empty" cells (lack cytoplasmic granules); former acidophils or basophils after release of hormone-containing granules

Anterior Pituitary Hormones

Prolactin

Prolactin (PRL) is a polypeptide hormone that functions in breast development, lactation, and ovulation inhibition. It is structurally homologous to growth hormone (GH) and human placental lactogen (HPL). All three hormones are synthesized in the RER.

- Suckling stimulates PRL secretion.
- Dopamine tonically inhibits PRL secretion.

TABLE 2-4. **Overview of Hypothalamic Hormones**

HORMONE	STRUCTURE	ACTIONS	REGULATED BY	CLINICAL NOTES
Corticotropin-releasing hormone (CRH)	Peptide	↑ ACTH	Cortisol (−)	↓ in chronic exogenous steroid use
Gonadotropin-releasing hormone (GnRH)	Peptide	↑ LH and FSH	Testosterone (−), progesterone (−), prolactin (−), estradiol (−)	Tonic GnRH suppresses HPG axis Pulsatile GnRH leads to puberty, fertility
Growth hormone-releasing hormone (GHRH)	Peptide	↑ GH	GHRH (−)	Analog (tesamorelin) used to treat HIV-associated lipodystrophy
Somatostatin (growth hormone–inhibitory hormone)	Peptide	↓ GH and TSH	Somatomedins (+), GH (+)	Analogs used to treat acromegaly
Dopamine (prolactin-inhibiting factor)	Amine	↓ prolactin	Prolactin (+)	Dopamine antagonists (eg, antipsychotics) can cause galactorrhea due to hyperprolactinemia
Thyrotropin-releasing hormone (TRH)	Peptide	↑ TSH and prolactin		

ACTH, adrenocorticotropic hormone; FSH, follicle-stimulating hormone; GH, growth hormone; HPG, hypothalamic–pituitary–gonadal; LH, luteinizing hormone; TSH, thyroid-stimulating hormone.

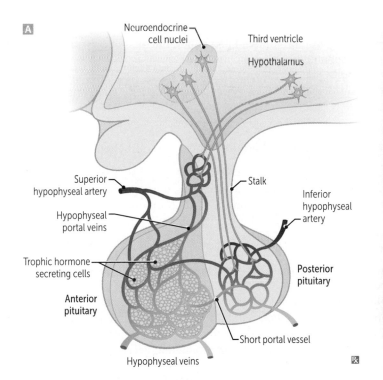

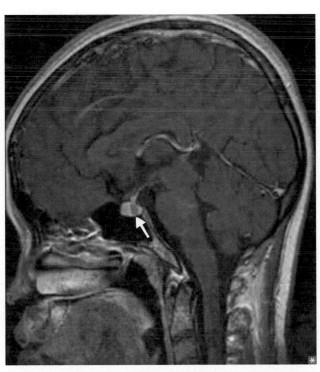

FIGURE 2-3. **Pituitary gland.** **A** Schematic of pituitary gland and **B** MRI of the brain showing pituitary microadenoma (arrow).

TABLE 2-5. Summary of Anterior Pituitary Hormone Function and Regulation

HORMONE	STRUCTURE	ACTIONS	REGULATED BY
Adrenocorticotropic hormone (ACTH)	Peptide	Induces synthesis of adrenal cortical hormones (cortisol, androgens, aldosterone)	Cortisol (–)
Follicle-stimulating hormone (FSH)	Peptide	Stimulates follicle growth in ovaries and spermatogenesis in testes	Inhibin (–), estrogen (–), progesterone (–), testosterone (–)
Luteinizing hormone (LH)	Peptide	Promotes testosterone synthesis in testes; promotes estrogen/progesterone synthesis in ovaries; surge causes ovulation and maintains the corpus luteum	Testosterone (–), estrogen (+/–), progesterone (–)
Growth hormone (GH)	Peptide	Promotes protein synthesis, tissue growth, and IGF-1 synthesis in liver	Somatomedins (eg, IGF-1) (–), somatostatin (–), glucose (–)
Thyroid-stimulating hormone (TSH)	Peptide	Stimulates growth of thyroid gland and synthesis and secretion of thyroid hormones	Thyroid hormones (–)
Prolactin (PRL)	Peptide	Stimulates enlargement of breast tissue and milk production	Dopamine (–), TRH (+)

IGF-1, insulin-like growth factor; TRH, thyroid-releasing hormone.

KEY FACT

Damage to the pituitary stalk can lead to decreased secretion of pituitary hormones secondary to disruption of the hypophyseal portal system (anterior pituitary) and hypothalamic neurons (posterior pituitary). The exception is prolactin (PRL) secretion, which is increased due to this same disruption, as dopamine from the hypothalamus usually inhibits PRL secretion.

FLASH FORWARD

FSH and LH are important reproductive hormones released by the anterior pituitary that control the menstrual cycle, ovulation, and spermatogenesis.

- PRL, in concert with other hormones, promotes additional breast development during pregnancy in preparation for milk production.
  - PRL stimulates lactation.
  - PRL inhibits ovulation by inhibiting gonadotropin-releasing hormone (GnRH) release.
  - PRL levels rise throughout the course of pregnancy, but their effects on lactation are inhibited by placental progesterone until birth.
- Excess PRL (eg, via a prolactinoma) causes galactorrhea and gynecomastia directly and infertility, hypogonadism, and amenorrhea by inhibiting GnRH secretion (Figure 2-4).

Growth Hormone

Growth hormone (GH) is a polypeptide hormone whose main function is to promote linear growth.

- GH may also be referred to as somatotropic hormone, or somatotropin.
- GH release is under hypothalamic regulation: Growth hormone-releasing hormone (GHRH) promotes and somatostatin inhibits GH release.
- GH also responds to exercise, trauma, sleep, and acute hypoglycemia (Figure 2-5).
- GH acts directly on tissues; its growth-promoting effect is primarily mediated via **insulin-like growth factor-1 (IGF-1)**, formerly known as somatomedin.
  - IGF-1 is produced by the liver in response to GH.
  - The metabolic effects of GH and IGF-1 include increased protein synthesis and fat utilization and decreased glucose uptake into tissues (Table 2-6).
- GH is secreted in a pulsatile pattern; at any moment in time, serum GH concentrations are usually low. After adolescence, overall production decreases and continues at a lower rate during adult life.
- GH, like glucagon, cortisol, and epinephrine, is a counterregulatory hormone that is released in response to hypoglycemia. Counterregulatory hormones increase serum glucose levels by promoting glycogenolysis, gluconeogenesis, lipolysis, and ketogenesis.

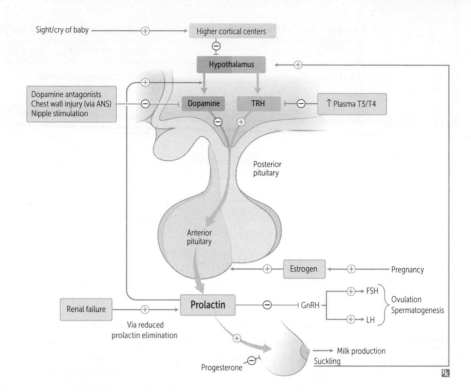

FIGURE 2-4. **Regulation of prolactin.** ANS, autonomic nervous system; FSH, follicle-stimulating hormone; GnRH, gonadotropin-releasing hormone; LH, luteinizing hormone; T$_3$/T$_4$, triiodothyronine/thyroxine; TRH, thyroid-releasing hormone.

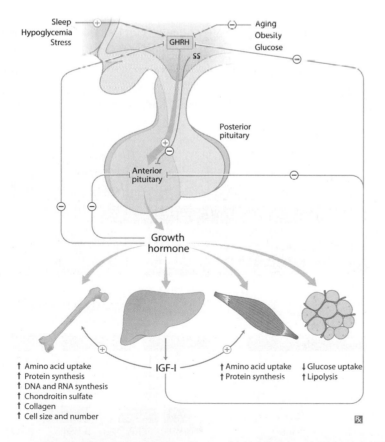

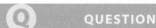

FIGURE 2-5. **Growth hormone regulation.** Factors that inhibit growth hormone (GH) secretion are insulin-like growth factor-1 (IGF-1) and somatostatin (SS). Factors that promote GH secretion are growth hormone-releasing hormone (GHRH), hypoglycemia, exercise, stress, sleep, and amino acids.

Q **QUESTION**

On examination of a pituitary adenoma biopsy, a pathologist observes extensive intracellular acidophilic granules. What hormone(s) might this adenoma be secreting?

TABLE 2-6.   **Effects of Growth Hormone and Insulin-like Growth Factor-1**

DIRECT EFFECTS OF GH	INDIRECT EFFECTS OF GH (THROUGH IGF-1)
Decreases glucose uptake (counterregulatory effects)	Stimulates protein synthesis at the organ level
Mobilizes fatty acids	Increases protein synthesis in chondrocytes (promotes linear growth)
Stimulates protein synthesis in muscle	Stimulates protein synthesis in muscle
Increases lean body mass	Increases lean body mass

IGF-1, insulin-like growth factor 1; GH, growth hormone.

Adrenocorticotropic Hormone

ACTH is a polypeptide hormone that stimulates corticosteroid production by the adrenal cortex.

FLASH FORWARD

Secondary and tertiary adrenal insufficiency (caused by pituitary or hypothalamic damage, respectively) cause cortisol deficiency but do not cause hyperpigmentation (decreased ACTH and thus decreased MSH). Because aldosterone secretion is primarily regulated by the renin-angiotensin-aldosterone system (RAAS), these patients with adrenal insufficiency do not typically have hypovolemia, hypotension, hyponatremia, or hyperkalemia.

- Synthesized by corticotropes in the anterior pituitary gland in response to stimulation by corticotropin-releasing hormone (CRH).
- Synthesized from a larger precursor, proopiomelanocortin (POMC); β-lipotropin and β-endorphin are also derived from POMC (Figure 2-6).
- A bioactive moiety, α-MSH (melanocyte-stimulating hormone), is present on the N-terminal end of ACTH.
- ACTH regulates the size, integrity, and synthetic function of the adrenal cortex.

Thyroid-Stimulating Hormone

TSH (also known as thyrotropin) is a glycoprotein hormone that stimulates the release of thyroid hormones (thyroxine [T_4] and triiodothyronine [T_3]) by the thyroid.

- Synthesized by thyrotropes in the anterior pituitary gland in response to stimulation by thyrotropin-releasing hormone (TRH).
- TSH secretion is stimulated by low thyroid hormone levels and inhibited by high levels.
- TSH also stimulates growth of the thyroid.

A   ANSWER

Growth hormone and/or prolactin.

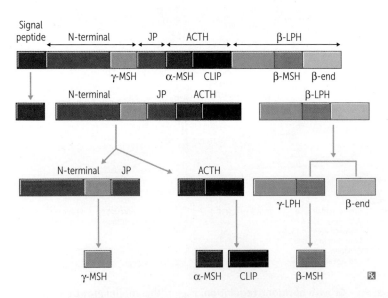

FIGURE 2-6.   **Composition of proopiomelanocortin (POMC).** ACTH, adrenocorticotropic hormone; end, endorphin; CLIP, corticotropin-like intermediate lobe peptide; JP, joining peptide; LPH, lipotropic hormone; MSH, melanocyte-stimulating hormone.

Anterior Pituitary Hormone Homology

The anterior pituitary gland produces six major hormones that can be classified into three groups based on structural homology.

- **Glycoproteins:** FSH, LH, and TSH are each composed of α- and β-subunits. They share an identical α-subunit, but each has a unique β-subunit.
- **Somatomammotropins:** GH and PRL are structurally related peptide hormones that belong to the same cytokine-hematopoietin family.
- **ACTH-related peptides:** ACTH, MSH, and lipotropin are formed by cleavage of a single large precursor molecule (POMC).

KEY FACT

Human chorionic gonadotropin (hCG) shares the same alpha subunit as FSH, LH, and TSH.

Posterior Pituitary

Hormones of the posterior pituitary are synthesized in hypothalamic neurons (named **magnocellular neurons** because of their large cell bodies) and transported via axoplasmic flow to axon terminals in the posterior lobe of the pituitary. These hormones include oxytocin and antidiuretic hormone (ADH; aka vasopressin). The hypothalamic nuclei responsible for hormone production are the paraventricular nucleus (oxytocin) and the supraoptic nucleus (ADH) (Figure 2-7).

Oxytocin and ADH are synthesized from larger precursors (prohormones) which are enzymatically cleaved within vesicles to produce active hormone. Release of oxytocin or ADH-containing granules is regulated by exogenous and endogenous stimuli, which are transformed into CNS signals.

Oxytocin

Two main actions (Figure 2-8):

- Promotes contractions of the uterine myometrium during labor.
- Stimulates contraction of myoepithelial cells in the breast, facilitating milk letdown to suckling infant.

Exogenous stimuli driving oxytocin secretion include suckling of an infant on the breast and dilation of the cervix in childbirth.

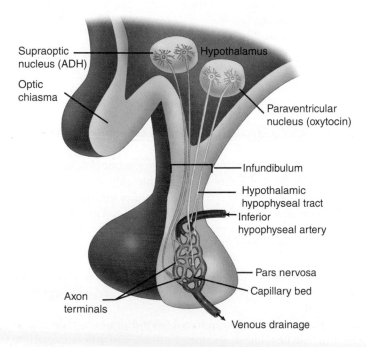

FIGURE 2-7.   Hypophyseal circulation and associated nuclei.

QUESTION

A patient with persistent headaches undergoes an MRI, and the radiologist notes a lesion in the hypothalamus. Upon questioning, the patient curiously notes that she is abnormally tan this winter. Why might this be?

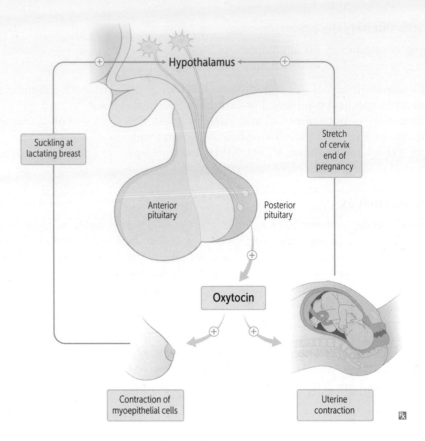

FIGURE 2-8. **Oxytocin effects and regulation.**

Antidiuretic Hormone

ADH plays a central role in osmoregulation by controlling water reabsorption in the kidney.

- The osmotic concentration of extracellular fluid (ECF) is sensed by specialized neurons within or adjacent to the hypothalamus. The size of these neurons changes with extracellular osmolality, resulting in nerve signals increasing or decreasing ADH secretion as appropriate.
- ADH secretion increases in hyperosmolar conditions.
- ADH increases permeability to water in the distal tubules and collecting ducts of the kidney, thereby increasing water reabsorption and decreasing plasma osmolality (Figure 2-9).
    - ADH stimulates membrane-bound V_2 receptors, triggering an increase in intracellular cAMP.
    - Special vesicles containing aquaporins insert into the luminal aspect of the cell membrane.
    - These permeable water channels allow for the free diffusion of water from tubule to peritubular fluid, decreasing ECF osmolality.
- At high concentrations, ADH constricts arterioles through the V_1 receptor. Consequently, ADH is also referred to as arginine vasopressin.
- In addition, ADH is secreted in response to large decreases (> 10%) in blood volume (Table 2-7). Secretion is stimulated by signals from atrial stretch receptors and baroreceptors.
    - Hypovolemia with resultant reduced atrial stretch results in decreased secretion of atrial natriuretic peptide (ANP). Low levels of ANP support increased secretion of ADH.
    - Baroreceptors of the aortic arch and carotid sinus sense decreased arterial pressure due to hypovolemia, resulting in decreased afferent signals to the medulla and consequent increase in ADH secretion and sympathetic stimulation.

ANSWER

A hypothalamic tumor releasing excess CRH induces synthesis of POMC in the anterior pituitary. POMC is cleaved into ACTH and MSH, the latter of which stimulates melanocytes and causes hyperpigmentation.

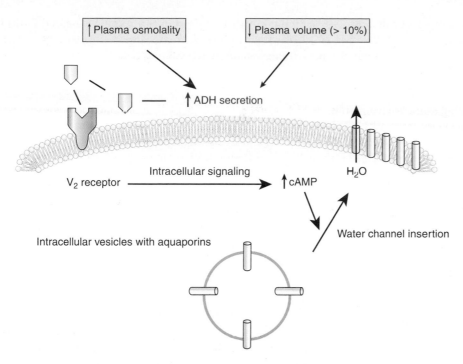

FIGURE 2-9.   **Antidiuretic hormone (ADH) signaling and aquaporin insertion.**

ANTERIOR PITUITARY DISEASE

Pituitary Tumors

Anterior pituitary disease can lead to both overproduction and underproduction of its hormones. Given the wide array of hormones produced by the anterior pituitary, these diseases present in a myriad of ways. To complicate matters, some diseases exhibit overproduction of certain hormones and underproduction of others.

Pituitary tumors are classified as functioning, in which they overproduce at least one hormone, or nonfunctioning, in which hormones are underproduced or produced at normal levels. Signs and symptoms of a pituitary tumor can be due to the effect of excess hormone if present, suppression of other hormone production due to mechanical compression, and/or elevated intracranial pressure due to mass effect. All pituitary tumors can cause bitemporal hemianopia due to compression of the optic chiasm. The most common pituitary tumor is a nonfunctioning, nonsecretory adenoma.

Prolactinoma

Prolactinomas are the most common functioning pituitary tumors, characterized by hypersecretion of PRL. The average age of onset is 20–40 years. The elevated PRL

TABLE 2-7.   **Factors Affecting Secretion of Antidiuretic Hormone**

INCREASE ADH SECRETION	DECREASE ADH SECRETION
↑ plasma osmolality	↓ plasma osmolality
Large ↓ in plasma volume (↓ ANP)	Large ↑ in plasma volume (↑ ANP)
↓ BP	↑ BP
Nicotine, opiates	Ethanol

ADH, antidiuretic hormone; ANP, atrial natriuretic peptide; BP, blood pressure.

characteristically induces lactation, but PRL also inhibits GnRH. Decreased GnRH leads to decreased FSH and LH, which in turn decreases levels of progesterone and estrogen (testosterone in males), causing amenorrhea/impotence.

DIFFERENTIAL

Dopamine tonically inhibits PRL secretion, so its depletion or pharmacologic antagonism increases PRL production. Excess PRL can arise from drugs that deplete or inhibit the synthesis/action of dopamine (reserpine, methyldopa, antipsychotics). In hypothyroidism, elevated TRH stimulates the anterior pituitary to upregulate PRL production.

PRESENTATION

- Headache, amenorrhea, infertility, galactorrhea; decreased libido and osteopenia due to decreased estrogen in women; impotence and gynecomastia in men.
- Bitemporal hemianopia due to the tumor's compressing the optic chiasm above.

DIAGNOSIS

- Serum chemistry: Elevated PRL. Rule out secondary causes by screening for primary hypothyroidism, pregnancy, confounding antiemetic/antipsychotic medications, renal failure, and cirrhosis. Marked psychological stress can also elevate PRL levels.
- Once secondary causes have been ruled out, MRI should be done to identify mass lesions.

TREATMENT

- **Dopamine agonists (bromocriptine, cabergoline)** are first-line treatment for any patient with hyperprolactinemia and are known to reduce the size and secretion of more than 90% of lactotroph adenomas.
- **Transsphenoidal surgery** is performed when dopamine agonists are ineffective in decreasing serum PRL concentration or in shrinking the adenoma as well as if the patient is pregnant and is suffering mass effect from the tumor.
- Asymptomatic patients without hypogonadism and with small tumors (< 1 cm) can be followed with serial PRL levels and MRIs.

Gigantism and Acromegaly

This disorder of excessive GH secretion presents as gigantism in children, in whom the epiphyses have not yet closed, or as acromegaly in adults. **Gigantism** refers to excess linear height of more than 2 standard deviations (SD) above the mean for a person's age, sex, and Tanner stage, which can occur in the setting of excess GH acting on the epiphyseal growth plates. **Acromegaly** is a related disorder resulting from GH acting on fused growth plate cartilage in adults.

DIFFERENTIAL

GH excess is most commonly caused by a pituitary adenoma composed of somatotroph cells. Less common causes include hypothalamic GHRH secretion or disruption of somatostatin tone. Gigantism can be a secondary feature of McCune-Albright syndrome and multiple endocrine neoplasia syndrome type I. Precocious puberty, normal genetics, and hyperthyroidism should be ruled out.

PRESENTATION

- Musculoskeletal and visceral overgrowth and deformity (gigantism) in children.
- Acromegaly (enlarged jaw, tongue, hands, feet; coarsening facial features; prognathism) in adults.
- Enlarged liver and heart (cardiomyopathy).
- Peripheral neuropathies such as carpal tunnel syndrome secondary to nerve compression.

FLASH FORWARD

Compression of the optic chiasm by a pituitary tumor causes bitemporal hemianopia, a specific visual field defect defined by loss of the left temporal field in the left eye and the right temporal field in the right eye. The fibers carrying the signal for these fields cross at the optic chiasm (see Figure 6-46).

KEY FACT

GH excess in children causes gigantism, whereas GH excess in adults causes acromegaly.

- Glucose intolerance and diabetes mellitus in one-sixth of cases.
- Amenorrhea and impotence.
- Headache due to mass effect, and bitemporal hemianopia.
- Mean age of onset for acromegaly is in the third decade. The onset of acromegaly is insidious, as opposed to the dramatic presentation of gigantism.

DIAGNOSIS

- Elevated serum IGF-1 (sensitive screening test).
- Oral glucose tolerance test (OGTT): Administer glucose, which normally suppresses GH, and then measure GH levels.
- MRI scans to localize the tumor after a positive OGTT.

TREATMENT

- **Transsphenoidal surgery** is the treatment of choice. Can be accompanied by radiotherapy.
- **Octreotide** is a long-acting somatostatin analog that can lower GH levels to normal.
- Bromocriptine, a dopamine agonist, can work synergistically with octreotide therapy.
- Pegvisomant (GH-receptor antagonist).

PROGNOSIS

Cardiac failure is the most common cause of death in acromegalic patients. They also suffer an increased risk of colon cancer and pituitary insufficiency.

Additional pituitary adenomas include ACTH-producing adenomas, which cause hypercortisolemia (Cushing syndrome). Rarely, the following adenomas occur: TSH producing adenomas, resulting in hyperthyroidism, and gonadotropin-producing adenomas (FSH or LH), resulting in reproductive dysfunction. All such adenomas can produce a mass effect, affecting the neighboring normal pituitary gland tissue, producing headache and bitemporal hemianopia.

Panhypopituitarism

This reduction in the release of all pituitary hormones may result from both primary and secondary causes. Primary causes directly affect the pituitary and include surgery, radiation, tumors, apoplexy (sudden hemorrhage into the gland, usually from adenoma), infection, infiltration by sarcoidosis or hemochromatosis, ischemia (Sheehan syndrome), carotid aneurysm, cavernous sinus thrombosis, and trauma. Secondary causes disrupt the hypothalamus or pituitary stalk and include hypothalamic tumors, hypothalamic hormone deficiency, surgery, infection, infiltration, and trauma.

PRESENTATION

Patients can present with signs and symptoms of any or all pituitary deficiencies. The most life-threatening pituitary deficiency is ACTH, followed by TSH, then FSH/LH, and lastly GH (Table 2-8).

DIAGNOSIS

Low or inappropriately normal levels of specific pituitary hormones in the setting of low target gland hormones. If neoplastic in etiology, MRI of the brain may localize the tumor for preoperative planning.

TREATMENT

Replacement of the missing hormones is required, with the most important being cortisol. Because most of the anterior pituitary hormones are proteins or glycoproteins that induce the secretion of other hormones, the target gland hormone is often used as replacement rather than the pituitary hormone (ie, TSH replaced with T_4, ACTH

KEY FACT

Ischemic necrosis of the pituitary **(Sheehan syndrome):** Postpartum hemorrhage causing hypovolemic shock results in ischemic necrosis of the pituitary. This is due to the increase in size and blood demand of the pituitary during pregnancy.

QUESTION

A 33-year old woman comes to your clinic complaining of decreased libido and an absent period for 3 months. After confirming that she is not pregnant, your comprehensive history reveals that she sideswiped two parked cars in the last month, her first accidents in 15 years. What are you concerned about and what tests would you order?

TABLE 2-8.   **Clinical Findings with Hypopituitarism**

HORMONE	NORMAL FUNCTION	CLINICAL FINDINGS IN HORMONE DEFICIENCY
GH	Growth and glucose homeostasis	Children: growth failure, dwarfism Adults: fatigue, osteoporosis, ↑ LDL, ↑ fat mass, ↓ muscle mass, ↑ risk of cardiovascular disease
Gonadotropin (LH/FSH)	Menstrual cycle and reproduction	Amenorrhea, impotence, genital atrophy, infertility, ↓ libido, ↓ axillary/pubic hair
TSH	Stimulates T_4 production from the thyroid gland	Resembles primary hypothyroidism without goiter (cold intolerance, lethargy); TSH inappropriately low in the setting of low T_4
ACTH	Stimulates glucocorticoid production from the adrenal gland	Resembles primary adrenal insufficiency but **without** skin hyperpigmentation from MSH or volume depletion, hypokalemia, and salt craving due to intact RAAS

ACTH, adrenocorticotropic hormone; FSH, follicle-stimulating hormone; GH, growth hormone; LDL, low-density lipoprotein; LH, luteinizing hormone; MSH, melanocyte-stimulating hormone; RAAS, renin-angiotensin-aldosterone system; T_4, thyroxine; TSH, thyroid-stimulating hormone.

replaced with hydrocortisone or another glucocorticoid, LH and FSH replaced with testosterone, estrogen, or progestin).

POSTERIOR PITUITARY DISEASE

Diabetes Insipidus

Diabetes insipidus (DI) is characterized by an ineffective ADH axis, resulting in inappropriately dilute urine. ADH (vasopressin), which is synthesized by the supraoptic nucleus and stored in the axon terminals of the posterior pituitary, functions to concentrate urine and conserve water. There are two types of DI.

- Central DI is due to absent or insufficient release of ADH from the posterior pituitary.
- Nephrogenic DI has normal ADH secretion, but the kidneys are unresponsive (renal resistance to the ADH). Causes are listed in Table 2-9.
- Primary polydipsia is a condition characterized by a marked increase in water intake, often seen in patients with psychiatric comorbidities, such as schizophrenia. It can also develop in patients with lesions affecting the hypothalamic thirst center.

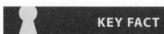

KEY FACT

Central DI is due to a lack of ADH. **Nephrogenic DI** is due to a failure to respond to ADH.

A   **ANSWER**

A prolactinoma could explain her symptoms, as well as the sudden decreases in driving ability. The tumor could be compressing her optic nerve, causing bitemporal hemianopia and significantly limiting her peripheral vision. You should obtain serum PRL levels and an MRI to look for a pituitary mass.

TABLE 2-9.   **Causes of Diabetes Insipidus**

Central DI	▪ Idiopathic (50% of cases) ▪ Trauma, surgery ▪ Tumors, sarcoidosis, TB ▪ Hand-Schüller-Christian disease ▪ Langerhans cell histiocytosis
Nephrogenic DI	▪ Hypercalcemia, hypokalemia ▪ Medications: Lithium, demeclocycline ▪ Polycystic kidney disease ▪ Aquaporin or vasopressin V_2 receptor gene mutations

DI, diabetes insipidus; TB, tuberculosis.

PRESENTATION

Excessive urination and thirst. In children, DI can present with fever, vomiting, and diarrhea.

- The high serum osmolality stimulates thirst, causing patients to drink large amounts of water.
- Hypernatremia is usually not significant if the patient has free access to water, but is often a problem in hospitalized or debilitated patients with unrecognized DI and reduced access to water.

DIAGNOSIS

- **ADH (vasopressin) challenge:** Complete fluid restriction + injection of ADH → increased urine osmolality (U_{Osm}) in central DI, but not nephrogenic DI (Table 2-10).
- Urinalysis: Low U_{Osm} and high plasma osmolality (P_{Osm}) in both central and nephrogenic DI, because the kidneys either do not receive ADH or cannot respond to ADH.
- Meanwhile, U_{Osm} and P_{Osm} are both low in primary polydipsia, since the medullary gradient of the kidneys is washed out and dilute urine is produced.

TREATMENT

- **Central DI:** Desmopressin, an ADH analog, is given subcutaneously, orally, or intranasally.
- Chlorpropamide increases the release of ADH in partial ADH deficiency.
- **Nephrogenic DI:** Thiazide diuretics (eg, hydrochlorothiazide [HCTZ]) or indomethacin (a nonsteroidal anti-inflammatory drug [NSAID])

PROGNOSIS

Patients who have access to water can usually keep up with the large urinary losses. When water is not readily available, the rising serum sodium concentration can cause weakness, fever, obtundation, and eventually death.

Syndrome of Inappropriate Secretion of Antidiuretic Hormone

In syndrome of inappropriate secretion of antidiuretic hormone (SIADH), excess ADH in the absence of hyperosmolarity leads to excessive free water retention and an inability to dilute urine. There is a net gain in free water over sodium, resulting in euvolemic hyponatremia. Causes of SIADH are listed in Table 2-11.

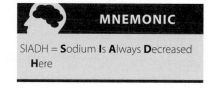

MNEMONIC

SIADH = **S**odium **I**s **A**lways **D**ecreased **H**ere

PRESENTATION

- Patients are often asymptomatic if SIADH is chronic. If onset is acute, brain swelling can result, leading to lethargy, weakness, seizures, and coma/death.

TABLE 2-10. Differentiating Between Central and Nephrogenic Diabetes Insipidus

	INCREASE IN U_{OSM} WITH WATER DEPRIVATION?	RESPONSE TO INJECTION OF ADH?
Central DI	No	Yes
Nephrogenic DI	No	No
Primary polydipsia	Yes	Yes

ADH, antidiuretic hormone; DI, diabetes insipidus; U_{Osm}, urine osmolality.

TABLE 2-11. **Common Causes of SIADH**

Neoplasms with ectopic ADH secretion	▪ Small-cell lung carcinoma ▪ Thymoma
Pulmonary diseases	▪ TB ▪ Lung abscesses ▪ Pneumonia
CNS disorders	▪ Skull fractures/trauma ▪ Subdural hematoma
Drugs	▪ Chlorpropamide ▪ Vincristine, vinblastine ▪ Cyclophosphamide ▪ Carbamazepine

ADH, antidiuretic hormone; CNS, central nervous system; TB, tuberculosis.

KEY FACT

Hyponatremia must not be corrected too quickly because this can result in central pontine myelinolysis. This potentially fatal disease is caused by damage to the myelin sheaths of nerves in the brain stem from rapid changes in osmolality. Patients can experience altered mental status, acute paralysis, and dysphagia, among other neurologic symptoms.

▪ SIADH causes volume expansion, but edema and hypertension are usually not present because of natriuresis (excreting excess sodium in urine).

DIAGNOSIS

SIADH exhibits hypotonic hyponatremia ($\downarrow$ serum Na and P_{Osm}) in the presence of increased U_{Osm} (> 300 mOsm/L).

▪ Blood urea nitrogen (BUN) and uric acid are also decreased, reflecting diluted fluid stores. Plasma creatinine (Cr) remains relatively normal.
▪ Need to rule out hypothyroidism ($\downarrow$ cardiac output, glomerular filtration rate [GFR]) and adrenal insufficiency ($\uparrow$ CRH and ADH).

TREATMENT

Fluid restriction in mild cases of SIADH. When fluid restriction is not feasible or not working, use **conivaptan** (a V_2 receptor antagonist) or **demeclocycline** (acts on collecting tubule to limit response to ADH). Hypertonic saline may be used if cerebral edema, convulsions, or coma develops.

PITUITARY/HYPOTHALAMIC PHARMACOLOGY

Leuprolide

MECHANISM

GnRH agonist: GnRH is normally secreted in a pulsatile fashion by the hypothalamus and stimulates the release of FSH and LH from the anterior pituitary. Leuprolide is a GnRH analog that has a longer half-life; it can be used in a pulsatile fashion to increase LH/FSH or continuously to suppress LH/FSH.

USES

When given in a pulsatile fashion, it is used to treat women with amenorrhea who desire fertility. When given in a continuous fashion, leuprolide suppresses the growth of prostate and breast cancer, leiomyomas, and endometriosis, and also halts precocious puberty. This occurs through the downregulation of GnRH receptors on prolonged stimulation.

SIDE EFFECTS

Bone pain, feet/ankle swelling, symptoms of hypogonadism.

Somatotropin

MECHANISM

GH analog: Increases lean muscle mass; promotes linear growth in children prior to closure of epiphyses.

USES

Dwarfism; treats wasting associated with AIDS or malignancy.

SIDE EFFECTS

Hand/foot edema, arthralgias, carpal tunnel syndrome, decreased insulin sensitivity, hyperglycemia.

Octreotide

MECHANISM

Somatostatin analog: Somatostatin is a hypothalamic hormone that normally inhibits the release of GH, glucagon, insulin, gastrin, and vasoactive intestinal peptide (VIP). Octreotide has a longer half-life than somatostatin.

USES

Esophageal varices, VIPomas, carcinoid syndrome, acromegaly, Zollinger-Ellison syndrome.

SIDE EFFECTS

Gallbladder disease, pancreatitis, hypo- or hyperthyroidism, hypo- or hyperglycemia.

Dopamine Agonists (Bromocriptine, Cabergoline)

MECHANISM

Dopamine receptor agonists. PRL secretion is normally inhibited by dopamine from the hypothalamus.

USES

Prolactinomas, Parkinson disease (high doses required).

SIDE EFFECTS

Psychotic symptoms, dizziness, headache, nausea, lightheadedness, confusion.

Desmopressin

MECHANISM

Vasopressin analog (ADH): Has minimal V_1 activity (minimal action on vascular smooth muscle). More effect on V_2 receptors, which act on the renal collecting tubules to increase water reabsorption. Also stimulates release of von Willebrand factor (vWF) from the endothelium in platelet dysfunction disorders.

USES

Central DI, von Willebrand disease.

SIDE EFFECTS

Hyponatremia, transient headache, flushing.

ADH Antagonists (Demeclocycline, Conivaptan, Tolvaptan)

MECHANISM

Conivaptan and tolvaptan inhibit ADH receptors (V_1 and V_2) directly, whereas demeclocycline inhibits the second messenger cascade through an unknown mechanism.

USES

Hyponatremia due to SIADH, congestive heart failure, or cirrhosis.

SIDE EFFECTS

Hypernatremia, hypokalemia, hypotension.

Oxytocin

MECHANISM

Posterior pituitary hormone that stimulates milk secretion and induces uterine contractions during labor.

USES

Induces labor; decreases postpartum bleeding by inducing contractions. Also used to stimulate breast milk letdown in new mothers.

SIDE EFFECTS

Chest pain, confusion, excessive vaginal bleeding, palpitations, seizures.

Thyroid and Parathyroid

THYROID

The thyroid gland regulates growth and metabolic rate through the actions of its two major hormones, **thyroxine (T_4)** and **triiodothyronine (T_3)**. Also, the parafollicular (C) cells of the thyroid gland produce **calcitonin,** a hormone that lowers serum calcium levels; however, in humans, it is not usually significant in maintaining calcium homeostasis.

Anatomy

Situated anterior to the trachea, the thyroid is a butterfly-shaped structure below the larynx extending from C5 to T1. It is composed of a right and left lobe united by a thin strip of thyroid tissue called the isthmus (Figure 2-10).

The thyroid is among the largest endocrine organs, weighing 10–20 g. It receives a disproportionately large share of cardiac output per gram of tissue. The rich blood supply of the thyroid is derived from two pairs of vessels: the superior and inferior thyroid arteries.

- **Superior thyroid artery:** This first branch off the external carotid artery supplies the superior half of the thyroid.
- **Inferior thyroid artery:** Stems from the thyrocervical trunk, which is a branch of the subclavian artery.
- Three sets of veins drain the thyroid: **Superior, middle, and inferior thyroid veins.** The superior and middle veins drain into the internal jugular veins, whereas the inferior thyroid veins empty into the brachiocephalic veins.

KEY FACT

A **goiter** is an enlarged thyroid gland due to any cause, such as inflammation, tumor, or autoimmune disease. Endemic goiter, caused by iodine deficiency, is the most common cause of goiter worldwide.

ANSWER

This patient likely has central DI, given her recent surgical history. Because she is not producing sufficient ADH, we would not expect her to respond to water deprivation, but her urine osmolality should increase upon injection of exogenous ADH.

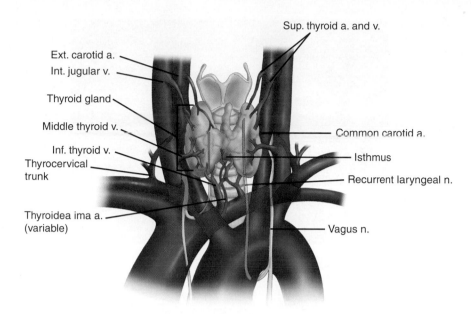

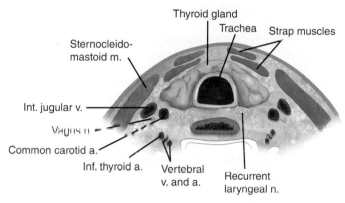

FIGURE 2-10. **Anatomy of the thyroid gland.**

Embryology

The thyroid is formed from an endoderm-derived epithelial outpouching, the **thyroid diverticulum,** which develops in the floor of the foregut at 3–4 weeks of gestation. The thyroglossal duct progenitor migrates caudally, and the thyroid gland eventually assumes its normal position below the larynx unless migration is disrupted. This duct remains patent during development, maintaining a connection between the foregut and thyroid. Ultimately, the thyroglossal duct closes, leaving the **foramen cecum** of the tongue as an adult remnant (Figure 2-11). The thyroid begins secreting hormone as early as the 18th week of fetal development.

Histology

At the microscopic level, the thyroid gland is made up of spherical, closed follicles that are lined with cuboidal epithelial cells.

- The basal surfaces of follicular cells are in contact with a rich blood supply that allows for the absorption of iodide to be used in hormone production (Figure 2-12).
- The apical membranes of follicular cells face a lumen filled with a secretory substance referred to as colloid. The major constituent of colloid is the glycoprotein **thyroglobulin,** which stores iodine and is a precursor of the thyroid hormones.
- Interspersed within the walls of thyroid follicles are small collections of parafollicular C cells that synthesize and secrete calcitonin.

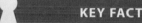

KEY FACT

A **thyroglossal duct cyst** develops when the thyroglossal duct does not close, persisting in the midline near the hyoid bone or at the base of the tongue (Figure 2-11). **Ectopic thyroid tissue** is most commonly found at the base of the tongue.

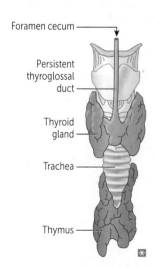

FIGURE 2-11. **Thyroglossal duct.**

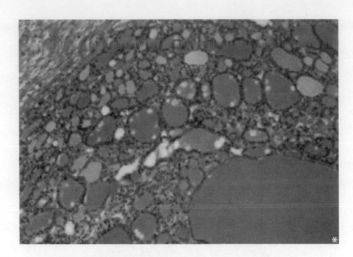

FIGURE 2-12.   **Thyroid follicular cells.**

Thyroid Hormone Synthesis

Iodide Extraction

The thyroid acquires iodide, a necessary factor for hormone synthesis, from the circulation. The following numbered steps (1–9) refer to Figure 2-13.

1. Follicular cells possess a sodium-iodide symporter on their basal surfaces that **actively transports** iodide out of the blood and into the cytosol of follicular cells. This process of intracellular accumulation is known as **iodide trapping,** and is inhibited by thiocyanate and perchlorate anions.
2. Intracellular iodide rapidly diffuses across the apical membranes of follicular cells and into the colloidal lumen. Here, it binds to tyrosine residues on thyroglobulin. TSH stimulates iodide transport.

Thyroglobulin Synthesis and Secretion

Thyroglobulin is a large glycoprotein produced by the thyroid that plays an important role in thyroid hormone synthesis. Thyroid hormones are synthesized from tyrosine residues in the protein structure of thyroglobulin. It serves as both a precursor and a storage form of thyroid hormone.

3. Thyroglobulin is synthesized by thyroid follicular cells and is secreted across the apical membrane. Thyroglobulin is the principal component of colloid.

Oxidation and Organification

Following thyroglobulin synthesis and iodide uptake, the next step in thyroid hormone synthesis is iodination of thyroglobulin, a process that requires oxidation and organification reactions.

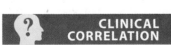

CLINICAL CORRELATION

Propylthiouracil (PTU) and methimazole, used to treat hyperthyroidism, inhibit thyroid peroxidase. PTU also inhibits 5'-deiodinase, which converts T_4 to active T_3.

4. **Thyroid peroxidase,** an apical membrane enzyme, binds an iodide atom and a tyrosine moiety, brings them into close apposition, and promotes **oxidation** of iodide and tyrosine. This leads to the generation of short-lived free radicals that enable the reaction between iodide and tyrosine residues on thyroglobulin. The antithyroid medications propylthiouracil (PTU) and methimazole inhibit thyroid peroxidase. PTU also inhibits 5'-deiodinase, which converts T_4 to active T_3.
5. In the process of **organification,** these free radicals (ie, iodine and tyrosine moieties) undergo an additional reaction to form monoiodotyrosine (MIT). A second organification reaction can take place, adding iodine to an MIT molecule to form diiodotyrosine (DIT).

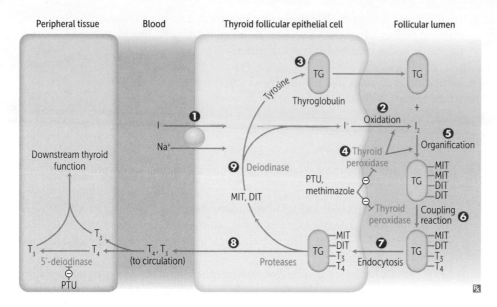

FIGURE 2-13. **Thyroid hormone biosynthesis.** DIT, diiodotyrosine; MIT, monoiodotyrosine; PTU, propylthiouracil; T_3, triiodothyronine; T_4, thyroxine; TG, thyroglobulin.

Coupling

The final step in thyroid hormone synthesis is the coupling of two iodotyrosine residues (MIT or DIT) to form iodothyronine.

6. With MIT and DIT still bound to thyroglobulin, they undergo coupling reactions to form T_4 and T_3. T_4 and T_3 remain attached to thyroglobulin as stored hormone awaiting TSH stimulation. Coupling, like oxidation, is performed by thyroid peroxidase.
   - T_3 is formed by the coupling of one MIT and one DIT moiety.
   - T_4 is formed by the coupling of two DIT moieties. T_4 makes up a majority of thyroid hormone synthesized in this process.

Thyroid Hormone Release

TSH binds to surface receptors on thyroid epithelial cells and serves as the chief stimulus for hormone release (see the asterisk in Figure 2-13).

7. TSH-mediated stimulation of the thyroid gland results in pinocytosis of luminal colloid.
8. Within the follicular cells, lysosomes fuse with pinocytic vesicles, and thyroglobulin is proteolytically digested. Products of protein breakdown include T_4 and T_3, both of which are transported across the basal membrane and into the circulation.
9. Continued cleavage of thyroglobulin produces a large proportion of MIT and DIT molecules within follicular cells. **Deiodinase** mediates iodine moiety cleavage from MIT/DIT and recycling for future thyroid hormone synthesis.

Thyroid Hormone Transport and Metabolism

T_4 and T_3 are principally bound to thyroxine-binding globulin (TBG), a protein secreted by the liver.

- **TBG** slows metabolic inactivation and urinary excretion of thyroid hormones, thereby extending their half-lives. T_4 is the major hormone secreted by the thyroid and carried in the circulation; however, T_3 is the physiologically active form of the hormone.
- **Activation:** 5′-Deiodinase catalyzes the conversion of T_4 to T_3 by the removal of an iodine atom. 5′-Deiodinase is present in the liver, kidneys, thyroid, and target organs.

KEY FACT

T_4 is the major hormone produced by the thyroid, but it needs to be activated by 5′-deiodinase in the periphery to T_3.

> **KEY FACT**
>
> Changes in TBG levels can alter the total levels of T_3 and T_4 but **will not change free, active T_3 and T_4 levels.** Thus, patients are euthyroid and do not show signs of hypo- or hyperthyroidism.

> **KEY FACT**
>
> **The Wolff-Chaikoff effect** is a protective downregulation of thyroid hormone production in the presence of large amounts of iodine (seen with cardiac catheterization and CT with contrast).
>
> In contrast, the **Jod-Basedow effect** is the overproduction of thyroid hormone, causing overt hyperthyroidism in the presence of large amounts of iodine in persons who fail to manifest the Wolff-Chaikoff effect.

- **Inactivation:** A separate deiodinase enzyme targets another site on the T_4 molecule, forming biologically inactive reverse T_3 (rT_3). Enzymatic inactivation of T_3 occurs primarily in the liver and kidneys (Figure 2-14).

Deiodination is a major mechanism by which thyroid hormone activity is enhanced or reduced, depending on whether active hormone (T_3) or inactive hormone (rT_3) is produced.

Thyroid Hormone Regulation

The hypothalamic-pituitary axis responds to changes in the levels of **free** T_4 and T_3 in the serum (Figure 2-15).

- Low levels of free thyroid hormone stimulate the release of TRH from the hypothalamus and TSH from thyrotropes in the pituitary gland.
- TRH enters the hypophyseal circulation and stimulates more release of TSH into the systemic circulation.
- TSH promotes increased thyroid hormone synthesis and secretion by upregulating the processes of iodide uptake, organification, coupling, and pinocytosis of colloid material.
- TSH also exerts trophic effects on the thyroid gland, increasing its size through continued protein synthesis.

Downstream Effects

Thyroid hormone contributes to growth, development, and metabolism.

- **Bone growth:** Thyroid hormone facilitates growth by stimulating GH release. Thyroid hormone also stimulates calcification and closure of cartilaginous growth plates throughout the body.
- **CNS maturation:** Thyroid hormone is vital for CNS development during the prenatal period and for the first three years of life. Thyroid hormone promotes neuronal differentiation and, ultimately, synapse formation.
- **Adrenergic effects:** Thyroid hormone renders β_1-adrenergic receptors in the heart more responsive to signaling molecules. Contractility, stroke volume, and heart rate are all increased, thereby increasing cardiac output.

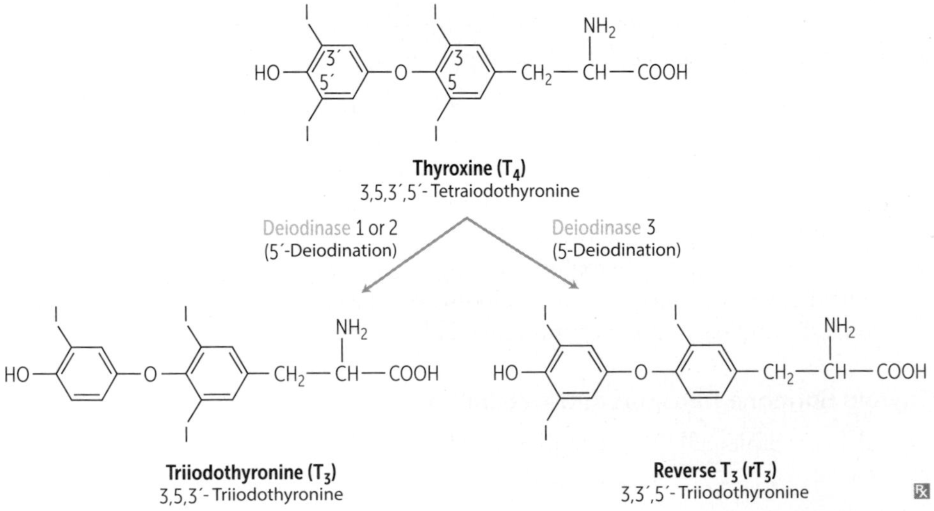

FIGURE 2-14. **Thyroid hormone structure.**

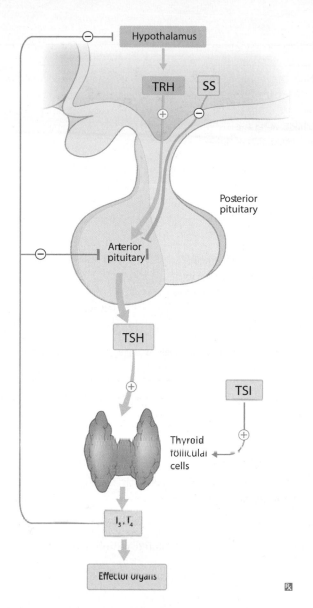

FIGURE 2-15. **Hypothalamic-pituitary-thyroid axis.** T₃, triiodothyronine; T₄, thyroxine; TRH, thyroid-releasing hormone; TSH, thyroid-stimulating hormone.

- **Basal metabolic rate (BMR):** Thyroid hormone promotes the synthesis of cytochromes, cytochrome oxidase, and Na⁺–K⁺ ATPase, while also increasing the number and activity of mitochondria. These actions ultimately increase O_2 consumption, the BMR, and body temperature.
- **Intermediary metabolism:** Thyroid hormone stimulates fuel mobilization and catabolism to support the body's increased BMR. Gluconeogenesis, glycogenolysis, and lipolysis are all enhanced to this end.

DISORDERS OF THE THYROID

Hyperthyroidism

Hyperthyroidism causes **thyrotoxicosis;** elevated thyroid hormones in the blood. Graves disease causes the majority of cases of hyperthyroidism. Other cases are due to miscellaneous causes, including thyroiditis, toxic thyroid adenomas, and, rarely, TSH-secreting pituitary tumors, struma ovarii, and hCG-secreting tumors. See Table 2-12 for causes and their unique presentations.

QUESTION

What is the difference between thyroglobulin and thyroid-binding globulin (TBG)?

MNEMONIC

T₃ functions—
4 B's:

Brain maturation
Bone growth
Beta-adrenergic effects
Basal metabolic rate increases

KEY FACT

Thyroid storm is a life-threatening form of thyrotoxicosis characterized by high fever, tachyarrhythmia, psychosis, confusion, diarrhea, and liver dysfunction. It is managed with intensive care unit-level support, antithyroid medications, glucocorticoids, and β-adrenergic blockers.

TABLE 2-12. **Causes of Hyperthyroidism**

CAUSE	ETIOLOGY	CLINICAL MANIFESTATIONS
Graves disease	■ Type II hypersensitivity: TSI binds TSH receptor on thyroid gland → ↑T$_3$/T$_4$ ■ Diffuse uptake on thyroid scan ■ Most common in women of childbearing age ■ Can be associated with other autoimmune disorders ■ Associated with HLA DR3, HLA B8	■ Diffuse nontender goiter with or without bruit ■ Infiltrative ophthalmopathy (exophthalmos, extraocular muscle dysfunction) ■ Pretibial myxedema
Toxic multinodular goiter (Plummer disease)	■ Hyperfunctioning areas that make ↑T$_3$/T$_4$ (patchy uptake on thyroid scan) ■ Due to a mutation in the TSH receptor ■ More common in the elderly	■ Nontender goiter with one or more nodules
Subacute granulomatous (de Quervain) thyroiditis	■ Inflammation of thyroid gland → spilling of preformed thyroid hormones → transient hyperthyroidism. Pituitary inhibition causes transient hypothyroidism before return to euthyroid state ■ Usually preceded by upper respiratory infection	■ Thyroid gland firm, painful, tender ■ Fever ■ ↑ESR ■ Pain radiating to ears, neck, and arm
Struma ovarii	This is a very rare condition in which ectopic thyroid tissue develops as part of an ovarian tumor, causing hyperthyroidism	

ESR, erythrocyte sedimentation rate; HLA, human leukocyte antigen; TSH, thyroid-stimulating hormone; TSI, thyroid-stimulating immunoglobulin.

ANSWER

Thyroglobulin is the thyroid hormone precursor produced by follicular cells and stored in the colloid. TBG is the circulating protein that binds thyroid hormone in serum.

PRESENTATION

Signs and symptoms are due to increased BMR and sympathetic tone:

■ Tremor, weight loss despite robust appetite, irritability, restlessness, insomnia, heat intolerance, diaphoresis, increased frequency of bowel movements or frank diarrhea, and tachycardia/palpitations.
■ Warm and moist skin due to peripheral vasodilatation and excessive sweating.
■ Increased risk of atrial fibrillation, isolated systolic hypertension, and high-output cardiac failure.

DIAGNOSIS

■ Increased T$_3$ and T$_4$.
■ Decreased TSH (except in TSH-secreting tumors).
■ Anti-TSH receptor antibodies for Graves disease (thyroid-stimulating immunoglobulins).
■ Radioactive iodine uptake (RAIU) scan: Localized uptake (toxic adenoma, multinodular thyroid), generalized uptake (Graves disease), or no uptake (thyroiditis, struma ovarii).

TREATMENT

Treatment for Graves disease and toxic multinodular goiter is as follows:

■ **Propylthiouracil (PTU)** and **methimazole:** Inhibit thyroid hormone synthesis by inhibiting the oxidation and organification of iodine by thyroid peroxidase; PTU also inhibits the peripheral conversion of T$_4$ → T$_3$ by 5′-deiodinase.
■ **Radioactive iodine ablation:** To destroy the thyroid follicular cells. Radioiodine is contraindicated for treatment of hyperthyroidism during pregnancy because it can cross the placenta and destroy the infant's thyroid gland, leading to hypothyroidism (cretinism).
■ **β-Blockers** such as propranolol: Control of adrenergic symptoms (sweating, tachycardia, tremor).

Subacute granulomatous thyroiditis is treated with NSAIDs or glucocorticoids in severe cases.

Hypothyroidism

Over 95% of cases of hypothyroidism result from failure of the thyroid gland itself. Primary hypothyroidism is characterized by decreased T_4 and elevated TSH as a result. The most common cause of primary hypothyroidism in the United States is **Hashimoto thyroiditis** (in the developing world, iodine deficiency is most common). Other causes can be seen in Table 2-13.

PRESENTATION

Signs and symptoms are due to decreased BMR and sympathetic tone (Table 2-14):

- Lethargy, fatigue, muscle weakness.
- Cold intolerance, constipation, weight gain, coarse/dry skin, macroglossia.
- Delayed recovery phase of deep tendon reflexes.
- Slow mentation.
- Diastolic hypertension.
- **Myxedema coma:** Stupor, coma, and hypoventilation coupled with hypothermia, bradycardia, and hypotension. A life-threatening hypothyroid condition that results from long-standing, untreated hypothyroidism. Triggered by trauma, infections, and cold exposure. Treatment is with hormone replacement and supportive measures; mortality is high.

DIAGNOSIS

- T_3/T_4/TSH/TRH: May be helpful for diagnosing and distinguishing among primary, secondary, and tertiary causes.
- Chemistries: Mild normocytic anemia, hyponatremia, hypoglycemia.
- Immunology: Antithyroid peroxidase antibody test for Hashimoto thyroiditis.
- Imaging: Pituitary or pelvic imaging for tumor, if evidence of TSH producing tumor or struma ovarii is discovered.

TREATMENT

Hypothyroidism is treated with **levothyroxine (T_4)** replacement.

> **KEY FACT**
>
> In newborns, hypothyroidism causes **cretinism** (mental retardation, short stature, coarse features, umbilical hernia). Thyroid hormone deficiency during fetal development may be due to a failure of thyroid gland formation, inability to synthesize hormone (T_3/T_4), lack of iodine, radioiodine taken by the mother, or untreated hypothyroidism in the mother.

TABLE 2-13. Common Causes of Hypothyroidism

PRIMARY CAUSES	
Hashimoto thyroiditis	Autoimmune in origin (HLA-DR3 and -DR5). Antithyroid peroxidase antibodies confirm the diagnosis. Lymphocytic infiltrate with germinal centers seen on histology, as well as Hürthle cells. Increased risk for B-cell lymphoma
Subacute granulomatous (de Quervain) thyroiditis	Self-limited hypothyroidism following a flu-like illness. May have elevated ESR, jaw pain, and a tender thyroid gland. Histology shows granulomatous inflammation. Hyperthyroid earlier in course
Iodine deficiency	Most common cause in the developing world
Riedel thyroiditis	Rare disease in which thyroid tissue is chronically replaced by fibrosis. Rock-hard, fixed, painless goiter
Lithium	Lithium toxicity may cause hypothyroidism
Surgical resection and ^{131}I treatment	Surgical removal or radioactive iodine ablation may cause hypothyroidism
SECONDARY CAUSE	
Sheehan syndrome	Postpartum pituitary necrosis secondary to postpartum hemorrhage. Decreased TSH

ESR, erythrocyte sedimentation rate; HLA, human leukocyte antigen; TSH, thyroid-stimulating hormone.

TABLE 2-14.   **Signs and Symptoms of Abnormal Thyroid Hormone Levels**

	HYPERTHYROIDISM	HYPOTHYROIDISM
Symptoms	Hyperactivity, irritability	Mental sluggishness
	Heat intolerance, sweating	Cold intolerance
	Palpitations	Dyspnea
	Fatigue, weakness	Fatigue, weakness
	Diarrhea	Constipation
	Hair loss, oily skin	Hair loss, dry skin
	Oligomenorrhea, loss of libido	Menorrhagia, loss of libido
	Weight loss, robust appetite	Weight gain, poor appetite
	Polyuria	Paresthesias
Signs	Tachycardia	Bradycardia
	Tremor	Delayed deep tendon reflex relaxation phase
	Goiter	
	Warm, moist skin	Goiter
	Proximal muscle weakness	Dry, doughy skin
	Exopthalmos (Graves only)	Carpal tunnel syndrome
	Lid retraction, lid lag	Periorbital edema
		Puffy face, hands, and feet (myxedema)
		Peripheral edema
Lab findings	$\uparrow T_3$ and T_4	$\downarrow T_3$ and T_4
	Primary: $\downarrow$ TSH	Primary: $\uparrow$ TSH, TRH
	Secondary: $\uparrow$ TSH	Secondary: $\downarrow$ TSH
		Tertiary: $\downarrow$ TRH
	Anti-TSH receptor antibodies in Graves	Anti-TPO antibodies in Hashimoto

TPO, thyroperoxidase; TRH, thyroid-releasing hormone; TSH, thyroid-stimulating hormone.

Thyroid Neoplasms

Thyroid cancer is the most common endocrine malignancy in the United States, with an annual incidence of approximately 2 cases per 100,000. Risk factors include childhood head and neck radiation exposure, male gender, young age, and positive family history.

PRESENTATION

Typically presents as a solitary nodule. Dyspnea, coughing/choking spells, dysphagia, and hoarseness may occur due to compression of the trachea or esophagus.

DIAGNOSIS

- **Chemistries:** TSH (usually normal).
- **Thyroid ultrasound:** Large size (> 1–1.5 cm), irregular borders, hypoechogenicity, intranodular hypervascularity, and intranodular microcalcifications indicate increased risk for malignancy. Radioactive iodine thyroid scintiscanning should only be used if the TSH is low and a toxic nodule is suspected.
- **Fine-needle aspiration:** Provides cytopathologic diagnosis of four varieties of cancer (Table 2-15). Fifteen percent of nodules have suspicious or malignant pathology; the remainder are benign or indeterminate.

TREATMENT

Thyroidectomy for all thyroid cancers except anaplastic carcinoma. Potential complications include hypothyroidism, hypoparathyroidism, and damage to the recurrent laryngeal nerve.

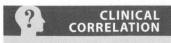

TABLE 2-15.   Types of Thyroid Cancer

TYPE	% (OF THYROID CANCERS)	CHARACTERISTICS	TREATMENT
Papillary carcinoma	70–80	■ History of radiation exposure increases risk ■ Slow-growing, spreads by lymphatics in the neck ■ "Orphan Annie" nuclei A (cells in papillary cancer have dispersed chromatin, giving appearance of empty nuclei) ■ Psammoma bodies (concentric calcification of individual necrotic tumor cells) ■ Related to *BRAF* activating mutation or *RET*/receptor tyrosine kinase activating mutations	Lobectomy or total thyroidectomy +/– radioiodine
Follicular carcinoma	10–20	■ More aggressive than papillary carcinomas ■ Tends to invade into blood vessels → spreads to bone, lung, and liver (lymph node involvement rare) ■ *RAS* oncogene mutation	Total thyroidectomy (prophylactic if *RET* mutation detected in childhood) +/– radioiodine
Medullary carcinoma	5	■ Arises from parafollicular "C" cells of thyroid ■ Produces calcitonin (can be used as tumor marker) ■ Amyloid deposits B (derived from altered calcitonin molecules) ■ Associated with the MEN 2A and MEN 2B syndromes ■ *RET* oncogene mutation	Total thyroidectomy (prophylactic if *RET* mutation detected in childhood)
Anaplastic carcinoma	5	■ Older patients ■ Highly aggressive. Poor prognosis (death within a few months)	Surgical resection of tumor in the neck, chemotherapy, and radiation

MEN, multiple endocrine neoplasia.

Multiple Endocrine Neoplasia

All the multiple endocrine neoplasia (MEN) syndromes are inherited in an autosomal dominant fashion. They are divided into three categories based on the oncogene and endocrine glands involved:

■ **MEN 1 (Wermer syndrome):** Tumors of the pancreas, pituitary, and parathyroid (the **3 Ps**) (Figure 2-16). May present with kidney stones secondary to hyperparathyroidism and GI ulcers secondary to gastrin-producing pancreatic adenomas (gastrinomas), which cause Zollinger-Ellison syndrome.
■ **MEN 2A (Sipple syndrome):** Medullary thyroid carcinoma, pheochromocytoma, and parathyroid adenoma.
■ **MEN 2B:** Medullary thyroid carcinoma, pheochromocytoma, and oral/GI ganglioneuromatosis (associated with marfanoid habitus).

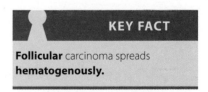

KEY FACT

Follicular carcinoma spreads **hematogenously.**

KEY FACT

MEN 1 arises from mutations in the self-named *men1* oncogene, whereas MEN 2A and 2B stem from mutations in the *ret* oncogene.

DRUGS FOR HYPOTHYROIDISM

Levothyroxine (T$_4$) is the principal pharmacologic agent used for hypothyroidism. Triiodothyronine (T$_3$) is not used routinely for the treatment of hypothyroidism because it is arrhythmogenic and can precipitate heart failure, although it may be used to treat myxedema coma.

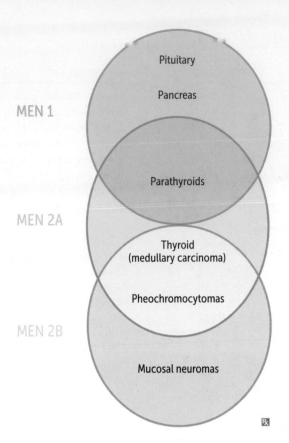

FIGURE 2-16. **Multiple endocrine neoplasias.** MEN 1 = 3 P's: pituitary, parathyroid, and pancreas. MEN 2A = 2 P's: parathyroids and pheochromocytoma. MEN 2B = 1 P: pheochromocytoma.

Levothyroxine

MECHANISM

T_4 analog, binds to nuclear receptors. Leads to increased protein synthesis, increased metabolic rate, and increased β-receptors → increased sensitivity to catecholamines.

USES

Hypothyroidism. Off-label/surreptitiously for weight loss.

SIDE EFFECTS

Signs and symptoms of hyperthyroidism (ie, tachycardia, heart failure, sweating, tremor, diarrhea).

ANTITHYROID DRUGS

Two main classes of drugs are used to treat hyperthyroidism: thioamides and iodine. Thioamides inhibit thyroid hormone synthesis. Excess iodine reduces thyroid synthesis and release (via the Wolff-Chaikoff effect) and radioiodine ablates cells that make thyroid hormone.

Thionamides (Methimazole, Propylthiouracil)

MECHANISM

Inhibit the enzyme **thyroid peroxidase,** which catalyzes the oxidation and organification of iodine in thyroid hormone synthesis; propylthiouracil (PTU) also inhibits peripheral conversion of T_4 to T_3 by 5′-deiodinase.

USES

Hyperthyroidism; PTU should be avoided as a first-line agent due to the potential for severe liver failure. In pregnant patients, PTU is used during the first trimester only. Methimazole is used only during the second and third trimesters in order to reduce its potential teratogenic effects in the first trimester.

SIDE EFFECTS

Rash, urticaria, fever, nausea; major effects include agranulocytosis, thrombocytopenia, acute hepatic necrosis, and vasculitis.

Iodine (Iodide and Radioiodine)

MECHANISM

Iodide is selectively concentrated in the thyroid gland for hormone synthesis; when given in large doses, it inhibits thyroid hormone release. Radioiodine (^{131}I) is also concentrated in the thyroid gland and emits beta and gamma radiation.

USES

Large doses of iodide are used for thyroid storm and before thyroidectomy for hyperthyroidism (to prevent thyroid storm). Radioiodine is used for hyperthyroidism and adjuvant treatment for some thyroid cancers.

SIDE EFFECTS

Metallic taste, excessive salivation, diarrhea, rash.

PARATHYROID GLAND

The parathyroid glands play an important role in calcium homeostasis and bone health, predominantly through involvement in calcium and phosphate metabolism.

- The main hormone that mediates these effects is **parathyroid hormone (PTH)**, which acts on the kidneys and bone. PTH increases serum calcium while decreasing serum phosphate concentrations.
- **Vitamin D** and **calcitonin** also play important roles in calcium homeostasis, as discussed later.

Anatomy

The parathyroid glands are four small, pea-sized structures attached to the posterior aspect of the thyroid gland, external to the fibrous thyroid capsule (Figure 2-17). The glands are anatomically separated into two superior and two inferior parathyroids. Both sets are supplied by the inferior thyroid arteries with venous drainage through the thyroid plexus of veins.

Embryology

The development of many parts of the head and neck stems from six branchial (or pharyngeal) arches, composed of mesoderm, that are lined by ectoderm and endoderm on opposite surfaces. These arches are divided by four invaginations of the ectoderm and endoderm; at these points, the ectoderm makes up branchial clefts, while the endoderm makes up branchial pouches (Figure 2-18). The point at which the ectoderm and endoderm meet is referred to as **branchial membranes.** All of these arches, clefts, and pouches develop into specific structures (Tables 2-16 through 2-18).

- Differentiation of the third branchial pouch takes place in the fifth and sixth weeks of gestation.
- The ventral wing of the third pouch gives rise to the thymus.

QUESTION

A 24-year-old man presents with weight loss, hyperactivity, diarrhea, and heat intolerance. Lab tests show high T$_3$ and T$_4$ and low TSH. A radioactive iodine uptake (RAIU) thyroid scan comes back negative, and the patient denies tenderness on thyroid palpation. What should you suspect is going on?

FLASH FORWARD

DiGeorge syndrome is a consequence of abnormal development of branchial pouches 3 and 4 due to chromosome 22q11.2 deletion. Clinical manifestations include hypocalcemia secondary to absence of the parathyroid glands, immune deficiency secondary to absence of thymic tissue leading to abnormal T-cell maturation, and congenital cardiac malformations.

KEY FACT

Branchial cysts are lesions found **lateral** to the midline of the neck. They result from failed obliteration of the temporary cervical sinuses. In contrast, **thyroglossal duct cysts,** found **medially,** result from failed obliteration of the thyroglossal duct as the thyroid gland migrates inferiorly during development.

ANSWER

The patient may be abusing levo-thyroxine. He is exhibiting signs of hyperthyroidism, which was confirmed by high thyroid hormones. Low TSH suggests a primary cause, but a negative RAIU scan and absence of a tender thyroid makes primary causes less likely (Table 2-12).

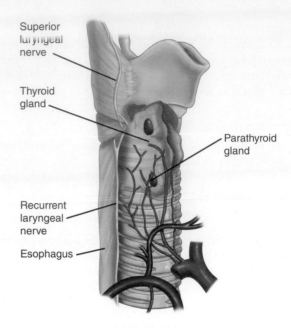

FIGURE 2-17. **Lateral view of trachea, thyroid gland, and parathyroids.**

KEY FACT

The **inferior** parathyroids are derived from the *third* branchial pouch, whereas the **superior** parathyroids are derived from the *fourth* branchial pouch, an apparent reversal of the rostrocaudal arrangement of these structures during development. This is due to the paired migration of the inferior parathyroids with the thymus, which facilitates enhanced caudal migration.

FLASH FORWARD

Ectopic parathyroid tissue results from abnormal migration. Ectopic parathyroids can be found in the anterior/posterior mediastinum, retroesophageal space, or even within the thyroid or thymus. Despite abnormal migration, the parathyroids typically remain symmetrical from side to side.

- The dorsal wing ultimately becomes the inferior parathyroids.
- By the seventh week of gestation, the third branchial pouch diverticulum elongates, ultimately allowing the developing thymus and inferior parathyroids to separate from the pharynx (Figure 2-19).
- The thymus migrates medially and caudally, pulling the inferior parathyroids until the thymus and parathyroids lose their connections to one another.
- The inferior parathyroids ultimately attach to the dorsal surface of the thyroid.
- The fourth branchial pouch, which gives rise to the superior parathyroids, follows a similar developmental course and timeline.
- The developing superior parathyroids do not migrate with another structure (ie, thymus), but rather travel a shorter distance before attaching to the dorsal surface of the thyroid.

Histology

The parathyroid glands are connective tissue–encapsulated structures that contain two populations of cells: **chief cells** and **oxyphil cells.**

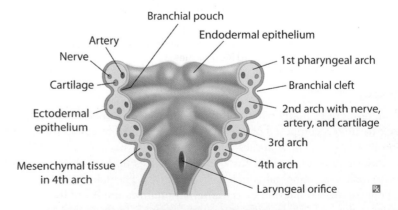

FIGURE 2-18. **Early development of branchial arches.**

TABLE 2-16. Branchial Pouch Derivatives

BRANCHIAL POUCH	DERIVATIVES
First pouch	Middle ear cavity (+ Eustachian tube), mastoid air cells
Second pouch	Epithelial lining of palatine tonsil
Third pouch (dorsal wing)	Inferior parathyroids
Third pouch (ventral wing)	Thymus
Fourth pouch	Superior parathyroids, thyroid gland C cells (derived from ultimobranchial body)

- Chief cells are predominant. They are small, polygonal cells with secretory granules containing PTH, arranged into curvilinear cords separated by capillaries.
- Oxyphil cells, which have an unknown function, are large cells containing abundant acidophilic mitochondria.

CALCIUM AND PHOSPHATE HOMEOSTASIS

Calcium plays an important role in numerous physiologic processes, ranging from muscle contraction to neuronal impulse transmission. Extracellular calcium concentrations are tightly regulated to protect against large fluctuations. Only 0.1% of total body calcium is found in the extracellular fluid (ECF). The vast majority of the remaining calcium, approximately 99%, is stored within bone (Figure 2-20).

- Forty percent of serum calcium is bound to plasma proteins. Hydrogen ions compete with calcium for binding sites on albumin and other proteins, so an increase in pH leads to increased calcium affinity.
- Ten percent of serum calcium is complexed with anions such as phosphate and citrate.
- Fifty percent of serum calcium is in a free, ionized form.

Only free calcium is biologically active. Like calcium, phosphate is involved in a range of physiologic processes. A very small quantity (1%) of total body phosphate is found in the extracellular space; most phosphate is in bone.

Calcium and phosphate homeostasis are regulated through the coordinated actions of three hormones: PTH, vitamin D, and calcitonin. These hormones control calcium and phosphate by acting on bone, intestine, and kidney.

TABLE 2-17. Branchial Clefts and Membranes

BRANCHIAL CLEFT	DERIVATIVES
First cleft	External auditory meatus
Second, third, and fourth clefts	Temporary cervical sinuses (normally obliterated)
BRANCHIAL MEMBRANE	**DERIVATIVES**
First membrane	Tympanic membrane
Second, third, and fourth membranes	Temporary structures (normally obliterated)

TABLE 2-18.   **Branchial Arches**

BRANCHIAL ARCH	DERIVATIVES (CARTILAGE)	DERIVATIVES (MUSCLE)	INNERVATION
1	Mandible, malleus, incus, sphenomandibular ligament	Muscles of mastication (temporalis, masseter, lateral/medial pterygoids), mylohyoid, anterior belly of the digastric, tensor tympani, tensor veli palatini, anterior two-thirds of the tongue	CN V_2 (maxillary) and V_3 (mandibular)
2	Stapes, styloid process, lesser horn of the hyoid, stylohyoid ligament	Stapedius, stylohyoid, posterior belly of the digastric, muscles of facial expression ("smilers")	CN VII
3	Greater horn of the hyoid	Stylopharyngeus, posterior one-third of the tongue	CN IX
4	Thyroid, cricoid, arytenoids, corniculate, cuneiform	Cricothyroid, levator veli palatini, pharyngeal constrictors	CN X (superior laryngeal branch)
5	No major developmental contributions		
6	Thyroid, cricoid, arytenoids, corniculate, cuneiform	All intrinsic muscles of larynx except the cricothyroid	CN X (recurrent laryngeal branch)

CN, cranial nerve.

Parathyroid Hormone

PTH is a polypeptide hormone synthesized and secreted by the parathyroid **chief cells.** The main function of PTH is to increase free serum calcium.

PTH is initially synthesized as a larger, inactive preprohormone. Proteolytic processing produces a final active hormone that is stored in secretory granules of chief cells. Despite

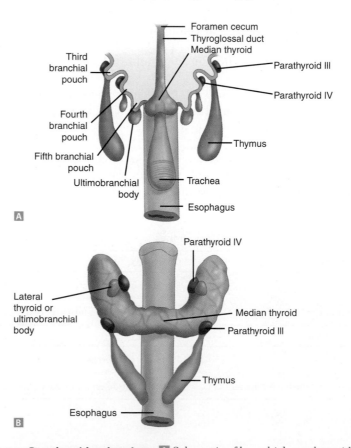

FIGURE 2-19.   Parathyroid embryology. **A** Schematic of branchial pouches with associated derivatives. **B** Migration of the inferior parathyroids.

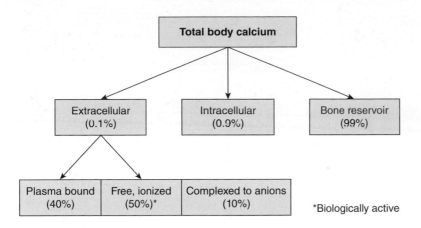

FIGURE 2-20.   **Distribution of total body calcium.**

rapid metabolism of PTH by the kidneys after secretion, smaller peptide fragments of the hormone retain full biological activity for hours.

PTH REGULATION

The stimuli for PTH release include serum calcium and magnesium levels.

- PTH secretion is inversely proportional to serum ionized calcium levels. Low serum calcium stimulates increased PTH secretion, whereas high serum calcium levels inhibit secretion.
- Mild decreases in magnesium stimulate PTH secretion. Severe hypomagnesemia, however, inhibits PTH secretion.

MECHANISMS OF ACTION

In order to affect serum calcium and phosphate levels, PTH alters bone turnover, renal tubule reabsorption, and vitamin D activation. Through these direct and indirect actions, PTH raises serum calcium levels and decreases serum phosphate levels (Figure 2-21). Because calcium and phosphate bind in serum, decreasing serum phosphate also increases free serum calcium. The specific actions include:

- **Increased bone resorption:** PTH stimulates both osteoclasts and osteoblasts (bone resorption > bone formation), leading to increased calcium and phosphate levels.
    - PTH enhances the activity of existing osteoclasts and also promotes the differentiation of new osteoclasts from progenitor cells by binding to receptors on osteoblasts, which then interact with osteoclasts via receptor activator of nuclear factor $\kappa\beta$ ligand (RANKL) and macrophage colony-stimulating factor (M-CSF).
    - Increased resorption from bone mineral leads to the release of both calcium and phosphate into the extracellular space.
- **Increased renal calcium reabsorption:** PTH stimulates the distal renal tubule to increase reabsorption of calcium.
- **Increased phosphate excretion:** In the proximal renal tubule, PTH inhibits phosphate reabsorption, leading to enhanced phosphate excretion.
- **Increased vitamin D activity increases intestinal Ca^{2+} absorption:** PTH increases the activity of 1α-hydroxylase in the kidney. This results in increased levels of $1,25\text{-}(OH)_2$ vitamin D (calcitriol). Calcitriol affects intestinal absorption of calcium and bone resorption (see next section). Thus, PTH, via its activation of vitamin D, also has an indirect effect on serum calcium levels.

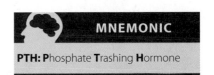

MNEMONIC

PTH: **P**hosphate **T**rashing **H**ormone

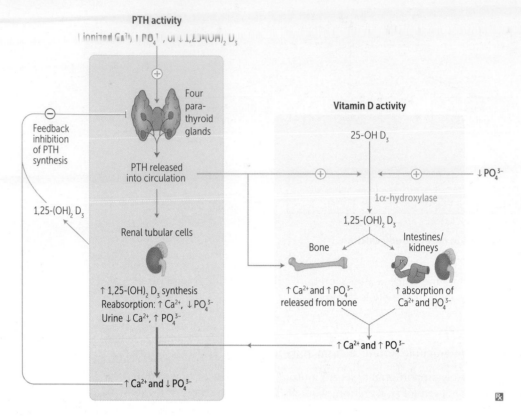

FIGURE 2-21.   **Actions of PTH and vitamin D in maintaining calcium and phosphate homeostasis.** $1,25\text{-}(OH)_2\, D_3$, 1,25-dihydroxyvitamin D_3; PTH, parathyroid hormone.

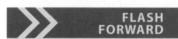

FLASH FORWARD

Vitamin D deficiency in children causes **rickets,** which is characterized by the inability to calcify newly formed bone matrix (osteoid) with consequent malformation (bowing) of long bones (Figure 2-22).

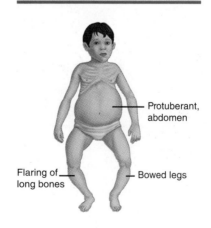

— Protuberant, abdomen

Flaring of long bones —

— Bowed legs

FIGURE 2-22.   **Clinical signs of rickets in a young boy.** Note the bowed legs, protuberant abdomen, and flaring of long bones.

Vitamin D

The chief forms of vitamin D are **ergocalciferol (vitamin D_2)** and **cholecalciferol (vitamin D_3).**

- Vitamin D_2 is produced by plant and fungal sources. It is not synthesized within the human body.
- Vitamin D_3 is produced by animal sources. Endogenous production also takes place in the skin. Specific wavelengths of UV light react with 7-dehydrocholesterol to produce vitamin D_3. Thus, sun exposure may help prevent vitamin D deficiency in certain individuals.

ACTIVATION

Following synthesis in the skin, cholecalciferol (vitamin D_3) is initially inactive. It must undergo a series of additional reactions in the liver and kidney to become biologically active (Figure 2-23).

- Cholecalciferol is first hydroxylated in the liver to form **25-hydroxycholecalciferol.** This is the storage form of vitamin D. It is also the level measured in clinical lab tests. 25-Hydroxycholecalciferol exerts negative feedback on this reaction in the liver.
- In the kidney, 25-hydroxycholecalciferol undergoes a second hydroxylation reaction catalyzed by **1α-hydroxylase.** The product of this reaction, **1,25-dihydroxychole-calciferol [$1,25\text{-}(OH)_2$ vitamin D],** is the active form of vitamin D, also referred to as **calcitriol.** 1α-Hydroxylase activity is upregulated by PTH, leading to increased vitamin D activity.
- Overall, PTH, low calcium, and low phosphate increase $1,25\text{-}(OH)_2$ vitamin D formation.

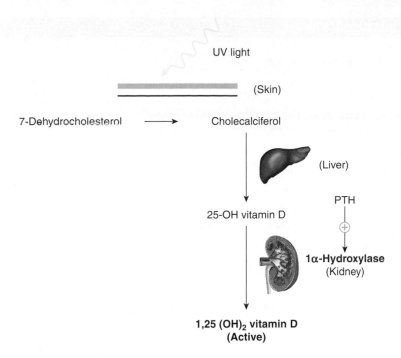

UV light

(Skin)

7-Dehydrocholesterol $\longrightarrow$ Cholecalciferol

(Liver)

25-OH vitamin D

PTH

1α-**Hydroxylase**
(Kidney)

1,25 (OH)$_2$ vitamin D
(Active)

FIGURE 2-23. **Activation of vitamin D.** PTH, parathyroid hormone; UV, ultraviolet.

ACTIONS

The active form of vitamin D (calcitriol) raises extracellular levels of calcium and phosphate and promotes the mineralization of bone. These metabolic changes are the result of effects on the intestine, kidneys, and bone:

- **Increases intestinal calcium and phosphate absorption:** 1,25-(OH)$_2$ vitamin D upregulates gene transcription of a calcium-binding protein (calbindin D-28K) in the intestinal brush border. This protein increases the absorption of dietary calcium.
- **Increases bone resorption of calcium and phosphate:** 1,25-(OH)$_2$ vitamin D is important for PTH-induced bone resorption. It is thought to facilitate this process by increasing calcium transport across membranes (similar to the mechanism in the intestine). Thus, at the level of bone, 1,25-(OH)$_2$ vitamin D promotes resorption of calcium and phosphate so they can be used for the mineralization of new bone.
- **Increases renal reabsorption of calcium and phosphate (minor effect):** 1,25-(OH)$_2$ vitamin D promotes increased reabsorption of both ions by the renal tubules. This effect is relatively minor and contributes little to the overall concentrations of extracellular calcium and phosphate.

Calcitonin

Calcitonin is a polypeptide secreted by the parafollicular, or C, cells of the thyroid gland. Although it promotes reduction in extracellular calcium through anti-PTH-like effects, calcitonin is not necessary for the maintenance of calcium homeostasis. Patients who have had their thyroid removed (eg, as treatment for thyroid cancer) show no changes in serum calcium concentrations despite the complete absence of calcitonin.

ACTIONS

Calcitonin is secreted in response to high serum calcium levels. It acts primarily on bone, decreasing the resorptive activity of osteoclasts. Calcitonin also has minor effects on the intestines and renal tubules aimed at decreasing extracellular calcium.

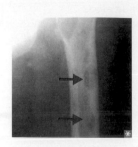

FIGURE 2-24. Osteitis fibrosa cystica.

MNEMONIC

Patients with hypercalcemia: "Stones, bones, groans, and psychiatric overtones."

MNEMONIC

Causes for hypercalcemia—
MISHAP
Malignancy
Intoxication with vitamin D
Sarcoidosis (see Chapter 5)
Hyperparathyroidism
Alkali (milk-alkali syndrome)
Paget disease (see Chapter 5)

CALCIUM DISORDERS

Primary Hyperparathyroidism

In primary hyperparathyroidism, excess secretion of PTH causes hypercalcemia. A benign parathyroid adenoma is responsible for 80% of cases, and parathyroid gland hyperplasia accounts for the remaining 20% of cases.

PRESENTATION

Usually asymptomatic. Incidentally discovered based on elevated calcium levels. When symptomatic, patient presents with renal, GI, or neurologic symptoms.

- **Renal:** Polyuria, hypercalciuria, renal calculi (calcium oxalate). If chronic, can lead to nephrocalcinosis, decreased GFR, and eventually renal failure.
- **Skeletal:** Bone pain. Increased PTH leads to increased osteoclastic activity → increased bone resorption and decreased bone mineral density. This can lead to osteitis fibrosa cystica, in which cystic spaces in bone are filled with brown fibrous tissue (Figure 2-24).
- **GI:** Nausea, vomiting, weight loss, constipation, anorexia, peptic ulcer disease, acute pancreatitis.
- **Neurologic:** Mental status changes, depression, fatigue.

In hypercalcemic crisis: Polyuria, dehydration, mental status changes.

DIAGNOSIS

- **Serum chemistry:** Increased Ca^{2+}, decreased phosphate; chloride is often elevated.
- **Endocrine:** Increased or inappropriately normal PTH.
- Also check PTH-related peptide (PTHrP), vitamin D levels, alkaline phosphatase, urine calcium. See below for other causes of hypercalcemia.
- **ECG:** Short QT interval.

TREATMENT

- Curative treatment is surgical exploration and parathyroidectomy of the adenomatous gland.
- If surgery is declined or not possible, treatment includes encouragement of adequate hydration. Can give diuretics (furosemide) to enhance calcium excretion. Avoid thiazide diuretics, as they can exacerbate hypercalcemia. Can also give bisphosphonates to inhibit bone loss, or calcitonin.

Other Causes of Hypercalcemia

- **Malignancy-induced hypercalcemia** can result from lytic bone metastases (eg, breast cancer) or tumor producing PTHrP, including squamous cell carcinoma of the lung and renal adenocarcinoma. PTH levels are low.
- **Vitamin D toxicity** secondary to granulomatous disease (sarcoidosis, tuberculosis), certain lymphomas or histoplasmosis. For example, in granulomatous disease, lymphocytes in the granulomas make 1α-hydroxylase → increased vitamin D → increased calcium resorption. PTH levels are low.
- **Familial hypocalciuric hypercalcemia (FHH):** Autosomal dominant disorder caused by a mutation in calcium-sensing receptors on the parathyroid glands → leads to inappropriate secretion of PTH → mild hypercalcemia. Unlike other causes of hypercalcemia, urinary calculi and renal failure are not seen in cases of FHH.
- **Thiazide diuretics:** Increase renal reabsorption of calcium in the distal tubule.
- **Milk-alkali syndrome:** Ingestion of excessive amounts of calcium-based antacids.
- **Increased bone turnover:** Vitamin A toxicity, hyperthyroidism, immobilization.

Primary Hypoparathyroidism

Causes, from most to least common: hypoparathyroidism following thyroid surgery, in which the surgeon accidentally removes or otherwise injures the parathyroid glands, autoimmune gland failure, gland infiltration, pseudohypoparathyroidism due to PTH end-organ resistance, and **DiGeorge syndrome** (failure of the third and fourth pharyngeal pouches to develop).

PRESENTATION

Neuromuscular excitability due to hypocalcemia.

- Muscle fatigue and weakness.
- Numbness and tingling around the mouth, hands, and feet.
- Tetany: **Chvostek sign** (tapping of the facial nerve in front of the ear → upper lip and facial muscles contract); **Trousseau sign** (inflation of a blood pressure (BP) cuff to a pressure higher than systolic BP → carpal spasms).
- Laryngeal spasm.
- Basal ganglia calcifications (can cause parkinsonian symptoms). The ocular lens can also be calcified, leading to cataracts.
- Depression, psychosis.

DIAGNOSIS

- **Serum chemistry:** Low or inappropriately normal PTH with low Ca²⁺. Check albumin, vitamin D, Mg²⁺, alkaline phosphatase, and urine calcium as well. See Table 2-19 for lab differential of hypocalcemia.
- **ECG:** Increased QT interval.
- **Imaging:** Basal ganglia calcifications.

TREATMENT

Calcium supplements, vitamin D supplements (calcitriol), and intravenous (IV) calcium gluconate for acute symptoms.

Other Causes of Hypocalcemia

- **Pseudohypoparathyroidism:** End-organ resistance to PTH (kidney and bones do not respond to PTH). Patients may have **Albright hereditary osteodystrophy,** characterized by short stature, shortening of the fourth and fifth metacarpals, and mild mental retardation.
- **Hypoalbuminemia** causes a decrease in total calcium, but ionized calcium levels are normal. There are no clinical signs of calcium deficiency.
- **Severe hypomagnesemia** leads to decreased PTH synthesis and release, as well as end-organ resistance to PTH.
- **Calcium sequestration:** Enzymatic fat necrosis uses up calcium. Most commonly a result of acute pancreatitis. Other conditions that lead to calcium sequestration

CLINICAL CORRELATION

In the case of parathyroid hyperplasia, the surgeon removes three of the four parathyroid glands and autotransplants (reimplants) the remaining gland into the patient's forearm to avoid hypoparathyroidism.

MNEMONIC

Chvostek sign: Tap the **ch**eek;
Trousseau sign: Cuff the **tr**iceps.

KEY FACT

Correcting for serum albumin is critical to interpreting total calcium levels.

Free calcium = 0.8 × (4.0 − serum albumin) + serum Ca²⁺

TABLE 2-19.   Summary of Calcium Disorders

	SERUM CALCIUM	SERUM PHOSPHATE	PTH
Primary hyperparathyroidism	↑	↓	↑
Malignancy-induced hypercalcemia (PTHrP)	↑	↓	↓
Primary hypoparathyroidism	↓	↑	↓
Pseudohypoparathyroidism	↓	↑	↑/normal

PTH, parathyroid hormone; PTHrP, PTH-related peptide.

include citrate excess after blood transfusions and acute increases in PO_4 due to rhabdomyolysis, tumor lysis, or acute renal failure.

■ **Renal osteodystrophy** is a consequence of **secondary hyperparathyroidism** resulting from the death of proximal tubule cells in renal failure patients.
  ■ Loss of these cells results in decreased vitamin D activation by 1α-hydroxylase.
  ■ The kidneys have decreased ability to excrete phosphate, resulting in hyperphosphatemia.
  ■ In response, the chief cells of the parathyroid glands produce excess PTH, resulting in excess bone resorption. Serum calcium levels are typically low or low-normal in secondary hyperparathyroidism.

CALCIUM DRUGS

Bisphosphonates (eg, Alendronate)

MECHANISM

Stabilizes bony matrix, coats hydroxyapatite to prevent osteoclasts from resorbing bone.

USES

Treatment of **postmenopausal osteoporosis** and in Paget disease to reduce bone turnover. Prevention of accelerated bone loss in patients on long-term, high-dose glucocorticoid therapy.

SIDE EFFECTS

Heartburn, erosive esophagitis, stomach upset, joint/back pain, osteonecrosis of the jaw.

Calcitonin

MECHANISM

Lowers serum calcium, has mild analgesic properties for bone pain.

ADMINISTRATION

Intranasal, subcutaneous.

USES

Hypercalcemic states.

SIDE EFFECTS

Runny nose, nasal discomfort, flushing.

Calcitriol

MECHANISM

Activated form of vitamin D; increases calcium absorption from intestines.

USES

Hypocalcemia, vitamin D replacement in patients with end-stage renal disease.

SIDE EFFECTS

Signs and symptoms of vitamin D intoxication include hypercalcemia, polyuria, weakness, headache, somnolence, and constipation.

Adrenal Gland

One important function of the adrenal (or suprarenal) gland is to coordinate the body's response to physiologic stress. The gland is anatomically and functionally divided into two parts: the adrenal medulla (core) and outer adrenal cortex.

The adrenal medulla is a functional extension of the sympathetic nervous system, secreting the catecholamines epinephrine and norepinephrine into systemic circulation.

In contrast, the adrenal cortex synthesizes steroid hormones, which have diverse functions, ranging from stress responses (**cortisol**) to control of water and electrolyte balance (**aldosterone**) to androgenizing effects (**testosterone, dehydroepiandrosterone [DHEA] sulfate**).

ANATOMY

The triangular-shaped adrenals sit atop the superoanterior aspects of the kidneys, where they are encased in a capsule of fat and connective tissue (Figure 2-25).

- The vascular supply to the adrenal glands consists of three sets of arteries:
  - **Superior adrenal arteries,** which branch off the inferior phrenic artery.
  - **Middle adrenal arteries,** which originate from the abdominal aorta adjacent to the celiac trunk.
  - **Inferior adrenal arteries,** which branch off the renal artery.
- The venous drainage of the adrenal gland differs between the two sides.
  - Left adrenal → left adrenal vein → left renal vein → inferior vena cava (IVC)
  - Right adrenal → right adrenal vein → IVC

EMBRYOLOGY

The adrenal cortex and medulla differ in their embryologic origins (Figure 2-26).

FLASH FORWARD

Corticotropin-releasing hormone (CRH) secreted from the hypothalamus regulates ACTH secretion from the anterior pituitary (basophils), which regulates adrenal gland size and steroid hormone synthesis. Cortisol negatively feeds-back to inhibit and thereby regulate the level of ACTH produced. CRH → ACTH → Adrenal gland size/ hormone synthesis Cortisol ⊣ ACTH.

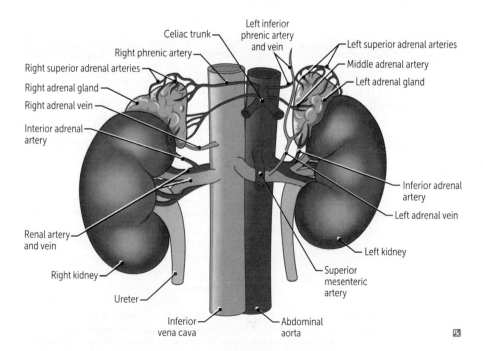

FIGURE 2-25.   Anatomy and blood supply of adrenal glands.

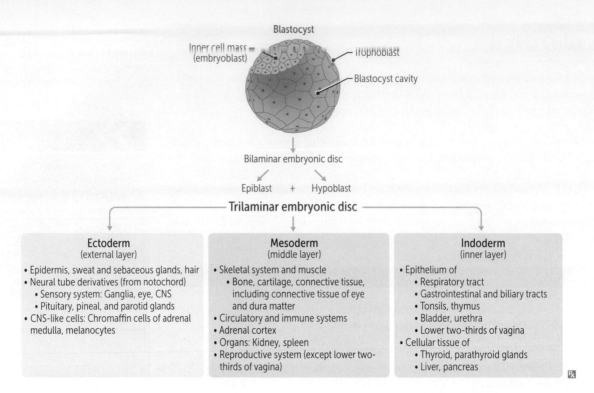

FIGURE 2-26. **Germ layer derivatives.** During week 1 of embryogenesis, the zygote mitotically divides to form the morula, then the blastocyst. The blastocyst consists of an outer and inner cell mass. The outer cell mass (ie, trophoblast) becomes the placenta, while the inner cell mass becomes the embryo. During week 3, the inner cell mass has divided into a trilaminar embryonic disc, consisting of three basic germ cell layers: ectoderm, mesoderm, and endoderm. Neuroectoderm (formed via the notochord's interaction with the ectoderm above it) forms the neural plate, which produces the neural tube and neural crest cells. Germ cell layers form all organs and tissue.

FLASH FORWARD

Pheochromocytoma is a rare neoplasm formed from chromaffin cells in the adrenal medulla (90%) or extra-adrenal sites (10%). It is the most common tumor of the adrenal medulla in adults.

- **Adrenal cortex:** Derived from mesoderm.
- **Adrenal medulla:** Derived from neural crest cells, which migrate to the adrenal medulla, where they differentiate into chromaffin cells; these neuroendocrine cells are similar to postganglionic sympathetic neurons (they secrete epinephrine and norepinephrine).

HISTOLOGY

The adrenal cortex is further divided into three distinct layers (Table 2-20).

- **Zona glomerulosa:** A relatively thin external layer (15% of the cortex) composed of cells containing the enzyme aldosterone synthase. Consequently, the zona glomeru-

TABLE 2-20.   Adrenal Gland Summary

REGION	HORMONE	CONTROLLED BY	LOSS LEADS TO . . .
Glomerulosa	Aldosterone	Angiotensin II, potassium	Hyponatremia, hypovolemia, hyperkalemia
Fasciculata	Cortisol	ACTH	Decreased ability to compensate for physiologic stress, decreased ability to mobilize glucose
Reticularis	Androgens	ACTH	Gynecomastia, delayed onset of puberty (in males); not a major androgen contributor

ACTH, adrenocorticotropic hormone.

losa is the only layer that is capable of producing appreciable quantities of the mineralocorticoid **aldosterone.**

- **Zona fasciculata:** The largest layer (75% of the cortex) composed of cells that primarily synthesize and secrete **glucocorticoids** (cortisol).
- **Zona reticularis:** The deepest layer (10% of the cortex) composed of cells that primarily synthesize adrenal **androgens** (dehydroepiandrosterone [DHEA] and androstenedione).

STEROID HORMONE SYNTHESIS

Cholesterol Acquisition

Steroid hormones of the adrenal cortex are synthesized using cholesterol as the precursor. Approximately 20% of this cholesterol is produced de novo within adrenal cortical cells; the remainder is acquired from circulating low-density lipoproteins (LDL). LDL molecules are internalized via endocytosis then hydrolyzed within lysosomes to produce free cholesterol within the cell.

Synthetic Pathways

Free cholesterol within adrenal cortical cells is transported to mitochondria.

- The initial step in steroid hormone synthesis is rate limiting and conserved across all layers of adrenal cortex. In this reaction, the rate-limiting enzyme (RLE), cholesterol desmolase, converts cholesterol to pregnenolone (Figure 2-27). ACTH and angiotensin II stimulate this conversion.
- 3-β-Hydroxysteroid dehydrogenase and **21-hydroxylase**, and 11-β-hydroxylase are all required for aldosterone and cortisol synthesis.

FLASH FORWARD

Neuroblastoma is a neoplasm formed from neural crest cells that may be found anywhere along the sympathetic chain, including the adrenal medulla. It is the most common tumor of the adrenal gland in children.

MNEMONIC

GFR (glomerulosa, fasciculata, reticularis) corresponds with **S**alt (Na⁺), **S**ugar (glucocorticoids), and **S**ex (androgens): "The deeper you go, the sweeter it gets."

Q   QUESTION

Recall the difference between the left and right adrenal gland blood supply.

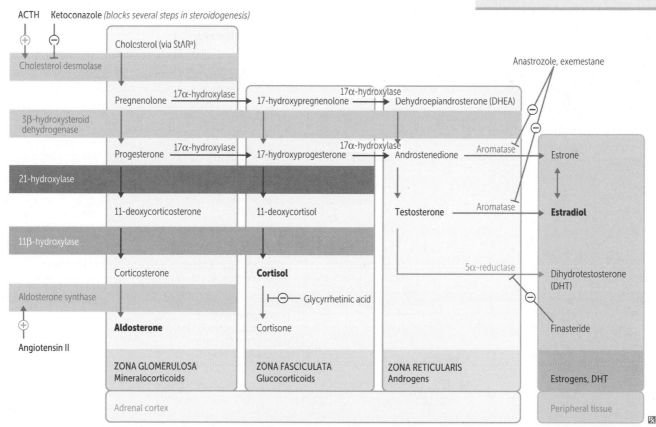

ªRate-limiting step.

FIGURE 2-27.   Steroid hormone synthetic pathways. ACTH, adrenocorticotropic hormone; StAR, steroidogenic acute regulatory protein.

- **17-α-Hydroxylase** and 17,20-lyase are both required to convert pregnenolone into DHEA and progesterone into androstenedione.
- The ultimate products are aldosterone (zona glomerulosa), cortisol (zona fasciculata), and weak androgens (zona reticularis).

GLUCOCORTICOIDS

Glucocorticoid Synthesis and Regulation

The hypothalamus, anterior pituitary, and adrenal cortex interact to coordinate glucocorticoid synthesis. Hypoglycemia, trauma, illness, fever, and physical exertion trigger the hypothalamus to secrete CRH.

- CRH stimulates corticotrophs of the anterior pituitary to release ACTH (Figure 2-28).
- ACTH upregulates desmolase, the RLE in cholesterol and pregnenolone synthesis, which, in turn, makes it the RLE in cortisol synthesis. ACTH also promotes gland hypertrophy.
- A negative feedback system is employed in which ACTH and CRH stimulate cortisol production and high cortisol levels feedback to inhibit ACTH and CRH secretion (Figure 2-28).

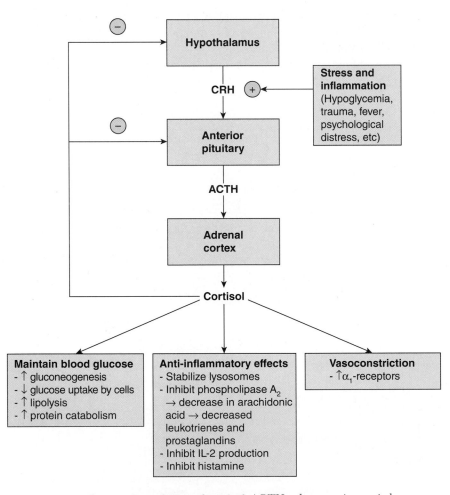

FIGURE 2-28. **Effects and regulation of cortisol.** ACTH, adrenocorticotropic hormone; CRH, corticotropin-releasing hormone; IL-2, interleukin-2.

Endogenous Glucocorticoids

Glucocorticoids, so named for their effects on blood glucose levels, are now recognized for a diverse set of actions including alterations of immune function, bone turnover, and cardiovascular function.

- **Cortisol:** Predominant glucocorticoid (provides 95% of endogenous glucocorticoid activity); chronic stress results in prolonged secretion; high potency; produced in zone fasciculata (see Table 2-21 for overview of stress hormones).
- **11-Deoxycortisol:** Immediate precursor to cortisol (provides < 5% of endogenous glucocorticoid activity); low potency.
- **Synthetic (exogenous) corticosteroids:** Hydrocortisone, prednisone, methyl-prednisolone, and dexamethasone. Synthetic glucocorticoids with various potencies relative to cortisol.

Actions of Cortisol

Cortisol plays multiple roles in maintaining homeostasis, influencing the immune response, intermediary metabolism, vascular tone, and, to a limited extent, renal function.

- **Promotes energy mobilization via gluconeogenesis:** Cortisol effectively increases blood glucose concentration. Cortisol reduces the uptake of glucose into cells, while increasing the amount of substrate (gluconeogenic amino acids and glycerol) for gluconeogenesis in the liver. Cortisol does so by stimulating lipolysis and protein catabolism, leading to the mobilization of fatty acids and amino acids, respectively (see Figure 2-28).
- **Anti-inflammatory effects:** Cortisol both prevents inflammation and reduces existing inflammatory conditions.
    - Inhibits production of leukotrienes and prostaglandins by promoting synthesis of lipocortin, an inhibitor of phospholipase A_2. Phospholipase A_2 normally supplies arachadonic acid for leukotriene and prostanglandin synthesis. As a result, there is a decrease in capillary permeability and leukocyte recruitment to inflamed tissue.
    - Stabilizes lysosomal membranes to prevent rupture and minimize release of proteolytic enzymes.
    - Decreases production of inflammatory cytokines (eg, tumor necrosis factor-alpha [TNF-α]), leading to reduction in macrophage activation.
    - Suppresses adaptive immune system function by inhibiting production of inter-leukin-2 (IL-2), a cytokine that encourages T-cell proliferation. Other cytokines are also disrupted in response to cortisol.

> **KEY FACT**
>
> Cortisol promotes gluconeogenesis and suppresses inflammation (via inhibition of phospholipase A_2 [PLA$_2$]) under conditions of physiologic stress.

TABLE 2-21. Stress Hormones

GH	<ul><li>Increases lipolysis in adipose tissue</li><li>Promotes protein synthesis</li></ul>
Glucagon	<ul><li>Increases lipolysis in adipose tissue</li><li>Stimulates glycogenolysis</li><li>Promotes gluconeogenesis</li></ul>
Cortisol	<ul><li>Increases lipolysis in adipose tissue</li><li>Stimulates gluconeogenesis</li><li>Upregulates vascular adrenergic (α_1) receptors</li></ul>
Epinephrine	<ul><li>Increases lipolysis in adipose tissue</li><li>Promotes glycogenolysis</li><li>Vasoconstriction (via α receptors)</li></ul>

GH, growth hormone.

- Blocks histamine release from mast cells and serotonin release from platelets, thereby inhibiting allergic reactions.
  - **Adrenergic receptor upregulation:** Cortisol helps smooth muscle maintain responsiveness to the vasoconstrictive effects of norepinephrine by upregulating α_1-adrenergic receptors on vascular smooth muscle cells. Cortisol also contributes to vascular tone through inhibition of nitric oxide synthase, decreasing the production of the vasodilator nitric oxide. Cortisol can increase blood pressure in these ways.
  - **Mineralocorticoid activity:** Its mineralocorticoid effects are normally negligible relative to its marked glucocorticoid activity (because it is inactivated by renal 11β-hydroxysteroid dehydrogenase); however, in disease states characterized by very high concentrations, cortisol can exert a potent mineralocorticoid effect by binding to mineralocorticoid (aldosterone) receptors (see Table 2-22 for an overview of abnormal cortisol states).

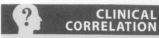

CLINICAL CORRELATION

11β-hydroxysteroid dehydrogenase type II may be inhibited by glycyrrhizic acid (found in licorice), leading to syndrome of apparent mineralocorticoid excess.

FLASH FORWARD

Cushing syndrome is characterized by a classic clinical picture: hypertension, central obesity, weight gain, moon facies, insulin resistance, skin thinning/purple striae, buffalo hump, hirsutism, osteoporosis, and amenorrhea.

MINERALOCORTICOIDS

Mineralocorticoid Synthesis and Regulation

ACTH promotes aldosterone synthesis (see Figure 2-27 for its synthetic pathway); however, it does not significantly affect the rate of secretion. The rate of aldosterone secretion is influenced by changes in ECF volume, arterial pressures, and sodium and potassium concentrations in the ECF. Key determinants of aldosterone secretion are:

- **High serum potassium** increases secretion.
- The **renin-angiotensin-aldosterone system** (RAAS) increases secretion.
- **High serum sodium** decreases secretion (minimally).

Actions of Aldosterone

Aldosterone has three major and related effects (Figure 2-29): Increased sodium reabsorption, increased BP, and increased potassium and hydrogen ion excretion.

- **Increased sodium reabsorption:** Aldosterone stimulates the synthesis of new sodium channels in the principal cells of the kidney's collecting tubules. These additional sodium channels promote sodium reabsorption and reduce sodium excretion in the urine.
- **Increased arterial pressure:** Aldosterone increases total sodium reabsorption, but does not significantly alter serum sodium concentration. This is because water is also reabsorbed by the collecting tubules. The net effect is an **increase in extracellular volume,** which, over time, can cause arterial pressure to rise.
- **Increased potassium secretion:** Aldosterone induces the opening of large numbers of sodium and potassium channels in the principal cells of the kidney's collecting ducts. Enhanced sodium reabsorption is accompanied by increased potassium secretion into the tubule lumen.

TABLE 2-22. Abnormal Cortisol States

DISORDER	CORTISOL	ACTH
Primary hypercortisolism (cortisol-producing tumor)	↑	↓
Pituitary hypersecretion of ACTH (Cushing disease)	↑	↑
Primary adrenal insufficiency (Addison disease)	↓	↑
Secondary adrenal insufficiency	↓	↓

ACTH, adrenocorticotropic hormone.

KEY FACT

Activation of the RAAS and high serum potassium are the major stimuli for the release of aldosterone from the adrenal cortex.

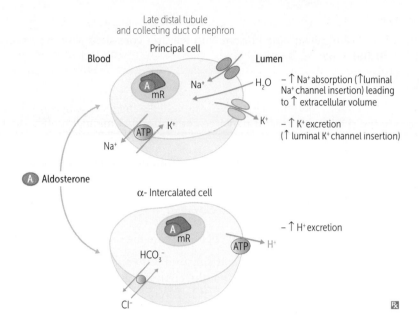

FIGURE 2-29. **Effects of aldosterone.** ATP, adenosine triphosphate.

- **Increased hydrogen (H⁺) secretion:** Aldosterone increases H⁺ secretion from α-intercalated cells into the lumen of distal tubules and collecting ducts for excretion (H⁺ dumping) by increasing H⁺ ATPase activity on the lumen side. This results in increased HCO_3^-/Cl^- exchanger activity on the interstitia/blood side, leading to increased HCO_3^- release into the blood (overall alkalinizing effect).

ADRENAL ANDROGENS

Adrenal androgens (androstenedione, DHEA, and dehydroepiandrosterone sulfate [DHEA-S]) play important roles during several periods of development:

- **Fetal development:** Androgens and estrogens are produced in the placenta from precursors (eg, DHEA-S) made by the maternal and fetal adrenal glands, since the placenta cannot synthesize cholesterol and therefore cannot produce sex steroids de novo.
- **Adrenarche:** Stage of adrenal maturation during which weak adrenal androgens are converted peripherally into the potent androgens, testosterone and dihydrotestosterone (DHT) (Figure 2-27). These androgens play important roles in secondary sexual differentiation and pubic and axillary hair growth.
- **Menopause:** Period after which ovaries no longer produce estrogen. However, androstenedione is produced by the ovaries and adrenal glands and is converted to estrone, a weak estrogen, via the enzyme aromatase (Figure 2-27).

DISORDERS OF THE ADRENAL GLAND

Cushing Syndrome

Cushing syndrome refers to the signs and symptoms of excess cortisol and is most commonly caused by exogenous glucocorticoid therapy. Other causes include pituitary adenomas (Cushing disease; excess ACTH from the pituitary → bilateral adrenal hyperplasia), adrenocortical tumors, and ectopic ACTH production (small-cell carcinoma of the lung, bronchial carcinoid tumors).

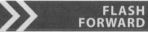

FLASH FORWARD

Hyperaldosteronism (Conn syndrome) is characterized by **hypertension** with hypernatremia, **hypokalemia,** and metabolic alkalosis (due to excessive H⁺ dumping). Primary hyperaldosteronism is usually due to an adrenal adenoma, while secondary hyperaldosteronism is related to pathology causing the upstream activation of RAAS.

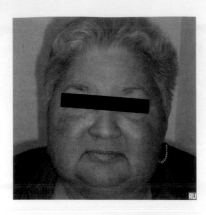

FIGURE 2-30. **Presentation of Cushing syndrome.** Note the swelling of the face into a rounded shape–Cushingoid "moon face."

FLASH FORWARD

Because patients with **11β-hydroxylase deficiency** lack an enzyme in the adrenal steroid synthetic pathway (see Figure 2-27), they cannot produce normal levels of cortisol and aldosterone. The steroid precursors are shunted into the production of excessive quantities of sex hormones. Consequently, patients with 11β-hydroxylase deficiency are **hypertensive,** and females are **virilized.**

PRESENTATION

Patients with Cushing syndrome present with features consistent with excess cortisol (Figure 2-30 and Table 2-23).

DIAGNOSIS

To screen for Cushing syndrome, a low-dose overnight dexamethasone (a cortisol analog) suppression test (DST), 24-urine urinary free cortisol, and/or midnight salivary cortisol may be performed.

- Normally, in a low-dose DST, ACTH release from the pituitary gland is decreased, resulting in suppression of cortisol release.
- In Cushing syndrome, cortisol levels are not suppressed. 24-hour urinary free cortisol and late night salivary cortisol are also elevated.

After hypercortisolemia is confirmed, ACTH levels are measured (Figure 2-31).

- Low ACTH levels indicate hypercortisolism due to an adrenal tumor secreting cortisol on its own and cause atrophy of the opposite tumor-free adrenal gland.
- High ACTH indicates ACTH-dependent hypercortisolism and results in bilateral adrenal hyperplasia.

If ACTH is high, a high-dose DST or CRH stimulation test is performed.

- Cortisol suppression with a high-dose DST indicates an ACTH-secreting pituitary adenoma (Cushing disease).
- If a high-dose DST does not suppress cortisol, ACTH is being produced ectopically (eg, small-cell lung cancer) and therefore does not respond/feed back to dexamethasone in the high-dose DST (Table 2-24).

TREATMENT

Tumor removal; ketoconazole or metyrapone to lower cortisol levels.

Primary Hyperaldosteronism (Conn Syndrome)

Conn syndrome is caused by excess secretion of aldosterone, resulting in increased sodium reabsorption and increased hydrogen (H^+) and potassium (K^+) secretion. Pri-

TABLE 2-23. **Cushing Syndrome Presentation**

SYMPTOMS	CAUSE
Central obesity, moon facies, buffalo hump, weight gain	Cortisol-induced increases in glucose leading to high insulin → increased fat storage
Hypertension	Cortisol-induced adrenergic receptor up-regulation and mineralocorticoid effects
Glucose intolerance, hyperglycemia	Decreased peripheral glucose utilization, increased hepatic gluconeogenesis
Purple striae, thinning skin	Cortisol-induced decreases in collagen synthesis
Proximal muscle wasting and weakness	Use of amino acids for cortisol-induced gluconeogenesis in the liver
Osteoporosis	Bone resorption > bone formation
Immunosuppresion	Cortisol-induced decreases in inflammatory responses
Depression, mania	Unknown, but likely due to high cortisol changing brain morphology

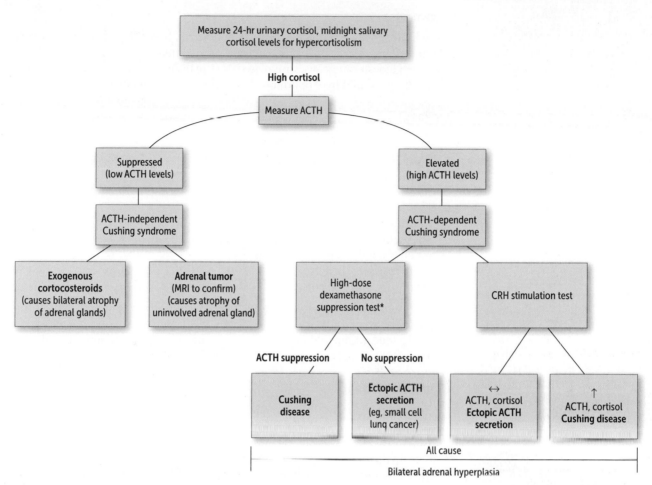

FIGURE 2-31. Diagnosis of Cushing syndrome. ACTH, adrenocorticotropic hormone; CRH, corticotropin-releasing hormone.

* A low-dose overnight dexamethasone suppression test can be performed initially to see if high morning cortisol levels are lowered.

mary aldosteronism is most commonly due to a benign adenoma in the zona glomerulosa. Secondary causes include:

- Renin-secreting tumors, renovascular disease such as renal artery stenosis, and malignant hypertension.
- Edematous state with decreased arterial volume (congestive heart failure [CHF], cirrhosis, nephrotic syndrome), leading to RAAS activation.
- Diuretics.
- Excess nonaldosterone mineralocorticoid due to exogenous mineralocorticoids, CAH, and excessive ingestion of licorice (leads to build-up of precursors of cortisol).

TABLE 2-24. Summary of Cushing Syndrome

	SERUM/URINE CORTISOL	ACTH	HIGH-DOSE DEXAMETHASONE TEST
Pituitary Cushing (Cushing disease)	↑	↑	Cortisol suppressed
Adrenal Cushing	↑	↓	Not performed (already know ACTH is low)
Ectopic Cushing (small cell lung cancer)	↑	↑	Cortisol not suppressed

PRESENTATION

- Sodium and water retention causes hypertension. Severe hypokalemia causes symptoms of muscle weakness and can cause arrhythmia.
- Excess aldosterone causes increased Na^+ reabsorption and increased K^+ and H^+ secretion → mild hypernatremia, hypokalemia, and metabolic alkalosis.

DIAGNOSIS

Screen for hypertension.

- **Serum chemistry:** Mildly increased Na^+, decreased K^+ and increased bicarbonate.
- **Hormones:** Aldosterone is elevated in both primary and secondary hyperaldosteronism. Renin is suppressed in primary hyperaldosteronism, but elevated in secondary hyperaldosteronism.
- **Sodium suppression test:** Sodium-load patient and then measure for appropriate aldosterone suppression. Infusion of saline normally decreases aldosterone levels but does not do so in Conn syndrome.

TREATMENT

Surgery to remove the adenoma in the adrenal gland. If the patient is a poor surgical candidate or suffers from bilateral adrenal hyperplasia, medical management is preferred. Spironolactone inhibits aldosterone action on the kidneys. Other antihypertensives can also be used to manage the patient's high BP.

Adrenal Insufficiency

Adrenal insufficiency results from adrenal gland failure and is most commonly due to autoimmune destruction of the adrenal glands. Primary adrenal insufficiency is termed **Addison disease.** Primary causes include infection (TB, cytomegalovirus, histoplasmosis, or disseminated meningococcemia in **Waterhouse-Friderichsen syndrome**), vascular disorders (hemorrhage or infarction), metastasis, infiltrative disease (hemochromatosis, amyloidosis, or sarcoidosis), and drugs such as ketoconazole and rifampin. Secondary adrenal insufficiency is characterized by decreased ACTH production as a result of hypopituitarism, whereas tertiary adrenal insufficiency results from the abrupt withdrawal of corticosteroids or from decreased CRH production.

PRESENTATION

- Most commonly manifests as weakness, fatigue, anorexia, nausea/vomiting, orthostasis, hyponatremia, and hypoglycemia, which stem from decreased cortisol and mineralocorticoid deficiency.
- Increased ACTH in primary adrenal insufficiency (due to lack of cortisol feedback) leads to skin and mucosal hyperpigmentation (due to increased MSH, derived from proopiomelanocortin [POMC], the precursor to ACTH synthesis); decreased aldosterone leads to hypotension (due to salt loss), hyponatremia, hypovolemia, hypoperfusion, and hyperkalemia.
- Tertiary adrenal insufficiency and decreased pituitary production of ACTH in secondary adrenal insufficiency do not cause skin/mucosal hyperpigmentation, or hyperkalemia, or affect aldosterone synthesis.

DIAGNOSIS

- **ACTH stimulation testing:** Administer ACTH IV to stimulate cortisol. Normally, the adrenal gland increases its production of cortisol in response to ACTH. In primary and chronic secondary or tertiary adrenal insufficiency, cortisol production does not increase considerably when ACTH is given.
- **Serum chemistry:** Decreased Na^+, increased K^+ (in primary adrenal insufficiency), decreased glucose.
- **Endocrine:** Decreased cortisol levels; ACTH may be elevated (primary), or normal/decreased (secondary or tertiary).

KEY FACT

Waterhouse-Friderichsen syndrome: hemorrhagic necrosis of the adrenal glands, usually due to disseminated intravascular coagulopathy (DIC) related to a *Neisseria meningitidis* infection (more frequently in children/young).

A ANSWER

Corticosteroids (treatment for SLE that suppresses the immune system/reduces inflammation and therefore many symptoms of SLE); bilateral adrenal atrophy.

- **Metyrapone stimulation test:** Administer metyrapone (blocks final step in cortisol synthesis) to lower cortisol in an attempt to increase ACTH response; in secondary and tertiary adrenal insufficiency, there is no change in ACTH levels.

TREATMENT

Treatment for Addison disease involves replacement of glucocorticoids and mineralocorticoids. Treatment of secondary and tertiary hypocortisolism requires only glucocorticoids.

Congenital Adrenal Hyperplasia

CAH is a group of autosomal recessive disorders that cause cortisol deficiency. This results in increased ACTH production and bilateral adrenal gland hyperplasia (Table 2-25).

TREATMENT

Glucocorticoids prevent excess ACTH secretion from the pituitary gland.

Pheochromocytoma

Pheochromocytoma is a catecholamine-producing tumor that arises from chromaffin cells, which are mainly located in the adrenal medulla (10% are extra-adrenal). Pheochromocytoma may be associated with multiple endocrine neoplasia (MEN) types 2A and 2B, neurofibromatosis, and von Hippel-Lindau syndrome.

PRESENTATION

Hypertension, palpitations, anxiety, weight loss, and headaches—all occurring in an episodic fashion.

DIAGNOSIS

- 24-h urinary metanephrines, vanillylmandelic acid, and catecholamines, or plasma free metanephrines and catecholamines.
- Clonidine suppression test → if above tests are equivocal, clonidine normally decreases catecholamines, but they remain elevated in patients with pheochromocytoma.

KEY FACT

Congenital adrenal hyperplasia:
- Hypertension → 17α-hydroxylase deficiency
- Increased sex hormones → 21-hydroxylase deficiency
- Increased sex hormones and hypertension → 11β-hydroxylase deficiency

(See Figure 2-27 and Table 2-25.)

QUESTION

A 25-year-old man presents with episodic hypertension and headaches. When asked about his family history, he mentions that his father had been diagnosed with medullary thyroid cancer years ago and was recently diagnosed with hyperparathyroidism. What is the most likely diagnosis for this young man, and what should he be monitored for in the future?

TABLE 2-25. Congenital Adrenal Hyperplasias

ENZYME DEFICIENCY	MINERALO-CORTICOIDS	CORTISOL	SEX HORMONES	BP	[K+]	LABS	PRESENTATION
17α-hydroxylase[a]	↑	↓	↓	↑	↓	↓ androstenedione	XY: pseudohermaphroditism (ambiguous genitalia, undescended testes) XX: lack secondary sexual development
21-hydroxylase[a]	↑	↓	↑	↓	↑	↑ renin activity ↑ 17-hydroxy-progesterone	Most common Presents in infancy (salt wasting) or childhood (precocious puberty) XX: virilization
11β-hydroxylase[a]	↓ aldosterone ↑ 11-deoxycorti-costerone (results in ↑ BP)	↓	↑	↑	↓	↓ renin activity	XX: virilization

[a]All congenital adrenal enzyme deficiencies are characterized by an enlargement of both adrenal glands due to ↑ ACTH stimulation (due to ↓ cortisol).

TREATMENT

The treatment of choice is surgical removal of the pheochromocytoma. Medical therapy involves use of α-blockers (phenoxybenzamine, phentolamine) and β-blockers. α-Blockade should be achieved before surgery to avoid a hypertensive crisis, as catecholamines can be released from the tumor during surgery.

Pancreas

The pancreas is a multifunctional organ of the endocrine and digestive systems. The endocrine pancreas plays a vital role in carbohydrate, lipid, and protein metabolism through the secretion of two hormones: insulin and glucagon.

ANATOMY

The pancreas is a retroperitoneal organ situated posterior to the stomach. It lies between the duodenum and spleen (Figure 2-32). It is divided into four segments: head, neck, body, and tail. The pancreatic head lies adjacent to the second segment of the duodenum, and the tail abuts the spleen. The body of the pancreas lies transversely across the retroperitoneum. (**The pancreatic ductal system is discussed in Chapter 3.**)

The **arterial blood supply** to the pancreas is composed of:

- **Pancreatic arteries:** Supply the body and tail of the pancreas; derived from the splenic artery.
- **Superior pancreaticoduodenal:** Supplies the head of the pancreas; derived from the gastroduodenal artery.
- **Inferior pancreaticoduodenal:** Supplies the head of the pancreas; derived from the superior mesenteric artery (SMA).

The **venous drainage** of the pancreas is provided by pancreatic veins that drain into the portal vein from tributaries of the splenic vein and superior mesenteric vein.

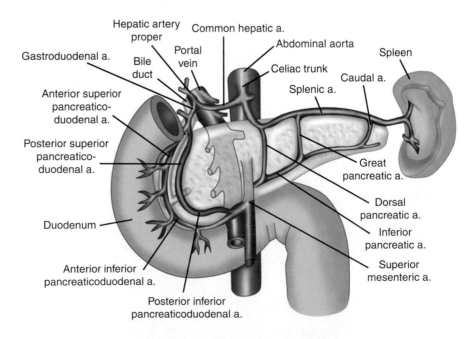

FIGURE 2-32.   **Anatomy of the pancreas with its arterial supply.**

EMBRYOLOGY

The primitive gut is composed of the foregut, midgut, and hindgut. Foregut derivatives include the esophagus, stomach, upper duodenum, liver, gallbladder, and pancreas.

The mature pancreas develops from two separate buds of tissue off the foregut: the ventral and dorsal pancreatic buds. The ventral bud gives rise to the pancreatic head and uncinate process, and the dorsal bud forms the remaining components of the pancreas. (See Chapter 3 for more details.)

During development, the buds rotate and fuse to form a complete pancreas derived primarily from endoderm (acinar cells, islet cells, and acinar epithelium are endoderm derivatives).

Pancreatic exocrine and endocrine functions begin at different stages of development. Exocrine function does not begin until shortly after birth, whereas endocrine signaling commences at weeks 10–15 of development. The developing fetus can begin to regulate blood glucose levels relatively early in development.

HISTOLOGY

The islets of Langerhans are clusters of hormone-producing endocrine cells interspersed within pancreatic exocrine tissue (Figure 2-33).

The three major cell populations within islets are shown in Table 2-26.

Autonomic nerve fibers innervate the blood vessels and endocrine cells of the pancreatic islets. The sympathetic and parasympathetic nervous systems influence insulin and glucagon secretion. Because nerve fibers are in close apposition with only 10% of islet endocrine cells, gap junctions between cell membranes play a role in the spread of signals to the remaining cells.

INSULIN

Biosynthesis

Insulin is a small protein composed of two polypeptide chains, A and B, joined by disulfide linkages. It is synthesized as a preprohormone, preproinsulin. A series of proteolytic reactions in the endoplasmic reticulum and Golgi complex generate the biologically active form of insulin (51 amino acids) and an inactive peptide referred to as **C-peptide** (31 amino acids). C-peptide is derived from the cleavage of proinsulin to form insulin. On stimulation of the β-cell, insulin and C-peptide are released from granules into the circulation in equimolar quantities.

FLASH FORWARD

During pregnancy, a woman with diabetes mellitus must strictly control her blood glucose levels. Maternal glucose crosses the placenta during pregnancy and causes fetal hyperinsulinemia. Hyperglycemia has adverse effects on the developing fetus, increasing the risk of fetal congenital anomalies. Following delivery, rapid withdrawal of high glucose levels in the setting of persistent hyperinsulinemia in the neonate may result in severe hypoglycemia.

FLASH FORWARD

In **type 1 diabetes mellitus (DM-1)**, autoimmune destruction of pancreatic β-cells leads to insulin insufficiency.

FLASH FORWARD

In patients with hypoglycemia secondary to high circulating insulin levels, C-peptide levels help distinguish between endogenous (eg, insulinoma) and exogenous (eg, surreptitious use) sources.
C-peptide levels can also be used to assess remaining endogenous insulin production in patients receiving exogenous insulin (eg, type 2 DM).

TABLE 2-26. **Islet Cell Types and Function**

CELL TYPE	QUANTITY (%)	LOCATION	HORMONE	FUNCTION
Alpha (α)	20	Peripheral	Glucagon	Increases blood glucose
Beta (β)	70	Central	Insulin	Decreases blood glucose
Delta (δ)	< 5	Variable	Somatostatin	Inhibits release of other islet cell hormones

(Adapted with permission from Junqueira LC, Carneiro J, *Basic Histology: Text & Atlas*, 11th ed, New York: McGraw-Hill, 2005: 408.)

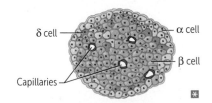

FIGURE 2-33. **Islets of Langerhans.**

Secretion

Glucose is the most powerful stimulus for insulin release (Table 2-27). Glucose enters β-cells via the glucose transporter **GLUT 2** via facilitated diffusion, meaning that intracellular glucose concentration equilibrates with serum glucose concentration. Increases in serum glucose within β-cells are shunted into the glycolytic pathway. Increased glucose catabolism leads to a rise in the intracellular ATP:ADP ratio, which causes the **ATP-sensitive potassium channel** on the surface of β-cells to close. Closure of this potassium channel leads to depolarization of the cell, resulting in opening of voltage-gated calcium channels. The subsequent rise in intracellular calcium facilitates fusion of insulin-containing vesicles with the cell membrane, releasing insulin from the cell (Figure 2-34).

Another mediator of insulin release is the second messenger cAMP. Serum glucose stimulates cAMP formation within the β-cell, which mobilizes intracellular calcium stores and stimulates insulin granule exocytosis.

Insulin Receptor Activation

Stimulation of the insulin receptor leads to downstream signaling cascades that result in alterations in metabolism and growth.

The insulin receptor (in the tyrosine kinase receptor superfamily) consists of two extracellular α-subunits and two transmembrane β-subunits with tyrosine kinase activity. Insulin binds to the α-subunits, leading to autophosphorylation of β-subunits and subsequent signaling pathway activation:

- **Mitogenic pathway:** Mitogen-activated protein (MAP) kinase cascade causes the growth-promoting effects of insulin.
- **Metabolic pathway:** Phosphatidylinositol-3-kinase activation leads to GLUT 4 transporter membrane insertion in skeletal muscle and adipose tissue cells and anabolic pathway stimulation.
- With continued exposure to insulin, insulin-bound receptors are down-regulated, desensitizing those tissues to insulin's effects.
- In response to low insulin levels, target tissues upregulate the number of insulin receptors on their surfaces.

Action

Insulin's actions on carbohydrate and lipid metabolism are mediated mainly by three types of tissues: liver, muscle, and fat. The coordinated actions of insulin at these tissues promote the storage of nutrients by the body.

- Effects on the liver:
  - Stimulates glycogen formation (upregulates activity of glucokinase and glycogen synthase).

MNEMONIC

GLUT-**2** is bi(**2**)-directional and is found on cells related to glucose regulation: B-islet cells, liver, kidney, small intestine.

KEY FACT

Insulin-independent glucose uptake occurs in the brain, red blood cells, intestine, cornea, kidney and liver; uses GLUT transporters 1, 2, and 3.

MNEMONIC

BRICK L cells do not need insulin:
Brain
RBCs
Intestine
Cornea
Kidney
Liver

TABLE 2-27. **Factors Affecting Insulin Release**

PROMOTE INSULIN SECRETION	INHIBIT INSULIN SECRETION
Glucose	α-Adrenergic stimulation
Amino acids	Somatostatin
Vagal stimulation	Drugs: Phenytoin, vinblastine, colchicine
Sulfonylureas	
CCK, GIP, glucagon-like peptide	
Secretin, gastrin	
β-Adrenergic stimulation	

CCK, cholecystokinin; GIP, gastric inhibitory polypeptide.

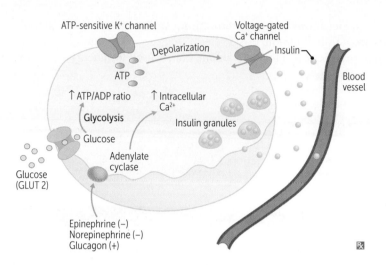

Q QUESTION

What do the alpha cells of the Islets of Langerhans secrete, and where are they located?

FIGURE 2-34. Pancreatic β-cell insulin secretion. ADP, adenosine diphosphate; ATP, adenosine triphosphate; GLUT 2, glucose transporter-2.

- Inhibits glycogenolysis (↓ glycogen phosphorylase activity).
- Inhibits gluconeogenesis (↑ phosphofructokinase-2 activity).
- Inhibits catabolism of fatty acids and amino acids.
- Promotes triglyceride synthesis.
- Effects on muscle:
  - Increases glucose uptake (promotes insertion of GLUT 4 on target cell membranes).
  - Stimulates glycogen formation (upregulates activity of glycogen synthase).
  - Increased amino acid uptake and protein synthesis.
  - Decreased protein degradation.
- Effects on fat:
  - Increased glucose uptake (promotes insertion of GLUT 4 on target cells).
  - Increased triglyceride storage (↑ lipoprotein lipase activity promotes triglyceride hydrolysis from lipoproteins).

GLUCAGON

Biosynthesis and Secretion

Glucagon is a counterregulatory polypeptide to insulin. It is secreted by pancreatic α-cells in response to stimuli including amino acids, catecholamines, gastric hormones, glucocorticoids, and most importantly, hypoglycemia (Table 2-28).

Action

The main action of glucagon is to promote elevations in blood glucose concentrations. Glucagon is a catabolic hormone that balances the energy-storing (anabolic) effects of insulin. The liver is glucagon's major site of action. It stimulates surface-bound receptors on hepatocytes, thereby activating adenylate cyclase and raising the levels of cAMP within cells. cAMP is the second messenger responsible for mediating the downstream effects of glucagon. The major actions of glucagon are:

- **Promotes increases in serum glucose:**
  - Increased glycogenolysis (secondary to ↑ glycogen phosphorylase activity).
  - Increased gluconeogenesis (secondary to ↓ phosphofructokinase-2 activity).
  - Increased amino acid uptake by liver (provides substrate for gluconeogenesis).
- **Stimulates increases in serum fatty acids:**
  - Activates adipose cell lipase, leading to lipolysis and free fatty acid release.
  - Inhibits storage of triglycerides in the liver.

KEY FACT

Glucagon's major physiologic actions take place in the liver: gluconeogenesis, glycogenolysis, and ketone production. A major stimulus for these actions is hypoglycemia.

TABLE 2-28. Factors Affecting Glucagon Secretion

↑ GLUCAGON SECRETION	↓ GLUCAGON SECRETION
Hypoglycemia	Hyperglycemia
Norepinephrine, epinephrine	Fatty acids
Amino acids	Somatostatin
CCK, gastrin	Insulin
Glucocorticoids	

CCK, cholecystokinin.

- **Leads to elevations in urea production:** Amino groups from catabolized amino acids are shunted into the urea cycle.
- **Ketone production:** The main ketone bodies used for energy are acetoacetate and β-hydroxybutyrate.

The minor actions of glucagon are:

- Increased bile secretion.
- Increased cardiac contractility.
- Decreased gastric acid secretion.
- Increased local blood flow in selected tissues.

SOMATOSTATIN

Somatostatin is a relatively small polypeptide (14 amino acids) secreted by the pancreatic δ-cells in response to high levels of blood glucose, amino acids, fatty acids, and gastric hormones. Somatostatin lengthens the period over which nutrients are incorporated into the circulation. Actions of somatostatin include:

- Decreased secretion of insulin and glucagon (paracrine effect).
- Decreased gastric, duodenal, and gallbladder motility.
- Decreased function of intestinal mucosa (decreased absorption and secretion).
- Decreased secretion of GH and TSH.

DISORDERS OF THE ENDOCRINE PANCREAS

Diabetes Mellitus

Hyperglycemia is the key feature in DM, which results either from reduced insulin secretion (type 1) or tissue resistance to insulin (type 2) (Table 2-29). Complications of DM can be divided into neuropathy, microvascular disease (retinopathy, nephropathy), and macrovascular disease (atherosclerosis).

TABLE 2-29. Type 1 and Type 2 DM

FEATURE	TYPE 1 DM	TYPE 2 DM
Percentage of cases (%); prevalence (%)	10; 0.9	90; 8.1
Age of onset	< 30 yr	> 40 yr
Pathogenesis	Family history uncommon; polygenic; HLA-DR3, DR4. Autoimmune islet β-cell destruction leading to decreased insulin production	Family history common (90% concordance rate in identical twins); polygenic. Insulin resistance, progressive β-cell failure
Histology	Leukocytic infiltrate in islets	Islet amyloid polypeptide
Symptoms and characteristics	Polyuria, polydipsia, polyphagia, and weight loss common; severe glucose intolerance, low serum insulin	Variable symptoms of polyuria, polydipsia, polyphagia; obese (fat reduces the number of insulin receptors); mild-moderate glucose intolerance; variable serum insulin
Treatment	Insulin (always required/high sensitivity to insulin)	Diet; hypoglycemic drugs; insulin (low sensitivity to insulin)
Severe complications	Diabetic ketoacidosis	Hyperosmolar nonketotic coma

DM, diabetes mellitus; HLA, human leukocyte antigen.

PRESENTATION

- Polyuria, polydipsia (glucose-induced osmotic diuresis → dehydration), hyperglycemia.
- Macrovascular complications:
    - Atherosclerosis: Nonenzymatic glycation produces advanced glycosylation end products, which cause changes in collagen composition in arterial walls and trap LDL, leading to increased lipid deposition.
        - Coronary artery disease.
        - Peripheral vascular disease.
        - Stroke—commonly due to carotid artery stenosis or arteriolosclerosis of the lenticulostriate arteries.
- Microvascular complications:
    - Diabetic nephropathy: Hyalinization in regions surrounded by glomerular capillary loops (Kimmelstiel-Wilson nodules), proteinuria/microalbuminuria due to hyalinization of the efferent arteriole causing glomerular hyperfiltration injury and later nephrotic syndrome.
    - Diabetic retinopathy (Figure 2-35).
    - Diabetic neuropathy: Peripheral neuropathy (loss of pain and vibratory sensation in the legs—characteristic "stocking" distribution), autonomic neuropathy (sexual impotence, delayed gastric emptying).
- Osmotic damage: Glucose is converted to sorbitol in organs via aldose reductase, leading to accumulation/damage.
    - Diabetic peripheral neuropathy (loss of pain and vibration senses with a characteristic "stocking" distribution in the legs; increased risk of infection/injury leading to amputation); related to glucose infiltration of myelinating Schwann cells, autonomic neuropathy (sexual impotence, delayed gastric emptying).
    - Cataracts.

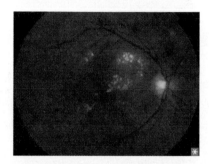

FIGURE 2-35. **Diabetic retinopathy.**

DIAGNOSIS (TABLE 2-30)

Non-enzymatic glycation of hemoglobin produces HbA_{1c}, which acts as a marker of glucose intake over the preceding 120 days (a red blood cell lives for 120 days). An HbA_{1c} of > 6.5% fulfills the criteria for the diagnosis of diabetes. HbA_{1c} is also used to monitor glucose control over time, with a goal HbA_{1c} of < 7.0%

TREATMENT

Insulin is usually given by subcutaneous injection; it can also be given IV for emergency situations (DKA). All DM-1 patients need insulin. For Type 2 DM diabetics, diet and exercise should be the first-line therapy. Most require pharmacologic treatment, including oral hypoglycemic drugs (metformin, sulfonylurea) and some also need insulin. Complications include fungal infections, particularly *Candida albicans*, and nonhealing ulcers and wounds.

Pathogenesis of Diabetic Ketoacidosis

Diabetic ketoacidosis (DKA) is a complication of DM-1. Events (eg, forgetting to take insulin, infections, illnesses, excess alcohol ingestion) that decrease insulin supply or

TABLE 2-30. **Diagnostic Criteria for Diabetes**

TEST	DIABETES CRITERIA
HbA_{1c}	≥ 6.5%
Fasting plasma glucose	≥ 126 mg/dL
Oral glucose tolerance test	≥ 200 mg/dL
Random plasma glucose	> 200 mg/dL + symptoms of hyperglycemia

 QUESTION

Insulin does which of the following?
A. decreases triglyceride storage
B. increases glucose uptake in tissues
C. increases protein degradation in muscle
D. decreases glycogen formation in the liver
E. all of the above

increase insulin demand precipitate ketoacidosis. Lack of insulin causes lipolysis and releases free fatty acids from adipose tissues. Patients present with:

- Elevated serum ketone levels
- Hyperkalemia (insulin normally drives K⁺ into cells)
- Kussmaul respirations (rapid, deep breathing)
- Acetone in breath (fruity odor), acidosis
- Dehydration, orthostatic hypotension
- Altered consciousness/coma

Decreased insulin → increased lipolysis → increased glycerol and free fatty acids → β-oxidation of free fatty acids → increased ketones → anion gap metabolic acidosis.

Insulinoma

An uncommon cause of hypoglycemia in nondiabetics, insulinomas result from tumors of β-cells in the pancreas. Often associated with MEN I syndrome. Other causes of hypoglycemia that must be ruled out include exogenous insulin, or sulfonylureas, or decreased glucose production secondary to adrenal insufficiency; liver or renal failure; alcoholism; glucagon deficiency; sepsis; autoimmune hypoglycemia; or postoperative complications of gastric bypass surgery.

PRESENTATION

Patients with insulinomas present with the Whipple triad:

- Fasting hypoglycemia.
- Symptoms of hypoglycemia (excessive epinephrine → sweating, tremor, tachycardia; CNS dysfunction → dizziness, headache, change in mental status).
- Relief of symptoms after IV glucose.

DIAGNOSIS

Increased insulin + C-peptide, decreased serum glucose.

- Chemistries: Check glucose level and C-peptide; if increased insulin but decreased C-peptide, then it is factitious hypoglycemia (Table 2-31).
- β-Hydroxybutyrate (low in insulin-mediated hypoglycemia).
- Blood urea nitrogen/creatinine, liver function tests (BUN/Cr, LFTs).
- Insulin-like growth factors (IGF-1, IGF-2).
- Serum cortisol +/– ACTH (cosyntropin) stimulation test.

TREATMENT

Surgical resection is used to treat insulinomas. For acute treatment for other causes of hypoglycemia, sugar-containing foods are given by mouth. If the patient cannot eat, either 50% dextrose in water ($D_{50}W$) is given IV or glucagon is administered IM.

Pancreatic endocrine tumors are often associated with MEN 1 (consists of a parathyroid tumor, pituitary tumor, and pancreatic endocrine tumor).

KEY FACT

Causes of hypoglycemia:
- Exogenous insulin
- Insulinomas
- Ethanol ingestion
- Postoperative complication of gastric surgery
- Reactive hypoglycemia
- Liver or renal failure
- Autoimmune hypoglycemia

A   ANSWER

B. Insulin is a "builder"; it increases glucose uptake in tissues, glycogen formation, amino acid uptake and protein synthesis, as well as triglyceride synthesis; it decreases gluconeogenesis, glycogenolysis, and the breakdown of fatty and amino acids.

TABLE 2-31.   Insulinoma Versus Factitious Hypoglycemia

	INSULINOMA	FACTITIOUS HYPOGLYCEMIA
Serum insulin	↑	↑
C-peptide	↑	↓

TUMORS OF ISLET CELLS

Gastrinoma (Zollinger-Ellison Syndrome)

A pancreatic or duodenal gastrin-secreting tumor, causing acid hypersecretion and resultant ulcers in the duodenum and jejunum. Can be associated with MEN 1 syndrome (Table 2-32).

PRESENTATION

- Abdominal pain (related to ulcers)
- Diarrhea (related to malabsorption)

DIAGNOSIS

High levels of gastrin despite secretin test (should inhibit gastrin release).

TREATMENT

Surgical resection of tumor, proton pump inhibitors to control acid hypersecretion.

Glucagonoma

Neuroendocrine tumor of α-islet cells; rarely associated with MEN 1 syndrome (Table 2-32).

PRESENTATION

- Hyperglycemia
- Rash: Necrolytic migratory erythema

DIAGNOSIS

Radioimmunoassay for glucagon levels.

TABLE 2-32. Other Tumors of the Pancreatic Islet Cells

TUMOR	FEATURES	DIAGNOSIS
Gastrinoma (Zollinger-Ellison syndrome)	Excess gastrin release leads to ↑ acid and peptic ulcer disease	▪ ↑ basal acid output ▪ IV secretin test shows ↑ gastrin (secretin normally inhibits gastrin)
Glucagonoma	▪ Tumor of α-cells ▪ Hyperglycemia ▪ Necrolytic migratory erythema (red, scaly rash)	↑ serum glucagon levels
VIPoma (Verner-Morrison syndrome)	Increase in vasoactive intestinal peptide (VIP); VIP inhibits gastric acid secretion; watery diarrhea, hypokalemia, achlorhydria	Clinical and ↑ serum VIP levels
Somatostatinoma	Increase in somatostatin; inhibits CCK, VIP, GIP, gastrin, secretin, motilin; achlorhydria, steatorrhea, cholelithiasis, DM	Clinical and serum somatostatin levels

CCK, cholecystokinin; DM, diabetes mellitus; GIP, gastric inhibitory polypeptide; VIP, vasoactive inhibitory peptide.

QUESTION

A thin, 15-year-old white girl complains of being extremely thirsty often and says that she needs to urinate all the time. Urinalysis reveals glucosuria. What histologic changes would likely be present in her pancreas?

TREATMENT

Octreotide (somatostatin analog), surgical resection.

VIPoma

Tumor-producing vasoactive intestinal peptide (VIP), 90% of which arise in the pancreas. VIP normally stimulates gastric motility and secretion; can be associated with MEN 1 syndrome (Table 2-32).

PRESENTATION

- Watery diarrhea despite fasting
- Hypokalemia
- Achlorhydria

DIAGNOSIS

Radioimmunoassay for VIP levels.

TREATMENT

Surgical resection, octreotide (somatostatin analog).

Somatostatinoma

Rare tumor of δ-islet cells arising in the pancreas or GI tract; can be associated with MEN 1 syndrome (Table 2-32).

PRESENTATION

- Diabetes mellitus (due to gastric inhibitory polypeptide inhibition)
- Cholelithiasis (due to cholecystokinin inhibition)
- Weight loss
- Steatorrhea
- Diarrhea (due to secretin inhibition)
- Hypochlorhydria or achlorhydria (due to gastrin inhibition)

DIAGNOSIS

Fasting serum somatostatin levels.

TREATMENT

5-Fluorouracil and streptozotocin, surgical resection.

DIABETES DRUGS

Type 1 DM requires insulin; type 2 DM can be managed by lifestyle modifications (exercise, diet), oral hypoglycemic drugs, and/or insulin. The goals of diabetic pharmacologic therapy are to control acute symptoms and limit future complications.

Insulin

Insulin is self-administered by subcutaneous injection, typically in the abdomen, arms, or legs. It can be given IV in emergency situations (ie, DKA). Dosing depends on the type of insulin (eg, short-acting vs long-acting) that is prescribed. New inhaled forms are also available.

MECHANISM

Supplies insulin in insulin deficiency (type 1 DM) or resistance (type 2 DM), leading to decreased plasma glucose.

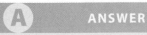

ANSWER

Leukocytic infiltrate in islets of Langerhans and destruction of β-cells.

USES

- Type 1 DM, type 2 DM, DKA.
- Insulin comes in short-, intermediate-, and long-acting forms that affect its dosing schedule (Table 2-33).

SIDE EFFECTS

Hypoglycemia, hypokalemia (K+-shift into intracellular compartment).

ORAL HYPOGLYCEMIC DRUGS

Sulfonylureas

MECHANISM

Inhibits potassium channels on β-cells and prevents hyperpolarization, thus leading to membrane depolarization, increased calcium influx, and insulin release; increased insulin leads to decreased glucagon release from α-cells and increased tissue sensitivity to insulin.

USES

Type 2 DM; for glucose control after failure of conservative diet and exercise regimen. Successful therapy requires ~ 30% of β-cell function (secondary failure of drug due to decreased β-cell function). Used in thin patients.

- **First-generation:** Tolbutamide (good in renal dysfunction), chlorpropamide (long-acting, may cause SIADH and disulfiram-like reactions).
- **Second-generation:** Glipizide, glyburide.

SIDE EFFECTS

Hypoglycemia, weight gain, type IV hypersensitivity reaction.

TABLE 2-33.   Types of Insulin

INSULIN TYPE	ONSET/DURATION OF ACTION	USES	NOTES
Rapid acting: ■ Lispro ■ Glulisine ■ Aspart	20 min/4 h	Type 1 DM Type 2 DM Gestational DM for postprandial glucose control	Can cause hypoglycemia; rare hypersensitivity reactions
Short acting: ■ Regular	1 h/6–8 h	Type 1 DM Type 2 DM Gestational DM DKA (IV) Hyperkalemia (+glucose) Stress hyperglycemia	The only insulin given IV
Intermediate-acting: ■ NPH	2–4 h/10–18 h	Type 1 DM Type 2 DM Gestational DM	Most commonly used insulin type
Long-acting: ■ Glargine ■ Detemir	1 h/12–24 h 1 h/8–24 h	Type 1 DM Type 2 DM Gestational DM for basal glucose control	Establishes basal insulin level

DKA, diabetic ketoacidosis; DM, diabetes mellitus; NPH, neutral protamine Hagedorn.

Metformin

MECHANISM

Decrease hepatic glucose production; increase peripheral insulin sensitivity. Exact mechanism of action unknown. Decreases postprandial glucose levels but does not cause weight gain or hypoglycemia (euglycemic).

USES

First-line treatment for obese diabetic patients; synergistic with sulfonylureas, in patients without renal failure. Contraindicated in patients with renal impairment (drug excreted by kidneys) or CHF.

SIDE EFFECTS

Lactic acidosis, GI distress (nausea, diarrhea), avoid IV contrast.

Acarbose

MECHANISM

Inhibits α-glycosidase → decreased carbohydrate absorption from the GI tract → decreased insulin demand.

USES

Type 2 DM.

SIDE EFFECTS

Flatulence, diarrhea, abdominal discomfort.

Thiazolidinediones (Rosiglitazone, Pioglitazone)

MECHANISM

Binds nuclear peroxisome proliferator-activated receptor (PPAR) to control transcription of insulin-responsive genes, leads to insulin sensitization and decreased hepatic gluconeogenesis and insulin receptor upregulation.

USES

Type 2 DM, in the absence of liver disease, CHF or coronary artery disease.

SIDE EFFECTS

Weight gain, edema (peripheral or macular), liver function abnormalities.

Repaglinide

MECHANISM

Works like sulfonylureas by stimulating release of insulin from the pancreas.

USES

Type 2 DM.

SIDE EFFECTS

Hypoglycemia, weight gain.

Glucagon-Like Peptide-1 (GLP-1) Analogs (Exenatide, Liraglutide)

MECHANISM

Increases insulin and decreases glucagon (eg, endogenous GLP-1).

USES

Type 2 DM.

SIDE EFFECTS

Nausea/vomiting, pancreatitis.

Dipeptidyl Peptidase 4 (DDP-4) Inhibitors (-gliptins [Linagliptin, Saxagliptin, Sitagliptin])

MECHANISM

Increases insulin and decreases glucagon via inhibition of DPP-4, the enzyme that degrades incretins.

USES

Type 2 DM.

SIDE EFFECTS

Mild urinary or respiratory infections.

Sodium-Glucose Cotransporter 2 (SGLT-2) Inhibitors (-gliflozins [Canagliflozin, Dapagliflozin])

MECHANISM

Blocks reabsorption of glucose in the proximal convoluted tubule by inhibiting SGLT-2.

USES

Type 2 DM.

SIDE EFFECTS

Glucosuria, UTIs, vaginal yeast infection.

NOTES

CHAPTER 3

Gastrointestinal

EMBRYOLOGY   172
   Overview of Gastrointestinal System Development   172
   Congenital Malformations of the GI Tract   174

ANATOMY   178
   Abdominal Wall   178
   Abdominal Planes and Regions   180
   Peritoneum and Abdominal Viscera   183
   Arterial Supply of the GI Tract   184
   Venous Drainage of the GI Tract   185
   Lymphatic Drainage of the GI Tract   188
   Nerve Supply of the GI Tract   189

PHYSIOLOGY   192
   Hypothalamus   192
   Mouth   192
   Esophagus   195
   Stomach   195
   Small Intestine   199
   Colon   204
   Exocrine Pancreas   205
   Liver and Gallbladder   206

PATHOLOGY   210
   Oral Cavity   210
   Esophagus   213

Stomach   219
Small and Large Intestine   224
Inflammatory Diseases of the Colon   229
Tumors of the Colon   232
Appendicitis   236
Abdominal Hernias   236
Liver Disease   238
Inborn Errors of Metabolism   247
Hepatic Tumors   248
Gallbladder Disease   250
Exocrine Pancreas   253
Enzyme Markers of GI Pathology   255

PHARMACOLOGY   258
   H$_2$ Blockers   258
   Proton Pump Inhibitors   259
   Bismuth and Sucralfate   260
   Octreotide   260
   Antacids   260
   Infliximab   260
   Osmotic Laxatives   261
   Sulfasalazine   262
   Ondansetron   262
   Metoclopramide   262
   Orlistat   262

Embryology

OVERVIEW OF GASTROINTESTINAL SYSTEM DEVELOPMENT

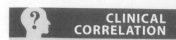
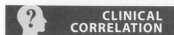
The development of the GI tract is divided into three main sections. These sections share common innervations and vascular supply (Figure 3-1):

- Cephalic foldings form the **foregut**: oral cavity, pharynx, esophagus, stomach, duodenum proximal to the bile duct, liver, pancreas, bile ducts, and gallbladder. Note that the cephalic foldings also give rise to the trachea and lungs, though these are not considered part of the foregut. Pain in the foregut is typically referred to the epigastric region.
- Lateral foldings form the **midgut**: duodenum distal to the bile duct, jejunum, ileum, cecum, appendix, ascending colon, and proximal two-thirds of the transverse colon. Pain in the midgut is typically referred to the umbilical region.
- Caudal foldings form the **hindgut**: distal third of the transverse colon, descending colon, sigmoid colon, rectum, and upper portion of the anal canal. Pain in the hindgut regions is typically referred to the suprapubic region.

Fourth Week

Embryonic foldings (cephalic, lateral, and caudal) form the primitive gut tube:

- Endoderm becomes intestinal epithelium and glands.
- Mesoderm becomes connective tissue, muscle, and wall of intestine.
- Migrating neural crest cells form the autonomic nervous system innervation.

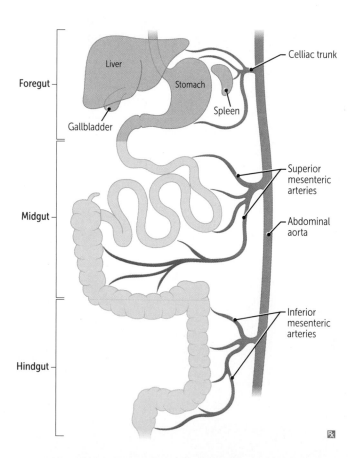

FIGURE 3-1. **Development of the GI tract: foregut, midgut, and hindgut.**

Sixth Week

The midgut loop has cranial (proximal to the superior mesenteric artery [SMA]) and caudal (distal to the SMA) limbs. The cranial loop undergoes rapid growth and is herniated out the umbilicus.

Tenth Week

The abdominal cavity enlarges and allows the herniated midgut loops to return while undergoing a counterclockwise rotation. After a total 270-degree rotation around the axis of the SMA, the organs begin to take their adult positions (Figure 3-2).

Embryologic Remnants

Postnatally, several vessels of the prenatal circulation form ligaments in the adult:

- Umbilical vein—ligamentum teres hepatis
- Umbilical arteries—medial umbilical ligaments
- Ductus venosus—ligamentum venosum
- Ductus arteriosus—ligamentum arteriosum
- Allantois–urachus—median umbilical ligament

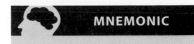

MNEMONIC

Umbi**L**ical arteries—media**L** umbilical ligaments
Alla**N**tois–urachus—media**N** umbilical ligament
Note there are two umbilical arteries and two medial umbilical ligaments, but only one allantois and one median umbilical ligament.

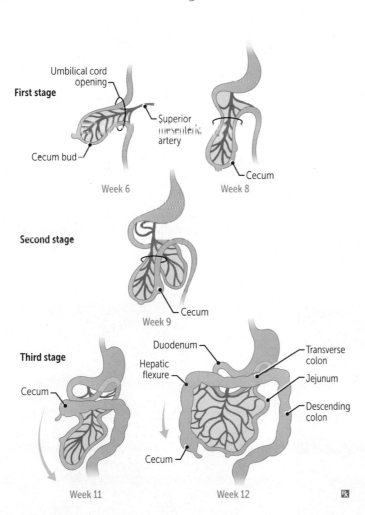

FIGURE 3-2. **Development of the midgut.** Herniation and rotation around the superior mesenteric artery.

CONGENITAL MALFORMATIONS OF THE GI TRACT

Omphalocele

Failure of herniated midgut to return to the abdominal cavity during the tenth week of embryonic development. The herniated intestine is **covered by peritoneal membrane** and is **midline** through the umbilicus (Figure 3-3A). Most commonly affects children of mothers at the extremes of reproductive age.

PRESENTATION

During the second-trimester ultrasound or when a herniated sac is found at birth. Twenty-five percent to 40% of affected infants have other birth defects, such as chromosomal abnormalities, congenital diaphragmatic hernia, or heart defects. Omphaloceles can be a part of **Beckwith-Wiedemann syndrome**, which is a collection of congenital defects that include macrosomia, macroglossia, midline abdominal wall defects (omphalocele, umbilical hernia), ear pits or creases, and hypoglycemia, hemihyperplasia, and visceromegaly.

DIAGNOSIS

Herniated sac can be visualized by ultrasound in 95% of cases. Serum **α-fetoprotein (AFP)** levels are elevated in 70% of cases. AFP levels remain elevated because the fetus cannot swallow amniotic fluid, which prevents normal destruction of AFP by fetal GI proteolytic enzymes. Acetylcholinesterase (AChe) testing also detects approximately 75% of ventral wall defects.

TREATMENT

Close monitoring of the fetus during pregnancy and prompt treatment following delivery, including surgical reduction of the herniated contents.

Gastroschisis

A full-thickness abdominal wall defect caused by vascular injury during development allowing small or large bowel to escape the abdominal cavity. **No protective peritoneal membrane** covers the herniated intestine, which protrudes lateral to the umbilicus (Figure 3-3B). Gastroschisis is more common in children born to women < 20 years of age.

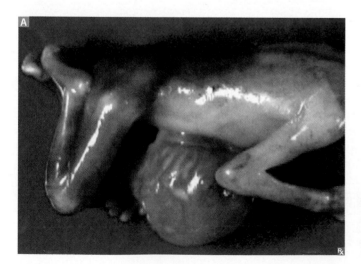
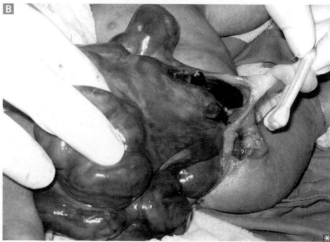

FIGURE 3-3. **Omphalocele and gastroschisis.** A Omphalocele in a newborn. Note the presence of a peritoneal membrane covering the herniated bowel defect and that the defect is midline. B Gastroschisis. Note the absence of a peritoneal membrane covering the exposed midgut and that most defects are to the right of midline.

PRESENTATION

Most often seen in the second-trimester ultrasound in combination with polyhydramnios and an elevated serum AFP. Extruded abdominal contents are noted at birth. The defect is usually to the right of the umbilicus and may be associated with intestinal atresia.

DIAGNOSIS

Herniated bowel resembles cauliflower on ultrasound. Elevated AFP on triple screen.

TREATMENT

Surgical correction of the abdominal wall defect with return of the herniated contents to the abdomen. **Artificial covering** may be used to minimize heat/fluid loss and assist with **temperature regulation** (exposed bowel causes increased heat loss). **Nasogastric tube (decompresses the stomach), broad-spectrum antibiotics,** and **total parenteral nutrition (TPN).**

Intestinal Malrotation and Volvulus

Develops as a result of abnormal midgut development and rotation (Figure 3-4).

- **Cecum** remains in the right upper quadrant (RUQ) or in the left abdomen, and the **duodenojejunal** junction remains to the right of the midline.
- Peritoneal attachments to the lateral abdominal wall normally fix the cecum retroperitoneally. In malrotation, they cross over the duodenum to reach the high, malrotated cecum and are called **Ladd bands.** They can cause partial or complete obstruction of the duodenum (which can manifest from infancy to early adulthood).
- **Midgut volvulus** occurs when the malrotated intestine twists on the axis of the SMA, compromising intestinal blood flow.

PRESENTATION

Midgut volvulus may occur at any time, often during the first year of life, and presents with sudden onset of severe **bilious** emesis, abdominal pain and distention, and rectal bleeding. Delay in recognition and treatment can lead to significant intestinal necrosis, resulting in shock and loss of viable intestine. Resection of the small bowel may lead to **short gut syndrome.**

DIAGNOSIS

- **Abdominal plain film:** Variable; may be normal (early) or gasless, may show pneumatosis intestinalis (air in the bowel wall), or free air.
- **Upper GI study:** Documents the position of the ligament of Trietz and intestinal rotation; may have a corkscrew appearance.
- **Ultrasound:** May show twisted superior mesenteric vessels ("whirlpool sign"), fixed midline bowel loops, and duodenal dilation. Near 100% sensitivity.

KEY FACT

Malrotation—Abnormality in development causing the intestines to take a different position in the abdomen than usual.
Volvulus—Twisting of a loop of bowel or other structure about its base of attachment, constricting venous outflow. The large intestine is predisposed to volvulus.

CLINICAL CORRELATION

Seventy percent of patients with malrotation have associated anomalies, including:
- Other abdominal defects: Situs inversus, septal defects, transposition of the great vessels, and anomalous systemic or pulmonary venous return.
- Asplenia or polysplenia.

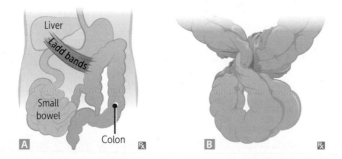

FIGURE 3-4. **A** **Malrotation and** **B** **volvulus.**

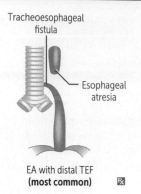

Tracheoesophageal fistula

Esophageal atresia

EA with distal TEF (most common)

FIGURE 3-5. **Esophageal atresia (EA) with distal tracheoesophageal fistula (TEF).** Ninety percent of cases of TEF result in a blind pouch end of the esophagus and a fistula between the distal esophagus and trachea. This is correlated with a very high risk of aspiration and suffocation.

TREATMENT

Urgent surgery consisting of Ladd procedure. Counterclockwise volvulus reduction, lysis of adhesive bands, bowel resection if needed, appendectomy, and repositioning of the small intestine and cecum. May lead to short-bowel syndrome or death if treatment is delayed due to bowel necrosis.

Esophageal Atresia with Tracheoesophageal Fistula

Maldevelopment of the upper GI tract may cause the esophagus to end in a blind pouch (atresia) associated with a fistula between the trachea and distal esophagus (Figure 3-5). There are multiple less common variants of atresia and fistula formation.

PRESENTATION

Most patients present with **cyanosis** (bluish skin due to poor oxygenation), **choking and vomiting with feeding,** drooling, and **poor feeding.** These patients may have VACTERL association: vertebral defects, anal atresia, cardiac defects, tracheo-esophageal fistula, renal anomalies, and limb abnormalities. People diagnosed with VACTERL association typically have at least three of these characteristic features.

DIAGNOSIS

- Prenatal ultrasound usually shows polyhydramnios, although the diagnosis is most commonly suggested based on an infant's **difficulty with feeding.** In this case, the examiner attempts to place a feeding tube but will not be able to reach the stomach.
- Radiography: Reveals an air bubble in the proximal esophagus and air in the stomach and intestines.

TREATMENT

Tracheoesophageal fistula (TEF) is considered a surgical emergency. The esophagus must be repaired immediately to protect the newborn's airway. Preoperatively, the baby is NPO (nil per os or nothing by mouth), and care is taken to prevent aspiration.

Duodenal Atresia

During weeks 5–8 of development, the duodenum becomes completely obstructed by proliferating endoderm. Failure of the duodenum to recanalize by week 10 results in duodenal atresia.

PRESENTATION

Vomiting (bilious) and abdominal distention appear within 48 hours of birth. If the biliary system is obstructed, physical exam may reveal an abdominal mass or jaundice. The newborn may be small for gestational age. Incidence is 1 in 2500 to 1 in 40,000 live births.

Nearly one third of affected newborns have **Down syndrome.** Of those affected, 30% also have:

- Gastroschisis.
- Imperforate anus or other intestinal atresia.
- Cardiac, renal, and vertebral malformations.

DIAGNOSIS

Duodenal atresia may be detected by prenatal ultrasound or may not become apparent until birth.

- **Prenatal ultrasound:** Polyhydramnios from inability to swallow amniotic fluid (seen in 50%) or dilated bowel.
- **Abdominal radiograph:** "Double-bubble" sign due to dilation of the stomach and proximal duodenum, separated by the pyloric sphincter (Figure 3-6).

TREATMENT

Definitive treatment is **duodenoduodenostomy** (anastomosis of the proximal and distal duodenum to bypass the obstruction) or **duodenojejunostomy.** Preoperative patients need a nasogastric tube, intravenous (IV) fluids, and correction of electrolyte abnormalities. Postoperative care may include TPN until oral feeds can be started.

Post-Duodenal Atresia

Intestinal atresia distal to the duodenum occurs owing to vascular accidents in utero. If the SMA is obstructed, "apple-peel" atresia occurs. This manifests as a blind-ending proximal jejunum with absence of a long length of small bowel and dorsal mesentery. The terminal ileum distal to the atresia assumes a spiral configuration around an ileocolic vessel.

Extrahepatic Biliary Atresia

Extrahepatic biliary system fails to recanalize, leading to bile flow obstruction. Presents with dark urine, pale stools, jaundice shortly after birth, and conjugated hyperbilirubinemia.

Pyloric Stenosis

Pyloric stenosis is of idiopathic cause and develops as a result of congenital hypertrophy of the pylorus, which in turn results in obstruction of the gastric outlet. Incidence is 1 in 600 live births; it is most commonly seen in firstborn males.

PRESENTATION

Usually between 3 and 6 weeks of age, patients present with difficulty feeding followed by projectile, **nonbilious** vomiting. **Signs of illness** (fever, diarrhea) are notably absent. Affected children are often hungry after the episodes and may develop abdominal pain, belching, and weight loss. Wavelike motions may be seen over the abdomen after feeding and just before vomiting occurs.

DIAGNOSIS

- Physical exam classically demonstrates a palpable "olive" mass in the epigastric region. Lab tests may demonstrate a hypochloremic, hypokalemic, metabolic alkalosis secondary to loss of hydrogen chloride (HCl) in emesis.
- **Ultrasound** shows an elongated and hypertrophic pylorus.
- Barium studies show:
    - **String sign:** Seen on barium swallow when barium moves through the pylorus.
    - **Shoulder sign:** The pylorus bulges into the antrum of the stomach.
    - **Double-tract sign:** Parallel streaks of barium seen in the narrow pylorus.

TREATMENT

Pyloromyotomy (longitudinal incision through the muscle of the pylorus with dissection to the submucosa) is definitive therapy.

Pancreas Divisum

A failure of the dorsal and ventral pancreatic buds to fuse during development. This forces the bulk of the pancreas (derived from the dorsal pancreatic bud) to drain through the minor papilla, causing a relative stenosis of pancreatic drainage (Figure 3-7). This is the **most common congenital defect of the pancreas,** with an incidence of 3–10% of live births.

PRESENTATION

Most patients are asymptomatic; however, those who develop pancreatitis (from failure of drainage through the minor papilla) present with epigastric pain radiating to the back and abdominal distention associated with nausea, vomiting, diarrhea, and jaundice. Symptoms may be worsened with ingestion of alcohol or fatty foods.

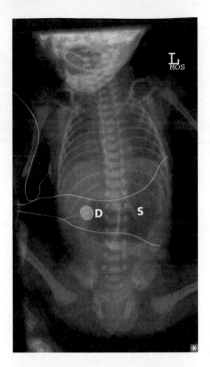

FIGURE 3-6. Double-bubble sign. An abdominal radiograph of a child with duodenal atresia showing dilation of the stomach and proximal duodenum. D, duodenal bubble; S, stomach bubble.

KEY FACT

DUODENAL ATRESIA	PYLORIC STENOSIS
Bilious vomiting	**Non-bilious** vomiting
Post-ampulla of Vater	**Pre-**ampulla of Vater
Double-bubble sign	"Olive mass"
Associated with Down syndrome	

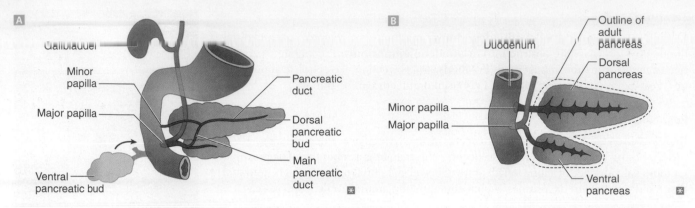

FIGURE 3-7. **Pancreas divisum.** **A** Note that the major papilla derives from the ventral pancreatic bud. This bud rotates around the duodenum to fuse with the dorsal bud. **B** When the buds fail to fuse, pancreas divisum results, forcing the bulk of the pancreas (the dorsal pancreatic bud) to drain through the minor papilla.

DIAGNOSIS

Most patients are asymptomatic, and no diagnosis is made. Those that have episodes of pancreatitis may undergo the following workup:

- Amylase and lipase: Usually elevated in acute episodes of pancreatitis.
- Endoscopic retrograde cholangiopancreatography (ERCP): Demonstrates two separately draining pancreatic ducts. Associated risk of causing pancreatitis.
- Magnetic resonance cholangiopancreatography (MRCP): Noninvasive method that shows direct continuity of the dorsal pancreatic duct and the minor papilla.

TREATMENT

- For acute episodes of pancreatitis: Rest, gastric suction, fluid and electrolyte replacement, and pain control.
- Definitive surgical treatment is poorly established, but endoscopic options include sphincterotomy (cutting of the minor papilla during ERCP to enlarge its opening) or an ERCP-guided stent of the minor papilla.

> **CLINICAL CORRELATION**
>
> Annular pancreas is a rare congenital anomaly (1 in 20,000 live births) in which the ventral pancreatic duct encircles the descending duodenum and fuses to the dorsal pancreatic duct, causing duodenal obstruction.

Anatomy

ABDOMINAL WALL

The abdomen is defined as the region of the trunk that lies between the diaphragm (superiorly) and the inlet of the pelvis (inferiorly).

Surface Anatomy

Landmarks of the abdominal wall are shown in Figure 3-8.

Linea Alba

A vertical fibrous band that extends from the symphysis pubis to the xiphoid process and lies in the midline. It is formed by fusion of the aponeuroses of the muscles of the anterior abdominal wall and is represented on the surface by a median groove.

Linea Semilunaris

Defines the lateral edge of the rectus abdominis muscle and crosses the costal margin at the tip of the ninth costal cartilage.

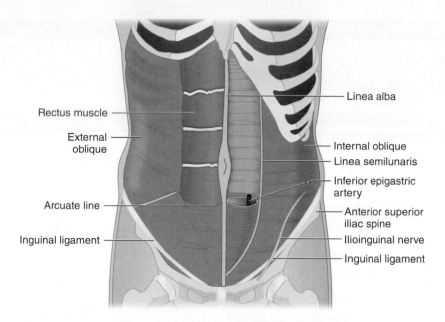

FIGURE 3-8.   Landmarks of the abdominal wall.

Arcuate Line

Defines the lower limit of the posterior aspect of the rectus sheath. Above the arcuate line, the aponeuroses of the internal oblique split and form a layer posterior to the rectus abdominis muscle along with the aponeuroses of the transversalis muscle (Figure 3-9). Inferiorly, the aponeurosos of the external, internal and transversalis muscles all form an anterior sheath, with only the transversalis fascia on the posterior aspect.

The arcuate line usually forms one third of the distance from the umbilicus to the pubic crest and is the landmark at which the **inferior epigastric arteries perforate the rectus abdominis muscles.**

Inguinal Groove

Formed by the inguinal ligament. It lies beneath a skin crease in the groin and is formed by the rolled-under margin of the aponeurosis of the external oblique muscle.

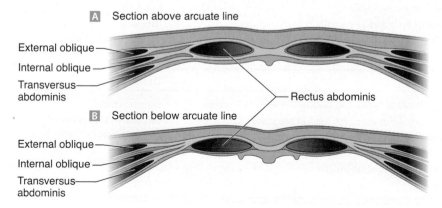

FIGURE 3-9.   Cross-section of the anterior abdominal wall. Note that above the arcuate line **A**, the aponeurosis of the internal oblique is split around the rectus abdominis muscle, whereas below the arcuate line **B**, the aponeuroses of all three muscle layers gather anterior to the rectus abdominis muscle. The inferior epigastric vessels pierce the abdominal sheath at this line.

ABDOMINAL PLANES AND REGIONS

Abdominal Regions

Anatomically, there are **nine** defined regions of interest (Table 3-1 and Figure 3-10). In clinical practice, however, these regions are defined imprecisely.

Abdominal Quadrants

The abdomen can be divided into **four** quadrants (Table 3-2), using a horizontal line and a vertical line that intersect at the umbilicus.

Layers of the Abdominal Wall

The anterolateral abdominal wall (Figures 3-8 and 3-9) is made up of the following:

- Skin
- Superficial fascia (fatty [Camper] and membranous [Scarpa])
- Deep fascia
- Aponeuroses of the muscle layers—anterior wall
- External oblique muscle—lateral wall
- Internal oblique muscle—lateral wall
- Transversus abdominis muscle—lateral wall
- Transversalis fascia
- Extraperitoneal fat
- Parietal peritoneum

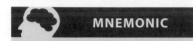

MNEMONIC

To remember the fascial layers:
You go **Camp**ing **Outside** (**Camp**er fascia is **external** to Scarpa).

TABLE 3-1. Contents of the Respective Abdominal Regions

RIGHT HYPOCHONDRIAC	EPIGASTRIC	LEFT HYPOCHONDRIAC
Liver and gallbladder	Esophagus and stomach	Stomach
Right kidney	Adrenal glands	Pancreas
Colon, hepatic flexure	Liver	Spleen
	(Transverse colon)	Left kidney
	Abdominal aorta and vena cava	Colon, splenic flexure
	Pylorus and duodenum (first part)	
RIGHT LUMBAR	**UMBILICAL**	**LEFT LUMBAR**
Kidney	(Transverse colon)	Kidney
Colon (ascending)	Duodenum and pancreas	Colon (descending)
Gallbladder	Abdominal aorta and vena cava	Pancreas
Small intestine	Small intestine	Small intestine (jejunum)
Duodenum (first part)	Iliac vessels	
RIGHT ILIAC	**HYPOGASTRIC**	**LEFT ILIAC**
Cecum	Distensible pelvic organs (eg, bladder in infants or in adults when full; uterus after 12th week of pregnancy)	Sigmoid colon
Right ovary/fallopian tube (female)		Left ovary/fallopian tube (female)
Appendix	Small intestine	Small intestine
Small intestine (ileum)	Iliac vessels	
	Spermatic cords, seminal vesicles	
	Rectum	

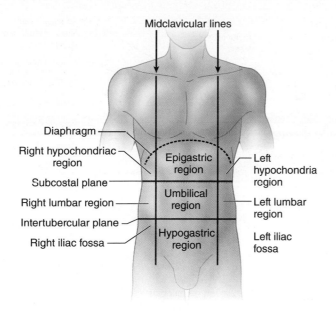

Midclavicular lines

Diaphragm

Right hypochondriac region

Subcostal plane

Right lumbar region

Intertubercular plane

Right iliac fossa

Epigastric region

Left hypochondria region

Umbilical region

Left lumbar region

Hypogastric region

Left iliac fossa

FIGURE 3-10.   Surface anatomy of the abdominal wall.

Inguinal Canal

The inguinal canal is an oblique passage through the inguinal region and a site of inguinal hernias (both direct and indirect; Figures 3-11 and 3-12). During embryonic development, the testes and spermatic cord (in males) and the round ligament (in females) descend through the inguinal canal.

TABLE 3-2.   Abdominal Quadrants

	RIGHT	LEFT
Upper	Liver (right lobe)	Liver (left lobe)
		Stomach
	Gallbladder (fundus where the linea semilunaris crosses the costal margin)	Spleen
		Pancreas (body, tail)
	Kidney and suprarenal gland	Kidney and suprarenal gland
	Colon (hepatic) flexure and right transverse	Colon (splenic) flexure and left transverse
	Duodenum (parts 1–3) with pancreas (head)	Small intestine (jejunum and proximal ilium)
	Small intestine	
	Pylorus	
Lower	Colon (ascending)	Colon (descending and sigmoid)
	Cecum	Small intestine
	Appendix (including McBurney point)	
	Small intestine (ileum)	Left ovary/Fallopian tube
	Right ovary/Fallopian tube	Left ureter
	Right ureter	

FLASH FORWARD

- **Direct inguinal hernia:** Protrudes **medial** to the epigastric artery and vein; directly through Hesselbach triangle.
- **Indirect inguinal hernia:** Protrudes **lateral** to the epigastric artery and vein through the deep inguinal ring, often by an incomplete obliteration of the processus vaginalis.
- **Femoral hernia:** Protrudes **below** the inguinal ligament in the femoral triangle.

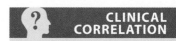

CLINICAL CORRELATION

Classic pain localized to:
- RUQ: gallbladder
- RLQ: appendix
- LLQ: diverticulitis

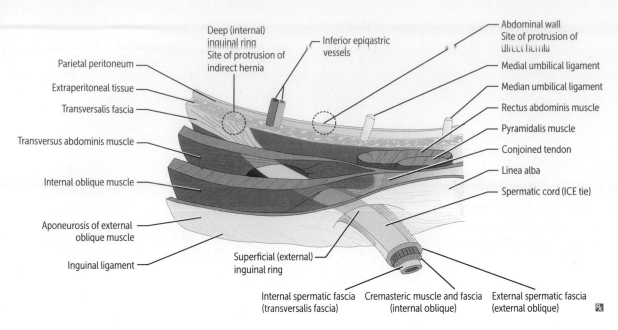

FIGURE 3-11. **Direct and indirect inguinal hernias.**

Boundaries of the inguinal canal:

- **Deep inguinal ring:** Oval opening in the fascia transversalis lateral to the inferior epigastric vessels.
- **Superficial inguinal ring:** Triangular defect in the aponeurosis of the external oblique muscle, lateral to the pubic tubercle.

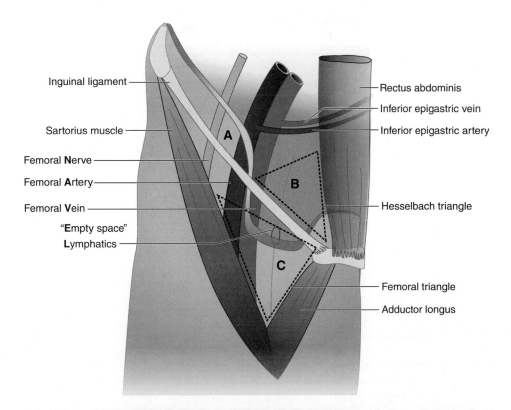

FIGURE 3-12. **Femoral canal and sites of herniation.** (A) Indirect hernias pass through the deep inguinal ring which overlies the external iliac vessels just lateral to the inferior epigastric vessels. (B) Direct hernias pass through Hesselbach triangle which is defined by the inferior epigastric artery, rectus abdominis muscle, and inguinal ligament. (C) Femoral hernias pass through the femoral ring, medial to the femoral vein, and bulge out of the femoral triangle.

- **Anterior wall:** Aponeurosis of the external oblique muscle with some of the internal oblique aponeurosis laterally.
- **Posterior wall:** Mainly transversalis fascia, with the conjoint tendon (falx inguinalis) medially. The conjoint tendon is the merger of the internal abdominal oblique and transverse abdominis aponeuroses.
- **Roof:** Internal oblique and transverse abdominal muscles.
- **Floor:** Inguinal and lacunar ligaments.

Hesselbach Triangle

Anatomic region bounded by inferior epigastric artery, rectus abdominal muscle, and inguinal ligament. Direct hernias pass **through** this triangle.

Femoral Triangle

The femoral triangle (Figure 3-12) is the anatomic region of the upper inner thigh bounded by the following:

- **Superiorly:** Inguinal ligament
- **Laterally:** Sartorius muscle
- **Medially:** Adductor longus muscle

Just below the inguinal ligament, there is a femoral sheath (fascial tube containing the femoral vein, artery, and canal, the last of which contains lymphatics). The femoral nerve (L2–L4) lies outside of the sheath.

PERITONEUM AND ABDOMINAL VISCERA

Abdominal and Pelvic Peritoneum

The peritoneum is a serous membrane that covers the abdominal organs and is composed of **two layers:** the parietal and visceral peritoneum.

Parietal Peritoneum

- The outer membrane that lines the deep surface of the abdominal walls and the inferior surface of the diaphragm.
- The nerve supply originates from the nerves of the surrounding abdominal muscles and skin, intercostal and phrenic nerves in the abdominal region, and obturator nerve in the pelvic region.

Visceral Peritoneum

The membrane that directly covers the abdominal organs. There is no somatic nerve supply to the visceral peritoneum.

Peritoneal Cavity

- The peritoneal cavity is a narrow, "potential" space between the opposing layers of the peritoneum, and it reflects the rotation of the GI tract during its embryonic development. Some abdominal organs are contained within the peritoneal cavity (Figure 3-13).
- **Normally, no space** exists between the parietal and visceral peritoneum (only ~50 mL of serous peritoneal fluid).
- In **pathologic conditions** (eg, ascites), more fluid can accumulate between the two layers of peritoneum. This phenomenon of extravascular fluid accumulation is known as **third spacing.**

As a "potential" space (meaning there is usually no significant amount of fluid within the space, although fluid can accumulate there in pathologic states), the peritoneal cavity can be divided into the greater and lesser peritoneal sacs.

CLINICAL CORRELATION

Failure of the processus vaginalis to obliterate leads to communication between the abdominal cavity and the scrotal sac. This allows a fluid collection called a hydrocele to accumulate in the scrotum.

MNEMONIC

Contents of the femoral triangle (from lateral to medial) include: **NAVEL**
Femoral **N**erve
Femoral **A**rtery
Femoral **V**ein
Empty space
Lymphatic
OR
Venous near the penis

CLINICAL CORRELATION

- Ascites is an accumulation of extra fluid in the peritoneal cavity (common causes include liver failure, right-sided heart failure, ovarian cancer).
- Pneumoperitoneum is air or other gas in the peritoneal cavity (due to intestinal or stomach perforation, or intentional insufflation for laparoscopy).
- Hemoperitoneum is an accumulation of blood within the peritoneal cavity (due to bleeding from intraperitoneal organs) and results in diffuse abdominal pain.

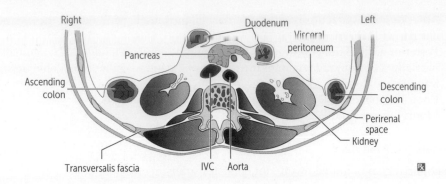

FIGURE 3-13. **Retroperitoneal structures.**

CLINICAL CORRELATION

Atherosclerosis can cause gradual occlusion at the bifurcation of the abdominal aorta, which may result in claudication and impotence.

CLINICAL CORRELATION

SMA syndrome: Compression of the transverse portion of the duodenum between the aorta and the superior mesenteric artery. This results in chronic, intermittent, or acute duodenal obstruction.

KEY FACT

Arteries supplying GI structures branch **anteriorly** and are unpaired. Arteries supplying non-GI structures branch **laterally** and are paired.

KEY FACT

Watershed zones:
- **Splenic flexure:** Receives dual blood supply from the terminal branches of the superior mesenteric and inferior mesenteric arteries.
- **Sigmoid colon:** Receives blood supply from terminal branches of the inferior mesenteric, pudendal, and iliac circulations.

- The **lesser sac** (omental bursa) is a pouch of peritoneum that lies posterior to the stomach, liver, and lesser omentum. It communicates with the greater sac through the **epiploic foramen** (omental, or **Winslow**, foramen).
- The anterior border of the Winslow foramen is the hepatoduodenal ligament, which contains the portal triad (hepatic artery, bile duct, and portal vein). It can be used surgically to control hemorrhage during a cholecystectomy.
- The **greater sac** encompasses the rest of the peritoneum and is subdivided by the transverse mesocolon into the supracolic compartment (above), and the infracolic and pelvic compartments below the mesocolon.

Mesentery

Mesentery is a double layer of peritoneum that wraps around abdominal organs, contains blood vessels, and attaches the organ to its major blood supply.

ARTERIAL SUPPLY OF THE GI TRACT

The arterial blood supply of the GI tract is derived from the abdominal aorta.

Abdominal Aorta

The abdominal aorta is the portion of the descending aorta inferior to the diaphragm. It gives off **three large branches** from the anterior surface that supply blood to the GI organs (Figure 3-14 and Table 3-3):

- Celiac trunk: Supplies derivatives of the foregut (esophagus through proximal duodenum [Figure 3-15]). It is located just inferior to the diaphragm and phrenic arteries.
- Superior mesenteric artery (SMA): Supplies derivatives of the midgut (distal duodenum to splenic flexure of the colon).
- Inferior mesenteric artery (IMA): Supplies derivatives of the hindgut (splenic flexure of the colon through proximal rectum).

The abdominal aorta also gives rise to the **inferior phrenic, middle suprarenal, renal, and gonadal** arteries. The abdominal aorta divides into the **left** and **right common iliac** arteries, which then descend into the pelvis.

Key Anastomoses of the Abdominal Arterial System

Anastomoses are connections of two vessels that can allow collateral flow around obstructions or infarcts (eg, thromboembolism), transfer of pressure from one system to another (eg, portal hypertension), or perfusion of a region with relatively stenotic blood supply (eg, watershed infarcts). Several key anastomoses occur in the abdominal arterial system (Table 3-4).

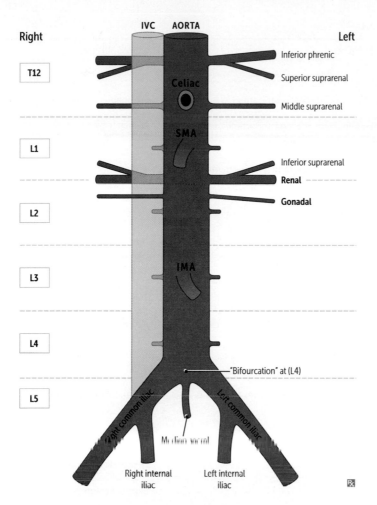

Right

IVC   AORTA

Left

T12 — Inferior phrenic

Celiac — Superior suprarenal

Middle suprarenal

L1

SMA

Inferior suprarenal

Renal

Gonadal

L2

L3

IMA

L4

"Bifourcation" at (L4)

L5

Right common iliac   Left common iliac

Median sacral

Right internal
iliac

Left internal
iliac

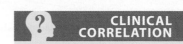

FIGURE 3-14. Abdominal aorta and its branches. IVC, inferior vena cava.

VENOUS DRAINAGE OF THE GI TRACT

Three major venous systems are responsible for the venous drainage of the GI tract are the azygos vein, inferior vena cava (IVC), and hepatic portal system.

Azygos Venous System

The azygos venous system is an anastamosis between the superior vena cava (SVC) and IVC. It is composed of:

- Azygos vein: Runs up the right side of the vertebral column and drains blood from the posterior walls of the thorax and abdomen.
- Hemiazygos vein: Runs up the left side of vertebral column.

Inferior Vena Cava Venous System

The IVC venous system (Figure 3-16) is responsible for draining the blood from the lower half of the body (below the diaphragm) into the right atrium. Drainage patterns:

- Formed by the left and right common iliac veins at L5.
- The **right** gonadal and suprarenal veins drain directly into the IVC; their **left** counterparts drain into the left renal vein, which then drains into the IVC.

> **CLINICAL CORRELATION**
>
> Left testicular varicocele may occur as a result of occlusion of the left renal vein (eg, compression by a left renal tumor).

TABLE 3-3. Main Branches of the Abdominal Aorta

PRIMARY BRANCHES	SECONDARY BRANCHES	ORGANS SUPPLIED
Celiac Artery		
Left gastric artery	Esophageal branch of the left gastric artery	Esophagus, stomach
Splenic artery	Dorsal pancreatic artery, short gastric arteries, left gastro-omental (gastroepiploic) artery	Stomach, pancreas, spleen[a]
Common hepatic artery	Gastroduodenal artery (then right gastro-omental and superior pancreaticoduodenal), right gastric artery, hepatic artery proper	Upper duodenum, liver, gallbladder, pancreas, stomach
Superior Mesenteric Artery		
Inferior pancreaticoduodenal arteries	Anterior and posterior inferior pancreaticoduodenal arteries	Head of the pancreas; second through fourth portions of duodenum
Middle colic artery	Marginal artery of Drummond	Transverse colon
Right colic artery		Ascending colon
Intestinal arteries (jejunal and ileal arteries)	Arterial arcades and vasa recta	Jejunum and ileum
Ileocolic artery	Colic and ileal arteries; ileal branch gives rise to the appendicular artery	Ileum, cecum, appendix
Inferior Mesenteric Artery		
Left colic artery	Marginal artery of Drummond	Descending colon
Sigmoid artery		Sigmoid colon
Superior rectal artery		Rectum (proximal portion)

[a]The spleen is not a foregut derivative. It is of mesodermal origin.

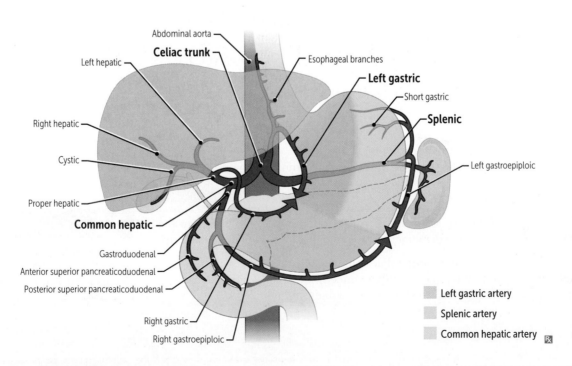

FIGURE 3-15. Celiac trunk.

TABLE 3-4. **Key Anastomoses of the Abdominal Arterial System**

MAJOR ANASTOMOSES	CONNECTING ARTERIES	CLINICAL CORRELATION
Celiac trunk–SMA	Superior and inferior branches of the pancreaticoduodenal arteries	Dual supply of the pancreatic head in case of infarct
SMA–IMA	Middle colic–left colic arteries	Severe hypotension can cause relative infarction and necrosis of the splenic flexure
IMA–internal iliac	Superior rectal–middle rectal arteries	Dual supply of the proximal rectum
Subclavian/Internal thoracic–external iliac	Superior epigastric–inferior epigastric arteries	Collateral flow around an aortic stenosis (eg, coarctation of the aorta)

IMA, inferior mesenteric artery; SMA, superior mesenteric artery.

Portal Venous System

The portal venous system is centered on the portal vein, which drains blood from the spleen, intestine, and colon into the liver, and is formed by the **superior mesenteric** and **splenic veins.** The **portal vein** is situated in the hepatoduodenal ligament.

The portal vein transports nutrient- (and toxin-) rich blood from the GI tract as well as products of lysed RBCs from the spleen to the sinusoids of the liver. The liver then drains through the hepatic veins into the IVC.

Portal to Inferior Vena Caval Anastomoses (Collaterals)

Pathologies that cause portal hypertension, such as cirrhosis from metabolic insults or infection, lead to collateral intra-abdominal venous flow pathways (anastomoses; [Figure 3-17 and Table 3-5]).

KEY FACT

Lymphatic drainage from organs almost always follows the arterial supply. For example, lymphatic drainage from the foregut passes through the celiac nodes (as the foregut is supplied by the celiac trunk).

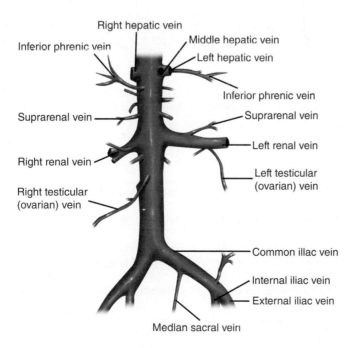

FIGURE 3-16. **Inferior vena cava.**

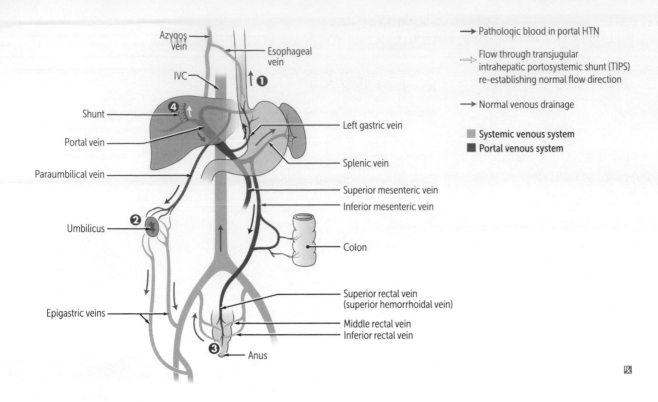

FIGURE 3-17. **Portosystemic anastomoses in portal hypertension.** HTN, hypertension; IVC, inferior vena cava.

LYMPHATIC DRAINAGE OF THE GI TRACT

The end point of lymphatic flow from the GI tract and its organs is the thoracic duct, which in turn empties into the venous system at the junction of the internal jugular vein and left subclavian vein. The thoracic duct collects most of the lymph in the body, **except** from the right thorax, arm, head, and neck, which drains into the right lymphatic duct.

Before passing into the thoracic duct, the lymph from the GI tract passes through the preaortic lymph nodes, which can be divided into the celiac, superior mesenteric, and inferior mesenteric nodes.

TABLE 3-5. **Key Portosystemic Venous Anastomoses in Portal Hypertension**[a]

REGION[a]	ANASTOMOSIS (PORTOSYSTEMIC)	CLINICAL SIGNIFICANCE
Esophagus ❶	Left gastric vein–esophageal venous plexus (to azygos vein)	Esophageal varices
Umbilicus ❷	Paraumbilical vein–superficial and inferior epigastric veins	Caput medusae (engorged veins that look like snakes around the umbilicus)
Rectum ❸	Superior rectal vein–middle and inferior rectal veins	Enlarged internal hemorrhoids and anorectal varices
Retroperitoneal	Visceral veins of Retzius–retroperitoneal parietal veins	Ascites

[a] Corresponding number on Figure 3-17.

Note: A transjugular intrahepatic portosystemic shunt (TIPS; ❹ in Figure 3-17, above) relieves portal hypertension, shunting blood to the systemic circulation by bypassing the liver.

Peyer Patches

Peyer patches, known as gut-associated lymphoid tissue (GALT), are conspicuous aggregates of lymphoid tissue located throughout the lamina propria and submucosa of the digestive tract. They play a critical role in immune function by acting as the first line of defense against pathogens invading the gut. This occurs through specialized epithelium that contains microfold cells (M cells), which directly sample antigen in the intestinal lumen and present it to antigen-presenting cells. Large concentrations are typically found in the ileum and, in certain pathologic states such as inflammatory bowel disease (IBD), can proliferate to the point at which they are visible to the naked eye (this may be associated with idiopathic intussusception).

- Peyer patches produce **secretory IgA** in germinal centers of B cells located in the lamina propria.
- Gastric mucosa-associated lymphoid tissue (**MALT**) lymphoma is frequently (80%) associated with chronic inflammation by *Helicobacter pylori*.

> **KEY FACT**
>
> Lymphadenopathy is often the first sign of GI infection or neoplasia.

NERVE SUPPLY OF THE GI TRACT

The GI tract has a complex nerve supply, divided into two major groups: extrinsic (parasympathetic and sympathetic innervation), and intrinsic (enteric) innervation.

Extrinsic Innervation

Extrinsic motor and sensory innervation is supplied by both parasympathetic and sympathetic nerves (Figure 3-18).

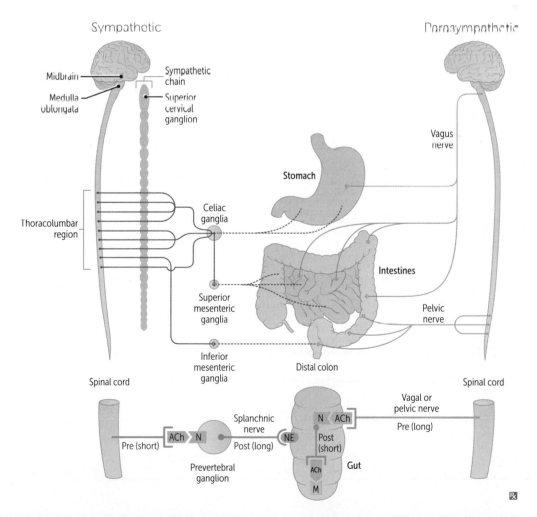

FIGURE 3-18. **Extrinsic nervous system of the GI tract.** ACh, acetylcholine; M, muscarinic; N, nicotinic; NE, norepinephrine.

Sympathetic Innervation

Preganglionic fibers arise at spinal cord levels T5–L1 and synapse with the prevertebral abdominal ganglia (celiac, superior, and inferior mesenteric). The **preganglionic** neurotransmitter is **acetylcholine.** The **postganglionic** fibers form **splanchnic nerves** to innervate the gut and communicate with the enteric nervous system.

The primary **postganglionic** neurotransmitter is **norepinephrine,** which acts as an **inhibitory neurotransmitter** in the GI tract, **decreasing motility** as well as secretory and digestive functions.

Parasympathetic Innervation

Supplied by the vagus and pelvic nerves:

- The **vagus** nerve (CN [cranial nerve] X) provides both **parasympathetic afferent** and **efferent** stimuli for the esophagus through the splenic flexure of the colon.
- **Pelvic nerves** arising at S2 and S3 innervate the hindgut (splenic flexure through proximal rectum).
- Preganglionic fibers of the parasympathetic (vagus and sacral) nerves **synapse directly** in the enteric nervous system on nicotinic receptors, whereas postganglionic neurons are shorter and use muscarinic receptors.
- The parasympathetic system **increases** the activity level of the enteric nervous system.

There are several key similarities and differences between the parasympathetic and sympathetic innervation of the GI tract:

- Both divisions use acetylcholine (ACh) and nicotinic receptors at the ganglion, whereas the enteric innervation by the parasympathetic nervous system (PNS) is muscarinic ACh and by the sympathetic nervous system (SNS) is norepinephrine.
- Preganglionic neurons are shorter in the SNS and longer in the PNS, whereas postganglionic neurons are longer in the SNS and very short in the PNS.
- The PNS originates cephalic and sacral, whereas the SNS is between in the thoracolumbar region.

Intrinsic Innervation

Also known as the **enteric nervous system,** or the "third division" of the autonomic nervous system. It is composed of a series of ganglionic nerve plexuses, contained entirely within the gut wall and running from esophagus to anus. Enteric neurons use many neurotransmitters, most notably **neuropeptides.**

The two principal components of the enteric nervous system are the **myenteric (Auerbach) plexus** and the **sub0mucosal (Meissner) nerve plexus** (Figure 3-19):

- The **myenteric (Auerbach) nerve plexus** is located between the **outer longitudinal** and **inner circular muscle layers.** Its main function is to coordinate **motility** along the full length of the gut wall.
- The **submucosal (Meissner) nerve plexus** is located in the **submucosa** between the innermost mucosal layer and the inner circular layer of smooth muscle. Its main function is to **regulate secretions, blood flow, and absorption.**

Visceral Sensation

- **Normal visceral sensation,** for the most part, is not consciously perceived, except for sensations such as hunger and rectal distention.
- **Abnormal visceral sensation,** however, is perceived as diffuse **pain.**

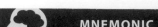

MNEMONIC

The parasympathetic system allows one to **rest** and **digest** (via the **vagus** nerve).

MNEMONIC

Parasympathetic **P**roduces secretions and **P**ropels food, but **S**ympathetic **S**uppresses GI function.

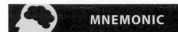

MNEMONIC

Auerbach is **A**uter or **M**yenteric is between the **M**uscle.
Myenteric is for **M**otility
Submucosal makes **S**ecretions

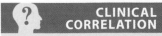

CLINICAL CORRELATION

Overdistention, ischemia, and chemical and mechanical irritation are examples of noxious stimuli resulting in abnormal visceral sensation, which tends to produce dull, achy, colicky discomfort.

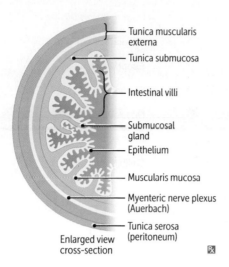

Tunica muscularis externa
Tunica submucosa
Intestinal villi
Submucosal gland
Epithelium
Muscularis mucosa
Myenteric nerve plexus (Auerbach)
Tunica serosa (peritoneum)

Enlarged view cross-section

FIGURE 3-19. **Cross-section of digestive tract wall.**

Visceral Versus Parietal Pain

- Due to the differential innervation of the viscera and the parietal peritoneum, visceral pain results in **cramping** pain, whereas parietal pain causes **sharp** pain.
- The pain fibers that originate in the **viscera** are transmitted via autonomic nerves, mainly sympathetic, **type C fibers**, which only transmit **colicky, cramping, poorly localized** types of pain.
- In contrast to the viscera and visceral peritoneum, the parietal peritoneum is innervated by extensions of the **peripheral spinal nerves**, which carry the same types of noxious pain sensations as those overlying the dermatomes. Therefore, parietal pain results in **sharp, localized** pain.
- If the pathologic process progresses from the visceral to the parietal region, the referred pain will become localized, corresponding to the dermatome overlying the affected organ.

Referred Pain

Many organs have an embryonic origination in one location of the body and then **migrate** to another area, pulling their vascular and nervous supply with them. Thus, **visceral pain** is often **referred** to the site of embryologic origin rather than the actual location of the organ.

Example: The embryologic origin of the diaphragm and its nerves is in the neck. When the diaphragm or the surrounding abdominal structures are inflamed and cause diaphragmatic irritation (ie, cholecystitis, ruptured spleen), the patient often feel pains in the shoulder because the corresponding dermatome shares a C3–C4 nerve root with the phrenic nerve. This phenomenon is known as **referred pain.**

The same concept holds true for other abdominal and thoracic organs (Figure 3-20).

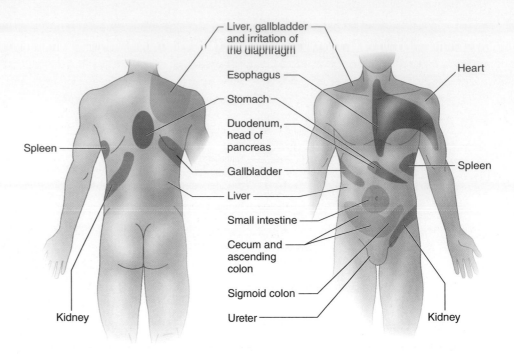

FIGURE 3-20.   **Location of pain referred from major abdominal and thoracic organs.**

Physiology

HYPOTHALAMUS

The hypothalamus controls the body's sense of hunger and fullness.

- **Lateral hypothalamic area (LHA):** Sensation of hunger (ie, stimulates feeding).
- **Ventromedial nucleus of the hypothalamus (VNH):** Sensation of fullness (ie, tells the person to stop feeding).

MOUTH

The mouth is the first site of digestion. It is the site of mechanical breakdown of the food by mastication (chewing).

- The **chewing reflex** causes the up-and-down movement of the lower jaw. This functions to mix the food bolus with lubricating saliva and salivary enzymes, as well as produce smaller particles for swallowing.
- Most of the muscles of mastication are innervated by the trigeminal nerve (CN V).

Salivary Secretions

The salivary glands produce approximately 1 L of saliva each day. Saliva helps buffer, dilute, moisten, and digest food, while also protecting the oral cavity from bacteria. Secretion is stimulated by the smell, sight, taste, or even thought of food, as well as vagal afferents.

The two major types of salivary protein secretions are **serous** (eg, α-amylase) and **mucous** (mucin).

- **Major salivary glands** include the parotid (serous), submandibular (or submaxillary; mixed serous and mucous), and sublingual glands (mixed).
- **Minor salivary glands** include a group of tiny glands located in the buccal mucosal area.

MNEMONIC

Lateral nuclei make one grow **laterally.**

FLASH FORWARD

Lesions of the LHA can cause anorexia.
- The "fat" lateral nuclei make you hungry.
VNH can cause obesity.
- The "skinny" medial nuclei make you feel full.

KEY FACT

Leptin is a protein hormone released from adipocytes. It acts on many parts of the hypothalamus, especially the arcuate and paraventricular nuclei. Leptin decreases appetite and increases metabolism.

KEY FACT

Peptide YY is produced by the small intestine and colon and reduces appetite in response to eating.

Salivary glands contain acinar cells that feed into salivary ducts. These structures are both surrounded by **myoepithelial cells,** which contract to express saliva.

- **Parasympathetic stimulation:** An **increase** in the secretion of **watery** saliva is mediated by **CN VII** (facial nerve) and **CN IX** (glossopharyngeal nerve) from the superior and inferior salivatory nuclei in the brain stem via **muscarinic receptors.**
- **Sympathetic stimulation** is mediated via **β-adrenergic receptors** and causes an **increase** in secretion of viscous saliva (via T1–T3 nerves of the superior cervical ganglion).

Composition of Saliva

- **Enzymes:**
  - **α-Amylase (ptyalin):** Begins digestion of carbohydrates, particularly starches, by hydrolyzing α-1,4 bonds to form disaccharides. It is **inactivated** by the **low pH** of the **stomach.**
  - **Lingual lipase:** Begins digestion of lipids; breaks down triglycerides into fatty acids and monoglycerides. It is capable of continued digestion within the stomach. **In contrast to pancreatic lipase,** it can cleave fatty acids from all three positions on a triglyceride.
- **Ions:**
  - High in HCO_3^- and K^+.
  - Low in Na^+ and Cl^-.
- **Tonicity:**
  - Slower flow rates allow more time for ductal cells to transport ions and adjust the tonicity of the secretions (Figure 3-21). The exception to this rule is HCO_3^-, which is selectively stimulated and is secreted in proportion to flow rate.
  - In low flow rate states (< 1 mL/min), saliva is **hypotonic** relative to plasma, with low Na^+ and Cl^- and high K^+.
  - In **high** flow rate states (~ 4 mL/min), saliva is **closer to isotonic** (relative to plasma), with high Na^+ and Cl^- and low K^+. **The exception to this rule is HCO_3^-.**
- The **pH** is between 6 and 8.

> **KEY FACT**
>
> The salivary glands are unique because they are stimulated by both the sympathetic and parasympathetic branches of the autonomic nervous system.

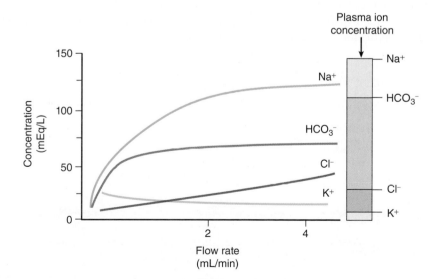

FIGURE 3-21. Salivary flow rates and secretory tonicity. Low flow rates provide more time for resorption of sodium and chloride, whereas potassium is secreted slightly more, resulting in a hypotonic solution. High flow rates are nearly isotonic due to less time provided for ion exchange. Bicarbonate is selectively stimulated and therefore increases secretion in proportion to flow rate (eg, parasympathetic stimulation increases both bicarbonate secretion and flow rate).

- **Antibacterial actions:** The flow of saliva and the presence of enzymes and antibodies help to fight dental caries:
  - Lysozyme attacks bacteria and digests food particles.
  - Lactoferrin.
  - Thiocyanate ions enter bacteria and become bactericidal.
  - Antibodies (IgA).
  - Defensins.

» FLASH FORWARD

Motility disorders of the esophagus:
Upper esophagus (striated muscle):
- Myasthenia gravis = dysphagia due to weakness

Lower esophagus (smooth muscle):
- Achalasia = dysphagia due to failure of the LES to relax
- Scleroderma = dysphagia due to fibrosis of the connective tissue

Swallowing (Deglutition)

Deglutition is a process regulated by the **swallowing reflex,** which is **coordinated in the medulla (swallowing center).** Simply stated, swallowing is propulsion of the food bolus through the pharynx while respiration is temporarily blocked. The **three stages** of swallowing are voluntary, pharyngeal, and esophageal (Figure 3-22).

- **Voluntary (oral) stage:** The bolus is pushed to the posterior of the pharynx, which has a high concentration of somatosensory receptors, by the tongue. This triggers the involuntary stages of swallowing.
- **Pharyngeal phase:** Initiated through the epithelial swallowing receptor reflex, this phase is carried out through the following steps:
  - **Upward movement of the soft palate** to prevent reflux of food into the nasal cavities.
  - **Constriction of the palatopharyngeal folds,** which creates a small passageway that permits only properly masticated food to pass into the posterior pharynx.
  - **Tightening of the vocal cords** and upward movement of larynx cause **closure of the epiglottis,** which swings backward over the opening of the larynx to prevent food from entering the trachea.
  - The upper esophageal sphincter (UES) relaxes in < 1 second.
  - Peristaltic waves move the bolus from the pharynx to the esophagus.
  - During this stage, **breathing is inhibited.**
- **Esophageal phase:** Controlled by both the swallowing reflex and the enteric nervous system. It involves movement of food toward the stomach, causing **relaxation of the lower esophageal sphincter (LES)** as a result of **vagal stimulation** (peptidergic neurons releasing vasoactive intestinal peptide [VIP]).
- As food passes the UES, it contracts to prevent reflux into the pharynx.
- **Primary peristalsis** is a continuous peristaltic wave controlled by the swallowing center in the medulla. Food movement is accelerated by gravity.

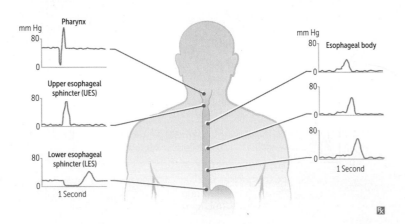

FIGURE 3-22.   Pressure tracings of the pharynx and esophagus during swallowing. Positive deflections are shown when muscle contracts, and negative deflections are shown when muscle relaxes. As the bolus travels down the tube, pushed by contractions, the deflections are positive. Note that the deflections are negative as the bolus passes through the superior and inferior esophageal sphincters as the muscle relaxes.

- **Secondary peristalsis** is a reflexive reaction mediated by the enteric nervous system. Distention of the esophagus triggers a peristaltic contraction that clears the esophagus of remaining food.

Receptive relaxation is the relaxation of the stomach in response to the relaxation of the LES. This occurs after the first primary peristaltic wave. After receptive relaxation, the LES closes to prevent gastroesophageal reflux.

ESOPHAGUS

The esophagus is a muscular tube lined with **nonkeratinized stratified squamous epithelium.** It connects the pharynx through the UES to the stomach via the LES.

- **Upper esophagus:** Mostly striated muscle; primarily controlled by the nucleus ambiguus.
- **Lower esophagus:** Predominantly smooth muscle; controlled by the dorsal nucleus of the vagus nerve.

The esophagus quickly propels food toward the stomach via **peristaltic contractions** controlled by:

- The **extrinsic nervous system:** The sympathetics and parasympathetics of the CNS.
- The **intrinsic nervous system** (enteric nervous system): Myenteric (**Auerbach**) plexus, which promotes motility of smooth muscle, and the submucosal (**Meissner**) plexus, which controls secretion and blood flow.
- The enteric nervous system uses **ACh, dopamine,** and **serotonin** as neurotransmitters.

Because the esophagus is located in the thoracic cavity, its pressure is equal to intrathoracic pressure, which is negative relative to the abdominal cavity and atmosphere. The UES prevents air from entering the esophagus, whereas the LES prevents reflux of gastric contents.

Vomiting

Vomiting (emesis) is controlled by the vomiting center of the medulla, which can be stimulated by afferents from:

- Gastric overdistention.
- Oropharyngeal stimuli.
- Chemoreceptor trigger of the area postrema of the medulla.
- Vestibular stimulus.

The vomiting reflex includes several sequential actions: reverse peristalsis (from the small intestine), relaxation of the stomach and pylorus, forced inspiration (increases abdominal pressure), relaxation of the LES, and forceful expulsion.

Retching is the initial phase of vomiting, but occurs against a closed UES. In this case, the bolus returns to the stomach through a patent LES.

STOMACH

Anatomy and Histology

The stomach functions as both a reservoir and site of digestion for the food bolus. It has three layers of smooth muscle: longitudinal, circular, and oblique, which churn the food bolus until the digestive contents eventually pass through the pyloric sphincter. It is also organized into several different functional regions (Figure 3-23).

FLASH FORWARD

Chronic gastroesophageal reflux disease (GERD) can lead to Barrett esophagus, which is metaplasia of stratified squamous epithelium of the lower esophagus into columnar epithelium similar to that of intestinal mucosa.

CLINICAL CORRELATION

GERD has many causes, including:
- **Inappropriate relaxation** of the **LES.**
- **Increased intra-abdominal pressure** (eg, obesity), which overwhelms the LES.
- **Hiatal hernia.**
- Ingestion of certain foods (eg, citrus, caffeine, fatty, or spicy).

CLINICAL CORRELATION

Damage to the myenteric plexus in the lower two-thirds of the esophagus causes **achalasia** (failure of the LES to relax).

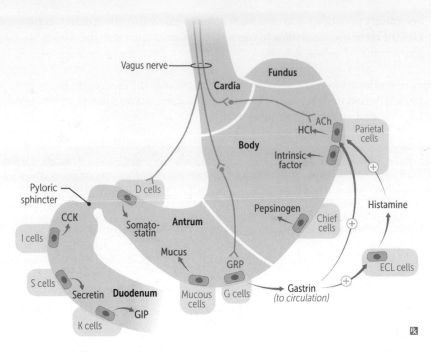

FIGURE 3-23. **Stomach anatomy, histology, and physiology.** ACh, acetylcholine; CCK, cholecystokinin; ECL, enterochromaffin-like; GIP, gastric inhibitory peptide; GRP, gastrin-releasing peptide; HCl, hydrochloric acid.

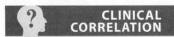

CLINICAL CORRELATION

Hiatal hernias are caused by a protrusion (herniation) of the cardia and/or fundus into the thorax.

- Cardia: Distal to the LES; does not secrete acid, has mucous glands.
- Fundus: Dilated region superior to a horizontal line drawn through the cardiac orifice.
- Body: Between the fundus and antrum, food reservoir and major site of gastric digestion. Both the body and the fundus contain multiple cell types:
  - **Parietal cells:** Secrete hydrogen ion (H^+) and intrinsic factor (IF).
  - **Chief cells:** Secrete pepsinogen, a key enzyme in protein digestion.
- Antrum: Distal region that is highly muscular, grinds food, and regulates gastric emptying through the pyloric sphincter. Contains multiple cell types:
  - **Mucus-secreting cells:** Release both mucus and bicarbonate.
  - **G cells:** Secrete gastrin, which stimulates gastric acid, motility, and growth of gastric mucosa.

Mechanical Contractions

The stomach's main motor functions include storing, mixing, and emptying.

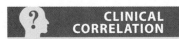

CLINICAL CORRELATION

Interstitial cells of Cajal are implicated in both gastrointestinal stromal tumors (GIST) and GI motility disorders.

Interstitial cells of Cajal (ICC) function as the pacemakers of the GI tract and generate spontaneous electrical slow waves. They also transduce signals from the enteric motor neurons through local smooth muscle to stimulate contractions. The stomach's baseline rate is 3–5 contractions per minute, also known as the **basal electrical rhythm.**

- **Parasympathetic** stimulation of the vagus nerve **increases** stomach contractions, whereas **sympathetic** stimulation via the celiac plexus **decreases** stomach contractions.
- **Migrating motility complex (MMC):** Contractions of the stomach and small intestine during fasting conditions. These contractions occur in a cyclic motor pattern and prevent bacterial overgrowth (housekeeping). They repeat every 90–120 minutes and are mediated by **motilin.**
- **Vagovagal reflex:** In response to esophageal distention, the fundus and body of the stomach relax. Cholecystokinin (CCK) further increases stomach distention.
- Food is stored for about 45 minutes before it is mixed and processed into **chyme** and squeezed out via the pyloric sphincter. Phasic waves of contraction can narrow the

pyloric sphincter and force **chyme** back into the stomach for more efficient mixing; this is also known as **retropulsion.**

- **Emptying** of the stomach is enabled by an intense contraction, which pushes chyme through the pyloric sphincter.

The **rate of stomach emptying** is controlled by the content of food.

- Hypotonic or hypertonic food delays gastric emptying.
- The presence of lipids and partially digested proteins in the food stimulates the release of CCK, which decreases gastric motility, thus delaying gastric emptying.
- Increase of H⁺ in the duodenum inhibits gastric emptying via direct neural reflexes.

General Regulation of Gastric Secretions

Gastric secretion occurs in three interrelated stages: **cephalic, gastric,** and **intestinal phases.**

- **Cephalic phase:** Parasympathetic stimulation from the appetite centers of the hypothalamus and/or amygdala to the stomach produces salivary and gastric secretions due to the sight, smell, or thought of food.
- **Gastric phase:** Initiated by distention of the stomach, the gastric phase uses long vagovagal and enteric reflexes to stimulate the **release of gastrin** and increase acid production.
- **Intestinal phase:** Further release of gastrin from the duodenum as a result of the presence of protein in the upper portion of the small intestine.

The **presence of chyme** in the intestines stimulates gastric secretion in the intestinal phase. However, it also **paradoxically inhibits gastric secretion** via the **reverse enterogastric reflex,** as well as through the release of several hormones, including secretin, gastric inhibitory peptide, VIP, and somatostatin.

The inhibition of gastric secretions helps regulate the amount of chyme entering the duodenum.

The secretory products of the stomach are depicted in Figure 3-23 and Table 3-6.

Mechanism of Hydrochloric Acid Secretion

Mechanism of gastric HCl secretion in parietal cells (Figure 3-24):

- $CO_2 + H_2O \rightarrow H^+ + HCO_3^-$ via the action of **carbonic anhydrase.**
- H^+–K^+ ATPase pump secretes H^+ into the stomach lumen, in exchange for K^+.
- HCO_3^- and Cl^- are exchanged at the basal (bloodstream) side of the parietal cell, adding bicarbonate to the bloodstream, while Cl^- follows H^+ into the stomach lumen. This bicarbonate is eventually secreted by the pancreas into the small intestine.

This influx of HCO_3^- into the venous system is called the "alkaline tide," reflecting an acute increase in pH; this can also raise the urine pH after a large meal.

Regulation of Hydrochloric Acid Secretion

The vagal system stimulates gastric acid secretion through both direct and indirect mechanisms.

- The **direct mechanism** uses vagal innervation of parietal cells to stimulate **muscarinic ACh receptors;** these subsequently activate the inositol 1,4,5-triphosphate (IP_3) second-messenger system and intracellular Ca^{2+} to promote H^+ secretion.
- The **indirect mechanism** functions by vagal nerve release of **gastrin-releasing peptide (GRP) at G cells** in the gastric antrum. GRP is released in response to the

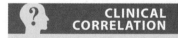

TABLE 3-6.   Gastric Secretions

PRODUCT	SOURCE	LOCATION	ACTION	REGULATION STIMULUS	REGULATION INHIBITION
Gastric acid (HCl)	Parietal (oxyntic) cells	Body, fundus	Aids in digestion Activates pepsin from pepsinogen Kills pathogens	Gastrin, ACh (vagus), histamine	Low pH, prostaglandins, GIP secretion (negative feedback), somatostatin
Intinsic factor (IF)	Parietal (oxyntic) cells	Body, fundus	Binds to vitamin B_{12}, leading to its uptake in the ileum	Gastrin, ACh (vagus), histamine	Low pH, prostaglandins, GIP secretion (negative feedback), somatostatin
Pepsinogen	Chief cells	Body, fundus	Precursor for pepsin. Digests protein at a pH between 1.0 and 3.0	ACh (vagus), increased local H^+	Somatostatin
Mucus	Mucous cells	Entire stomach (particularly antrum)	Protects mucosa from the acidic environment and pepsin	ACh (vagus)	
HCO_3^-	Mucous cells	Entire stomach (particularly antrum)	Neutralizes acid	ACh (vagus)	
Gastrin	G cells	Antrum (and duodenum)	↑ Secretion of: H^+, pepsinogen, histamine. Trophic on gastric mucosa. ↑ Gastric motility	Small peptides, amino acids, Ca^{2+} in gastric lumen, GRP (vagus), gastric distention	↑ H^+ in the gastric antrum

ACh, acetylcholine; GIP, gastric inhibitory peptide; GRP, gastrin-releasing peptide.

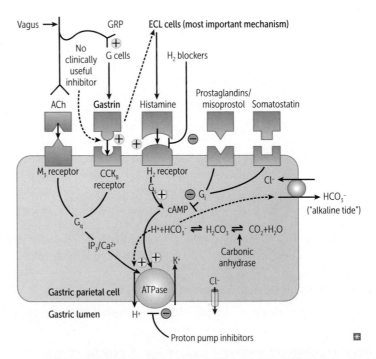

FIGURE 3-24.   **Acid secretion by parietal cells.** Demonstration of the regulatory mechanisms of HCl secretion by parietal cells, stimulated by histamine, acetylcholine, and gastrin, or inhibited by somatostatin and prostaglandins. ACh, acetylcholine; cAMP, cyclic adenosine monophosphate; CCK_B receptor, cholecystokinin B receptor; ECL cells, enterochromaffin-like cells; GRP, gastrin-releasing peptide; G_q, G_s, G_i, G proteins (stimulatory, inhibitory); H_2-receptor, histamine 2-receptor; IP_3, inositol triphosphate; M_3-receptor, muscarinic 3 receptor.

cephalic phase or gastric distention and stimulates the secretion of **gastrin** from G cells in both the gastric antrum and duodenum. Gastrin is secreted in response to small peptides, amino acids, or Ca^{2+} in the stomach lumen, gastric distention, and vagal stimulation. Gastrin stimulates parietal cells (H^+), chief cells (pepsinogen), enterochromaffin-like (ECL) cells (histamine), growth of gastric mucosa (trophic action), and gastric motility.

Histamine, stimulated by gastrin, is released from ECL cells in the gastric mucosa and stimulates the parietal cells through H_2 **receptors.** It is also released by vagal ACh.

Because these regulatory systems use different receptors and second messengers, they undergo **potentiation** (the response to two stimulants is greater than the sum of the two responses individually).

As the food bolus passes into the duodenum, several mechanisms begin to decrease the release of gastric H^+, including:

- **pH:** The lack of food in the stomach to buffer the H^+ secretion causes a decrease in pH. Below a pH of 3.0, gastrin release is inhibited.
- Fatty acids, amino acids, and glucose in the duodenum cause the release of **gastric inhibitory peptide (GIP)** from K cells in the proximal small intestine, which inhibits acid production (and increases insulin release).

Excess H^+ in the duodenum triggers **secretin** release from S cells, which increases the release of pancreatic and biliary HCO_3^- into the duodenum.

Absorption

The stomach is capable of absorbing alcohol and lipid-soluble drugs, such as aspirin.

SMALL INTESTINE

Anatomy and Histologic Characteristics

Approximately 6 m long, the small intestine is the primary site of digestion and absorption. It is divided into three regions: the duodenum, jejunum, and ileum.

The **duodenum** is mostly retroperitoneal (second, third, and fourth portions), begins at the gastroduodenal junction at the pyloric sphincter, and is divided into four parts:

- **Superior (first portion):** The only truly peritoneal segment of the duodenum; it is attached superiorly to the hepatoduodenal ligament and inferiorly to the greater omentum.
- **Descending (second portion):** Fixed retroperitoneal location; receives both the common bile duct and the main pancreatic duct through the hepatopancreatic ampulla (of Vater).
- **Horizontal (third portion):** Fixed retroperitoneal location at the level of L3; it runs between the divergence of the SMA and the aorta.
- **Ascending (fourth portion):** Retroperitoneal; meets the jejunum at the duodeno-jejunal flexure, located by the suspensory muscle of the duodenum (ligament of Treitz).

Following the duodenum, the small intestine is mobile and suspended in the peritoneal cavity by mesentery.

The **jejunum** accounts for the proximal three-fifths of the remaining small intestine. The **ileum** represents the remaining distal two-fifths, ending at the **ileocecal valve,** which marks the start of the large intestine.

FLASH FORWARD

The proton pump inhibitors (PPIs, eg, omeprazole) function to inhibit gastric acid secretion at the H^+–K^+ ATPase.

H_2-receptor antagonists, such as cimetidine, competitively inhibit histamine from binding to its receptors on parietal cells.

KEY FACT

Atropine can block the direct pathway (by blocking muscarinic ACh receptors).

Vagotomy decreases acid production by blocking both the direct and indirect pathways (Figures 3-23 and 3-24).

KEY FACT

The superior (first) portion of the duodenum is the most common site of duodenal ulcers based on its proximity to gastric acid.

KEY FACT

The horizontal (third) portion of the duodenum is the most common site of traumatic duodenal injuries (crushed against the L3 vertebra).

KEY FACT

The plicae circulares, intestinal villi, and microvilli all function to slow the progression of the food bolus through the small intestine and significantly increase the surface area for absorption.

The plicae circulares, intestinal villi, and crypts of Lieberkühn form the major histologic features of the small intestine and are composed of multiple cell types (Figure 3-25):

- **Plicae circulares:** Circular folds of submucosa that run one-half to two-thirds of the way around the lumen (Figure 3-25A). They begin in the duodenum, are most frequent in the proximal jejunum, and reduce in size and frequency toward the terminal ileum. Plicae circulares reach around the entire circumference of the intestine, in contrast to haustra of the colon (helps in distinguishing small intestine from colon on abdominal x-ray).
- **Intestinal villi:** Intraluminal projections of the lamina propria ~1 mm in height, each containing a single terminal branch of the arterial, venous, and lymphatic trees (lacteals).
- **Crypts of Lieberkühn:** Spaces between intestinal villi responsible for cell proliferation (putative multipotential stem cells in the crypts are thought to serve as progenitor cells of the four major cell types contained within the villi: enterocytes, goblet cells, enteroendocrine cells, and Paneth cells).
- **Enterocytes:** Surface epithelial cells responsible for absorption as well as secretion of some digestive enzymes (Table 3-7). Under electron microscopy, numerous microvilli are noted on each enterocyte, further increasing the absorptive surface of the intestine up to 600 times. They make up the **brush border** facing the intestinal lumen and are involved in H_2O and electrolyte balance in the small intestine.
- **Goblet cells** secrete mucus into the GI lumen; they increase in frequency from the duodenum to the terminal ilium.
- **Enteroendocrine cells** secrete endocrine (eg, CCK, secretin, GIP, motilin) and paracrine (eg, somatostatin, histamine) hormones into the bloodstream.
- **Paneth cells** secrete growth factors and antimicrobial substances (eg, lysozyme, α-defensin) into the lumen as a component of innate immunity.
- **M cells (microfold):** Modified epithelial cells that cover lymphatic nodules (ie, Peyer patches) in the lamina propria. They contain microfolds that take up microorganisms and macromolecules in endocytotic vesicles for presentation to CD4+ T lymphocytes.

The average life span of intestinal cells is 3–6 days.

Because digestive enzymes can only interact on the surface of chyme, the surface area of ingested food must be increased. The length and tubular structure of the intestines, as well as the endothelial brush border, plicae circulares, and intestinal villi, increase the surface area, aiding absorption.

The **basal electric rhythm of the small intestine is faster** than that of the stomach: 12 waves per minute in the duodenum and 8–9 waves per minute in the ileum.

- Chyme is **mixed** via **segmental** contractions and **propelled forward** with **peristaltic** contractions (which increase with parasympathetic stimulation from the vagus nerve and decrease with sympathetic stimulation from the mesenteric ganglion).
- Fasting migrating motor complex (MMC) occurs every 90 minutes.

Absorption

The primary location for absorption of nutrients is the small intestine (Table 3-8).

- **Nonfat, water-soluble** nutrients are absorbed through the small intestine into the portal vein, where they are transported to the liver for storage and processing.
- Oligo- and disaccharides (nonabsorbable) are broken down into monosaccharides (absorbable by enterocytes) by brush border enzyme oligosaccharide hydrolases.
- **Fat-based nutrients** enter into the mesenteric lymphatic system of the intestines via the terminal lacteals and use the thoracic duct to enter the bloodstream, bypassing the liver.
- **Water** and **ions** (ie, Na^+, Cl^-, K^+) are absorbed passively with solutes. Sodium can facilitate the absorption of other nutrients through a cotransporter, whereas a basolateral Na^+–K^+ ATPase maintains the sodium gradient.

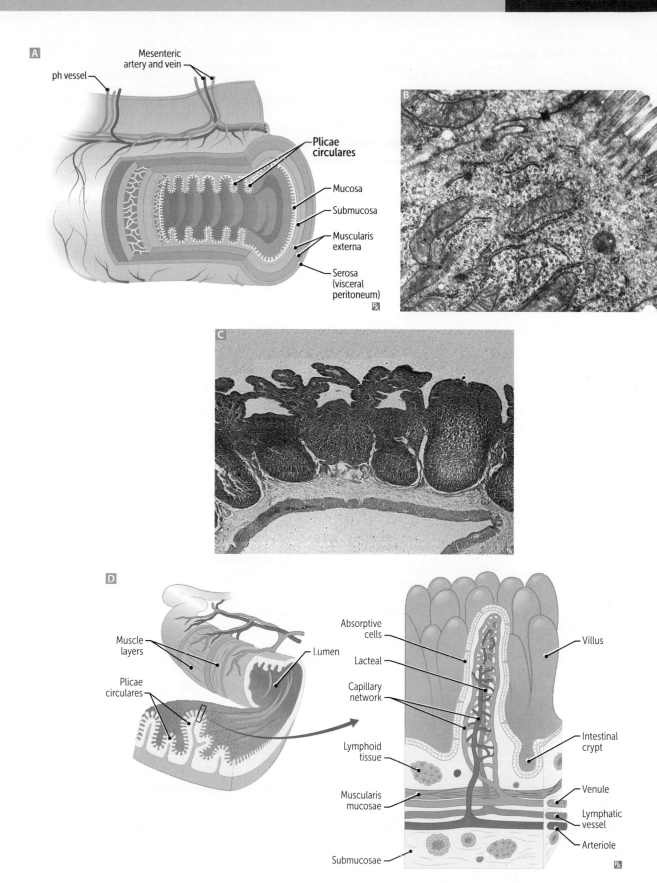

FIGURE 3-25. Small intestine anatomy and histology. **A** Diagram of cross-section of small intestine demonstrating plicae circulares. **B** Electron micrograph of the intestinal brush border. Note the numerous microvilli enhancing the surface area. **C** Peyer patches seen in a section of rabbit ileum. This is a major site of M cells. **D** Diagram of an intestinal villus with cell locations. Enteroendocrine cells are not shown, but migrate upward and can be found at all levels of each villus.

TABLE 3-7. Small Intestinal Secretions

SOURCE	PRODUCT	ACTION	REGULATION STIMULUS
Crypts of Lieberkühn	Cl⁻	Makes a watery fluid for easier absorption	CCK, secretin, enteric nervous reflexes
	HCO_3^-	Makes a watery fluid for easier absorption Helps neutralize gastric acids	
Brush border enterocytes	Peptidases	Hydrolysis of dipeptides and tripeptides into amino acids	Enteric nervous reflexes
	Sucrase	Hydrolysis of sucrose into fructose and glucose	
	Maltase	Hydrolysis of maltose into two glucoses	
	Isomaltase	Hydrolysis of saccharides not digested earlier	
	Lactase	Hydrolysis of lactose into galactose and glucose	
	α-Dextrinase	Hydrolysis of terminal α-1,4 bonds, to make glucose	
	Intestinal lipase	Breakdown of neutral fats into fatty acids and glycerol	
Brunner glands	Heavy alkaline mucus	Protects duodenum from the large amount of gastric acid	Secretin, tactile/irritating stimuli, ACh (vagus)
Goblet cells	Mucus	Lubricates and protects intestines	Enteric nervous reflexes

ACh, acetylcholine; CCK, cholecystokinin.

TABLE 3-8. Nutrient Digestion and Absorption

NUTRIENT	ABSORBED PRODUCTS	MECHANISM	CLINICAL CORRELATION

Carbohydrates	Monosaccharides:
	  Glucose
	  Galactose
		SGLT1 (Na⁺-dependent cotransport)	4 kcal/g; transported to liver through portal vein; associated with lactose intolerance; monosaccharides exit the cell into the blood through the GLUT 2 transporter (facilitated diffusion)

	Fructose	GLUT 5 (facilitated diffusion)	
Lipids	FFA Monoglycerides Cholesterol Lysolecithin	Diffusion (through micelles formed from bile salts)	9 kcal/g; transported to lacteals and through lymphatics to systemic circulation (bypass liver); facilitate absorption of fat-soluble vitamins (A, D, E, K); abetalipoproteinemia from lack of ApoB prevents absorption (Figure 3-26)
Protein	Di/Tripeptides	H⁺-dependent di/tripeptide cotransport	4 kcal/g; transported to liver through portal vein; deficient absorption associated with pancreatic disease (eg, chronic pancreatitis, cystic fibrosis); Hartnup disease is caused by a lack of the neutral AA cotransporter
	AA	Na⁺-dependent AA cotransport	
Vitamins	Fat-soluble	Via micelles with lipids	A, D, E, K are affected by anything that inhibits lipid absorption; B_{12} is absorbed by an independent mechanism involving intrinsic factor
	Water-soluble	Na⁺-dependent cotransport	
Calcium	Ca^{2+}	Calbindin-D28K (vitamin D-dependent Ca^{2+}-binding protein)	Needs active vitamin D (1,25-dihydroxycholecalciferol) from liver and kidney metabolism; deficiency of active vitamin D associated with rickets (children), osteomalacia (adults)

AA, amino acids; Apo B, apolipoprotein B; FFA, free fatty acids; GLUT, glucose transporter; SGLT, sodium-glucose transport protein.

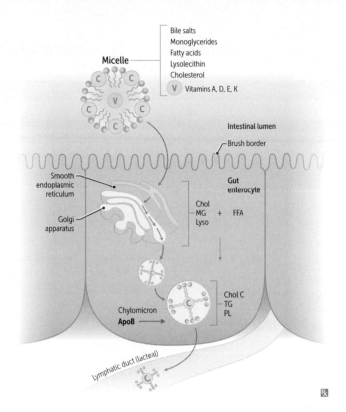

Micelle —
- Bile salts
- Monoglycerides
- Fatty acids
- Lysolecithin
- Cholesterol
- (V) Vitamins A, D, E, K

FIGURE 3-26. **Mechanism of lipid absorption.** ApoB, apolipoprotein B; Chol C, cholesterol ester; FFA, free fatty acids; Lyso, lysolecithin; MG, monoglyceride; PL, phospholipid; TG, triglyceride.

Certain key nutrients (Fe, folate, vitamin B_{12}) have individual mechanisms and locations of absorption (Table 3-9).

Lipids (Figure 3-26) are emulsified by bile acids in the small intestine and form micelles due to their hydrophobic nature. **Micelles** transport fatty acids, cholesterol, and monoglycerides to the brush border of the enterocytes. Glycerol is hydrophilic and is not part of the micelle body.

- Within the **enterocyte,** reesterification of the fatty acids, monoglycerides, and cholesterol takes place to form triglycerides, phospholipids, and cholesterol esters.
- Triglycerides and cholesterol esters are mixed with apoproteins to form **chylomicrons.**
- Chylomicrons then enter the lymphatic system and enter the bloodstream via the thoracic duct.

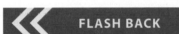

FLASH BACK

Vibrio cholerae produces the cholera toxin, which causes increased secretion of chloride, leading to osmotic diarrhea.

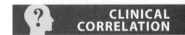

CLINICAL CORRELATION

Abetalipoproteinemia is an inability of chylomicrons to leave the enterocyte due to a lack of β-apolipoprotein.

TABLE 3-9. **Specific Nutrient Absorption**

NUTRIENT	LOCATION	MECHANISM	CLINICAL CORRELATION
Iron (Fe^{2+})	Duodenum	Absorbed as ferrous iron (Fe^{2+}, < 5% absorbed) or heme iron (~25%); digested in enterocytes, stored bound to ferritin and transported by transferrin	Iron deficiency anemia (microcytic, hypochromic), Plummer-Vinson syndrome, hemosiderosis
Folate	Proximal jejunum	Brush border splits polyglutamates into monoglutamates, which are absorbed and converted to the transport form, 5-methyltetrahydrofolate	Megaloblastic anemia, neural tube defects (congenital effect of maternal deficiency)
Vitamin B_{12} (cobalamin)	Terminal ileum	Gastric pepsin releases B_{12} from food, binds to R-protein (salivary secretion) in stomach, pancreatic proteases degrade R-protein in duodenum, binds intrinsic factor (from parietal cells), absorbed in terminal ileum	Associated with pernicious anemia (megaloblastic), gastrectomy (loss of parietal cells), deficiency masked by folate supplementation

Hormones and Peptides

GI hormones and peptides found in the small intestine are listed in Table 3-10.

COLON

The main function of the colon is the **reabsorption of electrolytes and water,** as well as short-term storage of undigested material (feces), followed by its excretion. The colon is larger in diameter than the small intestine and is inhabited by normal bacterial flora.

The colon is divided into several anatomic segments: the cecum and ascending, transverse, descending, and sigmoid colon. Overall length averages 1.5–1.8 m.

TABLE 3-10. Gastrointestinal Hormones and Peptides

HORMONE/PEPTIDE	SOURCE	ACTION	STIMULATION	INHIBITION
Gastrin	G cells (gastric antrum and duodenum)	Stimulates parietal cells (H$^+$), chief cells (pepsinogen), ECL cells (histamine); trophic on gastric mucosa; increases gastric motility	Small peptides, amino acids, or Ca^{2+} in gastric lumen, gastric distention, vagal stimulation	Low gastric pH
CCK	I cells (duodenum and jejunum)	Stimulates pancreatic enzyme secretion (amylase, lipase, proteases) and gallbladder contraction, relaxes sphincter of Oddi, trophic on exocrine pancreas and gallbladder, inhibits gastric emptying	Fatty acids and amino acids in the small intestine	Secretin
Secretin	S cells (duodenum)	Stimulates pancreatic and biliary HCO$_3^-$ secretion (neutralizes gastric acid to facilitate pancreatic enzymes) and production of bile, trophic on exocrine pancreas, inhibits gastric H$^+$ secretion	Decreased gastric pH, fatty acids in the duodenum	
Somatostatin	D cells (duodenum), delta cells (pancreatic islets)	Inhibits gastric acid and pepsinogen secretion, pancreatic and small intestine secretion, gallbladder contraction, and insulin and glucagon release	Decreased luminal pH	Vagal stimulation
GIP	K cells (duodenum and jejunum)	Stimulates insulin release (endocrine), inhibits gastric H$^+$ secretion (exocrine)	Amino acids, fatty acids, oral glucose	
Pancreatic polypeptide	F cells (PP cells; pancreas and small intestines)	Inhibits pancreatic enzyme and HCO$_3^-$ secretion	Ingestion of carbohydrates, proteins, or lipids	
GLP-1	L cells (small intestine)	Stimulates insulin release, inhibits gastric acid and glucagon secretion, decreased gastric motility	Oral glucose load	
Motilin	ECL cells (duodenum and jejunum)	Stimulates MMC in the stomach and small intestines and production of pepsin	Released by absence of food for > 2 h	
Histamine	ECL cells	Stimulates gastric acid secretion	Gastrin, ACh (vagus)	
VIP	Enteric neurons and pancreas	Stimulates receptive relaxation of the stomach, relaxation of intestinal smooth muscle, intestinal secretion of water and electrolytes, and increased release of pancreatic HCO$_3^-$	Intestinal distention and vagal activation	
GRP, or bombesin	Neurons of gastric mucosa (vagus)	Increases secretion of gastrin from G cells	Cephalic phase, gastric distention	

ACh, acetylcholine; CCK, cholecystokinin; ECL, enterochromaffin-like; GIP, gastric-inhibitory polypeptide; GLP-1, glucagon-like peptide-1; GRP, gastrin-releasing peptide; MMC, migrating motor complex; VIP, vasoactive intestinal peptide.

- In contrast to the small intestine, the colon has no villi and only a few folds.
- It contains goblet, endocrine, and absorptive cells.
- The colon is the **most efficient absorber of water** via actively transported sodium. It can also absorb chloride, potassium, and short-chain fatty acids.
- Its muscle layer has three longitudinal bands of smooth muscle (tenia coli) and typical haustrations (sacculated wall).
- The colonic bacteria synthesize **vitamin K,** B-complex vitamins, folic acid, and **short-chain fatty acids** (a preferred source of nutrition by colonocytes) and metabolize nitrogen from urea to NH_3.
- Peristaltic waves open the ileocecal valve and force chyme into the cecum. The colon has **slow waves** that slowly mix the feces, allowing fluid reabsorption in the ascending colon with **haustrations** (segmental contractions), which take about 8–15 hours and cause a net movement of feces to the transverse colon, where transit speed tends to increase.
- **Large contractions** of the colon (**mass movements**) occur one to three times per day and prepare stool to be eliminated by moving feces large distances toward the rectum. Distention of the rectum produces the urge to defecate and initiates the **rectosphincteric reflex** (both intrinsic and cord reflexes that relax the **internal anal sphincter**).
- **Contractions increase** with parasympathetic stimulation of the vagus and sacral nerves and **decrease** with sympathetic stimulation from the mesenteric ganglion.
- A full stomach can cause a parasympathetic reflex known as the **gastrocolic reflex,** which **increases** the frequency of **mass movements.**

The colon is capable of secreting **potassium** and bicarbonate.

Feces consist of water, bacteria, undigested plant products, and inorganic matter.

EXOCRINE PANCREAS

The bulk of pancreatic tissue (90%) is exocrine glandular tissue composed of acinar cells and a ductal system; approximately 2% is endocrine via the islets of Langerhans, and the remaining portion is supporting tissue. The acinar cells synthesize pancreatic enzymes in the rough endoplasmic reticulum (RER) and store the inactive enzymes, known as zymogens, in secretory granules.

Pancreatic Enzymes

The pancreas secretes about 1 L of fluid per day into the duodenum. This is composed of enzymes and high concentrations of bicarbonate. These enzymes digest carbohydrates, protein, fats, and nucleic acids (Table 3-11). The bicarbonate neutralizes gastric acid to create an optimal pH for pancreatic enzymes to function.

- The **release of pancreatic secretions** is stimulated by CCK, secretin, and ACh from the vagus nerve.
- Once the inactive and active enzymes are excreted out the pancreatic duct via the ampulla of Vater, the duodenal brush border enzyme **enterokinase (enteropeptidase)** activates **trypsinogen to trypsin.**
- Trypsin can activate the remaining zymogens and proenzymes into their active forms; it also autocatalyzes more trypsinogen to trypsin.
- The pancreas produces enzyme inhibitors to inactivate trace amounts of active enzymes within the pancreatic parenchyma.

GI hormones found in the pancreas include somatostatin, pancreatic peptide, and VIP (Table 3-10).

KEY FACT

No MMC occur in the colon or the esophagus.

KEY FACT

The colon can secrete excess potassium in diarrhea, resulting in hypokalemia.

CLINICAL CORRELATION

Cystic fibrosis:
- Causes pancreatic insufficiency.
- Inability to absorb fat-soluble vitamins A, D, E, K.

KEY FACT

Pancreatic insufficiency can lead to malabsorption, steatorrhea, and deficiency in fat-soluble vitamins.

TABLE 3-11. Pancreatic Enzymes

ENZYME	ZYMOGEN/PROENZYME	ENZYME CLASS	CATALYZING ACTIVITY
Pancreatic α-amylase	None (secreted as active form)	Polysaccharidase	Hydrolysis of starch to oligosaccharides and disaccharides Hydrolysis of glycogen Does **not** hydrolyze cellulose
Trypsin	Trypsinogen	Protease	Activates other pancreatic zymogens Hydrolysis of proteins into peptides
Chymotrypsin	Chymotrypsinogen	Protease	Hydrolysis of peptides into amino acids
Carboxypeptidase	Procarboxypeptidase	Protease	Hydrolysis of peptides into amino acids
Elastase	Proelastase	Protease	Hydrolysis of elastin
Pancreatic lipase	None (secreted as active form)	Lipase	Hydrolysis of neutral fats into fatty acids and monoglycerides
Colipase	Procolipase	Lipase	Assists lipase by displacing inhibitory bile salts
Cholesterol ester hydrolase	None (secreted as active form)	Lipase	Hydrolysis of cholesterol esters into cholesterol and fatty acids Also hydrolyses the ester bond of triglycerides to glycerol and fatty acids
Phospholipase A_2	Prophospholipase	Lipase	Hydrolysis of phospholipids into fatty acids and lysolecithin
Ribonuclease	None (secreted as active form)	Nuclease	Hydrolysis of RNA into ribonucleotides
Deoxyribonuclease	None (secreted as active form)	Nuclease	Hydrolysis of DNA into deoxyribonucleotides

LIVER AND GALLBLADDER

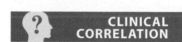

CLINICAL CORRELATION

On physical exam, the size of the liver can be determined by percussion dullness; usually it is not palpable below the costal margin.

Liver Overview

Located in the right upper quadrant, the liver typically spans from the fifth intercostal space in the midclavicular line to the right costal margin.

Anatomically, the liver is divided into **four lobes:** right, left, caudate, and quadrate. The **right and left lobes** are divided by the **falciform ligament,** making the right lobe significantly larger than the left.

Functionally, the liver is divided into eight segments (numbered I–VIII) based on blood supply. This division is significant for surgeons as liver resections are done based on this segmental division.

- **Hepatocytes** are polygonal epithelial cells arranged in long plates one to two cells thick, giving the histologic specimen a very uniform appearance.
- **Liver sinusoids** course between these plates of hepatocytes. They are composed of fenestrated endothelial cells and are in free communication with each other throughout the liver.
- The **liver lobule** (Figure 3-27) is an anatomic and functional structure created by the radial arrangement of plates of hepatocytes and the intervening sinusoids around the central vein. The lobules are separated by connective tissue. Traveling within this connective tissue in between the lobules are the **portal triads—branches of the hepatic artery, portal vein, and bile duct.**

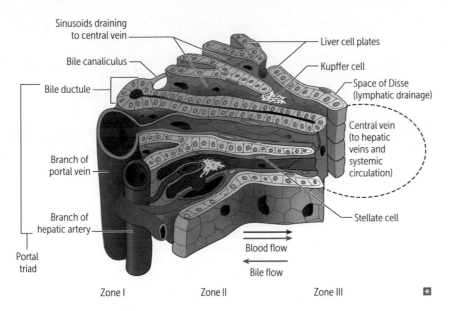

Sinusoids draining to central vein — Liver cell plates

Bile canaliculus — Kupffer cell

Bile ductule — Space of Disse (lymphatic drainage)

Branch of portal vein — Central vein (to hepatic veins and systemic circulation)

Branch of hepatic artery — Stellate cell

Portal triad

Blood flow →
← Bile flow

Zone I   Zone II   Zone III

FIGURE 3-27. **Detailed structure of the liver lobule.**

- Each hexagonally shaped lobule is divided into **three zones:** zone I encircles the portal triad, zone III is located around the central veins, and zone II is between the other zones.
- The **space of Disse** occurs between the endothelial cells of the sinusoids and the hepatocytes themselves.
- **Kupffer cells** are macrophages that are specific to the liver and reside in the liver sinusoids.

The liver has a dual blood supply, with 80% of the blood coming from the portal vein and the other 20% from the hepatic artery.

- The **portal venous blood** comes from the venous drainage of the GI tract; it is therefore rich in nutrients but lacks oxygen. This blood allows the liver to perform its metabolic functions.
- The **arterial supply** to the liver is responsible for oxygenating the hepatocytes and supporting liver cells.

Liver Function

- **Aids digestion:** Hepatocytes continuously secrete bile acids. Most of the **bile** produced by the liver is **recycled** through the ileum via a Na^+-dependent bile salt cotransporter and then travels up the portal vein into the liver as the **enterohepatic circulation.**
- Serves as the **first site of metabolism** of ingested substances absorbed from the small intestine.
- **Maintains the body's blood chemistry:** The liver is the site of many key biochemical processes, such as gluconeogenesis and glycolysis, pharmacologic metabolism (eg, cytochrome P-450 system), and protein synthesis (eg, hepatocytes synthesize coagulation factors, albumin, complement, transferrin, ceruloplasmin, lipoproteins, and cholesterol).
- **Storage:** Maintains a supply of glycogen, vitamins, iron, and copper.

Gallbladder

The main function of the gallbladder is to **store and concentrate bile.** After eating, vagal nerve stimuli cause the gallbladder to contract and relax, promoting the release of bile into the common bile duct.

CLINICAL CORRELATION

- Zone I of the liver lobule receives blood from the portal system first and is primarily affected by toxins; it is also the hepatic exit for bile and is most quickly affected by bile stasis.
- Zone III is located farthest from the hepatic artery and is most likely to be damaged by ischemia and fat accumulation.

KEY FACT

Functions of hepatocytes:
- Formation of bile and bile pigments
- Production of serum proteins (albumin)
- Uptake of chylomicrons
- Production of plasma lipoproteins
- Drug, vitamin, and hormone metabolism
- Vitamin and mineral storage

FLASH BACK

Drugs absorbed by the small intestine are subject to "first-pass metabolism" by the liver.

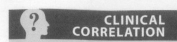

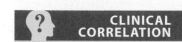

The gallbladder is located on the inferior surface of the liver. It is **divided into the fundus, body, and neck**; it drains through the **cystic duct** (Figure 3-28).

- The cystic duct joins with the **common hepatic duct** to form the **common bile duct.**
- The **common bile duct** descends and finally joins with the pancreatic duct at the **ampulla of Vater** to empty into the second portion of the duodenum.
- Histologically, the mucosa of the gallbladder is composed of **simple columnar epithelium** in which all of the cells are virtually identical; it resembles the small intestine and colon, but lacks goblet cells and crypts.
- The **absorptive epithelium** uses Na$^+$–K$^+$ ATPase to create electrolyte gradients that dehydrate and **concentrate the bile.**

Bilirubin

Bilirubin is a product of heme metabolism (Figure 3-29).

Reticuloendothelial System

The body produces approximately 250–300 mg of heme daily, chiefly from the breakdown of senescent RBCs. A smaller portion comes from turnover of hepatic heme, hemoproteins, and premature destruction of RBCs in the bone marrow (an important clinical consideration with hematologic disorders involving intramedullary hemolysis).

Normally, heme is oxidized to **biliverdin** by heme oxygenase, and then reduced to **bilirubin** by biliverdin reductase.

Liver and Gallbladder

- **Unconjugated bilirubin (indirect bilirubin)** is transported to the liver in the bloodstream bound to albumin, as it is insoluble at physiologic pH.
- **In the liver,** hepatocytes take up bilirubin by carrier-mediated processes. It is then transported to the endoplasmic reticulum and **conjugated** with glucuronic acid by bilirubin uridine diphosphate **(UDP)-glucuronyltransferase.**
- Conjugated bilirubin (**direct bilirubin;** bilirubin glucuronide), now in a water-soluble form, is excreted into bile.

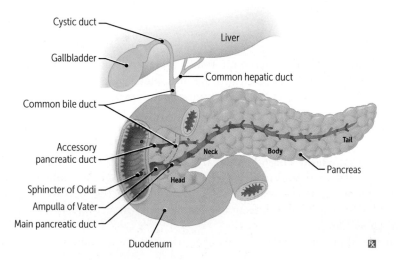

FIGURE 3-28.   The gallbladder and its structures.

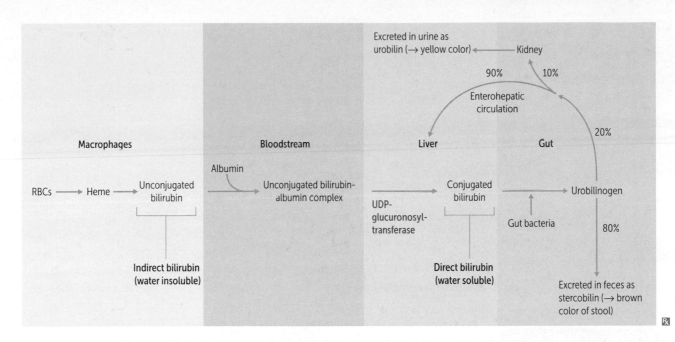

FIGURE 3-29. **Bilirubin pathway.** UDP, uridine diphosphate.

Colon

Normal gut bacteria **hydrolyze** the majority of conjugated bilirubin to an unconjugated form called **urobilinogen** (~80–90% is excreted in the stool; ~10–20% is passively absorbed in the terminal colon, where it enters the portal venous system and is recycled by the liver).

Kidneys

Approximately 10% of the resorbed urobilinogen is filtered and secreted by the kidney.

Bile

Produced by hepatocytes, bile is excreted into the bile canaliculi, where it travels down the bile ducts until it is either excreted or stored in the gallbladder. Bile has **two main functions:**

- Helps to **emulsify** large fats, thus aiding in their absorption by the small intestine.
- Serves as a means of excretion of excess cholesterol, bilirubin, and some pharmaceuticals. Bile salts and lecithin together increase the solubility of cholesterol several million times.

There are several steps in bile synthesis (Figure 3-30):

- **Primary bile acids** are synthesized in the liver from cholesterol.
- **Cholesterol** is first converted into **cholic acid** or **chenodeoxycholic acid** and then **conjugated** with either glycine or taurine to form bile salts.
- More than 95% of bile is **recycled in the ileum,** where it is transported back into the hepatocytes via the **enterohepatic cycle.**
- Approximately 0.2–0.6 mg of bile is lost in feces each day; this loss is balanced by de novo production in hepatocytes.

Secondary bile acids are the result of bacterial metabolism of primary bile acids that have been recirculated via the enterohepatic cycle.

FLASH FORWARD

Jaundice is a yellowing of the skin, and scleral icterus is a yellowing of the sclerae due to elevated bilirubin levels.

Increased indirect bilirubin can occur with excess hemolysis or severe liver damage.

Increased direct bilirubin may indicate a blockage of the bile ducts.

KEY FACT

Key regulatory factors:
- CCK is the primary stimulatory regulator of bile excretion.
- Somatostatin is the primary inhibitory regulator of bile excretion.
- Secretin also stimulates the liver to produce bile.

FLASH FORWARD

Bile acid sequestrants interrupt enterohepatic circulation by binding bile acids in the GI tract and preventing reabsorption; this forces increased de novo synthesis from cholesterol.

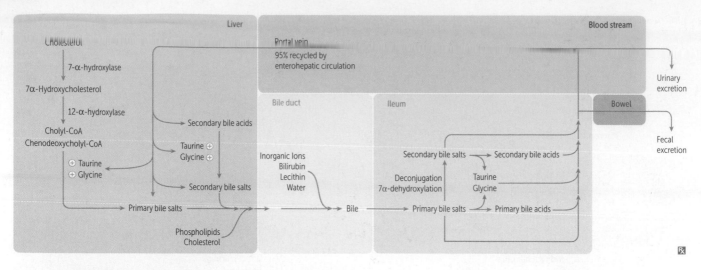

FIGURE 3-30.   Bile formation. Solid lines into the ductular lumen indicate active transport; dotted lines represent passive diffusion. CCK, cholecystokinin.

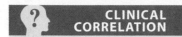

CLINICAL CORRELATION

Gallstones are composed of cholesterol, bile salts, and low levels of phosphatidylcholine (a phospholipid that renders cholesterol soluble).

FLASH BACK

Conditions associated with HIV/AIDS found in the mouth:
- Hairy leukoplakia, an inflammatory condition caused by Epstein-Barr virus.
- Oral candidiasis (thrush).
- Herpetic stomatitis and herpes esophagitis; caused by herpes simplex virus.

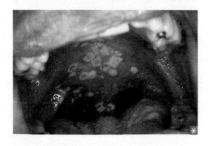

FIGURE 3-31.   Oral candidiasis (thrush). Extensive cottage cheese–like plaques indicative of *Candida* infection. Most frequently presents with odynophagia in immunocompromised patients.

Composition of bile:

- Bile salts
- Phospholipids
- Cholesterol
- Lecithin
- Water
- Bilirubin
- Ions

Pathology

ORAL CAVITY

Mouth and Jaw

Many lesions exist in the mouth and can be subdivided into benign, premalignant, and malignant categories. Certain nonmalignant and premalignant lesions exhibit similar characteristics and can be clinically difficult to differentiate. Premalignant lesions also are hard to identify because they lack the classic characteristics of advanced cancer: pain, ulceration, induration, and cervical lymphadenopathy.

Benign Lesions

- **Lichen planus** is a self-limited, nonmalignant disease of unknown cause that results in classic Wickham striae, which are white, lace-like patterns on top of papules or plaques. It commonly manifests on wrists, elbows, and oral mucosa and is associated with chronic hepatitis C.
- **Oral candidiasis** (Figure 3-31) is a yeast infection in the mouth; it is commonly seen in breast-feeding infants or **immunocompromised hosts.**

Premalignant Lesions

Leukoplakia (Figure 3-32) is **squamous cell hyperplasia,** which can develop into dysplasia, carcinoma in situ, and invasive carcinoma. It can also be seen in inflammatory conditions unrelated to malignancy. **Hairy leukoplakia** is a distinct inflammatory condition affecting immunocompromised patients (**pre-AIDS–defining condition**).

Malignant Lesions

Malignant lesions are the most common pathologic finding in the mouth. Smoking is the greatest risk factor for oral cancer. **Squamous cell carcinoma (SCC)** is the most common oral cancer. Risk factors include chronic cigarette smoking and alcohol use.

Characteristic pathologic findings and treatments are described in Table 3-12.

Salivary Glands

Sjögren syndrome, an autoimmune condition, is the most notable disease affecting the salivary glands. Other important conditions include salivary gland stones (sialolithiasis), benign and malignant tumors, and infections such as mumps (described in Table 3-13).

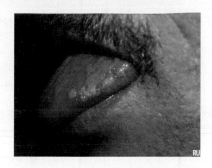

FIGURE 3-32. Hairy leukoplakia.

Sjögren Syndrome (Xerostomia; Keratoconjunctivitis Sicca)

Can occur independently or in conjunction with another autoimmune condition, such as rheumatoid arthritis or systemic lupus erythematosus (SLE).

TABLE 3-12. Most Common Pathologies Affecting the Mouth and Jaw

	PRESENTATION	DIAGNOSIS	TREATMENT	PROGNOSIS
MALIGNANT				
SCC	Persistent papules, plaques, erosions, ulcers	Biopsy with TNM staging	Combination of surgery, radiation, and chemotherapy, depending on stage	Related to stage; often diagnosed at a late stage and frequently recurs, even if caught early
Melanoma	Oral lesion with asymmetry, irregular borders, color changes, increasing diameter	Biopsy	Surgical resection with negative margins; radiation if negative margins are not obtained	Depends on stage, including tumor thickness and ulceration
PREMALIGNANT				
Leukoplakia	White patches or plaques on oral mucosa that cannot be scraped off	Biopsy	Surgery, cryotherapy ablation, carbon dioxide laser ablation	1–20% of lesions progress to malignancy in 10 years
HSV-1 herpetic stomatitis	Vesicular lesions with erythematous bases	Multinucleated giant cells on Tzanck smear	Acyclovir, pain management, fluids	Recurs; some patients have success with chronic suppression
BENIGN				
Aphthous ulcers	Localized, shallow, round ulcers with gray bases that heal in 7–14 days	Clinical presentation	Symptomatic relief with oral analgesics	Some patients have recurrent aphthous stomatitis
Oral candidiasis (thrush)	White plaques that **can be scraped off**	KOH prep	Nystatin mouthwash for 7–10 days	Can be recurrent if patient immunocompromised
Lichen planus	Wickham striae: white, lace-like patterns on top of papules or plaques	Biopsy	Symptomatic relief with topical corticosteroids	Self-limited, can recur

HSV, herpes simplex virus; SCC, squamous cell carcinoma; TNM, tumor, nodes, metastasis.

TABLE 3-13.   Most Common Diseases of Salivary Glands

	CAUSE/PRESENTATION	DIAGNOSIS	TREATMENT	PROGNOSIS
Mumps	Paramyxovirus (parotitis, fever, myalgias, headache, anorexia, orchitis)	Positive IgM mumps antibody, rise in IgG titers, isolation of mumps virus	Symptomatic: analgesics and antipyretics	Vaccination has decreased the incidence of mumps infections
Hypertrophy	Can be caused by eating disorders (bulimia), kwashiorkor, alcoholism, and metabolic disease	Clinical observation	Treat underlying disease	
Sialolithiasis (salivary stones)	▪ Submandibular glands; more common in men ▪ Forms when saliva rich in calcium is stagnant ▪ Some association with gout and nephrolithiasis	Palpation of salivary ducts or imaging studies if not palpable	Conservative therapy: hydration (and sucking on candy to increase salivation), moist heat, massaging the gland, and milking the duct	Secondary infection (sialadenitis), often by *Staphylococcus aureus* and unilateral; chronic sialolithiasis may indicate dysfunctional gland
Salivary gland tumors	▪ Risk factors: radiation and EBV ▪ Smoking has not been connected to malignant tumors, but is linked to Warthin tumor ▪ Most common tumor is pleomorphic **adenoma** (mixed tumor), affecting parotid glands	Fine-needle aspiration with TNM staging biopsy, CT, MRI	▪ Benign: surgical excision ▪ Malignant: Wide margin surgical excision with or without chemo- or radiation therapy	High rate of recurrence

EBV, Epstein-Barr virus; Ig, immunoglobulin; TNM, tumor, nodes, metastasis.

KEY FACT

Hallmarks of Sjögren syndrome are dry eyes (keratoconjunctivitis sicca) and dry mouth (xerostomia) along with multisystem involvement, including skin, lung, heart, and kidney.

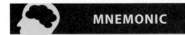

MNEMONIC

Sjögren syndrome is a **MMAPLE** tree:
Multisystem involvement
Mouth dry (xerostomia)
Arthritis
Parotid enlargement
Lymphoma
Eyes dry (keratoconjunctivitis sicca)

KEY FACT

Patients with Sjögren syndrome have an increased risk of lymphoma.

The hallmark of this syndrome is an abnormal lymphocytic infiltration of exocrine glands, most notably the salivary and lacrimal glands, resulting in the classic findings of dry mouth and dry eyes. This abnormal lymphocyte activity also leads to an increased risk of **B-cell lymphoma,** which presents as unilateral parotid swelling.

DIAGNOSIS

The presence of **anti-Ro/SSA** or **anti-La/SSB antibodies** is indicative of Sjögren syndrome. Additionally, the following tests may be used.

- **Schirmer test** is a measure of tear production.
- **Rose Bengal stain** can show areas of corneal or conjunctival epithelial cell damage.
- A **salivary gland biopsy** sample from the lip may show focal collections of lymphocytes.

TREATMENT

- **Symptomatic:** Eye drops for keratoconjunctivitis sicca and the use of sugarless candy or lozenges containing malic acid to stimulate the production of saliva.
- **Good oral hygiene and dental care** is important because of an increased risk of dental caries, gum disease, and halitosis due to decreased saliva production. May also help to prevent salivary calculi, dysphagia, and oral candidiasis.
- More severe cases may require **pilocarpine,** a muscarinic agonist that stimulates salivation, but has side effects of sweating, abdominal cramping, and flushing.

Salivary Gland Tumors

Pleomorphic Adenoma

Most common salivary gland tumor. Presents as painless, mobile mass. **Benign** but will recur if incompletely excised or ruptured intraoperatively.

Mucoepidermoid Carcinoma

Most common **malignant** salivary gland tumor. Painless, slow-growing mass with mucinous and squamous components.

Warthin Tumor

Benign, lymphocyte-rich tumor of parotid gland.

ESOPHAGUS

Esophageal Atresia and Tracheoesophageal Fistula

Esophageal atresia (EA) is the most common congenital anomaly of the esophagus, often associated with tracheoesophageal fistula (TEF) (connection between the trachea and esophagus).

There are several forms of EA, many with TEF (Figure 3-33). Each type depends on the anatomy of the esophagus and the presence or absence of a fistula.

PRESENTATION

Depends on the type of EA/TEF:

- Neonates typically present very early with frothing and bubbling at the nose and mouth as well as coughing, cyanosis, and respiratory distress exacerbated by feeding.
- Children who have TEF but no EA can present later in life with recurrent pneumonia from the aspiration of gastric contents.

DIAGNOSIS

- The diagnosis is confirmed by trying to pass a nasogastric tube into the stomach. If it does not pass easily, an anteroposterior chest radiograph will show the catheter coiled in the blind pouch.
- **Distal TEF** can be diagnosed by a gas-filled GI tract on plain film.

KEY FACT

In the most common form of EA/TEF, (type III; see Figure 3-33C), the proximal esophagus ends in a blind pouch, and the distal esophageal segment demonstrates a proximal TEF.

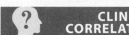

CLINICAL CORRELATION

Maternal polyhydramnios (excess accumulation of amniotic fluid): Develops as a consequence of EA, as a fetus cannot swallow amniotic fluid. Also found in duodenal atresia and Down syndrome.

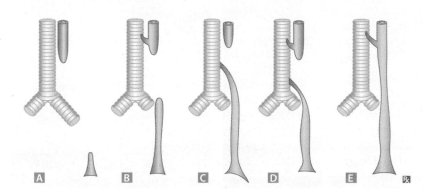

FIGURE 3-33.   The five varieties of esophageal atresia and tracheoesophageal fistula.
A Isolated esophageal atresia (EA). **B** EA with tracheoesophageal fistula (TEF) between proximal segments of esophagus and trachea. **C** EA with TEF between distal esophagus and trachea. **D** EA with TEF between both proximal and distal ends of esophagus and trachea. **E** TEF without EA (H-type fistula).

TREATMENT

Surgical correction.

Esophageal Diverticula

Saccular outpouchings that can be found in the esophagus just as they are found in the colon.

- **False diverticula:** Mucosal layers protruding through the muscularis; most common type.
- **True diverticula:** Contains all layers of the esophageal wall; less common type.

The three characteristic locations of the diverticula:

- **Pharyngoesophageal (Zenker) diverticulum** (Figure 3-34): Located immediately above the cricopharyngeus muscle of the upper esophageal sphincter (UES).
- **Midesophageal diverticula:** Usually located in the middle third of the esophagus. Typically associated with inflammatory conditions such as tuberculosis (TB).
- **Epiphrenic diverticula:** Located in the distal esophagus in the region of the lower esophageal sphincter (LES).

DIAGNOSIS

Patients typically present in their 60s. The earliest sign is transient dysphagia and/or malodorous breath. As the pouch enlarges, more debris is retained and patients can aspirate, complain of gurgling or **regurgitating undigested food,** or have a mass in the neck. The best diagnostic technique is a barium swallow.

TREATMENT

Surgical treatment depends on type and location.

- Zenker diverticula require division of the cricopharyngeus muscle without diverticulectomy (relaxation of the muscle corrects for the defect).
- Epiphrenic diverticula require distal esophageal myotomy with diverticulectomy.

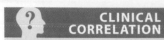

CLINICAL CORRELATION

Zenker and epiphrenic types of diverticula are commonly associated with motor abnormalities of the esophagus, such as spasm, achalasia, and UES/LES hyperactivity.

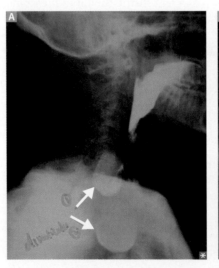
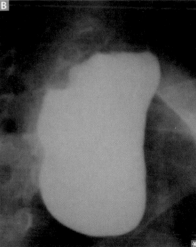

FIGURE 3-34.   **Large pharyngoesophageal diverticulum.** **A** Barium swallow showing two esophageal diverticula (arrows) and **B** compression of esophagus.

Esophageal Varices

Develops as a consequence of portal hypertension resulting in increased pressure in the left gastric vein. Veins have thinner walls in the distal esophagus and are thus more prone to dilation and bleeding. Variceal bleeding is often a cause of upper GI bleeds in patients with portal hypertension (eg, patients with cirrhosis). The resulting hematemesis is usually painless.

DIAGNOSIS

Via endoscopy; sometimes difficult to detect during active variceal hemorrhage.

TREATMENT

Medications can aid in stopping an acute bleed but are not curative.

KEY FACT

In **variceal bleeding,** hematemesis is **painless.** With a **Mallory-Weiss tear,** hematemesis is **painful.**

- **Vasopressin:** Vasoconstriction of mesenteric vessels, which decreases portal venous flow.
- **Proton pump inhibitors (PPIs):** Reduce risk and size of post-ligation ulcers.
- **Somatostatin** or **octreotide:** Inhibits release of vasodilating hormones, indirectly causing vasoconstriction.
- **Endoscopy:** Definitive treatment, either sclerotherapy or variceal band ligation.
- **Balloon tamponade** can provide short-term hemostasis.
- Transjugular intrahepatic portosystemic shunt (**TIPS procedure**—an artificial shunt from the portal vein to the hepatic vein, which reduces the pressure).
- **β-blockers** are drug of choice for prophylaxis.

Mallory-Weiss Tear

Longitudinal tear in the esophagus at the gastroesophageal junction. Associated with severe retching (alcohol intoxication) and bulimia (vomiting type). Accounts for 5–10% of upper GI bleeds; risk of Boerhaave syndrome. Hematemesis is painful.

Boerhaave Syndrome

Occurs in the setting of spontaneous esophageal rupture with exit of gastric contents into the mediastinum, as well as subcutaneous emphysema presenting with crepitus and retrosternal chest pain. Associated with overindulgence in food and alcohol. High mortality rate.

Esophageal Web

Thin mucosal membrane often found in upper esophagus, causing dysphagia and increased risk of esophageal SCC; associated with Plummer-Vinson syndrome (iron deficiency anemia, esophageal web, and atrophic glossitis).

Achalasia

Defined as **"failure to relax,"** achalasia is characterized by:

- Disordered peristalsis (required for diagnosis).
- Increased resting tone of the LES and incomplete relaxation of LES when swallowing.

Achalasia can be due to primary (most common) or secondary causes.

- **Primary/embryologic achalasia** develops as a result of the failed **migration of ganglionic cells** to the myenteric plexus; these cells are required for LES relaxation.
- **Secondary achalasia** occurs from any pathologic process that impairs esophageal motility. **Chagas disease** (principal cause of achalasia in South America) develops as a result of infestation with *Trypanosoma cruzi*, which destroys the myenteric plexus of the esophagus, duodenum, colon, and ureter.

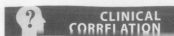

CLINICAL CORRELATION

Difficulty in swallowing both solid and liquid food indicates a motility (neuromuscular) problem.
Difficulty in swallowing solid food indicates an anatomic (mechanical) problem.`

- **Achalasia-like conditions** can occur with amyloidosis, sarcoidosis, or carcinoma.
- In achalasia, the narrowed portion of the esophagus has a lower density of ganglion cells than normal, but the upstream, dilated region is structurally normal

Always consider esophageal cancer in patients with swallowing difficulties and **systemic signs.** Endoscopy is warranted if cancer is considered.

PRESENTATION

Presents with progressive dysphagia beginning with solid foods and progressing to liquids, putrid breath, and frequent nocturnal regurgitation and/or aspiration of undigested food.

DIAGNOSIS

- Manometry shows normal or elevated resting LES pressure, decreased LES relaxation, and absence of peristalsis.
- Barium swallow classically shows a dilated esophagus with a distal **"bird-beak"** narrowing (Figure 3-35).

TREATMENT

Surgical treatment (myotomy) is curative; balloon dilation, botulinum toxin injection, and calcium channel blockers can be used for symptomatic treatment.

Hiatial Hernia

Herniation of part of the stomach into the thoracic cavity (Figure 3-36). Associated conditions include reflux, ulceration, bleeding, and perforation.

- **Sliding hernia (95%):** Protrusion of the stomach above the diaphragm, creating a bell-shaped dilation. GERD may be a manifestation. Treatment is the same as that for GERD (see following section).
- **Paraesophageal hernia:** Part of the greater curvature protrudes through the esophageal hiatus, next to the esophagus. More prone to strangulation than a sliding hernia. Treatment is surgical correction to prevent strangulation.

Gastroesophageal Reflux Disease

Gastroesophageal reflux disease (GERD) develops as a result of abnormal relaxation of the LES and/or delayed gastric emptying with increased pressure in the stomach (eg, hiatal hernia or pregnancy). These abnormalities allow gastric contents to reflux into the esophagus, thus leading to esophageal injury, and chronic inflammation that

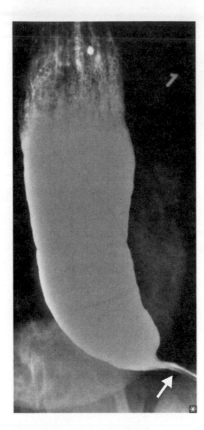

FIGURE 3-35. Bird-beak esophagus typical of achalasia. Aperistalsis of the esophagus associated with smooth narrowing at the lower end of the esophagus (arrow), suggesting achalasia of the esophagus.

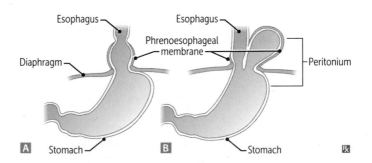

FIGURE 3-36. Hiatal hernias. A Sliding hiatal hernia; B paraesophageal hiatal hernia.

can progress to complications such as erosive esophagitis, esophageal stricture, Barrett esophagus, or esophageal adenocarcinoma.

PRESENTATION

Symptoms of GERD may include heartburn, water brash (an acidic taste in the mouth), dysphagia, hoarseness, globus sensation (lump in the throat), chronic cough (especially at night), and regurgitation.

DIAGNOSIS

Diagnosis is based on clinical history and response to antisecretory medications (PPI and/or H_2 blockers). For some patients, pH monitoring may be helpful. A **triad of histologic features** indicative of mucosal inflammation may be seen on endoscopic biopsy:

- Eosinophils
- Basal zone hyperplasia
- Elongation of the lamina propria papillae

TREATMENT

Lifestyle and diet changes (smoking cessation; avoidance of alcohol and caffeine, fatty foods, acidic foods, spicy foods, and chocolate), antacids, and over-the-counter histamine H_2-blockers for heartburn. More advanced disease requires pharmacologic acid suppression with histamine blockers or proton pump inhibitors. GERD that is incompletely controlled by medication and lifestyle changes can be treated surgically or endoscopically with antireflux procedures.

PROGNOSIS

Long standing reflux can predispose to Barrett esophagus, which can ultimately develop into adenocarcinoma of the esophagus (Figure 3-37).

Barrett Esophagus

Occurs when esophageal mucosa undergoes **intestinal metaplasia** from squamous to specialized columnar epithelium containing goblet cells (Figures 3-38 and 3-39). Goblet cells above the gastroesophageal junction are required for diagnosis. This is a complication of long-standing GERD and increases the risk for adenocarcinoma.

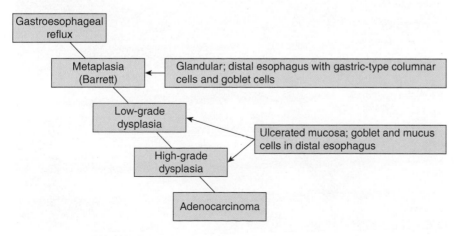

FIGURE 3-37.   **Progression from gastroesophageal reflux disease to Barrett esophagus and adenocarcinoma.**

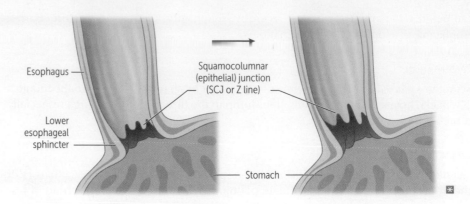

FIGURE 3-38.   **Changes seen with Barrett esophagus.**

PRESENTATION

Long-standing GERD. Advanced cases may present with progressive (weeks to months) dysphagia for solids, weight loss, cough, and/or regurgitation/aspiration (worse at night).

DIAGNOSIS

- **Endoscopy:** Salmon-colored esophageal mucosa extending upward from the gastro-esophageal junction, in contrast to the normal pale pink squamous epithelial mucosa of the esophagus.
- **Biopsy:** Intestinal-type goblet cells in the columnar mucosa of the esophagus.

TREATMENT

Regular endoscopic surveillance to ensure Barrett esophagus has not progressed to esophageal cancer, along with aggressive medical or surgical treatment of GERD. Dys-

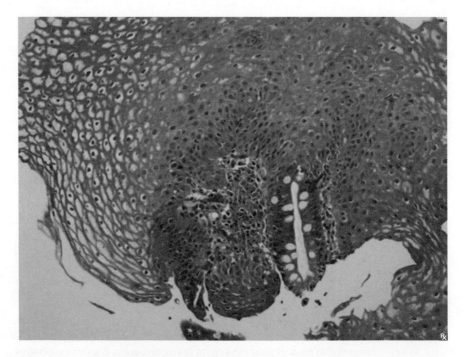

FIGURE 3-39.   **Histology of Barrett esophagus.** Histopathologic findings in nondysplastic Barrett esophagus. Note the glandular epithelium containing goblet cells (arrow).

plasia and limited adenocarcinoma can be treated with either endoscopic ablation (eg, radiofrequency ablation, cryoablation, endoscopic mucosal resection) or surgery.

PROGNOSIS

Complications of Barrett esophagus include strictures, peptic ulceration, and the potential for malignant transformation into adenocarcinoma.

Esophageal Cancer

The incidence varies greatly, depending on geographic region, suggesting environmental causative factors. In the United States, it is more common in African Americans, males, and those with lower socioeconomic status. There are two major types:

- **SCC:** Linked to smoking, alcohol consumption, nitrites, smoked opiates, fungal toxins, radiation, achalasia, very hot tea, and esophageal injury (eg, lye exposure).
- **Adenocarcinoma:** A result of chronic GERD leading to intestinal metaplasia of stratified nonkeratinized esophageal epithelium (Barrett esophagus), which leads to dysplastic changes in the columnar epithelium and adenocarcinoma.

PRESENTATION

Typically, **SCC** appears in the **upper** and **middle** esophagus, whereas **adenocarcinoma** appears in the **lower** esophagus. Most common presenting symptoms are dysphagia and weight loss. The disease is usually incurable once dysphagia is present, as > 60% of the esophageal circumference is involved. Other symptoms include odynophagia, emesis, and aspiration secondary to TEF formation.

Unlike most cancers that spread hematogenously, esophageal cancer typically spreads locally to surrounding tissue, lymph nodes, lungs, liver, and pleura.

DIAGNOSIS

- Periodic screening endoscopy is recommended in high-risk patients with biopsy of suggestive lesions. Endoscopy with biopsy is the gold standard for diagnosis.
- **Contrast radiography.** Identifies esophageal strictures, ulcerations, and mucosal abnormalities with a ragged, ulcerated appearance.

TREATMENT

Endoscopic or surgical resection for potentially curable lesions with or without preoperative chemotherapy and radiation therapy. Palliative treatment for symptomatic advanced-stage lesions (stricture balloon dilation and esophageal stent placement).

PROGNOSIS

Tumor resection, chemotherapy, and radiation therapy are used in some patients to reduce tumor burden, but these are rarely curative. Survival rate 5 years after diagnosis is around 25%.

STOMACH

Gastritis

Gastritis is an inflammation of the gastric mucosa. Depending on the cause, type, and duration of inflammation, it can be subdivided into acute and chronic types.

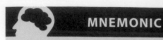
Acute Gastritis

Acute, transient mucosal damage with mucosal edema and inflammation. The injury can erode the mucosa and affect underlying epithelium, in which case **hemorrhagic gastritis** develops. Most common causes include:

- Nonsteroidal anti-inflammatory drug (NSAID) overuse (decreases prostaglandin E_2, which has protective effects on gastric mucosa).
- Alcohol consumption.
- **Cushing ulcers** are associated with head trauma (high intracranial pressure stimulates the vagus nerve, leading to parietal cell stimulation via ACh).
- **Curling ulcers** are associated with burns (fluid loss due to burn, resulting in decreased blood to mucosa).
- Uremia.
- Stress-induced gastritis.
- Corticosteroid use.

Chronic (Atrophic) Gastritis

Continuous inflammation of the gastric mucosa leads to mucosal atrophy and epithelial metaplasia (hence "chronic" and "atrophic"). Based on the location of the injury and the causative agent, chronic gastritis is divided into **types A** and **B**.

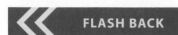
- **Type A:** Affects the fundus and body of the stomach and spares the antrum. Typically secondary to **pernicious anemia** (also known as autoimmune gastritis). It is associated with antibodies to parietal cells (specifically targeting the H^+–K^+ ATPase) and to the intrinsic factor (IF). It leads to achlorhydria with consequent hypergastrinemia.
- **Type B:** Antral-predominant, sparing the fundus and body. Typically secondary to chronic *Helicobacter pylori* infection.

PRESENTATION

Abdominal pain, dyspepsia, and visual changes noted on endoscopic inspection **do not reliably correlate** with the histopathologic diagnosis of gastritis.

DIAGNOSIS

Can be confirmed only histologically (biopsy).

- Diagnosis of *H pylori* infection is based on biopsy (specimen shows gram-negative rods), **urease breath test,** and **stool antigen and serum antibody testing** (see the section on peptic ulcer disease [PUD] for further discussion).
- Pernicious anemia is always suspected in patients with megaloblastic anemia, chronic neurologic changes, and an **abnormal Schilling test.**
- The **Schilling test** occurs in two stages:
  1. Radiolabeled vitamin B_{12} is injected intramuscularly to saturate liver B_{12} receptors and then given orally. If more than 10% is excreted in urine in the first 24 hours, the test result is normal, representing normal uptake in the intestine.
  2. If stage 1 was abnormal, oral radiolabeled B_{12} is given with intrinsic factor; if more than 10% is excreted in urine in first 24 hours, the diagnosis of pernicious anemia is made.

TREATMENT

- For treatment of *H pylori*, see the section on PUD.
- Patients with pernicious anemia need **parenteral** vitamin B_{12} supplementation.
- Proton pump inhibitors are normally given to patients in ICU, those started on corticosteroids, and those with head trauma or burns, as prophylaxis against acute erosive gastritis.

PROGNOSIS

All forms of gastritis have the potential to lead to adenocarcinoma of the stomach. Type B gastritis can lead to primary gastric lymphoma as well.

Ménétrier Disease

Hyperplasia of mucus-secreting cells resulting in rugal hypertrophy and **hypoproteinemia.** Also causes atrophy of parietal cells, thus resulting in achlorhydria. Patients are at risk for adenocarcinoma.

Peptic Ulcer Disease

Ulcer formation in the stomach or the first part of the duodenum. Gastric mucosal cells secrete mucus with large quantities of **bicarbonate** in order to maintain a **pH of 6–7 around the epithelial cells,** in contrast to the pH of 1–2 in the **gastric lumen.** When the mucus layer is breached, by drugs, bacteria, or systemic disorders, epithelial injury occurs, and ulcers can form. Malignant ulcers tend to be large with irregular, thick rolled borders, while benign ulcers tend to be smooth-rimmed circles.

Gastric Ulcers

Less common and occur later in life. Typically develop along the lesser curvature, in the **antral** and **prepyloric** regions (Figure 3-40). Malignant transformation is **more common** than with duodenal ulcers. They are primarily caused by *H pylori* and NSAIDs. Basal and nocturnal acid secretion is typically normal to **decreased.**

Duodenal Ulcers

More than 95% occur in the first portion of the duodenum. Ulcers are typically > 1 cm in size, and **malignancy is extremely rare.** Basal and nocturnal acid secretion tends to be **increased.** NSAIDs and *H pylori* and NSAIDs are also associated risk factors.

PRESENTATION

Burning, gnawing epigastric pain is typical but not specific for this diagnosis (Table 3-14).

- Patients with **duodenal ulcers** tend to give a history of pain **2–3 hours after meals** that is **relieved with food.**
- Patients with **gastric ulcers** have increased **pain with food,** as well as nausea and weight loss.

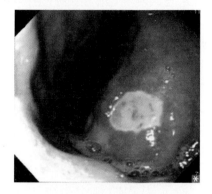

FIGURE 3-40. Gastric ulcer. Note sharply demarcated edges, clean base, and minimal elevation of the edges.

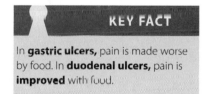

KEY FACT

In **gastric ulcers,** pain is made worse by food. In **duodenal ulcers,** pain is **improved** with food.

TABLE 3-14. The Most Common Characteristics of Peptic Ulcer Disease

	GASTRIC ULCER	DUODENAL ULCER
Percentage	25%	75%
Common causes	*Helicobacter pylori* (~80%), NSAID use	*H pylori* (90–95%), NSAID use
Presenting symptoms	Pain with food	Pain 2–3 h after meals and relieved by food
Complications	Perforation, bleeding, malignancy, gastric outlet obstruction	Perforation, bleeding, gastric outlet obstruction, pancreatitis
Malignancy	10%	Rare
Location	Type-dependent; typically lesser curvature	First portion of duodenum

On physical exam, patients can have tenderness to palpation in the epigastric region. Abdominal rigidity and peritoneal signs are concerning for perforation (most common with duodenal ulcers), which can lead to peritonitis. The most common complication is **upper GI bleeding,** which presents as melena and/or hematemesis.

Diagnosis

- **Endoscopy** is the gold standard for diagnosing gastric and duodenal ulcers.
- **Contrast radiography** can show defects in the gastric and duodenal epithelium caused by ulcers, although small erosions are typically missed.
- *H pylori* infection must also be excluded, as a large number of cases are secondary to this common bacterium. Tests include serum antibodies (**not useful in confirming successful treatment**), stool antigen (**useful in confirming eradication**), urease breath test, and biopsy of tissue via esophagogastroduodenoscopy.
- On endoscopy, the gross appearance is a clean, sharply demarcated ulceration; **unlike ulcerated cancers,** the edges are only slightly elevated.

Treatment

If secondary to chronic NSAID use, the medication should be discontinued or limited. Misoprostol can be added to protect the mucosa if NSAIDs cannot be stopped. Lifestyle changes such as discontinuing alcohol and tobacco are also helpful if these are thought to contribute. Antibiotics should be administered if the patient is found to be infected with *H pylori*.

- One well-accepted treatment recommendation is **clarithromycin + amoxicillin + proton pump inhibitor ± bismuth subsalicylate for 10–14 days.**
  - Metronidazole replaces amoxicillin in penicillin-allergic patients.
  - In areas with clarithromycin-resistant *H pylori*, PPI + bismuth subsalicylate + metronidazole + tetracycline is used.
- For gastric ulcer, biopsy should be performed at the margin of the ulcer to rule out malignancy.

Zollinger-Ellison Syndrome

This syndrome is associated with multiple peptic ulcerations in the stomach and duodenum due to excess gastrin secretion by a gastrinoma, leading to excess gastric acid production. It is associated with multiple endocrine neoplasia (MEN) type 1.

Gastric Cancer

Gastric cancer is a malignant tumor that is the second most common cause of cancer-related death worldwide. Histologically, about 85% are adenocarcinomas, and the remaining 15% are lymphomas and leiomyosarcomas.

Adenocarcinoma

There are two types of gastric adenocarcinoma:

- **Intestinal type:** Thought to arise from the intestinal metaplasia of gastric mucosal cells. Lesions are typically ulcerative and occur in the antrum and lesser curvature (Figure 3-41). Risk factors are a diet high in **salt** and **nitrates,** *H pylori* colonization, blood type A, and chronic gastritis.
- **Diffuse type:** Cells lack normal cohesion, resulting in an infiltrating, discrete mass in the stomach wall. They are more common in younger patients, involve all portions of the stomach, and result in decreased motility, hence, the term **linitis plastica,** or "leather bottle," appearance. **Signet ring cells** are commonly present (Figure 3-42). Prognosis is very poor.

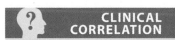

CLINICAL CORRELATION

Patients with perforated duodenal ulcer often present with epigastric pain radiating to the left shoulder as well as with air under the diaphragm on chest film.

CLINICAL CORRELATION

Gastric cancer is much more common in Japan than the United States, as the Japanese diet is significantly higher in salted, pickled, and smoked foods high in nitrates and salt.

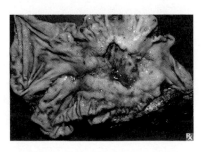

FIGURE 3-41. Gastric adenocarcinoma. Irregular ulcer with thickened rolled borders.

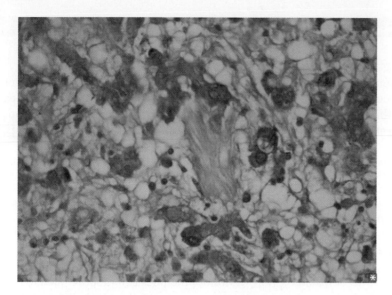

FIGURE 3-42.   **Signet-ring carcinoma cells with high degree of pleomorphism (vary in size and shape).** Intracellular mucin displaces the nuclei to the periphery of the tumor cells.

Primary Gastric Lymphoma

The stomach is the most common extranodal site for lymphoma formation, often associated with *H pylori* infection. Histology ranges from low-grade (mucosal-associated lymphoid tissue [MALT] lymphomas) to high-grade (large-cell non-Hodgkin lymphomas).

PRESENTATION

- Asymptomatic until metastasis or incurable extensive growth has occurred. Patients with **advanced cancer** present with insidious upper abdominal pain, postprandial fullness, early satiety, weight loss, and nausea.
- Typically spreads locally to adjacent organs (direct extension to porta hepatis and transverse colon) and peritoneum.
- Metastases to the left supraclavicular lymph node produce palpable lymphadenopathy (**node of Virchow**).
- Hematogenous dissemination to the ovaries (**Krukenberg tumor**).
- **Sister Mary Joseph sign:** Metastatic mass that protrudes into the umbilicus producing a bulging palpable nodule. Intestinal type occurs more frequently than diffuse type.
- **Leser-Trélat sign:** Multiple outcroppings of seborrheic keratosis.

DIAGNOSIS

Endoscopy is often the first test performed and can identify a majority of lesions. Radiographic examination with IV and oral contrast (double contrast) and CT scan imaging can identify very small lesions. Lack of distention is also a clue to diffuse-type gastric cancer. Definitive diagnosis is established based on biopsy.

TREATMENT

- Surgical resection of involved gastric tissue and adjacent lymph nodes, along with radiation and chemotherapy.
- *H pylori* antibiotic therapy is often enough to treat MALT lymphomas, but subtotal gastrectomy with chemotherapy and radiation is used for higher-grade lymphomas.

PROGNOSIS

- Prognosis for patients with **adenocarcinoma** is poor (5-year survival rate is 10–20%).
- Prognosis for patients with **primary gastric lymphoma** is somewhat better (5-year survival rate is 40–60%).

KEY FACT

Lipid-soluble vitamins are A, D, E, and K. Deficiencies cause:
A: Night blindness, dry skin, corneal degeneration
D: Rickets (children), osteomalacia (adults)
E: Posterior column/spinocerebellar tract demyelination, hemolytic anemia
K: Bleeding with prolonged PT and aPTT but normal bleeding time

QUESTION

A 43-year-old woman presents with an ovarian mass. The mass is resected and reveals signet ring cells. Where is the primary tumor site, and what is the name of this metastasis?

SMALL AND LARGE INTESTINE

Malabsorption Syndromes

This group of disorders is characterized by **decreased absorption,** most often in the small bowel, of essential nutrients. Patients can present with **chronic diarrhea** and/or **steatorrhea** (fatty stool) as well as with systemic effects, such as weight loss and specific vitamin and mineral deficiencies, particularly the **lipid-soluble vitamins A, D, E, and K.**

Underlying pathophysiologies include:

- Pancreatic insufficiency (exocrine deficiencies).
- Damage to the intestinal mucosal surface (surgical resection or pathologic insult to the intestinal villi).
- Liver deficiencies (inadequate bile salt production, abetalipoproteinemia).
- Decreased intestinal transit time (eg, after bariatric surgery).

The spectrum of malabsorption syndromes includes celiac sprue, lactate deficiency, Whipple disease, tropical sprue, short bowel syndrome, bacterial overgrowth syndrome, protein-losing enteropathy, pancreatic failure, and pernicious anemia.

Celiac Sprue (Gluten-Sensitive Enteropathy)

Autoimmune entity with antibodies against the water-insoluble **gliadin** fraction of **gluten,** a protein found in wheat, barley, and rye. Age at presentation varies, but it classically occurs in infants during the time of **cereal introduction.**

- Symptoms can be:
    - **Mild:** Single vitamin deficiency, bloating, and/or chronic diarrhea.
    - **Severe:** Characteristic **chronic diarrhea** with steatorrhea and pale, bulky, foul-smelling stools; multiple vitamin and mineral deficiencies; weight loss; **growth retardation;** and **failure to thrive.**
    - Associated with **dermatitis herpetiformis,** caused by IgA deposition in dermal papillae (Figure 3-43).
    - In 80–90% of cases, association with the human leukocyte antigens **HLA-B8, -DQ2, -DQ8,** or **-DW3.**
- **Classic pathohistologic findings:** Mucosal inflammation, villous atrophy (flattening), and crypt hyperplasia (Figure 3-44). Primarily affects the duodenum and jejunum.
- Can be diagnosed by identifying **antigliadin, antiendomysial,** or **anti–tissue transglutaminase** antibodies as well as a confirmatory small-bowel biopsy.
- **Treatment:** Elimination of gluten-containing foods from the diet is curative in 90% of cases. Remaining patients can be treated with steroids, which typically improve symptoms.

Lactase Deficiency

- Presents as dairy intolerance. It is rare as an inborn error but is common during adulthood as the lactase present in the immature brush border disappears, thus causing **acquired lactose intolerance.** There are no intestinal changes.
- **Treatment:** Avoidance of offending disaccharide or administration of oral enzyme supplements such as lactase.

Whipple Disease

Malabsorptive syndrome with associated systemic symptoms secondary to infection by the classically gram-positive, but often gram-variable organism *Tropheryma whippelii.*

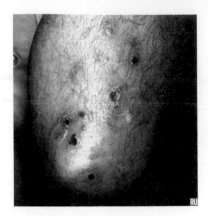

FIGURE 3-43. **Dermatitis herpetiformis in a patient with celiac sprue.** Characterized by pruritic, grouped vesicles in a typical location. The vesicles are often excoriated and may occur on the knees, buttocks, and posterior scalp.

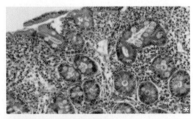
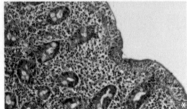

FIGURE 3-44. **Distal duodenum biopsy in a patient with celiac disease.** Note the characteristic features of blunting of villi, crypt hyperplasia, and increased intraepithelial lymphocytes of crypts.

 ANSWER

The patient has a **Krukenberg tumor** from a primary **gastric cancer** (likely diffuse type).

- **Symptoms:** Typical malabsorptive symptoms, such as weight loss and diarrhea, along with systemic signs of infection with fever, polyarthralgias, and abdominal pain. Can affect multiple organ systems, including the CNS.
- **Pathohistologic findings:** Distended lamina propria of the small intestine filled with distinctive **periodic acid-Schiff (PAS)-positive** macrophages with pale, foamy cytoplasm.
- *T whippelii* is best visualized with electron microscopy.
- **Treatment:** Antibiotics are necessary to eradicate the bacterial source. Drug of choice is **ceftriaxone** followed by oral double-strength **trimethoprim-sulfamethoxazole** for 1 year.

Other malabsorption syndromes (Table 3-15) include but are not limited to tropical sprue, abetalipoproteinemia, and intestinal lymphangiectasia.

TABLE 3-15. **Overview of Malabsorption Syndromes**

SYNDROME	MORPHOLOGY	CLINICAL MANIFESTATIONS	TREATMENT
Celiac sprue	<ul><li>Gluten-sensitive enteropathy</li><li>Biopsy: Mucosal</li><li>Inflammation, villous atrophy, and crypt hyperplasia</li><li>Can be diagnosed with anti-gliadin, anti-endomysial, or anti-tissue transglutaminase antibodies, as well as with biopsy</li></ul>	Diarrhea, vitamin/mineral deficiency, **dermatitis herpetiformis** rash	<ul><li>Avoid gluten-containing foods such as wheat, barley, and rye</li><li>Steroids (in ~10% of patients)</li></ul>
Tropical sprue	<ul><li>Unknown occult tropical bacteria</li></ul>	Diarrhea, steatorrhea, weight loss, **folate deficiency**	**Tetracycline** for 6 months. Folic acid replacement
Whipple disease	<ul><li>Caused by gram-positive bacterium *Tropheryma whippelii*</li><li>Flat, blunt villi</li><li>Foamy **macrophages (PAS-positive),** found in lamina propria</li></ul>	Fever, polyarthralgias, weight loss, diarrhea, abdominal pain	**Trimethoprim-sulfamethoxazole** for 1 year
Disaccharidase deficiency	Enzyme deficiency that causes malabsorption	Chronic diarrhea	Avoid offending foods
Abetalipoproteinemia	Congenital lack of apolipoprotein-B; autosomal recessive	Steatorrhea, acanthotic erythrocytes, serum lipid abnormalities, ataxia, atypical retinitis pigmentosa	Medium-chain triglycerides, vitamin E and fat-soluble vitamins
Intestinal lymphangiectasia	Ectatic lymphatics; either sporadic or secondary to cardiac disease	<ul><li>Nausea, vomiting, intermittent diarrhea, and occasionally steatorrhea</li><li>Peripheral edema from hypoalbuminemia</li></ul>	Low-fat, high-protein, medium-chain triglyceride diet
Pancreatic insufficiency	Pancreatic damage/cancer, cystic fibrosis leading to decreased pancreatic enzymes	Fat and ADEK vitamin malabsorption causing steatorrhea and vitamin deficiencies	Supplement pancreatic enzymes and vitamins; treat underlying condition
Bacterial overgrowth syndrome	Inflammatory infiltrate in bowel wall, causing malabsorption as bacteria compete for nutrients	Nonspecific GI symptoms, vitamin deficiencies	Antibiotic therapy, vitamin supplementation

PAS, periodic acid-Schiff.

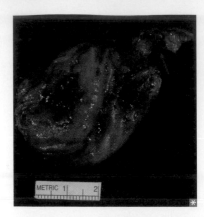

FIGURE 3-45. **Meckel diverticulum.** Gross pathology specimen of a patient's resected bowel reveals a Meckel diverticulum (arrow) with perforation at its tip, attached to the small intestine. Differential diagnosis: Benign ulcers of the small bowel are rare, and ulcerated malignancies are usually irregular in appearance.

MNEMONIC

For Meckel diverticulum, remember the rule of 2s:
2 inches long
2% of the population
2 feet from the ileocecal valve
2% are symptomatic

KEY FACT

Diverticulosis is the most common cause of painless hematochezia in patients > 60 years old.

Diverticular Disease

Diverticula, outpouchings in any hollow viscus such as the GI tract, can be either **congenital** (involving the entire thickness of the involved segment) or **acquired** (mucosal herniation through the muscular layer).

- **Diverticulosis** is the condition of having diverticula, typically implied as being colonic.
- **Diverticulitis** results when the diverticula in question become inflamed.

Meckel Diverticulum

Congenital true diverticulum (involving all three layers of bowel wall) (Figure 3-45) of the terminal ileum that results from incomplete closure of the **omphalomesenteric duct,** found in approximately 2% of the population, ~60 cm (2 ft) from the ileocecal valve, and normally 2 inches long. Mucosa can be ileal (50% of cases), **gastric,** pancreatic, duodenal, or colonic.

PRESENTATION

- Typically asymptomatic and discovered incidentally (patients are typically < 5 years of age).
- Patients can present with endocrine dysfunction due to gastric or pancreatic tissue hormonal production found in the Meckel diverticula.

DIAGNOSIS

- Abdominal pain and intestinal obstruction can result from intussusception or volvulus.
- **Bleeding** may result from mucosal ulcer formation in those with ectopic gastric tissue, which is often present.
- If gastric mucosa is present, a **Meckel scan** may be performed by IV injection of **technetium-99 (^{99}Tc),** which is taken up by parietal cells of the ectopic gastric mucosa.

TREATMENT

Once symptoms occur, surgical excision is curative.

Diverticulosis

Multiple acquired diverticula (Figure 3-46) found at the origin of a mesenchymal feeder artery and typically located in the sigmoid colon. It is thought to be related to a low-fiber diet, which results in increased luminal pressure due to increased colonic muscular contractions required to move stool. Incidence increases with age in Western populations, occurring in almost 50% of adults > 50 years of age. Complications include **hematochezia, diverticulitis** (often caused by fecalith), and **fistula formation** following rupture.

PRESENTATION

- Typically asymptomatic.
- Symptomatic patients can present with acute, painless, voluminous rectal bleeding.

DIAGNOSIS

Colonoscopic evaluation to rule out other lesions and assess the mucosa. Often identified incidentally on colonoscopy.

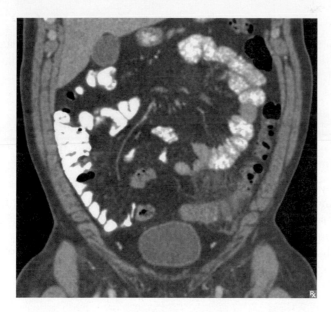

FIGURE 3-46. **Diverticulosis.** Coronal CT shows diverticulosis of the sigmoid and descending colon, with perisigmoid inflammatory changes.

TREATMENT

- **High-fiber diets** are typically suggested in order to increase stool bulk and decrease colonic intraluminal pressure.
- Diverticular bleeding is managed with fluid repletion and transfusion as necessary. With most mild to moderate cases, bleeding resolves spontaneously (~80% of cases)
- Severe cases can be treated with vessel cauterization or clipping during colonoscopic visualization.
- **Mesenteric angiography** is both **diagnostic and therapeutic,** as vasoconstriction and artificial blood clot formation can be induced.

Diverticulitis

Most common complication of diverticulosis, due to infection thought to be secondary to an impacted **fecalith,** resulting in lymphatic obstruction and localized ischemia, which can lead to bacterial overgrowth. Infection can also be secondary to a microperforation leading to contamination of local peritoneum of gut flora. Abscess formation and perforation with peritonitis are serious complications of diverticulitis.

PRESENTATION

Patients with diverticulitis typically present with left lower quadrant (LLQ) abdominal pain, guarding, or peritoneal signs (rebound tenderness), as well as **leukocytosis** and fever. Constipation or obstruction may develop secondary to localized swelling.

DIAGNOSIS

Care must be taken when obtaining imaging studies due to the risk of diverticular perforation during acute infection. Therefore, **barium enema** and **colonoscopy** are **contraindicated.**

- **Abdominal CT** scan can be used to assess for diverticular inflammation as well as pericolic abscess formation.
- An **upright abdominal plain film** should also be obtained to rule out free peritoneal air, which would suggest perforation.

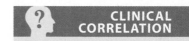

CLINICAL CORRELATION

Typical presentation of diverticulitis is similar to the symptoms of "left-sided appendicitis."

TREATMENT

When there are no signs of perforation, treatment is bowel rest, pain management, fluid resuscitation, and **broad-spectrum antibiotics.** Surgery is required for signs of perforation as well as for drainage of large abscesses.

Intussusception

A condition that typically develops in children < 2 years of age as a result of distal "telescoping" of a portion of the proximal bowel into a more distal one (Figure 3-47). Most common at the **ileocecal junction.**

- The majority of pediatric cases are idiopathic, although there is a seasonal and clinical relationship to certain viral infections, particularly **rotavirus,** in which lymphoid hyperplasia of Peyer patches, which act as lead points, occurs.
- Remaining cases are secondary and occur when a proximal "lead point" is pulled into the distal segment by peristaltic contractions; most commonly found in adults, in which case, cancer must be ruled out.

PRESENTATION

- Symptoms consist of sudden onset of episodic, crampy, severe abdominal pain lasting 10–20 minutes, followed by relatively symptom-free periods. Emesis and nausea can occur during these episodes.
- The classic triad is **pain, palpable sausage-shaped mass,** and **currant-jelly stools,** although all three symptoms are not typically present at the same time.

DIAGNOSIS

- Air contrast enemas are both **diagnostic and therapeutic** in most cases.
- On abdominal plain film, a filling defect in the large colon is diagnostic.
- Abdominal ultrasound can also be used to visualize the intussusception, revealing a **bull's-eye** or **coiled-spring** pattern due to invagination of the proximal segment.

TREATMENT

As mentioned, nonsurgical means are attempted first (**air contrast enema).** Surgery is indicated if enema fails or if perforation occurs.

? CLINICAL CORRELATION

Secondary causes of intussusception:
- Intestinal lymphomas
- Meckel diverticulum
- Vascular malformations
- Intestinal polyps

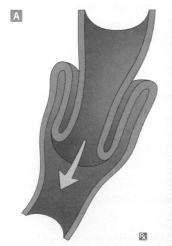 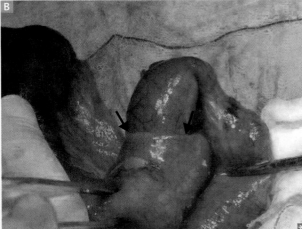

FIGURE 3-47. Intussusception. **A** Diagram of telescoping bowel seen in intussusception. **B** Intraoperative photograph showing telescoping of bowel.

Hirschsprung Disease (Congenital Megacolon)

Hirschsprung disease (HD) is characterized by **complete functional obstruction** of the large bowel due to the **absence of ganglion cells** of both the submucosal and myenteric neural plexuses.

- Aganglionic bowel **always** involves the **rectum** and then progresses proximally to varying degrees (the most severe disease involves the entire colon and even some small intestine).
- Obstruction leads to the characteristic **dilation** of normal bowel proximal to the aganglionic segment, hence, the name **congenital megacolon.**
- Several **genetic mutations** have been associated with HD, the most common of which is the *RET* proto-oncogene.
- HD has also been associated with Down syndrome, Waardenburg syndrome, cardiac defects, and several other congenital conditions. HD occurs in about 1 in 5000 live births, with a male-female ratio of 3:1 to 4:1.

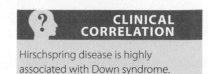

CLINICAL CORRELATION

Hirschspring disease is highly associated with Down syndrome.

PRESENTATION

Typically manifests in a newborn as a **failure to pass meconium** within the first 48 hours of life. Other symptoms of bowel obstruction can be present, such as bilious vomiting and abdominal distention.

DIAGNOSIS

- Rectal biopsy is considered the gold standard for diagnosis and reveals the absence of ganglion cells in the rectal tissue.
- Barium enema can suggest the diagnosis and shows severe dilation of the proximal colon that abruptly narrows into the aganglionic distal colon

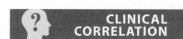

CLINICAL CORRELATION

Early differential diagnosis of HD includes cystic fibrosis, which may present similarly. Genetic testing can be used to make a definitive diagnosis.

TREATMENT

Surgical correction. The aganglionic section is resected, and the normal bowel is connected to the anus.

Omphalocele

The membranous, intestine-filled peritoneal sac that protrudes from the periumbilical abdominal wall during development fails to return to the abdominal cavity.. The defect is **midline.** Associated with other congenital malformations (see Figure 3-3A).

TREATMENT

Surgical correction.

Gastroschisis

Defect of the abdominal wall **lateral of midline** that is **not covered** with peritoneum. Usually an isolated congenital defect (see Figure 3-3B).

TREATMENT

Surgical correction.

INFLAMMATORY DISEASES OF THE COLON

By definition, *colitis* is an inflammation of the colon. There are several causes; the most common are discussed below.

Crohn Disease and Ulcerative Colitis

Crohn disease (CD) and ulcerative colitis (UC) are two major idiopathic types of inflammatory bowel disease (IBD) (Figures 3-48 and 3-49).

PRESENTATION

UC and CD share many features resulting from bowel inflammation, including **diarrhea with blood or mucus, crampy abdominal pain,** fever, tenesmus, weight loss, and blood loss; however, they also differ in important ways, as listed in Table 3-16. Consider IBD or colon cancer in any patient with rectal bleeding and systemic signs.

DIAGNOSIS

Diagnosis is made by colonoscopy with biopsy specimen showing characteristic histologic findings.

TREATMENT

The medical treatment for both IBDs is similar and includes 5-ASA medications (mesalamine) for milder forms; corticosteroids, biologics, and immunomodulators such as azathioprine for more severe cases.

PROGNOSIS

Surgical therapy (**colectomy**):

- In patients with uncontrolled UC, colectomy is **curative.**
- In patients with CD, surgery is **not curative** but is required to manage complications in 70% of patients.
- Both types of IBD are associated with an increased risk of colon cancer; this risk is higher in UC.

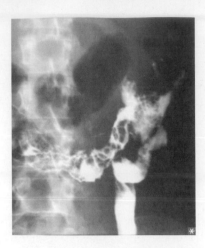

FIGURE 3-48.   Crohn disease. Barium enema showing narrowed colon with lacunar defects and fistulous tracks at the splenic flexure, two of which are spreading towards the left diaphragm.

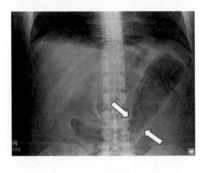

FIGURE 3-49.   Ulcerative colitis. X-ray depicts areas of thumbprinting (white arrow) that is suggestive of colonic bowel wall edema.

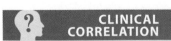

CLINICAL CORRELATION

In patients with Crohn disease, Ca^{2+} binds to the excess lipids in the intestinal lumen and is excreted in stool. This leads to an excess of oxalate that precipitates in the kidneys, forming calcium oxalate kidney stones.

TABLE 3-16.   Clinical and Pathologic Features of Crohn Disease and Ulcerative Colitis

	CROHN DISEASE	ULCERATIVE COLITIS
Location	May involve **any portion** of the GI tract (from mouth to anus), usually the terminal ileum and colon; **skip lesions,** with **rectal** sparing	**Colitis** only occurs in the **large intestine; continuous lesions,** always with rectal involvement
Gross morphology	**Transmural inflammation; cobblestone-like** mucosa, **creeping fat,** bowel wall thickening ("string sign" on barium studies), linear ulcers, fistulas	Mucosal and submucosal inflammation only; friable mucosal pseudopolyps, haustra loss leading to "lead pipe" appearance
Microscopic morphology	**Noncaseating granulomas** and lymphoid aggregates	Crypt abscesses and ulcers, bleeding, **no granulomas**
Complications	Strictures, fistulas, perianal disease, malabsorption, nutritional depletion, calcium oxalate kidney stones	Severe stenosis, toxic megacolon, **colorectal carcinoma**
Extraintestinal manifestations	Migratory polyarthritis, erythema nodosum, ankylosing spondylitis, uveitis, immunologic disorders	Pyoderma gangrenosum, **primary sclerosing cholangitis**

Pseudomembranous Colitis

Pseudomembranous colitis is an acute inflammation of the colon mediated by overgrowth of *Clostridium difficile*. Typically, this is precipitated by a course of antibiotics (classically, ampicillin, clindamycin, or a cephalosporin) that depletes the normal colonic bacterial flora (*Escherichia coli* and *Bacteroides fragilis*).

PRESENTATION

Symptoms are due to the *C difficile* toxins. Toxin A, an enterotoxin, binds to and damages brush border cells and attracts neutrophils to the site of infection. Toxin B, a cytotoxin, destroys the enterocyte cytoskeleton. Combined, this results in hypermotility, inflammation, and increased capillary permeability.

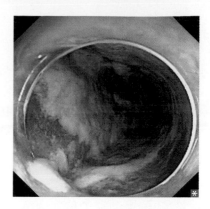

FIGURE 3-50. Pseudomembranous colitis. Colonoscopy shows a colonic wall covered by thick pseudomembranes.

- Typical symptoms include watery diarrhea, abdominal pain or cramping, and fever. It can also be associated with colonic bleeding. Leukocytosis is also common.
- In severe cases, the colonic mucosa becomes covered with yellow or gray exudates, hence the term **pseudomembranous colitis** (Figure 3-50). This can lead to toxic megacolon, volvulus, or colonic perforation, all of which can be life threatening.

DIAGNOSIS

A stool sample is tested for the A and B toxins of *C difficile*.

TREATMENT

The first step in treating pseudomembranous colitis is stopping the inciting antibiotic.

- As with many infectious diarrheas, **antidiarrheal agents** such as loperamide are **contraindicated,** as they will prolong production of toxins in the colon, thus worsening the condition.
- *C difficile* infection can be treated with metronidazole (first-line) or oral vancomycin.
- Fecal microbiota transplant can also be used in refractory cases of *C difficile* infection.

Infectious Colitis

Infectious causes of colitis can be viral, bacterial, or parasitic. Patients with infectious colitis typically present with severe diarrhea, fever, leukocytosis, and abdominal pain. Clues in the history may include travel, recent antibiotic use, specific food consumption, and immunodeficiency. Review specific organisms in the microbiology section. (See Table 3-17 for common causes of infectious diarrhea.)

TABLE 3-17. Causes of Diarrhea[a]

CAUSES OF BLOODY DIARRHEA	CAUSES OF WATERY DIARRHEA
Campylobacter	*Vibrio cholerae* (rice-water diarrhea)
Salmonella (undercooked poultry)	*Clostridium perfringens*
Shigella	*Giardia* (freshwater streams)
Enterohemorrhagic *Escherichia coli* (EHEC) (contaminated hamburger)	*Cryptosporidium* (in immunocompromised)
Enteroinvasive *E coli* (EIEC)	Enterotoxigenic *E coli* (ETEC)
Yersinia	Viruses (rotavirus, Norwalk, adenovirus)
C difficile (hospitalization, recent antibiotics)	*C difficile*
Entamoeba histolytica	*Bacillus cereus* (reheated rice)

[a] Common associations with each pathogen are shown in parentheses.

Typhoid Fever

Salmonella typhi is the agent responsible for typhoid fever, the symptoms of which include bacteremia, splenomegaly, and even **liver necrosis**, as well as ulceration of Peyer patches with intestinal bleeding and ulceration. If the gallbladder is colonized, the individual becomes a carrier. **Rose spots,** a classic rash on the skin, are pathognomonic.

Entamoeba histolytica

Entamoeba histolytica is a dysentery-causing protozoan parasite (Figure 3-51). Amebae invade the crypts of colonic glands and burrow down into the submucosa. The organisms fan out laterally, creating **flask-shaped ulcers.** They can penetrate the portal venous system and spread to the liver, causing **liver abcesses.** Diagnosis is by stool ova and parasites or stool *E histolytica* antigen.

Giardia lamblia

Giardia lamblia is an intestinal protozoan that attaches to the small intestinal mucosa but does not appear to invade. Therefore, fecal leukocyte tests are negative. Associated with greasy, **fatty stools** and **foul-smelling flatulence** consistent with malabsorption. Diagnosis is by *Giardia* antigen stool testing. Treatment is metronidazole.

Cryptosporidia

Cryptosporidiosis leads to diarrhea in immunocompromised people and is a potentially fatal complication of AIDS.

TUMORS OF THE COLON

Benign Polyps

These polyps have extremely low potential for malignancy (see Table 3-18 for types of polyps).

- **Hyperplastic polyps** are the most common type of benign polyp.
- **Juvenile polyps** are hamartomatous proliferations of the lamina propria enclosing widely spaced, dilated cystic glands. Usually seen in children < 5 years old but can be diagnosed at any age.
- **Other types** include mucosal polyps, submucosal lipomas, inflammatory pseudo-polyps, and other types of hamartomatous polyps.

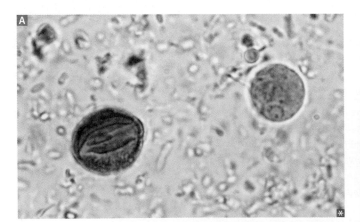
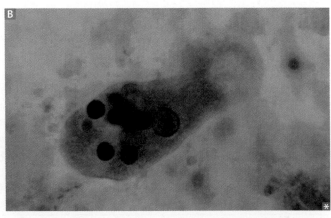

FIGURE 3-51. ***Entamoeba histolytica.*** **A** Photomicrograph shows *Entamoeba histolytica* cysts that when mature, will display four identifiable nuclei. **B** Trichrome-stained photomicrograph depicts an *Entamoeba histolytica* trophozoite within which a number of erythrocytes can be seen as dark inclusions.

TABLE 3-18. Types of Colonic Polyps and Syndromes

Cowden syndrome	Hamartomatous polyps in the GI tract. Increased risk of neoplasms of the thyroid, breast, uterus, and skin
Familial adenomatous polyposis	Patients develop 500–2500 colonic adenomas that carpet the mucosal surface. Most polyps are tubular adenomas. 100% risk of colonic cancer by midlife. Increased risk of duodenal cancer
Gardner syndrome and Turcot syndrome	Both of these syndromes share the same APC genetic defect as FAP, but differ in one regard: these two syndromes have extraintestinal tumors, whereas FAP does not
Hyperplastic polyps	No malignant potential when left-sided and small. Formed as the result of abnormal mucosal maturation, inflammation, or architecture
Juvenile polyps	Hamartomatous proliferations of the lamina propria enclosing widely spaced, dilated cystic glands. Usually seen in children < 5 y
Lynch syndrome (hereditary nonpolyposis colon cancer)	Early-onset colon cancer due to defects in mismatch repair genes. Also can develop extracolonic tumors
Peutz-Jeghers syndrome	Hamartomatous polyposis. Increases risk of pancreatic cancer and melanotic mucosal and cutaneous pigmentation

APC, adenomatous polyposis coli; FAP, familial adenomatous polyposis.

Adenomatous Polyps

By definition, adenomatous polyps are dysplastic and therefore are potentially malignant. There are three subtypes:

- **Tubular** adenomas are the most common of the three; can be pedunculated, sessile, flat, or depressed.
- **Tubulovillous** polyps are so named because they have characteristics of both tubular and villous adenomas; they have an intermediate rate of malignant conversion.
- **Villous** adenomas have the **highest rate of malignant conversion.** Histologically, they have a cauliflower-like appearance with fingerlike villi extending down into the center of the polyp.

Polyposis Syndromes

Several genetic disorders can cause multiple colonic polyps, usually at young ages.

Familial Adenomatous Polyposis (FAP)

- Autosomal dominant genetic disorder.
- Caused by mutation in adenomatous polyposis coli (APC) gene.
- Presents with numerous precancerous and cancerous colon polyps (Figure 3-52) in the second or third decade of life.
- Diagnosis confirmed with more than 100 polyps found on colonoscopy.
- Nearly 100% of patients develop colorectal cancer.
- Prophylactic total colectomy is indicated, often during childhood.

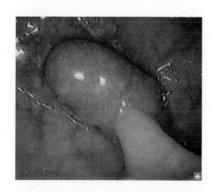

FIGURE 3-52. Colonic polyp.

Gardner Syndrome

Autosomal dominant genetic disorder characterized by multiple adenomatous colon polyps in conjunction with extraintestinal tumors, including osteomas, hepatoblastomas, papillary thyroid carcinoma, and periampullary adenomas.

Turcot Syndrome

Autosomal recessive disorder that causes colonic polyps and tumors of the central nervous system, especially glioblastoma multiforme and medulloblastoma.

Hereditary Nonpolyposis Colorectal Cancer (HNPCC)

Autosomal dominant disorder that causes colorectal adenomas and colorectal cancer. A mutation in a **DNA mismatch repair gene** (*hMLH1* or *hMSH2*) is thought to be the cause of the disease. This leads to a hypermutable state and also causes **microsatellite instability**.

Peutz-Jeghers Syndrome

Autosomal dominant disorder characterized by a combination of hamartomatous colon polyps and **mucocutaneous hyperpigmented lesions** on the lips (Figure 3-53), oral mucosa, hands, and genitals. The colon polyps rarely become cancerous, but they can cause symptoms such as obstruction, pain, and bleeding. Those affected have a higher likelihood of cancer in the stomach, pancreas, breast, and ovaries.

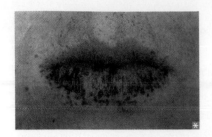

FIGURE 3-53. **Peutz-Jehgers syndrome.**

Colorectal Cancer

Histologically, colorectal cancer is **adenocarcinoma of the large intestine or rectum (or both)**. It is the third most common cancer, as well as the second leading cause of cancer-related death in both men and women in the United States.

- **Risk factors** include advanced age, family history, low-fiber diet, adenomas, IBD (especially UC), FAP, Peutz-Jeghers syndrome, and HNPCC.
- **Screening** should start at age 50 with colonoscopy every 10 years or fecal occult blood every year. Flexible sigmoidoscopy can be used instead of colonoscopy but must be done at least every 5 years.
- Colon cancer typically arises from adenomas in the colon. Research shows that, over time, underlying genetic mutations along with environmental influences lead to the stepwise conversion of normal colonic epithelium to dysplastic adenomas and, finally, to malignant adenocarcinoma (**adenoma-carcinoma sequence;** Figure 3-54).
- The most common mutations are in the **APC** gene, which occur **early** in the development of colon cancer, in the **K-RAS** gene, which is often the next gene mutated, and in the **p53** gene, which occur **later**. Many other gene mutations have been implicated and occur at various stages in the development of cancer.

KEY FACT

Mutated *RAS* remains in an activated state, continuously delivering mitotic signals and thus preventing apoptosis.

PRESENTATION

Colon cancer typically occurs in adults > 50.

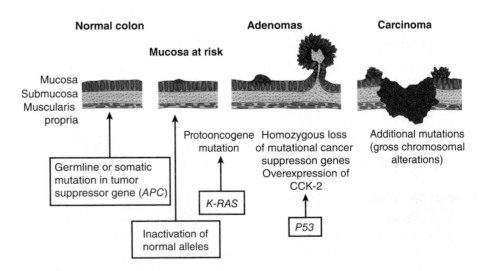

FIGURE 3-54. **Adenoma-carcinoma sequence.** The development of carcinoma from adenomatous lesions is referred to as the adenoma-carcinoma sequence.

- **Left-sided (sigmoid) colon cancer:**
  - **Early** symptoms of **obstruction** (the left side has a narrower lumen).
  - Tumors produce a "**napkin-ring,**" or "**apple-core**" constriction (encircling annular growth; Figure 3-55).
  - May complain of a change in bowel habits/stool consistency ("pencil-thin stools") due to obstruction, though most frequent symptom is rectal bleeding.
- **Right-sided colon cancer:**
  - **Anemia,** weight loss, and abdominal **pain.**
  - Stool is watery in the right colon; thus, obstruction seldom occurs.
- **Either side:**
  - Stool changes or hematochezia.
  - Abdominal discomfort.
  - Constitutional symptoms such as weight loss.
  - Unexplained anemia in men and postmenopausal women—think colon cancer.
  - Higher incidence of *Streptococcus bovis* endocarditis.

DIAGNOSIS

- Colonoscopy with tissue biopsy revealing adenocarcinoma is the gold standard for diagnosis. Once the diagnosis is made, CT scans are done to look for metastases.
- **Carcinoembryonic antigen (CEA)** is not recommended as a diagnostic serum marker for colon cancer; however, it can be very useful in evaluating the success of surgical resection, as well as in monitoring the recurrence of the cancer.

TREATMENT

Surgical resection and chemotherapy (usually involving fluorouracil and oxaliplatin) are the most common treatments.

- Colon cancer can **metastasize hematogenously** as well as through the **lymphatics.**
- The most common sites of **metastasis** are the regional lymph nodes, **liver,** lungs, and peritoneum; other possible sites for metastases are the bones and brain.

PROGNOSIS

Depends on the stage of the tumor at diagnosis. Favorable when the cancer is detected early, before metastasis has occurred. Once widespread, the 5-year survival rate drops to < 10%.

Carcinoid Tumors

Small, slow-growing neoplasms arising from neuroendocrine cells along the GI tract, which release a variety of substances into the bloodstream, often serotonin. This can result in carcinoid syndrome if the tumor metastasizes to or past the liver, as the liver can no longer metabolize the serotonin.

PRESENTATION

Carcinoid syndrome: Wheezing, flushing, diarrhea, and right-sided valvular and endocardial lesions. The left side of the heart is spared as the lungs are able to metabolize serotonin.

DIAGNOSIS

High urine levels of 5-hydroxyindoleacetic acid (5-HIAA) (serotonin metabolite).

TREATMENT

Surgical excision is curative if tumor is small. Octreotide can be used for symptomatic treatment.

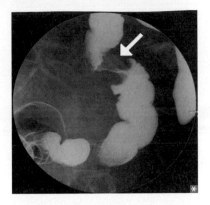

FIGURE 3-55. Annular, constricting adenocarcinoma of the descending colon. This radiographic appearance is referred to as an "apple-core" lesion and is always highly suggestive of malignancy.

? CLINICAL CORRELATION

CEA can be elevated in other conditions:
- Malignant: Cancers of the pancreas, stomach, breast, lung, and certain types of thyroid and ovarian cancers.
- Other: Chemotherapy and radiation therapy may lead to temporary elevation of CEA (massive death of tumor cells releases CEA into the circulation).

APPENDICITIS

Appendicitis is the most common indication for emergency abdominal surgery in children (commonly due to lymphoid hyperplasia related to infection), but it can occur in all age groups, peaking at 15–30 years (in adults, commonly related to a fecalith).

FLASH BACK

McBurney point is located one-third of the distance from the anterior superior iliac spine to the umbilicus.

PRESENTATION

Classic presentation is fever and periumbilical abdominal pain, later localizing to the right lower quadrant (**McBurney point**), accompanied by signs of peritoneal irritation (rebound tenderness, rigidity, guarding). Anorexia, vomiting, constipation, and diarrhea may also be present.

DIAGNOSIS

Diagnosis is **clinical.** It is better to take out a healthy appendix than to let one rupture.

- Leukocytosis, pyuria, and fecal leukocytes are the most common laboratory findings. Pregnancy testing is mandatory on premenopausal women to rule out ectopic pregnancy.
- Abdominal CT is generally diagnostic and should be performed in equivocal cases.

TREATMENT

Surgical appendectomy is necessary and curative. There is a 40% rate of perforation in the pediatric population, but the mortality rate is < 1%.

ABDOMINAL HERNIAS

Hernias are abnormal protrusions of the abdominal contents through a defect in the abdominal wall.

The **hernial mass** consists of three parts: covering tissues (formed by layers of the abdominal wall), a peritoneal sac, and any structure (including viscera) contained within the abdominal cavity.

Hernias are described as reducible, irreducible, or strangulated (Table 3-19).

TABLE 3-19.   Causes of the Most Common Abdominal Hernias

HERNIA TYPE	CAUSE	LOCATION
Indirect inguinal hernia	Congenital weakness in the fascial margin of the internal inguinal ring (patent processus vaginalis). Therefore, covered by all layers of spermatic fascia	Originates lateral to the inferior epigastric vessels
Direct inguinal hernia	Congenital or acquired weakness in the fascia of the inguinal canal floor, leading to protrusion of contents through the external inguinal ring. Therefore, covered by external spermatic fascia only	Originates medial to the inferior epigastric vessels (above and medial to the pubic tubercle)
Femoral hernia	Weakness of the femoral septum, allowing protrusion of the hernial sac through the femoral canal within the femoral sheath	Originates below and lateral to the pubic tubercle
Umbilical	Congenital (eg, infants) or acquired (eg, multiparous women) abnormality in the musculature around the umbilical cord	Originates at the umbilicus
Incisional	Acquired as a postoperative complication	Originates at surgical incision sites

- **Reducible:** Most common type, usually painless. The abdominal contents can be easily returned to the abdomen.
- **Irreducible (incarcerated):** Difficult to return the contents to the abdominal cavity. Can become painful if bowel is obstructed or incarcerated.
- **Strangulated:** The entrapped organ (usually bowel, sometimes fat) becomes incarcerated in the fascial defect, resulting in compromised blood supply. Strangulated hernias are intensely painful and very dangerous due to bowel obstruction and possible necrosis. They require **immediate surgical repair.**

PRESENTATION

- **Inguinal hernias** (Figure 3-56):
  - Most common type, more common in **men.**
  - Direct implies herniation through external inguinal ring only, medial to the inferior epigastric vessels.
  - Indirect implies herniation through internal and external inguinal rings, lateral to the inferior epigastric vessels; can enter scrotum.
  - Patients complain of painless bulge in inguinal area that is worse with cough or straining (or any other increase in intra-abdominal pressure).
  - Treatment is surgical.
- **Femoral hernias** (Figure 3-56):
  - More often seen in **women.**
  - More frequently incarcerated than inguinal hernias due to small area of femoral ring and nearby anatomy.
  - Can be painful, requiring prompt surgical repair.
- **Umbilical hernias:**
  - Often present in **infants** or **children.**
  - Often due to congenital defects in abdominal wall at umbilicus.
  - Can occur in adults, either in multiparous women or those with chronic cough or ascites (secondary to increased intra-abdominal pressure).
  - Patients complain of bulge at umbilicus that is worse with Valsalva maneuver.
  - Painless unless incarcerated bowel is present.
  - Treatment is surgical.

DIAGNOSIS

Based on clinical symptoms and physical exam.

- A **direct inguinal** hernia bulge should be felt on either side of the finger, and the **indirect inguinal** hernia bulge should be felt on the tip of the finger.
- **Femoral** hernias can often be palpated medial to the femoral pulse and inferior to the inguinal ring.
- CT scan or ultrasound may be necessary with patients who have hernias that are not easily palpable (ie, obese patients).

>
> **KEY FACT**
>
> Hesselbach triangle (a site of direct inguinal hernias):
> - Rectus abdominis muscle (medial)
> - Inguinal ligament (inferior)
> - Inferior epigastric blood vessels (superior and lateral)

>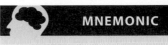
> **MNEMONIC**
>
> **MD**s don't **LI**e:
> **M**edial to the inferior epigastric vessels = **D**irect inguinal hernia
> **L**ateral to the inferior epigastric vessels = **I**ndirect inguinal hernia

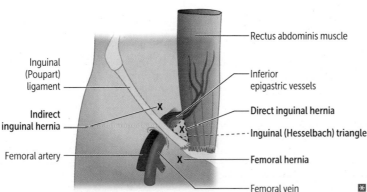

FIGURE 3-56. Sites of inguinal and femoral hernias.

TREATMENT

Surgical repair (herniorraphy). In low-risk cases in which the hernia is not causing the patient significant symptoms, nonoperative management may be used.

LIVER DISEASE

Jaundice

Patients with jaundice often present with yellowed skin or sclera that represents an underlying increase in serum bilirubin (Table 3-20 and Figure 3-57).

TABLE 3-20.   Jaundice: Underlying Causes[a]

JAUNDICE	DISEASES	SERUM BILIRUBIN	URINE BILIRUBIN	URINE UROBILINOGEN
Conjugated	Congenital hepatocellular disease: **Dubin-Johnson syndrome ❸:** Inherited defect in liver excretion of conjugated bilirubin that leads to a functionally normal glossy black liver **Rotor syndrome ❹:** Defect in hepatic storage of conjugated bilirubin, leading to a functionally normal liver without any discoloration Physical obstruction of the bile duct by: Gallstones Tumors, especially pancreatic tumors Primary sclerosing cholangitis Parasites	↑ Direct bilirubin (> 15%)	↑	Normal
Unconjugated	Hemolytic disease: Sickle cell Glucose-6-phosphate dehydrogenase deficiency Spherocytosis Microangiopathic hemolytic anemia Paroxysmal nocturnal hemoglobinuria ABO/Rh isoimmunization Autoimmune hemolytic anemia (warm and cold) Congenital hepatocellular conditions: **Crigler-Najjar type 1 ❷:** Absent UDP-glucuronyl transferase, unable to convert unconjugated to conjugated bilirubin, severe jaundice at birth, **does not respond to phenobarbital** **Crigler-Najjar type 2:** Less severe form of Crigler-Najjar type 1 and **responds to phenobarbital,** which induces hepatic enzymes, including UDP-glucuronyl transferase **Gilbert syndrome ❶:** Transient decrease in the activity of UDP glucuronyl transferase, which causes asymptomatic rise in indirect bilirubin, associated with stress; common, affecting about 5% of the population	↑ Indirect bilirubin	Absent (acholuria)	↑ (from heme metabolism)
Mixed	Acquired hepatocellular disease: Cirrhosis Hepatitis Drugs (ie, steroids, rifampin, probenecid, ribavirin) Liver failure (ie, sepsis)			

[a] Numbers refer to locations in Figure 3-57.

UDP, uridine diphosphate.

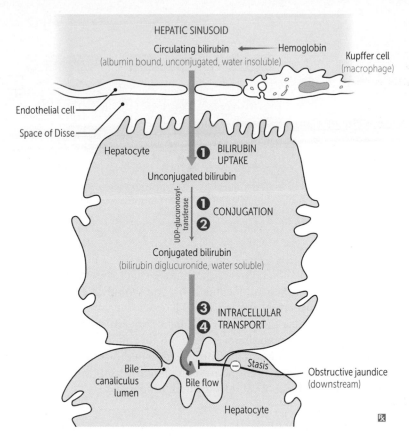

FIGURE 3-57. Hereditary hyperbilirubinemias. Numbered positions refer to the diseases listed in Table 3-20.

- **Physiologic jaundice:** Extremely common (50% of newborns). A condition in neonates that results from the relative deficiency in glucuronyl transferase in the immature liver in newborns. They also have a large red cell mass with a shorter cellular life span. **Hemolysis** resulting from mild trauma during the birth process can exacerbate the condition by increasing bilirubin production.
- **Adult jaundice:** A pathologic process due to overproduction (eg, hemolysis) or impaired excretion (eg, bile duct obstruction, hepatocellular dysfunction) of bilirubin.

PRESENTATION

- Scleral icterus typically appears first, generally at serum bilirubin levels of 2–3 mg/dL. Yellowing of the skin is seen at even higher levels of serum bilirubin.
- **Newborns:** Jaundice present **at birth** is **pathologic and is often due to an inherited hyperbilirubinemia.** In contrast, **physiologic jaundice** of the newborn is clinically benign and occurs **48–72 hours following birth.** Bilirubin levels rise at < 5 mg/dL/day and peak at < 15 mg/dL. Direct bilirubin comprises < 10% of the total.

DIAGNOSIS

The **most important step** in diagnosis is determining if the jaundice is secondary to conjugated (direct), unconjugated (indirect), or mixed hyperbilirubinemia (Figure 3-58). This can easily be determined by laboratory testing of patient blood samples.

- **Direct** hyperbilirubinemia is always pathologic.
- **Indirect** hyperbilirubinemia may be physiologic or pathologic.

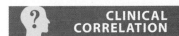
CLINICAL CORRELATION

Jaundice at birth is **always pathologic.** Jaundice that occurs 48–72 hours after birth is **physiologic jaundice** and clinically benign.

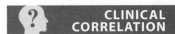
CLINICAL CORRELATION

In a patient presenting with painless jaundice, pancreatic cancer must be high on the differential diagnosis.

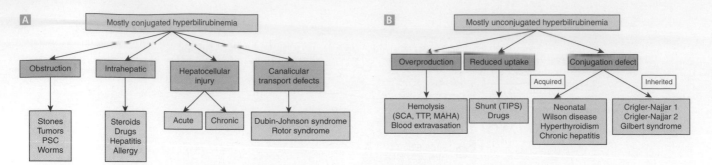

FIGURE 3-58. **Differential diagnosis for elevation of A direct and B indirect bilirubin.** PSC, primary sclerosing cholangitis; MAHA, microangiopathic hemolytic anemia; TIPS, transjugular intrahepatic portosystemic shunt; TTP, thrombotic thrombocytopenic purpura; SCA, sickle cell anemia.

TREATMENT

Address the underlying condition. Physiologic jaundice of the newborn typically resolves with normal maturation and breast-feeding/hydration within 1–2 weeks. More severe cases of unconjugated hyperbilirubinemia in the newborn can be treated with **phototherapy,** or exposure to blue-green light. The light converts bilirubin to its photoisomer, which is water-soluble and therefore easier to excrete. Prior to development of phototherapy, newborns with severe unconjugated hyperbilirubinemia were at risk of developing **kernicterus,** permanent neurologic damage from bilirubin crossing the blood-brain barrier, which is not yet fully formed in neonates.

Hereditary Hyperbilirubinemias

Rare conditions that can be differentiated by the predominant form of bile acids (conjugated or unconjugated) present in the bloodstream.

Hereditary Causes of Direct (Conjugated) Hyperbilirubinemia

Dubin-Johnson Syndrome

Rare inherited **autosomal recessive** condition caused by impaired intrahepatic bilirubin secretion.

- The absence of the canalicular protein **multidrug-resistant protein 2 (MRP-2)** impairs transport of conjugated bilirubin and other non–bile acid organic anions into the bile canaliculus.
- Grossly, the **liver** appears **pigmented and often enlarged,** but is functionally normal.

PRESENTATION

Mostly asymptomatic, but may present with chronic or recurrent jaundice of varying intensity.

DIAGNOSIS

- Elevated serum direct bilirubin
- Normal complete blood count (CBC)
- Normal liver enzymes
- Grossly black liver on biopsy

TREATMENT

No treatment is usually necessary. Individuals with this disorder have a normal life expectancy.

Rotor Syndrome

Similar to Dubin-Johnson syndrome, but now known to be a separate disorder. In Rotor syndrome, defects occur in the hepatic storage of conjugated bilirubin, which causes it to leak out. Grossly, however, the liver appears normal.

Hereditary Causes of Indirect (Unconjugated) Hyperbilirubinemia

Gilbert Syndrome

- Benign inherited condition causing mild, intermittent indirect hyperbilirubinemia. Present in approximately 5% of the population.
- Caused by transient reduction in hepatic glucuronyl transferase activity to about one-third normal levels, leading to a decrease in bile conjugation.

PRESENTATION

Usually an incidental finding in an otherwise healthy adolescent or young adult male (male-to-female predominance 2–7:1); manifests as **mild jaundice** during **periods of stress,** such as concurrent illness, strenuous exercise, or fasting.

DIAGNOSIS

- Elevated serum indirect bilirubin (usually two to three times normal, almost always < 6 mg/dL).
- Normal CBC.
- Normal liver enzymes.

TREATMENT

No treatment necessary; reassurance only.

Crigler-Najjar Syndrome (Type 1)

Rare autosomal recessive genetic condition. Type 1 is the more severe form and is caused by a **complete lack of hepatic glucuronyl transferase, the enzyme responsible for conjugation of indirect to direct bilirubin.** On gross inspection, the liver appears normal.

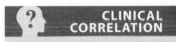

CLINICAL CORRELATION

Crigler-Najjar type 1 does not respond to phenobarbital, whereas Crigler-Najjar type 2 does respond to phenobarbital, which induces liver enzyme synthesis.

PRESENTATION

Suspect in **neonates** presenting with severe **jaundice at birth.** Due to the complete lack of glucuronyl transferase, bile is colorless and contains only traces of unconjugated bilirubin. Babies also may present with kernicterus, lethargy, and a high-pitched cry.

DIAGNOSIS

Severe jaundice and icterus in a newborn with severely elevated serum indirect bilirubin (**> 30 times normal values**).

TREATMENT

- Aggressive treatment with phototherapy and exchange transfusions in the immediate neonatal period.
- Heme oxygenase inhibitors, which inhibit the breakdown of heme, and cholestyramine.
- Liver transplant prior to onset of brain damage.
- Patients **do not** respond to **phenobarbital.**
- Fatal within 18 months after birth if untreated (due to severe kernicterus).

Crigler-Najjar Syndrome (Type 2)

Less severe than type 1, a nonfatal disorder caused by a **partial lack of hepatic glucuronyl transferase.** As with type 1, the liver is morphologically normal.

PRESENTATION

Suspect in neonates presenting with severe **jaundice at birth.** Babies have strikingly yellow skin due to high levels of unconjugated bilirubin.

DIAGNOSIS

Severe jaundice in a newborn and severely elevated serum indirect bilirubin.

TREATMENT

Phototherapy; patients **respond to phenobarbital.**

PROGNOSIS

Can lead to neurologic damage due to kernicterus if untreated. Excellent prognosis if treated; patients develop normally.

Infectious Hepatitis

Infectious hepatitis is caused by five distinct viruses. They cause a range of illnesses, from benign, self-limited disease to fulminant liver failure to chronic infections that progress to cirrhosis and death. See Tables 3-21 and 3-22 for further information.

Alcoholic Hepatitis

Alcoholic hepatitis is due to reversible inflammatory liver damage caused by a high level of alcohol consumption over time and is the most common cause of cirrhotic liver disease in most Western countries. Genetic and environmental factors both play an important role in the pathophysiology of this disease.

Direct toxicity from ethanol and its metabolites, in addition to oxidative damage, disrupts the function of cell and mitochondrial membranes, thus leading to lipid accumulation.

PRESENTATION

Can be asymptomatic in its mildest form or can present with fulminant hepatic failure and death in its most severe form.

- **Classic presentation:** Nausea, malaise, tachycardia, and low-grade fever in an individual with a history of heavy alcohol use.

TABLE 3-21. Types of Viral Hepatitis

	ROUTE OF TRANSMISSION	PROGNOSIS	UNIQUE CHARACTERISTICS
Hepatitis A	Contaminated food/water (fecal-oral)	Self-limited illness, usually benign	Does not cause a carrier state
Hepatitis B	All bodily fluids apart from stool (parenteral)	Acute illness with possible fulminant liver failure, can progress to a chronic symptomatic or asymptomatic state	Can be transmitted from mother to child
Hepatitis C	Blood transfusions, occupational exposure, IV drug use (parenteral), sexual transmission (rare)	Most progress to chronic infection and many progress to cirrhosis	Concurrent alcohol use accelerates the progression of disease
Hepatitis D	Must be encapsulated with the hepatitis B surface antigen to replicate (parenteral)		In the United States, mostly found among IV drug users
Hepatitis E	Contaminated water (fecal-oral)		A high rate of mortality among pregnant women

TABLE 3-22.   Hepatitis Serologic Markers

Anti-HAV (IgM)	IgM antibody to HAV; best test to detect acute hepatitis A
Anti-HAV (IgG)	IgG antibody indicates prior HAV infection and/or prior vaccination; protects against reinfection
HBsAg	Antigen found on surface of HBV; indicates hepatitis B infection
Anti-HBs	Antibody to HBsAg; indicates immunity to hepatitis B
HBcAg	Antigen associated with core of HBV
Anti-HBc	Antibody to HBcAg; IgM = acute/recent infection; IgG = prior exposure or chronic infection. IgM anti-HBc may be the sole ⊕ marker of infection during window period
HBeAg	Secreted by infected hepatocyte into circulation. Not part of mature HBV virion. Indicates active viral replication and therefore high transmissibility
Anti-HBe	Antibody to HBeAg; indicates low transmissibility

HAV, hepatitis A virus; HBc, hepatitis B core; HBcAg, hepatitis B core antigen; HBeAg, hepatitis B early antigen; HBsAg, hepatitis B surface antigen; HBV, hepatitis B virus; IgG, immunoglobulin G; IgM, immunoglobulin M.

- **Patients with concomitant hepatic failure or portal hypertension:** Ascites, coagulopathy, significant hematemesis from ruptured esophageal varices, or evidence of encephalopathy, such as asterixis and altered mental status. Right upper quadrant (RUQ) tenderness and hepatomegaly may be noted on physical exam.

DIAGNOSIS

Clinical diagnosis can be made based on presentation and history of alcohol abuse.

- **Lab tests** reveal elevated aspartate aminotransferase (AST) and alanine aminotransferase (ALT) in a ratio of 2:1, elevated alkaline phosphatase (ALP), and prolonged prothrombin time (PT; due to decreased coagulation factor production by liver).
- **Histology:** Steatosis, neutrophilic infiltrate, centrilobular balloon necrosis of hepatocytes, and eosinophilic inclusion bodies known as **Mallory bodies** (Figure 3-59). Eventually, alcoholic hepatitis may lead to irreversible fibrosis.

TREATMENT

Alcoholic steatosis and hepatitis can be reversible if the patient is able to achieve abstinence from alcohol, the most important goal of treatment.

- **Immediate treatment** should include first IV folate and thiamine, followed by caloric and fluid support with an IV glucose solution. Seizures and other symptoms of withdrawal can be fatal if left untreated.
- **Vitamin K** should be given in an attempt to reverse any coagulopathy that may be due to concurrent nutritional deficiencies. However, most often, fresh frozen plasma will be needed to reverse coagulopathy for significant bleeding or invasive procedures.
- A 4-week course of **prednisolone** may benefit patients with severe forms of the disease.

PROGNOSIS

If alcohol abuse continues, the patient risks progression to cirrhosis, which carries a much poorer prognosis.

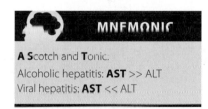

MNEMONIC

A Scotch and **T**onic.
Alcoholic hepatitis: **AST** >> ALT
Viral hepatitis: **AST** << ALT

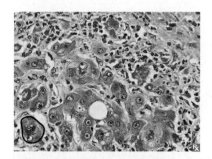

FIGURE 3-59.   Microscopic features of alcoholic hepatitis. Alcoholic hepatitis characterized by single or focal cell swelling (ballooning [outlined cell]) and cellular necrosis, as well as the presence of eosinophilic cytoplasmic inclusions known as Mallory bodies.

Reye Syndrome

Reye syndrome is a rare childhood hepatoencephalopathy. The pathogenesis is thought to be damage to mitochondria caused by **salicylate (aspirin)** metabolites or some other toxin in the milieu of a viral infection or underlying mitochondrial polymorphism, although cases also occur in the absence of salicylate use.

Mitochondrial dysfunction leads to elevation of short-chain fatty acids and hyperammonemia as well as cerebral edema.

PRESENTATION

Vomiting, lethargy, drowsiness, and progressive stupor, often preceded by a viral infection, often an upper respiratory infection (eg, influenza A or B or varicella) combined with **salicylate** (aspirin) use. Signs of increased intracranial pressure, such as hypercapnea, irregular respirations, and sluggish pupils, may also be present.

DIAGNOSIS

- Lab findings reflect liver damage and include:
  - Elevated **AST**
  - **Hyperammonemia**
  - Normal or slightly elevated **bilirubin**
  - Prolonged **PT**
- **Histology** of the liver shows diffuse microvesicular steatosis (nucleus is **not** dislocated) with **large, pleomorphic mitochondria.**

TREATMENT

Generally supportive. If cerebral edema is controlled, the liver usually is able to regenerate. **Elevated intracranial pressure** is managed with hyperventilation, mannitol, and barbiturates.

PROGNOSIS

At least 70% of patients survive, and the prognosis is related to the depth of coma and peak ammonia levels. Patients should be screened for fatty acid metabolism defects and should not be given aspirin.

Cirrhosis and Portal Hypertension

Cirrhosis is an **irreversible scarring** of the liver that occurs after years of chronic insult. In essence, cirrhosis is **chronic liver damage,** characterized by complete disarray of the hepatic cytoarchitecture, with progressive scarring (generalized fibrosis) and typical "regenerative" nodule formation (Figure 3-60). Morphologically, it can be divided into:

- **Micronodular cirrhosis:** Nodules < 3 mm, uniform in size.
- **Macronodular cirrhosis:** Nodules > 3 mm, with increased risk of hepatocellular carcinoma (HCC), usually due to significant liver injury leading to hepatic necrosis (postinfectious, or drug-induced).
- **Mixed:** Macromicronodular form.

Many etiologic agents are involved in the development of cirrhosis (Table 3-23). They are generally divided into four major groups:

- Infectious.
- Inherited/metabolic disorders.
- Drugs/toxins affecting the liver.
- Other causes: Underlying primary diseases that ultimately affect the liver.

Cirrhosis is a major risk factor for the development of HCC. Alcoholism is the most common cause of cirrhosis in the United States.

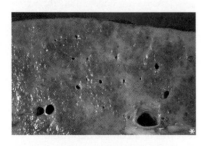
FIGURE 3-60. **Liver with end-stage cirrhosis.**

TABLE 3-23. **Causes of Cirrhosis**

TYPE OF CIRRHOSIS	CAUSES
Infectious	**Viral hepatitis,** brucellosis, capillariasis, echinococcosis, schistosomiasis, toxoplasmosis
Inherited/metabolic disorders	AAT, Alagille syndrome, biliary atresia, Fanconi syndrome, **hemochromatosis, Wilson disease,** glycogen storage diseases
Drugs/toxins	**Alcohol,** amiodarone, arsenic, oral contraceptive pills
Other	**Heart failure** with long-standing congestion of the liver, **biliary obstruction,** CF, graft-versus-host disease, nonalcoholic steatohepatitis (NASH), **primary sclerosing cholangitis,** sarcoidosis

AAT, α_1-antitrypsin; CF, cystic fibrosis.

PRESENTATION

Cirrhosis has a variety of manifestations:

- **Clinical presentation:** Complex, resulting from severely impaired liver function (hepatocellular damage), consequences of diffuse hepatic tissue scarring with portal hypertension, or a combination of both.
- **Jaundice** and **pruritus** resulting from the inability of the liver to excrete bilirubin.
- **Hypoalbuminemia** as a result of impaired albumin synthesis.
- **Hyperestrogenism,** which causes spider hemangiomas, palmar erythema, gynecomastia (in males), and hypogonadism.
- **Anemia** (multifactorial, folate deficiency can contribute).
- **Coagulopathies** from decreased production of clotting factors.
- **Portal hypertension,** leading to esophageal varices, caput medusae, and hemorrhoids as described earlier (Figure 3-61).
- **Splenomegaly** resulting in **thrombocytopenia.**

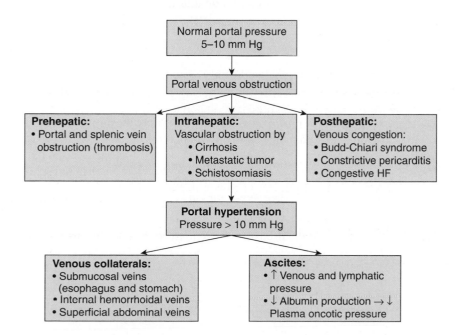

FIGURE 3-61. **Pathophysiology of portal hypertension.** HF, heart failure.

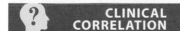

FLASH BACK

Hepatic portal vein to inferior vena cava (IVC) anastomoses (collaterals):
- Esophagus: Left gastric vein to azygos vein leads to esophageal varices.
- Umbilicus: Paraumbilical vein to superficial and inferior epigastric veins leads to caput medusae.
- Rectum: Superior rectal vein to middle and inferior rectal veins leads to hemorrhoids.

FLASH BACK

Portal hypertension in the context of congestive heart failure (CHF):
- Prolonged right-sided failure with retrograde transmission of venous pressure via the IVC.
- Liver sinusoids dilated/engorged with blood, leading to liver swelling and centrilobular fibrosis/alternating congestion ("nutmeg liver").
- Hepatic failure, pulsatile liver.
- Firm, enlarged liver with signs of chronic liver disease in patients with CHF.

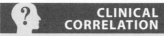

CLINICAL CORRELATION

Cirrhosis leads to a complete disarray of liver function, and thus elevated ALP, bilirubin, γ-glutamyl transferase, and PT, as well as anemia, thrombocytopenia, hypoalbuminemia, and hyponatremia.

CLINICAL CORRELATION

Budd-Chiari syndrome occurs when the hepatic vein is occluded via thrombosis or compression by an adjacent tumor, leading to an inability of the liver to drain blood, causing abdominal pain, ascites, hepatomegaly, and centrilobular necrosis.

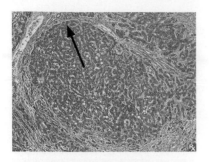

FIGURE 3-62. Histologic features of cirrhosis. Liver cell nodules of varying sizes are trapped in fibrous bands of tissue. Reactive bile duct proliferation is shown in the fibrous septae (arrow), with macrovesicular fatty change present in the hepatocytes.

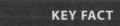

KEY FACT

β-blockers such as nadolol may be used as prophylaxis against variceal bleeding. Diuretics may be used to limit recurrence of ascites.

CLINICAL CORRELATION

Suspect PBC in women with a history of Sjögren syndrome, Raynaud disease, or scleroderma.

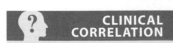

Additional sequelae include ascites, peripheral edema, and/or hydrothorax:

- **Hypoalbuminemia** leads to decreased intravascular oncotic pressure and, along with **portal hypertension,** contributes to the formation of **ascites.** Ascitic fluid can become infected, causing spontaneous bacterial peritonitis.
- **Hepatic encephalopathy:** Severe loss of hepatic function leads to **shunting** of blood around the liver, leading to accumulation of toxic metabolites in the blood (**ammonemia**) and causing brain toxicity, often manifested with **asterixis,** a hand-flapping tremor.
- **Hepatorenal syndrome:** Increased portal venous pressure leads to decreased effective intravascular volume and decreased renal perfusion pressure (due to intrarenal redistribution of blood flow). Renal failure can thus develop in the presence of liver failure without intrinsic renal problems.

PATHOHISTOLOGY

Bridging fibrosis and small **regenerative nodules** (Figure 3-62).

- Represent hepatocytic reaction to injury.
- Lack of normal liver cytoarchitecture (no portal triads and sinusoids).
- Contribute to increased intrasinusoidal pressure (intrasinusoidal hypertension).

DIAGNOSIS

- **Physical exam** may reveal any of the signs and symptoms mentioned above as evidence of liver disease.
- The **damaged liver** may be enlarged and tender.
- A **cirrhotic liver** is shrunken, firm, and nodular.
- **Lab tests** may reveal elevated AST and ALT, but normal values do not rule out cirrhosis, as these values return to normal as the hepatocytes "burn out."
- Although not used for diagnosis, **RUQ ultrasound** shows the nodules characteristic of cirrhosis. Ultrasound can also be used to evaluate for splenomegaly, ascites, portal vein thrombosis, and HCC.
- The **gold standard** for diagnosing cirrhosis remains **tissue biopsy.** However, biopsy is not necessary if the patient's presentation and workup are both consistent with cirrhosis.

TREATMENT

- For complications of cirrhosis: Sclerotherapy or banding for symptomatic esophageal varices, drainage of excess peritoneal fluid for ascites (called **paracentesis**), nutritional support.
- Treatment of hepatic encephalopathy: **lactulose** (reduces the ammonia production of colonic bacteria), rifaximin (decreases the colonic concentration of ammoniagenic bacteria).
- Procedures, such as portocaval shunting (more invasive) and transjugular intrahepatic portosystemic shunting (less invasive), that allow blood to bypass the portal venous system are also used, thus relieving the symptoms and complications of portal hypertension. However, these do not address the issue of cirrhosis or liver dysfunction and are typically used as a bridge to the only definitive treatment, liver transplantation.

PROGNOSIS

Can be fatal if it progresses to liver failure or HCC. Cirrhosis is not uniformly fatal.

Primary Biliary Cirrhosis

Primary biliary cirrhosis (PBC) is characterized by destruction of the small- and medium-sized bile ducts in the liver, resulting in **intrahepatic cholestasis.** PBC has a poorly understood pathophysiology; however, it is frequently associated with a variety of autoimmune disorders, thus suggesting an autoimmune cause. It primarily affects middle-aged women (35–60 years of age).

PRESENTATION

Most cases are asymptomatic for a prolonged period. **Symptoms develop gradually** as the disease progresses and reflect progressive liver damage due to cholestasis. Symptoms range from severe pruritus, jaundice, malabsorption, and fatigue to signs of hepatocellular failure and portal hypertension.

DIAGNOSIS

The **most classic lab abnormality** is an **extreme elevation in ALP (alkaline phosphatase)**, along with elevated AST and ALT, GGT (γ-glutamyl transferase), cholesterol (especially HDL), **IgM**, and cryoglobulins. **Antimitochondrial antibodies** are highly specific for this disease.

Liver biopsy confirms the diagnosis; positive findings include lymphocytic infiltrates in the portal regions, **granulomas**, and loss of bile ductules in the liver parenchyma (Figure 3-63).

TREATMENT

No therapies can halt or reverse PBC; it is possible only to provide symptomatic relief and slow the progression of disease. The most common drug used is **ursodiol** in an attempt to reduce cholestasis; whether it improves prognosis is controversial. Liver transplantation is the only life-saving treatment currently available.

PROGNOSIS

Progressive disease that ultimately leads to cirrhosis of the liver.

INBORN ERRORS OF METABOLISM

Hemochromatosis

- An inherited, **autosomal recessive**, male-predominant metabolic disorder of iron storage, characterized by increased intestinal iron absorption.
- Excessive serum levels of iron lead to deposition in and damage to several major organs, including the liver, pancreas, heart, joints, and pituitary gland.

PRESENTATION

Organ damage usually does not become apparent until patients are at least 40 years of age. Early signs include weakness, weight loss, abdominal pain, and loss of libido.

- **Cirrhosis** with iron deposits (Figure 3-64) affecting the hepatocytes and resulting in hepatomegaly and symptoms of chronic liver disease.
- Iron deposition in **pancreatic islet cells** can lead to type 1 diabetes mellitus (DM-1).
- **Iron deposition** in the skin and **increased melanin production** cause bronze skin discoloration (hence, combined with the risk of DM-1, the name **bronze diabetes**).
- Significant risk of **heart failure.**

DIAGNOSIS

- Clinical presentation.
- Elevated percentage of transferrin saturation (> 50%).
- Elevated serum iron and ferritin.
- Iron:total iron-binding capacity ratio > 50%.
- Urinary iron.
- Confirm with liver biopsy.

KEY FACT

Circulating antimitochondrial antibodies are detected in > 90% of PBC cases.

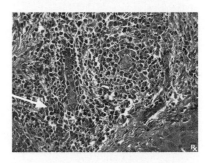

FIGURE 3-63. **Histologic features of primary biliary cirrhosis.** This slide shows a granuloma, a common feature of primary biliary cirrhosis, as well as inflammatory cells (arrow) attacking the bile ducts.

KEY FACT

- The clinical symptoms of hemochromatosis affect males >> females; partly because menses cause loss of iron.
- Females are clinically affected after menopause.

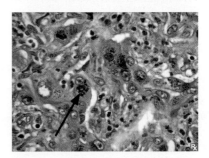

FIGURE 3-64. **Hemosiderin-laden hepatocytes (arrow) indicative of hemochromatosis.**

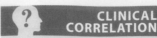

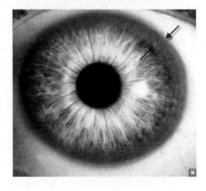

FIGURE 3-65. Kayser-Fleischer ring of Wilson disease.

TREATMENT

- **First line:** Intermittent phlebotomy to remove excess body iron
- **Second line:** Chelating agents (deferoxamine)
- Abstinence from alcohol consumption (increases iron absorption)
- Supportive treatment of common complications (ie, diabetes, congestive heart failure [CHF])

Wilson Disease (Hepatolenticular Degeneration)

An inherited **autosomal recessive** metabolic disorder characterized by excessive serum levels of **copper** with deposition in major organs (primarily the liver, brain, kidneys, and corneas).

Wilson disease develops as a result of a mutation in the **ATP7B gene** on **chromosome 13 (13q14.3)**, which codes for a **P-type ATPase** that transports copper into bile and incorporates it into ceruloplasmin. The mutant form of *ATP7B* inhibits the release of copper into bile.

PRESENTATION

Suspect Wilson disease in **young adult patients** who present with stigmata of liver disease along with neurologic changes.

- Classically, patients have **Kayser-Fleischer rings** (deposits of copper on the outer edges of the corneas; Figure 3-65) on **slit-lamp** examination.
- Liver disease can present in the form of hepatitis, cirrhosis, or decompensation.
- Personality and neurologic changes resulting from copper accumulation in the brain.

DIAGNOSIS

- Decreased serum ceruloplasmin levels.
- Increased serum and urine copper levels.
- Confirm with liver biopsy.

TREATMENT

- Avoid copper-rich foods (eg, shellfish, nuts, chocolate, mushrooms, or organ meats).
- Copper **chelators,** primarily **penicillamine.** Alternative agents include potassium sulfide, pyridoxine, and zinc acetate.
- Definitive treatment is liver transplantation, which is effective because the *ATP7B* gene is only active in the liver.

PROGNOSIS

Wilson disease is a chronic illness that can be fatal without treatment.

HEPATIC TUMORS

Hepatic tumors can be either primary tumors (derived from liver cells) or metastatic tumors. **The most common tumors of the liver are metastatic (ie, colon cancer).**

Benign Liver Tumors

The most common benign tumors include hepatic adenoma (HA) and focal nodular hyperplasia (FNH).

Hepatic Adenoma

Seen predominantly in women in the third and fourth decades. Risk factors include: the use of **oral contraceptives,** use of anabolic steroids, and type I glycogen storage diseases. HAs are usually benign and often regress after offending drug is discontinued, but they do have premalignant potential, and large adenomas can rupture.

Focal Nodular Hyperplasia

As with HA, **FNH** also occurs primarily in women but is **not associated** with the use of oral contraceptives.

PRESENTATION

- **HA:** Primarily in the right liver lobe and often large (> 10 cm). Clinical features include pain and palpable mass or signs of intratumor hemorrhage.
- **FNH:** Generally asymptomatic and incidental finding on imaging studies as a solid tumor in the right lobe consisting of a fibrous core with stellate projections.

HISTOLOGY

Both tumors consist of normal or slightly atypical hepatocytes; however, **FNH** also contains **biliary epithelium** and **Kupffer cells.** Hepatocytes contain increased glycogen, appearing paler and larger than normal.

DIAGNOSIS

CT, MRI, and selective hepatic angiography are used to make the diagnosis.

- Hypervascular appearance on angiography.
- Technetium scans typically show **uptake in FNH** due to the presence of Kupffer cells but lack of uptake in HA.

TREATMENT

Imaging to follow progression of small tumors. If the lesion is > 8–10 cm, near the surface, and resectable, then surgical removal may be appropriate.

- Patients with HA should stop taking oral contraceptives.
- Pregnancy increases the risk of hemorrhage in HA due to hormonal influence; women with large adenomas should be counseled to avoid pregnancy.

PROGNOSIS

In HA, the risk of malignant change is small, although it is increased with multiple tumors and tumors > 10 cm. In FNH, there is no evidence for malignant transformation.

Malignant Liver Tumors

The two most common types of liver carcinoma are primary HCC and metastatic carcinoma.

Hepatocellular Carcinoma

HCC is one of the most common tumors in the world, with the highest prevalence in Asia and sub-Saharan Africa due to the high prevalence of **hepatitis B and C;** it is less common in the United States and Western Europe. It is four times more common in men.

PRESENTATION

Symptoms are similar to those of chronic liver disease. The most common presenting symptoms are pain or mass in the RUQ. **Physical exam** may reveal friction rub or bruit over the liver. **Elevations** of **AFP** and **ALP** are common.

DIAGNOSIS

Based on imaging, and elevated serum AFP levels. A workup for HCC should be done on any solitary nodule seen on CT in a patient with cirrhosis.

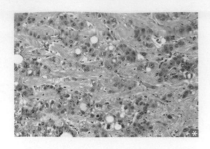

FIGURE 3-66. Hepatocellular carcinoma. Scirrhous growth pattern of hepatocellular carcinoma.

Liver biopsy may be performed but diagnosis can usually be made based on triple-phase CT scan showing arterial enhancement with rapid venous washout. **Histologically,** tumors can range from well differentiated (Figure 3-66) to poorly differentiated. Central areas of necrosis may exist in large tumors. Bile globules and acidophilic inclusions are sometimes present.

TREATMENT

Depending on tumor, node, metastasis (TNM) classification, treatment options include partial hepatectomy, liver transplantation, focal radiation, radiofrequency ablation, percutaneous acetic acid, and ethanol ablation.

PROGNOSIS

Usually diagnosed late, when distant metastases (lung, brain, bone, and adrenal) have already occurred. The median life expectancy after diagnosis is 6–20 months.

Metastatic Tumors

In the United States, the incidence of metastatic carcinoma is at least **20 times greater** than that of primary HCC. The most common metastases include tumors from the **GI tract, the lungs, the breast,** and **melanoma.**

PRESENTATION

Most symptoms can be attributed to the primary tumor; however, patients may also present with nonspecific symptoms of weakness, weight loss, fever, sweating, and loss of appetite. Liver biochemical tests are often abnormal, but mildly elevated and nonspecific.

DIAGNOSIS

Imaging to assess for metastatic disease to the liver should be sought for any patient with primary malignancy, especially of the lung, GI tract, or breast.

TREATMENT

Most metastatic carcinomas respond poorly to all forms of treatment, which is usually only palliative. The exception is metastatic colon cancer, which has a 5-year survival rate of at least 25% after resection when the disease is limited to the colon and liver alone.

Other Liver Tumors

- **Hemangioma:** Benign and generally left untreated.
- **Cholangiocarcinoma:** Tumor of biliary system elements within the liver. Increased risk associated with liver flukes *(Clonorchis sinensis),* often seen in immigrants.
- **Hepatoblastoma:** Most common primary liver tumor in **children.**
- **Cavernous hemangioma:** Common, benign tumor that typically begins at age 30–50 years. Biopsy is contraindicated because of risk of hemorrhage.
- **Angiosarcoma:** Malignant tumor of endothelial origin. Associated with exposure to arsenic and vinyl chloride.

GALLBLADDER DISEASE

Cholelithiasis

Gallstones are a common cause of RUQ pain and are classically found in patients who are overweight, middle-aged, and female. About 10–20% of Americans have gallstones, and about 50% of these people eventually have symptoms.

There are three types of stones, namely cholesterol, mixed, and pigment (bilirubin) (Table 3-24).

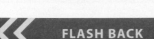

FLASH BACK

The liver is the most common site of metastasis for GI (and other) tumors due to its size, high rate of blood flow, unique dual blood supply, and cytoarchitecture.

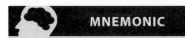

MNEMONIC

Metastases >> Primary liver tumors
Cancer **S**ometimes **P**enetrates **B**enign **L**iver
(**C**olon > **S**tomach > **P**ancreas > **B**reast > **L**ung)

TABLE 3-24. **Types of Gallstones and Typical Findings**

	COMPONENTS	RISK FACTORS	RADIOGRAPHY
Cholesterol stones	Cholesterol	Crohn disease (inhibits bile acid recycling in the terminal ileum), CF, clofibrate (decreases bile acid secretion), estrogen, multiparity, rapid weight loss, Native American heritage, advanced age	Mostly **radiolucent** (cannot be seen); **10–20%** are **opaque** due to calcifications
Mixed stones, most common types	Cholesterol and pigment	Most common	Radiolucent
Pigment	Pigment (bilirubin)	Chronic RBC hemolysis, alcoholic cirrhosis, advanced age, biliary infection	**Radiopaque** (seen on radiograph)

CF, cystic fibrosis.

Stones form when there is a disruption in cholesterol transport from the liver into the bile; this process is coupled with a simultaneous secretion of phospholipid and bile salts. Disruption of the **cholesterol:bile salt ratio** leads to cholesterol precipitation in the gallbladder, thus enabling the formation of stones.

- **Cholesterol load > bile salts:** Bile salts and lecithin are unable to solubilize the cholesterol.
- **Disrupted bile salt production** (decreased bile acid absorption from the intestine or hepatic failure) leads to increased cholesterol:bile salt ratio.

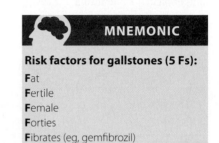

MNEMONIC

Risk factors for gallstones (5 Fs):
Fat
Fertile
Female
Forties
Fibrates (eg, gemfibrozil)

PRESENTATION

Gallstones are strongly suggested by RUQ pain, which occasionally radiates to the right shoulder. The pain is usually worse after fatty meals (**postprandial pain**) as the gallbladder contracts against the stone and can be associated with nausea/vomiting.

DIAGNOSIS

There are several ways to image the biliary system and gallbladder (Figure 3-67). **Ultrasound** is the best way to visualize gallstones and is the gold standard for diagnosis. **Radiography** can be deceiving because most gallstones are radiolucent and may not appear on abdominal plain film. Endoscopic retrograde cholangiopancreatography (**ERCP**) is both a diagnostic and therapeutic procedure that can visualize gallstones in the common bile duct and remove them. MRCP can be used for diagnosis prior to ERCP. Endoscopic ultrasound (EUS) can also be diagnostic.

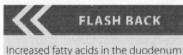

FLASH BACK

Increased fatty acids in the duodenum and jejunum stimulate I-cell production of CCK (cholecystokinin), which stimulates gall bladder contraction.

TREATMENT

Elective cholecystectomy (removal of the gallbladder) in symptomatic patients. Some patients may not require surgery but should modify their diet and avoid fatty food.

PROGNOSIS

The prognosis is good, but there are many potential complications:

- Recurrent biliary colic (intermittent pain).
- Acute cholecystitis (prolonged blockage of the cystic duct, causing gallbladder inflammation or infection).
- Choledocholithiasis (gallstone obstructing the common bile duct).
- Acute cholangitis (bacterial infection of the biliary tree).
- Gallstone ileus and gallstone pancreatitis.
- **Porcelain gallbladder** (calcified gallbladder due to chronic cholecystitis): Indication for surgical removal, as porcelain gallbladder can progress to gallbladder carcinoma.

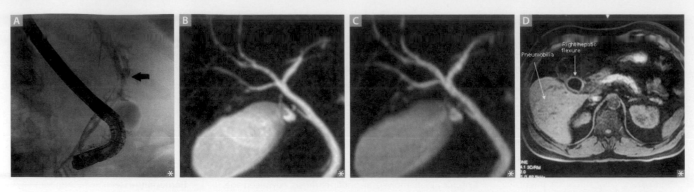

FIGURE 3-67. **Methods of bile duct imaging.** **A** Postoperative endoscopic retrograde cholangiopancreatography (ERCP) showing gastric tube anastomosed to proximal end of the common bile duct (CBD) (arrow). The inflated balloon catheter and stent can be seen within the reconstructed biliary tract. **B C** Maximum intensity projection (MIP) of **B** coronal and **C** axial acquired magnetic resonance cholangiopancreatography (MRCP) datasets of a patient with primary sclerosing cholangitis. **D** Spiral CT with evidence of pneumobilia and cholecystocolic fistula (arrows).

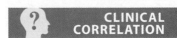

CLINICAL CORRELATION

Charcot triad (cholangitis): RUQ pain, fever, jaundice

Reynolds pentad = Charcot triad + Shock and altered mental status

KEY FACT

"Sonographic" Murphy sign when it is elicited by ultrasound probe.

KEY FACT

Positive HIDA scan = obstruction in passage (cystic duct) = nonvisualization of gallbladder confirms diagnosis.

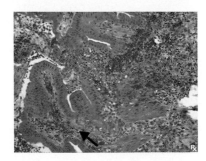

FIGURE 3-68. **Acute cholecystitis.** Neutrophilic and lymphocytic infiltrates (arrow) can be seen within the epithelium and muscular wall of the gallbladder.

Cholecystitis

Inflammation of the gallbladder is a common complication of cholelithiasis (Figure 3-68).

PRESENTATION

Very similar to that of cholelithiasis: Postprandial colicky RUQ pain radiating to the right scapula, as a result of intermittent blockage of the common bile duct. Nausea/vomiting and bloating can also be present.

- Jaundice may occur as a result of complete blockage of the common bile duct (choledocholithiasis), leading to infection or **cholangitis.**
- **Charcot triad:** Epigastric/RUQ pain, fever, and jaundice may indicate the presence of cholangitis.

DIAGNOSIS

- Classic physical exam feature is the **Murphy sign.**
    - **Elicitation:** Palpate the right subcostal area (gallbladder fossa) while the patient inspires deeply; the gallbladder descends toward the examiner's fingers.
    - **Positive response:** The patient feels increased discomfort and/or pain with this maneuver and will have disruption of deep inspiration.
- Ultrasound exam can show stones in the gallbladder, thickening of the gallbladder wall, and edema. Hepatobiliary iminodiacetic acid (**HIDA**) scan (cholescintigraphy) is more sensitive for cholecystitis and can confirm the diagnosis.

TREATMENT

Start antibiotics (usually against gram-negative bacteria, such as *E coli* and *Klebsiella*, empirically), and perform cholecystectomy once the patient is stable.

Gallbladder Carcinoma/Cholangiocarcinoma

Tumors of the gallbladder (**gallbladder carcinoma**) are much more common than tumors arising from within the bile ducts (**cholangiocarcinoma**). They usually manifest in the seventh decade of life and are more common in women than in men. Gallstones are present 60–90% of the time. The 5-year survival is < 1%, as the tumor has often already invaded the liver at the time of diagnosis.

Primary Sclerosing Cholangitis

Chronic cholestatic liver disease characterized by inflammation, fibrosis, and irregular dilation of obstructed intrahepatic and extrahepatic bile ducts. Increased risk of cholangiocarcinoma. Associated with ulcerative colitis.

PRESENTATION

Usually diagnosed in the context of IBD, although it can also present with abnormal liver function tests, pruritus, RUQ pain, and fatigue.

DIAGNOSIS

Elevated alkaline phosphatase. MRCP shows multiple strictures and dilation of the intra- and extrahepatic bile ducts.

EXOCRINE PANCREAS

Acute Pancreatitis

Caused by activation of pancreatic enzymes, which leads to **pancreatic autodigestion** with liquefactive hemorrhagic necrosis and fat necrosis of the pancreas.

PRESENTATION

Classically presents as sudden-onset epigastric abdominal pain radiating to the back and flanks accompanied by anorexia and nausea. May occur following a large meal or drinking binge.

DIAGNOSIS

Clinical symptoms and imaging:

- Leukocytosis and elevated serum amylase (> 3 times upper limit of normal) and lipase (more specific, persists longer) should be expected.
- **Histology:** Fat necrosis with pale basophilic calcium soaps (which can lead to hypocalcemia), hemorrhage, necrotic debris, and inflammatory response (Figure 3-69).
- Abdominal plain film may show localized ileus (**sentinel loop**) in C-loop of duodenum.
- Contrast-enhanced CT or MRI can be used in equivocal cases where the diagnosis is otherwise unclear.

TREATMENT

- Rest, gastric suction, fluid and electrolyte replacement, and pain control with opioids (**meperidine**).
- Surgical treatment is only for trauma, ductal stones, obstructive lesions, and infected pancreatic necrosis.

PROGNOSIS

- About 20% of patients may have complications of necrosis, organ failure, or both, including disseminated intravascular coagulation (DIC), acute respiratory distress syndrome (ARDS), diffuse fat necrosis, hypocalcemia, pseudocyst formation, hemorrhage, and infection.
- About 10% of patients with pancreatic cancer present with acute pancreatitis. Suspect it in older patients with no other risk factors.

KEY FACT

Primary sclerosing cholangitis is often associated with IBD, especially ulcerative colitis.

MNEMONIC

Causes of acute pancreatitis—
I GET SMASHED

Idiopathic
Gallstones
Ethanol
Trauma
Steroids
Mumps
Autoimmune disease
Scorpion sting
Hypercalcemia/Hyperlipidemia
ERCP
Drugs

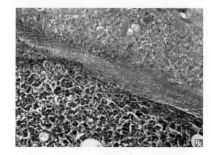

FIGURE 3-69. Acute pancreatitis with extensive necrosis. The entire upper portion of this photomicrograph shows extensive parenchymal necrosis, whereas the lower portion is relatively spared.

FLASH BACK

Morphine may cause spasm of the sphincter of Oddi and worsen pain.
Meperidine is the preferred analgesic for treating the pain of acute pancreatitis because it does not cause spasm of the sphincter of Oddi.

Chronic Pancreatitis

Chronic pancreatitis may present as episodes of acute inflammation in a previously injured pancreas or as chronic damage with persistent pain or malabsorption. The causes are similar to those of acute pancreatitis.

- In the United States, **alcoholism** is the most common cause in **adults.**
- **Cystic fibrosis (CF)** is the most common cause in **children.**

Presentation

- Epigastric pain radiating to the back is often absent in chronic disease.
- More common type of pain is persistent, deep-seated, and unresponsive to antacids; worsened by ingestion of fatty foods or alcohol.
- Symptoms of **pancreatic insufficiency** include **steatorrhea** (presenting as fatty, malodorous stools), weight loss, and deficiencies of fat-soluble vitamins (**A, D, E,** and **K**).

Diagnosis

- In **contrast to acute pancreatitis,** serum amylase and lipase are usually not elevated, as the pancreas is sufficiently damaged such that it can no longer produce excess amylase and lipase. The classic triad includes progressive parenchymal fibrosis with **pancreatic calcification, steatorrhea,** and **DM.**
- Radiographic hallmark is the presence of scattered calcifications (Figure 3-70).

Treatment

Address the two major problems: **pain and malabsorption.**

- **Pain:** Avoid alcohol and large meals. Use of narcotics can often lead to opiate addiction and has led to the use of palliative procedures (resection of strictures, stent placement, and ductal decompression).
- **Malabsorption:** Enzyme replacement and dietary fat restriction.

Prognosis

Patients who abstain from alcohol and use vigorous replacement therapy do reasonably well.

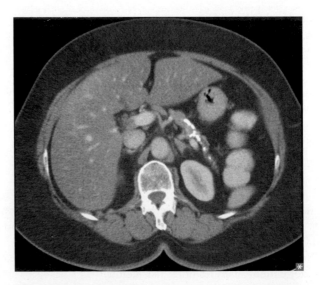

FIGURE 3-70. **Chronic pancreatitis and pancreatic calculi.** CT scan depicting stones and strictures exclusively located in the tail of the pancreas.

Pancreatic Adenocarcinoma

- Pancreatic adenocarcinoma is a malignancy of the exocrine portion of the pancreas; it is one of the most deadly cancers (5-year survival rate of < 5%).
- **Risk factors:** Age, smoking, family history, and chronic pancreatitis associated with alcohol abuse.

PRESENTATION

Tumors are located in the head of the pancreas 75% of the time, giving the classic presentation of **painless obstructive jaundice,** and are silent until late in disease progression. Common signs and symptoms include unexplained weight loss, malaise, epigastric pain that radiates to the middle of the back, and signs of obstructive jaundice. Other signs include **migratory thrombophlebitis (Trousseau sign)** and, occasionally, the onset of DM.

DIAGNOSIS

- No lab test is specific for pancreatic cancer, although elevated bilirubin, alkaline phosphatase, and abnormal imaging confirm biliary obstruction.
- The primary tumor marker for pancreatic cancer is **CA 19-9;** it cannot be used for screening, but can be used to monitor progression of the disease.
- CT scan is the most common imaging study used for diagnosing pancreatic cancer (Figure 3-71). EUS with fine needle aspiration is the primary method of tissue biopsy. Other studies include ERCP (during which a biopsy can be taken), MRI, and EUS.

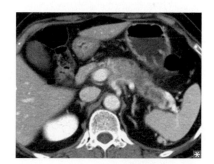

FIGURE 3-71. Pancreatic cancer. Abdominal CT showing pancreatic cancer involving the body of the pancreas.

TREATMENT

Surgical resection, called a pancreaticoduodenectomy (Whipple operation), is the primary treatment if resection is possible. Adjuvant chemotherapy and radiation are often used in combination as well.

PROGNOSIS

Pancreatic cancer has a dismal prognosis, with death usually occurring within 1 year of diagnosis.

ENZYME MARKERS OF GI PATHOLOGY

Commonly used laboratory assays (Table 3-25) available in most clinical practices include serum **AST, ALT, γ-glutamyl transferase,** bilirubin, **ALP, amylase, lipase,** and **PT.** Other, more specialized markers (ie, **ceruloplasmin** with Wilson disease) are used when rare conditions are suspected.

Many of these enzyme markers can be affected by pathologies outside the gut. Therefore, the differential diagnosis must include both extrinsic (outside the GI tract) and intrinsic (within the GI tract) pathologies.

Aspartate Aminotransferase

ANATOMIC SIGNIFICANCE

Intracellular **(cytosol and mitochondria)** enzyme found in liver cells, but also in skeletal muscle, heart, brain, and RBCs.

PHYSIOLOGIC ACTION

Catalyzes the transfer of amino groups to form pyruvate.

TABLE 3-25.   **Key Enzyme Markers of GI Pathologies**

ENZYME MARKER	RANGE OF NORMAL VALUES	KEY PATHOLOGIES INDICATED BY ABNORMALITY
AST	0–35 IU/L	Increased in liver damage (any cause)
ALT	0–35 IU/L	Increased in liver damage (any cause)
GGT	9–85 IU/L	Increase specific for liver disease (any cause)
Bilirubin		
Direct	0.1–0.4 mg/dL	
Indirect	0.2–0.7 mg/dL	
Total	0.1–1.2 mg/dL	
Alkaline phosphatase	41–133 IU/L	Nonspecific indicator of tissue damage (liver, bone, or intestinal); also increased in pregnancy
Amylase	20–110 IU/L	Increased in pancreatic pathologies, intestinal disease, and ruptured ectopic pregnancy
Lipase	0–160 IU/L	Increased in pancreatitis (acute and chronic); also increased in other pancreatic pathologies
PT	11–15 s	Increased in liver disease and warfarin therapy
Ceruloplasmin	20–35 mg/dL	Decreased in Wilson disease (hepatolenticular degeneration)

ALT, alanine aminotransferase; AST, aspartate aminotransferase; GGT, γ-glutamyltransferase; PT, prothrombin time.

LAB TEST INTERPRETATION

Increased concentration in the bloodstream with **tissue** (especially liver) **damage.** Tissue damage may occur with liver damage, or with cor pulmonale (right heart failure), myocardial ischemia, and extensive trauma.

Alanine Aminotransferase

ANATOMIC SIGNIFICANCE

Intracellular (**cytosol**) enzyme; relatively specific to the liver. Also found in kidney cells, skeletal muscle, and cardiac tissue.

PHYSIOLOGIC ACTION

Catalyzes the transfer of amino groups to form oxaloacetate.

LAB TEST INTERPRETATION

Increased along with AST in the bloodstream with **tissue** (especially liver) **damage.** Levels approximate the magnitude of liver damage. Also increased with right heart failure, myocardial ischemia, and extensive trauma.

AST AND ALT ELEVATIONS

Individually, abnormal values of AST or ALT are relatively nonspecific measures of liver damage. Certain characteristics in the pattern of elevation and the ratio of AST to ALT, however, enable clinical correlations to be made (Table 3-26).

γ-Glutamyl Transferase

ANATOMIC SIGNIFICANCE

Present in hepatic and biliary epithelial cells.

TABLE 3-26. **Level of AST and ALT Elevations**

MILD AST AND ALT ELEVATION (< 5× UPPER NORMAL LIMIT)	SEVERE AST AND ALT ELEVATION (> 15 × UPPER NORMAL LIMIT)	EXTREME AST AND ALT ELEVATION (AST AND ALT ≥ 5000)	NONHEPATIC CAUSES OF AST:ALT ABNORMALITIES
Wilson disease	Wilson disease	Acute viral hepatitis (with unusual viruses such as herpes simplex virus)	Drugs (ie, statins) Pregnancy
Chronic hepatitis (viral, alcoholic, etc)	Acute viral hepatitis	Acute toxic injury (ie, acetaminophen poisoning)	
Ethanol α_1-Antitrypsin deficiency Toxins/drugs	Ischemic injury Toxins/drugs Budd-Chiari syndrome Autoimmune hepatitis Hepatic artery ligation	Acute ischemic injury	Myocardial infarct Muscle disorders

Physiologic Action

Induced by alcohol intake.

Lab Test Interpretation

Increased in liver disease. Can be used to isolate liver pathology in cases of elevated alkaline phosphatase. γ-Glutamyl transferase is sensitive but **not specific** for liver disease. Best tool to assess recent alcohol use.

Alkaline Phosphatase

Anatomic Significance

Synthesized in liver, bone, intestine, and placenta.

Physiologic Action

Nonspecific indicator of tissue damage (liver, bone, intestine, and/or placenta).

Lab Test Interpretation

Increased in obstructive hepatobiliary disease. Also increased in bone disease (ie, Paget disease, bone metastases), hyperparathyroidism, **pregnancy (third trimester)**, and GI disease (ie, perforated ulcer).

Amylase

Anatomic Significance

Synthesized primarily in the pancreas and salivary glands; however, also produced by the ovaries, intestines, and skeletal muscle.

Physiologic Action

Hydrolyzes complex carbohydrates.

Lab Test Interpretation

Increased in **pancreatic disease** (pancreatitis, pseudocyst, pancreatic duct obstruction, malignancy), **bowel obstruction or infarction, mumps, parotitis, peritonitis, and ruptured ectopic pregnancy. Decreased in pancreatic insufficiency and CF.

> **KEY FACT**
>
> Check for γ-glutamyl transpeptidase (specific to the hepatobiliary system) to differentiate hepatobiliary involvement from other pathologies.

Lipase

ANATOMIC SIGNIFICANCE

Synthesized in the pancreas, liver, intestine, stomach, tongue, and other cells throughout the body.

PHYSIOLOGIC ACTION

Hydrolysis of glycerol esters and long-chain fatty acids.

LAB TEST INTERPRETATION

Increased in **pancreatic pathologies** (including acute/chronic pancreatitis, pseudocyst, and malignancy), **CF, intestinal malignancy, IBD, peritonitis, biliary disease, and liver disease.**

Prothrombin Time

ANATOMIC SIGNIFICANCE

Measures activity of clotting factors synthesized in the liver.

PHYSIOLOGIC ACTION

Screening test used to evaluate the **extrinsic pathway** of the coagulation system and monitor warfarin therapy. Also a relatively rapid and sensitive indicator of hepatic capacity for protein synthesis, since the half-lives of factors II and VII are relatively short (hours).

LAB TEST INTERPRETATION

Increased with **liver disease, warfarin therapy, vitamin K deficiency,** and **DIC.** The best test to identify level of liver dysfunction in patients with advanced cirrhosis, as the liver is no longer able to produce AST or ALT.

Ceruloplasmin

ANATOMIC SIGNIFICANCE

Synthesized in the liver.

PHYSIOLOGIC ACTION

Main copper-carrying protein in serum.

LAB TEST INTERPRETATION

Decreased in **Wilson disease,** malnutrition, nephrotic syndrome, and Menkes disease (X-linked disorder of copper deficiency).

> **CLINICAL CORRELATION**
>
> Measuring lipase levels is the most specific test to detect pancreatitis.

Pharmacology

This section describes the drugs used to treat the most common GI pathologies. Figure 3-72 summarizes the physiology of gastric secretions and the mechanism of action of respective compounds used in the treatment of certain GI diseases.

H₂ BLOCKERS

KEY DRUGS

Cimetidine, ranitidine, famotidine, nizatidine.

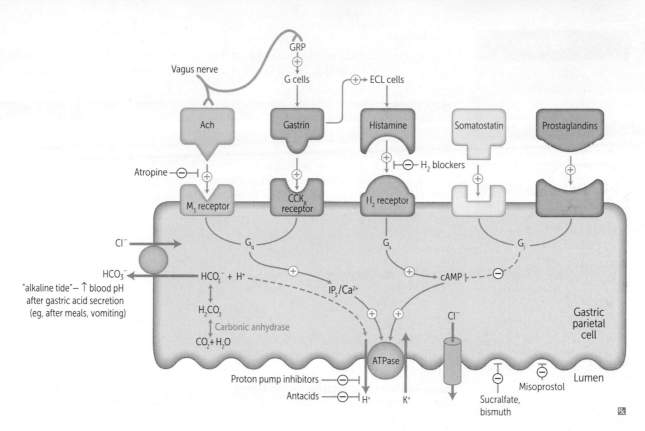

FIGURE 3-72. Summary of gastrointestinal therapies. ACh, acetylcholine; CCK_B, cholecystokinin-B receptor; ECL, enterochromaffin-like cell; GRP, gastrin-releasing peptide; H^+, hydrogen ion; HCO_3^-, bicarbonate.

MECHANISM

Reversibly blocks the histamine H_2 receptors responsible for stimulating the stomach parietal cells, leading to decreased H^+ secretion by these cells.

USES

Treatment and maintenance therapy of peptic ulcer disease (PUD), GERD, and dyspepsia.

SIDE EFFECTS

Cimetidine is a potent inhibitor of the cytochrome P450 system. It is also a potent antiandrogenic and can lead to decreased renal creatinine clearance. Ranitidine also inhibits the P450 system, although to a lesser degree than cimetidine. Both cimetidine and ranitidine decrease renal excretion of creatinine.

> **KEY FACT**
>
> Cimetidine inhibits the cytochrome P-450 system and increases the concentration of drugs cleared by this system. Caution should be taken when using these drugs simultaneously.

PROTON PUMP INHIBITORS

KEY DRUGS

Omeprazole, esomeprazole, lanoprazole, rabeprazole, pantoprazole, and dexlansoprazole.

MECHANISM

Irreversibly inhibits the $H^+–K^+$ ATPase pump in the stomach parietal cells.

USES

PUD, gastritis, GERD, Barrett esophagus, Zollinger-Ellison syndrome, and upper GI bleeds. Part of triple therapy for *H pylori* (a PPI, clarithromycin, and amoxicillin or metronidazole).

SIDE EFFECTS

Generally mild and include headache, nausea, and diarrhea. PPIs also confer increased risk of *C difficile* infection, pneumonia, and decreased serum Mg^{2+} with long-term use.

BISMUTH AND SUCRALFATE

MECHANISM

Bind to the ulcer base, providing a protective layer for the stomach, as well as allowing HCO_3^- secretion to restore the pH gradient in the mucus layer. Sucralfate suppresses *H pylori* and inhibits acid secretion in infected patients with duodenal ulcers. Bismuth lacks antiacidic properties.

USES

Binding agents commonly used to aid in ulcer healing as well as to treat traveler's diarrhea.

SIDE EFFECTS

Sucralfate has minimal adverse side effects other than possible aluminum toxicity. Bismuth toxicity can occur in patients with renal failure.

OCTREOTIDE

MECHANISM

Octreotide is a long-acting somatostatin analog that is a potent inhibitor of growth hormone, glucagon, and insulin. It also relaxes the splanchnic circulation.

USES

Acute variceal bleeds, acromegaly, pituitary tumors, carcinoid tumors, VIPomas.

SIDE EFFECTS

Headache, GI upset, cardiac conduction changes, hyperglycemia.

ANTACIDS

Antacids are weak bases that decrease gastric acidity by neutralizing gastric acid to form water and a salt. They also affect the action of pepsin, which requires a pH < 4.0. Agents are composed of sodium bicarbonate and aluminum, magnesium, or calcium salts. Aluminum and magnesium salts are most common and promote the healing of duodenal ulcers. However, all antacids can cause hypokalemia. Chronic use may lead to adverse effects (Table 3-27).

INFLIXIMAB

MECHANISM

IgG_1 monoclonal antibody with a high specificity and affinity for tumor necrosis factor alpha (TNF-α). Infliximab most likely works by destroying activated TNF-α cells through apoptosis or complement-mediated actions. TNF-α is found in the stool of patients with Crohn disease and may be correlated with disease severity.

TABLE 3-27.   Consequences of Antacid Overuse

ANTACID	CONSEQUENCES
Aluminum-containing antacids	Constipation Seizures Osteodystrophy Binds to tetracycline to form insoluble complex that is not absorbed Increases absorption of certain drugs such as levodopa Antacid binds to secreted and ingested phosphate to form insoluble salts; hypophosphatemia may lead to osteomalacia and myopathy
Sodium-containing antacids	Transient metabolic alkalosis Fluid retention Hypernatremia
Magnesium-containing antacids	Hypermagnesemia, fluid and electrolyte imbalance Hypophosphatemia Diarrhea Hypotension Hyporeflexia Cardiac arrest
Calcium-containing antacids	Milk-alkali syndrome may lead to hypercalcemia, renal stones, and metabolic alkalosis Constipation

USES

Indicated for Crohn disease. It is increasingly being used earlier in the disease presentation. Also used in a variety of rheumatologic conditions, including ankylosing spondylitis, psoriatic arthritis, rheumatoid arthritis, and ulcerative colitis.

SIDE EFFECTS

Infusion reactions, such as shortness of breath, hypotension, fever/chills, and urticaria, can occur. Delayed hypersensitivity reactions are marked by myalgia, fever, rash, and immunosuppression (infection, reactivation of latent tuberculosis).

OSMOTIC LAXATIVES

KEY DRUGS

Magnesium hydroxide, magnesium citrate, lactulose, polyethylene glycol, sorbitol.

MECHANISM

Osmotic laxatives draw water into the bowel lumen owing to their hypertonicity.

USES

Constipation. Lactulose is also used for hepatic encephalopathy.

SIDE EFFECTS

Diarrhea, dehydration. Use with caution in the elderly and in patients with renal impairment.

SULFASALAZINE

MECHANISM

5-Aminosalicylic acid (ASA) derivative, consisting of ASA (anti-inflammatory cyclo-oxygenase [COX] inhibitor) and sulfapyridine (antibacterial). Decreases inflammatory response in the colon and systemically inhibits prostaglandin synthesis.

USES

An enteric-coated tablet indicated for ulcerative colitis. It can also be used for rheumatoid arthritis.

SIDE EFFECTS

Contraindicated in patients with sulfa allergy. Most patients experience GI intolerance upon initiation of this drug. Folic acid needs to be coadministered with this medication.

ONDANSETRON

MECHANISM

Antiemetic selective serotonin (5-HT$_3$) receptor antagonist. Blocks serotonin on peripheral vagal nerve terminals and in the central chemoreceptor trigger zone.

USES

Prophylaxis for highly emetogenic chemotherapy and for prevention and treatment of postoperative nausea and vomiting.

SIDE EFFECTS

Should be used on a scheduled basis for chemotherapy, not as needed because it is indicated for the prevention of nausea. Side effects include headache, malaise, constipation, and prolongation of the QT interval (use caution in patients with QT prolongation).

METOCLOPRAMIDE

MECHANISM

Metoclopramide is a D$_2$ receptor antagonist and also a mixed 5-HT$_3$ receptor antagonist/5-HT$_4$ receptor agonist. It increases GI resting tone and motility.

USES

Gastroparesis; is an antiemetic.

SIDE EFFECTS

It can cause parkinsonian effects and tardive dyskinesia. It can also cause blood pressure changes, galactorrhea, and constipation. It can interact with many other medications. It is contraindicated in patients with Parkinson disease and bowel obstruction.

ORLISTAT

MECHANISM

A derivative of lipstatin, an inhibitor of lipase. It decreases the breakdown and absorption of fatty acids.

USES

It is used in the treatment of obesity and has been shown to achieve modest weight loss.

SIDE EFFECTS

Steatorrhea, decreased absorption of fat-soluble vitamins (A, D, E, K), loose bowel movements.

NOTES

CHAPTER 4

Hematology and Oncology

EMBRYOLOGY 266
Hematopoiesis 266
Types of Hemoglobin 266

ANATOMY 267
Blood 267

PATHOLOGY 272
Anemia 272
Blood Loss 288
Heme Pathology 288
Hemorrhagic Disorders 290
White Cell Disorders 295
Myeloproliferative Syndromes 300
Solid Tumors 308

PHARMACOLOGY 310
Chemotherapy Drugs: Alkylating Agents 310
Antimetabolites 312
Topoisomerase Inhibitors 313
Drugs That Target Tubulin 314
Hormonal Agents 315
Targeted Molecular Therapeutics 315
Native Cytokines Used in Cancer Treatment 318
Anticoagulants 318
Antiplatelet Agents 320
Thrombolytics 322

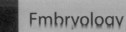

Embryology

HEMATOPOIESIS

Formation of Blood Cells

The outer layer of the **yolk sac,** derived from the extraembryonic mesoderm, is the major site for hematopoiesis in the embryo. The hematopoietic stem cells migrate into the yolk sac from **primitive ectoderm** or **epiblast** and leave the yolk sac to start populating the fetal **liver** between the fourth and the fifth weeks of gestation. As the fetus develops, other hematopoietic organs, including the spleen, lymph nodes, thymus, and bone marrow are also involved in the formation of blood cells (Figure 4-1).

- **Liver:** The major site of hematopoiesis in early embryonic life beginning at week 9.
- **Spleen:** Exclusively a hematopoietic organ until 14 weeks of gestation. At around 15–18 weeks, the spleen is populated with T-cell precursors. In the 23rd week, B-cell precursors enter the spleen and form B-cell regions.
- **Thymus:** Once completely developed, the thymus is populated by lymphocytes derived from stem cells elsewhere (in the yolk sac, liver, and omentum).

TYPES OF HEMOGLOBIN

- Adult hemoglobin (Hb $\alpha_2\beta_2$) is composed of two α and two β subunits and serves to transport O_2 and CO_2.
- Hemoglobin is an allosteric molecule and exhibits positive cooperativity, resulting in sigmoid-shaped dissociation (Figure 4-2).
- This allows efficient loading of O_2 for hemoglobin in an O_2-rich environment (ie, lung) versus unloading of O_2 for hemoglobin in O_2-poor environments (ie, peripheral tissues).
- Elevations in H^+, CO_2, 2,3-bisphosphoglycerate (2,3-BPG), and temperature favor a right shift on the dissociation curve, which facilitates O_2 unloading (Figure 4-2).
- T (taut; deoxygenated) form has low affinity for O_2 versus R (relaxed; oxygenated) form, which has high affinity for O_2 (300×).

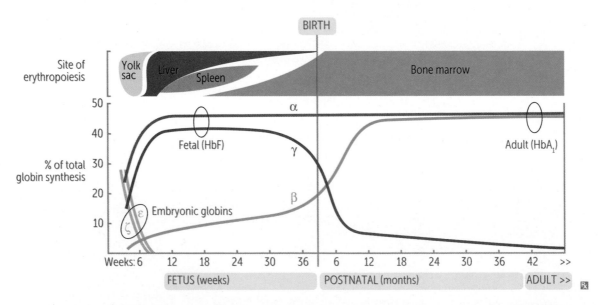

FIGURE 4-1. **Expression of globin isoforms during prenatal and postnatal development.**

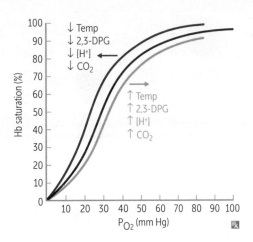

FIGURE 4-2. **Oxygen dissociation curve.** DPG, diphosphoglycerate.

Fetal Hemoglobin (Hb$\alpha_2\gamma_2$)

Produced from the fetal liver, it contains two α-chains and two γ-chains and has higher O_2 affinity than adult hemoglobin.

Adult Hemoglobin (Hb$\alpha_2\beta_2$)

The main type of adult hemoglobin contains two α-chains and two β-chains. The transition from fetal to adult hemoglobin concentrations is complete at approximately 6 months of age.

Anatomy

BLOOD

Blood is a specialized connective tissue containing red blood cells (RBCs), white blood cells (WBCs), and platelets suspended in plasma. See Figure 4-3 for a detailed hematopoietic tree.

Plasma

Plasma is yellow fluid (rich in proteins, hormones, electrolytes, and small molecules) that makes up approximately 55% of the total blood volume.

Cells

There are three major types of blood cells: erythrocytes (RBCs), leukocytes (WBCs), and platelets. Blood cells constitute about 45% of the total blood volume.

Erythrocytes

The erythrocyte is a biconcave, anucleated cell (Figure 4-4) specialized to carry oxygen. It has a diameter of 7.5–8.7 µm, a volume of 90 fL, and a surface area of 136 µm², providing a large surface area:volume ratio. See Table 4-1 for terms used in the evaluation of RBCs.

RBCs exclusively utilize glucose as a source of energy, with 90% **anaerobically** degraded to lactate and the rest metabolized through the hexose monophosphate (HMP) shunt in the production of reduced nicotinamide adenine dinucleotide phosphate (NADPH). They survive for an average of 120 days and are destroyed in the spleen by macrophages.

Reticulocytes are immature RBCs that can be identified by specific staining because they contain **polyribosomes** (Figure 4-4). They account for 0.5–1.5% of RBCs. The

FLASH FORWARD

Other pathologic forms of hemoglobin:
- HbA$_2$ (β-thalassemia)
- HbH (α thalassemia, all four α genes deleted)
- Hb Bart (α thalassemia, three α genes deleted)

FLASH BACK

Binding of 2,3-BPG causes ↓ affinity for O_2.
Fetal hemoglobin does not bind with 2,3-BPG, resulting in ↑ affinity for O_2.

KEY FACT

Serum = plasma without clotting factors.

KEY FACT

Corticosteroids inhibit polymorphonuclear neutrophil (PMN) migration from the circulation into the periphery, causing benign leukocytosis. They also cause apoptosis of lymphocytes and sequestration of eosinophils in lymph nodes.

KEY FACT

RBCs are the only cells without a nucleus, and they do not utilize aerobic metabolism.

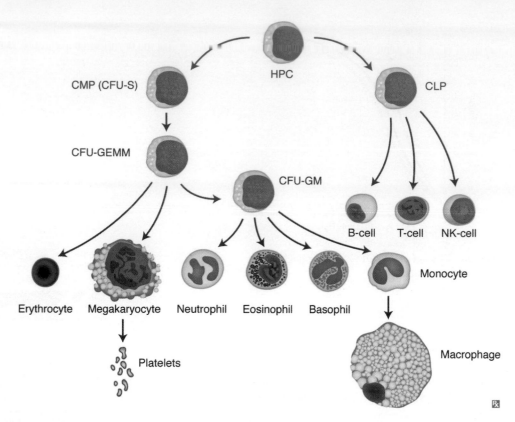

FIGURE 4-3. **Normal hematopoiesis.** CFU-GEMM, colony-forming unit that generates myeloid cells; CFU-GM, granulocyte-macrophage progenitor; CFU-S, spleen colony-forming unit; CLP, common lymphoid progenitor; CMP, common myeloid progenitor; HPC, hematopoietic progenitor cell; NK, natural killer.

reticulocyte count is increased in conditions in which RBC production is increased (eg, hemolytic anemia and blood loss); it is decreased in conditions in which RBC production is decreased (eg, aplastic anemia).

Leukocytes

Leukocytes lead the fight against infection or foreign invasion. The WBC count normally ranges from 4000 to 11,000/μL. WBCs can be divided into five different types of cells: neutrophils, basophils, eosinophils, monocytes, and lymphocytes (Table 4-2).

- **Neutrophils:** Can morphologically be divided into two groups.
    - Immature neutrophils (also known as bands) have a horseshoe shape and are seen during bacterial infections, leukemias, and other in-flammatory conditions.
    - **Hypersegmented** neutrophils (with more than five lobes) are older cells seen in macrocytic anemias associated with vitamin B_{12} and folate deficiencies.

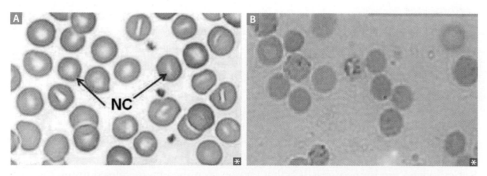

FIGURE 4-4. **A** Normal blood cells (NC) and stomatocytes (narrow central pallor). **B** Supravital stain showing increased reticulocytes.

TABLE 4-1.   Key Terms

Hematocrit	Represents the percentage of whole-blood volume composed of erythrocytes
Mean cell hemoglobin	The average content of hemoglobin per RBC
MCHC	The average concentration of hemoglobin in a given volume of packed RBCs. The MCHC is low if the RBCs are hypochromic
MCV	The average volume of an RBC. A normal value is 80–100 fL. More than 100 fL is a macrocytic anemia, whereas < 80 fL is microcytic
RDW	The coefficient of variation of RBC volume. An increased RDW means that the RBCs vary greatly in size

MCHC, mean corpuscular hemoglobin concentration; MCV, mean corpuscular volume; RDW, RBC distribution width.

- Multilobed (3–5), phagocytic cells with granules in the cytoplasm. They account for 60–70% of all leukocytes and are the prime mediators of acute inflammation.
    - Primarily two groups of granules are present in the cytoplasm: Specific granules are peroxidase-negative, small, and pale-looking, whereas azurophilic granules are lysosomes that are peroxidase-positive, large, and dense, and contain myeloperoxidase enzymes (see Table 4-2, image A).
    - After phagocytosis, neutrophils consume O_2, producing free radicals that help kill bacteria (most effective mechanism).
    - Neutrophils also contain lactoferrin, which avidly binds with iron, robbing bacteria of this essential nutrient and leading to bacterial death.
    - Important neutrophil chemostatic agents are C5a, interleukin (IL)-8, LTB4, kallikrein, and platelet-activating factor.
- **Lymphocytes:** Small, round cells with scant cytoplasm and densely staining nuclei (Table 4-2, Image B). There are four different types of lymphocytes:
    - **B lymphocyte:** Matures in **B**one marrow and migrates to peripheral lymphoid tissues (follicles of lymph nodes, white pulp of spleen, and unencapsulated lymphoid tissue). B lymphocytes mediate humoral immunity and express monomeric molecules of **IgM and IgD as the receptors for the antigen.** Recognition of the antigen leads to differentiation into plasma cells and production of antibodies (including IgG, IgA, and IgM). They function as memory cells and APCs and express MHC class II. They are CD19, CD20, and CD21 positive.
    - **T lymphocyte:** Matures in **T**hymus. Precursor cells of T lymphocytes originate in the bone marrow. After maturation, T lymphocytes leave the thymus and redistribute in lymphoid tissues. They induce cell-mediated immunity and express **T-cell receptors.** T lymphocytes differentiate into cytotoxic T cells (major histocompatabilty complex I [MHC I] and CD8), helper T cells (**MHC II, CD4, T-cell receptor, and CD3**), suppressor T cells, and delayed hypersensitivity T cells. Mechanisms of T-cell activation include binding of the antigen to MHC complex as a first step, then addition of co-stimulatory signal (CD28 or CD40L).
    - **Plasma cells:** Normally only present in the bone marrow and not in the peripheral blood. Eccentric cells with purple "clock-faced" nuclei. Cytoplasm has abundant blue rough endoplasmic reticulum and well-developed Golgi apparatus. They differentiate from B lymphocytes and produce large amounts of antibodies specific for a particular antigen.
    - **Natural killer (NK) cells:** NK cells are a type of cytotoxic lymphocyte that mediates both adaptive immunity and innate immune response. They express both CD16 and CD56. The cytoplasm contains small granules filled with perforin and granzyme (induces apoptosis) that help target and kill cells lacking MHC I, including tumor-derived cells and cells infected with viruses.
- **Monocytes:** Cells with kidney-shaped nuclei (Table 4-2, Image C). The cytoplasm contains fine azurophilic granules (lysosomes) and appears basophilic with a "frosted-

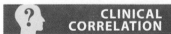

CLINICAL CORRELATION

Leukocyte adhesion deficiency is an autosomal recessive defect of integrins (CD18 subunits), resulting in delayed separation of the umbilical cord, increased circulating PMN, recurrent bacterial infections (that lack pus formation), severe gingivitis, and poor wound healing.

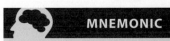

MNEMONIC

Causes of eosinophilia—
NAACP

Neoplasia
Asthma
Allergic processes
Collagen vascular diseases
Parasites

TABLE 4-2.   Leukocytes

LEUKOCYTE	PERCENTAGE	CHARACTERISTICS	FUNCTION
Neutrophil	60–70	Multilobed (3–5), specific and azurophilic granules, lactoferrin	Phagocytic cell, mediator of acute inflammation
Lymphocyte	20–30		
B lymphocyte		Small, round cell, scant cytoplasm, dense nuclei	Humoral immunity
T lymphocyte		Small, round cell, scant cytoplasm, dense nuclei	Cell-mediated immunity
Plasma cell		Eccentric cell, purple nuclei	Produces antibodies
Natural killer cell		Small granules of perforin and proteases	Cell-mediated immunity
Monocyte	2–10	Kidney-shaped nuclei, basophilic and azurophilic granules	Precursor for macrophages and APCs
Eosinophil	1–6	Bilobed nuclei, large eosinophilic granules	Phagocytic cell, defends against parasites and allergic reactions
Basophil	< 0.5	Bilobed nuclei, basophilic granules	Mediates allergic reactions by release of histamine and other vasoactive substances
Mast cell	—	Basophilic granules IgE cross-linking to allergens trigger Degranulation (eg, histamine release)	Mediator of allergic diseases and other Type I hypersensitivity reaction

TABLE 4-2. **Leukocytes** *(continued)*

LEUKOCYTE	PERCENTAGE	CHARACTERISTICS	FUNCTION
Macrophage	2–8	Oval nuclei	Phagocytoses bacteria, aged RBC, and other cell debris Granuloma formation
Dendritic cell	—	Express MHC class II and Fc receptors on surface	Innate and adaptive immunity

APCs, antigen-presenting cells.

glass" appearance. Monocytes are precursor cells for macrophages and antigen-presenting cells (APCs). They account for 2–10% of all leukocytes.

- **Eosinophils:** Bilobed cells with large eosinophilic granules (Table 4-2, Image D). Eosinophils comprise 1–6% of all leukocytes.
- Eosinophils function as phagocytic cells and defend against parasitic infections (via major basic protein). They are capable of releasing a variety of chemical mediators including cytokines, chemokines, arachidonic metabolites (eg, leukotrienes, prostaglandins E_1 and E_2 and thromboxane B_2), and platelet-activating factor.
- Eosinophils can also downregulate allergic reactions by inactivating basophil-derived histamine (via histaminase).
- **Basophils:** Cells with bilobed nuclei that mediate allergic reactions. Basophils stain with **B**asic stain (**B**lue) and have deeply basophilic granules (Table 4-2, Image E). Basophils account for < 0.5% of all leukocytes and express **IgE** receptors that, when triggered, release histamine, heparin, prostaglandins, leukotrienes, and other vasoactive amines. They have a causative role in allergic diseases, including asthma and hay fever, and are frequently elevated in myeloproliferative diseases.

Mast Cells

Granulocytes that are derived from bone marrow precursors and mature in tissues (Table 4-2, Image F). They are especially abundant near blood vessels and in tissues exposed to the external environment (eg, skin, respiratory, gastrointestinal, and urogenital systems). Similar to basophils, they express IgE receptors and counter parasitic infections and chronic allergic diseases.

Macrophages

Cells with oval nuclei and blue-gray to pale cytoplasm (Table 4-2, Image G). Macrophages are derived from monocytes and reside in the tissues. They serve as tissue scavengers (Figure 4-5) and are phagocytic, consuming bacteria, aged RBCs, and cell debris. Macrophages also serve as APCs and are activated by γ-interferon. Macrophages are also important in granuloma formation (eg, TB and sarcoidosis), where they are converted to epitheloid histocytes and giant cells.

KEY FACT

Mast cell activation:
1) Cross-linking of cell surface IgE by antigen
2) Complement C3a/C5a
3) Tissue trauma: Histamine (from immediate response) vs leukotrienes (delayed response)

FLASH FORWARD

Cromolyn sodium prevents mast cell degranulation. Used for asthma prophylaxis. Omalizumab inhibits IgE binding to mast cells. Used for severe allergic asthma.

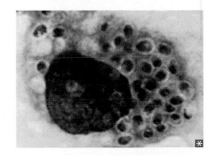

FIGURE 4-5. **Active macrophage.** Histiocyte macrophage containing numerous yeast cells of *Histoplasma capsulatum.*

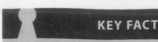

KEY FACT

Macrophage derivatives in various organs and tissues:
- Kupffer cells in the liver
- Microglial cells in the brain
- Osteoclasts in the bone
- Mesangial cells in the kidney (derived from monocytes)

Dendritic Cells

Dendritic cells are sentinels, adjuvants, and controllers of the immune system (both innate and adaptive immunity) and are present in various tissues (Table 4-2, Image H). They serve as APCs and express major histocompatibility complex (MHC) II and crystallizable fragment (Fc) receptors on their surface. They are the main inducers of the primary antibody response. Dendritic cells are called Langerhans cells in skin.

Pathology

ANEMIA

Classification and Appearance

An anemia is a reduction in the O_2-transporting capacity of blood. Anemias can be classified mainly by RBC size, measured by mean corpuscular volume (MCV): microcytic (MCV < 80), macrocytic (MCV > 100), and normocytic (MCV = 80–100) (see Figure 4-6). Other classification systems for anemia include the underlying mechanism (increased destruction versus impaired production), RBC shapes (Table 4-3), and hemoglobinization (normochromic versus hypochromic). Relevant signs and symptoms for anemia include:

- Hypoxia generated: General weakness or fatigue, dyspnea or angina on exertion, syncope, pale conjunctiva or skin, and koilonychias.
- Due to increased cardiac demand: Tachycardia or palpitation, systolic murmur, or high-output heart failure.

Microcytic Anemias

Microcytic anemias are smaller in size, from an extra RBC division to maintain hemoglobin concentration due to deficiency or defects in heme (iron + protoporphyrin), or globin.

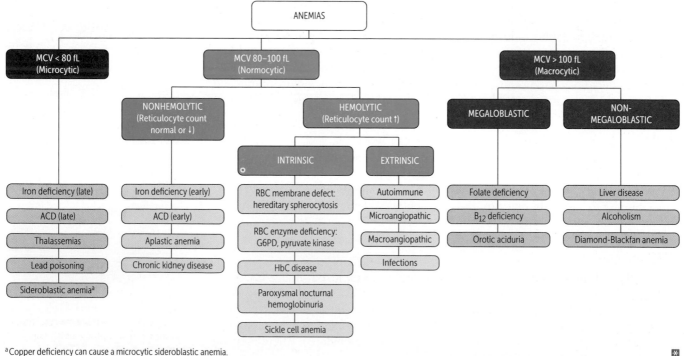

^{a} Copper deficiency can cause a microcytic sideroblastic anemia.

FIGURE 4-6. Categorization of anemias. On a peripheral blood smear, a lymphocyte nucleus is approximately the same size as a normocytic RBC. If RBC is larger than lymphocyte nucleus, consider macrocytosis; if RBC is smaller, consider microcytosis.

TABLE 4-3. **Red Blood Cell Forms**

TYPE	EXAMPLE	ASSOCIATED DISEASE EXAMPLES
Acanthocyte Spiny processes protrude from cell surface		Abetalipoproteinemia, liver disease
Basophilic stipping Numerous small purplish dots		Lead poisoning, thalassemia
Dacrocyte ("teardrop cell")		Myelofibrosis
Degmacyte ("bite cell")		Glucose-6-phosphate dehydrogenase deficiency
Elliptocyte		Hereditary elliptocytosis, iron deficiency
Heinz body		Glucose-6-phosphate dehydrogenase deficiency
Howell-Jolly bodies		Asplenia, functional hyposplenia

TABLE 4-3.   **Red Blood Cell Forms** *(continued)*

TYPE	EXAMPLE	ASSOCIATED DISEASE EXAMPLES
Macro-ovalocyte		Megaloblastic anemia
Ringed sideroblast		Lead poisoning
Schistocyte		Disseminated intravascular coagulation, thrombotic thrombocytopenic purpura
Sickle cell		Sickle cell anemia
Spherocyte		Hereditary spherocytosis, autoimmune hemolysis
Target cell		Thalassemia, liver disease, hemoglobin C disease, asplenia

Iron Deficiency Anemia

Iron is necessary for the **production of heme;** therefore iron deficiency decreases the O_2-carrying capacity of RBCs. Deficiency can be caused by:

- Increased requirement: **Pregnancy,** infants, and preadolescents.
- Dietary deficiency: Exclusively breast-fed infants after 6 months of age, elderly.
- Chronic blood loss: **Menorrhagia, gastrointestinal bleeding.**

PRESENTATION

Pallor (Figure 4-7A), **fatigue**, angina pectoris in persons with coronary artery disease (CAD), glossitis, kolionychias, and pica. Iron deficiency anemia can also be associated with **Plummer-Vinson syndrome.**

DIAGNOSIS

Decreased hemoglobin and hematocrit. Peripheral smear shows **microcytic, hypochromic RBCs** microcytic, hypochromic RBCs (Figure 4-7B). Patients are often normocytic for a while before developing symptoms. Their laboratory findings consist of **decreased serum iron, increased total iron-binding capacity (TIBC),** and **decreased ferritin.**

TREATMENT

Iron supplementation; management of blood loss, if present.

Thalassemia

Genetic syndrome resulting from decreased synthesis of one of the globin chains in HbA (normally $\alpha_2\beta_2$). Clinical abnormalities are caused by both the low concentration of hemoglobin and the excess of the other chain. There are two types of thalassemias, β- and α-thalassemias:

β-Thalassemia

Point mutations in either the promoter region or the splicing sites of the β-globin gene (on chromosome 11). These result in either premature stop condon (β_0) or reduced production of (β_+) globin. Also known as Mediterranean, or Cooley, anemia. Three forms exist:

- **Minor (β/β_+):** Heterozygote with underproduced β-globin chain. These patients are clinically asymptomatic, but laboratory studies show elevated hemoglobin A2 (HbA2).
- **Major (β_0/β_0):** Homozygote with absent β-globin chain, resulting in severe anemia.
- **HbS/β-thalassemia:** Combination of sickle cell and β-thalassemia. Most common form in the United States and in the Mediterranean. Patients present with sickle cell disease that is mild to moderate, depending on the amount of β-globin production.

β-Thalassemia major lacks HbA and is characterized by **α-chain aggregation.** Aggregation leads to **decreased RBC life span** and apoptotic death of RBC precursors, resulting in ineffective erythropoiesis. **Fetal hemoglobin is increased** as a compensatory mechanism but is inadequate.

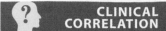

CLINICAL CORRELATION

Plummer-Vinson syndrome presents with the triad of upper esophageal web (dysphagia), iron deficiency anemia, and atrophic glossitis.

KEY FACT

Thalassemia is common among African, Indian, Southeast Asian, and Mediterranean populations.

KEY FACT

Thalassemias cause underproduction of normal globin proteins. Hemoglobinopathies (eg, sickle cell disease) involve structural abnormalities in globin proteins.

MNEMONIC

β-ThalaSSemia— 3 S's

Splenomegaly
Hemo**S**iderosis
Skeletal deformities

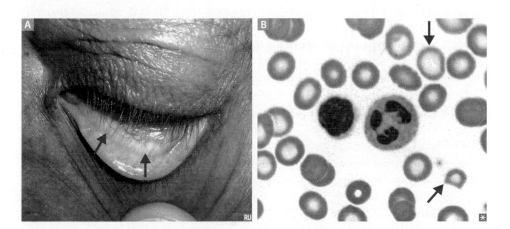

FIGURE 4-7. **Iron deficiency anemia.** **A** Conjunctival pallor and **B** and microcytosis and hypochromia in anemia.

PRESENTATION

- Anemia: Severe anemia a few months after birth (HbF is protective at birth).
- Splenomegaly: Massive extramedullary hematopoiesis (due to increased erythropoietin [EPO]).
- Skeletal deformities: Thinning of cortical bone and peripheral new bone formation; classic examples are "crew cut" appearance of skull on x-rays and "chipmunk face" appearance of facial bones.
- Hemosiderosis: Repeated blood transfusion resulting in iron overload.

In addition, these patients are at an increased risk for aplastic crisis (induced by parvovirus B19 infection).

DIAGNOSIS

Hemoglobin electrophoresis. **Microcytic, hypochromic** RBC morphology on peripheral blood smear (Figure 4-8).

TREATMENT

Blood transfusions (increased risk of secondary hemochromatosis).

PROGNOSIS

Complications may include growth retardation, death at an early age, cardiac failure, and other organ damage from hemosiderosis.

α-Thalassemia

Decreased production of α-globin due to either a gene mutation or deletion in one or more of the four α-globin genes (on chromosome 16). There is no compensatory increase in any other chains, but there is a relative excess of other chains including β, γ, and δ.

- α-Thalassemia is prevalent among **Asian** and **African** populations.
- Hb Bart: Excess γ-globin chains form stable tetramers, which are lethal in utero, resulting in hydrops fetalis.

PRESENTATION

Depends on the number of genes mutated or deleted.

- **Silent carrier state:** Only **one** α-globin gene affected; **asymptomatic.**
- **α-Thalassemia trait: Two** genes deleted; similar to β-thalassemia minor with **minimal anemia.**
- **Hemoglobin H disease: Three** α-globin genes affected; **HbH** (tetramers of β-globin chains) form; HbH has high O_2 affinity and also damages RBCs, leading to hemolysis; **anemia disproportionate** to the amount of hemoglobin.
- **Hydrops fetalis:** Deletion of **all four** genes; **Hb Bart** (stable tetramers of γ-globin chains) has extremely high O_2 affinity; severe anemia; leads to **intrauterine death** unless intrauterine transfusion is performed; fetus shows edema, pallor, and hepatosplenomegaly.

DIAGNOSIS

Hemoglobin electrophoresis. Based on **microcytic, hypochromic** cells on blood smear and clinical or molecular genetic studies (α-thalassemia traits).

Lead Poisoning

Lead inhibits aminolevulinic acid dehydrase (ALAD) and ferrochelatase. Individuals who live in older houses with lead paint, miners, and industrial workers exposed to lead batteries are at an increased risk of lead poisoning.

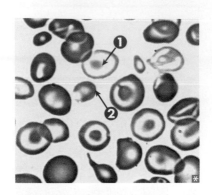

FIGURE 4-8. β-Thalassemia major. Note anisocytosis, poikilocytosis, ❶ target cells, and ❷ microcytosis.

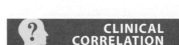

CLINICAL CORRELATION

Cis **deletion on the same chromosome:** Common in Asian patients, who present with an increased risk of spontaneous abortion and severe thalassemia in offspring.

Trans **deletion on each of the separate chromosomes:** Common in African-American patients, who present with no increased risk of spontaneous abortion or severe thalassemia in offspring.

PRESENTATION

Patients usually present with abdominal pain, peripheral neuropathy (eg, wrist and foot drop), encephalopathy, and characteristic Burton lines on gingiva and metaphyses of long bone (Figure 4-9).

DIAGNOSIS

Peripheral blood smear shows basophilic stippling (aggregate of rRNA) and hypochromic microcytic anemia or sideroblastic anemia.

TREATMENT

Succimer for children; dimercaprol and ethylenediaminetetraacetic acid (EDTA).

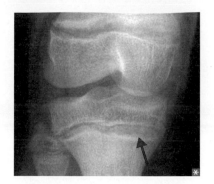

FIGURE 4-9. **X-ray showing lead lines on metaphyses of long bone.**

Sideroblastic Anemia

Sideroblastic anemia is anemia due to defective protoporphyrin synthesis. Etiology includes genetic (congenital defects of aminolevulinic acid synthetase [ALAS], x-linked) and acquired causes (eg, alcoholism, lead poisoning and vitamin B_6 [cofactor for ALAS] deficiency).

DIAGNOSIS

Special staining of bone marrow aspirate for iron shows ringed sideroblasts (trapped iron in mitochondria) (Figure 4-10). Laboratory studies show increased ferritin, decreased total iron-binding capacity (TIBC), increased serum iron saturation.

TREATMENT

Pyridoxine (B_6), cofactor for ALAS.

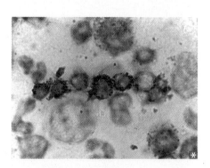

FIGURE 4-10. **Refractory anemia with ringed sideroblasts.** Iron stain of bone marrow aspirate showing numerous ring sideroblasts.

Macrocytic Anemias

In macrocytic anemias, the RBCs are larger than normal (MCV > 100) due to impaired DNA synthesis. The RBCs are larger in size because of fewer RBC divisions.

Megaloblastic Anemia

Deficiency in vitamin B_{12} or folate (coenzymes in DNA synthesis) leads to **delayed DNA replication,** although cytoplasmic maturation is normal. Causes of nonmegaloblastic, macrocytic anemias include alcoholism, liver disease, hypothyroidism, and anticancer drugs (eg, 5-fluorouracil [5-FU]). Enlargement of erythroid precursors gives rise to large RBCs (macrocytes). The bone marrow is hypercellular.

- Vitamin B_{12} deficiency can be caused by:
  - Decreased intake (especially in **vegans**).
  - Impaired absorption (proton pump inhibitor, pancreatic insufficiency, **pernicious anemia,** gastrectomy, malabsorption, **ileal resection,** *Diphyllobothrium latum*/fish tapeworm infection, **blind loop syndrome,** broad-spectrum antibiotics) (Figure 4-11).
  - Increased requirement (**pregnancy,** hyperthyroidism).
- Folic acid deficiency can be caused by:
  - Decreased intake (**alcoholics** and elderly).
  - Impaired absorption (sprue, phenytoin, oral contraceptives).
  - Increased loss (hemodialysis).
  - Increased requirement (**pregnancy,** infancy, increased hematopoiesis).
  - Folic acid antagonist chemotherapy (methotrexate).

PRESENTATION

Anemia, glossitis; **subacute combined degeneration** (due to impaired myelination from elevated toxic methylmalonic acid buildup) of the spinal cord in vitamin B_{12} deficiency, but not in folate deficiency.

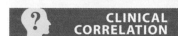

FLASH BACK

Subacute combined degeneration of the spinal cord: Vitamin B_{12} deficiency leads to demyelination of the dorsal and lateral columns of the spinal cord. As a result, patients exhibit ataxia (spinocerebellar tract), hyperreflexia (lateral corticospinal tract), and decreased position and vibration sensation (dorsal column).

CLINICAL CORRELATION

Orotic aciduria: Genetic mutation in uridine monophosphate synthase (converts orotic acid to uridine in pyrimidine synthesis). Often presents in children with megaloblastic anemia untreatable with folate or B_{12} supplementation; orotic acid in urine. Treatment is uridine monophosphate.

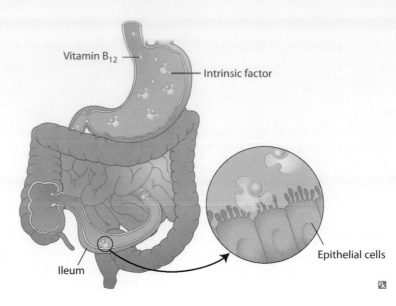

FIGURE 4-11.   **Mechanism of vitamin B$_{12}$ absorption.**

DIAGNOSIS

Peripheral blood smear may show **pancytopenia, oval macrocytosis,** and **hypersegmented neutrophils** (> 5 lobes) (Figure 4-12); bone marrow shows **megaloblastic hyperplasia.** In folate deficiency, there is decreased serum folate, elevated homocysteine, and normal methylmalonic acid. In contrast, in B$_{12}$ deficiency, there is decreased serum B$_{12}$, elevated homocysteine, and increased methylmalonic acid.

In pernicious anemia, **anti-intrinsic factor antibodies** are present and the **Schilling test** shows that the absorption of vitamin B$_{12}$ improves with administration of intrinsic factor.

TREATMENT

Requires vitamin B$_{12}$ with or without folate supplementation.

Normocytic Anemias

Glucose-6-Phosphate Dehydrogenase Deficiency

Glucose-6-phosphate dehydrogenase (G6PD) is an enzyme that normally protects RBCs from oxidants. In G6PD deficiency, this enzyme is **abnormally folded** and thus subject to proteolysis in older RBCs, leading to reduced ability to withstand **oxidative stress** (Figure 4-13). The oxidation of sulfhydryl groups causes hemoglobin to precipitate as **Heinz bodies** (Table 4-3, Image F).

G6PD deficiency is **X-linked** recessive and common in **black and Middle Eastern/ Mediterranean populations.** It is associated with resistance to malarial infection. Women may have both normal and abnormal cells if they are heterozygous. Episodes are usually self-limited, as normal cycling of erythropoiesis replaces the older RBCs with new RBCs that have normal G6PD enzyme activity. Hemolysis from G6PD deficiency can be both **intravascular and extravascular.**

PRESENTATION

Often asymptomatic. History of neonatal jaundice and cholelithiasis. Episodic fatigue, pallor, hemoglobinuria, and back pain (hemoglobin is nephrotoxic) a few days after oxidant stress. Exam may reveal jaundice and splenomegaly. Hemolysis often results from exposure to oxidative stress such as:

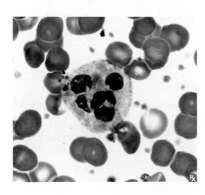

FIGURE 4-12.   **Hypersegmented neutrophil.**

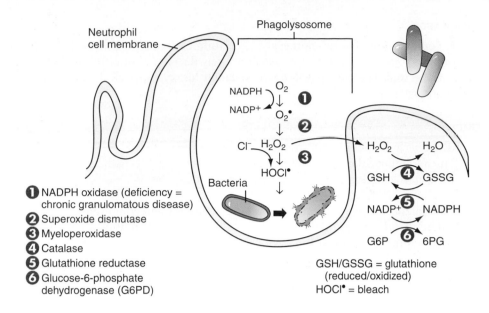

- **①** NADPH oxidase (deficiency = chronic granulomatous disease)
- **②** Superoxide dismutase
- **③** Myeloperoxidase
- **④** Catalase
- **⑤** Glutathione reductase
- **⑥** Glucose-6-phosphate dehydrogenase (G6PD)

GSH/GSSG = glutathione (reduced/oxidized)
HOCl• = bleach

FIGURE 4-13. Red blood cells and oxidative stress. G6P, glucose-6-phosphate; NADP, nicotinamide adenine dinucleotide phosphate; NADPH, reduced nicotinamide adenine dinucleotide phosphate; 6PG, 6-phosphogluconate.

- **Drugs:** Sulfonamides, dapsone, primaquine, chloroquine, and nitrofurantoins, among others.
- **Infections:** Viral hepatitis, typhoid fever, pneumonia.
- **Other:** Fava beans.

DIAGNOSIS

Measure **G6PD enzyme activity** after resolved hemolytic episodes (is normal at time of hemolysis due to presence of young cells but is decreased when no hemolysis is present)

- ↑ indirect bilirubin, ↓ serum haptoglobin from hemolysis
- ↓ hematocrit and hemoglobinemia in complete blood count (CBC).
- Heinz bodies and bite cells (results from splenic removal of Heinz bodies) on peripheral blood smear (Table 4-3, Images D and F).
- Hemoglobinuria in urinalysis.
- Splenomegaly and gallstones (from ↑ indirect bilirubin) in abdominal ultrasound.

TREATMENT

- Avoid precipitating factors.
- Provide O_2 and rest during episodes.
- Exchange transfusions if severe.
- Phototherapy in infants.

PROGNOSIS

Patients can remain healthy if they avoid precipitating factors, but complications include neonatal jaundice that may lead to kernicterus, a type of brain damage caused by pathologically high levels of bilirubin.

Hereditary Spherocytosis

Autosomal dominant deficiency of spectrin, ankyrin, or other membrane tethering cytoskeletal proteins leads to RBC fragility, forcing the RBCs into a spherical shape (Figure 4-14). Spherical cells are less deformable, become trapped within the spleen, and are then phagocytosed.

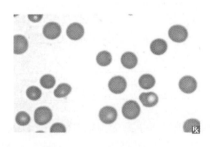

FIGURE 4-14. Hereditary spherocytosis.

PRESENTATION

Stable course of anemia, splenomegaly, and jaundice (predominantly extravascular hemolysis). Some are asymptomatic. Patients may develop **cholelithiasis** (bilirubin gallstones) as well. There is typically a positive family history, especially in an **autosomal dominant** pattern.

DIAGNOSIS

- RBC lysis in **hypotonic salt** (osmotic fragility test).
- ↑ mean corpuscular hemoglobin concentration (MCHC) (pathognomonic, but also seen in cold-agglutinin anemia) due to cell dehydration.
- Spherocytes in peripheral blood smear.
- Minimal anemia with reticulocytosis in CBC, and ↑ indirect bilirubin.
- Differential diagnosis includes anemia, biliary disease, hyperbilirubinemia, and autoimmune hemolytic anemia (which may also have spherocytes).

TREATMENT

- Splenectomy.
- Transfusion if severe.
- Phototherapy in infants.
- Supplemental folic acid and iron for increased RBC turnover.

PROGNOSIS

Possible complications include aplastic crisis triggered by B19 parvovirus infection, infections after splenectomy, cholelithiasis (bilirubin gallstones), and hemosiderosis from multiple blood transfusions.

Immunohemolytic Anemias

Antibodies are produced that lead to destruction of RBCs. Due to the presence of antibodies, these anemias are **Coombs-positive** (Figure 4-15). Three types of immunohemolytic anemias—warm antibody, cold agglutinin, and erythroblastosis fetalis—are discussed in the following sections.

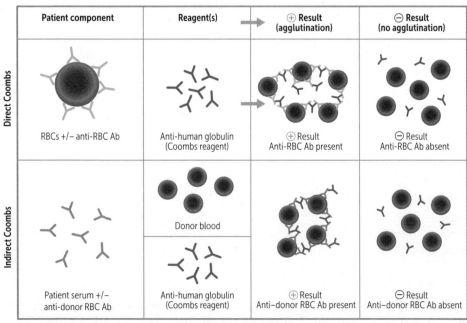

FIGURE 4-15. **Direct and indirect Coombs test.**

Warm Antibody Hemolytic Anemia

IgG autoantibodies bind RBCs under warm temperature of the central body (warm agglutinin), leading to spheroidal transformation. Spherocytes are sequestered and then phagocytosed in the spleen (extravascular hemolysis).

PRESENTATION

Elevated bilirubin (jaundice, pigment gallstones), reticulocytosis, and splenomegaly. Often associated with systemic lupus erythematosus (SLE), Hodgkin lymphoma, chronic lymphocytic leukemia (CLL), or certain drugs (α-methyldopa, penicillin, cephalosporins).

DIAGNOSIS

Spherocytosis, positive direct Coombs test (anti-Ig antibody added to patient's RBCs leads to agglutination if RBCs have IgG attached).

TREATMENT

Drug cessation, steroids, and splenectomy if necessary.

Cold Agglutinin Immune Hemolytic Anemia

IgM autoantibodies (pathologic cold agglutinins) occur at high titers and react at 28–31°C, and sometimes at 37°C. Some **intravascular hemolysis** is seen, especially in distal body parts. IgM is released when cells warm, leaving **C3b** bound to membrane. Thus, RBCs are also subject to **extravascular hemolysis.**

PRESENTATION

Episodic hyperbilirubinemia. May also have hemoglobinemia and hemoglobinuria. Laboratory results include a positive Coombs test and elevated C3.

- **Acute:** Often in recovery phase after infectious **mononucleosis** or **mycoplasmal pneumonia.**
- **Chronic:** Associated with lymphoproliferative neoplasms; may be associated with Raynaud phenomenon (Figure 4-16) due to vascular obstruction.

TREATMENT

Steroids, IVIG, and plasmapheresis.

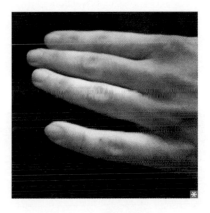

FIGURE 4-16.   Raynaud phenomenon.

Erythroblastosis Fetalis

Maternal alloimmunization to **fetal D antigen (Rh factor)** leads to destruction of fetal RBCs. Usually, the mother is D (Rh) negative and the fetus is D (Rh) positive. This sensitizes the mother to produce alloantigen, causing fetal RBC destruction in the subsequent D (Rh) positive fetus. May also occur in setting of **ABO incompatibility;** in these cases, the mother is O and the fetus is A or B.

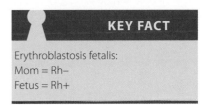

KEY FACT

Erythroblastosis fetalis:
Mom = Rh–
Fetus = Rh+

PRESENTATION

Fetal hemolytic anemia.

DIAGNOSIS

Test maternal and fetal blood for presence of antibodies (Table 4-4).

PROGNOSIS

Stillbirth, **hydrops fetalis** (fetal heart failure), **kernicterus** (unconjugated bilirubin damages basal ganglia and other central nervous system [CNS] structures, leading to neurologic damage).

TABLE 4-4.   Blood Groups

	ABO CLASSIFICATION				RH CLASSIFICATION	
	A	B	AB	O	RH⊕	RH⊖
RBC type						
Group antigens on RBC surface	A	B	A & B	None	Rh (D)	None
Antibodies in plasma	Anti-B IgM	Anti-A IgM	None	Anti-A Anti-B IgM	None	Anti-D IgG
Clinical relevance	Receive B or AB → hemolytic reaction	Receive A or AB → hemolytic reaction	Universal recipient of RBCs; universal donor of plasma	Receive any non-O → hemolytic reaction. Universal donor of RBCs; universal recipient of plasma	Universal recipient of RBCs	Treat mother with anti-D Ig (RhoGAM) during and after each pregnancy to prevent anti-D IgG formation

Reproduced with permission from Le T, et al. *First Aid for the USMLE Step 1 2017*. New York, NY: McGraw-Hill Education, 2017.

Anemia of Chronic Disease

Usually characterized by marrow hypoproliferation as a result of impaired responsiveness to erythropoietin (EPO) or impaired iron reutilization. In the setting of chronic inflammation and infections, increased hepcidin sequesters and limits iron release from macrophage to erythroid precursors and suppresses EPO release. Common causes include the following:

- **Chronic infections:** Osteomyelitis and bacterial endocarditis, among others.
- Chronic immune disorders: **Rheumatoid arthritis**, SLE.
- Renal disease.
- **Neoplasms:** Hodgkin disease and lung carcinoma, among others.

Mechanisms include the following:

- Increased hepcidin (produced from liver) limits iron release from marcophage to erythroid precursors and suppresses erythropoietin (EPO) release.
- Hepcidin is a master regulator in iron metabolism and normally limits iron transport by binding to ferroportin (iron transporter present in intestinal mucosal cells and macrophages).
- In the setting of inflammation or infection, increased hepcidin sequesters iron to keep it away from microorganisms.

PRESENTATION

Symptoms of the chronic disease along with mild anemia (fatigue, pallor).

DIAGNOSIS

- ↓ **TIBC**, ↓ **serum iron**, ↑ **serum ferritin** and iron storage in macrophages.
- Normocytic, normochromic RBCs (**early** stage) and microcytic, hypochromic RBCs (**late** stage) on peripheral smear.
- ↓ hemoglobin and hematocrit in CBC.

TREATMENT

Anemia may be resolved by administering erythropoietin and treating the underlying condition.

PROGNOSIS

Overall prognosis depends on the underlying condition.

Hemolytic Anemias

Result of **premature RBC destruction** causing a build-up of **hemoglobin metabolites** and an increase in **erythropoiesis.** Classified by location of destruction (intravascular vs extravascular), cause of destruction (extrinsic vs intrinsic to RBCs), and origin of defect (hereditary vs acquired), as summarized in Table 4-5.

- **Intravascular:**
  - Due to complement fixation, mechanical injury, or toxins.
  - Look for **hemoglobinemia,** methemalbuminemia, mild jaundice/elevation in **unconjugated bilirubin, hemoglobinuria** (early stage), hemosiderinuria, methemoglobinuria, decreased serum haptoglobin, hemosiderosis of renal tubules (**chronic** stage), and increased fecal urobilin.
- **Extravascular:**
  - Due to RBC injury, antibody attachment, structural or membrane defects leading to abnormal shape, and decreased ability to leave cords of Billroth and enter sinusoids of spleen.

TABLE 4-5. Hemolytic Anemia

INTRINSIC	EXTRINSIC
Hereditary	**Acquired**
Enzyme deficiencies (IV and EV)	**Antibody mediated (IV)**
HMP shunt: G6PD, glutathione synthetase	Transfusion reactions
Glycolytic enzymes: pyruvate kinase, hexokinase	Erythroblastosis fetalis
	Systemic lupus erythematous
Membrane disorders (EV)	Malignant neoplasms
Elliptocytosis	Mycoplasmal infection, mononucleosis
Spherocytosis	Drug-associated
Hemoglobin synthesis derangements (EV)	Idiopathic
Thalassemias	**Mechanical injury (IV)**
Sickle cell anemia (can also have IV)	Microangiopathic hemolytic anemias (TTP, DIC)
Acquired	Cardiac traumatic hemolytic anemia
Membrane disorders (EV)	**Infection (IV)**
Paroxysmal nocturnal hemoglobinuria	Malaria, babesiosis
	Chemical injury (IV)
	Lead poisoning
	Excessive destruction by spleen (EV)
	Hypersplenism

DIC, disseminated intravascular coagulation; EV, extravascular; G6PD, glucose-6-phosphate dehydrogenase; HMP, hexose monophosphate; IV, intravascular; TTP, thrombotic thrombocytopenic purpura.

■ Hemolysis usually occurs in mononuclear phagocytic cells in the spleen (reticuloendothelial system).

■ Look for jaundice/elevation in unconjugated bilirubin (increased risk of bilirubin gallstones), some decrease in serum haptoglobin, and **splenomegaly**. Minimal **hemoglobinemia** and **hemoglobinuria**.

Sickle Cell Disease

Point mutation (substitution of **valine** for glutamic acid at position 6) in the β-**globin chain gene** leads to production of abnormal hemoglobin, **HbS**. Common in populations of African heritage (approximately 10% of Africans are carriers of this mutation, which is protective against *Plasmodia falciparum* malaria).

Many variants of sickle cell exist including:

■ **Sickle cell trait:** Heterozygotes with an HbA and an HbS allele (HbSA); results in resistance against malarial infection. Patients usually are **asymptomatic** without anemia and only present with microscopic hematuria. However, they have an increased risk of renal microinfarctions and renal papillary necrosis. Labs show a **positive metabisulfate** screen, and Hb electrophoresis shows 55% HbA, 43% HbS, and 2% HbA2 (Figure 4-17).

■ **Sickle cell disease:** Homozygotes have two HbS alleles (HbSS).

■ **Others:** Heterozygotes (HbSC) with an HbS and an HbC (glutamic acid to lysine substitution) allele.

■ **Order of severity:** HbSS > HbSC > HbSA.

■ **Sickle β-thalassemia:** Heterozygotes with an HbS and β-thalassemia (HbS/[β]Th)

HbS undergoes aggregation and polymerization when **deoxygenated**, leading to **sickle-shaped cells** (Figure 4-18), which are subject to **splenic destruction**. These cells make the blood **hyperviscous,** which can lead to **microvascular occlusion.** Sickling may also occur as a result of **hypoxia or a fall in pH,** which reduces the O_2 affinity of hemoglobin. This is worsened by **dehydration,** which increases MCHC and aggregation of HbS molecules.

Presentation

Because HbF prevents polymerization of HbS, disease may not manifest until newborns are 6 months old. Patients usually present with a variety of symptoms, which can be divided into four different groups:

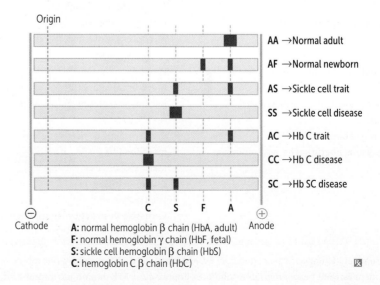

FIGURE 4-17.   **Hemoglobin electrophoresis.**

1. **Vaso-occlusion symptoms:**
   - Pallor from chronic hemolytic anemia.
   - Strokes, acute chest syndrome (associated with fever, hypoxia, and pulmonary infiltrate, most common cause of death in adults with sickle cell anemia), hand and feet swelling (dactylitis), and aseptic necrosis of femoral or humeral head.
   - Painful episodes in joints, abdomen, viscera, lung, liver, and penis.
   - Infarctions of lung and spleen (Figure 4-19), as well as autosplenectomy (most common cause of death from bacterial infections in sickle cell children), is completed by 6 years of age.
   - Increased susceptibility to encapsulated bacteria (patients require prophylactic vaccinations), such as *Streptococcus pneumoniae*, *Neisseria meningitidis*, and *Haemophilus influenzae*, as well as to *Salmonella* osteomyelitis secondary to asplenia.
   - Renal papillary necrosis, which leads to gross hematuria and proteinuria.

2. **Sequestration symptoms:**
   - Acute pooling of erythrocytes in the spleen, usually post infection (eg, from encapsulated *N meningitidis*).
   - Patients present with acute splenomegaly and septic shock-like state and hypovolemia.

3. **Hemolytic symptoms:**
   - Mostly intravascular hemolysis, leading to jaundice from unconjugated bilirubinemia (increased risk for bilirubin gallstones).
   - Massive erythroid hyperplasia due to expansion of hematopoiesis into skull ("crewcut"), facial bone ("chipmunk face"), and extramedullary hematopoiesis with hepatomegaly.

4. **Aplastic symptoms:**
   - ↑ risk of Parvovirus B19 infection.

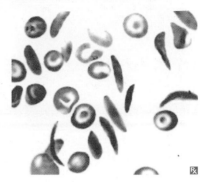

FIGURE 4-18.   Sickle cell anemia.

> **FLASH FORWARD**
>
> Fetal hemoglobin has lower affinity for 2,3-BPG than does adult hemoglobin and, as a result, has higher affinity for O_2.

DIAGNOSIS

- **Hb electrophoresis** (Figure 4-17) reveals high levels of HbS (approximately 90% HbS in sickle disease).
- Mixing blood with a **reducing agent** (metabisulfate screen) causes sickling; positive in both sickle cell trait and disease.
- CBC shows anemia, reticulocytosis, leukocytosis, thrombocytosis.

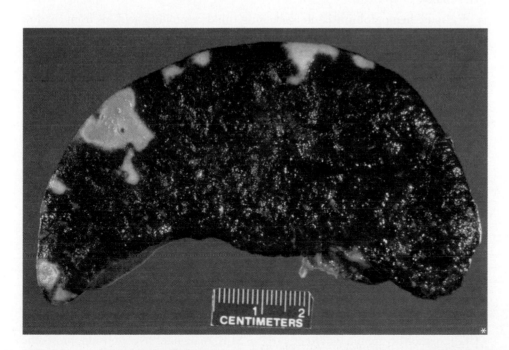

FIGURE 4-19.   Splenic infarction.

- Peripheral smear (Figure 4-18) reveals sickled RBCs, polychromasia, nucleated RBCs, and **Howell-Jolly bodies** (basophilic nuclear remnants due to autosplenectomy [Table 4-3, Image G]).
- Serum bilirubin and fecal/urinary urobilinogen are elevated (due to extravascular hemolysis); low haptoglobin level (due to intravascular hemolysis).
- Skull radiograph shows "**crew cut**" pattern due to extramedullary hematopoiesis.

TREATMENT

- Hydration
- Folic acid supplementation
- Blood transfusion
- Penicillin prophylaxis
- Pneumococcal, *H influenzae*, and meningococcal vaccines
- Pain control
- Bone marrow transplantation
- **Hydroxyurea** (increases concentration of HbF)

Pyruvate Kinase Deficiency

Autosomal recessive enzyme dysfunction leading to anemia that is **chronic** rather than episodic.

- Results from chronic decreased adenosine triphosphate (ATP), leading to membrane damage (Na^+/K^+ ATPase cannot be maintained).
- Presents with neonatal jaundice, extravascular hemolysis, and splenomegaly.
- Mild symptoms of anemia because 2,3-BPG buildup induces right shift (lower O_2 affinity), promoting O_2 release into tissues.

KEY FACT

Glycosylphosphatidylinositol (GPI)-anchoring decay-accelerating factor **(CD55),** a C3 convertase inhibitor, to inactivate complement destruction.

Paroxysmal Nocturnal Hemoglobinuria

Rare, **acquired** clonal hematologic disorder that arises from a mutation in the *PIGA* gene, which is essential for the synthesis of the glycosylphosphatidylinositol (GPI) anchors used for surface protein attachment. Many of the GPI-linked proteins inactivate complement, so without them, RBCs are subject to lysis by endogenous complement. Platelets and granulocytes can be affected also.

PRESENTATION

- Episodic **hemoglobinuria** on awakening (mild respiratory acidosis from shallow breathing at sleep increases CO_2 and activates complement); **hemosiderinuria** can lead to iron deficiency.
- **Pancytopenia** (RBCs, WBCs, and platelets are lysed).
- Increased risk of **venous thrombosis** and acute myeloid leukemia.

DIAGNOSIS

Based on clinical presentation. Flow cytometry to detect lack of CD55 decay-accelerating factor (DAF) on blood cells, and sucrose test or acidified serum test (activates complement).

PROGNOSIS

This can evolve into aplastic anemia and acute leukemia.

TREATMENT

Eculizumab (terminal complement inhibitor).

Microangiopathic Hemolytic Anemia

Mechanical trauma caused by narrowed vessels leads to **intravascular** hemolysis seen in disseminated intravascular coagulation (DIC), thrombotic thrombocytopenic purpura (TTP), hemolytic-uremic syndrome (HUS), SLE, malignant hypertension, prosthetic heart valves, and aortic stenosis.

PRESENTATION

Related to clinical syndrome causing hemolysis. Hemolysis is usually clinically irrelevant except in TTP and HUS.

DIAGNOSIS

Schistocytes (helmet cells; see Table 4-3) on peripheral blood smear (Figure 4-20).

Cardiac Traumatic Hemolytic Anemia

Shear stress due to the turbulent blood flow and abnormal pressures that occur with **prosthetic valves** leads to RBC damage.

Aplastic Anemia

Pancytopenia characterized by severe **anemia, neutropenia, and thrombocytopenia.** Failure or destruction of **multipotent myeloid stem cells** leads to inadequate production or release of differentiated cell lines. Common causes include the following:

- Radiation.
- Chemicals: Benzene.
- Drugs: Chloramphenicol, sulfonamides, alkylating agents, antimalarial drugs, antimetabolites.
- Viral agents (parvovirus B19, Epstein-Barr virus [EBV], HIV, hepatitis C virus [HCV]).
- Fanconi anemia.
- Idiopathic (immune-mediated or primary stem cell defect).

PRESENTATION

Onset usually gradual:

- Anemia → fatigue, malaise, pallor.
- Thrombocytopenia → purpura, mucosal bleeding, petechiae.
- Neutropenia → infection.

DIAGNOSIS

- **CBC:** Decreased RBC, WBC, and platelet count.
- **Marrow biopsy: Hypocellular bone marrow** without atypical cell morphology (Figure 4-21), decreased erythrocytic and granulocytic precursors, decreased megakaryocytes, and **fatty infiltration.**
- **Peripheral smear: Pancytopenia,** normochromic, normocytic, no reticulocytosis, and no splenomegaly.

TREATMENT

- Withdrawal of offending agent.
- Immune therapy: Antithymocyte globulin, cyclosporine.
- Allogenic bone marrow transplantation.
- RBC and platelet transfusion.
- Granulocyte colony-stimulating factor (G-CSF), granulocyte-macrophage colony-stimulating factor (GM-CSF).

PROGNOSIS

- If adverse effect of drug, withdrawal may lead to recovery.
- If idiopathic, poor prognosis.

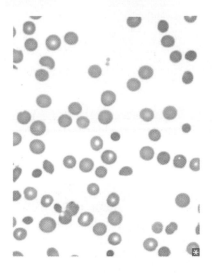

FIGURE 4-20. Schistocytes.

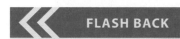

FLASH BACK

Aplastic anemia is a common adverse effect of chloramphenicol; it may or may not be reversed with discontinuation of the drug.

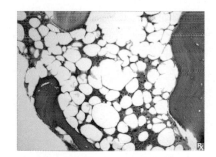

FIGURE 4-21. Bone marrow biopsy specimen of aplastic anemia. Note the hypocellular bone marrow (predominantly fat) with rare hematopoietic precursor cells but no atypical cells.

BLOOD LOSS

Acute Blood Loss

Loss of blood volume leads to a decrease in RBCs; other blood components are also affected.

PRESENTATION

Sudden weakness, fatigue, pale skin, malaise, dyspnea, cardiac failure, headache, presyncope/syncope, and shock. Patients may have history of **trauma** or bleeding. Bleeding may be external or internal.

DIAGNOSIS

CBC, peripheral blood smear. Differential includes other anemias (especially hemolytic anemias), hypothyroidism, myelofibrosis, acute porphyria, and SLE. **Hematocrit is initially normal but decreases** as interstitial fluid shifts into the vascular compartment, causing hemodilution. **Reticulocyte count increases** as erythropoiesis peaks at around 1 week. If hemorrhage is external, iron deficiency occurs over time. Peripheral smear is **initially normochromic and normocytic,** but reticulocytes appear later as polychromatophilic macrocytes.

TREATMENT

- Fluids
- Blood transfusion
- Elimination of cause of hemorrhage
- Other measures to prevent shock

Chronic Blood Loss

May lead to anemia when **loss exceeds erythropoiesis** or when **iron stores are diminished** (eg, GI bleeding from elderly patients who are at risk of developing colorectal cancer). Presentation, diagnosis, treatment, and complications are similar to those for anemias caused by impaired RBC production. Vitamin B_{12} and folate supplementation is appropriate.

HEME PATHOLOGY

Heme production occurs via the synthetic pathway (Figure 4-22). A defect in any of these steps can result in **porphyrias,** a group of diseases that result from the accumulation of heme intermediates.

Acute Intermittent Porphyria

AIP is autosomal dominant, leading to a deficiency in **porphobilinogen deaminase** with subsequent accumulation of upstream metabolites—**porphobilinogen** and coporphobilinogen (**urinary**), and **δ-aminolevulinic acid (ALA).** These intermediates lead to degeneration of myelin.

PRESENTATION

May be induced by certain medications (sulfa drugs and barbiturates, in addition to other P450 inducers, which increase heme synthesis). Symptoms include dark, foul-smelling urine, abdominal pain, hallucinations, blurred vision, and peripheral motor neuropathy (eg, foot drop) that mimics Guillain-Barré syndrome, such as foot drop.

DIAGNOSIS

Genetic testing; increased urinary secretion of porphobilinogen and porphyrins is pathognomonic. Measuring the activity of porphobilinogen deaminase is of little value, as some patients have normal levels.

KEY FACT

Corrected reticulocyte count (CRC) = actual hematocrit/45 × reticulocyte count. If > 3%, then a good bone marrow response to anemia is present. If < 2%, then erythropoiesis is diminished or a marrow disorder, such as iron deficiency anemia, occurs.

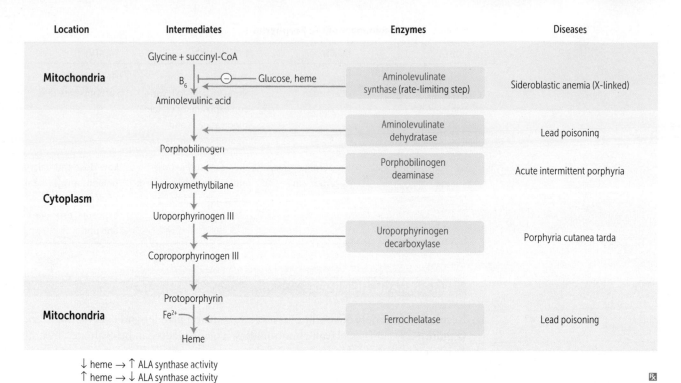

Location	Intermediates	Enzymes	Diseases

Glycine + succinyl-CoA

Mitochondria B_6 ─⊖── Glucose, heme   Aminolevulinate synthase (rate-limiting step)   Sideroblastic anemia (X-linked)

Aminolevulinic acid

Aminolevulinate dehydratase   Lead poisoning

Porphobilinogen

Porphobilinogen deaminase   Acute intermittent porphyria

Hydroxymethylbilane

Cytoplasm

Uroporphyrinogen III

Uroporphyrinogen decarboxylase   Porphyria cutanea tarda

Coproporphyrinogen III

Protoporphyrin

Mitochondria Fe^{2+} Ferrochelatase   Lead poisoning

Heme

↓ heme → ↑ ALA synthase activity
↑ heme → ↓ ALA synthase activity

FIGURE 4-22.   Heme synthetic pathway.

TREATMENT

Goal is to decrease heme synthesis, thereby reducing the production of porphyrin precursors. Patients should eat a high-carbohydrate diet during acute attacks. Severe attacks should be treated with hematin (inhibits ALA synthase).

Porphyria Cutanea Tarda

Part of the porphyria spectrum that results from deficient activity of the heme synthetic enzyme **uroporphyrinogen decarboxylase (UROD)**. This leads to elevated porphyrin by-products, including elevated **uroporyphyrin** (large insoluble molecule and photosensitive), iron, and transferrin.

PATHOLOGY

Accumulation of iron leads to siderosis, affecting liver function. Accumulated uroporphyrins lead to bullae and skin lesions that form upon exposure to sunlight.

PRESENTATION

Patients present with cutaneous bullae and skin lesions that form upon exposure to sunlight (due to accumulation of photosensitive uroporphyrin). Additional organ damage from iron accumulation includes liver siderosis and eventual fibrosis. Urine turns dark upon standing. The disease is exacerbated by consumption of alcohol, iron, and estrogens.

DIAGNOSIS

Plasma and urine analysis for elevated uroporyphyrin. The activity of the UROD can also be tested in red blood cells.

TREATMENT

- Low-dose antimalarial medications, phlebotomy.
- The porphyria syndromes are summarized in Table 4-6.

> **KEY FACT**
>
> AIP differs from other porphyrias because it has no sun-induced lesions.

TABLE 4-6.   **Summary of the Porphyrias**

DISEASE	DEFICIT	PRESENTATION	TREATMENT
Acute intermittent porphyria	Porphobilinogen deaminase	Dark, foul-smelling urine (usually following sun exposure or certain medications), and neurologic deficits	Hematin, high-carbohydrate diet
Porphyria cutanea tarda	Uroporphyrinogen decarboxylase	Bullae on sun-exposed areas, liver siderosis, dark urine upon standing	Low-dose antimalarials, phlebotomy. Avoidance of alcohol, sun exposure, estrogens and iron

HEMORRHAGIC DISORDERS

Result from a variety of conditions, including mixed platelet and coagulation disorders (Figure 4-23), and vessel wall abnormalities. The disorders can be evaluated by a variety of laboratory tests (Tables 4-7 and 4-8).

Platelet Disorders

Platelet disorders are defects in primary hemostasis (platelet plug formation) (Figure 4-24). The etiology includes quantitative (thrombocytopenia) and qualitative disorders (platelet dysfunction).

Patients usually present with skin bleeding, which ranges from petechiae (1–2 mm, typically not seen in qualitative disorders), purpura (> 1 mm), ecchymoses (> 3 mm), to easy bruising. Mucosal bleeding includes epistaxis, hemoptysis, GI bleeding, hematuria, and menorrhagia. Severe thrombocytopenia may lead to life-threatening intracranial bleeding.

Labs show increased bleeding time and decreased platelet count (thrombocytopenia). However, platelet count may be **normal** in qualitative disorders.

Thrombocytopenia

Reduction in number of platelets leads to decreased ability to form clots. Results from decreased production, decreased survival, sequestration, or dilution of platelets. Specific causes include:

FLASH FORWARD

Heparin-induced thrombocytopenia (HIT) results from acquired immunoglobulin G (IgG) antibodies to platelet factor IV/heparin complexes. Antibody binding results in thrombosis despite thrombocytopenia. Cessation of therapy is curative:

- Type I occurs rapidly and is clinically insignificant, resulting from platelet aggregation.
- Type II develops after 5–14 days; life-threatening thrombosis; immune reaction against complex of heparin and platelet factor IV. Can occur earlier if previously exposed to heparin.

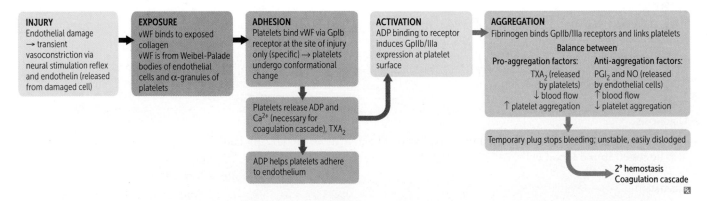

FIGURE 4-23.   **Primary hemostasis.** ADP, adenosine diphosphate; PGI$_2$, prostacyclin I$_2$; TXA$_2$, thromboxane A$_2$; vWF, von Willebrand factor.

TABLE 4-7.   **Laboratory Findings in Bleeding Disorders**

	PLATELET COUNT	BLEEDING TIME (PFA-100 TEST)[a]	PT	PTT	THROMBIN TIME/ FIBRINOGEN
Vessel abnormalities	—	↑	—	—	—
Thrombocytopenia	↓	↑	—	—	—
Qualitative platelet defects	—	↑	—	—	—
Hemophilia A and B	—	—	—	↑	—
Vitamin K deficiency	—	—	↑	↑	—
von Willebrand disease	—	↑	—	—/↑	—
DIC	↓	↑	↑	↑	↑
Liver disease	↓	↑	↑	↑	↑
Multiple transfusions	↓	↑	↑	↑	↑

[a]Platelet function test (PFA)-100 has replaced bleeding time test in many institutions.

DIC, disseminated intravascular coagulation; PFA, platelet function assay; PT, prothrombin time; PTT, partial thromboplastin time.

- Bone marrow diseases such as **aplastic anemia** and **acute leukemia.**
- Drugs: Alcohol, quinidine, **heparin,** sulfa, **cytotoxic drugs,** and thiazide diuretics.
- Infections such as measles, **HIV,** infectious mononucleosis, cytomegalovirus (CMV), *Haemophilus influenzae* type B.
- Increased destruction and sequestration of platelets from hypersplenism
- Transfusions result in dilution of platelets and clotting factors.
- **Immune-mediated thrombocytopenia:** Autoantibody production leads to platelet destruction (eg, SLE).

TREATMENT

Treat underlying cause and provide supportive therapy.

- **Idiopathic thrombocytopenic purpura:** Thrombocytopenia with normal or increased megakaryocytes. **Antiplatelet antibodies** attach to platelets (anti-GpIIb/IIIa antibodies) and lead to removal by splenic macrophages. No splenomegaly. Splenectomy is curative in two-thirds of patients.
  - **Children: Acute,** self-limited reaction to viral infection or immunization; treat only if severe.
  - **Adults: Chronic,** autoimmune condition; occurs more often in **females** (may cause short-lived thrombocytopenia in offspring, since antiplatelet IgG can cross

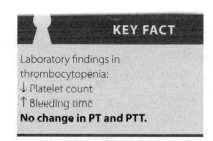

KEY FACT

Laboratory findings in thrombocytopenia:
↓ Platelet count
↑ Bleeding time
No change in PT and PTT.

TABLE 4-8.   **Tests of Bleeding Disorders**

TEST	DESCRIPTION
Bleeding time	Time (in minutes) taken for a standardized skin puncture to stop bleeding. Tests platelet function. Prolonged if platelet abnormality is present
Prothrombin time (PT)	Tests the adequacy of the extrinsic and common coagulation pathways. Prolonged when deficient in factors V, VII, or X, prothrombin, or fibrinogen
Partial thromboplastin time (PTT)	Tests the adequacy of the intrinsic pathway. Prolonged in heparin therapy
Mixing studies	In cases in which bleeding is prolonged, the patient's blood is mixed with blood that contains all the factors necessary for clotting. If the bleeding time corrects, the patient has a deficiency in one or more clotting factors. If the bleeding time does not correct, the patient has antibody to one or more clotting factors

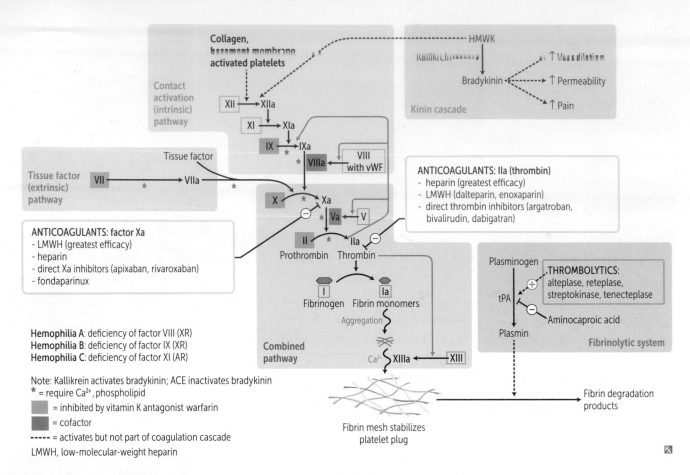

FIGURE 4-24. **Coagulation cascade.** HMWK, high-molecular-weight kininogen; tPA, tissue plasminogen activator; vWF, von Willebrand factor.

placenta). Initial treatment is corticosteroids, IVIG for symptomatic bleeding, and splenectomy in refractory cases.

■ **Thrombotic microangiopathies:** Result from **hyaline microthrombi** (platelet aggregates surrounded by fibrin) leading to **thrombocytopenia** and microangiopathic anemia (peripheral blood smear shows **schistocytes** and **helmet cells**).

   ■ **TTP:** Associated with a lack of metalloproteinase enzyme, (**ADAMTS13**) which normally degrades von Willebrand factor (vWF). The resulting multimeric form of vWF causes platelet aggregation with the pentad of microangiopathic hemolytic anemia, thrombocytopenia, renal failure, fever, and **neurologic deficits.** Usually in **adult** females.

   ■ **HUS:** Usually in **children** following *Escherichia coli* O157:H7 infection; Shiga toxin damage of endothelium results in the triad of microangiopathic hemolytic anemia, thrombocytopenia, and **renal failure.**

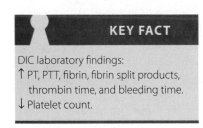

KEY FACT

DIC laboratory findings:
↑ PT, PTT, fibrin, fibrin split products, thrombin time, and bleeding time.
↓ Platelet count.

PRESENTATION

Characterized by bleeding from small vessels, which leads to **petechial, purpural, mucosal, and intracranial hemorrhage** (Figure 4-25). Platelet count below 100,000/mm³ is considered pathologic, though spontaneous bleeding does not typically occur until the platelet count falls below 20,000/mm³.

DIAGNOSIS

■ **Decreased platelet count** is the main diagnostic finding.
■ Prolonged bleeding time occasionally seen; is often normal and rarely used in diagnosis.
■ Bone marrow aspiration: Megakaryocytes decreased if decreased platelet production, increased if increased platelet destruction; usually not performed.

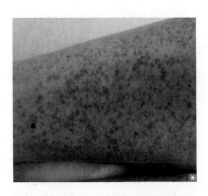

FIGURE 4-25. **Petechiae on lower extremity.**

PROGNOSIS

Varies with underlying cause.

Platelet Function Abnormalities

Qualitative platelet dysfunction that takes place in the setting of normal platelet counts. Caused by:

- Defects in platelet adhesion:
  - **von Willebrand disease:** Most common hereditary bleeding disorder; **autosomal dominant** deficiency of vWF, which normally carries and stablizes **factor VIII.** Patients usually present with mild mucosal and skin bleeding. However, deep tissue and joint bleeding that are characteristic in secondary hemostasis are not usually seen. Disease is characterized by normal platelet counts with:
    - Impaired adhesion → prolonged bleeding time.
    - Mild quantitative deficiency of factor VIII → prolonged activated partial thromboplastin time (aPTT).
  - **Bernard-Soulier disease:** Autosomal recessive disorder in which platelets are abnormally large and lack platelet-surface **glycoprotein Ib,** which is needed for platelet adhesion.
- Defects in platelet aggregation:
  - **Aspirin:** Acetylates and irreversibly inactivates cyclooxygenase (COX), an enzyme necessary for the production of **thromboxane A_2,** a platelet aggregant.
  - **Glanzmann thrombasthenia:** Hereditary deficiency of platelet-surface **glycoproteins IIb and IIIa,** which are required for forming fibrinogen bridges between platelets (platelet aggregation). Blood smear shows no platelet clumping and agglutination with ristocetin cofactor assay. Therefore, increased bleeding time.

PRESENTATION

Mucocutaneous bleeding.

DIAGNOSIS

↑ bleeding time in the setting of normal platelet count, PT, PTT (except vWF disease). Platelet aggregation studies, if a specific platelet disorder is suspected.

PROGNOSIS

Depends on underlying cause.

Clotting Factor Deficiencies

Lack of clotting factors leads to easy bruising and bleeding. Spontaneous bleeding into joints (hemarthrosis), muscle, and other tissues is common, as is postsurgical bleeding. These deficiencies are described below.

Hemophilia A

X-linked deficiency of factor **VIII;** also known as classic hemophilia. Prolonged PTT that corrects with mixing studies. Treatment is with infusion of factor VIII and demopressin to release additional factor VIII from endothelial stores.

Hemophilia B

X-linked deficiency of factor **IX;** also known as Christmas disease. Prolonged PTT that corrects with normal plasma mixing, but treatment with factor VIII produces no response. Treatment is with factor IX replacement.

Hemophilia C

Autosomal recessive disorder due to deficiency of factor XI. Laboratory tests show prolonged PTT that corrects with normal plasma mixing.

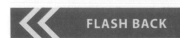

Vitamin K Deficiency

Leads to deficiency of **factors II, VII, IX, X,** and **proteins C and S.** In adults, caused by fat malabsorption due to pancreatic or small-bowel disease. In infants, caused by deficient exogenous vitamin K (not present in breast milk; therefore, prophylactic vitamin K is given to all newborns at birth to prevent hemorrhagic disease of newborn) and incomplete intestinal colonization by bacteria that synthesize vitamin K.

Coagulation Factor Inhibitor

Coagulation factor inhibitors are acquired autoantibodies against a coagulation factor resulting in impaired factor function (anti-factor VIII antibodies are most common). Clinical presentation is similar to hemophilia A; however, PTT **does not** correct with normal plasma mixing (due to the autoantibodies' binding).

Liver Disease

Hepatocellular damage prevents the production of **all coagulation factors except vWF** and **factor VIII,** and reduces activation of vitamin K by epoxide reductase, as they are exclusively formed in the liver. Liver disease may lead to **hypersplenism** and **overt thrombocytopenia.** As a result, PT, PTT, thrombin time, and bleeding time are prolonged.

PRESENTATION

Macrohemorrhage leads to **hemarthroses** (bleeding into joints), **easy bruising,** and large hematomas rather than petechiae.

DIAGNOSIS

Laboratory test results for PT, aPTT, and thrombin time.

TREATMENT

Vitamin K or fresh frozen plasma.

PROGNOSIS

Depends on severity and type of condition.

Disseminated Intravascular Coagulation

DIC: Activation of coagulation cascade leads to **microthrombi** and consumption of platelets and coagulation factors **(especially II, V, VIII, and fibrinogen);** characterized by both thrombosis (may result in tissue ischemia and infarction) and hemorrhage; results from the release of tissue thromboplastin or activation of the intrinsic pathway. Common causes include **obstetric** complications (preeclampsia, amniotic fluid emboli, retained fetus, or abruptio placentae), **gram-negative sepsis** (eg, *E coli, N meningitidis*), transfusion, trauma, **malignancy** (especially adenocarcinoma of the lung, pancreas, prostate, and stomach), acute pancreatitis, nephrotic syndrome, and **acute promyelocytic leukemia** (degranulation).

DIAGNOSIS

- Increased prothrombin time (PT), partial thromboplastin time (PTT), fibrin, D-dimers (fibrin split products), thrombin time and bleeding time.
- Decreased fibrinogen, platelet count.
- Bone marrow: Occasional helmet shaped cell and schistocytes (Table 4-3, Image J).

PROGNOSIS

Can lead to organ damage and shock; poor prognosis.

Vessel Wall Abnormalities

Disruption of the vessel wall leads to hemorrhage. Causes include:

- **Aging:** Atrophy of collagen leads to decreased vessel wall strength.
- **Scurvy:** Vitamin C deficiency results in collagen abnormality and decreased wall strength. Gingival hemorrhages and cutaneous petechiae (around hair follicles) are common, and bleeding into muscles and subcutaneous tissue may also be seen.
- **Ehlers-Danlos syndrome:** Inherited fibrillin defect results in elastin abnormality and decreased vessel wall strength, leading to skin hyperelasticity, joint hypermobility, and tissue fragility (increased risk of **aortic dissection** and **berry aneurysm**).
- **Cushing syndrome:** Protein wasting leads to loss of perivascular support.
- **Henoch-Schönlein purpura:** Hypersensitivity vasculitis (often associated with upper respiratory infection) results in immune complex deposition on vessel walls. Symptoms include palpable purpura, polyarthralgias, fever, painful focal GI hemorrhages, and acute glomerulonephritis.
- **Hereditary hemorrhagic telangiectasia (Osler-Weber-Rendu syndrome):** Autosomal dominant mutation leads to dilated, tortuous blood vessels with thin walls in skin and mucous membranes.
- **Waldenström macroglobulinemia:** Hyperviscous blood damages vessels.
- **Amyloidosis:** Deposition of amyloid in vessel walls.
- **Infections:** Meningococcemia, septicemia, infective endocarditis, rickettsiosis, and others lead to vasculitis and/or DIC.

PRESENTATION

Usually mild (petechiae, purpura in skin or mucous membranes); occasionally more severe (hemorrhages into joints and muscles, menorrhagia, epistaxis, GI bleeding, hematuria).

DIAGNOSIS

Platelet count, PT, and PTT are usually **normal.** Bleeding time is occasionally prolonged.

Note: Platelet function assay (PFA)-100 has replaced bleeding time tests in many institutions.

PROGNOSIS

Depends on specific cause.

WHITE CELL DISORDERS

Leukopenia

Decreased white blood cell count. Can reflect decreased number of granulocytes (eg, decreased number of neutrophils in **neutropenia**) and/or decreased number of lymphocytes **(lymphopenia).**

Neutropenia

Neutropenia (circulating neutrophils less than 1500) can result from:

- Decreased production:
  - Aplastic anemia
  - Certain adverse drug reactions
  - Inherited conditions
- Increased destruction:
  - Immunologic disorders (eg, SLE)
  - Certain adverse drug reactions (eg, chemotherapy can damage bone marrow stem cells)
  - Splenic sequestration
  - Reduction in numbers due to overwhelming infection (eg, gram-negative sepsis)

Lymphopenia

Lymphopenia (circulating lymphocytes < 1500 in adults, < 3000 in children) may result from:

- Immunodeficiency (eg, DiGeorge syndrome and HIV)
- Corticosteroids: Induce apoptosis of lymphocytes
- Cytotoxic drugs
- Viral infections
- Malnutrition
- Autoimmune destruction (eg, SLE)
- Whole-body radiation

PRESENTATION

- **Neutropenia:** Bacterial or fungal infections; malaise, chills, and fever; other signs of specific infections.
- **Lymphopenia:** Viral infections.

DIAGNOSIS

CBC with WBC count and differential.

PROGNOSIS

Depends on degree of reduction in number of cells and cause.

Reactive Proliferation

Leukocytosis

Circulating neutrophils are higher than 7000. Increased number of circulating WBCs, usually due to infection or inflammation.

- **Neutrophilic** → bacterial infection and tissue necrosis.
- **Eosinophilic** → allergies/asthma, parasitic infections, drugs, neoplasms (eg, Hodgkin lymphoma), collagen vascular diseases.

Lymphocytic Leukocytosis

Circulating lymphocytes are higher than 4000 in adults and 8000 in children. Increased number of WBCs in lymph nodes (Figure 4-26), usually due to infection or inflammation. For example: **infectious mononucleosis—EBV** and **CMV**, especially in young adults—infects B lymphocytes and leads to generalized lymphadenopathy. It is characterized by **atypical lymphocytes** (antigen-stimulated reactive CD8+ cells), anti-EBV

KEY FACT

Cortisol can sequester eosinophils in the lymph nodes, resulting in eosinopenia in hypercortisolism. This contrasts with eosinophilia in Addison disease (decreased cortisol).

KEY FACT

Corticosteroids induce a benign neutrophilic leukocytosis (due to impaired leukocyte adhesion, which results in release of marginal pool of neutrophils).

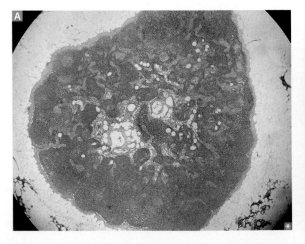

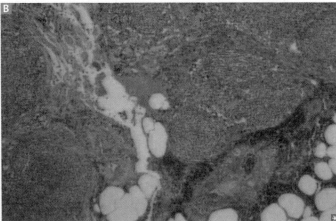

FIGURE 4-26. **Lymph nodes.** A Normal and B reactive.

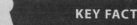

antibodies, and **heterophile antibodies.** It can be associated with sore throat, fever, and hepatosplenomegaly and is usually self-limited. Complications include risk of splenic rupture, recurrence, and B-cell lymphoma.

Neoplastic Proliferation

Neoplastic proliferation of WBCs can be classified into lymphomas and leukemias. Many are characterized by a specific chromosomal translocation (Table 4-9).

Lymphomas

Lymphomas are proliferations of lymphoid cells commonly found in the lymph node or extranodal tissues. These can be divided into **Hodgkin lymphomas** and **non-Hodgkin lymphomas (NHLs).**

Hodgkin Lymphoma

Malignant proliferation of WBCs featuring characteristic **Reed-Sternberg cells** (bi- or multinucleated giant cells with eosinophilic nucleoli or "owl eyes"; also CD30 and CD15 positive but lacking CD20) in addition to reactive lymphocytes (Figure 4-27). The majority of cases can be cured. There are four histologic variants: **nodular sclerosing, mixed cellularity, lymphocyte predominant,** and **lymphocyte depleted** (Figure 4-28 and Table 4-10).

PRESENTATION

Constitutional ("B") symptoms: Low-grade fever, night sweats, and weight loss often present. Typically presents with painless to progressive lymphadenopathy, usually involving the neck and anterior mediastinum. About half of cases are associated with **EBV infection.** Age distribution is bimodal (young and old). All types affect men more than women except for the nodular sclerosing type, which affects women more. Spread is contiguous.

DIAGNOSIS

Based on biopsy.

TREATMENT

Chemotherapy, radiotherapy.

COMPLICATIONS

Increased risk of **secondary malignancy** after radiation therapy (eg, secondary lung and breast cancer with radiation therapy to thyroid, mediastinal Hodgkin disease), whereas intensive chemotherapy may lead to secondary leukemia and infertility.

KEY FACT

Hodgkin lymphomas:
- Reed-Sternberg cells
- Single groups of axial nodes
- Contiguous spread
- Constitutional symptoms
- Bimodal (young and old)

Non-Hodgkin lymphomas:
- No Reed-Sternberg cells
- Multiple groups of peripheral nodes
- Noncontiguous spread
- Fewer constitutional symptoms
- Usually seen in those 20–40 years old
- Associated with HIV and autoimmune diseases

KEY FACT

Reed-Sternberg cells secrete cytokines, causing 1) constitutional symptoms and 2) recruitment of reactive lymphocytes, plasma cells, macrophages, and eosinophils that make up bulk of tumor mass; may lead to fibrosis.

TABLE 4-9.   Common Chromosomal Translocations

DISEASE	TRANSLOCATION
CML	t(9;22) Ph chromosome
Burkitt lymphoma	t(8;14) c-*myc*
Follicular lymphoma	t(14;18) *bcl*-2
AML M3 type	t(15;17) APL: RARA
Ewing sarcoma	t(11;22)
Mantle cell lymphoma	t(11;14)

AML, acute myelogenous leukemia; CML, chronic myelogenous leukemia.

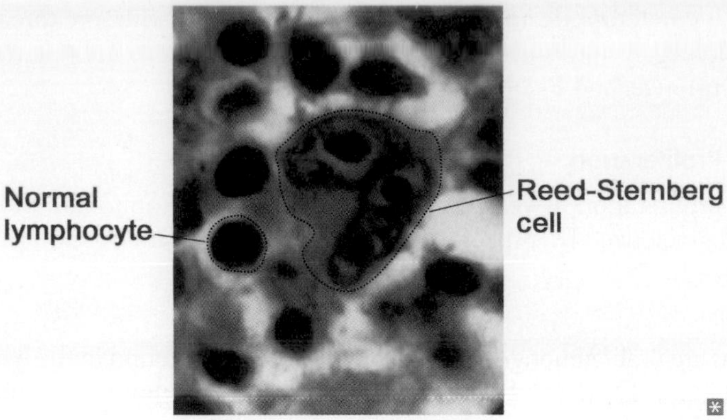

Normal lymphocyte

Reed-Sternberg cell

FIGURE 4-27. **Reed-Sternberg cells.** Photomicrograph shows normal lymphocytes compared with a Reed-Sternberg cell.

PROGNOSIS

Staging, the best predictor of prognosis, is based on the number of lymph node regions involved, involvement of extralymphatic sites, and extent of dissemination. Because of the high rate of cure with chemotherapy and radiotherapy, survivors often develop secondary cancers.

Non-Hodgkin Lymphoma

Malignant lymphoid proliferations of B cells (and occasionally T cells). Often these cases are associated with HIV and immunosuppression. Cells are often located in multiple groups of nodes, and **extranodal** involvement is common. Spread of malignant cells is **noncontiguous.** Can be classified by clinical behavior (low-, intermediate-, or high-grade), by nodular versus diffuse (follicular lymphoma is the only nodular type), by cytogenetic translocations, and by cytology of small versus large cells.

PRESENTATION

Lymphadenopathy in multiple groups of peripheral nodes. Constitutional symptoms occur less frequently than in Hodgkin lymphomas.

DIAGNOSIS

Based on clinical presentation and histologic findings on biopsy (see Table 4-11 for histologic classifications).

PROGNOSIS

Depends on type. Although average survival is better in low-grade lymphomas, they are rarely cured. Follicular lymphomas have better survival rates than diffuse forms. The prognosis for small-cell lymphomas is better than that for large-cell types.

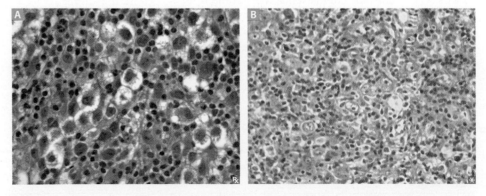

FIGURE 4-28. **Histologic types of Hodgkin lymphoma.** A Nodular sclerosing and B mixed cellularity.

TABLE 4-10. Histologic Types of Hodgkin Lymphoma and Their Characteristics

TYPE	PREVALENCE	NO. OF REED-STERNBERG CELLS	NO. OF LYMPHOCYTES	PROGNOSIS
Nodular sclerosing ▪ More common in women than men ▪ Cells are grouped into nodules surrounded by **fibrous bands** ▪ Usually located in cervical, supraclavicular, or mediastinal nodes ▪ **Lacunar cells** (Reed-Sternberg nucleus surrounded by empty space) ▪ Can be related to EBV infection	Most common (70%)	+	+++	Excellent
Mixed cellularity ▪ Typically seen in young men ▪ Also often related to EBV infection ▪ Complete effacement, multiple nodes ▪ Eosinophils, plasma cells, histiocytes, and Reed-Sternberg cells with regions of fibrosis	25%	++++	+++	Intermediate
Lymphocyte predominant ▪ Lymphocytes and histiocytes ▪ < 35-year-old men ▪ Popcorn cells (Reed-Sternberg cells)	6%	+	++++	Excellent
Lymphocyte depleted ▪ Few lymphocytes with large number of Reed-Sternberg cells and fibrosis ▪ Older men with disseminated disease, HIV patients	Rare	High relative to lymphocytes	+	Poor

EBV, Epstein-Barr virus.

Cutaneous T-Cell Lymphomas

Neoplastic mature T cells proliferate in the dermis and epidermis in **mycosis fungoides**. In a second, leukemic form of the disease known as **Sézary syndrome**, neoplastic cells circulate as well as concentrate in the skin, resulting in a physical presentation termed **leonine facies**.

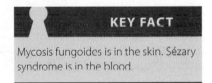

KEY FACT

Mycosis fungoides is in the skin. Sézary syndrome is in the blood.

PRESENTATION

Erythematous lesions develop on the skin in the inflammatory premycotic phase, progress along a typical path to the plaque phase, and finally enter the tumor phase (Figure 4-29).

DIAGNOSIS

Biopsy reveals CD4+ T cells with characteristic **cerebriform nuclei** proliferating in the dermis. Often there are focal concentrations of neoplastic cells in the epidermis known as **Pautrier microabscesses**.

PROGNOSIS

Indolent, median survival of 8–9 years; can progress to diffuse large-cell lymphoma.

Extranodal Marginal Zone Lymphoma (MALT Lymphoma)

Low-grade B-cell tumors arising most commonly in **Mucosal-Associated Lymphatic Tissue (MALT)** (salivary glands, small and large bowel, and lungs). May occur in the setting of *Helicobacter pylori* infection; in this case, treatment with antibiotics and eradication of the organism leads to tumor regression. MALT lymphoma is associated with other chronic inflammatory conditions, such as Hashimoto thyroiditis and Sjögren syndrome. Patients usually present with delayed lymphoma in the post–germinal center B cells.

TABLE 4-11. **Histologic Types of Non-Hodgkin Lymphoma and Their Characteristics**

TYPE	EXAMPLE	EPIDEMIOLOGY	CELL TYPE	GRADE	GENETICS	HISTOLOGY
Small lymphocytic lymphoma A ■ Appears as a focal mass of **chronic lymphocytic leukemia** ■ **Richter syndrome** or **prolymphocytic transformation** into diffuse B-cell lymphoma occurs in a quarter of cases		Adults	B	Low		Small, mature-looking lymphocytes; lymph nodes are effaced
Follicular lymphoma B ■ Common adult form; indolent and difficult to cure ■ Presents with painless "waxing and waning" lymphadenopathy ■ Treatment is low-dose chemotherapy or rituximab		Adults	B	Low	**t(14;18),** translocation of *BCL-2* to Ig heavy-chain locus on chromosome 14 leads to *BCL-2* overexpression and prevents apoptosis	Angulated grooved cells typical of those in normal lymphoid follicular center; **arranged in nodules** Complications include progression to diffuse large B-cell lymphoma
Diffuse large cell C ■ **Most common** type of non-Hodgkin lymphoma in adults ■ Often presents with extranodal mass ■ Aggressive, but about half are curable		Adults: 80%; children: 20%	B: 80%; mature T: 20%	Intermediate	Associated with *BCL-6*	Large B-cells (CD20+) that grow diffusely in sheets
Mantle cell lymphoma D ■ Poor prognosis ■ Frequent involvement of the GI tract causing lymphomatoid polyposis		Adults	B		t(11:14)—Translocation of cyclin D1 (11) and heavy-chain Ig (14) leads to overexpression of cyclin D1, which promotes G1/S transition in the cell cycle and facilitates neoplastic proliferation	Resemble cells in the **mantle zone** of lymph nodes

TABLE 4-11.   **Histologic Types of Non-Hodgkin Lymphoma and Their Characteristics** *(continued)*

TYPE	EXAMPLE	EPIDEMIOLOGY	CELL TYPE	GRADE	GENETICS	HISTOLOGY
Lymphoblastic lymphoma E ■ **Most common childhood** form ■ Very aggressive; 80% cured, but high relapse rate ■ Often presents with **acute lymphocytic leukemia** and **mediastinal mass**		Children and adults	Immature T	High		**Cell nuclei appear convoluted; arise from thymic lymphocytes**
Burkitt lymphoma F ■ Associated with **EBV, HIV** ■ **Very rapidly growing mass** ■ Jaw involvement common in endemic African form G ■ Pelvic/abdominal involvement often occurs in sporadic form		Children and adults	B	High	t(8;14). Translocation of *c-myc* (8) and heavy chain (14) leads to overexpression of *c-myc* oncogene, which drives excessive cell growth	**Starry-sky** appearance (sheets of lymphocytes with interspersed nonneoplastic macrophages) High mitotic index

EBV, Epstein-Barr virus.

Leukemias

Leukemias involve the malignant spread of granulocytic or lymphocytic precursors in the bone marrow and the circulation. Cells also frequently infiltrate liver, spleen, and lymph nodes. They can be separated into acute and chronic leukemias. **Acute** forms involve blasts (immature cells), affect children or the elderly, and have a short and drastic course. **Chronic** forms usually involve the proliferation of more mature cells, affect people in mid-life, and have a longer and less devastating course. Leukemias can also be classified by whether they involve **lymphocytic** or **myelogenous** cell types. Often, marrow failure can cause anemia, infections, and hemorrhage by reducing the numbers of RBCs, WBCs, and platelets.

Acute Lymphoblastic Leukemia

Neoplasm of lymphoblasts (immature B or T cells).

PRESENTATION

Pre-B-cell leukemias usually affect children. Pre-T-cell leukemias often occur with lymphoblastic leukemia; typical clinical picture is an adolescent male with a mediastinal mass that may spread to trachea (causing dyspnea or stridor), esophagus (causing dysphagia), or superior vena cava (SVC) syndrome. **Onset is sudden,** and patients usually present within days or weeks of symptom onset. **Marrow failure** usually results in fatigue, infection, and bleeding due to anemia, neutropenia, and thrombocytopenia. Bone pain, **lymphadenopathy, splenomegaly, hepatomegaly,** meningeal spread, and testicular spread are also common. Relapses often occur in the **CNS** and **testis.**

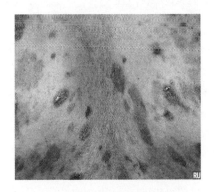

FIGURE 4-29.   **Skin lesions in Sezary syndrome.**

KEY FACT

Leukemia = proliferation in the bone marrow and bloodstream; divided into acute versus chronic and myelogenous versus lymphocytic. Common leukemias in each age group:
■ < 15 yrs: ALL
■ 15–39 yrs: acute myelogenous leukemia (AML)
■ > 40–60 yrs: AML, chronic myelogenous leukemia (CML)
■ 60+: CLL

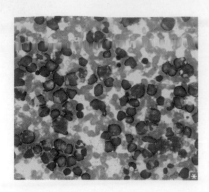

FIGURE 4-30. **Acute lymphoblastic leukemia.**

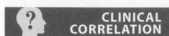

CLINICAL CORRELATION

Tumor lysis syndrome:
- Due to rapid cell turnover or lysis from chemotherapy
- Results in hyperuricacidemia, hyperphosphatemia, hyperkalemia
- Often associated with ALL

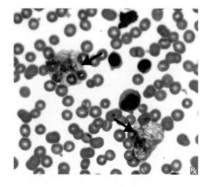

FIGURE 4-31. **Chronic lymphocytic leukemia (arrows).**

MNEMONIC

Acute promyelocytic leukemia—

A pro's engine **RARs (roars)** at 1715 **myels (miles)** per **Auer (hour).**

DIAGNOSIS

Based on flow cytometry, peripheral smear and bone marrow biopsy. Monomorphic cells with condensed chromatin, **minimal cytoplasm,** and no granules (Figure 4-30). Surface markers (TdT⁺ [marker of pre-T and pre-B cells], CD10⁺ [marker of pre-B cells only]) are also assessed to differentiate from acute myeloid leukemia.

TREATMENT

Chemotherapy.

PROGNOSIS

Almost all pediatric patients go into remission after chemotherapy, and in children about **two-thirds are cured.** This leukemia in pediatric patients is the most responsive to therapy. Prognosis is worst for those younger than age 2, those who present in adolescence or later, and those with the Philadelphia translocation, t(9;22). The WBC and platelet counts on admission are also important diagnostic indicators.

Chronic Lymphocytic Leukemia

Neoplastic proliferation of lymphoid cells, usually **CD5+ B cells.** This disease is the same as **small lymphocytic lymphoma (SLL)** except that the majority of the neoplastic cells in CLL are in the circulation and marrow as opposed to nodal or extranodal masses. Cells do not differentiate into antibody-secreting plasma cells.

PRESENTATION

Males are affected twice as often as females, and the average age of presentation is **60 years.** Patients are often asymptomatic or have nonspecific symptoms of weight loss and fatigue. Lymphadenopathy and hepatosplenomegaly are common. Bacterial infections are common as a result of **hypogammaglobulinemia.** Autoantibodies that develop in reaction to the tumor cells can lead to **warm antibody autoimmune hemolytic anemia** or thrombocytopenia. **Prolymphocytic transformation** into diffuse B-cell lymphoma occurs in one-quarter of cases (Richter transformation).

DIAGNOSIS

Small, round lymphocytes are visible in peripheral smears and bone marrow biopsies. **Smudge cells,** the result of the fragility of the neoplastic cells, are frequently seen (Figure 4-31). Some patients may have a monoclonal Ig "spike."

PROGNOSIS

Survival is typically 4–6 years. If prolymphocytic transformation occurs, survival is less than 1 year.

Acute Myelogenous Leukemia

Acquired genetic mutations in stem cells lead to proliferation of undifferentiated myeloid blasts. Also known as acute granulocytic leukemia. Classified as arising from myelodysplasia versus de novo.

One specific type of acute myelogenous leukemia (AML) is **acute promyelocytic leukemia (APL),** which results from a translocation of the retinoic acid receptor-α (*RAR*-α) gene from chromosome 17 to the promyelocytic leukemia (*PML*) gene on chromosome 15 [t(15;17)(q22;q12)]. The result is an abnormal receptor that prevents cell differentiation and maturation.

PRESENTATION

AML may occur at any age but is most common in older adults (median age at diagnosis is approximately 65 years). Cases arising from myelodysplasia usually affect people in the sixth decade or beyond. Patients have symptoms of fatigue, infection, and bleeding because of anemia, neutropenia, and thrombocytopenia; cutaneous lesions are common, including leukemia cutis, gingival hypertrophy, and chloromas. Risk factors for AML include prior exposure to alkylating agents or topoisomerase inhibitors, radiation, and myeloproliferative disorders.

DIAGNOSIS

Based on peripheral smear and bone marrow biopsy. Biopsy reveals > 20% myeloid blasts in marrow. On smear, myeloblasts have delicate chromatin, peroxidase-positive granules, and **abundant cytoplasm** compared with lymphoblasts (Figure 4-32).

Cells often contain **Auer rods** (peroxidase-positive cytoplasmic inclusions) in the cytoplasm, especially in APL. The lack of surface markers TdT and CD10 can be assessed to differentiate from ALL.

TREATMENT

Chemotherapy (7+3+3 – cytarabine, daunorubicin, etoposide); high-dose **all-trans-retinoic acid** can overcome the blockade caused by the abnormal protein in APL with a t(15;17) translocation.

PROGNOSIS

Chemotherapy is successful in producing complete remission in approximately 60% of patients, however, more than half of these people have recurrence of disease within 5 years. Specific genetic alteration influences prognosis. Also of note, treatment of APL may release large numbers of **Auer rods,** which can result in **DIC.**

Chronic Myelogenous Leukemia

Proliferation of pluripotent cells producing myeloid cells that are capable of terminal differentiation; also known as **chronic myelocytic** or **chronic granulocytic leukemia.** Note that this is both a leukemia and a myeloproliferative disorder. Production of normal cells is prevented because of overcrowding. Can be associated with the **Philadelphia (Ph) chromosome,** in which the **c-abl** gene is moved from **chromosome 9 to 22,** next to the *bcr* gene. The result is a fusion protein, *BCR-ABL,* with tyrosine kinase activity that leads to uncontrolled proliferation.

PRESENTATION

Insidious onset with nonspecific symptoms such as mild anemia and weight loss, typically in middle-aged patients. **Splenomegaly** is common. An **accelerated phase** with increasing anemia and thrombocytopenia often occurs after approximately 3 years. Whether or not there is an accelerated phase, all untreated patients eventually enter a **blast crisis with > 20% blasts on peripheral smear,** a condition similar to acute leukemia (two-thirds of patients progress to AML; one-third of patients progress to ALL). Risk factors include ionizing radiation and benzene.

DIAGNOSIS

Chromosomal analysis, or polymerase chain reaction (PCR), can be used to definitely detect the *BCR-ABL* fusion gene. Initial bone marrow biopsy and peripheral smear also show leukocytosis with mixed neutrophils, metamyelocytes, myelocytes (Figure 4-33), and absolute basophilia. The marrow is entirely filled with cells, especially mature granulocytic precursors. Can be differentiated from leukemoid reactions because **leukocyte alkaline phosphatase is not as elevated in CML.**

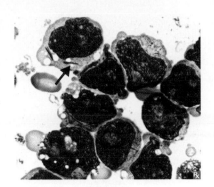

FIGURE 4-32. Acute myelogenous leukemia. Auer rods (arrow).

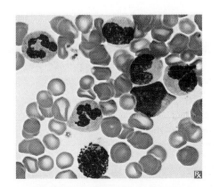

FIGURE 4-33. Chronic myelogenous leukemia.

TREATMENT

- **Gleevec (imatinib mesylate,** a small molecule inhibitor of the *BCR-ABL* tyrosine kinase): Induces apoptosis of leukemic cells; has almost completely replaced other therapies.
- **Allogenic bone marrow transplantation:** Cures up to 75% of cases; most effective in the stable phase.

PROGNOSIS

With or without treatment, initial progression is slow until accelerated phase and blast crisis.

Hairy Cell Leukemia

Uncommon leukemia distinguished by the presence of leukemic cells that have fine, hair-like cytoplasmic projections (Figure 4-34). Cells are CD103+ and tartrate-resistant acid phosphatase positive (TRAP+). The hairy cells can usually be seen in the peripheral blood smear. Pathology shows "dry tap" on bone marrow aspiration (hairy cell leukemia can lead to marrow fibrosis). Treatment is cladribine and adenosine deaminase inhibitor.

Adult T-Cell Leukemia/Lymphoma

T-cell neoplasm caused by infection with a retrovirus (human T-cell leukemia virus type 1 [**HTLV-1**]). Characterized by skin lesions, generalized lymphadenopathy, hepatosplenomegaly, hypercalcemia, and an elevated leukocyte count with multilobed CD4 lymphocytes. May cause progressive demyelinating disease of the CNS.

Plasma Cell Disorders

Include **multiple myeloma, Waldenström macroglobulinemia,** and **monoclonal gammopathy** of undetermined significance. These disorders are caused by clonal neoplastic transformation of Ig-secreting, terminally differentiated B cells. Monoclonal Ig is referred to as the **M component.** The balance between light-chain and heavy-chain production is lost, and excess free light chains (Bence Jones proteins) are excreted in the urine.

Multiple Myeloma

Neoplastic proliferation of small lymphoid cells leads to clonal expansion of plasma cells. The proliferation and survival of myeloma cells depends on multiple factors, most notably upon interleukin 6 (IL-6).

PRESENTATION

Usually presents in patients **50–60 years old.** Characteristics include:

- **Punched-out bone lesions**—due to osteoclast activating factor or IL-1 stimulation on the RANK receptor from osteoclasts, resulting in bone destruction—especially in the vertebrae and skull. Fractures of the vertebral column and bone pain are common (Figure 4-35).
- **Hypercalcemia** from bone destruction (plasma cells activate osteolytic factors).
- **Myeloma kidney,** or renal insufficiency with azotemia, because of excretion of Bence Jones proteins; tubular casts of Bence Jones protein (IgG light chains), giant cells, and metastatic calcification may be evident.
- **Marrow failure** leading to anemia and, rarely, leukopenia and thrombocytopenia.
- **Infections,** especially with *Streptococcus pneumoniae, Staphylococcus aureus,* and *Escherichia coli,* as a result of clonal Ig, leading to decreased production of normal Ig.
- **Amyloidosis** from IgG light chain.
- **Hyperviscosity syndrome** in a minority of cases.

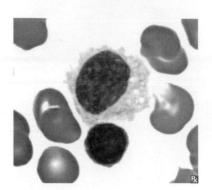

FIGURE 4-34. Hairy cell leukemia.

KEY FACT

Tartrate-resistant acid phosphatase (TRAP) is a marker for hairy B-cell leukemia.

MNEMONIC

Clinical manifestations of multiple myeloma—

CRAB

Hyper**C**alcemia
Renal involvement
Anemia
Bone lytic lesions/Back pain

Multiple **M**yeloma: **M**onoclonal
M protein spike

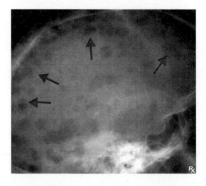

FIGURE 4-35. Punched-out lesion in multiple myeloma (arrows).

DIAGNOSIS

Hyperglobulinemia may lead to **rouleaux formation** of red cells (an aggregate of erythrocytes stacked like a pile of coins of coins [Figure 4-36]). Electrophoresis usually reveals increased Ig in blood and/or Bence Jones proteins in the urine. **IgG** is the M component in about half of cases; IgA in about one-quarter. Radiography usually reveals **punched-out round skeletal lesions,** but sometimes findings are more consistent with generalized osteoporosis. Cells have a characteristic **"fried-egg"** appearance (plasma cells with "clock-face" chromatin and intracytoplasmic inclusions containing immunoglobulin [Figure 4-37]).

PROGNOSIS

Survival varies, with an average of **3–5 years.** Some forms are indolent, but others have a survival of 6–12 months. Death usually occurs from infection or renal insufficiency. Chemotherapy leads to remission in about half of patients. **Bisphosphonates** can inhibit bone resorption. Bone marrow transplantation can improve survival but is not curative.

Waldenström Macroglobulinemia

Neoplasm of **plasmacytoid lymphocytes** (cells between B lymphocytes and plasma cells in terms of maturity) with monoclonal **IgM** secretion.

PRESENTATION

Typically affects **older individuals.** Nonspecific symptoms of fatigue and weight loss are common, as are lymphadenopathy, hepatomegaly, and splenomegaly. Anemia occurs as a result of marrow failure and is sometimes due to IgM **cold antibody autoimmune hemolysis. Hyperviscosity syndrome** often develops and presents with visual impairment such as retinal vascular dilation, neurologic issues, bleeding, and Raynaud phenomenon

DIAGNOSIS

Electrophoresis of serum reveals a clonal IgM spike, and 10% of cases show Bence Jones proteinuria; no bone lesions.

PROGNOSIS

Incurable and progressive with a median survival of 4 years. Plasmapheresis can treat hyperviscosity and hemolysis. Rarely transforms to large-cell lymphoma.

Monoclonal Gammopathy of Uncertain Significance

Some healthy, older adults may have benign M proteins with no symptoms or disease. Some, however, may go on to develop multiple myeloma or other plasma cell dyscrasias after 10–15 years. Amyloidosis can also develop.

Langerhans Cell Histiocytosis

Histiocytosis refers to the proliferation of histiocytes or macrophages. In Langerhans cell histiocytosis there is a clonal proliferation of **dendritic cells** known as Langerhans cells.

PRESENTATION

Various forms of this disease include the following:

- **Letterer-Siwe disease:** Acute disseminated histiocytosis; usually before age 2 years; characterized by cutaneous lesions on trunk and scalp; marrow failure, hepatosplenomegaly, and osteolytic lesions.
- **Hand-Schüller-Christian disease:** Triad of calvarial lesions, diabetes insipidus, and exophthalmos.
- **Multifocal Langerhans cell histiocytosis:** Affects children; patients develop fever, eruptions on the scalp and in the ear canals, recurrent infections, hepatosplenomegaly, and diabetes insipidus from posterior pituitary involvement.

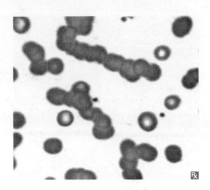

FIGURE 4-36. Rouleaux formation.

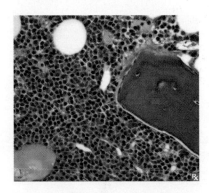

FIGURE 4-37. Multiple myeloma. Bone marrow replaced by sheets of plasma cells with eccentric nuclei and a clockface chromatin pattern.

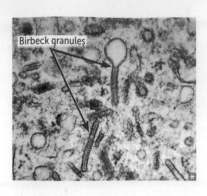

FIGURE 4-38. **Birbeck granules (arrows).**

- **Eosinophilic granuloma:** Unifocal or multifocal expansion of Langerhans cells, usually in marrow space and occasionally in lung, often asymptomatic and benign, but may present with fracture in adolescence (without skin involvement). Biopsy shows Langerhans cell with increased eosinophils and mixed inflammatory cells.

DIAGNOSIS

Electron microscopy reveals **Birbeck granules** (CD1a and S-100 positive) in the cytoplasm, which appear like **tennis rackets** (Figure 4-38).

PROGNOSIS

Depends on type. The acute disseminated presentation is rapidly fatal if untreated; with chemotherapy, half survive for about 5 years. Unifocal lesions can be excised or irradiated and occasionally heal without treatment. Multifocal histiocytosis can be treated with chemotherapy, although this may also heal without treatment. It has a better prognosis than the acute disseminated form.

MYELOPROLIFERATIVE SYNDROMES

Neoplastic proliferation of myeloid stem cells. Includes CML, polycythemia vera (PCV), and essential thrombocythemia (Table 4-12).

Polycythemia Vera

Neoplasm of multipotent myeloid stem cells leading to excessive production of **erythrocytes, granulocytes,** and **megakaryocytes.**

PRESENTATION

Insidious onset at median age of 60. Erythrocytosis causes stagnation of blood flow and cyanosis. Increased risk of **bleeding and thrombosis** leads to deep venous thrombosis, myocardial infarction, ischemic and hemorrhagic stroke, Budd-Chiari syndrome, splenic infarction, and mesenteric infarction. Headache, pruritus (itching after hot shower due to increased basophils), peptic ulceration, and hyperuricemia are common. The **spent phase** of the bone marrow has prominent fibrosis, resulting in extramedullary hematopoiesis. The clinical picture of myelofibrosis with myeloid metaplasia develops. **Splenomegaly** may occur from congestion early on or as a result of extramedullary hematopoiesis.

DIAGNOSIS

Increased hematocrit, decreased EPO (due to *JAK2* V617F mutation) (Table 4-13). Bone marrow is hypercellular until the spent phase, when fibrosis is prominent. To differentiate from CML, leukocyte alkaline phosphatase levels are **elevated,** and polymerase chain reaction (PCR) does not reveal the *BCR-ABL* gene.

TREATMENT

Involves frequent **phlebotomy** to maintain normal red cell mass; lengthens survival by approximately 10 years.

KEY FACT

Polycythemia/erythrocythemia can be:
- Relative: Due to decreased plasma volume (volume contraction) caused by **H_2O deprivation** (eg, prolonged vomiting, diarrhea, or diuretics).
- Absolute: Increased total RBC mass due to polycythemia vera (PCV), increased sensitivity of erythropoietin (EPO) receptor, increased levels of EPO, physiologic changes (lung disease, high altitude, cyanotic heart disease), or EPO secreting tumors.

TABLE 4-12. Laboratory Values for Myeloproliferative Syndromes

SYNDROME	RBCS	PLATELETS	GENE
Polycythemia vera	↑	↑	*JAK2* mutation (eg, V617F)
Essential thrombocytosis	Normal	↑	30–50% have *JAK2* mutation (eg, V617F)
Myelofibrosis	↓	Variable	30–50% have *JAK2* mutation (eg, V617F)

TABLE 4-13. Laboratory Values for Polycythemia/Erythrocythemia, Hypoxia, and Renal Cell Carcinoma

	PLASMA VOLUME	RBC MASS	SAO₂	ERYTHROPOIETIN (EPO) LEVELS
Relative polycythemia/erythrocythemia	↓	—	—	—
Absolute polycythemia/erythrocythemia	↑	↑	—	↓
Hypoxia (eg, high altitude or lung disease)	—	↑	↓	↑
Renal cell carcinoma (with ectopic EPO secretion)	—	↑	—	↑

SAO₂, arterial O₂ saturation.

PROGNOSIS

Without treatment, death occurs within months.

Myelofibrosis with Myeloid Metaplasia

Neoplastic changes in multipotent stem cells lead to proliferation of cells, including megakaryocytes (Figure 4-39). The **megakaryocytes** release platelet-derived growth factor (PDGF) and transforming growth factor-β (TGF-β), which encourage growth of non-neoplastic fibroblasts. The fibroblasts produce significant amounts of collagen, and the result is **prominent fibrosis** occurring early in the course of the disease. Similar to the spent phase of polycythemia vera (PCV)

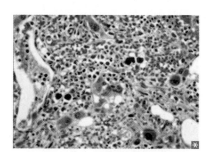

FIGURE 4-39   **Myeloid dysplasia.**
Dysplastic megakaryocytes with mononuclear and hypolobulated forms.

PRESENTATION

Usually affects individuals **60+ years of age,** who present with anemia, bleeding, thrombosis and recurrent infections (due to defective hematopoiesis); other nonspecific symptoms, hyperuricemia (due to high cell turnover), and hepatosplenomegaly (marrow fibrosis necessitates extramedullary hematopoiesis) are also common.

DIAGNOSIS

Marrow is initially hypercellular but progressively becomes hypocellular and fibrotic (Figure 4-40). Eventually, the marrow is converted to bone by osteosclerosis. Peripheral smear shows **leukoerythroblastosis,** increased numbers of nucleated erythroid progenitors and early granulocytes, as fibrosis leads to the abnormal release of these cells. **Teardrop erythrocytes,** or **dacrocytes,** are common as well (Figure 4-41). Lab tests reveal normochromic normocytic anemia and thrombocytopenia as the disease advances.

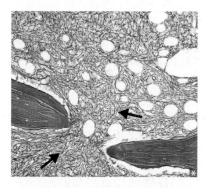

FIGURE 4-40.   **Bone marrow fibrosis in myelofibrosis (arrows).**

TREATMENT

JAK2 kinase inhibitors.

PROGNOSIS

Survival ranges from 1 to 15 years.

Essential Thrombocythemia

Neoplastic proliferation of myeloid stem cells, which leads to production of megakaryocytes.

PRESENTATION

Indolent course, usually asymptomatic except for episodes of prominent thrombosis and hemorrhage.

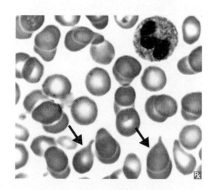

FIGURE 4-41.   **Teardrop cells (arrows) in myelofibrosis.**

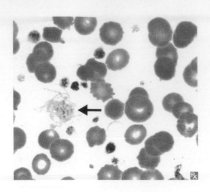

FIGURE 4-42. **Megakaryocyte (arrow) in essential thrombocytosis.**

DIAGNOSIS

JAK2 mutations. Marrow is moderately hypercellular, and large numbers of normal and **abnormally large megakaryocytes** are seen (Figure 4-42). No fibrosis develops. Peripheral smear shows extremely large platelets.

TREATMENT

Aspirin and hydroxyurea for high-risk patients (older individuals, history of thrombosis).

PROGNOSIS

Survival is variable (5–30 years).

SOLID TUMORS

Tumor Nomenclature

- **Hyperplasia** (reversible): Increase in number of cells. Distinct from hypertrophy (increase in cell size).
- **Metaplasia** (reversible): One adult cell type is replaced by another. Often secondary to irritation (eg, Barrett esophagus) and/or environmental exposure (eg, smoking-induced tracheal/bronchial squamous metaplasia). Also occurs where two different epithelial tissues meet (eg, squamocolumnar junction of the uterine cervix).
- **Dysplasia** (reversible): Abnormal growth with loss of cellular orientation, shape, and size in comparison to normal tissue maturation. Dysplasia commonly is neoplastic.
- **Anaplasia** (irreversible): Loss of structural differentiation and function of cells, resembling primitive cells of the same tissue. Often equated with undifferentiated malignant neoplasms. May see "giant cells" with a single large nucleus or several nuclei.
- **Neoplasia** (irreversible): An uncontrolled and excessive clonal proliferation of cells. Neoplasia may be benign or malignant.
- **Desmoplasia** (irreversible): Fibrous tissue formation in response to a neoplasm (eg, linitis plastica in diffuse stomach cancer).

Tumors are often classified by their tissue of origin and their ability to spread beyond the primary site (metastasis) (Table 4-14).

Benign

Tumor shows microscopic and gross evidence that it will remain localized and not metastasize. It is amenable to surgical resection.

- **Fibroma:** A benign tumor of fibrous or connective tissue.
- **Chondroma:** A benign tumor of cartilaginous cells.
- **Adenoma:** A benign tumor of glandular cells.

TABLE 4-14. **Benign and Malignant Tumor Nomenclature from Different Tissue Origins**

TISSUE ORIGIN	BENIGN	MALIGNANT
Epithelium (*adeno* or *papil*)		
eg, Lung	Lung *adeno*ma	Lung *adenocarcinoma*
eg, Breast	Breast *papill*oma	Breast *papillary carcinoma*
Mesenchyme		
Blood vessels (*angio*)	Hem*angio*ma	*Angio*sarcoma
Smooth muscle (*leiomyo*)	*Leiomyo*ma	*Leiomyo*sarcoma
Striated muscle (*rhabdomyo*)	*Rhabdomyo*ma	*Rhabdomyo*sarcoma
Connective tissue (*fibro*)	*Fibro*ma	*Fibro*sarcoma
Bone (*osteo*)	*Osteo*ma	*Osteo*sarcoma
Fat (*lipo*)	*Lipo*ma	*Lipo*sarcoma

- **Papilloma:** A benign tumor of epithelial tissue that typically has a stalk or pedicle.
- **Polyp:** Similar to a papilloma, any growth, benign or malignant, that has a stalk or pedicle.
- **Cystadenoma:** A tumor of epithelial glandular origin but with production of a substrate, producing cysts within the neoplasm.
- **Hamartoma:** Mass of disorganized tissue elements, not necessarily a neoplasm.

Malignant

Cells that tend to adhere, infiltrate, and destroy surrounding tissue, with characteristics of clonality and abnormal proliferation. Prone to metastasize to distant sites.

- **Sarcoma:** Malignant tumor arising from mesenchymal tissue.
- **Carcinoma:** Malignant tumor of epithelial origin.
- **Teratoma:** Tumor that contains more than one germ cell layer and typically contains immature and mature elements.
- **Leukemias and lymphomas:** See previous section.

Tumor Grading Versus Staging

Grading and staging of tumors guides medical and surgical therapy and provides information on prognosis.

Grading

Tumors can be graded 1–4 in levels of increasing severity and **differentiation** based on their microscopic appearance. However, note some grading systems range from 1 to 3. Well-differentiated tumors are grade 1 and tend to be less aggressive. Grade 4 tumors tend to be poorly differentiated and highly aggressive.

Staging

The extent to which a primary tumor has **spread,** which helps determine treatment and **prognosis.** Typically described in the **TNM** staging system, which refers to (**T**) Tumor: the extent of tumor growth; (**N**) Nodes: which and how many lymph nodes are involved; and (**M**) Metastasis: has the tumor metastasized.

Oncogenes

Genes derived from mutations in "proto-oncogenes" to "oncogenes," which promote cell growth in cancer cells. Oncogenes classically contribute to persistent expression of cellular growth factors (eg, cyclin-dependent kinases).

- **MYC gene:** Oncogene most commonly found in human tumors.
- **Others:** *MYB, JUN, FOS,* and *REL* oncogenes.

Tumor Suppressor Genes

Genes that suppress continued cell growth. Inhibition of these genes makes cells refractory to inhibition of growth. Typically requires "two hits" on both chromosomes to be oncogenic, with exceptions in haploinsufficiency genes (eg, *BRCA1, NF1*).

- **Retinoblastoma (RB):** First tumor suppressor gene to be discovered. Retinoblastoma is a neoplasm of the retina that typically occurs in young children with an abnormal *Rb* gene located on chromosome 13. Findings include leukocoria and loss of red light reflex in infants.
- **Others:** *APC* gene, TGF-β, and *TP53.*
- **Two-hit hypothesis:** In order for a tumor suppressor gene to be rendered inactive both normal alleles must be inactive.

Oncogenic Viruses

Viral infection of cells can lead to unchecked proliferation and tumor development (Table 4-15).

TABLE 4-15.   Oncogenic Viruses

TUMOR VIRUS	VIRUS TYPE AND ASSOCIATED TUMOR
Human T-cell leukemic virus type 1	RNA oncogenic virus. Associated with T-cell leukemia and lymphoma
Epstein-Barr virus	DNA oncogenic virus. Associated with Burkitt lymphoma, AIDS-related lymphomas, Hodgkin lymphoma, nasopharyngeal carcinoma
Human papillomavirus	DNA oncogenic virus. Associated with cervical carcinoma
Human herpesvirus-8	DNA oncogenic virus. Associated with Kaposi sarcoma
Hepatitis B virus	DNA oncogenic virus. Associated with hepatocellular carcinoma

Paraneoplastic Syndromes

Complex of symptoms that cannot be explained by the spread of tumor cells. Occur in 10–15% of cancer patients. Certain cancers cause specific paraneoplastic syndromes (Table 4-16).

Pharmacology

CHEMOTHERAPY DRUGS: ALKYLATING AGENTS

These drugs are cell cycle nonspecific (Figure 4-43). They act by interfering with nucleic acid function in various ways. All are contraindicated in pregnancy and cause myelosuppression and nausea. Antiemetic medications are frequently used in conjunction with chemotherapy. Please refer to Pharmacology section in Chapter 3 (Gastrointestinal).

Cyclophosphamide and Ifosfamide

MECHANISM

Nitrogen mustard alkylating agents that covalently cross-link DNA at guanine N-7. They require activation by the CYP-450 enzyme system in the liver. Cyclophosphamide is also a potent immunosuppressive agent.

USES

Solid tumors and hematologic malignancies.

TABLE 4-16.   Paraneoplastic Syndromes

SYNDROME	ASSOCIATED CANCER
Cushing syndrome	Small-cell cancer of the lung, pancreatic carcinoma
SIADH	Small-cell cancer of the lung, intracranial neoplasm
Hypercalcemia	Squamous cell cancer of the lung, breast cancer, renal cell carcinoma
Myasthenia gravis	Thymoma
Hypertrophic osteoarthropathy	Lung cancer
Migratory venous thrombosis (Trousseau syndrome)	Pancreatic carcinoma
Cancer cachexia	Progressive loss of lean body mass and body fat, weakness, anorexia, and anemia

SIADH, syndrome of inappropriate secretion of antidiuretic hormone.

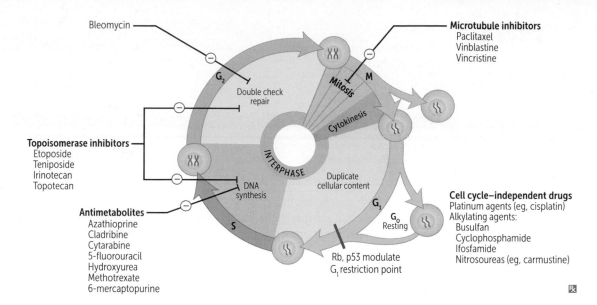

FIGURE 4-43. **Classes of chemotherapy drugs.**

SIDE EFFECTS

Hemorrhagic cystitis caused by urotoxic metabolite acrolein (seen mainly with ifosfamide). Prevented by hydration and **coadministration of mesna.**

Nitrosoureas (Carmustine, Lomustine, Streptozocin)

MECHANISM

Interfere with DNA and RNA synthesis by alkylation and protein modification. These agents require bioactivation. They are **lipid-soluble** and are able to cross the **blood-brain barrier.**

USES

Used in a variety of malignancies, including **CNS tumors** (due to its lipophilic properties), hematologic malignancies, adenocarcinomas and hepatomas, and breast and ovarian cancers.

SIDE EFFECTS

CNS toxicity (dizziness and ataxia), myelosuppression and dose-related nephrotoxicity, hepatotoxicity, and pulmonary toxicity (infiltrates or fibrosis).

Cisplatin, Carboplatin, Oxaliplatin

MECHANISM

Cross-link DNA strands, thus inhibiting DNA replication.

USES

Testicular, bladder, ovary, and lung carcinomas.

SIDE EFFECTS

Anaphylactic-like reactions, nephrotoxicity, neurotoxicity, ototoxicity, vomiting. Prevent nephrotoxicity with **amifostine** (free radical scavenger) and chloride (saline) diuresis.

Busulfan

MECHANISM

Alkylates DNA.

USES

Leukemias/lymphomas. Also used to ablate patient's bone marrow before bone marrow transplantation.

SIDE EFFECTS

Pulmonary fibrosis, hyperpigmentation, seizures, and severe myelosuppression.

ANTIMETABOLITES

These drugs are cell cycle specific (predominantly for the synthesis [S] phase) (Figure 4-44). They structurally resemble purines, pyrimidines, or other endogenous compounds, but are nonfunctional and therefore block nucleic acid synthesis. All are **contraindicated in pregnancy** and tend to **cause myelosuppression.**

Methotrexate

MECHANISM

Folic antimetabolite inhibiting **dihydrofolate reductase,** therefore impairing DNA and protein synthesis.

USES

Leukemias/lymphomas, choriocarcinomas, and sarcomas. Also used for abortion, ectopic pregnancy, rheumatoid arthritis, Crohn disease, psoriasis, inflammatory bowel disease, and vasculitis.

SIDE EFFECTS

Myelosuppression, which is reversible with **leucovorin** (folinic acid). Also causes fatty change in liver (similar to ethanol and amiodarone). Skin rash, mucositis (eg, mouth ulcers), nephrotoxicity, and pulmonary fibrosis.

Pemetrexed

MECHANISM

A pyrrolopyrimidine antifolate analog with activity in the S phase. It is transported into the cell via the reduced folate carrier and requires activation. Its main mechanism of action is inhibition of **thymidylate synthase.**

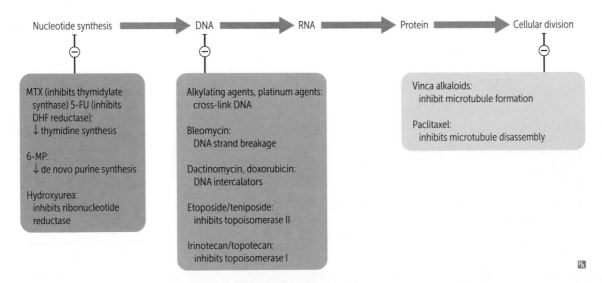

FIGURE 4-44. Cancer drugs—targets. 6-MP, 6-mercaptopurine; MTX, methotrexate.

USES

Mesothelioma and other lung cancers.

SIDE EFFECTS

Myelosuppression, skin rash, mucositis, diarrhea, fatigue. Vitamin supplementation with **folic acid** and **vitamin B$_{12}$** appear to reduce these toxicities.

6-Mercaptopurine (6-MP)

MECHANISM

Blocks purine synthesis. Must be activated by hypoxanthine guanine phosphoribosyl transferase (HGPRTase).

USES

Leukemias/lymphomas. Prevents organ rejection. Treatment for rheumatoid arthritis, inflammatory bowel disease, and SLE.

SIDE EFFECTS

6-MP is **metabolized by xanthine oxidase,** so toxicity is increased with coadministration of allopurinol (xanthine oxidase inhibitor). Myelosuppression, hepatotoxicity, nausea and vomiting.

Cytarabine

MECHANISM

Pyrimidine antagonist, terminates chain elongation. Also inhibits DNA polymerase.

USES

Leukemias/lymphomas.

SIDE EFFECTS

Potent myelosuppressive agent: leukopenia, thrombocytopenia, megaloblastic anemia, neurotoxicity, and nephrotoxicity.

5-Fluorouracil

MECHANISM

Pyrimidine analog that is bioactivated to 5-fluoro-deoxyuridine monophosphate (5F-dUMP). 5F-dUMP binds folic acid, and this complex **inhibits thymidylate synthase,** thus inhibiting nucleic acid synthesis.

USES

Solid tumors (eg, colon cancer, pancreatic cancer). Used topically for basal cell carcinoma of the skin.

SIDE EFFECTS

"Hand-foot syndrome" (dermopathy after extended use), mucositis, GI toxicity (diarrhea).

TOPOISOMERASE INHIBITORS

Etoposide, Teniposide

MECHANISM

Inhibits **topoisomerase** II (increases DNA damage).

USES

Solid tumors (particularly testicular and small cell lung cancer), leukemias, lymphomas.

SIDE EFFECTS

Myelosuppression, GI upset, alopecia.

Irinotecan, Topotecan

MECHANISM

Inhibit **topoisomerase I** (prevent DNA unwinding and replication).

USE

Colon cancer (irinotecan); ovarian and small cell lung cancers (topotecan).

SIDE EFFECTS

Severe myelosuppression, diarrhea.

DRUGS THAT TARGET TUBULIN

Vinca Alkaloids (Vincristine, Vinblastine)

MECHANISM

Prevent microtubule formation by **interfering** with tubulin binding. The **mitotic spindle** cannot form, and the M phase does not proceed.

USES

Leukemias/lymphomas, and solid tumors.

SIDE EFFECTS

ViNcristine causes Neurotoxicity. VinBlastine causes Bone marrow toxicity.

Taxanes (Paclitaxel, Docetaxel)

MECHANISM

Prevent microtubule breakdown by **stabilizing** tubulin already bound in **mitotic spindles.** M phase cannot complete.

USES

Solid tumors (eg, ovarian and breast carcinomas).

SIDE EFFECTS

Myelosuppression, alopecia, and hypersensitivity.

Ixabepilone, Epothilone

MECHANISM

Microtubule inhibitors active in the M phase of the cell cycle.

USES

Breast cancers.

SIDE EFFECTS

Myelosuppression, hypersensitivity reactions, and neurotoxicity (peripheral sensory neuropathy).

HORMONAL AGENTS

Selective Estrogen Receptor Modulators (Tamoxifen, Raloxifene)

MECHANISM

Estrogen agonist and antagonist properties depending on the individual target organ.

USES

Estrogen-sensitive breast cancers, especially in postmenopausal women. Raloxifene additionally stimulates the bone to increase density (useful to prevent osteoporosis), but is used less.

SIDE EFFECTS

Tamoxifen activates estrogen receptors on other types of tissue such as endometrium, increasing endometrial cancer risk, whereas raloxifene **does not** increase the risk of endometrial carcinoma (raloxifene is not an estrogen receptor antagonist in endometrial tissue). All can cause mild hot flashes and nausea.

Leuprolide and Goserelin

MECHANISM

Agonists of luteinizing hormone-releasing hormone (LHRH). Shuts off LH release when given continuously, thereby inhibiting testosterone or estrogen production.

USES

Infertility (pulsatile use), prostate cancer (continuous use after androgen receptor blockade with flutamide), uterine fibroids (continuous use), and precocious puberty (continuous use).

SIDE EFFECTS

Hot flashes, decreased bone density, decreased libido.

TARGETED MOLECULAR THERAPEUTICS

Anti-EGRF Antibodies (Cetuximab, Panitumumab)

MECHANISM

The epidermal growth factor receptor (EGFR) is a member of the erb-B family of growth factor receptors. Its signaling pathway is involved in cellular growth and proliferation, invasion and metastasis, and angiogenesis. Cetuximab is an antibody directed against the extracellular domain of the EGFR. Panitumumab is a human monoclonal antibody directed against the EGFR and works through inhibition of the EGFR signaling pathway.

USES

Colorectal cancer and some head and neck cancers.

SIDE EFFECTS

Cetuximab is associated with an acneiform skin rash, hypersensitivity infusion reaction, and hypomagnesemia. Infusion-related reactions are seen only rarely with panitumumab, and its main side effects are acneiform skin rash and hypomagnesemia.

Anti-EGFR Agents (Gefitinib, Erlotinib)

MECHANISM

Small molecule inhibitors of the tyrosine kinase domain associated with EGFR.

USES

Non–small cell lung cancer. Erlotinib has also been approved for use in the treatment regimen of pancreatic cancer.

SIDE EFFECTS

Both drugs have the potential to interact with other drugs metabolized by the liver CYP3A4 system and grapefruit. Acneiform skin rash, diarrhea, and anorexia and fatigue are often seen.

Trastuzumab

MECHANISM

Antibody against *HER2/neu* receptor may facilitate T-cell cytotoxicity against cancer cells with *erbB2* amplification or *HER2* overexpression.

USES

Breast cancers that have *HER2* overexpression or *erbB2* gene amplification.

SIDE EFFECTS

Cardiotoxicity, especially when combined with doxorubicin.

Anti-VEGF Antibodies (Bevacizumab)

MECHANISM

Antiangiogenic. Vascular endothelial growth factor (VEGF) is an important angiogenic growth factor. **Bevacizumab** is a recombinant monoclonal antibody that targets all forms of VEGF-A, binding and preventing interactions with target VEGF receptors.

USES

Colorectal cancer, non–small-lung cancer and breast cancer.

SIDE EFFECTS

Hypertension, increased incidence of arterial thromboembolic events (transient ischemic attack, stroke, angina, and myocardial infarction), wound healing complications and gastrointestinal perforations, and proteinuria.

Anti-VEGF Agents (Sorafenib, Sunitinib)

MECHANISM

Antiangiogenic. Small molecule inhibitors of the tyrosine kinase domain associated with VEGF.

USES

Sorafenib is approved for use in renal cell cancer and hepatocellular cancer. **Sunitinib** is used in renal cell cancer and gastrointestinal stromal tumors (GIST).

SIDE EFFECTS

Can have potential interactions with drugs metabolized by the CYP3A4 system, grapefruit, and St. John's wort. Hypertension, bleeding complications, and fatigue are also seen. Skin rash and the hand-foot syndrome are commonly seen with sorafenib use. There is an increased risk of cardiac dysfunction with sunitinib.

Anti-*BCR-ABL* Agents (Imatinib, Dasatinib, Nilotinib)

MECHANISM

Imatinib inhibits *BCR-ABL* tyrosine kinase specific to CML by blocking the binding site of ADP substrate. Nilotinib is a more potent *BCR-ABL* inhibitor, and dasatinib inhibits both *BCR-ABL* and Src kinases.

USES

CML with the t(9:22) Philadelphia chromosomal translocation and GI stromal tumors (GISTs).

SIDE EFFECTS

Mild. Potential interactions exist with other drugs, grapefruit, and St. John's wort, which are also metabolized by the CYP3A4 system.

Anti-CD20 Antibody (Rituximab)

MECHANISM

An antibody against the surface receptor CD20 expressed on most B cells.

USES

Non-Hodgkin lymphoma, CLL, inflammatory bowel disease, and rheumatoid arthritis.

SIDE EFFECTS

Infusion reactions, tumor lysis syndrome, skin and mouth reactions, infections. Increased risk of progressive multifocal leukoencephalopathy

Anti Proteasome (Bortezomib)

MECHANISM

Interferes with proteasomes, which normally control the degradation of proteins regulating cell proliferation. Causes apoptosis in tumor cells.

USES

Multiple myeloma, mantle cell lymphoma.

SIDE EFFECTS

Gastrointestinal effects, asthenia, peripheral neuropathy, and myelosuppression.

Cancer Immunotherapy (Nivolumab)

MECHANISM

Monoclonal antibody targeting **PD-1** (cell surface receptor expressed on activated T cells) to overcome **immune checkpoint blockade** exhibited in many cancer cells (expressing the ligand PD-L1, which binds to PD-1 and inhibits T cells from attacking the tumor).

USES

Metastatic melanoma. Second-line treatment for renal cell carcinoma and squamous non-small-cell lung cancer.

SIDE EFFECTS

Skin rash, peripheral edema, immune-mediated inflammation in multiple organs (eg, lung, liver, and kidney), and immune mediated hypo- or hyperthyroidism.

NATIVE CYTOKINES USED IN CANCER TREATMENT

Interferon-Alpha

MECHANISM

Enhances cell-mediated immunity against some cancers and viruses, possibly by upregulating expression of antigen in tumor cells. May also have direct apoptotic activity.

USES

Melanoma, renal cell carcinoma, CML.

SIDE EFFECTS

Flulike symptoms and aggravation of psychiatric disorders.

Interleukin-2

MECHANISM

Stimulates T-cell survival and activation, enhancing cell-mediated immunity against cancer cells.

USES

Kidney cancers and **melanoma.**

SIDE EFFECTS

Capillary leak syndrome (triad of hypotension, low vascular resistance, and high cardiac output similar to septic shock).

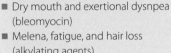

CLINICAL CORRELATION

Common side effects of chemotherapy drugs (Figure 4-45):

- Finger numbing/tingling (vincristine)
- Burning urination/increased frequency (cyclophosphamide)
- Leg swelling and orthopnea (doxorubicin)
- Dry mouth and exertional dysnpea (bleomyocin)
- Melena, fatigue, and hair loss (alkylating agents)
- Abdominal pain and jaundice (mercaptopurine, methotrexate)

ANTICOAGULANTS

Anticoagulants are used for the treatment and prevention of unwanted blood clotting. Examples include deep venous thrombosis (DVT), pulmonary embolism (PE), and embolic stroke. They prevent clot formation by interrupting either the intrinsic (heparin) or extrinsic (warfarin) coagulation cascade. It is very important to understand the similarities of and differences between heparin and warfarin (Table 4-17).

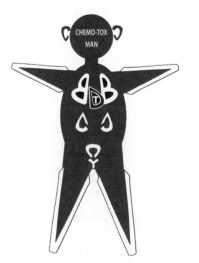

Cisplatin/Carboplatin → ototoxicity (and nephrotoxicity)

Vincristine → peripheral neuropathy
Bleomycin, Busulfan → pulmonary fibrosis
Doxorubicin → cardiotoxicity
Trastuzumab (Herceptin) → cardiotoxicity
Cisplatin/Carboplatin → nephrotoxicity (and ototoxicity)

CYclophosphamide → hemorrhagic cystitis

FIGURE 4-45. **Common chemotoxicities.**

TABLE 4-17.   Comparison of Heparin and Warfarin

DRUG	HEPARIN	WARFARIN
Structure	Large anionic polymer	Small lipid-soluble molecule
Route of administration	IV, SC	Oral
Site of action	Blood	Liver
Onset of action	Rapid (seconds; acute management)	Slow, dependent on half-life of clotting factors (chronic management)
Mechanism of action	Activates antithrombin III, reduces action of thrombin and factor Xa	Vitamin K antagonist (impairs synthesis of factors II, VII, IX, and X)
Duration of action	Acute (hours)	Chronic (weeks)
Treatment of overdose	Protamine	Vitamin K, fresh-frozen plasma
Method of monitoring	PTT (intrinsic pathway)	PT/INR (extrinsic pathway)
Cross placenta	No	Yes (teratogenic, eg, fetal hemorrhage)

INR, international normalized ratio; IV, intravenous; PT, prothrombin time; PTT, partial thromboplastin time; SC, subcutaneous.

Heparin

MECHANISM

Catalyzes the activation of **antithrombin III,** thus decreasing the activity of thrombin (factor IIa) and factor Xa. Heparin activity is monitored with the **partial thromboplastin time (PTT)** because of its effects on the **intrinsic coagulation pathway.** Newer low-molecular-weight heparins (eg, enoxaparin) do not have to be monitored by laboratory tests.

> **KEY FACT**
>
> The treatment for heparin overdose is protamine.

SITE OF ACTION

Blood.

USES

Immediate anticoagulation for DVT, PE, myocardial infarction (MI). DVT/PE prophylaxis in hospitalized patients.

SIDE EFFECTS

Bleeding. Overdose is treated with **protamine sulfate** (binds heparin and inactivates it). Rarely causes heparin-induced thrombocytopenia (HIT), which paradoxically increases the risk of thrombosis (due to autoantibodies to heparin-platelet factor 4 complex). Avoid low-molecular-weight heparin in patients with elevated creatinine.

Direct Factor Xa Inhibitors (Apixaban, Rivaroxaban)

MECHANISM

Direct oral anticoagulants bind to and inhibit factor Xa in the coagulation cascade, bypassing antithrombin as a mediator.

USES

Treatment and prophylaxis for DVT and PE, and stroke prophylaxis in patients with atrial fibrillation.

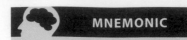
SIDE EFFECTS

Bleeding (reverse with **andexanet alfa**).

Warfarin

MECHANISM

Inhibits γ carboxylation of vitamin K-dependent clotting factors (factors II, VII, IX, and X, and proteins C and S). Warfarin affects the **extrinsic coagulation pathway** and is monitored clinically with the **prothrombin time (PT)**.

SITE OF ACTION

Liver (site of synthesis of clotting factors).

USES

Chronic anticoagulation (eg, DVT prophylaxis and in atrial fibrillation for stroke prophylaxis).

SIDE EFFECTS

Bleeding. Also, warfarin crosses the placenta, so it is **contraindicated in pregnancy** (heparin is used instead). Overdose is treated with fresh-frozen plasma (to supply fresh clotting factors) and IV vitamin K.

ANTIPLATELET AGENTS

Drugs that have antiplatelet activity either inhibit platelet adherence to the vascular endothelium (adhesion) or platelet adherence to other platelets (aggregation). Their major applications are to prevent MI and stroke (see Figure 4-46 for an overview of platelet activation).

Aspirin

MECHANISM

Acetylates and irreversibly inhibits cyclooxygenase (COX-1 and COX-2). This action prevents conversion of arachidonic acid to prostaglandins and thromboxane A_2. The result is decreased platelet aggregation (increased bleeding time), no effect on PT or PTT.

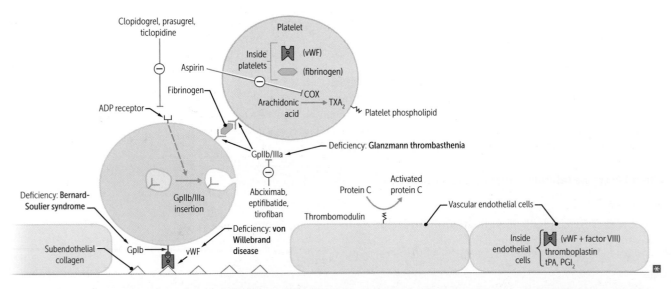

FIGURE 4-46. **Factors influencing platelet activation.** ADP, adenosine diphosphate; COX, cyclooxygenase; GP, glycoprotein; PGI, prostacyclin; tPa, tissue plasminogen activator; TXA_2, thromboxane A_2; vWF, von Willebrand factor.

SITE OF ACTION
In the platelet.

USES
Prevention of MI.

SIDE EFFECTS
Gastric ulcers, bleeding, Reye syndrome in children, tinnitus at very high doses.

Clopidogrel and Ticlopidine

MECHANISM
Irreversibly block ADP receptors on platelet membranes, thereby inhibiting platelet aggregation.

SITE OF ACTION
Platelet membrane.

USES
Prevention of thrombosis following coronary artery stent placement; stroke prevention.

SIDE EFFECTS
Bleeding. Ticlopidine can cause severe neutropenia.

Dipyridamole, Cilostazol

MECHANISM
Inhibit adenosine uptake by the platelet (secondary to blocking intraplatelet phosphodiesterase and increasing cAMP levels). The result is decreased platelet aggregation.

SITE OF ACTION
In the platelet.

USES
In combination with aspirin to prevent stroke. Cilostazol used for claudication symptoms.

SIDE EFFECTS
Bleeding, nausea, headache, facial flushing, hypotension, abdominal pain.

Glycoprotein IIb/IIIa Inhibitors: Abciximab, Eptifibatide, Tirofiban

MECHANISM
Binds to the glycoprotein IIb/IIa receptor on platelets and prevents interaction between fibrinogen and the IIb/IIIa receptor. The result is decreased platelet aggregation. Abciximab is made from monoclonal antibody Fab fragments.

SITE OF ACTION
Platelet membrane.

USES
Prevention of thrombosis during coronary artery angioplasty and stenting.

SIDE EFFECTS
Bleeding, thrombocytopenia.

THROMBOLYTICS

Thrombolytics are used to lyse active clots in the circulation. Their basic mechanism is to increase formation of plasmin, the intrinsic enzyme responsible for degrading fibrin clots. The two most common applications for thrombolytic agents are early MI and early thromboembolic (ischemic) stroke.

Streptokinase

MECHANISM

Indirectly activates plasminogen. Streptokinase first binds plasminogen, forming a 1:1 complex. This complex then catalyzes the formation of plasmin from another molecule of plasminogen. Streptokinase is **not fibrin-specific** (it activates free plasminogen that is not bound to fibrin clots).

SITE OF ACTION

Free plasminogen and fibrin-bound plasminogen.

USES

Acute MI, stroke, PE.

SIDE EFFECTS

Bleeding (contraindicated in patients with active bleeding, recent surgery, or history of intracranial bleeds); **allergic response** (since it is isolated from bacteria); it also loses efficacy after initial administration because patients become sensitized; a repeat dose is much less effective than the initial dose.

Tissue Plasminogen Activator (tPA)

MECHANISM

In contrast to streptokinase, **tPA is fibrin-specific.** Therefore it only activates plasminogen molecules that are bound to fibrin clots. It directly activates plasminogen.

SITE OF ACTION

Plasminogen bound to fibrin clots.

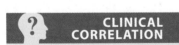

CLINICAL CORRELATION

There is a 3-hour window in patients with suspected ischemic stroke in which tPA can be administered. Hemorrhagic stroke must first be ruled out with a CT scan before tPA is given.

USES

Acute MI (if percutaneous coronary intervention is not available), stroke, PE.

SIDE EFFECTS

Bleeding; does not lose efficacy after initial dose (in contrast to streptokinase). **Note:** Fibrinolysis can be reversed with **aminocaproic acid.**

CHAPTER 5

Musculoskeletal, Skin, and Connective Tissue

EMBRYOLOGY   324
- Skeletal System   324
- Muscular System   332

ANATOMY   335
- Skeletal System   335
- Joints   343
- Muscular System   346

PHYSIOLOGY   354
- Muscle Types   354
- Metabolism   358
- Skin Physiology   360
- Important Laboratory Values   361

PATHOLOGY   362
- Skeletal Oncology   362
- Nononcologic Musculoskeletal Disease   367
- Connective Tissue Disorders   377
- Dermatology   389
- Vasculitides   396

PHARMACOLOGY   402
- Drugs Used to Treat Disorders of Bone   402
- Drugs Used to Treat Gout   404
- Drugs Used to Treat Connective Tissue Diseases   406
- Drugs Used to Treat Pain   406

Embryology

SKELETAL SYSTEM

Osteogenesis

Development

Bone develops from two sources: mesenchyme (intramembranous ossification) and cartilage (endochondral ossification). The biology of osteogenesis involves a number of different factors that are displayed in Figure 5-1.

- **Intramembranous ossification:** Flat bones (eg, skull, carpal bones) develop directly from mesenchyme found in preexisting membranes. The tissue becomes woven bone, which consists of bone spicules that become trabeculae and interconnect. This is eventually remodeled to lamellar bone. As opposed to endochondral ossification, there is no cartilage precursor.
- **Endochondral ossification:** Most bones, including long bones in the appendicular skeleton, develop from mesenchyme that has condensed into cartilage first. The **primary center of ossification** in the cartilaginous model forms the shaft of the bone (diaphysis). The ends of the bone (epiphyses) remain cartilaginous for several years after birth, during which time the **secondary centers of ossification** appear. Bone lengthening occurs in the epiphyseal cartilage plate at the diaphyseal-epiphyseal junction until it ossifies by about 20 years of age (Figure 5-2). Calcified bone matrix

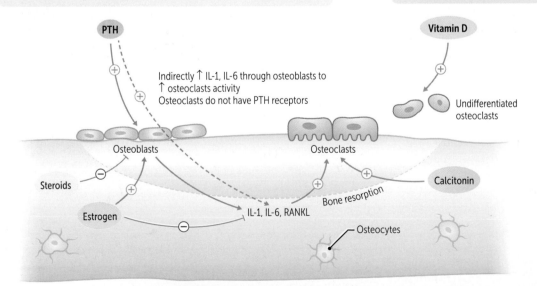

Systemic factors

PTH:
- Stimulates osteoblasts to secrete IL-1, IL-6, RANKL
- IL-1 and Il-6 activate osteoclasts + ↑ resorption of bone
- Goal: ↑ Ca²⁺, ↓ phosphate

Estrogen:
- Inhibits bone resorption
- Suppresses IL-1, IL-6
- Prolongs osteoblast lifespan
- Clinical correlation with ↓ estrogen after menopause with ↑ risk of femoral neck fractures

Calcitonin:
- Inhibits osteoclasts
- Goal: ↓ Ca²⁺ levels

Vitamin D:
- Differentiation of osteoclasts

Steroids: ↓ bone formation
- Inhibit osteoblast activity

Local cellular factors

Osteoblasts:
- Form bone by producing non-mineralized matrix
- Stimulate osteoclasts via cytokines (IL-1, IL-6, RANKL)

Osteoclasts:
- Resorb bone

Osteocytes:
- Former osteoblasts trapped in the matrix
- Maintain bone + cellular matrix

Osteochondroprogenitors:
- Mesenchymal stem cells that can differentiate into osteoblasts or chondrocytes

FIGURE 5-1. **Bone metabolism.** Actions of different cells involved in bone metabolism. IL, interleukin; PTH, parathyroid hormone; RANKL, receptor activator of nuclear factor κβ ligand.

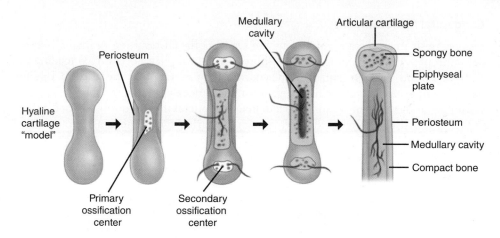

FIGURE 5-2. **Bone growth.** Primary ossification center in the diaphysis; secondary ossification center in the epiphyses.

is ultimately composed of 70% **hydroxyapatite** (calcium-phosphate crystals), 25% organic matrix (collagen, chondroitin sulfate, and hyaluronic acid), and 5% water.

Bone Cell Biology

Osteoblasts

Mononuclear cells that differentiate from mesenchymal stem cells in the periosteum. They are responsible for the synthesis of the calcium and phosphate bone collagen matrix.

Osteoclasts

Multinucleated cells that differentiate from hematopoietic lineage. They secrete acidic and lytic enzymes that function to degrade and subsequently resorb the bone.

Osteocyte

Star-shaped cell that begins as an osteoblast and is trapped in the matrix that it secretes. Osteocytes are connected by long cytoplasmic extensions that are in canals called **canaliculi.**

Parathyroid Hormone

Parathyroid hormone (PTH) is secreted by the parathyroid gland, which functions to increase serum levels of calcium and decrease serum levels of phosphate. At low and intermittent levels, PTH has an anabolic effect by directly activating osteoblasts to lay down bone and indirectly activating osteoblasts via various cytokines. In chronic hyperparathyroidism it causes catabolic effects (osteitis fibrosa cystica).

Estrogen

Estrogen inhibits bone resorption by inhibiting apoptosis in osteoblasts and indirectly inhibiting osteoclasts by suppressing interleukin (IL)-1, IL-6, and receptor activator of nuclear factor κβ ligand (RANKL). Estrogen deficiency due to a postmenopausal state or surgery can lead to excessive bone resorption and eventually osteoporosis.

Cytokines

Both IL-1 and IL-6 are cytokines produced by osteoblasts and a number of other cells. They have a positive effect on osteoclast differentiation by inducing the expression of RANKL on the surface of osteoblasts. RANKL induces osteoclast differentiation via the RANK signaling pathway.

KEY FACT

Achondroplasia is a disorder that affects endochondral ossification at the epiphyseal cartilage plates in long bones, resulting in premature closing of the epiphyses and short limbs.

KEY FACT

Larson syndrome is another form of dwarfism. It is an **autosomal recessive** disorder in which a **defect in the growth hormone receptor (GHR)** causes a lack of responsiveness to increased levels of GH in the body.

Congenital Malformations

Osteogenesis imperfecta is a deficiency in type I collagen resulting in fragile bones, achondroplasia is a signaling defect of fibroblast growth factor-3 (FGF-3) leading to disrupted bone development, Marfan syndrome is a mutation of the fibrillin 1 gene causing abnormal connective tissue, gigantism/acromegaly are due to excessive growth hormone, and cretinism is caused by a deficiency in fetal thryoid hormone. See Table 5-1 for a full list of congenital malformations. Marfan syndrome is associated with

TABLE 5-1.   Genetic Pathology

DISEASE	ETIOLOGY	CLINICAL PRESENTATION	LABORATORY TESTING
Osteogenesis imperfecta	AD disorder resulting from mutations of COL1A1 and COL1A2 genes that affect the synthesis and structure of type I collagen	Extremely fragile bones (multiple fractures), blue sclerae, poor wound healing, hearing loss	Multiple fractures are often noted on radiographs with exuberant healing of the callus
Achondroplasia	AD disorder caused by mutation in fibroblast growth factor (FGFR3), receptor is constitutively activated, which inhibits chondrocyte proliferation and endochondral ossification, preventing proper long bone growth	Short lives, increased spinal curvature, distorted skull growth	
Osteopetrosis	Mutation in carbonic anhydrase II impairs ability of osteoclasts to generate acidic environment necessary to resorb bone. This leads to thick, dense bone that is prone to fracture	Fractures, cranial nerve impingement, palsies (as a result of narrowed foramina) Bone marrow transplant is potentially curative, as osteoclasts are derived from hematopoietic cells	Pancytopenia Diffusely dense bones on radiograph
Marfan syndrome	AD disorder affecting the fibrillin gene. This causes abnormal elastin fibers, which affects the skeletal, cardiac, and ocular systems	Tall stature, long limbs, hyperextendable joints, long and tapering digits (Figure 5-3), pectus excavatum, and scoliosis Diagnosed with the Ghent diagnostic nosology	Aortic dilatation or dissection may be seen on echocardiogram
Endocrine Pathology			
Rickets	Deficiency of vitamin D during childhood; causes softening of bones due to defective bone mineralization	Bone pain, skeletal deformities (bowed legs, rachitic rosary), muscle weakness	Hypocalcemia
Osteomalacia	Deficiency of vitamin D during adulthood; causes softening of bones due to defective bone mineralization	Weak bones, bone pain, muscle weakness, pathologic fractures	Hypocalcemia
Osteoporosis	Decrease in bone mineral density leading to disrupted bone architecture; commonly seen in elderly women due to lack of estrogen in a postmenopausal state	Vertebral compression fractures; acute back pain, loss of height Femoral neck fractures Distal radius fractures	Bone mineral density test (DEXA scan) with T-score ≤ -2.5 Normal calcium and phosphate levels
Osteitis fibrosa cystica	Skeletal disorder caused by chronically high levels of PTH due to hyperparathyroidism. Osteoclasts are constantly active and resorbing bone	Bone pain/tenderness, fractures, skeletal deformities	Bone cysts will be evident on radiographs

TABLE 5-1.   Genetic Pathology *(continued)*

DISEASE	ETIOLOGY	CLINICAL PRESENTATION	LABORATORY TESTING
Dwarfism	Often due to deficiency in GH, but can have other causes; 70% due to achondroplasia, Turner syndrome, poor nutrition, stress (psychogenic dwarfism)	Short stature, delayed puberty	May see low GH levels
Gigantism	Hyperpituitarism causing excessive amounts of GH causes gigantism in infants and acromegaly in adults	Infants: Increased height and excessive body proportions Acromegaly (adults): Increased bone growth in the jaw, hands, and feet with increased soft tissue and visceral organ growth	IGF-1 levels are usually elevated Oral glucose tolerance test: GH levels should decrease after oral glucose load; if not, it is diagnostic of pituitary GH excess
Cretinism	Deficiency in fetal thyroid hormone due to lack of dietary iodine, mutations in thyroid hormone synthesis, or agenesis of the thyroid gland	Mental retardation, short stature, impaired bone growth, neurologic disorders of muscle tone and coordination	Iodine levels may be low
Hyperparathyroidism	Chronically increased parathyroid hormone results in excessive bone resorption via actions of PTH Primary can be due to idiopathic or parathyroid hyperplasia, adenoma or carcinoma. Secondary is often a compensation for ESRD	Weakness, fatigue, depression, bone pain, kidney stones, muscle soreness (myalgias), decreased appetite. Mnemonic: "**R**enal **S**tones, abdominal **G**roans, painful **B**ones and psychiatric **M**oans"	Primary hyperparathyroidism: Increased Ca, ALP, PTH, decreased phosphate Secondary hyperparathyroidism: Decreased Ca, Increased phosphate, ALP, PTH
Other			
Osteonecrosis	Infarction of the bone and marrow, usually very painful. Causes include alcoholism, sickle cell disease, exogenous/endogenous corticosteroids, pancreatitis, trauma, idiopathic (Legg-Calve Perthes disease), Caisson ("the bends," seen in divers)	Will usually present as pain in the affected area Most common site is the femoral head (due to insufficiency of the medial circumflex femoral artery)	Presents on radiographs as irregular serpiginous sclerosis and in late states mimics end-stage arthritis. MRI is the gold standard for diagnosing it in acute and subacute stages.
Osteoarthritis	Wear down of the cartilage in the joint space; develops with age and increasing impact on joints	Pain in the affected joints More common in weight-bearing joints (hips, knees)	Four key characteristics seen on radiographs: joint space narrowing, subchondral sclerosis, osteophytosis, and subchondral cysts
Paget disease of the bone (osteitis deformans)	Increased osteoclastic bone resorption followed by increased osteoblastic activity. The accelerated speed of new bone formation results in disorganized new bone that consists of a mosaic of woven and lamellar bone	Increased hat size Can see high-output heart failure from increased AV shunts Increased risk of osteogenic sarcoma Hearing loss is common due to narrowing of the auditory foramen	Increased ALP Histology will show a mosaic pattern of woven and lamellar bone

AD, autosomal dominant; ALP, alkaline phosphatase; AV, atrioventricular; ESRD, end-stage renal disease; GH, growth hormone; IGF-1, insulinlike growth factor-1; PTH, parathyroid hormone.

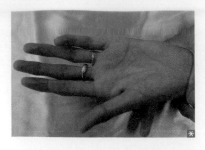

FIGURE 5-3. **Marfan syndrome.** Note the long slender fingers.

FLASH FORWARD

Ocular findings in Marfan syndrome include **ectopia lentis** (lens dislocation) in 50% of patients. Dislocation is usually upward and toward the temples. This is in contrast to ectopia lentis in homocystinuria, which is usually downward and into the anterior chamber.

FLASH FORWARD

Marfan syndrome is associated with ascending aortic dissection, mitral valve prolapse, and cerebral berry aneurysms. The Steinberg sign a thumb that projects out the ulnar border when completely opposed in a clenched hand.

KEY FACT

A **keloid** is a an excess production of type III collagen in scar tissue far larger than the initial wound, whereas a **hypertrophic scar** is an excess production of mainly type I collagen scar tissue.

ascending aortic dissection, mitral valve prolapse, and cerebral berry aneurysms. The Steinberg sign is a thumb that projects out of the ulnar border when completely opposed in a clenched hand. Collagen formation is a multi-step process (Figure 5-4). Preprocollagen is processed to triple helix procollagen by hydroxylation and glycosylation, followed by cleavage and cross-linking to form collagen fibrils. Defects in collagen synthesis can cause a variety of disorders, including scurvy, osteogenesis imperfecta, Ehlers-Danlos syndrome, and Menkes disease.

Skull

Development

The flat bones in the skull are separated by five connective tissue **sutures** that allow expansion of the skull while the brain grows:

- Frontal suture
- Sagittal suture
- Lambdoid suture
- Coronal suture
- Squamosal suture

Fontanelles are areas between the flat bones of the skull where the sutures meet. Fontanelles allow room for the brain to finish growing. All fontanelles usually close by about 2 years of age. Exam of the fontanelles can indicate dehydration (sunken fontanelle) or increased intracranial pressure (bulging fontanelle). There are six fontanelles (Figure 5-5; *note:* only the anterior and posterior fontanelles are shown):

- Anterior fontanelle: Closes by the end of the second year and is the last to close.
- Posterior fontanelle.
- Sphenoid fontanelles (one on each side of head).
- Mastoid fontanelles (one on each side of head).

Congenital Malformations

- **Microcephaly:** Failure of the brain, and subsequently the skull, to grow. Affected children are severely mentally retarded. The etiology may be an autosomal recessive genetic mutation or in-utero infection.
- **Craniosynostoses:** Premature closure of the sutures may lead to abnormal shape of the skull.

In rough endoplasmic reticulum of fibroblasts

Synthesis
Preprocollagen = Gly-X-Y
X, Y = proline or lysine
α chains

Hydroxylation -(OH)
Hydroxylation of proline & lysine residues
Vitamin C required
Deficiency → scurvy

Glycosylation
Glycosylation of pro-α-chain hydroxylysine residues
Triple helix formation (3 α-chains)
→ procollagen
Poor triple helix formation
→ osteogenesis imperfecta

Exocytosis

Proteolysis & Cross-linking
Peptide cleavage & covalent lysine-hydroxylysine cross-linking
→ collagen fibrils
Poor cross-linking → Ehlers Danlos syndrome → Menkes disease

FIGURE 5-4. **Collagen synthesis.**

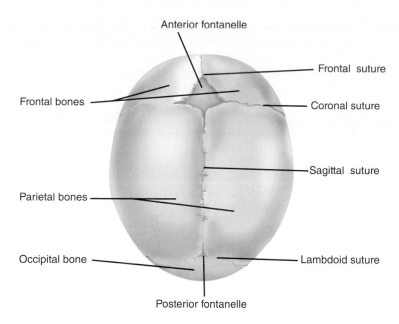

Anterior fontanelle

Frontal suture

Frontal bones

Coronal suture

Sagittal suture

Parietal bones

Occipital bone

Lambdoid suture

Posterior fontanelle

FIGURE 5-5. **Normal skull of a newborn with sutures and fontanelles.**

Vertebral Column

Development

In weeks 4–6 of embryonic development, mesenchymal cells surround the notochord, neural tube, and body wall to form significant structures of the vertebral column. The notochord eventually develops into the nucleus pulposus of the intervertebral disc. After puberty, secondary ossification centers appear at the tips of the spinous and transverse processes, which fuse completely by age 25.

The following vertebrae do not ossify in the previously described manner:

- Atlas (C1): Has no vertebral body.
- Axis (C2): Has a **dens** (odontoid process) that is the developmental remnant of the body of the atlas.
- Sacrum: These five vertebrae fuse together to form a wall of the pelvic cavity.
- Coccyx: Four rudimentary vertebrae fuse into a small triangle at the base of the spine.

The four main spinal areas are associated with four specific curvatures: cervical, thoracic, lumbar, sacral. These curvatures reverse themselves when moving to the next contiguous spinal segment. The cervical and lumbar segments have lordotic curves, but the thoracic and sacral segments are kyphotic.

Congenital Malformations

- **Chordoma:** This is a **remnant of the notochord.** One-third of chordomas become slow-growing, malignant tumors that infiltrate surrounding tissues, including bone. The most common location for a chordoma is the skull base, where it can infiltrate adjacent structures and cause cranial nerve palsies (prepontine cisterns) or cardiorespiratory disorder (brainstem). The second most common location is the lumbosacral region, where it can erode in the spinal canal or neural foramina, leading to lumbosacral nerve and/or cauda equina compression. The prognosis is poor, with only half of patients surviving past 5 years.
- **Variations in the number of vertebrae:** The vast majority of people have a total of 33 vertebrae: 7 cervical, 12 thoracic, 5 lumbar, 5 sacral, and 4 fused in the coccyx.

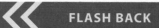
FLASH BACK

In embryonic development, the neural tube becomes the spinal cord, and the notochord eventually forms the vertebrae. The notocord is the embryologic origin of the nucleus pulposus.

KEY FACT

The annulus fibrosus is made of types I and II collagen.

QUESTION

A basketball player is quite thin, with very long legs and long, slender fingers. When he makes a fist with his thumb under his fingers, his thumb sticks out the other side. About what three vascular complications are you worried?

FLASH BACK

When a similar bony defect occurs at the base of the skull, a meningocele (protrusion of the meninges and cerebrospinal fluid [CSF]), meningoencephalocele (protrusion of the meninges and brain), or meningohydroencephalocele (protrusion of meninges, brain, and ventricle) may occur.

KEY FACT

The "triple screen" is a blood test done at weeks 16–18 of pregnancy that measures α-fetoprotein (AFP), β-human chorionic gonadotropin, and unconjugated estriol. Elevated **AFP** may indicate **spina bifida** or another congenital disorder such as anencephaly. In contrast, Down syndrome may cause a low ("down") AFP level.

KEY FACT

All pregnant women should take folic acid supplements to help prevent neural tube defects.

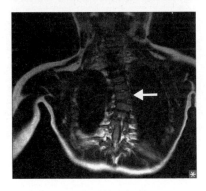

FIGURE 5-6. Hemivertebra. Note development of half of the vertebra and subsequent curving of the vertebral column (scoliosis).

ANSWER

Marfan syndrome is associated with ascending aortic dissection, mitral valve prolapse, and cerebral saccular (berry) aneurysms. The Steinberg sign is a thumb that projects out the ulnar border when completely opposed in a clenched hand.

- **Klippel-Feil syndrome (brevicollis):** A syndrome of unclear etiology caused by fusion of the cervical vertebrae. Typically involves the following constellation of symptoms:
  - Decreased range of motion in the cervical spine
  - Defects in the thoracic and lumbar spine causing **scoliosis**
  - Renal anomalies
  - Hearing loss
  - Short neck with low hairline

Spina Bifida

This spinal defect occurs when the **two halves of the vertebral arch fail to fuse, most commonly in the lumbosacral region** (L5 and/or S1). Because of the defect, the vertebral arch consists of two parts and is hence "bifid." There are many variations of spina bifida, ranging from mild to severe, depending on how much of the spinal cord and/or meninges protrude through the defect. See the Variations of Spina Bifida section and Table 6-1 in the Neurology chapter for further discussion.

Hemivertebra

One of the two chondrification centers in the central part of the vertebrae fails to appear, so only half of the vertebral body is able to form. This produces a lateral curvature and rotation of the spine and is one potential cause of **scoliosis** (Figure 5-6).

Spondylolysis and Spondylolisthesis

The vertebral arch pedicles fail to fuse with the vertebral body (spondylolysis: the connection is "lysed"), which may lead to displacement of a vertebral body relative to the vertebral body below it (spondylolisthesis). The displaced vertebral bodies may move anteriorly (anterolisthesis) or posteriorly (posterolisthesis; Figure 5-7).

Ribs

Development

Mesenchymal cells that surround the body wall form the costal processes that develop into ribs. Though costal processes occur at all vertebrae, only the thoracic vertebrae develop ribs. The "true ribs" are the first seven that attach to the sternum. The "false ribs," ribs 8–12, attach to the sternum via other ribs. The last two ribs are "floating ribs" that do not attach to the sternum at all.

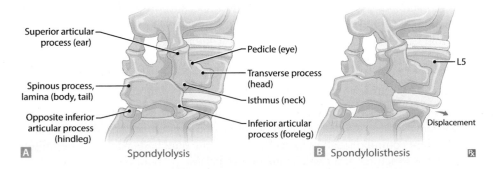

FIGURE 5-7. A comparison of spondylolysis and spondylolisthesis. Ⓐ Posterior oblique lumbar view mimics shape of a Scotty dog (see outline). In simple spondylolysis, Scotty dog appears to be wearing a collar. Ⓑ In spondylolisthesis, Scotty dog appears decapitated. L5 vertebral body and/or disk can be displaced anteriorly or posteriorly. Generally, the body goes anteriorly but the disk causes posterior pseudoprotrusion and/or protrusion.

Congenital Malformations

- **Accessory ribs:** An extra rib can develop from the costal processes of a cervical or lumbar vertebral body. A lumbar rib is more common; however, a cervical rib arising from C7 can cause **thoracic outlet syndrome,** in which the extra rib compresses the neurovascular bundle at the thoracic outlet.
  - The lower nerve roots of the brachial plexus (C8 and T1) are affected most commonly, leading to neurologic symptoms such as pain and tingling in the ulnar nerve distribution.
  - The upper nerve roots (C5, C6, and C7) can also be compressed, causing similar symptoms in the radial nerve distribution as well as the neck, ear, and torso.
  - A compressed subclavian vein can lead to swelling and cyanosis in the upper extremity of the affected side, and a compressed subclavian artery can cause pallor, pulselessness, low blood pressure, coolness, and rare small infarcts in the affected upper extremity.

Limbs

Development

Development of the limb bones begins when the early limb buds form at about the fourth week of embryonic development. By the fifth week, mesodermal cells from the lateral plate migrate into the limb buds.

- A thickened region of ectoderm called the **apical ectodermal ridge (AER)** develops at the edge of the limb bud; it produces **FGF** that induces the mesodermal cells to grow outward and form cartilage.
- The **zone of polarizing activity** at the base of the limb bud produces the **sonic hedgehog protein,** which activates homeobox-containing (*Hox*) genes to direct the patterned organization of the limbs and digits.

The rest of limb development follows this general timeline:

- Week 6: Digital rays develop in the hands and feet; digit formation involves selective **apoptosis** within the AER. By the end of week 6, the cartilaginous models of the limb bones are complete.
- Weeks 7–12: The long bones undergo endochondral ossification as discussed previously, and most of the primary ossification centers develop.
- Adult age: The primary ossification in the diaphysis does not fuse with the secondary ossification in the epiphysis until adult age, allowing for complete bone growth. At this time, the epiphyseal plate between the two finally ossifies, and bone growth ends.

Congenital Malformations

Limb anomalies range from issues with limb bud development, resulting in the complete absence of the limb, to problems in the growth or differentiation of limbs, causing shortened or deformed extremities. The limb anomalies listed below may be caused by genetic factors, environmental factors, or both.

- **Amelia:** Complete absence of one or more limbs, often due to maternal ingestion of a teratogen, such as **thalidomide.**
- **Meromelia:** Partial absence of one or more limbs.
- **Cleft hand and foot:** Also known as "lobster-claw deformities." Several of the digital rays fail to develop centrally; the lateral digits fuse, causing a claw-shaped hand or foot.
- **Congenital clubfoot:** A common anomaly occurring about once in every 1000 births, involving any deformity in the ankle bone (talus) of the foot. The most common type of clubfoot is **talipes equinovarus,** in which the foot is inverted and turned in medially. A genetic predisposition seems to be involved. The majority of cases involve abnormal positioning of the feet in the uterus.

KEY FACT

When testing a patient for thoracic outlet syndrome, look for a positive Adson sign: Have the patient maximally extend the neck and rotate the head toward the side being tested. Look for a decrease in the ipsilateral radial pulse and listen for a subclavian bruit.

FLASH BACK

The **interscalene triangle** is bordered anteriorly by anterior scalene, posteriorly by middle scalene, and inferiorly by medial surface of the first rib. An accessory cervical rib can compress this small area, causing thoracic outlet syndrome.

FLASH BACK

Many trisomy syndromes are associated with limb defects.
- Trisomy 21 (Down syndrome): **Clinodactyly** (curving of the fingers).
- Trisomy 18 (Edwards syndrome): Flexed digits (or overlapping) and "rocker-bottom" feet.
- Trisomy 13 (Patau syndrome): **Polydactyly.**

KEY FACT

The critical period of limb development occurs during the third to fifth weeks. Teratogens ingested early in this period may cause severe defects. In the late 1950s and early 1960s, many mothers took **thalidomide,** a sedative and antiemetic that caused severe teratogenic limb defects including amelia.

FLASH BACK

Today, the only FDA-approved uses for thalidomide are pain relief from erythema nodosum leprosum, the skin manifestation of leprosy, and newly diagnosed multiple myeloma.

- **Polydactyly:** An autosomal dominant trait that causes extra fingers or toes to develop, usually medially or laterally. More common in blacks. In whites, polydactyly is associated with heart disorders.
- **Syndactyly:** The most common limb anomaly. Cutaneous syndactyly involves simple webbing of the digits, usually in the toes. A more severe form is osseous syndactyly in which the bones of the digits fuse (as in the lateral digits in clubfoot) when the divisions between the digital rays fail to develop.
- **Brachydactyly:** Hypoplasia of the fingers or toes. It is uncommon and typically inherited as an autosomal dominant (AD) trait and associated with short stature.
- **Holt-Oram syndrome:** Also known as **heart-hand syndrome.** Due to mutations in the *TBX5* gene on chromosome 12, which is important in both cardiac and upper limb development. Major manifestations include:
  - Cardiac: **atrial septal defects,** ventral septal defects, atrioventricular block, atrial fibrillation.
  - **Abnormalities of the thumb:** Hypoplasia, elongation, or absence of the thumb.
- **Congenital hip dislocation:** A very common disorder, affecting about one in every 1000 infants. Predisposing factors include female gender, Native American heritage, first-born status, and breech birth. **Diagnosed by physical exam and/or hip ultrasound:**
  - Positive Ortolani test: One hears or feels a low-pitched click when abducting the hip.
  - Positive Barlow maneuver: While keeping hips in the adducted position, one hears a click when applying gentle pressure posteriorly.
  - Positive Galeazzi sign: One leg appears longer than the other. This may be more reliable for diagnosis in older infants.

  Treatment includes a Pavlik harness; if this fails, then open or closed reduction with spica casting is appropriate (depending on the age and severity of disease).

MUSCULAR SYSTEM

Almost all muscles in the human body develop from mesoderm (the notable exceptions being the dilator pupillae and sphincter of the iris that develop from the neuroectoderm). Cardiac and smooth muscles develop from **splanchnic mesoderm,** whereas most skeletal muscles develop from regions of the somites called **myotomes.** Developmental anomalies can lead to the absence of or variation in muscles (generally benign).

Skeletal Muscle

Mesenchymal cells in the myotome areas of the somites differentiate into **myoblasts** that then elongate and fuse into tubular structures called **myotubes.** Fibroblasts and external laminae that form around the muscle tubules encase the muscle in a fibrous sheath during its development. Myofilaments, myofibrils, and other muscle-specific organelles develop early. Skeletal muscle starts to grow as myotubes fuse together; after the first year, the increase in myofilaments leads to muscle growth.

Different myotomes give rise to different muscles in the body, generally depending on location.

Muscular Development of the Head and Neck

- **Preoptic myotomes** give rise to extraocular muscles.
- **Occipital myotomes** give rise to the tongue muscles.

Muscular Development of the Trunk

Each myotome of each somite in the trunk region divides into two parts: an **epaxial division** on the dorsal side and a **hypaxial division** on the ventral side. Each developing spinal nerve splits to innervate both areas: a **dorsal primary ramus** to the former and a **ventral primary ramus** to the latter.

KEY FACT

The dilator pupillae and sphincter muscles of the iris originate from neuroectoderm, not mesoderm.

- **Epaxial myotomes** develop into intrinsic back muscles and extensor muscles of the neck and vertebrae.
- **Hypaxial myotomes** develop into limb, abdominal, and intercostal muscles, as well as the following based on location:
  - Cervical myotomes form the prevertebral, geniohyoid, infrahyoid, and scalene muscles.
  - Thoracic myotomes form the flexor muscles of the vertebrae.
  - Lumbar myotomes form the quadratus lumborum muscle.
  - Sacrococcygeal myotomes form pelvic diaphragm muscles.

Muscular Development of the Limbs

Mesenchyme from the myotomes in the limb buds condense into two areas: posterior and anterior condensations.

The posterior condensations form:

- Extensor and supinator muscles in the upper limbs.
- Extensor and abductor muscles in the lower limbs.

The anterior condensations form:

- Flexor and pronator muscles in the upper limbs.
- Flexor and adductor muscles in the lower limbs.

Development of the Diaphragm

The diaphragm arises from several different parts of the developing body cavity; its embryonic components include:

- Septum transversum
- Pleuroperitoneal folds
- Body wall
- Dorsal mesentery of the esophagus

Smooth Muscle

Splanchnic mesenchyme around the primordial gut endoderm develops into the smooth muscle in the gastrointestinal (GI) tract. Somatic mesoderm gives rise to the smooth muscle in the walls of blood and lymphatic vessels.

Cardiac Muscle

Mesenchyme around the heart tube migrates from the lateral splanchnic mesoderm and then develops into cardiac myoblasts. Unlike skeletal muscle, cardiac muscle fibers do not fuse together but rather differentiate and grow as single cells. By week 4 of development, heart muscle can be recognized in the embryo.

Congenital Malformations

Congenital Diaphragmatic Hernia

Incomplete development of the diaphragm, usually a posterolateral defect on the left, allows abdominal contents to herniate into the thorax (Figure 5-8). The lungs are not able to expand fully, resulting in pulmonary hypoplasia and possibly pneumothorax. Poly-hydramnios is often associated with congenital diaphragmatic hernia. Prenatal diagnosis requires MRI or ultrasound evidence of abdominal organs displaced into the thorax.

Prune Belly Syndrome

Abdominal musculature is severely underdeveloped or even absent, most likely due to the involvement of myoblasts in the hypaxial myotomes. **Urinary tract defects** are commonly associated, including tortuous and dilated ureters, prostatic hypoplasia, and a thick-walled bladder. Cryptorchidism is extremely common (Figure 5-9). **Pulmonary**

QUESTION

When abducting the right hip of a first-born female neonate whose presentation was breech, you hear a low-pitched click. When the hips are adducted, you hear a click when applying pressure posteriorly. What do these signs indicate? What is the initial imaging test of choice?

MNEMONIC

Several **P**arts **B**uild **D**iaphragm

Septum transversum
Pleuroperitoneal folds
Body wall
Dorsal mesentery of esophagus

FLASH BACK

Heart muscle (and central nervous system [CNS]) can be recognized in the embryo by 4 weeks of gestation.

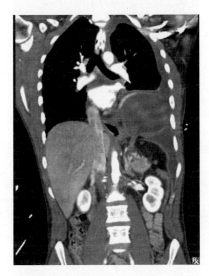

FIGURE 5-8. Diaphragmatic hernia. Coronal CT demonstrates the stomach passing upwards through a discontinuous diaphragm in a diaphragmatic hernia.

ANSWER

The Ortolani and Barlow maneuvers, respectively, indicate possible congenital hip dislocation (developmental dysplasia of the hip [DDH]). It is commonly seen in girls, first-borns, babies born in breech position, families with a history of DDH, and pregnancies complicated by oligohydramnios. The radiologic study of choice is an ultrasound. For infants 6 months or older, an X-ray is most appropriate.

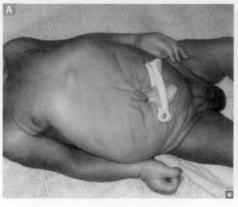
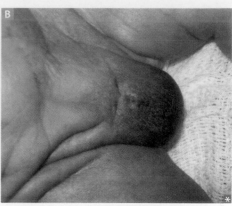

FIGURE 5-9.   **Prune belly syndrome.** **A** Wrinkled abdomen characteristic of prune belly syndrome secondary to absent abdominal musculature. **B** Undersized, underdeveloped scrotum with absent testes (cryptorchidism).

hypoplasia is also seen due to the pressure of the abdominal contents on the thorax. Diagnosis is made with neonatal ultrasound, and treatment includes surgical repair for severe cases.

Poland Syndrome

Uncommon anomaly with complete or partial (often just the sternal head) absence of the **pectoralis major** muscle. There may also be partial absence of the ribs and sternum, mammary gland aplasia, nipple hypoplasia, and absence of the serratus anterior and latissimus dorsi muscles (Figure 5-10). Does not usually cause disability, as the shoulder muscles are able to compensate for the missing muscle.

Congenital Torticollis

The **sternocleidomastoid (SCM)** muscle is either injured at birth or congenitally shortened, such that the infant's head is rotated and tilted in a fixed position. Contraction of one SCM tilts the head ipsilaterally, but due to the attachment of the SCM to the mastoid process posterior to the fulcrum of the head, **rotation is in the contralateral direction** (Figure 5-11). So, if the head is turned **right,** the **left** SCM is involved.

Accessory Muscles

Generally benign, accessory muscles can occur virtually anywhere in the body. One of the more common (about 6% of the population) and occasionally clinically significant cases is an **accessory soleus muscle,** which can cause pain in the posteromedial area of the ankle after strenuous exercise.

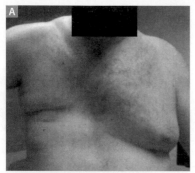
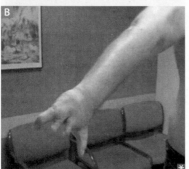

FIGURE 5-10.   **Poland syndrome.** **A** Absence of right breast and right pectoralis major muscles. **B** Right hand symbrachydactyly, often associated with Poland syndrome.

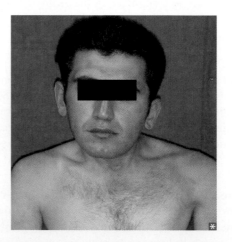

FIGURE 5-11   **Congenital muscular torticollis in a 25-year-old man.**

Anatomy

SKELETAL SYSTEM

Two types of connective tissue make up the skeletal system: bone and cartilage. All bones are made up of an outer layer of **compact** bone and an inner mass of **spongy** bone (mainly replaced by a **medullary cavity**), with different bones having different relative amounts of each. Compact bone is primarily for weight bearing, while the medullary cavity and areas around the spongy bone spicules house the formation of blood cells and platelets (Figure 5-12). Cartilage forms in the areas of the skeletal system where movement is required. Unlike bone, cartilage does not have its own blood supply and receives nutrition via diffusion.

There are two main divisions of the skeletal system:

- **Axial skeleton:** skull, vertebrae, hyoid bones, ribs, and sternum.
- **Appendicular skeleton:** limb bones, shoulders, and pelvic girdles.

Major Bones

Skull

Eight flat bones connected by sutures house the brain, associated blood vessels, cranial nerves, and meninges:

- Frontal bone
- Parietal bones (2)
- Temporal bones (2)
- Occipital bone
- Sphenoid bone
- Ethmoid bone (along with parts of the temporal and occipital bones, makes up the base of the skull)

The major sutures (see Figure 5-5) connecting these bones are as follows:

- Coronal suture: Connects the frontal bone with the parietal bones.
- Sagittal suture: Connects the two parietal bones.
- Squamosal sutures: Connect the temporal bones with the parietal bones.
- Lambdoid suture: Connects the occipital bone with the parietal and temporal bones.

Fourteen bones make up the face of the skull—namely, the orbits, nasal cavities, and jaw (Figure 5-13):

- Nasal bones (2)
- Lacrimal bones (2)
- Zygomatic bones (2)
- Vomer
- Palatine bones (2)
- Inferior nasal conchae (2)
- Maxillae (2)
- Mandible

The inner surface of the cranial base contains three depressions: the **anterior fossa, middle fossa,** and **posterior fossa.** Through each fossa various nerves and blood vessels are transmitted through holes in the skull called **foramina** (Figure 5-14).

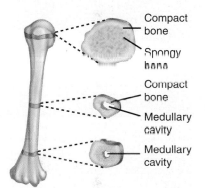

FIGURE 5-12. Humerus with transverse sections. Compact bone, spongy bone, and the medullary cavity are shown.

FLASH FORWARD

The **pterion** is the area where four of the bones of the neurocranium meet: frontal, parietal, temporal, and sphenoid. It is at this structurally weak point that the **middle meningeal artery** is easily ruptured in the event of trauma to the side of the head, **causing an epidural hematoma.**

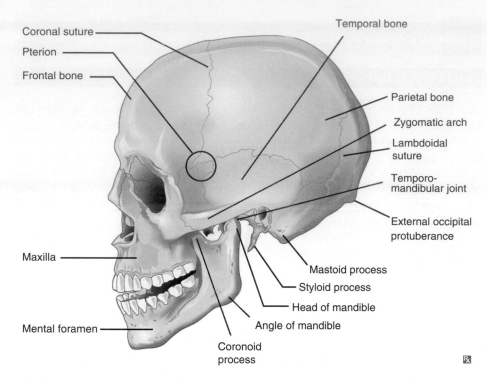

FIGURE 5-13. **Lateral view of the skull.**

Vertebral Column

The vertebral column is made up of 33 vertebrae (Figure 5-15). A typical vertebra has a **vertebral body** anteriorly (to support body weight), a **vertebral arch** posteriorly (made up of pedicles and laminae that serve to protect the spinal cord), and seven processes that serve different functions:

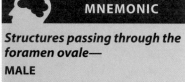

MNEMONIC

Structures passing through the foramen ovale—

MALE

Mandibular nerve (CN V₃)
Accessory meningeal artery
Lesser petrosal nerve
Emissary veins

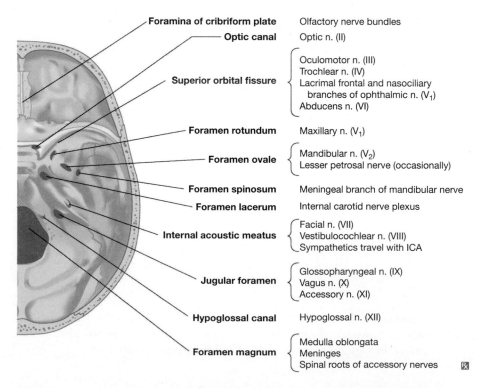

FIGURE 5-14. **Foramina of the skull.** Anatomic representation of the base of the skull with labeled foramen and its contents. ICA, internal carotid artery.

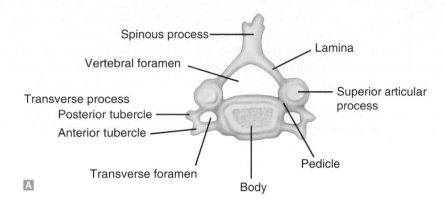

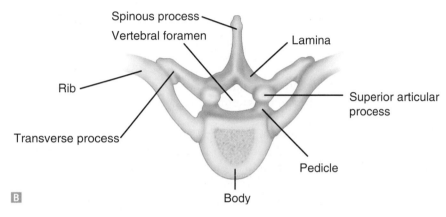

FIGURE 5-15.   **A typical cervical and a thoracic vertebra** A Cervical vertebra B thoracic vertebra.

- The **spinous process** projects posteriorly and allows for muscle attachment and movement.
- The two **transverse processes** project posterolaterally and function like the spinous process.
- Four **articular processes** (two superior, two inferior) project from the same place as the transverse processes but serve to guide some movement as well as prevent anterior movement of the superior vertebrae over the inferior vertebrae.

These 33 vertebrae are divided into five areas, each area with a specific curvature:

- Cervical:
  - C1–C7
  - Secondary curve resulting from the infant lifting its head
- Thoracic:
  - T1–T12
  - Primary curve from fetal development
  - Accentuated **kyphosis**—exaggeration of this (forward) curve—can be due to wedge vertebral compression fractures (from osteoporosis) or endplate and/or disk degeneration
- Lumbar:
  - L1–L5
  - Secondary curve resulting from walking
  - **Lordosis** is an exaggeration of this (backward) curve that can be due to pregnancy, excess abdominal fat, or spondylolisthesis (see below)
- Sacral:
  - S1–S5
  - Primary curve from fetal development
- Coccyx = 4 fused vertebrae

Q   QUESTION

A 15-year-old boy presents after being hit in the head with a bat. His parents report that he was unconscious for about 1 minute after the blow but regained consciousness quickly, and although he seems confused, he is able to talk to you in the ED. After getting the history, you return to your attending, confident this was a simple concussion. As you talk with him, a nurse runs up and informs you that the patient is unresponsive. What is your diagnosis?

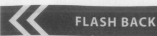

FLASH BACK

Spondylolisthesis is a cause of **lordosis.** It results from the failure of the pedicles to form properly or from stress fractures, which cause one or more of the lumbar vertebral bodies to freely move anteriorly, causing exaggerated curvature.

FLASH FORWARD

Dystocia, or abnormal/difficult labor, can be caused by the inability of the infant to pass through the pelvic inlet. The pelvic inlet may be too small (especially in android and platypelloid shaped pelvis) or the baby too large (macrosomia).

CLINICAL CORRELATION

The **ischial tuberosity** is a landmark for pudendal nerve block (S2–S4 dermatome anesthesia). The injection site is in the pudendal nerve, which crosses behind the sacrospinous ligament medial-inferior to the ischial tuberosity.

The top of the **iliac crest** is a landmark for the L4 vertebrae and is used to identify a lumbar puncture site.

McBurney point identifies the location of the appendix. It falls one-third the length away from the anterior superior iliac spine (ASIS) along an imaginary diagonal line running from the **ASIS** to the umbilicus.

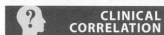

 ANSWER

Alteration in consciousness is often a presenting sign of an epidural hematoma. Patients are usually initially unconscious, recover to what is referred to as a "lucid interval," and then return to an unconscious state. It is crucial to identify these quickly, as rapidly increasing pressure within the brain can result in a herniation with severe neurologic sequelae.

Excessive lateral curvature of the vertebral column is called **scoliosis.** The vertebrae also rotate such that the spinous processes move toward the abnormal curvature. Scoliosis can result from different lengths of the lower limbs, hemivertebra (in which half of a vertebra does not develop), and weakness of intrinsic back muscles on one side (known as myopathic scoliosis). The most common form of scoliosis is idiopathic and may have a genetic contribution.

Between each pair of vertebrae (except the C1–C2 space) is an intervertebral disk that serves as a shock absorber and distributes weight. Each disk is made up of an outer fibrous ring known as the **annulus fibrosus** and an inner gelatinous mass known as the **nucleus pulposus.**

The spinal cord ends most commonly at or just below L1. A lumbar puncture is performed midline between spinous processes L3/L4 or L4/L5 to collect CSF from the subarachnoid space.

Pelvis

The pelvis is made up of the ischium, ilium, and pubis that join to form the **acetabulum,** which articulates with the femur, the sacrum, and the coccyx.

The pelvis is divided into the **greater pelvis** (false pelvis) and **lesser pelvis** (true pelvis) by the pelvic inlet. The **pelvic inlet** is the plane passing through the S1 vertebral body (the **sacral promontory**) and the **terminal lines** (including the pubic crest, iliopectineal line, and arcuate line of the ilium). The **pelvic outlet** is the plane passing through the pubic symphysis anteriorly, the inferior pubic rami and ischial tuberosities laterally, and the coccyx posteriorly.

The greater pelvis is superior to the pelvic inlet and contains abdominal organs such as the ileum and sigmoid colon. It is bound by the abdominal wall anteriorly, the iliac crests laterally, and L5/S1 posteriorly.

The lesser pelvis lies between the pelvic inlet and pelvic outlet. It contains the pelvic viscera (thus making it the "true pelvis") including the urinary bladder, uterus, and ovaries. The pelvic diaphragm lies inferiorly (Figure 5-16).

Upper Limbs

Each upper limb is made up of four basic skeletal segments:

- Pectoral girdle: Scapula, clavicle
- Arm: Humerus
- Forearm: Ulna (medial), radius (lateral)
- Hand: Carpus (Figure 5-17), metacarpus, phalanges

The **axillary nerve** runs along the **surgical neck** of the humerus. The **radial nerve** runs in the **radial groove,** as the name suggests. The **median nerve** runs along the **distal humerus.** The **ulnar nerve** runs posterior to the **medial epicondyle** (making this nerve responsible for the "funny bone" sensation).

Lower Limbs

Like the upper limbs, each lower limb is made up of four basic segments:

- Pelvic girdle: Hip
- Thigh: Femur
- Leg: Tibia (anteromedial), fibula (posterolateral)
- Foot: Tarsus, metatarsus, phalanges

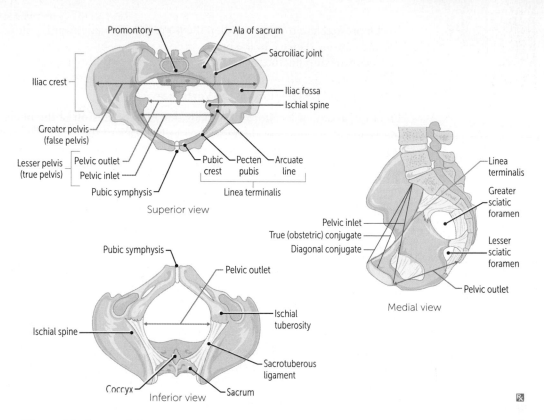

FIGURE 5-16.   **Views of the bony pelvis.**

Common Injuries and Disorders

Fractures of the Skull

There are several different types of skull fractures.

- **Linear** skull fractures are the most common and usually result from blunt trauma.
- **Basilar** skull fractures are usually linear and most often involve the temporal bone. Signs of basilar skull fractures are "**raccoon eyes**" (blood collecting in the orbits), **Battle sign** (blood collecting behind the ears), blood in the sinuses, and CSF leakage through the nose and ears. These fractures often involve the petrous segment of the temporal bone.
- **Comminuted** fractures occur when the bone is broken into several pieces, some of which can lacerate the brain.

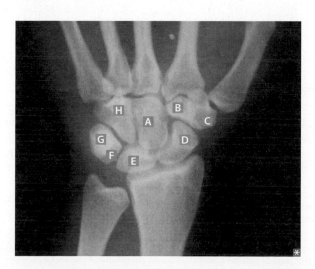

FIGURE 5-17.   **Carpal bones of the wrist. A** Capitate, **B** trapezoid, **C** trapezium, **D** scaphoid, **E** lunate, **F** triquetrium, **G** pisiform, **H** hamate.

QUESTION 1

A 1-year-old girl with a history of deafness presents to the ED with left leg pain. Physical exam reveals blue sclera. Her right leg is tender to palpation and radiographs reveal a right femoral shaft fracture. This is an unusual fracture for a child of her age. Why may it be incorrect to call child protective services?

QUESTION 2

A 20-year-old presents with hand numbness on the dorsal side. He had slept in a chair the night before. He can't extend his wrist, thumb, or metacarpal phalangeal joint. What is the diagnosis?

- **Depressed** fractures occur when the bone is depressed inward, putting pressure on and causing damage to the brain.
- A **contrecoup** fracture occurs at the side opposite of the impact.

Fractures and Dislocations of the Vertebrae

Fractures and/or dislocations are usually due to **hyperflexion of the neck,** often resulting from car accidents or direct trauma to the back of the head. The most common injury is a crush or compression fracture of the vertebral body. Because the articular surfaces of cervical vertebrae are inclined horizontally, anterior dislocations can occur in this region of the spine without concomitant fractures. On the other hand, in the thoracic and lumbar regions, articular surfaces are arranged vertically, so dislocations are usually seen with fractures.

Atlantoaxial Dislocation

The dens of the axis (C2) interlocks with the atlas (C1) through a foramen and is normally held in place by the transverse, alar, and apical ligaments, as well as the tectorial membrane (a continuation of the posterior longitudinal ligament). When trauma or rheumatoid arthritis causes a tear or degradation in the cruciform ligament, the dens may not move in tandem with the anterior arch of C1. This results in instability at the C1-C2 interval and potential posterior subluxation causing cervical cord compression or anterior subluxation resulting in compression of the medulla and respiratory depression.

Herniation of the Nucleus Pulposus

Also known as a "herniated disk" or "slipped disk," the nucleus pulposus actually pushes into or through the annulus fibrosus (Figure 5-18). This commonly occurs at the lumbar level but may occur in the cervical region as well. Posterolateral herniation compresses spinal nerve roots, whereas posterior herniation may compress the spinal cord. Herniated disks can result in weakness which would be seen in the myotome corresponding to the injured nerve root, as shown in Table 5-2.

- In the elderly, degeneration and wear at the posterior longitudinal ligament and posterior aspect of the annulus fibrosus in the lumbar region may allow the nucleus pulposus to herniate. Nerve root impingement at the L5/S1 intervertebral foramen level can result in radiating low back pain down the back of the thigh into the leg to the foot, called **sciatica.**
- Similar injuries in the cervical spine are also very common. **Hyperflexion** of the neck during head-on traffic collisions may cause rupture of the posterior ligaments

ANSWER 1

Osteogenesis imperfecta is often confused with child abuse because of the appearance of multiple healing fractures on radiographs. In addition to fractures, deafness and blue sclera are common signs.

ANSWER 2

This is a radial nerve palsy due to the compression that can occur when a person falls asleep with an arm on a chair back, hence the name "Saturday Night Palsy." Extension at the interphalangeal joints still can be done by the interosseous muscles (innervated by the ulnar nerve).

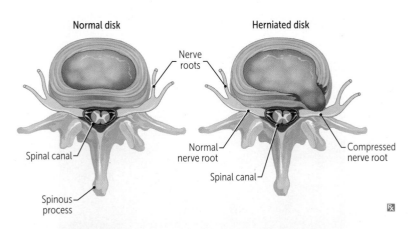

Normal disk / Herniated disk

Nerve roots

Spinal canal

Normal nerve root / Compressed nerve root

Spinal canal

Spinous process

FIGURE 5-18. Herniated disk. Note the tear of the annulus fibrosus and subsequent extrusion of the nucleus pulposus and subsequent irritation of the outgoing nerve roots.

TABLE 5-2.   Quick Lower Extremity Motor Exam

ACTION	MUSCLE	NERVE ROOT	NERVE	REFLEX
Hip flexion	Iliopsoas	L2,3	Femoral/lumbar plexus	None
Knee extension	Quadriceps	L4	Femoral	Patellar
Ankle dorsiflexion	Tibialis anterior	L5	Deep peroneal	None
Ankle plantarflexion	Gastrocnemius, soleus	S1	Tibial	Achilles
Toe plantarflexion	Flexor hallucis longus	S2	Tibial	None

and subsequent nucleus pulposus herniation at the C5–C7 levels, resulting in pain in the neck radiating to the shoulders and arms. Hyperextension of the neck, or **whiplash,** may stretch the anterior ligaments and cause fractures and dislocations of the vertebrae as well.

Spondylolysis

Defect or fracture in the **pars interarticularis** (ie, the part of the vertebral arch lamina that connects the inferior and superior articular processes). Though frequently asymptomatic, it can cause lower back pain at the L5 level. Although genetics probably plays a role, it is thought that repeated microtrauma to this region may cause stress fractures (occurs in gymnasts). If the defects are bilateral, this condition can progress to **spondylolisthesis,** in which the affected vertebra becomes displaced (Figure 5-7) (males more than females). Spondylolysis on plain radiographs is best demonstrated with oblique views of the spine.

Fractures of the Pelvis

May occur from anteroposterior compression, lateral compression, and acetabular fractures.

- Anteroposterior compression (ie, compression between the steering wheel and seat in automobile accidents) results in fractures of the pubic symphysis and pubic rami. These fractures can frequently damage pelvic organs, especially the urethra and/or bladder. Signs of pelvic fracture on exam include pelvic tenderness, palpable instability, and vaginal or urethral bleeding.
- Lateral compression can also involve the pubic rami as well as the ala of the ilium.
- Acetabular fractures can result from falls onto the feet with extended legs, causing the head of the femur to push through (protrusio acetabuli). These fractures are associated with fractures of the femoral neck and pubic rami.

Fractures of the Upper Limb

Fractures can occur at many places along the arm, often with concurrent damage to important arteries and nerves.

- **Clavicle:** The most common mechanism of injury is a fall directly on the shoulder with the arm at the side, as seen frequently in contact sports such as rugby and football. The fracture usually occurs in the middle one-third of the clavicle. The proximal piece is lifted superiorly by the SCM and the distal fragment is pulled inferiorly by the arm. The treatment is usually nonoperative.
- **Greater tuberosity:** Fractures often occur in conjunction with an anterior shoulder dislocation or separation of the shoulder. As such, they are often associated with rotator cuff tears, as three of the four rotator cuff muscles attach here (supraspinatus, infraspinatus, teres minor).
- **Surgical neck of the humerus:** May injure the axillary nerve.

> **KEY FACT**
>
> In the lumbar spine, posterolateral disk herniation impinges the spinal nerve numbered for the inferior vertebrae at that disk level (eg, the L5/S1 disk impinges the S1 nerve). Over 90% of clinically evident herniated disks occur at L4/L5 and L5/S1.

- **Distal half of the humerus:** Fractures of the humeral shaft occur in young patients with high-energy trauma and in low-energy trauma in elderly, osteopenic patients. The radial nerve is at risk, as it runs posteriorly on the humeral shaft along the radial/spiral groove.
- **Humerus, just superior to the elbow (ie, supracondylar fracture):** Most common fracture in children age 5–7, usually occurring as a result of a fall on an outstretched hand. The brachial artery, median nerve (specifically, the anterior interosseous nerve), and radial nerve are all at risk. Volkmann ischemic contracture is the dreaded complication, in which ischemia from brachial artery disruption leads to scar tissue formation and hand and forearm muscle flexion contractures.
- **Medial epicondyle:** Fracture is usually the result of an avulsion injury, which occurs with a fall on an outstretched arm and sudden traction on the flexor pronator muscle group of the forearm. This ulnar nerve is vulnerable in this type of injury, as it runs posteriorly to the medial epicondyle.
- **Distal radius:** Often associated with fractures of the ulna (styloid process). A common finding is a "dinner fork" deformity (dorsal displacement of the bone fragments distal to the fracture). Three primary types include
  - **Colles:** low energy, dorsally displaced fragment, extra-articular.
  - **Smith:** low energy, volarly displaced, extra-articular.
  - **Chauffer:** radial styloid fracture.
- **Scaphoid:** Also usually occurs due to a fall on an outstretched hand. Very little displacement of the bones with pain in the anatomic snuff box (medial border is the extensor pollicis longus [EPL]; lateral borders are the abductor pollicis longus [APB] and extensor pollicis brevis [EPB]; and proximally the radial styloid); often missed on x-rays and misdiagnosed as a sprain. It is often missed because it is a hairline fracture that is not seen initially but can be seen as a sclerotic line on x-ray 7 days later. If there is a high suspicion, an MRI is the most sensitive test in the acute setting. Whereas a sprain can be treated with rest and ice, fractures usually require casting or operative treatment. Improperly treated fractures may progress to a nonunion, avascular necrosis, and early arthritis.

Fractures of the Lower Limb

As in the upper limb, fractures may occur throughout the lower limb.

- **Femoral neck:** Occur most commonly in elderly patients (especially post-menopausal women, malnourished, or men on anti-androgen therapy) after a low-energy fall. Depending on the displacement of the fracture, the blood vessels (primarily the medial circumflex femoral artery) that supply the femoral head can be disrupted, which results in avascular necrosis of the femoral head. On presentation, the lower limb is usually shortened and laterally rotated.
- **Tibial fractures:** Several types of fractures can occur at the midshaft of the tibia. Low-energy fractures are often a result of a torsional (twisting) injury and have diagonal fractures. High-energy mechanisms, such as car accidents and falls when skiing, can result in compound fractures of the tibia and fibula or "boot-top" transverse fractures. Stress fractures are transverse and usually occur in sedentary people who become more active.
- **Pott fracture:** The medial (deltoid) ligament is overly stretched during severe foot eversion. The strong medial ligament does not tear, but causes fractures of the medial malleolus (transverse avulsion) and fibula (oblique at the level of the joint).
- **Fracture of the fifth metatarsal (Jones fracture):** Often occurs in sports with extreme lateral inversion of the foot. This can tear the lateral ligament and fracture the lateral malleolus. The fifth metatarsal is the attachment site of the peroneus brevis.
- **Lisfranc fracture:** Occurs in patients who fall on their foot in a hyper-plantar-flexed position. The Lisfranc ligament, which goes from the base of the second metatarsal to the medial cuneiform, can be disrupted with fractures of those bones or with a tear of the ligament. These are commonly treated operatively because, if left untreated, can result in midfoot collapse.

Coxa Valga and Coxa Vara

The angle between the shaft of the femur and the head of the femur varies among people of different ages and genders. When this angle is large, it is termed **coxa valga** and when it is too acute, it is called **coxa vara**. The latter can lead to a shortening of the leg, making it difficult to completely abduct the leg.

Legg-Calvé-Perthes Disease

Idiopathic avascular necrosis of the capital femoral epiphysis of the femoral head (can be bilateral) that causes decreased range of motion and upper leg pain, typically in male children aged 3–12 years. The cause is unknown. It is self-limited because the bone eventually revascularizes, but the prognosis may be complicated by osteoarthritis (OA).

Slipped Capital Femoral Epiphysis (SCFE)

This condition commonly occurs in obese adolescents during their growth spurt. It can present with hip pain or knee pain referred from the hip. It is due to a weakened epiphyseal plate as a result of acute trauma or chronic microtrauma, which causes the femoral head epiphysis to slowly slip away from the femoral neck, causing a coxa vara. The diagnosis is made by X-ray.

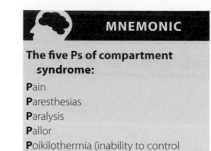

MNEMONIC

The five Ps of compartment syndrome:
Pain
Paresthesias
Paralysis
Pallor
Poikilothermia (inability to control temperature)

JOINTS

Types of Joints

Joints are simply defined as those areas where bones meet. There are three main types of joints: **synovial, cartilaginous,** and **fibrous.**

Synovial Joints

The most common in the body; allow for free movement between the two articulating bones. Lubricating fluid high in hyaluronic acid content known as **synovial fluid** is found between the two bones and facilitates movement. This cavity is enclosed by two structures: **articular cartilage** made from hyaline cartilage (type II collagen) at the surface of the bone ends and a **synovial membrane** that, in conjunction with an outer **fibrous capsule,** makes up the **articular capsule.** The periosteum of the two meeting bones blends together with the articular capsule. These joints are often strengthened by surrounding ligaments, which are especially important when considering common joint injuries.

There are six main types of synovial joints (Table 5-3).

Cartilaginous Joints

Two types of cartilaginous joints exist in the body throughout development. **Primary cartilaginous joints** are typically temporary articulations of bone made up of **hyaline**

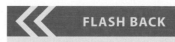

FLASH BACK

The hyaline cartilage in primary cartilaginous joints is made up predominantly of type II collagen.

TABLE 5-3. Types of Synovial Joints

TYPE OF SYNOVIAL JOINT	EXAMPLES	TYPE OF MOVEMENT
Plane joints	Acromioclavicular joint	Gliding in one axis
Hinge joints	Elbow joint	Flexion/extension
Saddle joints	Carpometacarpal joints	Flexion/extension, abduction/adduction, circumduction
Condyloid joints	Metacarpophalangeal joints	Same as saddle joints, with one axis usually greater than the other
Ball and socket joints	Hip joint	Flexion/extension, abduction/adduction, circumduction, medial/lateral rotation
Pivot joints	Atlantoaxial joint	Rotation (pronation/supination as in the radius; rotation of the atlas around the dens in the atlantoaxial joint)

cartilage; these are present during development of the long bones and at epiphyseal plates. **Secondary cartilaginous joints** are made up of **fibrocartilage.** An example of this joint type is the intervertebral disks that join the vertebrae together and allow for limited movement of the spine.

Fibrous Joints

The articulating bones are connected by ligaments or fibrous membranes. Movement in these joints may be limited or nonexistent, depending on the fibrous limitations connecting the bones. Examples include the sutures of the skull, the pubic symphysis, and the joint connecting the radius and the ulna.

Major Joints and Common Injuries

Vertebra

- **Atlanto-occipital:** Synovial joint between the atlas (C1) and the occipital condyles that allows the head to nod "yes."
- **Atlantoaxial:** Synovial joint between the atlas (C1) and the axis (C2) that allows the head to shake "no."
- **Facet joints:** Synovial joints between the inferior and superior articular facets of the spine.

Shoulder

- **Acromioclavicular joint:** A plane type of synovial joint between the lateral end of the clavicle and acromion of the scapula. Despite the strong ligaments keeping it in place, this joint may become separated following a fall onto the shoulder or outstretched arm.
- **Glenohumeral:** Ball-and-socket type of synovial joint between the humeral head and glenoid fossa. Because this fossa is shallow, the humeral head may be dislocated anteriorly or posteriorly. Anterior dislocation may result in damage to the axillary nerve. Posterior dislocations are more rare and are often caused by seizures and electrocution injuries.

Elbow

This hinge-type synovial joint is actually made up of three different joints:

- **Ulnohumeral:** Reinforced by the medial collateral ligament.
- **Radiohumeral:** Reinforced by the lateral collateral ligament.
- **Radioulnar:** Reinforced by the **annular ligament.** A **pulled elbow,** or nursemaid's elbow, may occur when a child is lifted forcibly by the arms while the forearm is pronated. This tears the annular ligament and causes subluxation of the radial head. Pain results from pinching of the annular ligament in the elbow joint, and pronation/supination becomes very limited. The elbow is reduced by supinating the forearm while the elbow is flexed.

Wrist

Radiocarpal joint. A condyloid type of synovial joint between the radius and carpal bones. The most common type of fracture at this site is from a **FOOSH (Fall On Outstretched Hand),** which leads to a **Colles fracture** ("dinner fork" deformity; Figure 5-19).

Hip

A ball-and-socket joint between the femoral head and acetabulum. Fractures involving this area have been discussed previously.

KEY FACT

Force from the hand to the humerus is transferred from the radius to the ulna through the interosseous ligaments, which are oriented in an inferomedial direction to transfer these pulling forces.

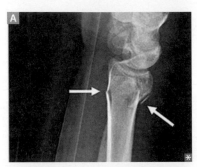

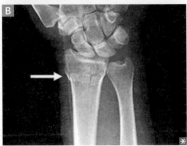

FIGURE 5-19. Dinner fork deformity of a distal radius fracture. **A** Lateral and **B** anteroposterior radiographs of the wrist. The distal fragment of the fracture is displaced dorsally (arrows), giving the impression of a dinner fork.

KEY FACT

Colles fracture involves the distal radius and frequently the styloid process of the ulna as well. Bone fragments are displaced dorsally distal to the fracture, causing what is known as the dinner fork deformity.

MNEMONIC

Varus: Distal end is medial to the joint.
VaLgus: Distal end is Lateral to the joint.

Knee

A hinge-type synovial joint between the tibia, femur, and patella, with multiple associated ligaments.

- **Medially:** The fibrocartilaginous **medial meniscus** is firmly attached to the **medial (tibial) collateral ligament.** Trauma to the lateral side of the knee causing excessive valgus deformity will often result in injury to both of these structures.
- **Laterally:** The **lateral meniscus** is fibrocartilage that is **not** firmly attached to the **lateral (fibular) collateral ligament.** Trauma to the medial side of the knee causing excessive varus deformity may result in injury to the lateral ligament. Tears of the lateral meniscus are less common since it has fewer points of attachment.
- **Anteriorly:** The **anterior cruciate ligament (ACL)** starts at the anterior tibia and extends posterolaterally to the lateral condyle of the femur. This ligament prevents excessive anterior movement of the tibia when the knee is flexed. A tear of this ligament can be demonstrated with a positive **anterior drawer sign,** in which the examiner flexes the knee and pulls on the tibia, causing abnormal anterior displacement. The Lachman test is a test similar to the anterior drawer, which tests for a tear of the ACL.
- **Posteriorly:** The **posterior cruciate ligament** starts at the posterior tibia and extends anteromedially to the medial condyle of the femur; it prevents excessive posterior movement of the tibia when the knee is flexed. A tear can be demonstrated with a positive **posterior drawer sign,** in which the examiner flexes the knee and pushes on the tibia, causing abnormal posterior displacement.

A common sports injury, called the "**unhappy triad,**" occurs when an athlete is hit from the lateral side or suddenly stops with a twist of the knee. The **medial collateral ligament** tears first, followed closely by the **medial meniscus,** and finally the **anterior cruciate ligament.** In this case, one would see abnormal passive abduction (valgus deviation) and a positive anterior drawer sign.

Ankle

Talocrural joint. A hinge-type synovial joint between the ends of the tibia/fibula and the talus. **Inversion** (foot rolls in) results in sprain (tearing) of the **lateral ligament** (**anterotalofibular ligament, ie, ATFL**) (Figure 5-20). Extreme **eversion** (foot rolls out)

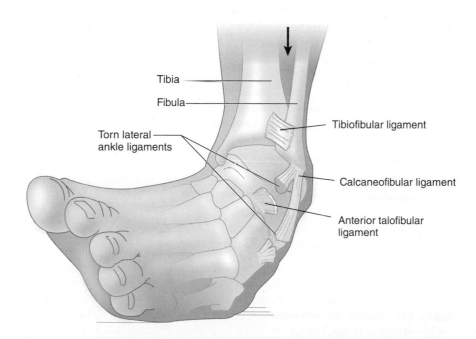

Tibia

Fibula

Torn lateral
ankle ligaments

Tibiofibular ligament

Calcaneofibular ligament

Anterior talofibular
ligament

FIGURE 5-20. **Ligament injury of ankle.** With typical inversion ankle injury, the antero-talofibular ligament is sprained or torn.

places stress on the **medial ligament (deltoid)** and may result in a **Pott fracture** of the fibula and medial malleolus, as discussed previously.

MUSCULAR SYSTEM

Types of Muscle

There are three basic types of muscle fibers that allow the human body to move, as well as provide form and heat: **skeletal, smooth,** and **cardiac.**

Skeletal Muscle

Skeletal muscle is composed of large, elongated, multinucleated fibers that show strong, quick, voluntary contractions.

Most skeletal muscles produce movements of the skeleton and are attached to bone or cartilage either directly or via tendons. There are many exceptions to this, however, such as eye muscles, superficial facial muscles, and the diaphragm. Nerve impulses in the somatic nervous system innervate muscle fibers to cause contraction. This is often under voluntary control, though some skeletal muscles, such as the diaphragm, are under involuntary control.

Though new muscle cells can be formed to a limited degree, the primary growth response (ie, to exercise) is through hypertrophy (increase in size, not number).

Skeletal muscle fibers of humans are classified into three types based on their physiologic, biochemical, and histochemical characteristics:

- **Type I** or slow, red oxidative fibers contain many mitochondria and abundant myoglobin, a protein with iron groups that bind O_2 and produce a dark red color. Red fibers derive energy primarily from aerobic oxidative phosphorylation of fatty acids and are adapted for slow, continuous contractions over prolonged periods, as required, for example, in the postural muscles of the back.
- **Type IIa** or fast, intermediate oxidative-glycolytic fibers have many mitochondria and much myoglobin, but also have considerable glycogen. They utilize both oxidative metabolism and anaerobic glycolysis and are intermediate between the other fiber types both in color and in energy metabolism. They are adapted for rapid contractions and short bursts of activity, such as those required for athletics.
- **Type IIb** or fast, white glycolytic fibers have fewer mitochondria and less myoglobin, but abundant glycogen, making them very pale in color. They depend largely on glycolysis for energy and are adapted for rapid contractions, but fatigue quickly. They are typically small muscles with a relatively large number of neuromuscular junctions, such as the muscles that move the eyes and digits.

Smooth Muscle

Smooth muscle is composed of grouped, mononucleated fusiform cells with weak, involuntary contractions.

Smooth muscle lacks the striations of skeletal and cardiac muscles and is found mainly within the walls of visceral organs and the tunica media of blood vessels.

- Unlike skeletal muscle, their contractions are slow and rhythmic, helping to move food (**peristalsis**) and regulate the flow of blood (**vasoconstriction**), in addition to other functions (**sphincteric activity**).
- Like cardiac muscle, smooth muscle is innervated by the autonomic nervous system, and contraction is involuntary.

ANSWER 1

Compartment syndrome can occur in open and closed tibial shaft fractures, owing to swelling in a compartment enclosed by fascia. Increased pressure presses on muscles, blood vessels, and nerves and blocks further blood flow. Immediate surgery is needed to cut open the fascia and release the pressure in the compartment.

ANSWER 2

A slipped capital femoral epiphysis commonly occurs in overweight adolescents. It usually has a gradual onset but can worsen suddenly with minor trauma. Hip radiographs are best to identify this condition, which often requires surgery.

Smooth muscle cells can undergo hypertrophy (increase in size) and hyperplasia (increase in number).

Cardiac Muscle

Cardiac muscle is composed of irregular branched cells bound together longitudinally by intercalated disks and shows strong, involuntary contractions.

The muscle of the heart (ie, myocardium) is composed of cardiac muscle. The cells are striated and contain a single (sometimes two) central nuclei. Actions of these cells are involuntary but are also under the control of specialized intrinsic pacemaker cells (in the sinoatrial [SA] and atrioventricular [AV] nodes) that are influenced by the autonomic nervous system.

Unlike skeletal or smooth muscles, cardiac muscle cannot regenerate, though hypertrophy can result from increased demand on the heart (ie, hypertension).

Important Muscles

Head and Neck Muscles

Mastication Muscles

There are four main muscles that move the mandible for chewing, all of which are innervated by various branches of CN V_3 (the mandibular branch of the trigeminal nerve):

- **Temporalis:** Elevates and retracts the mandible (closes the jaw).
- **Masseter:** Elevates and protrudes the mandible (closes the jaw).
- **Medial pterygoid:** Elevates and helps (slightly) to protrude the mandible (closing and grinding the jaw).
- **Lateral pterygoid:** Depresses (slightly) and protrudes the mandible as well as moves it from side to side (opening and grinding the jaw).

The main force that opens the jaw is gravity, though the lateral pterygoid as well as suprahyoid and infrahyoid muscles assist.

Muscles with "Glossus" and "Palat"

As a general rule, all of the muscles that end in "glossus" are innervated by CN XII (hypoglossal nerve), and all of the muscles that have "palat" in them are innervated by CN X (vagus nerve). The following muscles follow these rules:

- **Genioglossus:** CN XII; depresses and protrudes the tongue.
- **Hyoglossus:** CN XII; depresses and retracts the tongue.
- **Styloglossus:** CN XII; retracts and elevates the tongue for swallowing.
- **Levator veli palatini:** CN X; elevates the soft palate for swallowing/yawning.
- **Palatopharyngeus:** CN X; tenses the soft palate and moves the pharynx for swallowing.

There is one exception to each rule: The **palatoglossus** muscle, which elevates the posterior tongue *and* brings the soft palate to the tongue, follows the "palat" rule ("palat" is first in palatoglossus) and is innervated by the vagus nerve. The **tensor veli palatini,** which tenses the soft palate and opens the auditory tube during swallowing/yawning, does **not** follow the "palat" rule, but instead is innervated by a branch of CN V_3 (mandibular branch of the trigeminal nerve).

Sternocleidomastoid (SCM)

Attaches superiorly to the mastoid and divides inferiorly into two heads that form attachments to the sternum and clavicle. Contraction of one sternocleidomastoid (SCM) tilts the head to the ipsilateral side, while flexing and rotating the head to the contralateral side. The SCM is important for both anatomic and clinical reasons:

KEY FACT

Smooth muscle is also found at the base of hair follicles (erector pili muscles) and in the iris and ciliary body of the eye.

MNEMONIC

Three muscles CLOSE the jaw (the **M**s **M**unch): **M**asseter, **M**edial pterygoid, and te**M**poralis.
One muscle OPENS the jaw (the **L** Lowers): **L**ateral pterygoid.

MNEMONIC

All muscles that end with **GLOSSUS** (except the palatoglossus—"palat" is first!) are innervated by the hypo**GLOSSAL** nerve.
All muscles with **PALAT** are innervated by the **VAGUS** (except the tensor veli palatini, which is too **TENSE** to be with the rest).

FLASH BACK

The second through fourth branchial clefts usually merge and involute; when the second branchial cleft persists, a fistula can be formed between the pharynx and skin. This fistula is usually located along the anterior border of the upper third of the SCM.

- It divides the neck anatomically into anterior and posterior triangles.
- It is an important landmark for branchial anomalies that may occur during embryologic development.
- Congenital torticollis occurs when the SCM is congenitally shortened or injured at birth, causing a fixed tilted, rotated, and flexed position.
- Spasmodic torticollis (aka "cervical dystonia" or "wry neck") occurs with abnormally increased tone in the SCM. It is often associated with spasms of intense neck pain.

Larynx

Muscles are divided first into extrinsic and intrinsic groups. The **extrinsic muscles** function to **move the hyoid bone and larynx superiorly or inferiorly,** while the **intrinsic muscles** make fine adjustments to the **vocal folds** and **rima glottidis** to aid in speaking, whispering, and respiration.

The extrinsic laryngeal muscles are further divided into **suprahyoid** (mylohyoid, geniohyoid, tylohyoid, digastric) and **infrahyoid** (sternohyoid, omohyoid, sternothyroid, thyrohyoid) muscles. The suprahyoid muscles and **stylopharyngeus** elevate the hyoid and larynx, while the infrahyoid muscles depress these structures.

The intrinsic laryngeal muscles work together to alter the shape and tension of the vocal folds in order to change the size and shape of the space between the folds, called the rima glottidis. Dividing them into functional groups is helpful:

- Adductors (close the rima glottidis for phonation):
    - Lateral cricoarytenoid muscles: Main adductors.
    - Transverse and oblique arytenoid muscles: Adductors and sphincters to protect during swallowing.
    - Aryepiglottic muscles: Sphincters.
- Abductors (open the rima glottidis for breathing): Posterior cricoarytenoid muscles: The **only abductors** of the intrinsic muscles of the larynx (without these muscles, we would be unable to breathe!).
- Tensors (raise the pitch of the voice): Cricothyroid muscles. Both the motor and sensory innervation for these muscles come from above via branches of the superior laryngeal nerve: the external branch for motor and the internal branch for sensory.
- Relaxers (decrease the pitch of the voice, and used for singing):
    - Thyroarytenoid muscles.
    - Vocalis muscles (for fine adjustments).

KEY FACT

In rheumatoid arthritis hoarseness can be the product of synovitis involving the cricoarytenoid joints, in the absence of nerve damage, as these joints are always used in the production of the voice.

Almost all motor innervation of the inner laryngeal muscles comes from **below** via the **recurrent laryngeal nerve** (a branch of the **inferior** laryngeal nerve). Damage to the recurrent laryngeal nerve therefore causes hoarseness (if unilateral), and possible breathing difficulties and aphonia (if bilateral). Damage may occur following surgery, including thyroidectomy or compression or infiltration from cancer.

All sensory innervation comes from **above** via the **internal laryngeal nerve** (a branch of the **superior** laryngeal nerve). Damage to the superior laryngeal nerve therefore causes anesthesia of the laryngeal mucosa. This is dangerous as foreign bodies are more likely to pass, but this nerve is often temporarily blocked in order to pass an endotracheal tube. Laryngeal elevation is the primary mechanism for preventing aspiration during swallowing.

Upper Limb Muscles

Rotator Cuff Muscles

Four muscles collectively known as the rotator cuff muscles help to stabilize the humeral head in the glenohumeral joint while the shoulder moves. Subscapularis inserts onto lesser tuberosity; remaining muscles insert on greater tuberosity.

- **Supraspinatus:** Innervated by the suprascapular nerve; also helps the deltoid muscle to abduct the arm for the first 15°.
- **Infraspinatus:** Innervated by the suprascapular nerve; externally rotates the arm.
- **Teres minor:** Innervated by the axillary nerve; externally rotates the arm.
- **Subscapularis:** Innervated by subscapular nerves; internally rotates the arm.

Arm/Forearm Muscles

The muscles of the arm and forearm are divided into anterior and posterior compartments. Knowing the innervation and actions of these muscles enables clinicians to predict how patients will present following different types of trauma.

The **anterior compartment of the arm** contains three flexor muscles, all innervated by the musculocutaneous nerve:

- **Biceps brachii:** Flexes and supinates the forearm.
- **Brachialis:** Flexes the forearm.
- **Coracobrachialis:** Flexes and adducts the arm.

The **posterior compartment of the arm** contains only one extensor muscle, innervated by the radial nerve: the **triceps brachii**—extends the forearm.

The **anterior compartment of the forearm** contains **pronators** of the forearm and **flexors** of the forearm, hand, and fingers. All are innervated by the **median nerve,** except the flexor carpi ulnaris and the medial part of the flexor digitorum profundus, which are innervated by the **ulnar nerve.**

The **posterior compartment of the forearm** contains **extensors** and **supinators** (with the exception of the brachioradialis, which flexes the forearm). All are innervated by the **radial nerve.**

Medial epicondylitis (golfer's elbow): Repetitive flexion leads to pain in the medial part of the elbow.

Lateral epicondylitis (tennis elbow): Repetitive extension leads to pain in the lateral part of the elbow.

Upper nerve damage is discussed in Table 5-4 and its anatomy described in Figure 5-21.

Thenar/Hypothenar

Thenar muscles control actions of the thumb and are innervated by the recurrent branch of the median nerve (**except** the adductor pollicis, which is innervated by the ulnar nerve):

- Abductor pollicis brevis: Abduction
- Opponens pollicis: Opposition
- Flexor pollicis brevis: Flexion
- Adductor pollicis: Adduction

Hypothenar muscles control actions of the fifth digit and are innervated by the ulnar nerve:

- Opponens digiti minimi: Opposition
- Flexor digiti minimi: Flexion
- Abductor digiti minimi: Abduction

MNEMONIC

Rotator cuff muscles— **SItS**

Supraspinatus, **I**nfraspinatus, **t**eres minor, **S**ubscapularis (small "t" for teres **minor;** also the only rotator cuff muscle not innervated by a scapular nerve).

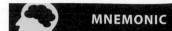

FLASH FORWARD

It may be helpful to review the brachial plexus (in Chapter 6) at this time.

MNEMONIC

THenar muscles for the **TH**umb.

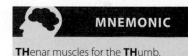

KEY FACT

The adductor pollicis has different innervation than the rest of the thenar muscles (the ulnar nerve instead of the recurrent median nerve).

TABLE 5-4. **Upper Limb Nerve Damage**

INJURY	NERVE AFFECTED	CLINICAL FINDING	ETIOLOGIES
Fracture of the surgical neck of the humerus	Axillary n.	Impaired shoulder abduction (deltoid) and lateral rotation (teres minor); flattened deltoid and loss of sensation over deltoid/lateral arm	Trauma
Shoulder dislocation	Axillary n.	Impaired shoulder abduction (deltoid) and lateral rotation (teres minor); flattened deltoid and loss of sensation over deltoid/lateral arm	Occurs during sports (overhead reaching) and electrocutions
Midhumerus fracture	Radial n.	Wrist drop (triceps is spared because innervation by radial n. is above this area of injury)	Trauma
Radial head dislocation	Radial n.	Wrist drop (triceps is spared because innervation by radial n. is above this area of injury)	Falling on outstretched arm or pulling on child's arm
Bullet shot to anterior biceps	Musculocutaneous n.	Impaired elbow flexion and forearm supination	Trauma
Supracondylar fracture (elbow)	Median n.	Impaired wrist flexion, flexion of digits 1–3, and pronation of the forearm → deficits make "hand of benediction"; can cause interruption of brachial artery and subsequent Volkmann ischemic contracture of the forearm/arm	Fall on outstretched arm
Fracture of lateral epicondyle of humerus	Median n.	Impaired wrist flexion, flexion of digits 1–3, and pronation of the forearm → deficits make "hand of benediction"	
Carpal tunnel	Median n. (superficial branch spared)	Sensory/muscular deficits in digits 1–3, impaired thenar muscles, palm sensation intact	Wrist overuse, obesity, pregnancy, volume overload, synovitis
Fracture of medial epicondyle of humerus	Ulnar n.	Impaired interossei muscles, impaired digit 4–5 flexors and lumbricals, impaired hypothenar; impaired wrist flexion on ulnar side, leading to a claw-hand deformity	
Fracture of hook of hamate	Ulnar n.	Impaired interossei muscles, impaired digit 4–5 flexors and lumbricals, impaired hypothenar	Fall onto hand
Guyon canal syndrome	Ulnar nerve	Clawing of ring and little fingers. Pain and paresthesias in ring and little fingers	Entrapment of the ulnar nerve at the wrist, often seen in cyclists due to pressure from the handlebars
Saturday night palsy	Radial nerve	Wrist drop: loss of elbow, wrist, and finger extension. Loss of sensation over posterior arm/forearm and dorsal hand	Midshaft disruption of radial nerve, either due to compression or fracture of the humerus
Erb palsy	C5-C6 roots	Impaired shoulder abduction (loss of deltoid/supraspinatus), impaired lateral rotation of arm (loss of infrapsinatus), loss of flexion and supination (loss of biceps brachii)	Lateral traction on neck during delivery in infants, trauma in adults
Klumpke palsy	C8-T1 roots	Total claw hand (loss of intrinsic hand muscles; lumbricals, interossei, thenar, hypothenar)	Upward force on arm during delivery in infants, trauma in adults
Winged scapula	Long thoracic nerve	Inability to anchor scapula to thoracic cage so it sticks out (loss of serratus anterior)	Axillary node dissection after mastectomy, stab wounds

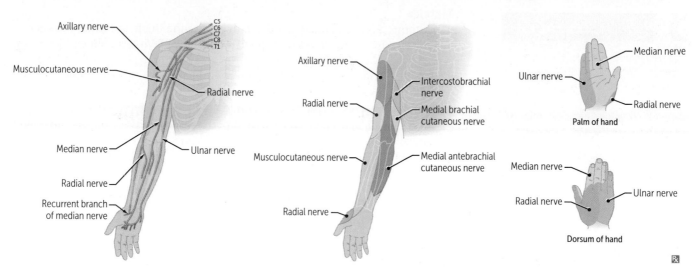

FIGURE 5-21. **Anatomy of brachial plexus and dermatomes of the hand.**

Intrinsic Muscles of the Hand

The intrinsic muscles of the hand include the interossei and the lumbricals. All the interossei and the third and fourth lumbricals are innervated by the ulnar nerve. The first and second lumbricals are innervated by the median nerve.

- Dorsal interossei: Abduct (DAB)
- Palmar interossei: Adduct (PAD)
- Lumbricals: flex metacarpophalangeal (MCP) joint, extend proximal interphalangeal (PIP)/distal interphalangeal (DIP) joints

Lower Limb Muscles

Gluteal Muscles

This region of the body contains two main groups of muscles.

The glutei mainly extend and abduct the thigh and are innervated by the gluteal nerves:

- Gluteus maximus: Inferior gluteal nerve; extends thigh.
- Gluteus medius and minimus: Superior gluteal nerve; abducts and medially rotates the thigh.

The smaller muscles of the gluteal region are covered by the gluteus maximus and help to **laterally rotate** the thigh:

- **Piriformis:** Ventral rami of S1 and S2.
- **Obturator internus:** Nerve to obturator internus (L5, S1).
- **Gemelli superior and inferior:** L5 and S1.
- **Quadratus femoris:** Nerve to quadratus femoris (L5, S1).

Thigh/Leg Muscles

Like the arm/forearm muscles, the thigh and leg muscles are organized into compartments. The thigh muscles are organized into three compartments: Anterior, medial, and posterior; the leg muscles are organized into anterior, lateral, and posterior compartments.

The **anterior compartment of the thigh** contains **flexors of the hip** and **extensors of the knee.** Most of them are innervated by the **femoral nerve,** though there are exceptions noted below. The **femoral artery** courses in this compartment as well.

> **KEY FACT**
>
> In 12% of people, the sciatic nerve splits, and one branch pierces the piriformis. Compression leads to symptoms of sciatica termed **piriformis syndrome,** which is common in mountain climbers who develop hypertrophic piriformis muscles.

- Muscles:
  - Sartorius: Flexes, abducts, and laterally rotates the thigh and flexes the knee.
  - Quadriceps (rectus femoris, vastus lateralis/medialis/intermedius): Flexes hip and extends knee.
  - Iliopsoas: Innervated by ventral rami of lumbar nerves (psoas) along with the femoral nerve (iliacus); flexes the hip.
  - Pectineus: Flexes, adducts, and helps to medially rotate the thigh.
  - Tensor fascia lata: Innervated by the superior gluteal nerve; flexes, abducts, and medially (internally) rotates the thigh, and keeps the knee extended. Becomes the iliotibial (IT) band.
- Artery: Femoral artery.
- Nerve: Femoral nerve, superior gluteal nerve (tensor fascia lata).

The **medial compartment of the thigh** contains the **adductors:**

- Muscles: Adductor longus/brevis/magnus, gracilis, obturator externus (laterally rotates thigh).
- Artery: Obturator artery.
- Nerve: Obturator nerve.

The **posterior compartment of the thigh** contains the **hamstrings,** which are extensors of the thigh and flexors of the leg. From medial to lateral:

- Muscles: Semitendinosus, semimembranosus, biceps femoris (long and short head).
- Artery: Profunda femoral artery, inferior gluteal artery, and the perforating arteries.
- Nerve: Sciatic nerve, common peroneal/fibular (short head of biceps femoris).

The anterior compartment of the leg contains dorsiflexors of the ankle and extensors of the toes:

- Muscles: Tibialis anterior, extensor hallucis longus, extensor digitorum longus, peroneus tertius.
- Artery: Anterior tibial vessels.
- Nerve: Deep peroneal/fibular nerve.

The lateral compartment of the leg contains the ankle evertors:

- Muscles: Peroneus longus and brevis
- Nerve: Superficial peroneal/fibular nerve

The posterior compartment of the leg (superficial and deep posterior) contains the plantar flexors of the ankle and flexors of the toes (exceptions noted below):

- Superficial posterior:
  - Muscles: Gastrocnemius, soleus, plantaris.
  - Artery/Veins: Posterior tibial artery, small (short) and great (long) saphenous veins.
  - Nerve: Sural nerve.
- Deep posterior:
  - Muscles: Flexor hallucis longus, flexor digitorum longus, tibialis posterior, popliteus.
  - Arteries: Peroneal and posterior tibial arteries.
  - Nerve: Tibial nerve.

Nerve Damage Affecting the Muscles of the Lower Limb

- **Piriformis syndrome:** The sciatic nerve enters the greater sciatic foramen very closely related to the piriformis muscle (usually the nerve is inferior to the muscle, though it can occasionally pierce the muscle or run superiorly). Some people who use the muscles in the gluteal region extensively (eg, skaters, mountain climbers, and cyclists) can overdevelop their piriformis muscle, resulting in pinched-nerve, sciatica-like symptoms. Women are more susceptible.

- The **Trendelenburg sign** occurs following damage to the **superior gluteal nerve** (affecting the gluteus medius and minimus), which can occur iatrogenically during an intramuscular (IM) injection to the upper medial gluteal region. To test for this, observe the patient's back while the patient raises each foot off the ground. If the right pelvis falls when the right foot is lifted, the **left** superior gluteal nerve is damaged; if the left pelvis falls when the left foot is lifted, the **right** superior gluteal nerve is damaged.
- Trauma in the femoral triangle region may damage the **femoral nerve**, causing weakened ability to flex the thigh (weak iliacus and sartorius), as well as loss of extension of the thigh (quadriceps femoris muscle).
- Injury to the **tibial nerve** is uncommon in the popliteal region because it runs deep (though deep knife wounds can injure it). Symptoms include loss of flexion of the leg, loss of plantar flexion of the ankle, and loss of flexion of the toes and inversion of the foot. There may also be loss of sensation on the sole of the foot.
- The **common fibular (peroneal) nerve** is the most commonly injured nerve in the lower leg because of its superficial course around the fibular neck, a common fracture site. Damage results in loss of function of all muscles in the anterior and lateral compartments, resulting in inability to dorsiflex the foot, evert the foot, and extend the toes. This is known as a **footdrop**, and the patient will develop a high-stepping gait to compensate. In addition, syphilis and granulomatous disease (eg, GPA) can cause footdrop.
- **Obturator nerve:** Can be injured during pelvic surgery. Results in decreased medial thigh sensation and decreased adduction.
- **Inferior gluteal nerve:** Can be injured in posterior hip dislocations (often seen in unrestrained car accidents). Results in loss of hip extension; hence, the patient reports difficulty climbing stairs and rising from a seated position.

Common Pathology of the Knee

- **Prepatellar bursitis:** Inflammation of the bursa in front of the kneecap. It is referred to as "housemaid's knee" because it is often caused by pressure from constant kneeling. Patients present with pain with activity, swelling in front of the kneecap, and tenderness and warmth to touch.
- **Baker cyst:** Popliteal fluid collection that results from swelling in the knee; often due to arthritis or meniscal tears. Patients do not present with pain but have a large swelling behind the knee. It is important to distinguish between a cyst and a ruptured deep vein thrombosis (DVT). Ultrasound is the gold standard to make the definitive diagnosis.
- **Pes anserine bursitis:** Inflammation of the bursa between the tibia and the insertion of the hamstrings at the pes anserinus. It is usually a result of overuse or constant friction and therefore is common in athletes. Patients report pain with exercising and climbing stairs and will have pain medially 2–3 inches below the knee joint.

Anatomic Landmarks of the Lower Extremity

Diaphragm

The diaphragm separates the thoracic and abdominal cavities and is the most important muscle for inspiration. Important structures pass through the diaphragm at various levels.

- T8: The inferior vena cava (IVC) passes through.
- T10: Esophagus and vagus nerve.
- T12: The aorta, thoracic duct, and azygos vein.

Cervical nerves C3, C4, and C5 make up the somatic **phrenic nerve.** Irritation of the diaphragmatic pleura or peritoneum causes pain that is referred to the shoulder. There are many etiologies including intra-abdominal abscess, fluid (secondary to perforated organ or abdominal trauma), and air (secondary to a perforated organ or following laparoscopic abdominal surgery) near the diaphragm.

MNEMONIC

What muscles insert on the medial tibia via the pes anserinus?
"**S**er**G**ean**T** pes": **S**artorius muscle, **G**racilis muscle, semi**T**endinosus muscle

KEY FACT

What courses behind the lateral malleolus?
Peroneus longus and brevis muscles, small saphenous vein

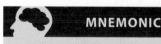

MNEMONIC

I 8 (ate) 10 EGGs AT 12
IVC at T**8**.
T**10**: **E**sopha**G**us and va**G**us.
Aorta/**A**zygos and **T**horacic duct at T**12**.

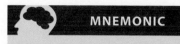

MNEMONIC

C3, 4, 5 keep the diaphragm alive!

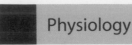

Physiology

MUSCLE TYPES

Skeletal Muscle

Overview

Each skeletal muscle fiber receives neural input from a motor neuron via the **neuromuscular junction.** A single motor neuron and the muscle fiber it innervates are known as a **motor unit.** Large motor units in large muscle groups execute coarse movements (eg, the quadriceps muscles), and small motor units control fine movements (eg, extraocular muscles).

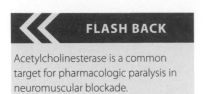

FLASH BACK

Acetylcholinesterase is a common target for pharmacologic paralysis in neuromuscular blockade.

In the synaptic cleft, the action potential (AP) that has propagated along the neuron is transferred to the **myocyte,** or muscle cell. The neurotransmitter **acetylcholine (ACh)** is released from the axonal bouton (Figure 5-22). The myocyte's postsynaptic membrane, known as the **motor end plate,** contains specialized **nicotinic ACh receptors.** These receptors are transmembrane cation channels (Na^+ and K^+) that open when bound to ACh. Activation of these ligand-gated channels results in increased local cation flux, leading to membrane depolarization that is propagated to the nearby **transverse tubule (T-tubule)** system (Figure 5-23). Excess ACh is hydrolyzed by the enzyme **acetylcho-**

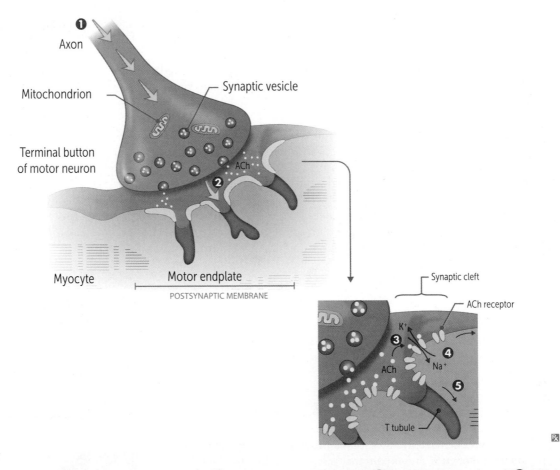

FIGURE 5-22. **Structure of the motor end plate.** ❶ Action potential is generated. ❷ Acetylcholine is released. ❸ ACh binds to postsynaptic receptors (sodium channels). ❹ Sodium ions flow across the plasma membrane. ❺ The flow generates an action potential resulting in muscle contraction.

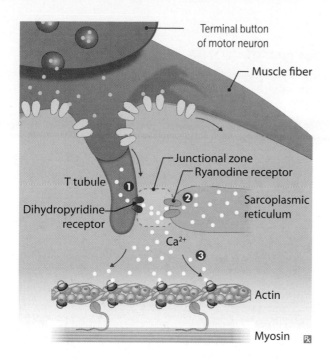

FIGURE 5-23.   Schematic of transverse tubule system. ❶ Action potential depolarizes dihydropyridine receptor. ❷ Ryanodine receptor on sarcoplasmic reticulum opens, releasing Ca^{2+}. ❸ Ca^{2+} binds to troponin on sarcomere, initiating contraction.

linesterase, which resides on the postsynaptic or postjunctional membrane, into acetate and choline. Choline is reabsorbed by the presynaptic neuron, via Na^+-coupled transport, for production of more ACh.

Excitation-Contraction Coupling

Myofibrils are the functional components of contraction. Depolarizations travel along the muscle cell and down the T-tubule (see Figure 5-23). This promotes depolarization of the voltage-sensitive dihydropyridine receptor, which is mechanically coupled to the ryanodine receptor on the sarcoplasmic reticulum (SR). This induces a conformational change that causes Ca^{2+} release from the SR. This increase in intracellular calcium triggers **excitation-contraction coupling** among longitudinally arranged intracellular contractile proteins in the **sarcomere**. Repeating units of sarcomeres comprise **myofibrils** within a single multinucleate myocyte (Figure 5-24).

The sarcomere is the most basic contractile unit. Under light microscopy, it appears as a series of bands and lines (Figures 5-25 and 5-26), spanning the space between **Z lines**.

Each myofibril contains interdigitating **thick** and **thin myofilaments**.

- Thick filaments contain a large-molecular-weight protein, **myosin**, which itself is made of heavy and light chains. The light chains contain **actin-binding sites** and an **ATP** cleavage site.
- Thin filaments have three components:
  - **Actin:** Bound by myosin, it contributes to **cross-bridge** formation that allows for movement of myosin filaments and change in myofibril length.
  - **Tropomyosin:** At rest, this protein occupies potential **myosin-binding sites** on the actin protein, preventing contraction.

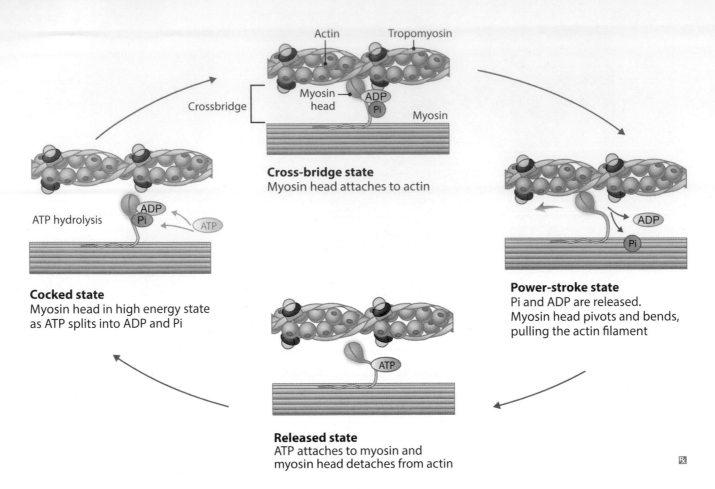

FIGURE 5-24. **Myofibrils and excitation-contraction coupling.** Arrangement of thick and thin filaments in the sarcomere.

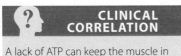

- **Troponin:** Ca^{2+} released from the sarcoplasmic reticulum binds troponin, inducing a conformational change that consequently moves tropomyosin, freeing actin's myosin-binding sites for contraction.

Once tropomyosin uncovers actin's myosin-binding sites, actin binds myosin light chains, creating **cross-bridges.** The myosin light chains pivot, and the myosin heavy chain slides along the actin filament. This event is known as a **twitch** and develops the tension that exerts force (proportional to the number of cross-bridges) during muscle contraction. Returning the pivoted or flexed myosin light chains to their original state requires the cleavage of ATP to ADP + P_i (inorganic phosphate). Once regenerated, the myosin light chain binds a new molecule of ATP for future cross-bridge coupling (see Figure 5-24).

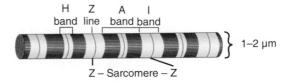

FIGURE 5-25. **Myofibril.**

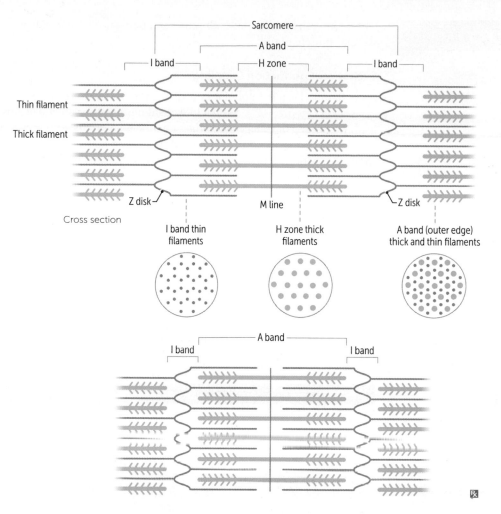

FIGURE 5-26.   **Arrangement of thick and thin filaments in the sarcomere.**

This process continues as long as the cytoplasmic Ca^{2+} concentration remains high. The Ca^{2+}-ATPase functions to ensure Ca^{2+} reuptake into the sarcoplasmic reticulum, thus reducing the cytoplasmic Ca^{2+} concentration. When the calcium concentration has returned to low levels, troponin returns to its original state and tropomyosin again blocks the myosin-binding sites on actin. If a muscle fiber is stimulated repeatedly without allowing sufficient time for Ca^{2+} to reaccumulate in the sarcoplasmic reticulum, the sustained high cytoplasmic Ca^{2+} concentration leads to sustained muscle contraction, or **tetanus.**

Within a given muscle, the maximum force or tension that can be produced is dependent upon the length of the muscle. The tension a muscle is able to produce is proportional to both the number of cross-bridges formed and the number that *could* be formed. At the extremes of myofibril length (very long and very short) either the number of existing cross-bridges or the number of available new cross-bridges is limited, thus reducing the tension the muscle fiber can produce.

Smooth Muscle

Overview

Smooth muscle differs from skeletal muscle in at least three important ways.

- First: Myofilaments are not organized into sarcomeres and do not appear striated.
- Second: Innervation is primarily via autonomic nervous sytem, not somatic.
- Third: Excitation-contraction cascade within smooth muscle differs from that of skeletal muscle.

FLASH BACK

Clostridium tetani induces tetanus via an exotoxin that maintains high intracellular Ca^{2+}.

MNEMONIC

Contraction results in HIZ shrinkage:

H, I, and **Z** bands shorten during muscle contraction, while the

A = Always stays the same length.

KEY FACT

Smooth muscle locations:
- Vasculature (larger than capillaries)
- Airways (larger than terminal bronchioles)
- GI tract
- Urinary bladder and ureters
- Uterus
- Muscles within the eye

These differences allow smooth muscle to perform its functions more efficiently than skeletal muscle could.

Excitation-Contraction Coupling

Smooth muscle lacks troponin. Instead, the protein **calmodulin** acts as the cross-bridging gatekeeper (Figure 5-27). Similar to skeletal muscle, the cascade begins with an AP. This leads to opening of voltage-gated Ca^{2+} channels and an increase in the intracellular Ca^{2+} concentration. Calmodulin then binds Ca^{2+} and activates **myosin light-chain kinase (MLCK),** which in turn phosphorylates myosin. Activated myosin is able to bind and release actin, repeatedly forming and breaking cross-bridges. Like skeletal muscle, each cycle consumes one molecule of ATP.

However, when the Ca^{2+} concentration decreases (again due to a Ca^{2+}-ATPase), and myosin is dephosphorylated via **myosin light-chain phosphatase,** the dephosphorylated form of myosin can still interact with actin via **latch-bridges.** These are residual attachments that allow for the maintenance of tonic tension within smooth muscle without consuming energy. In this way, (unlike skeletal muscle) smooth muscle can maintain tonic contraction without continually cleaving ATP. When combined with **gap junctions,** these capabilities allow smooth muscle to produce the coordinated tonic contractions necessary for aiding digestion, maintaining blood pressure (BP), voiding urine, and accomplishing labor and delivery.

METABOLISM

Cross-bridging of skeletal muscles requires a constant supply of ATP. At rest, muscles may be responsible for 30% of the body's O_2 consumption, while during exercise this number tops off at around 90%. The major energy source that fuels muscle contrac-

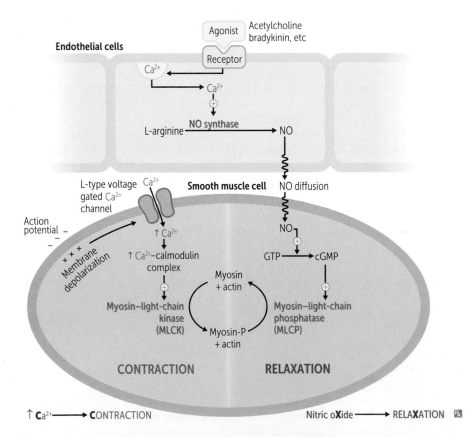

FIGURE 5-27. **Molecular events in smooth muscle contraction.**

tion is **carbohydrate metabolism.** Secondary sources of energy include **fatty acid** and **amino acid metabolism.**

Glucose

In the well-fed state, glucose is readily available to supply the energy needs of muscle. Therefore, simple glycolysis, coupled with the Krebs cycle, can meet the needs of muscles. Following a carbohydrate-rich meal, an increase in the intracellular transport of glucose occurs via insulin signaling. Each glucose molecule is immediately phosphorylated (to glucose-6-phosphate) upon entering the cell and then shuttled into glycolysis.

Glycogen

As the major storage form of glucose, glycogen is essential to **anaerobic glycolysis** in active muscle. The main storage sites of glycogen are the liver and skeletal muscles. Hepatic glycogen sustains the blood glucose level while muscle glycogen provides a readily available source of glucose during muscle contraction.

Regulation of glycogen metabolism occurs on two levels:

- Allosteric enzymatic regulation.
- Hormonal regulation by insulin.

Allosteric Regulation

Glycogen synthase, the enzyme responsible for intramuscular glycogen production, is allosterically favored by increased levels of the substrates of glycogen synthesis, such as glucose-1-phosphate. Simultaneously, **glycogen phosphorylase,** responsible for glycogen catabolism, is inhibited by glucose-6-phosphate and ATP, products of glycolysis and successful glycogen degradation.

In contrast, glycogen degradation occurs in the presence of molecules and messengers of muscle activity. Specifically, increased intracellular Ca^{2+} and **AMP** (a product of ATP hydrolysis) lead to enhanced glycogen phosphorylase activity. Once the muscle relaxes and Ca^{2+} returns to the sarcoplasmic reticulum or AMP is consumed to produce ATP, these effects are lost. The end result is that active muscle sends signals that increase the breakdown of glycogen into glucose, thus increasing available energy substrates.

Insulin Regulation

In the fed state, the body increases serum insulin levels. Specifically, in the liver, insulin depresses gluconeogenesis and increases glycogen production. Within skeletal muscle, insulin increases glucose transport into cells, where it is phosphorylated and enters metabolic pathways ending in ATP production. The absence of insulin exerts opposite effects. In this state, the liver mobilizes glycogen and adipose tissues mobilize fatty acids in order to maintain systemic glucose levels. Within muscles, a decrease in insulin-mediated glucose transport leads to glycogenolysis. More information on insulin's actions can be found in the endocrine physiology section in Chapter 2.

Lipid and Protein Metabolism

In a state of starvation, muscle is able to use fatty acids and ketones for energy. By the third week of starvation, muscle is able to operate almost entirely on mobilized fatty acids.

At the onset of a state of starvation, rapid muscle protein turnover occurs, resulting in the release of amino acids to the liver for gluconeogenesis. As the brain begins to use alternative sources of energy, thus reducing its need for glucose, protein breakdown decreases.

Exercise

During strenuous activity, skeletal muscle's metabolic needs are the greatest. Depending on the intensity of the activity, potential energy sources (glucose, glycogen, fatty acids,

QUESTION

Two days after a marathon and CrossFit competition, a 27-year-old man presents with fever and diffuse muscle pain, tenderness, and swelling. His urine is very dark. His potassium and creatinine kinase levels are elevated. What is the diagnosis?

and protein) are utilized in different proportions. When energy demands are greatest (ie, during sprinting), anaerobic metabolism predominates. Intracellular glucose and glycogen are the primary fuels for rapid energy requirements. In fact, anaerobic metabolism can begin sustaining ATP stores before O_2 delivery to muscle increases. When energy needs are low, however (ie, during walking), oxidation of circulating glucose and fatty acids is favored. This form of metabolism extracts far more energy from fuel (~38 ATP molecules per glucose molecule) and therefore can sustain muscle activity much longer than inefficient substitutes like anaerobic metabolism.

At the onset of aerobic exercise, hepatic glycogenolysis supplies ~40% of the increased energy needed by muscles. In these early stages, there is an exercise-induced translocation of glucose transporter (GLUT) 4 glucose transporters to the muscle plasma membrane. As time progresses, hepatic gluconeogenesis becomes more important in the maintenance of circulating glucose. In fact, resting muscle can transform glycogen stores into lactate for systemic release, leading to hepatic conversion to glucose and redistribution to active muscle.

At later stages of lengthy exercise, glucose use within skeletal muscle decreases and fatty acid oxidation increases from its original ~60% share to provide nearly all of the necessary substrates for aerobic exercise metabolism.

Nutritional Deficiency

Scurvy

Vitamin C deficiency leading to bone disease in growing children and to hemorrhages and healing defects in both children and adults.

Rickets (Children)/Osteomalacia (Adults)

Vitamin D deficiency leading to hypocalcemia and activation of parathyroid hormone (PTH). This causes loss of bone mass in adults (osteopenia) and bowing of the legs in children.

SKIN PHYSIOLOGY

Skin Anatomy

The skin is composed of five distinct layers (Figure 5-28):

- **Stratum corneum:** Most superficial layer, exposed to the outside environment. Dead, dry layer prevents penetration of microbes and dehydration of underlying tissues and provides mechanical protection from abrasion of the more-delicate underlying layers.
- **Stratum lucidum:** Thin layer of skin found on the palms, soles, and digits.
- **Stratum granulosum:** Composed of keratinocytes with, essentially, cells without nuclei or organelles.
- **Stratum spinosum:** Composed of keratinocytes that join via desmosomes. Contains Langerhans cells, which function as macrophages that engulf bacteria, foreign particles, and damaged cells in that layer.
- **Stratum basale:** Single layer of cells that constantly undergo mitosis to produce new cells that push away old cells. Two cell types are found in this layer: Merkel cells, which stimulate sensory nerves, and melanocytes, which produce melanin.

Wound Healing

Tissue repair involves two distinct steps:

1. Formation of granulation tissue via fibroblast deposition of type II collagen, capillary formation, and myofibroblast migration to contract the wound.
2. Fibrous scar formation as type II collagen is replaced with type I collagen.

ANSWER

Potentially life threatening, rhabdomyolysis may be caused by overexertion, crush injury, alcohol abuse, and certain medications. Patients usually present with fever, malaise, muscle pain, and tea-colored urine. Quick identification is important to prevent hyperkalemia (which results in cardiac complications) and acute renal failure.

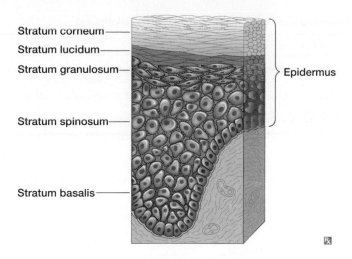

FIGURE 5-28.   **Skin anatomy.**

Important factors in tissue repair and wound healing:

- **Angiogenic growth factors:** Vascular endothelial growth factor (VEGF) and fibroblast growth factor (FGF)
- **Fibroblast growth factors:** Platelet-derived growth factors, transforming growth factor (TGF)-α, TGF-β
- **Copper:** Cofactor for lysyl oxidase, which cross links lysine and hydroxylysine in collagen stabilization
- **Vitamin C:** Cofactor for proline and lysine procollagen residue hydroxylation, which is necessary for collagen cross linking
- **Zinc:** Cofactor for collagenase, which is necessary for the replacement of type III collagen with type I collagen

IMPORTANT LABORATORY VALUES

Several key laboratory values can be used in the diagnosis of musculoskeletal or connective tissue disease. Erythrocyte sedimentation rate (ESR) and C-reactive protein (CRP) are markers of inflammation, including in diseases of autoimmunity. There are also several autoantibodies that are associated with autoimmune disease (see Table 5-5). Creatine kinase (CK) is a muscle-specific protein, and its elevated presence in the blood can indicate muscle injury.

TABLE 5-5.   **Laboratory Values Pertinent to Musculoskeletal and Connective Tissue Disorders**

LAB TEST	ABBREVIATION	MARKER FOR . . .
Erythrocyte sedimentation rate	ESR	Systemic inflammation
Creatine kinase	CK	Muscle injury
CK isoenzyme (myocardial bound)	CK-MB	Cardiac injury or regenerating muscle
Antineutrophil cytoplasmic antibody (ANCA)	c-ANCA (cytoplasmic)	Granulomatosis with polyangiitis (Wegener granulomatosis)
	p-ANCA (perinuclear)	Microscopic polyangiitis, Churg-Strauss vasculitis **or** focal necrotizing and crescentic glomerulonephritis
C-reactive protein	CRP	Direct marker for systemic inflammation

(continues)

TABLE 5-5. Laboratory Values Pertinent to Musculoskeletal and Connective Tissue Disorders *(continued)*

LAB TEST	ABBREVIATION	MARKER FOR . . .
Antinuclear antibody	ANA	Nonspecific; numerous autoimmune diseases and falsely positive in 5–10%
Rheumatoid factor	RF	Rheumatoid arthritis and other autoimmune and chronic inflammatory diseases; falsely positive in 5–10%
Anticyclic citrullinated peptide	Anti-CCP	Rheumatoid arthritis
Alkaline phosphatase	ALP	Bone turnover (therefore, increased in osteopetrosis, osteomalacia/rickets, osteitis fibrosa cystica, Paget disease)
Serum calcium	Ca^{2+}	Disordered calcium homeostasis
Parathyroid hormone	PTH	Parathyroid gland function
Parathyroid hormone-related peptide	PTHrP	Protein secreted by neoplastic cells, mimics PTH; its activity may lead to disordered calcium and/or phosphate homeostasis

Pathology

SKELETAL ONCOLOGY

Bone tumors can be classified as either primary tumors, which derive from bone tissue, or secondary tumors, which represent metastases from another organ system. Secondary tumors are far more common. Prostate, breast, and lung carcinomas account for 80% of bony metastases. The majority of these metastases spread hematogenously; rarely, however, these cancers can invade through local infiltration. Bony metastases can be further characterized as causing lesions that are **osteolytic, osteoblastic,** or both. Osteolytic lesions cause bone destruction by activating osteoclasts, usually through **parathyroid hormone-related peptide (PTHrP)** or through cytokines like interleukin-1 (IL-1) and tumor necrosis factor-alpha (TNF-α). Conversely, osteoblastic tumors stimulate the increased production of new bone tissue.

PRESENTATION

Although they are often **asymptomatic,** bony metastases may present with pain (from sweeping, nerve compression, or pathologic fracture). Marrow infiltration by lymphomas can present with symptoms of bone marrow suppression known as **myelophthisis.** Pain usually develops gradually over several weeks and is most intense at night, often waking the patient. Sudden onset of severe pain may indicate pathologic fracture. If neurologic symptoms such as numbness, weakness, or radiculopathy accompany back pain, an emergent spinal cord and cauda equina compression.

DIAGNOSIS

All patients should be screened with plain films and serum calcium levels. Osteolytic lesions > 1 cm in size, common with metastatic renal cancer, can regularly be detected with plain radiographs and often cause **hypercalcemia.** Osteoblastic lesions, commonly seen in breast and prostatic metastases, are best detected with radionucleotide bone scans, which will show increased uptake. In these instances, plain films may reveal focal sclerosis. These patients often have increased serum **alkaline phosphatase** levels and, if disease is widespread, hypocalcemia. Potential compressive lesions in the spine are best evaluated by MRI.

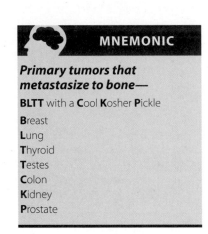

MNEMONIC

Primary tumors that metastasize to bone—

BLTT with a **C**ool **K**osher **P**ickle

Breast
Lung
Thyroid
Testes
Colon
Kidney
Prostate

KEY FACT

The three most common bony sites for metastases (in descending order):
- Vertebrae
- Proximal femur
- Pelvis

TREATMENT

The therapeutic approach depends on the source of the underlying malignancy and symptomatology. Bisphosphonates, agents that inhibit osteoclast function, are adjuvant medications used to preserve bone health and relieve pain. Severe bone pain in the terminal stages of cancer is very common, and adequate attention to pain symptoms may require relatively high doses of narcotic analgesics to maintain patient quality of life. Pain from bone cancer is one of the most difficult types of pain to treat and should never be neglected.

PROGNOSIS

Overall survival varies greatly, depending on the primary diagnosis.

Primary Neoplasms

Primary bone neoplasms can be classified as benign or malignant, and each tumor type has a characteristic location and morphology (Figure 5-29).

Benign

There are five important primary benign tumors of bone (Table 5-6):

- **Giant-cell tumor:** Benign tumor composed of spindle-shaped cells with multinucleated giant cells (osteoclasts). It is most commonly found at epiphyseal ends of long bones, such as the distal femur or proximal tibia. The peak incidence is in females between the ages of 20 and 40 years. It carries a distinct histologic appearance (Figure 5-30) and has a characteristic "soap-bubble" radiographic appearance.
- **Enchondroma:** Benign cartilage cyst found within the bone marrow, often affecting the smaller bones of the hands and feet. Multiple lesions can occur in patients with enchondromatosis (Ollier disease). On plain film, this tumor appears as a lytic area in the bone marrow with stippled calcification. On MRI, this tumor has a popcorn appearance.

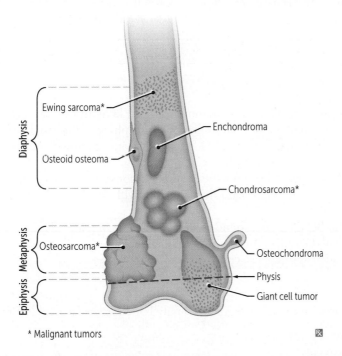

Diaphysis
- Ewing sarcoma*
- Enchondroma
- Osteoid osteoma

Metaphysis
- Chondrosarcoma*
- Osteosarcoma*
- Osteochondroma
- Physis

Epiphysis
- Giant cell tumor

* Malignant tumors

FIGURE 5-29. **Diagram of primary bone tumors.** Primary tumors of the bone occur at characteristic locations and have typical morphological appearances. Note the "soap bubble" appearance of giant cell tumors; marrow cavity location of endochondromas; cartilage cap of osteochondromas; central nidus of osteoid osteomas; central location of malignant chondrosarcomas; "onion skin" periosteal reaction of Ewing sarcomas; and lifting of the cortex in osteosarcomas.

TABLE 5-6.   Common Bone Tumors

TYPE	EPIDEMIOLOGY	LOCATION	DESCRIPTION
Benign			
Giant-cell tumor	Females 20–40 years of age	Epiphysis of distal femur and proximal tibia	Locally aggressive; multinucleated giant-cell tumor "Soap-bubble" appearance on radiograph
Enchondroma	No special incidence	Small distal bones of hands and feet	Risk for chondrosarcoma Can have multiple tumors
Osteochondroma	Most common benign tumor Males < 25 years of age	Long bones; especially metaphysis of the distal femur	Outgrowth of mature bone capped by benign cartilage
Osteoid osteoma	Males < 25 years of age	Cortex of long bones	Central nidus surrounded by sclerotic bone tissue
Osteoma	Males of any age	Facial bones and skull	Associated with Gardner syndrome (FAP) Mature bone continues growing on itself
Osteoblastoma	Males < 25 years of age	Vertebral column	Similar to osteoid osteoma except for location
Malignant			
Chondrosarcoma	Men 30–60 years of age	Pelvis, proximal femur	Malignant cartilage tumor May be primary or from osteochondroma Metastasizes to lungs
Ewing sarcoma	Males < 15 years of age	Pelvis and long bones	Anaplastic small blue-cell tumor "Onion-skin" appearance of bone on plain film Associated with 11;22 translocation
Osteogenic sarcoma (osteosarcoma)	Most common primary bone tumor Males 10–20 years of age and adults > 65 years Risk factors: Paget disease, familial retinoblastoma, irradiation	Metaphysis of distal femur and proximal tibia	Malignant osteoid formation "Sunburst" appearance on radiograph from elevation of periosteum

FAP, familial adenomatous polyposis.

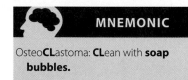

MNEMONIC

Osteo**CL**astoma: **CL**ean with **soap bubbles.**

- **Osteochondroma:** The most common benign bone tumor, usually occurring in young males. It often arises from the long metaphysis of the distal femur. On plain film, the tumor appears as a cartilage-capped bony outgrowth. Malignant transformation to chondrosarcoma is rare.
- **Osteoid osteoma:** A benign bone-forming tumor seen in adolescent males. It typically presents with night pain that improves with nonsteroidal anti-inflammatory drug (NSAID) use.
- **Osteoma:** Benign tumor found in the facial bones of males. There is a strong association with Gardner syndrome (familial adenomatous polyposis with extracolonic tumors, such as osteomas, epidermal cysts, and fibromas).

Malignant

There are three important malignant primary bone tumors (see Table 5-6):

- Chondrosarcoma
- Ewing sarcoma
- Osteosarcoma

Chondrosarcoma

One-quarter of all bone sarcomas are chondrosarcomas, with a peak incidence in the fourth to sixth decades. Primarily arising in flat bones like the shoulder and pelvic girdle,

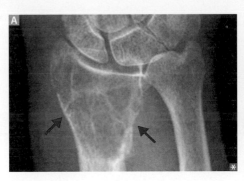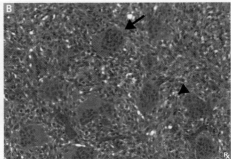

FIGURE 5-30.   **Giant-cell tumor pathology.** A Radiograph of a giant-cell tumor at the proximal head of the tibia. Bone destruction by this locally aggressive tumor causes the classic "soap bubble" appearance on X-ray. B Histology of giant-cell tumor of bone, showing osteoclast-like giant cells (arrow) and small spindle cells (arrowhead).

these tumors typically develop de novo by sporadic mutation. Rarely, they deviate from this pattern and appear in the diaphyses of long bones or arise by malignant transformation of enchondromas or osteochondromas.

PRESENTATION

Like other bone sarcomas, pain and swelling are the principal symptoms. New-onset pain, inflammation, and/or a gradually growing mass, especially in the scapula or pelvis, are commonly associated with this tumor.

DIAGNOSIS

Radiography reveals a lobular mass with mottled, punctate, or annular calcifications of the cartilaginous matrix.

TREATMENT

Surgical resection is the mainstay of therapy, as nearly all chondrosarcomas are resistant to chemotherapy.

PROGNOSIS

Chondrosarcomas follow an indolent course, eventually metastasizing to the lungs if not treated.

Ewing Sarcoma

Comprising only 10–15% of bone sarcomas, this anaplastic blue-cell tumor has its peak incidence in adolescents. The underlying genetic abnormality is expression of the **EWS-FLI1** fusion gene, resulting from a **t(11;22) translocation.** This genetic abnormality is often found in other primitive neuroectodermal tumors (PNETs), the family of tumors to which Ewing sarcoma belongs.

PRESENTATION

Most often found in diaphyses of long bones, pelvis, scapula, or ribs. Patients can complain of fever and anemia.

DIAGNOSIS

Radiography reveals a characteristic **"onion-peel"** periosteal reaction with a soft tissue mass. Pathologic examination uncovers sheets of small, round, undifferentiated blue cells (Figure 5-31) that can be confused with lymphoma or small-cell carcinomas.

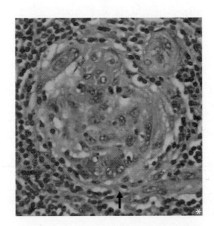

FIGURE 5-31.   **Histology of Ewing sarcoma.** Small blue cells typical of Ewing sarcoma, with a high nucleus-to-cytoplasm ratio and increased mitotic rate. Necrosis (arrow, pink area) is observed in the center of these tumors.

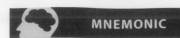

TREATMENT

The foundation of treatment is systemic chemotherapy to shrink the size of the tumor, followed by surgery.

PROGNOSIS

This condition is very aggressive and is treated as a systemic disease due to the high probability of early metastases. Common sites of metastasis include the lungs and other bones. Patients with disease of the distal extremities have a 5-year survival rate of 80%.

Osteosarcoma

The most common primary bone malignancy, this cancer results in the production of unmineralized bone (**osteoid**) and is therefore also known as **osteogenic sarcoma** (Figure 5-32). Osteosarcoma occurs in a bimodal age distribution and is most commonly found in male adolescents and the elderly. Tumors that occur late in life are often secondary to predisposing risk factors such as radiation exposure, familial retinoblastoma, or benign transformation (as in Paget disease). These tumors often metastasize to the **lungs.**

PRESENTATION

Osteosarcoma has an affinity for the metaphysis of long bones, specifically the distal femur, proximal tibia, and proximal humerus. Patients usually complain of pain and swelling of the affected region.

DIAGNOSIS

A plain film reveals osteolysis with a "moth-eaten" appearance and a periosteal "sunburst" reaction. New bone formation at the margin of the soft tissue mass leads to elevation of the periosteum known as the characteristic **Codman triangle.** Chest radiography and CT are employed to rule out lung metastases, whereas a bone scan can uncover bony metastases.

TREATMENT

Preoperative chemotherapy, limb-sparing surgery, and postoperative chemotherapy are the usual regimen.

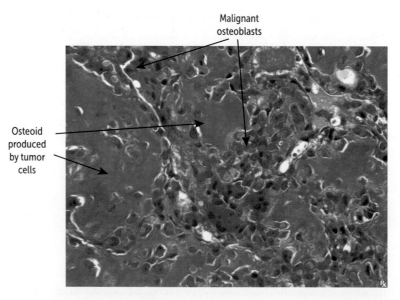

FIGURE 5-32. Histology of malignant osteosarcoma. Histology showing small malignant osteoblastic cells surrounded by osteoid, which appears as a homogeneous material between the malignant cells.

PROGNOSIS

The most important prognostic indicator is response to chemotherapy. Long-term survival in extremity sarcoma lies in the range of 60–80%.

NONONCOLOGIC MUSCULOSKELETAL DISEASE

Osteoporosis

The primary pathology of osteoporosis is a reduction of bone mass in spite of normal bone mineralization. Osteoporosis is defined by the World Health Organization as a reduction in bone mass of ≥ 2.5 standard deviations below the mean for young, healthy females. This measure, also known as a **T-score,** is clinically useful because it correlates with fracture risk as a sequela of reduced bone density. Risk factors for osteoporosis include increasing age, female gender, history of fractures, low body mass index, family history, poor calcium intake, steroid use, and smoking.

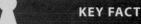

KEY FACT

T-score classifications:
≤ 2.5 to −1.0 = Low bone density (osteopenia), with an increased risk for osteoporosis
−1.0 to 1.0 = Normal

Bone density maintenance is a balance between bone deposition (osteoblastic activity) and resorption (osteoclastic activity). These two opposing components of **bone remodeling** serve to repair microfractures, maintain skeletal strength, and regulate serum calcium levels. However, any factor favoring resorption over deposition leads to an overall loss in bone mass.

Several key hormones influence the remodeling process:

- **Estrogens:** Deficiency results in increased osteoclast differentiation and activity, leading to increased rates of resorption. Postmenopausal women have significantly decreased estrogen levels and thus are at much higher risk for osteoporosis.
- **Vitamin D:** The active form, 1,25-dihydroxyvitamin D, is produced by coordinated chemical modifications in the skin, liver, and kidney. It increases GI absorption of dietary calcium. Adequate vitamin D intake (by dietary supplements if necessary) is an important component of both osteoporosis treatment and prevention.
- **PTH:** PTH increases bone resorption and reduces renal calcium excretion in order to raise serum calcium levels. PTH also causes increased phosphate excretion in the urine.
- **Thyroid hormone:** Hyperthyroidism is associated with increased bone loss.
- **Locally produced growth factors:** These include insulin-like growth factors (IGFs), ILs, transforming growth factor beta (TGF-β), and PTHrP.

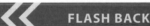

FLASH BACK

Parathyroid hormone–related protein (PTHrP) is secreted by several types of cancer and mimics the function of PTH, causing increased bone resorption and hypercalcemia of malignancy.

PRESENTATION

Reduced bone density does not produce specific symptoms; therefore, osteoporosis is often undetected until the patient fractures an affected bone. For this reason, the physician's index of suspicion must be elevated, especially in elderly women. **Bone mineral density (BMD)** should be determined in all postmenopausal women with risk factors or all women aged **65 and older.** Extra vigilance should be practiced with anyone at increased risk for falls (eg, impaired strength, coordination, or mentation), which are the most common precipitants of fracture.

Older patients who present with sudden-onset back pain may have suffered a vertebral compression fracture (Figure 5-33). These patients may also show loss of height and kyphosis. Hip fractures typically fit a history of a recent fall with pain and weakness in the affected hip and the inability to bear weight. Distal radius (Colles) fractures are also common.

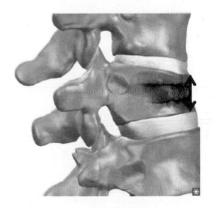

FIGURE 5-33. **Vertebral compression fracture.**

DIAGNOSIS

Dual-energy X-ray absorptiometry (DEXA) scans have become the most popular method of measuring bone density, although quantitative CT provides helpful information regarding vertebral trabecular bone. Typically, DEXA scans of the hip and lumbar spine define clinical BMD measures. If BMD is reduced, modifiable risk factors should be sought and treated appropriately.

TREATMENT

When osteoporosis is discovered, a variety of therapies are available. First, calcium and vitamin D deficiencies should be corrected, and if possible, moderate weight-bearing exercise should be incorporated into the patient's lifestyle.

Bisphosphonates (alendronate, ibandronate, risedronate, and zoledronic acid) are chemical analogs of pyrophosphate and act to reduce osteoclast number and function, allowing the balance between bone deposition and resorption to be restored. **Denosumab** is a monoclonal antibody against receptor activator of nuclear factor $\kappa\beta$ ligand (RANKL), a protein that promotes osteoclast activity, and can be offered as an alternative option. **Calcitonin** and the recombinant human PTH-analog teriparatide both have anabolic effects on bone, but are typically reserved for patients at a very high risk for fracture or who have failed treatment with a bisphosphonate.

For postmenopausal women, estrogen replacement therapies can be effective. However, they carry increased risks for cardiovascular disease, stroke, deep vein thrombosis, and breast cancer, and these possible risks must be weighed against the benefits for each patient. Alternatively, **selective estrogen receptor modulators (SERMs)** are available. These medications (**tamoxifen** and **raloxifene**) activate estrogen receptors on bone but act as partial agonists or antagonists on other estrogen tissues, somewhat reducing the risks associated with hormone replacement therapy.

PROGNOSIS

Disease progression depends greatly on severity at diagnosis and intensity of intervention. Most patients can do well, though risk increases with age.

Osteopetrosis (Marble Bone Disease)

Marble bone disease refers to a class of disorders sharing the common feature of defective osteoclastic bone resorption, leading to abnormally dense and fragile bone. The infantile form of the disease is more severe and arises from autosomal recessive mutations, while the less-severe adult forms are autosomal dominant. Several mutations have been linked to osteopetrosis, including one notable genetic defect involving mutations in carbonic anhydrase II. Deficiency of this enzyme prevents osteoclasts from producing carbonic acid for bone dissolution, and it also results in renal tubular acidosis due to decreased bicarbonate reabsorption.

PRESENTATION

Infantile osteopetrosis usually presents early in life with delayed growth, frequent fractures, and other sequelae of abnormal bone production. The failure in bone remodeling can lead to cranial nerve paralysis due to foraminal narrowing. Inadequate marrow space can lead to pancytopenia with extramedullary and splenic hematopoiesis. The adult forms are typically discovered incidentally by radiography during evaluation of a fracture, but can also present with complications such as deafness (due to compression of cranial nerve VIII) and osteomyelitis.

Due to a carbonic anhydrase II mutation, renal tubular acidosis also occurs, because there is a decrease in tubular HCO_3^- reabsorption.

DIAGNOSIS

Radiographic changes indicative of increased thickness of both cortical and trabecular bone include:

- Thickened cranium.
- Decreased size of paranasal and mastoid sinus cavities.
- Bone-in-bone appearance (endobone; Figure 5-34).
- Alternating bands of lucency and sclerosis.

TREATMENT

The infantile form is best treated with HLA-matched bone marrow transplantation to repopulate functional osteoclast progenitors (of the monocyte lineage). The adult form, if mild, requires no specific therapy.

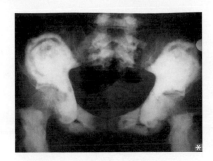

FIGURE 5-34. **Osteopetrosis (marble bone disease).**

Osteomalacia/Rickets

Calcium and vitamin D deficiencies result in hypocalcemia and hypophosphatemia, leading to impaired bone mineralization. Alternatively, chronic hypophosphatemia due to renal phosphate wasting can trigger osteomalacia. The key feature is a poorly mineralized bone matrix that is mechanically inferior to normal bone. In children, vitamin D deficiency leads to similar impairments in osteoid mineralization in a condition called **rickets.**

PRESENTATION

The defective bone mineralization in osteomalacia can result in diffuse bone pain and increased fractures. Due to the importance of vitamin D in maintaining muscle function, patients may present with decreased muscle tone, weakness, and abnormal gait. Children with rickets, in addition to these symptoms, may present with a variety of skeletal deformities. These include bowed legs, rachitic rosary (bead-like osteoid deposits on ribs), and pigeon breast (forward protrusion of sternum).

DIAGNOSIS

A serum 25-hydroxyvitamin D level < 15 ng/mL is associated with hypocalcemia and increased serum PTH. The elevated PTH causes increased bone resorption and decreased serum phosphate levels. Alkaline phosphatase levels are often elevated due to the increased activity of osteoblasts attempting to compensate for poor bone formation.

Radiologically, thinned cortical bone and widespread lucency are apparent. In addition, pseudofractures—radiolucent lines having the appearance of a fracture but lacking any clinical signs—are common in the scapula, pelvis, and femoral neck.

TREATMENT

Supplementation with vitamin D and calcium is integral, though therapy should certainly address the underlying disorder (eg, poor dietary intake, poor vitamin D absorption due to celiac sprue). If renal vitamin D activation is impaired, active forms of vitamin D must be given. If the patient is taking medications that increase vitamin D metabolism or lead to resistance, pharmacologic rescue doses (> 5000 IU for 3–12 weeks) may be required.

Paget Disease of Bone

Paget disease, also known as osteitis deformans, is a bone remodeling disorder characterized by increased osteoclastic and osteoblastic activity, leading to regions of high bone turnover. These lesions go through several sequential stages:

- **Lytic stage:** First, an area of normal bone accumulates abnormal osteoclasts that dissolve bone at accelerated rates.
- **Mixed stage:** Osteoblasts are activated to replace bone tissue, and now osteoclasts and osteoblasts act in rapid cycles of bone resorption and deposition.
- **Sclerotic stage:** Osteoblast-mediated bone formation becomes the dominant process, but this new bone is deposited in a disorganized manner.

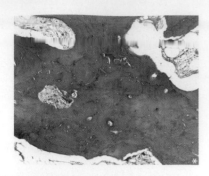

FIGURE 5-35. **Paget disease of bone.** H&E-stained micrograph shows thickened trabeculae with characteristic mosaic pattern.

■ **Quiescent stage:** Cell activity "burns out," and bone metabolism diminishes to a minimum.

The result of all this activity is to leave behind a disorganized mosaic of woven and lamellar bone that is weaker than normal bone.

PRESENTATION

The majority of patients with Paget disease are not symptomatic, and the condition is usually discovered incidentally based on abnormal laboratory values. Those with symptoms will often have bone pain, arthritis, or increased fractures, with the skull, spine, and long bones being the most common sites. Skull involvement can lead to hearing loss or cranial deformities, which may present simply as a change in hat size (Figure 5-35). Patients with extensive Paget disease may also develop **high-output heart failure** due to increased bone vascularity and formation of arteriovenous shunts. Rarely, a lesion will progress to a tumor, typically an **osteosarcoma** or fibrosarcoma.

DIAGNOSIS

Serum **alkaline phosphatase** levels are almost always elevated, and the degree of elevation can be used as a measure for the extent and intensity of disease. Notably, calcium, phosphate, and PTH levels are all normal. Radiographic images will have various findings depending on the stage of the bone lesions. During the early stages, lesions may appear as lytic, while bone in later stages may display cortical thickening. Bone scanning can also be helpful in identifying active lesions.

TREATMENT

Patients with symptomatic or active Paget disease are usually treated with **bisphosphonates,** which act to inhibit the osteoclasts that begin the cycles of bone turnover. Calcium and vitamin D should be supplemented to prevent bisphosphonate-induced hypocalcemia. Surgery may be indicated in cases of bone deformity or cancer.

Osteitis Fibrosa Cystica

A result of unchecked hyperparathyroidism, osteitis fibrosa cystica (also known as von Recklinghausen disease of bone) is marked by localized areas of excessive bone resorption that create cyst-like defects in the bone. These cystic spaces often contain disorganized osteoid stroma and old blood, earning them the name "brown tumors." Although osteitis fibrosa cystica can result from primary hyperparathyroidism, it is particularly common among patients with secondary hyperparathyroidism due to end-stage renal disease (ESRD).

PRESENTATION

Patients may experience bone pain or tenderness, bowing of bones, and pathologic fractures.

DIAGNOSIS

In patients with disease due to primary hyperparathyroidism, serum calcium is elevated and phosphate is decreased, whereas calcium is decreased and phosphate increased among those with secondary hyperparathyroidism. Alkaline phosphatase is elevated in both types. Radiographic examination will reveal well-demarcated lytic lesions corresponding to the brown tumors.

TREATMENT

The best therapy is to correct the underlying hyperparathyroidism, via vitamin D supplementation for patients with ESRD or surgical resection of hypersecreting parathyroid glands.

Fibrous Dysplasia

Fibrous dysplasia is a sporadic genetic disorder in which expanding lesions composed of mesenchymal cells arise within medullary bone, leading to skeletal abnormalities. In addition, patients may suffer from disordered pigmentation (café-au-lait spots) and endocrine excess (precocious puberty). Together, this triad is known as **McCune-Albright syndrome.** The specific genetic mutation leads to constitutive activation of the $G_s\alpha$ G-protein subunit. This causes autonomous activation of several cellular processes, including bone resorption, pigmentation, and ovarian hormone release.

PRESENTATION

Whereas fibrous dysplasia occurs equally across both genders, the McCune-Albright triad predominates in women (10:1). More frequently, patients suffer only a single skeletal lesion (mono-ostotic form) arising in the third decade. However, patients with multiple lesions (polyostotic form) typically present at < 10 years of age. Early onset generally correlates with greater severity. The polyostotic form afflicts the bones of the face, ribs, proximal femur, and tibia (Figure 5-36). Expansion of lesions, often exacerbated during pregnancy or hormonal therapy, leads to pain, deformity, fracture, and possible nerve entrapment.

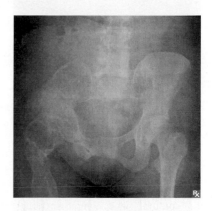

FIGURE 5-36. **Radiograph of polyostotic fibrous dysplasia of the pelvis.**

DIAGNOSIS

Patients presenting with bone pain and café-au-lait spots with rough borders should have plain films taken. Skeletal lesions appear as radiolucent regions with a ground-glass appearance and a thin cortex. Patients may also display symptoms of other endocrinopathies, such as thyrotoxicosis, acromegaly, hyperprolactinemia, hyperparathyroidism, or Cushing syndrome. Typically, serum **alkaline phosphatase** may be elevated, but calcium, PTH, and 25-hydroxyvitamin D levels are normal

TREATMENT

There is no definitive therapy. Surgical intervention is employed to prevent fractures, maintain threatened joints, or decompress nerves.

Osteomyelitis

Whether acute or chronic, osteomyelitis begins as a phagocytic response to a bacterial infection of the bone, leading to osteolysis. Causes include direct inoculation of bacteria into the bone during trauma, spread from nearby skin infection, and hematogenous spread. Many organisms can serve as the causative pathogens:

- *Staphylococcus aureus*—most common cause in adults, hematogenous spread.
- *Pseudomonas aeruginosa* and *Serratia*—more common in IV drug users.
- *Salmonella* species—increased susceptibility among sickle cell patients.
- *Mycobacterium tuberculosis*—predilection for the vertebrae (Pott disease).

PRESENTATION

Osteomyelitis often presents with nonspecific symptoms, such as fever, chills, and fatigue. There may be dull pain at the site or signs of inflammation including cutaneous erythema and swelling. The bone may be tender, and nearby joints may exhibit limited range of motion. History or examination findings consistent with common risk factors should be noted (eg, blunt trauma, IV drug use, diabetes, and hemodialysis).

Chronic osteomyelitis is marked by fluctuating activity with periodic exacerbations. Sinus tracts between bone and skin often drain purulent fluid and necrotic bone fragments. Increased pain and erythrocyte sedimentation rate (ESR) accompany exacerbations. Chronic immune system activation may lead to a positive rheumatoid factor (RF).

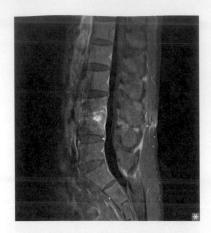

FIGURE 5-37. Vertebral osteomyelitis. MRI of osteomyelitis of the thoracic spine. At L3-L4, there is involvement of the adjacent vertebral bodies and intervening disk. Abnormally enhancing inflamed tissue extends from the disk space anteriorly as well as posteriorly into the epidural space, compressing the thecal sac.

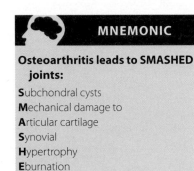

MNEMONIC

Osteoarthritis leads to SMASHED joints:

Subchondral cysts
Mechanical damage to
Articular cartilage
Synovial
Hypertrophy
Eburnation
DIP joints = Heberden nodes

DIAGNOSIS

In addition to these clinical findings, most patients have a normal or only mildly elevated white count. Elevated ESRs (> 100 mm/h) and C-reactive protein (CRP) levels are also common. Only 20–30% of blood cultures return positive. Radiographically, plain films may show soft tissue swelling or periosteal reaction. MRI imaging is also useful in detecting and mapping the extent of osteomyelitis (Figure 5-37).

TREATMENT

Early diagnosis and high-dose antibiotic therapy are essential for preventing bone necrosis. ESR and CRP levels can be monitored to assess response to treatment. Antibiotics are typically administered IV and given for 4–6 weeks. Chronic osteomyelitis can be treated with surgical debridement and long-term antibiotic therapy.

Osteoarthritis

Arising from "cartilage failure" of the diarthrodial (movable, synovium-lined) joints (Figure 5-38), osteoarthritis (OA) is the most common form of joint disease. Although age is the strongest risk factor, other systemic factors (genetics, nutritional and metabolic factors) and biomechanical factors (obesity, malalignment, joint injury or overuse, muscle weakness) contribute to the risk for degradation of articular cartilage. Cartilage loss occurs when the limited reparative capacity of hyaline cartilage is overcome by degradative processes. Loss of cartilage may be accompanied by new bone formation in and around the joint. Joint pathology may include some or all of the following changes:

- **Loss of articular cartilage:** As the cartilage degrades, it is unable to sufficiently repair itself, leading to changes in joint stress and architecture. Progressive cartilage loss may ultimately expose subchondral bone.
- **Sclerosis:** Increased mechanical stress transmitted to bone beneath degrading articular cartilage causes increased subchondral sclerosis, which appears as polished, ivory-like bone (eburnation).
- **Osteophytes:** Increased stress causes bone to remodel, producing bone spurs at the edges of articular surfaces.
- **Bone cysts:** Microfractures beneath the cortex form due to increased stress. The bone gets resorbed, and the cyst fills with fluid and fibrous tissue.

Soft tissue pathology may also include synovitis with mild hypertrophy and thickening of the joint capsule, usually near the site of cartilage injury. Cellular and inflammatory mediators from the synovitis serve to perpetuate cartilage degeneration.

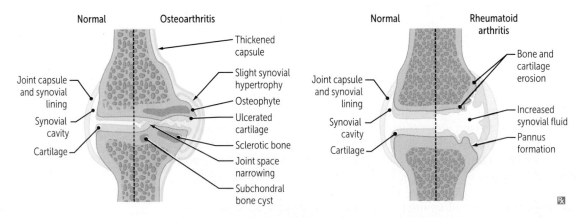

FIGURE 5-38. Comparison of joint abnormalities in rheumatoid and osteoarthritis. Osteoarthritis is characterized by joint space narrowing with cartilage loss, and most visibly by formation of osteophytes. Biomechanical stresses responsible for these changes can also promote bone sclerosis and cyst formation in affected joints. Meanwhile, the inflammatory processes in rheumatoid arthritis most notably cause fluid accumulation and erosion of both bone and cartilage.

PRESENTATION

Patients complain of a deep aching pain in weight-bearing diarthrodial joints after prolonged use. This pain often **improves with rest, and stiffness in the morning usually resolves within 15 minutes of awakening.** On physical examination of the hands, pain and bony swelling are most pronounced in the distal and proximal interphalangeal (DIP and PIP) joints. Swelling and bony crepitus may be evident in affected joints (Figure 5-39). Advanced disease may result in gross deformity, noticeable bony hypertrophy, partial dislocation (known as **subluxation**), and loss of joint motion. There are **no associated systemic symptoms (these symptoms should increase suspicion for autoimmune arthritis).**

DIAGNOSIS

Diagnosis is made using a combination of clinical and radiographic findings. The most frequent finding on plain film imaging is asymmetric joint space narrowing. Other common features on X-ray include sclerosis or osteophytes. An altered joint contour or subluxation can also be seen. Despite this list of possible changes, however, radiographic appearance often does not correlate with symptom severity. MRI or ultrasound can be useful in the evaluation of soft tissue, such as for the detection of synovitis. Laboratory tests are usually normal in primary OA, though synovial fluid analysis may be helpful to rule out other causes of arthritis, such as infection or inflammatory processes. Common characteristics of OA as compared with rheumatoid arthritis (RA) are shown in Table 5-7.

TREATMENT

Treatment goals include reducing pain, maintaining mobility, and preventing disability. Reducing joint loading through improved posture, assistive devices (orthotics), exercise, and weight loss are often the first steps in mild OA. NSAIDs and acetaminophen are palliative pain relievers but do not prevent disease progression. Other short-term interventions include glucocorticoid or hyaluronic acid injections. Generally used in patients

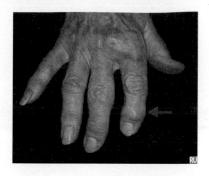

FIGURE 5-39. Osteoarthritic changes in the hand. Common anatomic changes include bony enlargements of the distal (DIP) and proximal interphalangeal (PIP) joints. The red arrow marks bony outgrowth at the DIP joint, often referred to as a Heberden node.

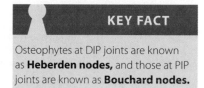

KEY FACT

Osteophytes at DIP joints are known as **Heberden nodes,** and those at PIP joints are known as **Bouchard nodes.**

TABLE 5-7. Differences Between Osteoarthritis and Rheumatoid Arthritis

	OSTEOARTHRITIS	RHEUMATOID ARTHRITIS
Epidemiology	Men = Women People > 40 years of age ~10% prevalence	Women > Men Usually people 20–60 years of age but can occur anytime ~1–2% prevalence
Mechanism of injury	Biomechanical: Cartilage failure (degradation exceeds repair)	Autoimmune: Immune system attacking the synovium and other intra-articular structures
Symptoms and signs	Joint pain, bony enlargement, crepitus Morning stiffness lasting < 30 min	Joint pain, synovitis, and systemic symptoms Morning stiffness > 1 hour
Joint distribution	PIPs, DIPs, first CMCs C/L/S spine Hips, knees, midfoot, 1st MTP	Wrists, MCPs, PIPs C-spine but spares T/L spine Ankles, MTPs
Radiology	Joint space narrowing Osteophytes usually present	Marginal erosions and subluxations Osteophytes usually absent
Treatment	NSAIDs, acetaminophen, joint replacement	DMARDs, NSAIDs

CMC, carpometacarpal; DIP, distal interphalangeal; DMARD, disease-modifying antirheumatic drug; MCP, metacarpophalangeal; MTP, metatarsophalangeal; NSAID, nonsteroidal anti-inflammatory drug; PIP, proximal interphalangeal.

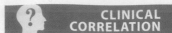

CLINICAL CORRELATION

Watch out for GI complications (peptic ulcer disease and/or hemorrhage), renal insufficiency, and aggravation of hypertension in patients regularly taking NSAIDs!

FLASH BACK

Rheumatoid arthritis exhibits elements of both type III (antibody complexes) and type IV (CD4+-mediated immune response) hypersensitivities.

who fail conservative therapy or are not surgical candidates, injections provide only limited-duration relief.

PROGNOSIS

The natural history of OA is progressive joint degeneration and decreasing range of motion that worsens with age, use, and wear. End-stage OA can be relieved with total joint arthroplasty, most commonly done for hips and knees.

Rheumatoid Arthritis

Rheumatoid arthritis (RA) is characterized by a chronic autoimmune process resulting in inflammatory synovitis of diarthrodial joints. It is more common in women and has a strong genetic association with **HLA-DR4** haplotypes. Smoking is a recently described risk factor. Chronic inflammation leads to encroachment of synovial hypertrophy, referred to as **pannus,** over bone and cartilage leading to erosion within the affected joint.

The inciting cause of RA is unknown. The initiation and propagation of synovitis is complex, involving T and B cells, synovial fibroblasts, and a network of cytokines, chemokines, and degradative enzymes. Synovitis includes B-cell production of **rheumatoid factor (RF).** RF complexes are IgM RF-autoantibodies directed against the F_c portion of an IgG. This is therefore a Type III hypersensitivity reaction. Proliferation of chronically inflamed synovial tissue results in pannus formation. If not treated, the end result is reactive fibrosis in the affected joints leading to deformity and loss of function.

PRESENTATION

Characteristically affecting small to medium joints at onset (proximal interphalangeal [PIP], metacarpophalangeal [MCP], wrist joints, ankles, and metatarsophalangeal [MTP] joints), RA is marked by morning stiffness lasting > 1 hour but **improving with use.** Joint involvement is symmetrical and may be associated with systemic complaints: fever, fatigue, and/or anorexia. Affected joints become swollen, tender, and warm, with a reduced range of motion.

As the disease progresses, joint laxity, subluxation, and cartilage degradation develop. In late stages, joint fibrosis and soft tissue contractures may predominate. Specifically, MCP joint subluxation with ulnar deviation of the fingers is common, as are finger deformities. Hyperextension of the PIP joint with DIP joint flexions is referred to as a "swan-neck" deformity (Figure 5-40), whereas hyperextension of the DIP joint with PIP joint flexions is known as a **"boutonnière" deformity**. Knee involvement can result in inflamed synovium within the popliteal fossa, creating the characteristic **Baker cyst.**

Patients often suffer from a variety of extra-articular symptoms. Muscle weakness and atrophy are common adjacent to affected joints. Twenty percent of patients may develop **rheumatoid nodules:** centralized zones of necrotic tissue surrounded by macrophages and granulation tissue, appearing in areas of mechanical pressure. Although the prevalence of rheumatoid vasculitis has declined due to aggressive RA management, pleuritis and pericarditis can be seen with active disease.

DIAGNOSIS

RA is primarily a clinical diagnosis, although laboratory evaluation may reveal an elevated erythrocyte sedimentation rate (ESR) and C-reactive protein (CRP), a positive RF test (in up to 80% of RA patients) and/or anti–cyclic citrullinated peptide (CCP) antibody (more specific lab finding than the other tests). Patients also often exhibit an anemia of chronic disease (normochromic, normocytic) with reactive thrombocytosis. Joint aspiration yields opaque watery (inflammatory) fluid with a WBC count of > 2000.

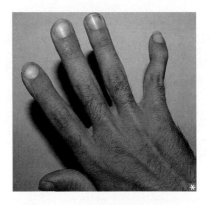

FIGURE 5-40. Rheumatoid arthritis in the hand. Swan-neck deformity and ulnar deviation in the fifth finger due to previous attacks of rheumatoid arthritis.

Radiography may show osteopenia adjacent to the joint and bone erosion typically at the margins of the joint (Figure 5-41).

TREATMENT

Therapeutic goals include (1) pain relief, (2) reduction of inflammation, (3) anatomic preservation, (4) functional maintenance, and (5) systemic control. Physical therapy and rest are effective for pain relief, and orthotics can be used to support weakened joints.

Medical management includes five modalities:

- **Aspirin and NSAIDs:** Alleviate pain of inflammation but do not stop disease progression.
- **Low-dose oral or intra-articular glucocorticoids:** Reduce inflammation and bone erosion but may cause many systemic side effects.
- **Disease-modifying antirheumatic drugs (DMARDs):** These include methotrexate, leflunomide antimalarials, and sulfasalazine. They slow disease progression by decreasing inflammatory mediators. DMARDs may inhibit or reduce the progression of bony erosions.
- **Biologic agents:** Proteins (antibodies, fusion proteins) engineered to target proinflammatory cytokines (TNF-α, IL-1, IL-6), T-cell activation (CD28), or pre-plasma cell B-cells (CD-20). Best in combination with DMARD therapy.
- **Immunosuppressive and cytotoxic agents:** Azathioprine, cyclosporine, and cyclophosphamide can be used but are often reserved for more resistant cases.

PROGNOSIS

RA varies greatly in prognosis, ranging from mild disease with minimal joint injury to progressive polyarthritis and significant disability. Often, the common clinical characteristics develop within 1–2 years of disease onset. Although not practically considered to be curable, disease can be put into remission, particularly with early, aggressive management.

Gout

Most commonly affecting middle-aged men and postmenopausal women, intra-articular **monosodium urate** crystal deposition can result in the significant arthropathy that defines gout. This pathology arises from hyperuricemia, which can be caused by either increased production or decreased excretion of uric acid. Dietary excess, physical stressors (eg, trauma, surgery, or myocardial infarction), excess alcohol ingestion, and diuretics can all precipitate an acute attack. Eventually, periodic episodes of acute gout give way to a chronic polyarticular synovitis.

PRESENTATION

Acute monarticular arthritis, often of the first metatarsophalangeal (MTP) joint of the great toe, is the most common presentation. Classically, acute episodes occur at night, waking patients from sleep to find a warm, red, tender, swollen toe (**podagra**). These acute attacks may be associated with large meals (increased uric acid from high-purine foods) or alcohol consumption (metabolites compete with uric acid for renal excretion). Chronic tissue deposition of excess urate may present clinically as subcutaneous foci (**tophi**), for example in the Achilles tendon, at the olecranon, or on the external ear.

DIAGNOSIS

Diagnosis must be confirmed by joint aspiration and examination of the fluid for **negatively birefringent needle-shaped crystals** (Figure 5-42). Synovial white counts are also elevated (~60,000 cells/µL). Synovial fluid cultures should be performed if there is clinical suspicion of simultaneous septic arthritis. A 24-hour urinary uric acid level may help delineate an underlying metabolic cause.

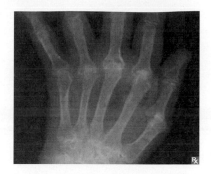

FIGURE 5-41. Joint destruction in rheumatoid arthritis. X-ray of a hand affected by rheumatoid arthritis, demonstrating diffuse erosions in the metacarpophalangeal (MCP) and carpal joints. Destruction of bone and cartilage can be great enough to cause joint space narrowing, as in this patient.

KEY FACT

Conditions predisposing patients to gout:
- **Decreased uric acid excretion (90%)**
  Thiazide diuretic use
  Renal failure
  Glucose-6-phosphatase deficiency
- **Overproduction of uric acid (10%)**
  Lesch-Nyhan syndrome
  Phosphoribosyl pyrophosphate (PRPP) synthetase excess
  Tumor lysis syndrome

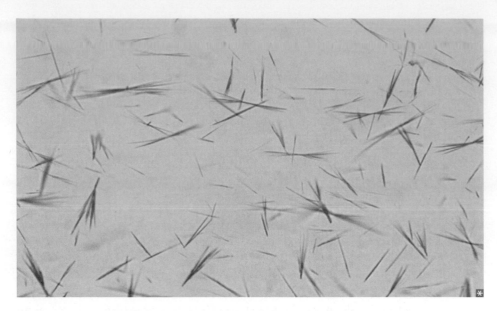

FIGURE 5-42. **Monosodium urate (MSU) crystals.** Extracellular and intracellular MSU crystals, as seen in a fresh preparation of synovial fluid, illustrate needle- and rod-shaped strongly negative birefringent crystals (compensated polarized light microscopy; 400 × magnification).

TREATMENT

Anti-inflammatory medications (**colchicine**, NSAIDs, and intra-articular or systemic glucocorticoid injections) are employed during acute episodes for pain relief. Notably, colchicine and NSAIDs can be toxic to elderly patients and those with renal insufficiency or GI disorders. Once acute attacks have subsided, urate-lowering therapies are used to prevent recurrence. **Probenecid** increases uric acid excretion and is especially useful in patients with poor uric acid excretion but preserved renal function. **Allopurinol** is best for uric acid overproduction, underexcretion from renal failure, or when a uricosuric is either contraindicated or not tolerated by the patient.

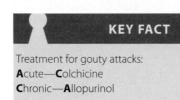

KEY FACT

Treatment for gouty attacks:
Acute—**C**olchicine
Chronic—**A**llopurinol

Pseudogout

Calcium pyrophosphate dihydrate deposition disease (CPPD), also known as pseudogout, results in the precipitation of crystals in the joint space through an unknown mechanism. Neutrophil phagocytosis of crystals leads to chemotactic recruitment of more inflammatory cells, as in true gout, perpetuating tissue injury.

Pseudogout occurring in patients < 50 years old should prompt a search for a metabolic basis. Possible culprits include the "four **H**s":

- Hyperparathyroidism
- Hemochromatosis
- Hypophosphatasia (low activity of alkaline phosphatase)
- Hypomagnesemia

PRESENTATION

Though often asymptomatic, many individuals with CPPD suffer from acute and chronic arthritis resembling true gout. However, chronic CPPD can lead to a **symmetrical** proliferative synovitis (more common in familial forms) resembling RA ("pseudo-RA"), or intervertebral disk calcification that mimics ankylosing spondylitis. In spite of these peculiar traits, the most common presentation is knee pain ("pseudo-OA"), although the wrist, shoulder, elbow, and ankle can also be affected (unlike in classic OA). Pseudogout attacks may be accompanied by fevers.

DIAGNOSIS

Just as with true gout, joint aspiration is necessary for definitive diagnosis. Phagocytosed **basophilic, rhomboid crystals with weak positive birefringence** are present (Figure 5-43). Radiographically, the finding of radiodense CPPD crystal deposits in menisci or hyaline cartilage is termed **chondrocalcinosis** and may be present in asymptomatic joints.

TREATMENT

Colchicine, joint aspiration, NSAIDs, and intra-articular glucocorticoid injections are the mainstays of therapy during acute attacks, sometimes shortening episodes from 1 month to 10 days in duration. Low-dose colchicine prophylaxis may aid those suffering from frequent attacks. Severe polyarticular attacks are best treated with steroids, but progressive large-joint destructive disease may necessitate surgical treatment.

CONNECTIVE TISSUE DISORDERS

Seronegative Spondyloarthropathies

These diseases are characterized by RF-negative inflammatory arthritis of the spine and/or extremities (asymmetrical, oligoarticular distribution). They occur more commonly in males and are strongly associated with **HLA-B27,** which is a gene that encodes for **human leukocyte antigen (HLA) major histocompatibility complex (MHC) I.**

Ankylosing Spondylitis

Ankylosing spondylitis (AS) is a seronegative spondyloarthropathy (Table 5-8) that targets the spine and sacroiliac joints in young men. Ninety percent of patients with AS are HLA-B27 positive, although only approximately 1–2% of HLA-B27 positive patients will develop AS.

The underlying cause of AS is unknown; inflamed sacroiliac joints have CD4+ and CD8+ T-cell infiltrates with high levels of TNF-α. Inflammation at this site leads to adjacent marrow edema, bony erosions, fibrous progression, and eventual ossification.

PRESENTATION

Symptomatic disease onset occurs in early adulthood, beginning with insidious dull lumbar or gluteal pain. Morning stiffness that improves with movement but returns at night and disrupts sleep is also typical. Bony pain may predominate at sites of enthesitis (inflammation at sites of tendinous or ligamentous insertion), including the major bony prominences of the trunk, girdle, and pelvis.

Several extra-articular symptoms can accompany AS. **Acute unilateral anterior uveitis** occurs in 30% of patients and may precede ankylosis. Up to 60% of patients suffer symptoms of bowel inflammation. **Aortitis, leading to aortic valve insufficiency** and sometimes precipitating congestive heart failure, is a rare but serious extra-articular manifestation of severe and prolonged disease. Interstitial lung disease may occur in upper lung fields.

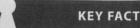

KEY FACT

Gout—Crystals are yellow when parallel to polarized light. Pseudogout—Crystals are blue when parallel to polarized light.

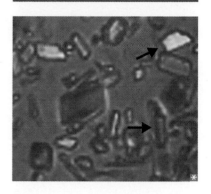

FIGURE 5-43. **Calcium pyrophosphate dehydrate (CPPD) crystals.** CPPD crystals from the joint space of pseudogout patients typically appear rhomboid (arrows) and display weak birefringence under polarized light.

TABLE 5-8. **Synopsis of Spondylolysis, Spondylolisthesis, and Ankylosing Spondylitis**

SPONDYLOLYSIS	SPONDYLOLISTHESIS	ANKYLOSING SPONDYLITIS
Defect/fracture in the pars interarticularis; uncommonly symptomatic	Displacement of a vertebra commonly caused by spondylolysis or degenerative disk disease	Inflammatory arthritis of spinal joints, causing back stiffness, pain, and limited range of motion; moves cephalad and eventually affects the cervical spine

At later stages, decreased lumbar range of motion leads to loss of lordosis and decreased flexion and extension of the torso. Restriction of chest expansion becomes significant, leading to a restrictive pulmonary defect. End-stage spinal involvement may result in fracture of brittle, osteoporotic vertebrae, leading to spinal cord injury.

Diagnosis

Definitive diagnosis is established by radiographic evidence of sacroiliitis in addition to one of the three following criteria:

- History of inflammatory back pain.
- Limitation of lumbar range of motion (frontal and sagittal planes).
- Limited chest expansion.

Patients may have an asymmetrical, oligoarticular (medium to large joint) arthritis.

Radiographically, sacroiliitis is revealed by blurred cortical margins, bony erosions, and sclerosis. "Pseudo-widening" of the joint space, due to erosive disease, may be seen before joint obliteration by fusion occurs. Osteitis of vertebral corners leads to "squaring" on plain films and eventual fusion of vertebrae, resulting in the pathognomonic **"bamboo" spine** seen on radiography (Figure 5-44). Early changes (bone marrow edema and enthesitis) are best seen on CT or MRI.

No specific laboratory test is diagnostic of AS; however, many nonspecific tests are positive, including elevated ESR and CRP as markers of inflammation and a low RBC count from anemia of chronic disease.

Treatment

Immunomodulation with anti-TNF-α therapies has revolutionized AS therapy. Traditional therapy has included NSAIDs and physical therapy, although these show little effect on disease progression. Traditional DMARDs, such as methotrexate, may improve extremity joint disease but have little to no effect on spinal involvement. Uveitis, specifically, is treated with local glucocorticoids. Surgery, in the form of total hip arthroplasty,

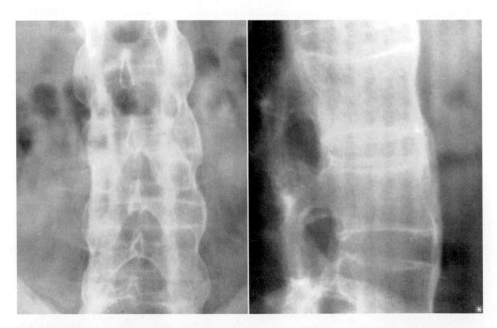

FIGURE 5-44. **Ankylosing spondylitis.** Frontal (left) and lateral (right) radiographs demonstrating "bamboo spine" deformity due to fusion of the vertebral bodies and posterior elements.

is reserved for patients with severe hip arthritis, and often results in immediate resolution of pain.

PROGNOSIS

End-stage AS is a chronic progressive disease, significantly reducing patient quality of life. Most patients suffer increasing pain, stiffness, and disability despite traditional therapy as they age and the disease progresses.

Reactive Arthritis

The **reactive arthritides (ReAs)** are a group of seronegative inflammatory arthritides in which up to 85% of sufferers share the **HLA-B27** antigen. It is thought that patients with this haplotype have a genetic susceptibility to arthritis if infected with certain enteric and genital pathogens. In addition, HIV-positive individuals are susceptible to these infections and subsequent ReAs. Several pathogens have been implicated, including:

- *Campylobacter* (most common enteric bacteria causing ReAs)
- *Chlamydia trachomatis*
- *Salmonella*
- *Shigella*
- *Yersinia*

Reactive arthritis most commonly affects 18- to 40-year-old males. The gender difference is attributed to the fact that men are much more likely than women to develop ReAs after sexually transmitted illnesses.

PRESENTATION

Reiter syndrome was the term used for the symptom triad of **arthritis, urethritis,** and **conjunctivitis.** Usually, patients report an antecedent GI or genitourinary (GU) infection less than 1 month prior to the onset of an asymmetrical progressive arthritis. Lower extremities (knees, ankles, and feet) are more commonly involved, though wrists and hands may also be affected. Joint effusions, dactylitis, tendinitis, and fasciitis are all common. Associated pathology may include ocular disease (which ranges from conjunctivitis to uveitis), mucosal and urethral ulcers, or sores of the palms and soles.

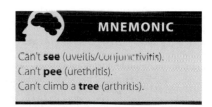

MNEMONIC

Can't **see** (uveitis/conjunctivitis).
Can't **pee** (urethritis).
Can't climb a **tree** (arthritis).

DIAGNOSIS

As a clinical diagnosis, reactive arthritis should be considered in patients suffering from inflammatory back pain and/or an oligoarticular, usually asymmetrical extremity joint arthritis occurring in close temporal proximity to an episode of dysuria or diarrhea.

TREATMENT

Acute arthritic symptoms are alleviated to varying degrees by NSAIDs, although chronic resistant disease may require immunomodulators such as sulfasalazine and methotrexate. Prompt treatment of concomitant GU infection may prevent the development of subsequent ReA in susceptible individuals.

Psoriatic Arthritis

Psoriatic arthritis is characterized by the development of both polyarthritis and psoriasis, occurring in roughly 5–10% of patients with psoriasis. As with the other seronegative spondyloarthropathies, there is a strong association with the HLA-B27 antigen. Psoriasis usually precedes any arthritic symptoms, but symptoms can appear in any order or even simultaneously.

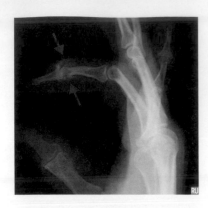

FIGURE 5-45. Pencil-in-cup deformity in psoriatic arthritis. X-ray imaging of patients with psoriatic arthritis may reveal deforming changes, particularly at the DIP joint, which typically appears as a pencil in a cup.

PRESENTATION

The first symptoms usually develop during the first decade of life, often with the scaly rash characteristic of psoriasis. Joint symptoms manifest as asymmetric, polyarticular pain and stiffness, with a predilection for the distal interphalangeal (DIP) joints that can lead to severe finger deformities. Patients may exhibit **dactylitis** (described as "sausage digits"), which is painful inflammation of an entire finger or toe. Also characteristic of this disease is the presence of nail changes, including pitting or discolorations. Extra-articular manifestations, such as uveitis or aortitis, are sometimes found in patients but are less frequent than in ankylosing spondylitis or reactive arthritis.

DIAGNOSIS

Diagnosis of psoriatic arthritis is primarily clinical, though laboratory or radiographic studies may aid in differentiation from other arthropathies. Patients will be negative for rheumatoid factor and may have elevated inflammatory markers. Plain films may show bone erosion in symptomatic joints. Involvement of the DIP joint is common and can display the classic "pencil-in-cup" appearance (Figure 5-45).

TREATMENT

Traditionally, psoriatic arthritis has been treated with NSAIDs to reduce inflammation and alleviate pain. DMARDs, such as methotrexate, can be used for more aggressive or resistant disease, though patients early in the disease course may be started on DMARDs to prevent any deforming effects. TNF-alpha inhibitors have also been shown to have marked efficacy against psoriatic arthritis, though these therapies are often reserved for cases refractory to DMARD treatments.

Systemic Lupus Erythematosus

Systemic lupus erythematosus (SLE) is an autoimmune connective tissue disease mediated by autoantibodies and immune complexes, causing inflammation and injury primarily to joints, skin, blood, and internal organs. Immune complexes of antibodies directed against double-stranded DNA may circulate and deposit in tissues or form in situ. Tissue injury occurs through immune complex activation of complement, and complement- and Fc-receptor-mediated recruitment and activation of inflammatory cells. SLE is a disease driven by T_H2 cytokines, particularly interferon-alpha (IFN-α).

Ninety percent of SLE patients are women between the ages of 14 and 45. This disease is three times more common in blacks than whites. Infection is the leading cause of death among younger patients, while deaths among patients older than 35 years are most commonly caused by cardiovascular involvement.

PRESENTATION

Definitive classification of a patient as having SLE requires the documentation of 4 of 11 criteria over the course of the patients' medical history (specificity and sensitivity: ~95% and 85%, respectively) (Table 5-9). In addition, **antinuclear antibodies** (ANAs) are positive in > 95% of patients; thus, repeated negative results make the diagnosis less likely. The most common symptoms over time include constitutional symptoms, rash, arthritis, and serositis (pleuritis and/or pericarditis). Less clinically prevalent symptoms include glomerulonephritis, nonbacterial verrucous endocarditis, and Raynaud phenomenon.

With the potential to affect nearly every organ system, SLE sequelae are quite diverse. Descriptions of high-yield major organ system manifestations are shown in Table 5-10.

- **Cutaneous: Lupus dermatitis** (Figure 5-46) can be discoid, systemic, or subacute. Most commonly, this occurs as a photosensitive and erythematous **malar rash** over the cheeks and nose (sparing the nasolabial fold).

KEY FACT

In a young female with fever, fatigue, rash, and joint pain, always think of SLE.

MNEMONIC

Symptoms of SLE—

RASH OR PAIN

Rash (malar or discoid)
Arthritis
Serositis
Hematologic disorders (eg, cytopenias)
Oral/nasopharyngeal ulcers
Renal disease, Raynaud phenomenon
Photosensitivity, positive Venereal Disease Research Laboratory (VDRL)/ rapid plasma reagin (RPR)
Antinuclear antibodies (ANAs)
Immunologic abnormalities (eg, anti-ds-DNA)
Neurologic disorders (eg, seizures, psychosis)

TABLE 5-9. Classification Criteria for the Diagnosis of Systemic Lupus Erythematosus

A patient must have 4 of the following 11 criteria at any time during disease history in order to be diagnosed with SLE.	
Immunologic disorder	**Anti-ds-DNA,** anti-Sm, and/or aPLs
Malar rash	Rash on cheeks, flat or raised
Discoid rash	Erythematous circular raised patches on skin; may result in scarring
Antinuclear antibody	An abnormal ANA titer (in the absence of drugs known to induce ANAs)
Mucositis (oral ulcers)	Oral and nasopharyngeal ulcers
Neurologic disorder	Seizures or psychosis
Serositis	Pleuritis or pericarditis
Hematologic disorder	Hemolytic anemia or leukopenia, lymphopenia, or thrombocytopenia in the absence of offending drugs
Arthritis	Nonerosive arthritis of $\geq$ 2 peripheral joints (tenderness, swelling, and/or effusion)
Renal disorder	Proteinuria (> 0.5 g/d or 3+) and/or cellular casts
Photosensitivity	Rash resulting from exposure to ultraviolet light

ANAs, antinuclear antibodies; aPL, antiphospholipid (antibodies).

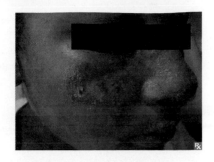

FIGURE 5-46. Cutaneous manifestation of systemic lupus erythematosus. Erythematous sharply demarcated plaques with scale in a butterfly pattern on the face of a 14-year-old girl with arthritis, chest pain, and facial rash.

TABLE 5-10. Organ System Manifestations of Systemic Lupus Erythematosus

ORGAN SYSTEM	MANIFESTATION	NOTES
Cutaneous	Lupus dermatitis	Most commonly a photosensitive, red, scaly **malar rash** over the cheeks and nose sparing the nasolabial folds
Musculoskeletal	Polyarthritis and synovitis	Symmetrical, small and medium extremity joint swelling and tenderness without bony erosions
	Myalgias and weakness	Must be distinguished from steroid side effect, metabolic causes, and pain syndromes
Renal	**Lupus nephritis**	Can be nephritic (ie, diffuse proliferative glomerulonephritis leading to hematuria) or nephrotic (ie, membranous glomerulonephritis leading to proteinuria); may progress to ESRD
Nervous	Cognitive dysfunction	Decreased memory and reasoning
	Headaches	Intensify with SLE flares; may simulate meningitis
	CNS vasculitis	May lead to stroke
	Psychosis	Must be distinguished from steroid side effect
Pulmonary	Pleuritis	With or without pleural effusion
	Interstitial inflammation	Dyspnea, with reduced D$_{LCO}$ on pulmonary function testing
Cardiovascular	Accelerated atherosclerosis	Inflammatory state and thrombotic and embolic disease lead to increased MI and stroke risks
	Myocarditis	Can result in arrhythmias
	Libman-Sacks endocarditis (subacute endocarditis)	Leads to valvular insufficiency and embolic CVAs

TABLE 5-10.   **Organ System Manifestations of Systemic Lupus Erythematosus** *(continued)*

ORGAN SYSTEM	MANIFESTATION	NOTES
Hematologic	Anemia of chronic disease	Normochromic, normocytic
	Hemolytic anemia	Low haptoglobin, high LDH, Coombs-positive
	Thrombocytopenia	Immune mediated
	Leukopenia	Primarily lymphocytopenia
Gastrointestinal	Vasculitis	Leads to perforations, ischemia, and bleeding
	Lupus pancreatitis	Disease-related vs drug-induced
Ocular	Sicca syndrome	aka secondary Sjögren syndrome
	Retinal vasculitis	May be vision threatening; treated with aggressive steroid therapy
	Optic neuritis	

CNS, central nervous system; CVA, cardiovascular accident; D$_{LCO}$, diffusion capacity of the lung for carbon monoxide; ESRD, end-stage renal disease; LDH, lactate dehydrogenase; MI, myocardial infarction; SLE, systemic lupus erythematosus.

- **Musculoskeletal:** Most patients experience intermittent polyarthritis, synovitis, and swelling or tenderness, often in the limbs. Bony erosions are rare; if seen, consider RA as an alternative diagnosis. Persistent pain in any one joint should increase clinical suspicion for **avascular necrosis,** especially in those patients receiving systemic glucocorticoid therapy.
- **Renal: Lupus nephritis** is a common cause of morbidity in SLE, and renal function should be checked regularly in every patient with SLE. Blacks are more likely than whites to progress to end-stage renal disease (ESRD).
- **Immunologic:** Increased infections may occur due to leukopenia and/or steroid-induced immunosuppression. Patients may also develop **antiphospholipid antibodies (aPLs),** which can cause widespread vasculitis or recurrent miscarriages. These aPLs may also lead to false-positive results on syphilis rapid plasma reagin/Venereal Disease Research Laboratory (RPR/VDRL) tests.
- **Cardiovascular:** Accelerated atherosclerosis in SLE leads to significantly increased risk of stroke and myocardial infarction. Inflammatory pericarditis or myocarditis can also be seen. Particularly worrisome is the development of **Libman-Sacks** endocarditis, which may lead to mitral and aortic valve insufficiency, as well as an increase in stroke risk secondary to emboli from the damaged valves.
- **Gastrointestinal:** Nausea, vomiting, and diarrhea can be manifestations of SLE, typically resulting from vascular disease within the abdomen. Vasculitis involving the intestine is an uncommon yet very serious complication and may result in perforation, ischemia, GI bleeds, diffuse abdominal peritonitis and, potentially, sepsis.

DIAGNOSIS

The most important laboratory test is the antinuclear antibody **(ANA),** which is positive in > 95% of patients with SLE. ANA is very sensitive, but it is not specific for SLE and can also be elevated in other inflammatory states, such as RA or chronic infections. High anti-double-stranded DNA **(anti-ds-DNA)** and anti-Smith **(anti-Sm)** titers are both specific for lupus and, when present, make it very likely the patient has SLE.

Antiphospholipid antibodies, although not specific for SLE, fulfill 1 of 11 classification criteria for diagnosis and thus should be tested for, particularly in women with recurrent spontaneous abortions. Women of childbearing age should receive a screen for anti-Ro antibodies because of a correlation with increased risk of fetal congenital heart block.

Antihistone antibodies are found in drug-induced lupus and are helpful in distinguishing this from SLE.

TREATMENT

NSAIDs are the front-line therapy for patients with arthritis and myalgias. **High-dose systemic steroids to control acute symptoms** are recommended for short periods of time only so as to reduce the incidence of steroid side effects. Some patients (eg, those with lupus nephritis) may require long-term low-dose therapy with glucocorticoids, azathioprine, mycophenolate, or other immunosuppressive agents. These agents include both traditional DMARDs, like methotrexate and antimalarials, and newer biologic therapies.

PROGNOSIS

Most patients experience a disease course with relatively quiescent stretches punctuated by acute exacerbations, but complete regression is rare. Most patients are affected chronically by varying degrees of skin and joint disease. ESRD is also common.

Sarcoidosis

A chronic disorder of waxing and waning course, sarcoidosis affects men and women from age 20 to 40 years. Most commonly found in black women, it is characterized by immune-mediated **noncaseating granulomas** and elevated serum angiotensin-converting enzyme (ACE) levels. Arising from disordered immune responses of unknown etiology, these granulomas form when mononuclear phagocytes infiltrate tissues in response to released IL-2. In the tissue, the phagocytes differentiate and fuse to produce the multinucleated giant cells that reside in the center of noncaseating granulomas (Figure 5-47). Local tissue inflammation, fibrosis, and functional deficits lead to patient symptomatology.

Pathology includes epithelial granulomas containing microscopic **Schaumann bodies** (calcium + protein) and **multinucleated giant cells.** These epithelioid giant cells are believed to produce elevated levels of 1,25-dihydroxyvitamin D, leading to enhanced calcium absorption in the gut and hypercalciuria, with or without hypercalcemia.

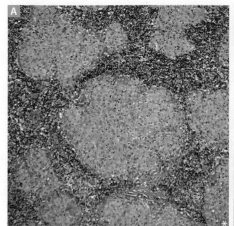
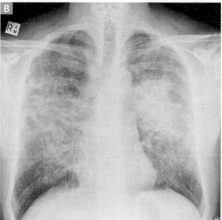
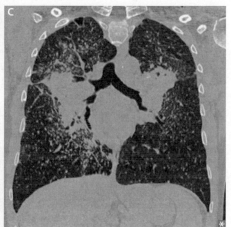

FIGURE 5-47.   Pathology and imaging of sarcoidosis. **A** This histological sample from a patient with sarcoidosis exhibits classic noncaseating granulomas. These circular structures consist of central giant cells composed of fused phagocytic immune cells, surrounded by elongated macrophages called "epithelioid" cells. **B** Typical findings on chest X-ray include bilateral hilar adenopathy and reticulonodular opacities. Long-standing sarcoidosis can also lead to fibrosis and calcifications visible on X-ray. **C** CT of patients with sarcoidosis can be helpful in more precisely determining nodal involvement and the extent of fibrosis, as evidenced by the large nodal and linear opacities in this image.

PRESENTATION

Although sarcoidosis is a systemic disease, the lungs are most commonly and severely affected. Pulmonary symptoms may develop over weeks to months and include cough, dyspnea, retrosternal chest discomfort, and occasionally hemoptysis. Many patients also present with constitutional symptoms of fatigue, low-grade fever, night sweats, malaise, and weight loss. Nontender lymphadenopathy is very common as well, often due to the widespread formation of granulomas.

Other common symptoms include uveitis, **erythema nodosum** (tender nodules or plaques, usually on the lower extremities), and salivary and lacrimal gland inflammation (causing sicca syndrome). Other cutaneous manifestations include infiltrated papules about the nose and erythematous or violaceous papules on the upper extremities (Figure 5-48). The combination of erythema nodosum, hilar lymphadenopathy, and arthritis/periarthritis (typically in and around the ankle) is called **Lofgren syndrome.**

DIAGNOSIS

Sarcoidosis should be considered in any patient between the ages of 20 and 40 who has respiratory complaints (dyspnea, cough), blurry vision, and/or erythema nodosum. Laboratory tests for lymphocytopenia, eosinophilia, increased ESR, hyperglobulinemia, and elevated **ACE** levels all can support the diagnosis. Patients may also have **hypercalcemia** associated with increased 1,25-dihydroxyvitamin D, which is produced by cells in noncaseating granulomas.

Radiographic imaging of the lungs is usually essential for diagnosis. Chest x-rays can reveal bilateral hilar and mediastinal adenopathy (termed "potato nodes"), diffuse infiltrates, and fibrosis (Figure 5-47). Pulmonary function tests may reveal a restrictive pattern with decreased lung volumes and diffusing capacities. Definite diagnosis requires biopsy evidence of the typical pathologic changes.

TREATMENT

The therapy of choice is a high-dose glucocorticoid taper. Methotrexate, antimalarials, TNF-α inhibitors, and immunosuppressants have all been used in refractory cases.

PROGNOSIS

Most patients suffering from acute disease achieve remission with no significant long-term sequelae. Half of all patients experience mild permanent organ damage that rarely progresses; 20% are left with intermittent recurring disease, and only 10% succumb to direct sequelae of sarcoidosis.

MNEMONIC

Findings in sarcoidosis—
GRAIN

Gammaglobulinemia
Rheumatoid factor
ACE increase
Interstitial fibrosis
Noncaseating granulomas

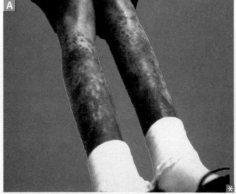 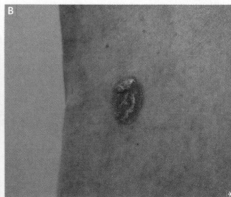

FIGURE 5-48. **Cutaneous manifestations of sarcoidosis.** A Skin rash on a 12-year-old girl with sarcoidosis. Both lower extremities show elevated, diffuse purplish-colored nodular and scaly rash. B Scaly annular violaceous plaque diagnosed as cutaneous sarcoidosis on the left calf of a 54-year old man.

Scleroderma/Systemic Sclerosis

Systemic sclerosis (SSc) is a disease characterized by excessive production of collagen, primarily in the skin, that results in sclerosis (hardening of tissue), thickening, and tightening. Also known as scleroderma, it is a heterogeneous disorder in terms of both the involvement of internal organs and joints and of the pace and severity of its clinical course. SSc is most commonly seen in women (female-to-male ratio of 3:1) between the ages of 35 and 64 years. It is slightly more common in blacks.

PRESENTATION

In **localized scleroderma** (eg, morphea, linear scleroderma), cutaneous changes consistent with dermal fibrosis are seen without organ involvement. **Systemic sclerosis** is classified as either diffuse or limited based on the extent of skin disease, but patients with either form are at risk for internal organ involvement. **Diffuse systemic sclerosis** includes extensive fibrotic skin changes with early internal organ involvement including pulmonary, renal, and cardiac systems. **Limited SSc** presents a slowly progressive course over years with fibrotic skin limited to the hands (Figure 5-49), forearms, feet, neck, and face. Patients usually present with Raynaud phenomenon and over time may develop telangiectasias, GI involvement (esophageal dysmotility/dysphagia), skin calcifications, and late pulmonary hypertension.

DIAGNOSIS

Diagnosis is based on clinical symptoms and confirmed with laboratory tests. A positive ANA is seen in over 90% of cases. Anticentromere antibody is present and very specific in patients with limited SSc, whereas patients with diffuse systemic sclerosis are characterized by antitopoisomerase I (or antiscleroderma-70) antibody.

Complications can be detected using pulmonary function testing (for restrictive lung disease) and barium swallow to look for esophageal dysmotility. Echocardiogram can indirectly screen for the presence of pulmonary hypertension.

TREATMENT

Treatment is primarily symptomatic as no therapy has been definitively successful in reversing the course of disease. Calcium channel blockers are useful in treating Raynaud phenomenon and pulmonary hypertension. Unfortunately, no effective therapy currently exists for skin involvement. The only medication known to reduce the mortality of patients with scleroderma are ACE inhibitors, used for patients with renal crisis.

PROGNOSIS

The major cause of mortality and morbidity is involvement of internal organ systems, specifically, renal failure and pulmonary hypertension. Though the average survival time following diagnosis is 12 years, this prognosis is strongly affected by the disease subtype. The limited cutaneous form has a much better prognosis than the diffuse cutaneous type.

Mixed Connective Tissue Disease

Mixed connective tissue disease (MCTD) is an autoimmune disorder wherein the patient may show clinical and lab features of more than one connective tissue disease, including SLE, RA, myositis, and progressive SSc. The exact pathophysiologic mechanism of MCTD remains unknown. It is much more common in women than in men.

PRESENTATION

Patients generally present with arthralgias or arthritis, commonly associated with skin changes. Raynaud phenomenon is seen in 90% of patients, and myositis with proximal

KEY FACT

CREST syndrome was the older terminology for limited SSc, and stood for **C**alcinosis, **R**aynaud phenomenon, **E**sophageal dysmotility, **S**clerodactyly, and **T**elangiectasias.

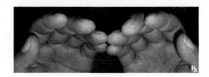

FIGURE 5-49. Scleroderma acrosclerosis. Rat-bite necrosis and ulceration of fingertips.

muscle weakness is also a common finding. Involvement of the lungs is common in MCTD, although most patients do not initially present with pulmonary symptoms.

DIAGNOSIS

Diagnosis is primarily made clinically, and generally requires the presence of Raynaud phenomenon or hand swelling, plus clinical features representative of at least two connective tissue diseases (eg, SLE, scleroderma, myositis). Importantly, a high level of anti-U1 ribonucleoprotein autoantibodies (**anti-RNP Ab**) in the absence of the anti-Smith autoantibody (**anti-Sm Ab**) is required for diagnosis.

TREATMENT

Generally, SLE-like features, arthritis, and pleuritis are treated with **NSAIDs**, antimalarials (**hydroxychloroquine**), low-dose **corticosteroids**, and methotrexate. Raynaud phenomenon is treated symptomatically with **calcium channel blockers.**

PROGNOSIS

The major cause of mortality is progressive pulmonary hypertension and its cardiac sequelae. MCTD rarely affects the kidneys and is generally considered to have a better prognosis than SLE.

Sjögren Syndrome

A systemic disease caused by autoimmune destruction of exocrine glands by lymphocytic infiltrates. It predominantly affects middle-aged women. The most frequent manifestations include dry mouth (**xerostomia**), dry eyes (**xerophthalmia**), and **bilateral parotid enlargement** (Figure 5-50). Patients with Sjögren syndrome are at increased risk for developing non-Hodgkin lymphomas, most commonly mucosa-associated lymphoid tissue (**MALT**) lymphomas.

PRESENTATION

In addition to **sicca** (dryness)—of the eyes, mouth, upper respiratory tract, and vagina—patients may present with constitutional symptoms, neuropathies, dental caries, and inflammatory joint pain.

DIAGNOSIS

Primary Sjögren syndrome is diagnosed in a patient with dry eyes, dry mouth, and lymphocytic infiltration of the salivary glands seen on histology. Secondary Sjögren syndrome presents with the same symptoms but is diagnosed when the patient already has another connective tissue disease.

Abnormal serologies include positive RF, positive ANA, and/or positive anti-SSA (anti-Ro) or anti-SS-B (anti-La). Lab abnormalities may include cytopenias, cryoglobulinemia, distal renal tubular acidosis, and a polyclonal hypergammaglobulinemia. Yearly laboratory testing to screen for transition to a lymphoproliferative disorder includes serum and urine protein electrophoresis and blood cell counts.

TREATMENT

Treatment is mainly symptomatic. Artificial tears and saliva preparations can be used to relieve dryness. Cholinergic drugs (ie, pilocarpine) can increase exocrine secretion. The complications of xerostomia and xerophthalmia are best prevented by good dental and ophthalmologic care, respectively. Severe extraglandular disease may require high-dose systemic corticosteroids. In patients with secondary Sjögren, treatment of the underlying connective tissue disease is often key.

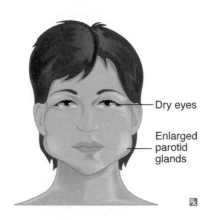

Dry eyes

Enlarged parotid glands

FIGURE 5-50. **Sjögren syndrome.** A representation of the clinical appearance of Sjögren syndrome, which is notable for parotid gland enlargement and sicca symptoms, or dryness, of the eyes.

PROGNOSIS

Typically, patients have a normal life expectancy. In patients who have associated disorders, the prognosis generally depends on those diseases.

Polymyositis and Dermatomyositis

Polymyositis (PM) and dermatomyositis (DM) are inflammatory muscle disorders characterized primarily by proximal muscle weakness. The most dramatic clinical distinction between these two disorders is the **prominent rash that occurs in DM,** though they also differ in their underlying pathophysiology. Humoral autoimmunity leads to microangiopathy and muscle fiber ischemia through antibody-mediated damage in DM. In contrast, cytotoxic T-cell-mediated damage is associated with PM, leading to muscle necrosis.

PRESENTATION

Most commonly, the myopathies present with **subacute, symmetrical, proximal, and girdle muscle weakness** that progresses over weeks and months. It is significant enough to inhibit daily activities (rising from a chair, combing one's hair, lifting objects, and climbing stairs). Fine motor movements are affected only late in disease progression, and extraocular and facial muscles are generally spared in both syndromes. **Myalgia is uncommon.**

The photosensitive rash of DM clinically distinguishes it from PM. Most commonly, it appears as puffy, purple eyelids **(heliotrope rash),** but it can also be seen as a macular red rash on the face and trunk, or as a purple papular eruption on the knuckles **(Gottron papules)** (Figure 5-51).

DIAGNOSIS

Serum muscle enzyme levels aid in diagnosis. Increases in **creatine kinase (CK)** usually indicate increased disease activity. In addition, electromyography **(EMG)** may help rule out neurogenic disorders.

Ultimately, muscle biopsy is definitive. PM is a primary inflammatory condition in which CD8+ T-cell infiltrates are found among muscle fibers, eventually leading to necrosis. In DM, endomysial inflammation occurs in the immediate vicinity of the small vessels. The resulting angiopathy leads to ischemic injuries within the muscle and perifascicular atrophy.

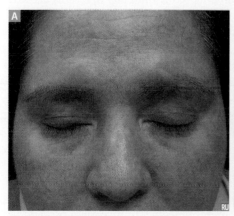
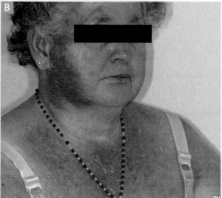
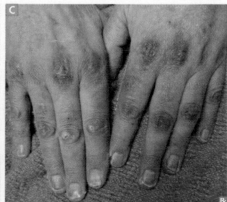

FIGURE 5-51. **Rashes of dermatomyositis.** **A** Heliotrope erythema of upper eyelids and edema of the lower lids. **B** Rash in sun-exposed areas, including in a V-pattern around the neck and upper chest ("shawl sign"). **C** Gottron papules on the dorsa of the hands and fingers, especially over the metacarpophalangeal and interphalangeal joints.

Myositis-specific autoantibodies may be helpful to define disease subsets. Patients who have antisynthetase antibodies (anti-Jo-1) have a higher prevalence of pulmonary and arthritic symptoms. Anti-signal-recognition particle (SRP) is associated with a severe PM phenotype, while anti-Mi-2 is a highly specific diagnostic indicator for DM.

TREATMENT

Immunosuppressive therapy is employed to improve muscle strength and relieve extra-muscular symptoms. Plasma CK levels can be followed as evidence of response to treatment, but improvement in muscle strength is the primary end point. Patients usually begin on high-dose (1 mg/kg) oral prednisone, tapering over months. Azathioprine, methotrexate, and cyclophosphamide are common second-line agents if treatment with glucocorticoids fails or the patient cannot tolerate the side effects.

PROGNOSIS

Most patients improve with therapy and achieve meaningful functional recovery through maintenance therapy. PM morbidity usually results from interstitial lung disease, respiratory muscle involvement, or cardiac complications. DM can be indicative of an underlying malignancy, and age-appropriate cancer screening, as well as a symptom-based investigation into a possible source, should be undertaken.

Muscular Dystrophy

Muscular dystrophy denotes a group of genetic disorders that lead to progressive muscle fiber degeneration. Most forms of muscular dystrophy predominantly affect proximal muscle groups, leading to weakness, poor gait, and ultimately cardiac and/or respiratory dysfunction. There exists a diversity of specific phenotypes with different underlying mutations, but the two most common variants are caused by deleterious mutations in the X-linked gene for the protein **dystrophin:**

- **Duchenne muscular dystrophy:** Complete loss of dystrophin (which is essential for membrane integrity in skeletal muscle) causes a severe phenotype.
- **Becker muscular dystrophy:** Mutations involving truncation of dystrophin, leading to a functional though less-active protein, cause a milder disease variant.

PRESENTATION

Duchenne muscular dystrophy typically manifests within the first few years of life, and affected children are noted to lag behind their peers in motor skills development. By age 4–5, patients are observed having marked difficulty with stairs and often develop a waddling gait. The vast majority of patients with Duchenne muscular dystrophy become wheelchair-bound by age 13. In the Becker variant, meanwhile, many of the same symptoms occur but are milder and can be delayed by decades.

Physical examination of these patients generally reveals proximal muscle weakness that gradually spreads distally. They may also exhibit the **Gower sign,** in which patients stand from a sitting position by first getting on their hands and feet. Atrophy and fatty replacement of muscle tissue can become pronounced in areas such as the calf, leading to the false appearance of muscle enlargement, or pseudohypertrophy.

DIAGNOSIS

Elevated creatinine phosphokinase (CPK) is specific for muscular dystrophy and can be as high as 250 times normal. CPK values rise due to leakage of the enzyme from skeletal muscle cells with disrupted plasma membranes. Definitive diagnosis can be accomplished by polymerase chain reaction (PCR) and genotyping of patients to identify the precise causative mutations. Biopsy is no longer essential to diagnosis, but histologic analysis may show muscle fiber degeneration and proliferation of adipose tissue.

Treatment

No truly effective treatment for muscular dystrophy has been yet described. Steroids can be helpful in delaying progression or even restoring strength, but these gains are inevitably short-lived. Surgery is sometimes warranted for skeletal deformities in severe disease.

Prognosis

Patients with Duchenne muscular dystrophy can survive to their thirties with good medical care, but ultimately succumb to complications of cardiac or respiratory failure. In milder forms, such as Becker muscular dystrophy, patients may survive well into their fifth or sixth decade of life.

DERMATOLOGY

Terminology

Many specific terms are used to describe skin lesions (Table 5-11).

Skin Disorders and Dermatitis

Common

The following represent commonly found skin lesions and rashes that are generally considered to be benign. Common skin lesions are shown in Figure 5-52.

Acne

Inflammation of pilosebaceous units caused by obstruction of hair follicles and subsequent bacterial colonization. Commonly occurs in adolescents and is usually found on the face and trunk (Figure 5-52A).

Allergic Contact Dermatitis

Delayed-type hypersensitivity (type IV) reaction to a topical irritant (often poison ivy, cosmetics, or jewelry). The rash appears in a distribution mirroring the site of contact with the irritant (Figure 5-52B).

FLASH BACK

■ Atopic dermatitis results from type I hypersensitivity—fast (minutes), IgE-mediated reaction
■ Allergic contact dermatitis results from type IV hypersensitivity—delayed (hours to days), T cell-mediated reaction

TABLE 5-11.   Key Terms in Dermatology

LESION NAME	DESCRIPTION
Bulla	Fluid-filled raised lesion > 5 mm across
Excoriation	Traumatic lesion characterized by breakage of the epidermis, causing a raw linear area (ie, a deep scratch); often self-induced
Macule	Circumscribed lesion ≤ 5 mm in diameter characterized by flatness and usually distinguished from surrounding skin by its coloration
Nodule	Elevated lesion with spherical contour > 5 mm across
Papule	Elevated dome-shaped or flat-topped lesion ≤ 5 mm across
Patch	Flat lesion (like a macule) > 5 mm
Plaque	Elevated flat-topped lesion usually > 5 mm across (may be caused by coalescent papules)
Pustule	Discrete, pus-filled, raised lesion
Scale	Dry, horny, platelike excrescence; usually the result of imperfect cornification
Vesicle	Fluid-filled raised lesion ≤ 5 mm across

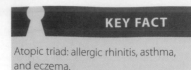

Atopic Dermatitis (Eczema)

Immune-mediated skin disease (type I hypersensitivity) causing scaly and vesicular eruptions, which rupture and crust over on flexor surfaces (Figure 5-52C). The rash is pruritic. It is often associated with other allergic conditions.

Melanocytic Nevus

A benign common mole (Figure 5-52D).

Psoriasis

Caused by unregulated proliferation of keratinocytes, psoriasis is identified by well-demarcated papules and plaques with silvery scales (Figure 5-52E). These areas are usually nonpruritic and found on extensor surfaces, such as knees and elbows. The rash may also exhibit Auspitz sign, which signifies small areas of bleeding from exposed dermal papillae when scales are scraped off. Biopsy often shows parakeratosis, which is characterized by stratum corneum that has retained nuclei. Approximately 10% of patients have associated psoriatic arthritis.

Rosacea

An inflammatory condition predominantly affecting the central face, leading to telangiectasias, central redness, and superficial pustules (Figure 5-52F). This is a chronic condition predominantly affecting women and may involve facial flushing in response to certain stimuli (ie, alcohol, embarrassment, heat).

Seborrheic Keratosis

A common benign epidermal growth that arises spontaneously (mainly on the trunk) and is clinically described as round, flat, coinlike plaques that look "pasted on" (Figure 5-52G). The lesions are tan to dark brown (due to melanin pigmentation of basaloid cells) and show a velvety to granular surface. It is usually seen in the elderly and is easily treated by excision. Usually a benign finding, but the sudden appearance of multiple lesions, known as the **Leser-Trélat** sign, can indicate an occult malignancy.

Urticaria

More commonly known as hives, this is an intensely pruritic skin elevation that can occur anywhere on the body. It is described as a "wheal-and-flare reaction" in which mast

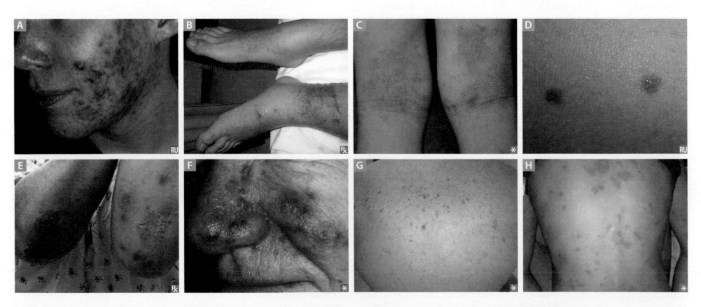

FIGURE 5-52. **Common skin lesions.** Physical appearance of A acne; B allergic contact dermatitis; C atopic dermatitis; D melanocytic nevus; E psoriasis; F rosacea; G seborrheic keratosis; and H urticaria.

cell release of histamine causes edema (the wheal) with surrounding erythema (flare) (Figure 5-52H). Urticaria can also be due to IgE-mediated reactions following exposure to certain foods, insect bites, and drugs. Treatment of urticaria includes antihistamines and removal of the causative agent. **Hereditary angioedema** is an inherited deficiency of C1 esterase inhibitor that results in uncontrolled activation of the early components of the complement cascade and is similar in presentation to hives.

Pigmented Lesions

These lesions involve aberrations in the pigmentation of the skin (Figure 5-53).

Albinism

Patients with albinism have a normal melanocyte count, but these melanocytes have decreased melanin production secondary to a deficiency of tyrosinase. Clinically, patients may present with silvery white hair and lightly pigmented or nonpigmented skin (Figure 5-53A). Albinism is a risk factor for future skin cancer development, and patients should be closely monitored.

Melasma

Hyperpigmentation of the skin around the face or on the abdomen that is associated with increased estrogen exposure (Figure 5-53B). Thus, it is commonly seen in women who are pregnant or using oral contraceptive pills.

Vitiligo

Autoimmune destruction of melanocytes, leading to patchy areas of complete depigmentation (Figure 5-53C).

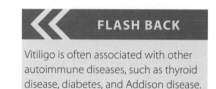

FLASH BACK

Vitiligo is often associated with other autoimmune diseases, such as thyroid disease, diabetes, and Addison disease.

Infectious

Skin infections have diverse manifestations, ranging from contained rashes to life-threatening conditions (Figure 5-54).

Cellulitis

An infection of the dermis and subcutaneous tissue, cellulitis is usually caused by gram-positive organisms, especially *Streptococcus pyogenes* or *Staphylococcus aureus*. Patients usually present with an acute and extremely painful erythematous region of skin that demonstrates progressive spread (Figure 5-54A). Treatment is with antibiotics.

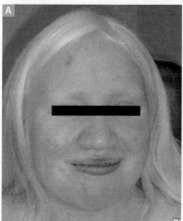
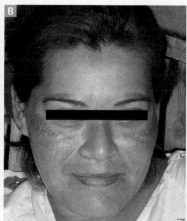
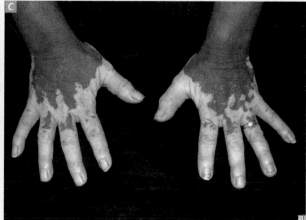

FIGURE 5-53.   **Pigmented skin lesions.** Physical appearance of **A** albinism; **B** melasma; and **C** vitiligo.

Impetigo

Impetigo is a highly contagious, superficial skin infection that is most often caused by *S aureus* or *S pyogenes*. It usually begins on the face and is characterized by vesicles and pustules that rupture and form a **honey-colored crust** (Figure 5-54B). Treatment is with antibiotics.

Necrotizing Fasciitis

Unlike cellulitis, necrotizing fasciitis involves the deeper layers of tissue down to the deep fascia. Usually caused by anaerobic bacteria or group A streptococci, it often manifests with fever and an area of erythema. If not treated, the tissue begins to turn gray/black, and crepitus can be elicited due to CO_2 and methane production during tissue destruction (Figure 5-54C). Amputation, shock, and death can result. Treatment includes **urgent surgical exploration** and debridement and IV antibiotics.

Staphylococcal Scalded Skin Syndrome

S aureus releases certain exfoliative toxins that bind to a cell adhesion molecule (desmoglein 1) and cleave it, leading to a loss of cell-to-cell adhesion. Desmoglein 1 is only found in the upper part of the epidermis; thus, the epidermolysis occurs between the stratum spinosum and stratum granulosum. Staphylococcal scalded skin syndrome is usually seen in newborns or children. It begins with fever and generalized rash, followed by sloughing of the upper layers of the dermis (Figure 5-54D).

Verrucae

More commonly known as warts, verrucae are caused by human papillomavirus (a DNA virus). Epidermal hyperplasia leads to cauliflower-like lesions that are more commonly found on children's hands and feet (Figure 5-54E). No extensive diagnostic testing is required, and treatment involves cryotherapy, salicylic acid, or cantharidin.

Conditions With Blisters

Autoimmune diseases can target connective components within skin tissue and lead to blisters (Figure 5-55).

> **MNEMONIC**
>
> The **bull**ae and antibodies responsible for **bull**ous pemphigoid are located **bull**ow the epidermis.

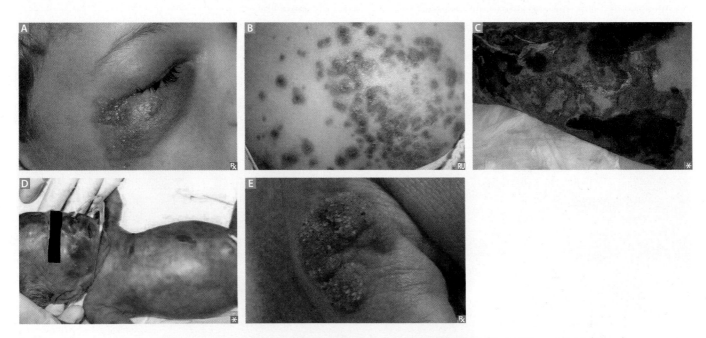

FIGURE 5-54. **Infectious skin lesions.** Physical appearance of **A** periorbital cellulitis; **B** impetigo; **C** necrotizing fasciitis; **D** staphylococcal scalded skin syndrome; and **E** verrucae.

Bullous Pemphigoid

A type II hypersensitivity reaction caused by autoantibodies targeting hemidesmosomes at the basement membrane. The bullae are below the epidermis and do not tend to rupture when touched. They can be found throughout the body but usually spare the oral mucosa (Figure 5-55A). Bullous pemphigoid shows linear immunofluorescence but only at the basement membrane.

Dermatitis Herpetiformis

Rare disorder characterized by extremely pruritic urticaria and grouped vesicles that are mainly along the extensor surfaces (Figure 5-55B). This disease is associated with **celiac disease** and responds to a gluten-free diet. The IgA antibodies developed against gluten cross-react with reticulin (a component of the anchoring fibrils that tether the epidermal basement membrane to the superficial dermis).

> **KEY FACT**
>
> Treatment for dermatitis herpetiformis is a gluten-free diet, or dapsone in non-responders.

Erythema Multiforme

An uncommon, self-limited disorder that appears to be a hypersensitivity response to certain infections (eg, *Mycoplasma* or herpes simplex virus [HSV]) and drugs. It is distinguishable by its target lesions—red papules that have a pale central area (Figure 5-55C).

- **Stevens-Johnson syndrome:** A febrile version of erythema multiforme that is marked by erosions and crusting of the mucosal surfaces of the lips, conjunctivae, oral cavity, urethra, and anogenital region along with bulla formation (Figure 5-55D). Less than 10% of the body surface area must be covered in order to make the diagnosis. It is commonly associated with drug reactions and carries a high mortality rate.
- **Toxic epidermal necrolysis:** Results in diffuse necrosis and sloughing of cutaneous and mucosal epithelial surfaces, producing a clinical situation analogous to an extensive burn (Figure 5-55E). This is the most severe version, affecting > 30% of the body surface area. Prognosis is poor, with a high mortality rate.

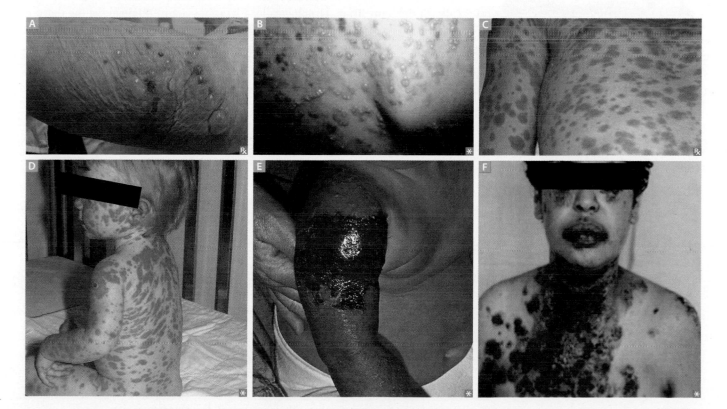

FIGURE 5-55.   Skin conditions with blisters. Physical appearance of **A** bullous pemphigoid; **B** dermatitis herpetiformis; **C** erythema multiforme; **D** Stevens-Johnson syndrome; **E** toxic epidermal necrolysis; and **F** pemphigus vulgaris.

Pemphigus Vulgaris

Pemphigus vulgaris is a rare autoimmune blistering disorder affecting the mucosa and skin (scalp, face, groin, and trunk) that, like bullous pemphigoid, is a type II hypersensitivity reaction. Early lesions appear as superficial vesicles and bullae that are suprabasal and easily rupture when touched (Figure 5-55F). It is caused by targeting of IgG antibodies against desmoglein in desmosomes, resulting in loss of integrity of normal intercellular attachments.

Acantholysis is the term for dissolution, or lysis, of the intercellular adhesion sites within a squamous epithelial surface. This is common to all forms of pemphigus. In contrast to bullous pemphigoid, pemphigus vulgaris is marked by reticular staining of antibodies under immunofluorescence.

Miscellaneous

Patients can be afflicted by many other skin conditions (Figure 5-56).

Acanthosis Nigricans

Caused by hyperplasia of the stratum spinosum. Patients present with a velvety, light-brown patch often in the axilla or on the back of the neck (Figure 5-56A). It is almost always associated with insulin resistance or underlying malignancy. Treatment involves eliciting the underlying cause and treating appropriately.

Lichen Planus

Pruritic, purple, polygonal papules are the presenting signs of this disorder of skin and mucous membranes. Resolving spontaneously in 1–2 years, it often leaves zones of postinflammatory hyperpigmentation (Figure 5-56B). Typically, there are multiple lesions on the flexor surface of extremities, mucous membranes, and genitalia. These lesions (especially in the oral mucosa) can sometimes have characteristic thin, white lines called **Wickham striae.** Histologically, a lymphocytic infiltrate along the dermo-epidermal junction gives the junction a zigzag contour known as a "saw-tooth" appearance. There is an association between lichen planus and hepatitis C.

Pityriasis Rosea

Self-resolving condition that begins with a single **"herald patch"** appearing on the trunk (Figure 5-56C), followed by multiple lesions on the chest and back, developing along the rib lines in a "Christmas tree" pattern. The lesions are usually oval in shape and may have a scaly border, called a "collarette scale." The rash usually resolves within 6–8 weeks.

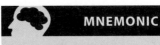

KEY FACT

A positive **Nikolsky sign** (rubbing of the skin results in complete separation of the outermost layer) is associated with pemphigus vulgaris and erythema multiforme. This sign is absent in bullous pemphigoid.

MNEMONIC

The 6 Ps of lichen planus:

Pruritic
Purple
Polygonal
Planar
Papules
Plaques

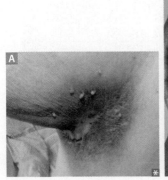
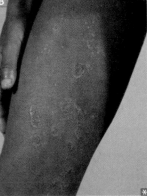
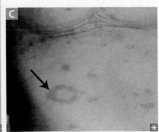

FIGURE 5-56.   Miscellaneous skin conditions. Physical appearance of **A** acanthosis nigricans; **B** lichen planus; and **C** herald patch (arrow) in pityriasis rosea.

Skin Cancer

The skin can be the site of both benign and malignant tumors (Figure 5-57).

Actinic Keratosis

Premalignant (dysplastic) lesions to squamous cell carcinoma that result from chronic sun exposure and are associated with a build-up of excess keratin. Lesions are < 1 cm in size and skin-colored with a sandpaper consistency. If too much keratin is deposited, "cutaneous horns" can develop.

Squamous Cell Carcinoma

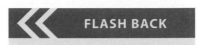

FLASH BACK

Patients with xeroderma pigmentosum cannot repair damaged DNA and are at increased risk for developing SCC and melanoma, as well as BCC.

Squamous cell carcinoma (SCC) is the second most common form of skin cancer, usually found on the face, lower lip, ears, and hands. Exposure to UV light with subsequent unrepaired DNA damage is the most frequent cause, although others exist. Prior to breaking through the basement membrane, SCC appears as a sharply defined, red, scaling plaque, which can ulcerate and/or develop chronic draining sinuses. It can become invasive or nodular, may develop hyperkeratosis, and may ulcerate. Histologically, atypia is present in all layers of the epidermis, and keratin "pearls" can be seen. Precursor lesions include actinic keratosis and **keratoacanthoma,** a rapidly growing, dome-shaped tumor with a keratinized cap. Only 5% metastasize.

Basal Cell Carcinoma

These common, slow-growing tumors also arise from chronic sun exposure. Clinically, they present as pearly papules, often containing prominent, dilated subepidermal blood vessels (telangiectasias). Basal cell carcinoma (BCC) tumors can also present with ulceration or as a superficial variant that appears as a scaling plaque. The cells forming the periphery of the tumor cell islands tend to be arranged radially with their long axes in approximately parallel alignment (palisading nuclei).

Malignant Melanoma

Melanoma is an aggressive cancer associated with sunlight exposure that can develop from dysplastic nevi. Activating mutations in the BRAF kinase are common driving forces in the transformation to malignancy. Clinical warning signs include a mole that

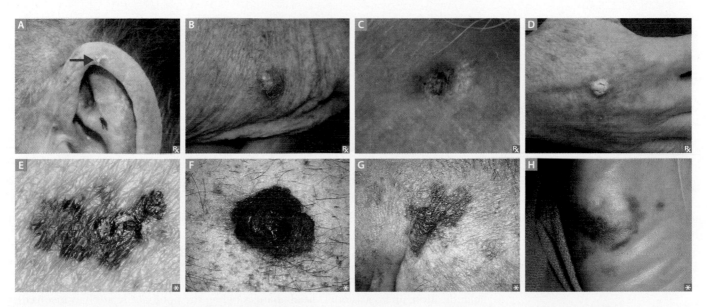

FIGURE 5-57. **Skin cancer lesions.** **A** Physical appearance of actinic keratosis (arrow); **B** squamous cell carcinoma; **C** basal cell carcinoma; **D** keratoacanthoma; **E** superficial spreading melanoma; **F** nodular melanoma; **G** lentigo maligna melanoma; and **H** acral lentiginous melanoma.

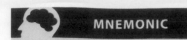

has enlarged, begins itching, or becomes painful; development of newly pigmented lesions in adults; irregular borders; and variation of color within a pigmented lesion. The depth of the tumor correlates directly with the risk of metastasis.

There are multiple types of melanoma, including **superficial spreading** (the most common type), **lentigo maligna** (raised papule on a dark patch in sun-exposed areas), **nodular** (dome-shaped lesion that grows vertically), and **acral lentiginous** (occurs on hands and mucosal surfaces, usually of Asian and black patients). Treatment consists of excision of the primary tumor. Metastatic disease is treated with chemotherapy; patients with the common *BRAF* V600E mutation may particularly benefit from a *BRAF* inhibitor such as vemurafenib.

VASCULITIDES

Goodpasture Syndrome

Goodpasture syndrome is an autoimmune disorder of unknown origin, characterized by a triad of diffuse **pulmonary hemorrhage, glomerulonephritis,** and antiglomerular basement membrane **(anti-GBM) antibodies.** Anti-GBM antibodies are specifically targeted against type IV collagen, which makes up most of the basement membrane. The disease is associated with **HLA-DR2;** there is a male predominance.

PRESENTATION

Most patients present with hemoptysis, cough, and dyspnea. Fever, chills, nausea, and vomiting can often accompany the pulmonary symptoms. Renal symptoms may rapidly progress to include azotemia and volume overload. The disease is most commonly seen in young men and elderly women, and generally represents a medical emergency.

DIAGNOSIS

A diagnosis is made by demonstrating circulating anti-GBM antibodies based on suspicion raised by the clinical picture. Chest X-rays may initially show bilateral perihilar or basilar consolidations, but ultimately progress toward a pattern consistent with interstitial lung disease. A lung or renal biopsy may be needed to demonstrate the presence of anti-GBM antibodies in the tissues.

TREATMENT

Aggressive treatment for Goodpasture syndrome includes corticosteroids, cyclophosphamide, and plasmapheresis in order to remove the circulating anti-GBM antibodies. Patients in acute renal failure may require dialysis.

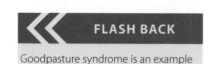

PROGNOSIS

Goodpasture syndrome is a medical emergency, and prognosis depends on the progression of the disease at diagnosis. Currently, the 5-year survival rates are about 80%. However, most patients who survive develop end-stage renal disease (ESRD), with approximately 30% requiring long-term dialysis.

Giant-Cell Arteritis (Temporal Arteritis)

Giant-cell arteritis (GCA) is primarily a large-vessel vasculitis, characterized by granulomatous inflammation of the internal elastic lamina. It typically affects the temporal artery but can involve any of the large branches of the carotids or arteries originating from the aorta. Clinically, GCA is manifested by temporal headache and tenderness, jaw claudication, and occasional visual changes (when the ophthalmic artery is involved). Approximately 50% of patients have symptoms of polymyalgia rheumatica (myalgias of the neck, shoulders, and hip girdle).

PRESENTATION

Patients usually complain of headaches (sometimes with scalp tenderness), vision disturbances, jaw claudication, and constitutional symptoms. In more severe cases, the patient may experience stroke symptoms or complete and sometimes permanent blindness. The disease affects older individuals (rarely < 50 years of age); with increasing age, the incidence of GCA rises. It is predominantly reported in white women (female-to-male ratio of 2:1) of Northern European descent.

DIAGNOSIS

The vast majority of patients present with an ESR > 50 mm/h, making this the most useful laboratory test, although it has low specificity. The diagnosis is usually suspected based on the clinical syndrome, but definitive diagnosis requires positive findings on temporal artery biopsy, including fragmentation of the intima with mononuclear and giant-cell infiltrates. However, the arteritis may have segmental involvement, so a negative biopsy does not exclude the diagnosis.

TREATMENT

High-dose prednisone remains the cornerstone of therapy and is begun based on high clinical suspicion rather than awaiting the results of biopsy. Treatment with slowly tapering doses of steroids usually continues for 12–18 months. Some patients are chronically maintained on very low dose (< 5 mg/day) prednisone or may require steroid-sparing medication (eg, methotrexate). Long-term steroid therapy requires prophylaxis against steroid-induced osteoporosis.

PROGNOSIS

The most dreaded complication, and a major source of morbidity, is loss of vision. This occurs in up to 15% of patients and is due to ischemic optic neuritis. Patients not treated for GCA generally develop widespread vasculitis leading to high rates of myocardial infarction and stroke. Steroid therapy can drastically reduce the risk of serious complications and often leads to complete resolution of the disease within several years, but side effects of treatment may also be significant.

Polyarteritis Nodosa

Polyarteritis nodosa (PAN) is characterized by inflammation of small and medium-sized arteries and typically affects the vessels of skin, peripheral nerves, kidneys, joints, and the GI tract. Histologically, the findings involve a transmural necrotizing inflammation, which can lead to arterial wall weakening, luminal obstruction, and aneurysm formation with resultant downstream ischemic damage. There is a strong association between PAN and hepatitis B, with pathogenesis attributed to immune complex formation.

PRESENTATION

PAN is a rare disorder that primarily affects individuals 40–60 years of age. It is more common in males, with a male-to-female ratio of 2:1. Key clinical features suggestive of PAN include skin lesions (palpable purpura, tender nodular lesions, **livedo reticularis**, and infarcts of the fingertips), peripheral neuropathy, hypertension with renal sediment abnormalities, orchitis in males (swelling of the testicles), and constitutional symptoms. GI involvement due to mesenteric arteritis is seen in 30% of the patients.

DIAGNOSIS

Elevated ESR, normocytic anemia, and decreased complement are usually present but findings are nonspecific. Hepatitis B surface antigen is present in 10–50% of the cases. Antineutrophil cytoplasmic antibodies (ANCA) are generally absent in PAN. Definitive diagnosis requires obtaining a biopsy specimen from accessible involved tissue (eg, skin, muscle, nerve) or imaging (ic, angiography) showing aneurysms and occlusions. The

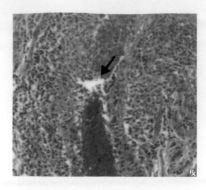

FIGURE 5-58. Polyarteritis nodosa (PAN). Histologic appearance (hematoxylin and eosin stain) of a typical acute lesion of PAN in a medium-sized artery. Note the presence of crowded blue nuclei representing immune cell infiltration and fibrinoid necrosis in the vessel wall (arrow).

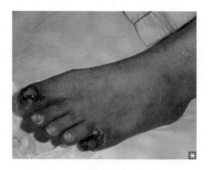

FIGURE 5-59. Buerger disease. Clinical appearance of a foot in a patient with Buerger disease.

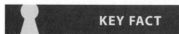

KEY FACT

Treat Buerger disease with smoking cessation!

pathologic feature defining classic PAN is a focal segmental necrotizing vasculitis of medium-sized and small arteries (Figure 5-58).

TREATMENT

High-dose corticosteroids remain the standard of care. Cytotoxic medications, such as cyclophosphamide, are added to corticosteroids in patients with major organ involvement.

PROGNOSIS

Outcome depends on the presence and extent of visceral and central nervous system (CNS) involvement. Most deaths occur within the first year, and nearly one-half of all untreated patients die within 3 months. However, corticosteroid therapy drastically improves prognosis, raising the 5-year survival rate to more than 50%.

Buerger Disease

Buerger disease, also known as thromboangiitis obliterans (TAO), is a vasculopathy of small- and medium-sized arteries. Characterized by segmental vascular inflammation and the absence of atheromas, it is most notable for a strong association with **heavy tobacco smoking.** Most people affected are 20–45 years of age and generally male. However, this gender discrepancy is thought to be due to the higher prevalence of smoking among males.

PRESENTATION

Usually presenting in younger patients who smoke, Buerger disease is characterized by distal extremity ischemia, claudication, and pain at rest (Figure 5-59). Persistent ischemic ulcers or gangrene of the digits and Raynaud phenomenon are also commonly present.

DIAGNOSIS

No specific laboratory tests or definitive histologic findings are helpful in establishing the diagnosis, which is based on clinical (including angiographic) findings. TAO is a diagnosis of exclusion, as many conditions, including atherosclerosis, emboli, autoimmune disease, hypercoagulable states, and diabetes, can mimic the symptoms.

TREATMENT

The only proven treatment for Buerger disease is the **complete discontinuation of tobacco use,** which has been shown to stop disease progression. Calcium channel blockers can be used to treat the vasospasm of Raynaud phenomenon. Limb amputation is sometimes necessary if the degree of damage is severe.

PROGNOSIS

There is a stark difference in prognosis for those patients who completely discontinue tobacco use and those who do not. More than 94% of patients who quit smoking avoid amputation, whereas among those who do not, 8-year amputation rates approach 43%. Of note, even when amputations are not required, claudication and Raynaud phenomenon often persist in those unwilling to abstain from tobacco use.

Takayasu Arteritis

Takayasu arteritis (TA), or **pulseless disease,** is a granulomatous inflammatory vasculitis of large arteries, including the aorta and its branches. Its mortality and morbidity arise from inflammation leading to aneurysm formation, stenosis, and thrombosis of large arteries.

PRESENTATION

Patients are typically young women, ranging in age from teens to thirties. The disease is particularly common in Asian populations. The presenting symptoms are usually constitutional (malaise, fever, and weight loss), and diagnosis is often delayed. Not uncommonly, the diagnosis is made when a mediastinal mass suspected to be a tumor turns out to be an aortic aneurysm. Physical examination may reveal arterial bruits, **unequal blood pressures between extremities, diminished pulses** ("pulseless disease"), or hypertension. In severe cases, inflammation of vessels may cause ischemic changes leading to visual disturbances, chest pain, or stroke.

DIAGNOSIS

There are no specific markers for TA. Arteriography and magnetic resonance angiography (MRA) are imaging modalities commonly used for diagnosing TA. The lesions are most often long-segment stenoses or arterial occlusions of the aorta and visceral vessels at their aortic origin. Due to the involvement of large arteries, biopsies are not performed.

TREATMENT

The main treatment for TA is high-dose systemic steroid therapy. Methotrexate and cyclophosphamide are used in patients who do not respond or in those patients in whom the minimally effective steroid dose is inappropriately too high for chronic use.

PROGNOSIS

Given the chronic relapsing-remitting nature of TA, patients require long periods of steroid treatment, which carries significant risks and side effects. Although the overall 15-year survival rate is reported to be as high as 90%, the morbidity and mortality depend on the degree of vascular and organ damage.

Granulomatosis With Polyangiitis (Wegener Granulomatosis)

Granulomatosis with polyangiitis (GWP) is a small-vessel necrotizing vasculitis of the upper and lower respiratory tracts with extravascular granulomatous inflammation, glomerulonephritis, and variable involvement of other organ systems (Table 5-12). Renal involvement is usually asymptomatic until advanced uremia develops—a very poor prognostic sign.

PRESENTATION

GWP affects patients of all ages, both sexes, and all races, although it is more commonly seen in whites. Patients usually present with constitutional symptoms, chronic sinusitis, epistaxis, mucosal ulcerations, and visual changes. Care must be taken in diagnosis, as the initial presentation is often misinterpreted as allergic or infectious in origin.

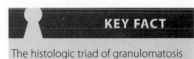

KEY FACT

The histologic triad of granulomatosis with polyangiitis is
(1) Focal necrotizing vasculitis
(2) Necrotizing granulomas of the lungs and upper airway
(3) Necrotizing glomerulonephritis

TABLE 5-12. Comparison of Granulomatosis with Polyangiitis (formerly Wegener Granulomatosis) and Goodpasture Syndrome

	GRANULOMATOSIS WITH POLYANGIITIS	GOODPASTURE SYNDROME
Pathogenesis	Autoimmune destruction of medium- and small-sized blood vessels	Antibodies against the basement membrane
Systems affected	Upper respiratory, lung, and renal involvement	Lung and renal involvement
Diagnosis	(+) c-ANCA	(+) Anti-GBM Linear staining on immunofluorescence

c-ANCA, cytoplasmic antineutrophilic antibody; GBM, glomerular basement membrane.

Pulmonary manifestations range from a complete lack of symptoms to chronic cough, alveolar hemorrhage, and pneumonitis. Renal disease is present in approximately 15% of patients initially and ultimately affects 50%.

DIAGNOSIS

In addition to clinical findings, diagnosis of GWP is suspected by demonstrating the presence of cytoplasmic antineutrophilic antibody (**c-ANCA**) that specifically is directed towards proteinase 3 (anti-PR3). Diagnostic biopsy results include small-vessel vasculitis, focal necrosis, and granulomatous changes. Chest radiographs or CT scan may show pulmonary nodular opacities, some of which may show cavitations.

TREATMENT

The mainstay of treatment is initially high-dose systemic steroids and an additional immunosuppressive. Additional treatments include methotrexate for disease limited to the upper respiratory tract and cyclophosphamide for more aggressive disease involvement. Trimethoprim-sulfamethoxazole (TMP-SMX) is used for maintenance therapy and while on cyclophosphamide to prevent *Pneumocystis jiroveci* pneumonia (PJP). IV immunoglobulins and plasmapheresis have been used in cases refractory to immunosuppressive therapy and in those with rapidly progressive glomerulonephritis.

PROGNOSIS

When left untreated, GWP is a rapidly fatal disease. Mortality is usually caused by renal failure and pulmonary complications within 5 months of diagnosis. However, aggressive immunosuppressive therapy leads to improvement in more than 90% of patients, with about 75% achieving remission.

Churg-Strauss Vasculitis

Churg-Strauss syndrome is a necrotizing vasculitis with eosinophilia affecting both medium and small vessels. It is often characterized by constitutional symptoms, prominent involvement of the respiratory tract with asthma-like symptoms, and skin lesions, including palpable purpura and subcutaneous nodules.

PRESENTATION

Patients usually present with new-onset **allergies** and **asthma** or sudden worsening of preexisting allergic conditions. They may also have increased cough, arthralgias, or asymmetric peripheral neuropathy. GI symptoms include bleeding, diarrhea, and colitis. Cardiac and renal manifestations are also seen.

DIAGNOSIS

Churg-Strauss is generally diagnosed based on clinical criteria, which include asthma, paranasal sinusitis, and peripheral neuropathy. Eosinophilia in blood, pulmonary nodular opacities on chest X-ray, and histologic evidence of vasculitis with eosinophils can be additional positive findings in support of a diagnosis. Serum levels of IgE also may be elevated. Unlike patients with GWP, patients with Churg-Strauss have a positive perinuclear antineutrophilic antibody (**p-ANCA**) that is specifically directed toward myeloperoxidase (anti-MPO).

TREATMENT

Treatment consists of high-dose steroids and immunosuppressives, as with many of the other vasculitides.

PROGNOSIS

Unfortunately, even with steroids, prognosis is poor. The 5-year survival rate is only 50%, with death occurring primarily due to cardiac and pulmonary complications.

Kawasaki Disease

Kawasaki disease (KD) is a febrile vasculitis of childhood characterized by fever, rash, conjunctivitis (usually unilateral), cervical adenopathy, mucocutaneous symptoms, and coronary artery aneurysms. Currently, KD is the leading cause of acquired cardiac disease in young children.

PRESENTATION

Diagnosis of KD is challenging due to its nonspecific and general presentation. It is a disease of young children with a peak incidence during the first 2 years. Children with KD typically present with fever that is unresponsive to antibiotics, and they are often found to be disproportionately irritable. Presenting signs also include erythema, desquamation and edema of the extremities, conjunctivitis, rash, lymphadenopathy, strawberry tongue, and swollen/fissured lips (Figure 5-60). KD is more common in the Japanese population and slightly more prevalent in males but can occur in any race and both genders.

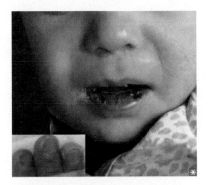

FIGURE 5-60. **Kawasaki disease.** Young patient presenting with cherry-red lips with hemorrhagic fissures, as well as erythema and edema of the fingertips.

DIAGNOSIS

Criteria for the diagnosis of KD include:

- Prolonged high-grade fever > 5 days.
- Conjunctivitis.
- Cracking and fissuring of lips with inflammation of mucosal membranes (strawberry tongue)
- Unilateral cervical lymphadenopathy.
- Rash involving the trunk and extremities.
- Erythema and edema of the hands and feet, progressing to desquamation.

To meet the diagnosis, four of the above criteria plus prolonged fever must be present.

TREATMENT

Treatment of KD is aimed at the prevention of coronary artery aneurysm formation and the resultant cardiac sequelae. IV immunoglobulins and high-dose aspirin are used as anti-inflammatory agents. For those patients who do develop coronary artery complications, surgical stenting, bypass, and even heart transplantation may be necessary.

PROGNOSIS

Acute KD is self-limiting; however, the main source of long-term morbidity and mortality is the development of cardiac complications. These include myocarditis, pericarditis, congestive heart failure, myocardial infarction, and aortic insufficiency. Twenty percent of untreated patients develop **coronary artery aneurysms,** which are associated with increased risk of fatal thrombosis or rupture. Therefore, follow-up imaging is advised for patients with KD.

Henoch-Schönlein Purpura

This small-vessel vasculitis is characterized clinically by palpable purpura, colicky abdominal pain, arthritis, and hematuria. Histologically, it involves **IgA,** C3, and immune complex deposition in arterioles, venules, and capillaries. Henoch-Schönlein purpura (HSP) is a multisystem disease and tends to involve skin, connective tissues, joints, kidneys, the GI tract, and the scrotum. Importantly, HSP and IgA nephropathy are related disorders, with the key difference being that IgA nephropathy only involves the kidneys in young adults, whereas HSP has other organ involvement and predominantly affects younger children.

PRESENTATION

The median age at presentation is 4 years, and the male-to-female ratio is about 1.5:1. Close to 50% have a history of preceding upper respiratory tract infection. The classic triad for HSP involves skin findings (**palpable purpura**) on buttocks and lower extremities, arthralgias, and GI symptoms (abdominal pain or intussusception). Palpable purpura refers to large areas of raised bruising stemming from extravasation of RBCs from injured vessels. Renal involvement is usually mild, but patients may present with hematuria. Testicular swelling and a history of bloody stools may also be elicited.

DIAGNOSIS

HSP is a clinical diagnosis, as most laboratory values tend to be within normal ranges. Renal tests and urinalysis may be abnormal if the kidneys are involved.

TREATMENT

Treatment is mainly conservative and symptomatic. NSAIDs are used to relieve joint pain. Even though NSAIDs do not seem to result in further platelet inhibition or increased purpura, caution must still be taken in patients with affected kidney function. Although no data exist to support their effectiveness, corticosteroids are occasionally used.

PROGNOSIS

Most (97%) children have a self-limited course lasting 1–2 weeks. However, approximately 20% have a recurrence during the first year. A small percentage of patients have persistent purpura, with or without renal involvement. Less than 1% of all cases progress to ESRD.

See Table 5-13 for high-yield features of each of the previously discussed vasculitides.

Pharmacology

DRUGS USED TO TREAT DISORDERS OF BONE

Bisphosphonates (Risedronate, Alendronate, Clodronate, Etidronate, Ibandronate, Pamidronate, Tiludronate, Zoledronate)

MECHANISM

Bind to bone, inhibit osteoclast-mediated bone resorption, and indirectly stimulate osteoblast activity.

USES

Osteoporosis, Paget disease, hypercalcemia, metastatic bone disease.

SIDE EFFECTS

GI disturbances (dyspepsia, reflux esophagitis, peptic ulcers), pill/corrosive esophagitis, and bone pain.

Calcitonin

MECHANISM

Inhibits bone resorption, leading to decreased blood calcium and phosphate. Calcitonin binds to receptors on osteoclasts and inhibits their action. In the kidney, calcitonin decreases the resorption of both calcium and phosphate in the proximal tubules.

MNEMONIC

Calci**ton**in **tones** down serum calcium levels by inhibiting osteoclast action and calcium phosphate resorption.

TABLE 5-13. **Common Symptoms and Findings in High-Yield Vasculitides**

DISORDER	VASCULITIS	EPIDEMIOLOGY	CLINICAL/LAB FINDINGS
Large artery			
Takayasu arteritis ("pulseless disease")	Granulomatous thickening of aortic arch and associated vessels	Asian women < 40 years old	Absent/weak upper extremity pulses, ocular disturbances, fever, arthritis, stroke
Medium artery			
Giant-cell (temporal) arteritis	Most common vasculitis affecting medium and large arteries. Granulomatous vasculitis commonly involving the superficial temporal artery	Elderly women > 50 years of age	Unilateral temporal headache, jaw claudication and impaired vision from ophthalmic artery occlusion Associated with polymyalgia rheumatica and ↑ ESR
Polyarteritis nodosa	Necrotizing immune complex inflammation of medium arteries (typically renal and visceral vessels)	Middle-aged men Associated with hepatitis B in 30% of patients	Vessels at all stages of inflammation Organ infarctions in kidneys, heart, bowels, and skin lead to renal failure, acute MI, bloody diarrhea, ischemic ulcers
Kawasaki disease	Necrotizing vasculitis involving coronary arteries	Self-limiting disease in children < 4 years of age	Fever, congested conjunctiva, desquamating rash, swelling of hands and feet, cervical adenopathy Abnormal ECG
Thromboangiitis obliterans (Buerger disease)	Idiopathic, segmental, thrombosing vasculitis	Seen in heavy smokers	Intermittent claudication, Raynaud phenomenon, may lead to gangrene
Small artery			
Granulomatosis with polyangiitis (Wegener granulomatosis)	Focal necrotizing vasculitis and granulomas in the upper airways, lungs, and kidneys	Children and adults	Perforation of nasal septum, sinusitis, otitis media, cough, hemoptysis, hematuria c-ANCA/anti-PR3 (+)
Microscopic polyangiitis	Similar to Wegener granulomatosis but lacking granulomas	Children and adults	Vessels at same stage of inflammation p- or c-ANCA (+)
Churg-Strauss syndrome	Granulomatous vasculitis with eosinophilia	Often seen in atopic patients	Allergic rhinitis, asthma, and eosinophilia p-ANCA/anti-MPO (+)
Henoch-Schönlein purpura	Involves skin, GI tract, renal vessels Related to IgA immune complex deposition	Most common form of childhood vasculitis	Palpable purpura of buttocks and lower extremities, polyarthritis, glomerulonephritis, and GI bleeding, often after URI

c-ANCA, cytoplasmic antineutrophilic antibody; ECG, electrocardiogram; ESR, erythrocyte sedimentation rate; MI, myocardial infarction; p-ANCA, perinuclear antineutrophilic antibody; URI, upper respiratory infection.

USES

Hypercalcemia, neoplasia, Paget disease, postmenopausal osteoporosis, corticosteroid-induced osteoporosis.

SIDE EFFECTS

Nausea, vomiting, tingling sensation in the hands, unpleasant taste in the mouth.

Teriparatide (Recombinant Parathyroid Hormone [Forteo])

MECHANISM

Stimulates Ca^{2+} absorption in the renal distal convoluted tubules and the release of calcium from bone through a G protein-coupled receptor.

USES

Osteoporosis.

SIDE EFFECTS

Nausea, headache, dizziness, hypercalcemia, leg cramps.

Selective Estrogen Receptor Modulators (SERMs) (Raloxifene, Tamoxifen)

MECHANISM

Activate estrogen receptors in bone and the cardiovascular system but have antagonist activity on estrogen receptors in mammary tissue or the uterus. SERMs also inhibit cytokines, recruit osteoclasts, and block PTH's bone-resorbing, calcium-mobilizing action.

USES

Osteoporosis prevention, breast cancer.

SIDE EFFECTS

Hot flashes, postmenopausal vasomotor symptoms, flushing, and increased risk of deep vein thrombosis and pulmonary embolism—tamoxifen is contraindicated in patients with a history of either. Tamoxifen may increase the risk of endometrial carcinoma via partial agonist effects.

TNF-α Antagonists (Adalimumab, Certolizumab, Etanercept, Golimumab, Infliximab)

MECHANISM

Block inflammatory cytokine TNF-α.

USES

RA, psoriasis, psoriatic arthritis, ankylosing spondylitis.

SIDE EFFECTS

Hypersensitivity, infection, exacerbation of heart failure, neuropathy, and risk of malignancy (skin cancer, possibly development of lymphoproliferative diseases).

Need to test for tuberculosis (TB) before starting, as these drugs can reactivate latent TB.

DRUGS USED TO TREAT GOUT

Colchicine

MECHANISM

Prevents neutrophil and leukocyte migration into the joint by binding to tubulin, depolymerizing microtubules, and interfering with motility and degranulation.

USES

Prophylaxis or relief of **acute** gout attack.

SIDE EFFECTS

GI disturbances, nausea, vomiting, abdominal pain, hepatic toxicity, and rarely neuro-myotoxicity. Severe diarrhea and GI hemorrhage may be a problem with large doses or standard doses in the setting of renal insufficiency. Since NSAIDs and steroids are potentially less toxic, they are more commonly used in acute attacks.

Xanthine Oxidase Inhibitors (Allopurinol, Febuxostat)

MECHANISM

Reduce the synthesis of uric acid by inhibiting the enzyme xanthine oxidase (Figure 5-61). For chronic use to prevent gout by lowering serum urate levels, but ineffective, and may aggravate acute gout.

USES

Both agents are used in the long-term prevention of gout. Allopurinol is additionally used for prevention of urate nephrolithiasis and tumor lysis syndrome.

SIDE EFFECTS

- Allopurinol: GI disturbances, liver function test abnormalities, and allergic skin reactions.
- Febuxostat: GI disturbances, liver function test abnormalities.

Probenecid

MECHANISM

Inhibits the absorption of uric acid in the proximal convoluted tubule, thus increasing uric acid excretion (see Figure 5-61). Be careful prescribing penicillins for patients on probenecid, as coadministration can lead to increased penicillin levels. Must have adequate renal function and is contraindicated if the patient has a history of nephrolithiasis.

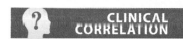

> **CLINICAL CORRELATION**
>
> Allopurinol is also used in lymphoma and leukemia to prevent tumor lysis syndrome and is associated with urate neuropathy.

> **CLINICAL CORRELATION**
>
> Probenecid promotes plasma penicillin levels.

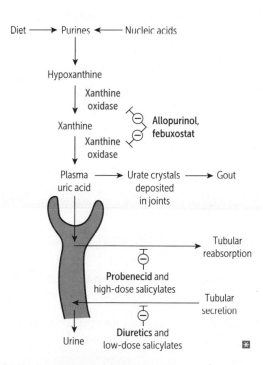

FIGURE 5-61.   Pharmacologic interventions in gout.

USES

Chronic gout.

SIDE EFFECTS

Dyspepsia and peptic ulceration. Hypersensitivity reactions occur occasionally as skin rashes. Drug-induced nephritic syndrome has been reported.

DRUGS USED TO TREAT CONNECTIVE TISSUE DISEASES

Corticosteroids

MECHANISM

By complexing with cytosolic receptors, corticosteroids can enter the nucleus and alter gene expression through tissue-specific nuclear response elements. This leads to inhibition of inflammatory cytokine production and relief of mucosal inflammation. Corticosteroids also reduce bronchial reactivity, increase airway caliber, and reduce the frequency of asthma exacerbations.

USES

Reduction of disease flare-ups, acute inflammation, and asthma.

SIDE EFFECTS

With short-term use, these can include sleeping difficulties, dyspepsia, increased appetite, tremulousness, and anxiety/psychosis. Long-term use can lead to Cushing syndrome, obesity, diabetes, osteoporosis, and infections due to immune suppression.

Cyclophosphamide

MECHANISM

The liver metabolizes cyclophosphamide into its active form, phosphoramide mustard. This form cross-links DNA and inhibits T- and B-cell function.

USES

Severe disease in patients with SLE, RA, vasculitis syndromes, and certain cancers (breast, ovarian and non-Hodgkin lymphoma).

SIDE EFFECTS

Ovarian failure, infertility, bone marrow suppression, **hemorrhagic cystitis,** increased risk for malignancy.

KEY FACT

A major side effect of cyclophosphamide is cystitis. Mesna is used to prevent cyclophosphamide-induced cystitis by binding to the metabolite acrolein in the bladder.

DRUGS USED TO TREAT PAIN

Opioids

MECHANISM

Opiates facilitate the opening of potassium channels, causing hyperpolarization that inhibits calcium channel opening and transmitter release. There are three different types of opioid receptors: μ (morphine), δ (enkephalin), and κ (dynorphin). All opioid receptors are linked through G proteins and inhibition of adenylate cyclase.

USES

Pain relief, cough suppression (dextromethorphan), diarrhea (loperamide and diphenoxylate), acute pulmonary edema, and as maintenance for opioid addicts (methadone).

SIDE EFFECTS

Sedation, respiratory depression, constipation, nausea, miosis (pinpoint pupils), and additive CNS depression with other drugs. Opioid antagonists such as naloxone and naltrexone can be given for overdose, as these drugs occupy the opioid receptors without exerting any effect.

Aspirin

MECHANISM

Acetylates and **irreversibly** inhibits cyclooxygenase (both COX-1 and COX-2) to prevent conversion of arachidonic acid to prostaglandins. Aspirin may increase bleeding but has no effect on prothrombin time (PT) or partial thromboplastin time (PTT).

USES

Antipyretic, analgesic, anti-inflammatory, antiplatelet activity, Kawasaki disease, OA, and inflammatory arthritides.

SIDE EFFECTS

Gastric ulceration, bleeding, hyperventilation, Reye syndrome, tinnitus.

Nonsteroidal Anti-inflammatory Drugs (Ibuprofen, Naproxen, Indomethacin, Ketorolac, and Others)

MECHANISM

Reversibly inhibit arachidonic acid and cyclooxygenase (COX-1 and COX-2), thus inhibiting production of prostaglandins and thromboxanes (Figure 5-62). COX-1 is a constitutive enzyme expressed in most tissues, including platelets. COX-2 is induced in inflammatory cells upon activation. NSAIDs increase bleeding time but have no effect on prothrombin time (PT) or partial thromboplastin time (PTT).

USES

Anti-inflammatory, analgesic, antipyretic, and antiplatelet effects. Indomethacin is used to close a patent ductus arteriosus.

SIDE EFFECTS

Renal damage, aplastic anemia, GI distress, ulcers, fluid retention, and hypertension.

Cyclooxygenase-2 Inhibitors (Celecoxib)

MECHANISM

Selectively inhibit cyclooxygenase-2 (COX-2) found in inflammatory cells. Unlike non-specific NSAIDs, COX-2 inhibitors spare the gastric mucosa from the corrosive effects of COX-1 inhibition.

USES

Anti-inflammatory and analgesic effects, often in such chronic conditions as RA.

SIDE EFFECTS

Side effects are similar to those of other NSAIDs but with less GI mucosa toxicity (ie, lower incidence of ulcers and bleeding). There is a small, but potentially clinically relevant, increased risk of cardiovascular events with COX-2 inhibitors when compared with nonselective NSAIDs, although all NSAIDs may increase risk.

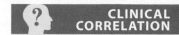

CLINICAL CORRELATION

Supplemental O_2 is contraindicated in morphine overdose in the patient with chronic obstructive pulmonary disease (COPD), as it might further suppress the patient's respiratory drive and contribute to respiratory failure.

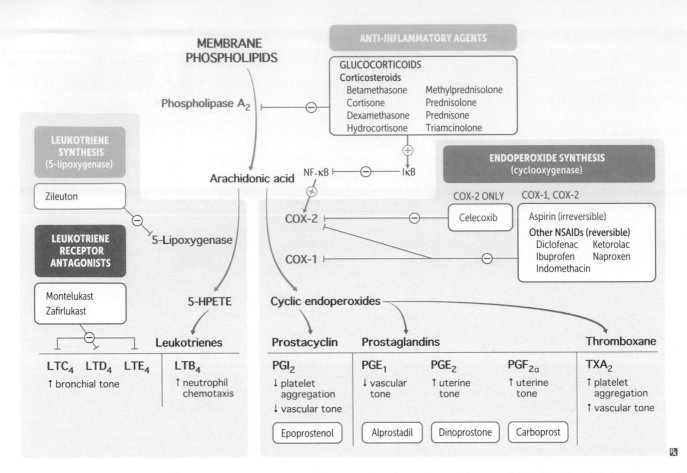

FIGURE 5-62. **Mediators derived from arachidonic acid.** Summary of mediators derived from arachidonic acid and their actions, and sites of action for anti-inflammatory drugs.

Acetaminophen

MECHANISM

Reversibly and weakly inhibits cyclooxygenase and is peripherally inactivated. Most of the effects are centered in the CNS.

USES

Antipyretic and analgesic but no effect on inflammation.

SIDE EFFECTS

Significant hepatic necrosis can occur with high doses, as hepatic metabolism of acetaminophen creates a highly toxic intermediate called N-acetyl-p-benzoquinone imine (NAPQI). This metabolite must be detoxified by conjugation to glutathione, but glutathione can be depleted when processing high doses of acetaminophen. Liver damage can be prevented if **N-acetylcysteine** is given to quickly regenerate glutathione (Figure 5-63).

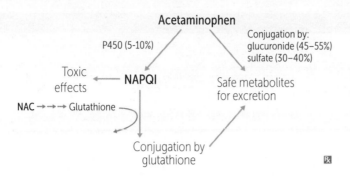

FIGURE 5-63. **Acetaminophen metabolism.** Acetaminophen is metabolized by the liver via conjugation with glucuronide or sulfate to create non-toxic metabolites. Alternatively, the P450 system can metabolize acetaminophen into cysteine or mercapturic acid, especially when the conjugation pathway becomes saturated by high drug doses. This process involves the formation of the toxic NAPQI intermediate, which must be detoxified by conjugation to glutathione. N-acetylcysteine (NAC) can replenish glutathione to prevent accumulation of NAPQI in the case of overdose.

NOTES

CHAPTER 6

Neurology and Special Senses

EMBRYOLOGY, ANATOMY, AND PHYSIOLOGY 412

Nervous System Development 412

Brain Development 414

Deep Brain Structures 431

Cerebellum 437

Brain Stem 440

Neurotransmitters 446

Spinal Cord 446

Cranial Nerves 457

Sensory Pathways 459

HISTOLOGY 464

Cells of the Nervous System 464

Intercellular Communication 466

PATHOLOGY 468

Neural Tube Defects 468

Ventricular System Malformations 468

Noncommunicating Hydrocephalus 469

Communicating Hydrocephalus 470

Hydrocephalus Mimics 473

Cerebrovascular Disorders 473

Dyskinesias 478

Aphasias 479

Degenerative Diseases 480

Demyelinating Diseases 481

Seizures 488

Cerebral Edema 488

Cerebral Contusion 489

Primary Brain Neoplasms 490

Neurocutaneous Disorders 492

Spinal Cord and Peripheral Nerve Lesions 494

Peripheral Neuropathy 499

Cranial Nerve Palsy 499

Central Nervous System Infections 503

Herniation Syndromes 503

Headache Syndromes 505

PHARMACOLOGY 507

Central Nervous System Neurotransmitters 507

Autonomic Drugs 508

Seafood Toxins 512

Anxiolytics and Hypnotics 513

Antidepressants 516

Neuroleptics 520

Mood Stabilizers and Anticonvulsants 521

Treatments for Neurodegenerative Disease 527

Clinical Anesthetics and Analgesics 530

Embryology, Anatomy, and Physiology

NERVOUS SYSTEM DEVELOPMENT

The nervous system is one of the first systems to develop. In the third gestational week, following gastrulation, the neural tube forms, and neural crest cells emerge and migrate, beginning the precisely controlled development of the central and peripheral nervous systems, respectively.

Gastrulation

During week 3 of embryogenesis, the three layers of embryonic tissue form through a process known as gastrulation (Figure 6-1):

- Ectodermal cells detach from the epiblast, the surface layer of the embryo, invaginate inward into a groove known as the primitive streak, and form the mesoderm and endoderm.
- Mesodermal cells in the primitive streak then migrate toward the head until blocked by the fused buccopharyngeal membrane at the primitive node (the most rostral part of primitive streak).
- In parallel, prenotochordal cells also invaginate and move rostrally, forming a line known as the **notochord** from the primitive node to the prechordal plate.

Neurulation

The primitive streak regresses and disappears, dragging the notochord toward the buccopharyngeal membrane.

The steps of neurulation are summarized in Figure 6-2.

- The notochord induces the overlying region of the ectoderm to form the **neural plate.**
- The neural plate begins to invaginate along the longitudinal axis and forms the **neural groove.**
- The neural groove continues to invaginate until the surrounding neural folds meet to form an open **neural tube,** the precursor to the central nervous system (CNS).
- The open neural tube then closes, starting in the center (at the middle of the future body) and progressing caudally and rostrally.

Neural Tube Defects

Failure of the neural tube to close at either end leads to birth defects.

- Failure of rostral neuropore closure leads to anencephaly, a condition characterized by the absence of the scalp, skull, and large portions of the forebrain.
- Failure of caudal neuropore closure leads to spina bifida (Figure 6-3).

KEY FACT

2 weeks = 2 layers (epiblast, hypoblast)
3 weeks = 3 layers (ectoderm, mesoderm, endoderm)

KEY FACT

Remnants of the **primitive streak** can become *sacraococcygeal teratomas.* Remember, teratomas include all three germ layers.

KEY FACT

The **notochord** becomes the nucleus pulposus, which lies within the vertebral column in the adult. Herniation of the nucleus pulposus through the annulus fibrosus may result in spinal root impingement and pain.

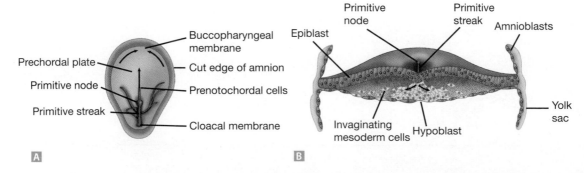

FIGURE 6-1.   **Gastrulation.** **A** Topographical view of migrating cells during gastrulation. Invaginating mesoderm cells (prenotochordal cells) detach from the epiblast and migrate along the longitudinal axis to form the notochord. **B** Cross-sectional view of mesodermal cells detaching from the epiblast.

Spina Bifida

Spina bifida occurs when the two halves of the vertebral arch fail to fuse, most commonly in the lumbosacral region (L5 and/or S1). Thus, the vertebral arch consists of two parts and is hence "bifid." Variations of spina bifida range from mild to severe. The clinical manifestations and severity of spina bifida vary depending on the degree of closure of the caudal/rostral neuropore as well as the location of the fusion defect (Table 6-1). Elevated levels of α-fetoprotein and acetylcholinesterase in maternal serum or amniotic fluid are suggestive of fetal neural tube defects.

Causes of neural tube defects include genetic factors, increased alcohol intake during pregnancy, and certain drugs taken during the first trimester, most notably valproic acid, an anticonvulsant. All pregnant women should take folic acid supplements to help prevent neural tube defects.

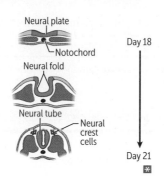

FIGURE 6-2. **Neurulation (in cross-section).**

Cross-Section of the Neural Tube

- The **neural tube** gives rise to the CNS, including the brain, brain stem, and spinal cord. In the brain stem and spinal cord, the dorsal alar plate, the ventral basal plate, and the intervening sulcus limitans develop within the central canal of the neural tube.
    - **Alar plate:** Gives rise to sensory neurons (lateral).
    - **Basal plate:** Gives rise to motor neurons (medial).
    - **Sulcus limitans:** Separates the two plates.
- **Neural crest cells** are derived from ectodermal cells. Ectoderm at the edges of the neural folds is induced by the neural tube to form neuroepithelia. These neural crest cells then migrate and give rise to multiple adult derivatives (see Figures 6-2 and 6-4), including:
    - Peripheral nervous system (PNS) ganglia and neurons.
    - Schwann cells.
    - Chromaffin cells of the adrenal medulla.
    - Melanocytes in the skin.
    - Connective tissue and skeletal tissue of the pharyngeal arches.
    - C cells (parafollicular cells) of the thyroid, which produce calcitonin.
    - Aortic arch and aorticopulmonary septum.
    - Enterochromaffin cells of the intestines (Auerbach and Meissner plexuses).
    - Odontoblasts.
    - Leptomeningeal cells (pia and arachnoid mater).
    - Sclera, cornea, and ciliary muscle.

Common disorders of neural crest cell migration are listed in Table 6-2.

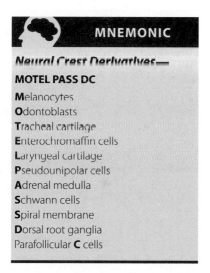

MNEMONIC

Neural Crest Derivatives—

MOTEL PASS DC

Melanocytes
Odontoblasts
Tracheal cartilage
Enterochromaffin cells
Laryngeal cartilage
Pseudounipolar cells
Adrenal medulla
Schwann cells
Spiral membrane
Dorsal root ganglia
Parafollicular **C** cells

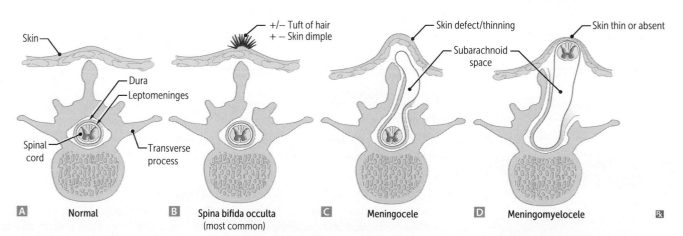

FIGURE 6-3. **Types of spina bifida.** The severity of spina bifida correlates with the degree of herniation of the contents: **B** none, **C** meninges, and **D** meninges and spinal cord.

TABLE 6-1. Neural Tube Defects

NEURAL TUBE DEFECT	ABERRANT ANATOMY	CLINICAL MANIFESTATION
Spina bifida occulta	Failure of vertebral arches to close without herniation of intraspinal contents	Small tuft of hair overlying the defect without any visible herniated contents. Spinal cord and nerves are usually normal. Occulta is the mildest version of spina bifida
Meningocele (*meningo* = meninges)	Failure of vertebral arches to close with herniation of meninges but not spinal cord	Herniated lumbosacral sac contains CSF and meninges, forming a lumbosacral cyst
Meningomyelocele (*myelo* = cord)	Failure of vertebral arches to close with herniation of both meninges and spinal cord	Herniated lumbosacral sac contains CSF, meninges, and spinal cord. Depending on the location, paralysis and loss of deep tendon reflexes and sensation in the lower extremities, as well as incontinence, may be seen. Associated with type II Arnold-Chiari syndrome
Meningoencephalocele (*encephalo* = brain)	Occipital bone is most commonly missing	Mental retardation
Meningohydroencephalocele (*hydro* = fluid)	Herniation of meninges, brain, and CSF-containing ventricles	Mental retardation

CSF, cerebrospinal fluid.

BRAIN DEVELOPMENT

Formation of Brain Vesicles

From week 6 onward, the neural tube forms three primary brain vesicles that give rise to five secondary vesicles. These secondary vesicles develop into various structures in the adult brain and associated cerebrospinal fluid (CSF)–filled cavities (Figure 6-5).

The three primary vesicles are:

- Forebrain (prosencephalon).
- Midbrain (mesencephalon).
- Hindbrain (rhombencephalon).

The five secondary vesicles are:

- Telencephalon (derived from the prosencephalon).
- Diencephalon (derived from the prosencephalon).
- Mesencephalon.
- Metencephalon (derived from the rhombencephalon).
- Myelencephalon (derived from the rhombencephalon).

Congenital Malformations

Chiari Malformation

Chiari malformation involves congenital herniation of the cerebellum through the foramen magnum, due to impaired development of posterior fossa.

- Occurs in 1 in 1000 live births.
- Type I: Herniation of cerebellar tonsils only (Figure 6-6).
- Type II (aka Arnold-Chiari malformation): Breaking of the tectal plate, aqueductal stenosis, herniation and unrolling of the vermis into the vertebral canal, and stretching of cranial nerves (CN) IX, X, and XI. May also present with syringomyelia in C8–T1 and lumbar meningomyelocele.

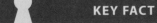

KEY FACT

Syringomyelia = fluid-filled cavity (cyst) within the spinal cord that often manifests with a "capelike" distribution of sensory loss.

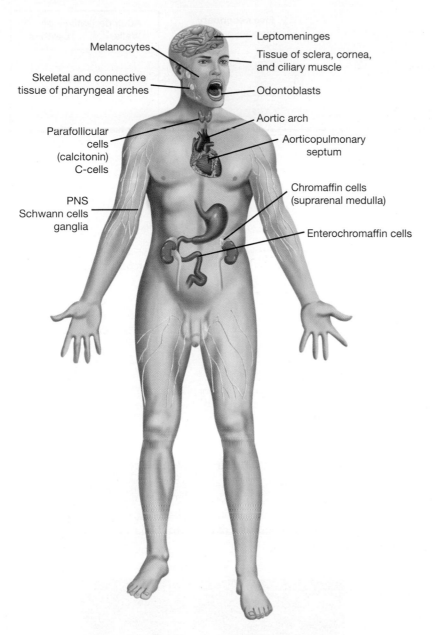

FIGURE 6-4.   Neural crest derivatives. The neural crest cells migrate peripherally from the neural tube to develop into the peripheral nervous system (PNS) and other important structures.

PRESENTATION

■ Type I may not show neurologic symptoms until adolescence or adult life and may include cerebellar ataxia, obstructive hydrocephalus, brain stem compression, and syringomyelia.

TABLE 6-2.   Neural Crest Derivatives and Their Corresponding Defects

NEURAL CREST DERIVATIVE	DEFECT
Aortic arch/aorticopulmonary septum	Great-vessel deformities
Pharyngeal pouches 3 and 4	DiGeorge syndrome
Enterochromaffin cells	Hirschsprung disease, achalasia
Melanocytes	Albinism

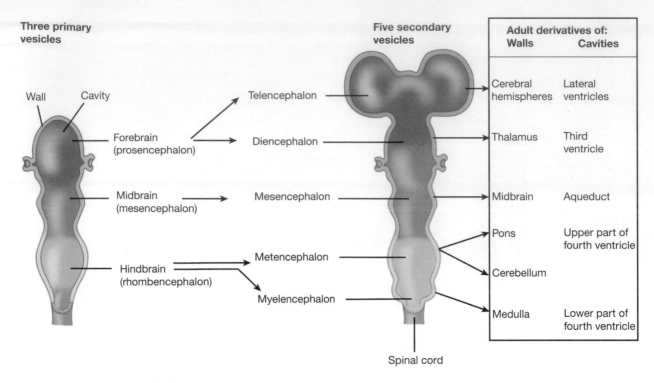

Three primary vesicles		Five secondary vesicles	Adult derivatives of:	
			Walls	Cavities
	Telencephalon		Cerebral hemispheres	Lateral ventricles
Forebrain (prosencephalon)	Diencephalon		Thalamus	Third ventricle
Midbrain (mesencephalon)	Mesencephalon		Midbrain	Aqueduct
			Pons	Upper part of fourth ventricle
Hindbrain (rhombencephalon)	Metencephalon		Cerebellum	
	Myelencephalon		Medulla	Lower part of fourth ventricle

Wall Cavity

Spinal cord

FIGURE 6-5. **Development of brain vesicles.**

- Type II may manifest with:
  - Difficulty swallowing (due to compression of the nucleus ambiguus).
  - Loss of pain/temperature sensation along the back of the neck and shoulders secondary to syringomyelia, which interrupts the ascending afferent sensory fibers in the spinothalamic tract.
  - Mental retardation secondary to coincident meningomyelocele, a visible cyst containing spinal cord matter protruding from the dorsum of the spine.
  - Hydrocephalus due to occlusion of cerebrospinal fluid (CSF) flow through the foramen magnum.

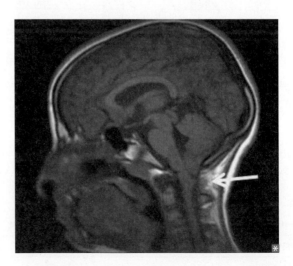

FIGURE 6-6. **Arnold-Chiari malformation type I.** The cerebellar tonsils (arrow) herniate through the foramen magnum.

PROGNOSIS

Depends on the degree of severity.

- Type I: Normal life span.
- Type II: Fifteen percent die within 1 year of birth. Death is usually due to cranial nerve and brain stem dysfunction resulting in respiratory failure.

Dandy-Walker Syndrome

Dandy-Walker syndrome occurs in 1 in 25,000 births, far less common than Arnold-Chiari syndrome. It is characterized by cerebellar vermis hypoplasia and failure of the foramina of Luschka and Magendie to open, resulting in dilation of the fourth ventricle (Figure 6-7).

PRESENTATION

Hydrocephalus, ataxia, and mental retardation.

PROGNOSIS

Varied; some may lead normal lives, and others die soon after birth. Overall, it carries a 12–50% mortality rate.

Hydrocephalus

Hydrocephalus is defined as an abnormal accumulation of CSF in the ventricles, which in turn may lead to an increased intracranial pressure (ICP). The most common congenital cause is aqueductal stenosis, a consequence of maternal infection (eg, cytomegalovirus [CMV] or toxoplasmosis).

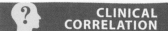

CLINICAL CORRELATION

Arnold-Chiari malformation:
- Aqueductal stenosis
- Herniation and unrolling of vermis into vertebral canal

Type I:
- May not show neurologic symptoms until adolescence or adulthood
- More common (1:1000)
- Only tonsils herniate

Type II:
- Small posterior fossa
- True herniation of brain stem
- Psychomotor retardation and developmental delays are frequently observed
- Cervical syringomyelia and lumbar meningomyelocele often associated

Dandy-Walker syndrome:
- Cerebellar vermis hypoplasia
- Dilation of the fourth ventricle

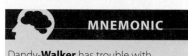

MNEMONIC

Dandy-**Walker** has trouble with **walking**

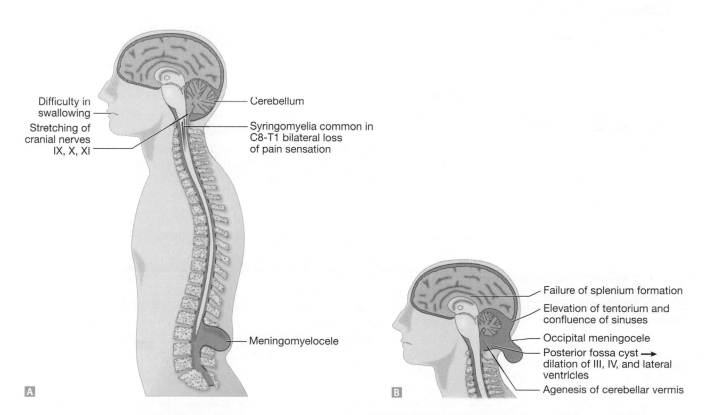

FIGURE 6-7.   Comparison of Arnold-Chiari syndrome types I and II and Dandy-Walker syndrome. A Arnold-Chiari syndrome is much more common and involves a "falling through" of the cerebellum. B Dandy-Walker syndrome entails agenesis of the cerebellum and expansion of the posterior fossa.

PRESENTATION

Enlarged cranium with thinning of the skull bones and cerebral cortex. Cranial sutures (fissures between skull bones) do not close until after birth. The increased ICP pushes the bones apart, enlarging the skull and head circumference.

TREATMENT

Placement of an extraventricular shunt (eg, from the ventricle to the peritoneum).

PROGNOSIS

Depends on the degree of increased pressure. In severe cases, brain tissue is compressed and cannot form properly, resulting in mental retardation.

Microcephaly

Microcephaly is characterized by small brain size. Growth of the skull depends on growth of the brain, so the head circumference is decreased secondary to defective brain development. This may be due to genetic causes, prenatal infection, or exposure to teratogens (eg, toxoplasmosis, alcohol, radiation).

PRESENTATION

Small head size; 50% of patients have some degree of mental retardation.

PROGNOSIS

Depends on the severity and degree of mental retardation.

Holoprosencephaly

Failure of midline cleavage of the forebrain. This can be seen in severe fetal alcohol syndrome and Patau syndrome (trisomy 13). The forebrain may lack midline features, including the corpus callosum, resulting in a single ventricle in the middle of the brain rather than bilateral ventricles (Figure 6-8).

PRESENTATION

Clinical symptoms can range from mild to severe. Extremely mild cases may only be identified via a single incisor. Severe cases, however, can present with cyclopia (single midline eye), a lack of central midline structures, and a single ventricle. The degree of mental retardation depends on the extent to which structures are affected.

PROGNOSIS

Depends on severity. In mild cases, individuals may lead a normal life; in more severe cases, the condition may result in mental retardation and early death.

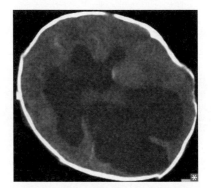

FIGURE 6-8. Holoprosencephaly. Note the lack of brain matter dividing the two hemispheres.

 KEY FACT

Fetal alcohol syndrome is the most common cause of mental retardation. It is characterized by microcephaly, congenital heart disease, abnormal facies, and, in severe cases, holoprosencephaly.

 KEY FACT

Patau syndrome (trisomy 13) is characterized by holoprosencephaly, microcephaly, polydactyly, cleft palate, narrow fingernails, and apneic spells. It is the rarest form of the viable trisomies (21, 18, and 13). Death occurs within 1 year.

Key Terms

- Gyrus (pl. *gyri*) = outpouching fold of the brain.
- Sulcus = groove between gyri.
- Cortex = layers of gray matter that overlie the deeper white matter of the brain.
- Sylvian fissure = oblique groove that divides the temporal lobe from the parietal and frontal lobes.
- Central sulcus = major sulcus that runs coronally, dividing the frontal lobe from the parietal lobe.
- Nuclei = collections of neuron cell bodies (as opposed to axons) in the CNS, usually sharing a common function.

Meninges

Connective tissue that surrounds the CNS, including the brain and spinal cord. The meninges consist of **three** membranes:

- **Pia mater:** Delicate and highly *vascular*; closely adheres to the surface of the brain and spinal cord. Derived from neural crest.
- **Arachnoid:** Delicate, *nonvascular* layer with **granulations** that absorb CSF. Derived from neural crest.
- **Dura mater:** Dense, tough exterior layer. Derived from mesoderm.

The membranes form several potential and real spaces:

- **Subarachnoid space:** Lies between the pia and the arachnoid and contains CSF. It is a relatively narrow space over the surface of the cerebral hemispheres, but it becomes much wider at the base of the brain. It terminates at the S2 vertebrae.
- **Subdural space:** Lies between the arachnoid and the dura and is traversed by **bridging veins** in the brain.
- **Epidural space:** Potential space outside the dura that contains meningeal arteries. In the spinal cord, it contains fatty areolar tissue, lymphatics, and venous plexuses.

Pathology of the Meninges

Meningeal tissues can be involved in several pathologic processes, including congenital malformation, bleeding, infection, and cancer. Bleeding in the meningeal spaces manifests differently depending on the source and location of the bleed.

Epidural Hemorrhage

Usually due to blunt head trauma resulting in rupture of the middle meningeal artery. Imaging shows a biconvex collection of blood bordered by suture lines with lens-shaped enhancement and smooth borders.

Subdural Hemorrhage

Usually due to deceleration injury resulting in rupture of the bridging veins. Venous bleeding accumulates slowly. Often accompanied by intracranial bleeds or contusions and presents as decline in mental status over days to weeks. Imaging shows enhancement of a crescent-shaped area that does *not* cross the midline but does cross dural attachments (suture lines), unlike **epidural hemorrhage.** Subdural hemorrhage is seen most often in the elderly as cortical atrophy puts increasing tension on bridging veins but can also be seen in alcoholics and shaken babies.

Subarachnoid Hemorrhage

Usually due to a ruptured berry aneurysm in the circle of Willis. Presents as the sudden onset of the "worst headache of my life." Imaging may show enhancement in the area of the hemorrhage. Risk factors include hypertension, smoking, connective tissue disorders, autosomal dominant polycystic kidney disease (ADPKD), and older age.

Meningitis

Inflammation of the meninges is often caused by bacterial, viral, or fungal infections.

- Bacterial meningitis: High fever, headache, nuchal rigidity, Kernig and Brudzinski signs present. The organism involved depends on the age of the patient.
- Viral meningitis (aseptic meningitis): Similar to bacterial, but less acute in onset with less severe symptoms.
- Fungal meningitis: Seen in immunocompromised patients, often due to *Cryptococcus,* organism highly dependent on geography.
- Diagnosis made by lumbar puncture (Figure 6-9 and Table 6-3).

MNEMONIC

The meninges **PAD** the brain from inside out:
Pia mater
Arachnoid
Dura mater

CLINICAL CORRELATION

Epidural hematoma:
- Lucid interval in 50% ("talk and die" syndrome).
- Middle meningeal artery is most commonly ruptured.

Subdural hematoma:
- More common than epidural.
- Cortical atrophy in elderly puts tension on bridging veins.
- May be associated with contusion, subarachnoid, and other hemorrhages.
- Seen in shaken baby syndrome. Look for associated retinal hemorrhages in newborn.

Subarachnoid hemorrhage:
- Ruptured berry aneurysm
- High intensity. "Worst headache of my life."
- Sudden onset: "thunderclap headache."
- Marfan, Ehlers-Danlos type 4.
- Autosomal dominant polycystic kidney disease, hypertension, smoking, blacks, ↑ age.

Intracerebral/parenchymal hemorrhage:
- Trauma, infarct, amyloid angiopathy, diabetes, hypertension (Charcot-Bouchard aneurysm), premature birth).
- Many localize to basal ganglia or thalamus.

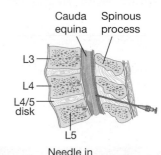

FIGURE 6-9. Lumbar puncture. The correct position may be located by finding the space between the spinous processes at the level of the iliac spine.

KEY FACT

Meningismal signs manifest when the inflamed meninges are stretched.
- **Kernig sign:** Pain elicited while straightening knee with hip flexed at 90 degrees.
- **Brudzinski sign:** Patient flexes knees in response to passive flexion of the neck.

KEY FACT

In a lumbar puncture, the needle encounters the following layers:
- Skin
- Subcutaneous tissue
- Supraspinous/interspinous ligaments
- Ligamentum flavum
- Epidural fat
- Epidural space
- Dura mater
- Arachnoid mater
- Subarachnoid space

TABLE 6-3. **Cerebrospinal Fluid Characteristics of the Different Types of Meningitis**

	BACTERIAL	FUNGAL	VIRAL
Cell Type	PMN predominant	Lymphocyte predominant	Lymphocyte predominant
Glucose	Decreased	Decreased	Normal
Protein	Elevated	Slightly elevated	Slightly elevated

PMN, polymorphonuclear neutrophil.

Meningioma

Benign, well-circumscribed, slow-growing tumor. Meningiomas occur more commonly in women than men. The patient often presents with headache or sudden paralysis and can be treated by resection or, rarely, radiation. These tumors are slow-growing and carry a favorable prognosis.

Carcinomatous Meningitis

The meningeal space is a common site for metastatic spread from cancer outside the CNS. This condition is life threatening and may manifest with mental status changes and headaches. Cranial nerve deficits may be found on clinical exam. Treatment consists of chemotherapy delivered to the CSF (intrathecal).

Ventricles

Ventricles are interconnected spaces in the skull that contain CSF. CSF buffers the brain from impact, transports hormones, and removes waste products. CSF is produced by the **choroid plexus,** a tissue rich in blood vessels and covered with ciliated ependymal cells. It projects into the lateral, third, and fourth ventricles, and contributes to the **blood-brain barrier (BBB),** a tight barrier that separates circulating blood from the CSF (Figure 6-10). Other components of the BBB combine to form a functional "neurovascular unit":

- Tight junctions between capillary endothelial cells.
- Basement membrane.
- Astrocyte foot processes.

The permeability of the BBB is characterized by:

- Increased permeability to nonpolar/lipid-soluble substances versus polar/water-soluble substances.
- Permeability to glucose and amino acids via carrier-mediated transport.
- Specialized circumventricular organs have an incomplete BBB and therefore can directly sense the concentrations of many compounds in the bloodstream without the need for specialized transport systems (eg, **area postrema, basal hypothalamus, organum vasculosum of the lamina terminalis**).
- Infarction leads to vasogenic edema due to destruction of BBB.

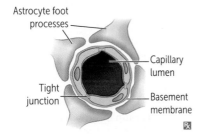

Astrocyte foot processes

Capillary lumen

Tight junction

Basement membrane

FIGURE 6-10. **Blood-brain barrier.**

Ventricular System

- Two lateral ventricles communicate with the third ventricle through the foramen of Monro (Figure 6-11).
- The third ventricle communicates with the fourth ventricle through the cerebral aqueduct (of Sylvius).
- The **fourth ventricle** communicates with the subarachnoid space via three outlet foramina: two **foramina of Luschka** and one **foramen of Magendie.** The foramina of Luschka drain laterally, and the foramen of Magendie drains in the midline (see Figure 6-11).

KEY FACT

The aqueduct is the most common site of stenosis.

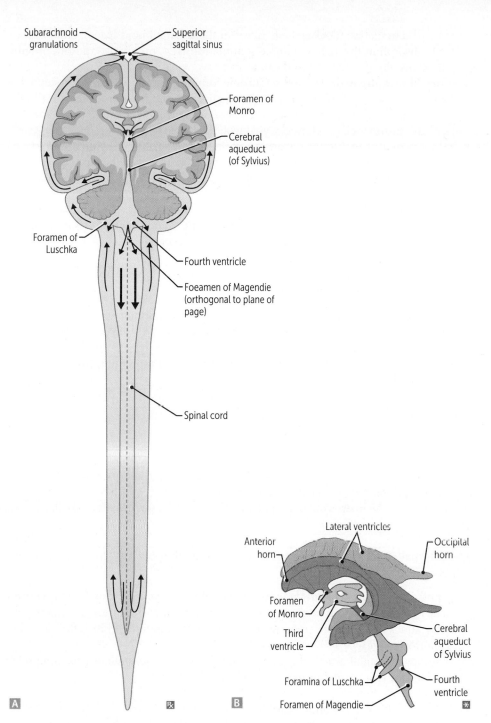

FIGURE 6-11.   Ventricular system. A Note the flow of CSF from the lateral ventricles through the foramen of Monro to the third ventricle, through the aqueduct to the fourth ventricle, into the subarachnoid space through the foramina of Luschka and Magendie, and back into the dural venous sinuses via arachnoid granulations. B The same structures shown in sagittal view.

Hydrocephalus develops as a result of an excess accumulation of CSF in the ventricles, which in turn causes ventricular dilation. There are several forms:

- **Noncommunicating hydrocephalus:** Ventricles **do not** communicate with subarachnoid space, but CSF production remains constant. Obstruction between or within the ventricles (eg, congenital aqueductal stenosis).
- **Communicating hydrocephalus:** Ventricles **do** communicate with subarachnoid space. Can arise from three causes: (1) CSF oversecretion (eg, choroid papilloma);

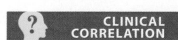

CLINICAL CORRELATION

Noncommunicating hydrocephalus is often seen in patients with myelomeningocele due to relationship with Arnold-Chiari malformation and impaired development of posterior fossa.

(2) CSF circulation blockage (eg, tumor in the subarachnoid space); and (3) poor CSF absorption through arachnoid granulations (eg, meningitis, postmeningitis adhesions, dural venous sinus thrombosis).

- **Normal-pressure hydrocephalus:** Chronic form of communicating hydrocephalus with equilibration of CSF formation and absorption. Often preceded by a high-pressure phase. Classic triad of symptoms includes urinary incontinence, dementia, and gait disturbance ("wet, wacky, and wobbly").
- **Hydrocephalus ex vacuo:** Expansion of ventricular volume secondary to loss of brain tissue, as seen in neurodegenerative conditions such as Alzheimer disease.
- **Pseudotumor cerebri** (benign/idiopathic intracranial hypertension): Increased resistance to CSF outflow. Seen most commonly in young obese women who present with headache, visual changes, and, less frequently, menstrual abnormalities or a history of oral contraceptive use. Exam reveals papilledema, increased ICP (detected by lumbar puncture), and slitlike ventricles on neuroimaging.

The site of ventricular dilation can indicate the site of mechanical obstruction in CSF flow:

- Obstruction in the **foramen of Monro** leads to dilated **lateral** ventricles.
- Obstruction in the **aqueduct of Sylvius** leads to a dilated **third** ventricle and **lateral** ventricles.
- Obstruction in the **fourth ventricle** leads to a dilated **aqueduct, third ventricle,** and **lateral ventricles.**

Blood Supply

Circle of Willis

The circle of Willis is a network of arteries that sits at the base of the brain in the area encircling the optic chiasm and pituitary gland. Provides a source of collateral flow and allows for equilibration of pressure and blood flow to entire brain. It is fed by two major arterial systems: the internal carotids (anterior circulation) and the vertebrobasilar system (posterior circulation; Figure 6-12).

The internal carotid artery gives rise to several branches before joining the circle of Willis:

- Ophthalmic artery: The first branch of the ophthalmic artery gives rise to the **central artery of the retina.** Its occlusion leads to sudden-onset blindness. Transient ischemic attack (TIA) due to embolic occlusion and restoration of blood flow is called **amaurosis fugax.**
- Anterior choroidal artery: Supplies the lateral geniculate nucleus (thalamic relay nucleus for vision), globus pallidus, and internal capsule.

Major components of the circle of Willis:

- Anterior cerebral artery (ACA): Supplies the medial aspect of the frontal lobes, including the lower extremity regions of the motor and sensory cortices.
- Anterior communicating artery: Most common site of **aneurysm** in the circle of Willis, giving rise to **bitemporal hemianopia.**
- Middle cerebral artery (MCA): Supplies the lateral aspect of the hemispheres, including the trunk–face–upper extremity area of the motor and sensory cortices, as well as Broca and Wernicke speech areas. It is the most commonly involved artery in embolic stroke.
- The lateral striate branches of the MCA, which supply the internal capsule and basal ganglia, can be involved in nonembolic lacunar infarctions and commonly lead to pure motor hemiparesis, pure sensory hemiparesis, or mixed sensorimotor hemiparesis (Table 6-4).

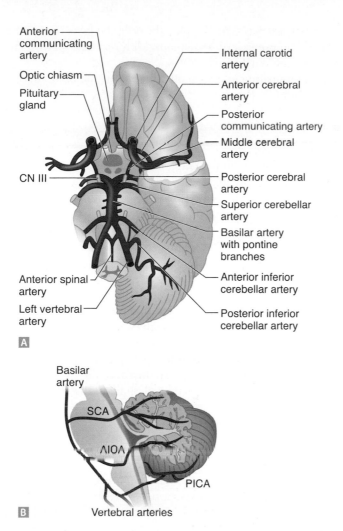

FIGURE 6-12.   An inferior view of the circle of Willis and a sagittal view of cerebellar blood supply. A At the center are the optic chiasm and the pituitary gland. Note how the basilar artery sprawls over the pons and how CN III emerges between the posterior cerebral artery (PCA) and the superior cerebellar artery (SCA). The location of CN III predisposes it to compression by PCA aneurysms. B Note the three regions of the cerebellum supplied by the SCA, anterior inferior cerebellar artery (AICA), and posterior inferior cerebellar artery (PICA).

TABLE 6-4.   Neurologic Deficits Associated with Common Strokes

RELEVANT CEREBRAL ARTERY	ASSOCIATED NEUROLOGIC DEFICIT
ACA	Contralateral lower extremity hemiplegia and/or sensory deficits
MCA	Upper branch: face and arm hemiparesis, hemisensory loss, and nonfluent (Broca) aphasia Lower branch: Fluent (Wernicke) aphasia
PCA	Contralateral homonymous hemianopia
PICA	Lateral medullary (Wallenberg) syndrome: ipsilateral facial and contralateral body pain/temperature sensory loss, nystagmus, ataxia, vocal cord paralysis, and Horner syndrome

ACA, anterior cerebral artery; MCA, middle cerebral artery; PCA, posterior cerebral artery; PICA, posterior inferior cerebellar artery.

■ Posterior cerebral artery (PCA): Supplies the occipital lobe; hypoperfusion may lead to contralateral homonymous hemianopia with macular sparing. Aneurysms may be associated with CN III palsy.

■ Posterior communicating artery: Another common site of aneurysms, which may be associated with CN III palsy.

Vertebrobasilar system:

■ Anterior (ventral) spinal artery (ASA): Supplies the ventral portion of the spinal cord; hypoperfusion manifests with weakness, loss of pain and temperature sensation, but sparing of position and vibratory sensation.

■ Posterior inferior cerebellar artery (PICA): Supplies the medulla and the posterior inferior cerebellum; hypoperfusion manifests with lateral medullary (Wallenberg) syndrome.

■ Anterior inferior cerebellar artery (AICA): Supplies the pons, CN VII, and the anterior inferior surface of the cerebellum; hypoperfusion manifests with lateral pontine syndrome.

■ Pontine arteries (from basilar artery): Supply the base of the pons, including the corticospinal fibers and CN VI; hypoperfusion presents with "locked-in" syndrome in which the patient is aware but suffers from paralysis of all muscles except for those controlling blinking and vertical eye movement.

■ Superior cerebellar artery (SCA): Supplies the pons, the superior surface of the cerebellum, and CN VII and VIII; an aneurysm of the SCA can lead to compression of CN III, which manifests as a dilated pupil on the affected side.

Dural Veins and Sinuses

Superior cerebral ("bridging") veins drain into the superior sagittal sinus to the confluence of sinuses. Meanwhile, the **great cerebral vein of Galen** drains deep cerebral veins into the **straight sinus,** and then the confluence of sinuses (Figure 6-13). The superior sagittal sinus, great cerebral vein, and occipital sinus all drain into the confluence of sinuses, which in turn empties into the transverse sinus, the sigmoid sinus, the internal jugular vein, and finally into the superior vena cava. The cavernous sinuses drain into the superior and inferior petrosal sinuses, which drain into the transverse sinuses and sigmoid sinuses, respectively.

The **cavernous sinus** is a collection of venous sinuses surrounding the pituitary gland. It drains blood from the eye and superficial cortex and feeds into the jugular vein (Figure 6-14).

KEY FACT

The dural venous sinuses provide pathogens and neoplastic cells with a valveless path from the face/sinuses through bridging veins to the brain.

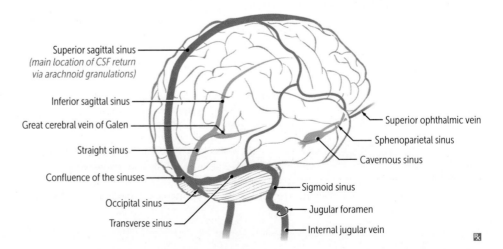

FIGURE 6-13. **Venous sinuses of the brain.**

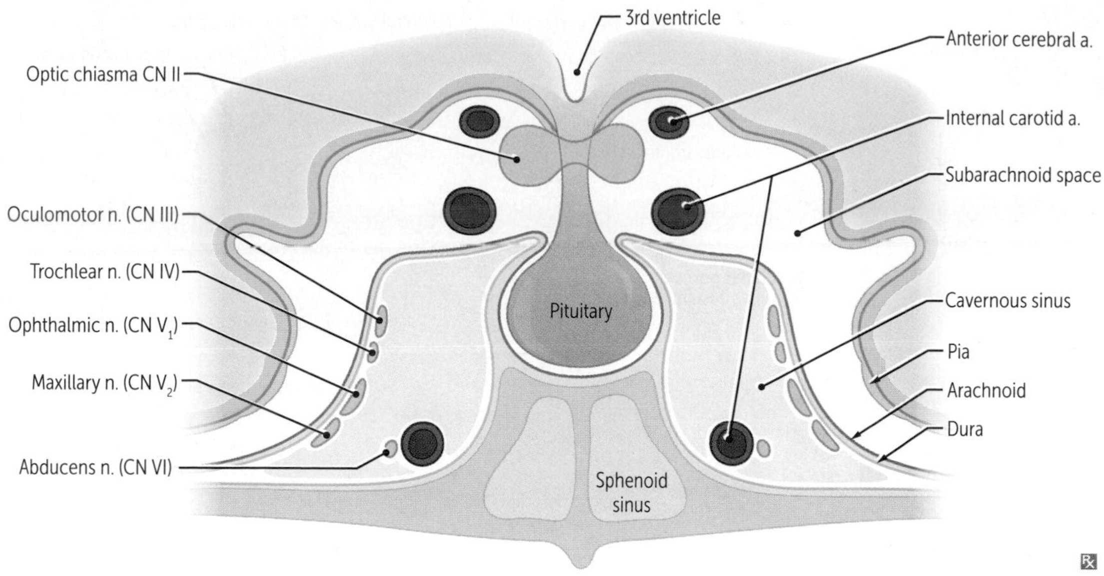

FIGURE 6-14.   **Cavernous sinus.** Coronal cut through the cavernous sinus showing passage of cranial nerves and internal carotid through the sinus. Note that the relatively medial position of CN VI makes it the cranial nerve most susceptible to impingement by an expanding pituitary tumor.

The cavernous sinus contains several structures.

- CN III, IV, V$_1$, V$_2$, VI, and postganglionic sympathetic fibers that supply the orbit.
- CN III, IV, V$_1$, and V$_2$ are attached to the wall of the sinus; CN VI is free floating and is most susceptible to impingement by an enlarging pituitary tumor.
- The internal carotid arteries pass through both sides of the sinus.
- Venous drainage from the face drains to the cavernous sinus, providing a route through which skin infections can reach the brain.

> **CLINICAL CORRELATION**
>
> **Cavernous sinus syndrome** results from increased pressure in the cavernous sinus and leads to **ophthalmoplegia and facial sensory loss.**

Cerebral Cortex

The cortex is composed of specialized regions that are responsible for specific functions. Thus, injury and lesions in different areas of the brain produce deficits appropriate to the function of that area (Figure 6-15). Brodmann labeled different areas of the brain by number; some of these areas are still referred to by these numbers (Figure 6-16).

ORGANIZATION

The cerebral cortex is composed of six layers of cells; the relative size of each layer varies among regions of the brain. Each layer consists of different types of cells and is specialized to send and receive input to and from different areas of the brain. Layer 5 in the primary motor cortex is known for the large motor neurons of the corticospinal tracts known as **Betz cells.**

The cortex is divided into the frontal, parietal, temporal, and occipital lobes (see Figure 6-15). Major fissures and sulci (grooves) separate the different lobes.

- The **sylvian (lateral) fissure** divides the temporal lobes from the frontal and parietal lobes.
- The **central sulcus** divides the frontal lobe from the parietal lobe.
- The **sagittal sulcus** divides the brain into the left and right hemispheres.

Frontal Lobe

LOCATION

Anterior to the central sulcus and superior to the sylvian fissure.

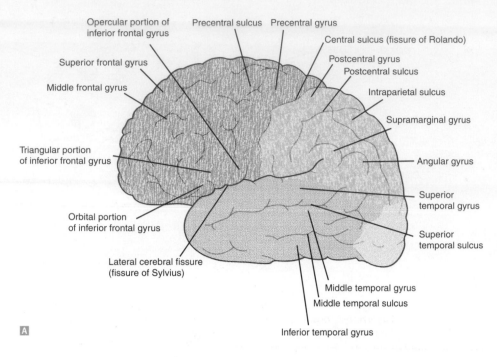

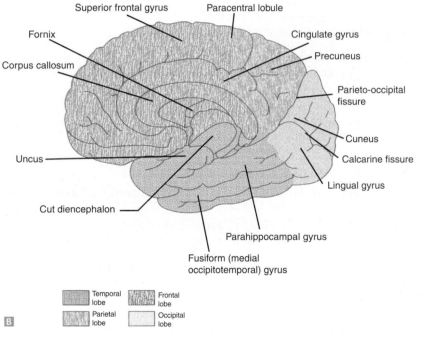

FIGURE 6-15. Basic surface anatomy of the cerebrum. **A** **B** Major structures of note are the four major lobes, precentral sulcus/gyrus, central sulcus, sylvian fissure, cingulate gyrus, corpus callosum, uncus, and hippocampal gyrus.

MAJOR AREAS

Prefrontal cortex, premotor cortex, primary motor cortex, frontal eye fields, Broca area.

FUNCTIONS

■ **Movement (primary motor and premotor cortex):** Areas in charge of movement include the primary motor cortex and premotor cortex, located anterior to the central sulcus. The primary motor cortex is closest to the central sulcus, and the premotor cortex is located more anteriorly. The **premotor cortex** plans movements in response

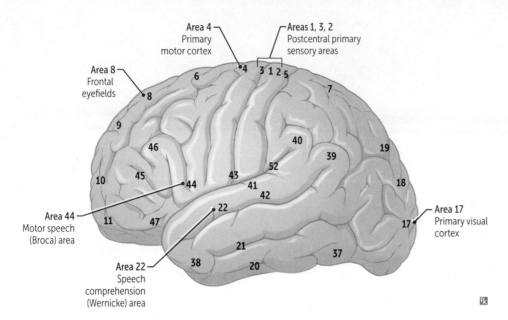

FIGURE 6-16. **Brodmann areas of the brain.** Areas of note include areas 3–1–2 = primary sensory cortex; area 4 = primary motor cortex; area 8 = frontal eye fields; area 44 = Broca area; area 22 = Wernicke area; and area 17 = primary visual cortex.

to external cues and is particularly active when sequential movements follow visual cues. The **primary motor cortex** executes the planned movement via the descending motor neurons of the corticospinal tract. Areas of the motor cortex correspond geographically to the body parts they control, as mapped out by the motor homunculus (Figure 6-17). Lesion of a motor strip causes spastic paralysis of the contralateral region corresponding to the region depicted on the motor homunculus (see Figure 6-17A).

- **Eye movements (frontal eye fields):** The frontal eye fields (also known as area 8) control eye movements. Lesions of the frontal eye fields:
  - Ischemic lesion (ie, stroke): Eyes drift toward the side that is injured.
  - Hyperactivity (ie, seizure): Eyes drift away from the side of hyperactivity.
- **Social judgment (prefrontal cortex):** The frontal lobe is responsible for inhibiting impulsive thoughts to tailor behavior to fit social norms. Lesion of the prefrontal cortex may result in disinhibition. For example, Phineas Gage, a formerly mild-mannered man who survived severe frontal lobe damage, became rude, obnoxious, and defiant of social norms.
- **Language production (Broca area):** Broca area, or area 44 (Figure 6-16), is involved in language production. Lesion in the Broca area results in an inability to produce coherent speech and writing. Patients appear to have difficulty forming words and speak very slowly and laboriously. Comprehension is intact, however.
- **Executive functions:** Concentration, orientation, abstraction, judgment, mood, and inhibition of primitive reflexes. Lesion can lead to unmasking of primitive reflexes such as suckling, grasp, and rooting reflexes.

MNEMONIC

Gaze deviates toward an ischemic stroke and away from a seizure.

BLOOD SUPPLY

ACA and MCA.

Parietal Lobe

LOCATION

The parietal lobes are located lateral to the sagittal sulcus and posterior to the central sulcus.

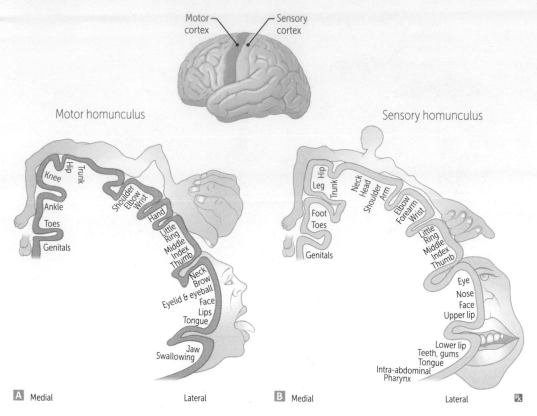

FIGURE 6-17. **A** Motor and **B** sensory homunculi.

MAJOR AREAS

Primary sensory cortex.

FUNCTIONS

- **Sensation (primary sensory cortex):** The primary sensory cortex is just posterior to the central sulcus. Like the motor cortex, a sensory homunculus represents the anatomic correlations (see Figure 6-17B). The ascending spinothalamic and dorsal columns synapse in the thalamus and project to the primary sensory cortex. The primary sensory cortex then sends projections to the secondary and association cortices that integrate sensory components into a cohesive interpretation. Lesion leads to loss of tactile sensation in regions corresponding to the region depicted on the sensory homunculus.
- **Spatial relationships:** Determination of right and left. Lesion causes **Gerstmann syndrome** (inferior parietal lobe of the dominant hemisphere).
  - Right-left confusion.
  - Finger agnosia: Inability to name and recognize one's own fingers or others' fingers.
  - Agraphia and alexia: Inability to write and read.
  - Acalculia: Inability to make arithmetic calculations.
- **Vision:** Contralateral inferior quadrantanopia due to injury to the superior optic tract that passes through the parietal lobe on the way to the occipital lobe.
- **Attention:** Visual and cognitive attention.
  - Unilateral lesion: **Contralateral neglect,** for example, an individual with a right parietal lesion may fail to put clothes on his left side (eg, will only put on the right shoe). May also reproduce the classic drawing of a clock with all the numbers on one side.

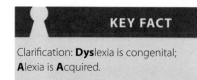

KEY FACT

Clarification: **Dys**lexia is congenital; **A**lexia is **A**cquired.

- Lesion of the dominant hemisphere: **Apraxia,** or inability to carry out learned movements (combing hair, brushing teeth). Patients often are unable to perform an action when commanded to, but are able to imitate or perform the action in response to other triggering stimuli.
- Bilateral lesions: **Balint syndrome,** a form of visual agnosia, in which patients are unable to scan visual space and to grasp an object in space.

BLOOD SUPPLY

ACA and MCA.

Occipital Lobe

LOCATION

Most posterior region of the brain.

MAJOR AREAS

Primary visual cortex, association visual cortex.

FUNCTIONS

- **Vision (primary and association visual cortices):**
  - Visual pathway: Retina → fibers cross at the optic chiasm → synapse at the lateral geniculate nucleus (LGN) → primary visual cortex within the occipital lobe.
  - Visual signals are processed through inputs from the primary visual cortex to the visual association cortex in the occipital lobe.
- **Visual recognition (association cortices):**
  - Lesion results in visual agnosia, the inability to recognize objects one sees.
  - Lesion causes alexia without agraphia, the acquired inability to read while retaining the ability to write.

BLOOD SUPPLY

PCA.

Temporal Lobes

The temporal lobes contain structures vital for hearing, memory, and emotion.

LOCATION

Inferior to the sylvian fissure.

MAJOR AREAS

Primary auditory cortex, hippocampus, amygdala, Wernicke area.

FUNCTIONS

- **Hearing (primary auditory cortex):** Located within the superior temporal gyrus and transverse temporal gyrus (Heschl gyrus).
- **Auditory pathway:** Cochlea → CN VIII → medullary cochlear nuclei → fibers cross just prior to the superior olivary nuclei, travel along the lateral lemniscus tract → synapse in the medial geniculate nucleus (MGN) → primary auditory cortex (see Figure 6-48 in the later discussion of the auditory pathway).
  - Lesion proximal to the CN VIII decussation and superior olivary nuclei leads to unilateral hearing loss with potential deafness.
  - Lesion distal to the CN VIII decussation and medullary cochlear nuclei causes bilateral diminished hearing without deafness.
- **Memory (hippocampus):** The hippocampus is responsible for learning and consolidation of short-term memory, before memories are later integrated diffusely throughout

the cortex. The hippocampus is part of the Papez circuit, an important pathway in the limbic system, which contains structures presumed to play a role in memory and emotion (Figure 6-18). Hippocampal lesion results in anterograde memory loss (inability to form new memories) and a temporally graded retrograde amnesia.

- **Emotion:** The temporal lobe is part of the limbic system. Memory and emotion are intimately related, both structurally and functionally.
    - Fear: Emotional responses, such as the fear response, are mediated by the amygdala.
    - Lesion leads to ablation of the fear response, or **Klüver-Bucy syndrome:**
        - Psychic blindness (visual agnosia)
        - Personality changes (abnormal docility)
        - Hyperorality (puts everything in one's mouth)
        - Hypersexuality and loss of sexual preference (mounts anything in sight).
- **Seizure activity** is commonly associated with vivid hallucinations. The temporal lobe is one of the common foci for epilepsy.
- **Language comprehension (Wernicke area):** Wernicke area, or area 22, is responsible for comprehension of language. It is also critical for production of *coherent* language.
    - Lesion in Wernicke area: Patients are unable to understand what is spoken to them. They produce speech fluently that consists of either real or made-up words (neologisms) and phrases, but it does not make any sense.
    - The aphasia square (Figure 6-19) summarizes the various forms of aphasia.
        - Broca aphasia: Inability to produce speech or repeat sentences. Also has trouble with written expression. Comprehension is intact.

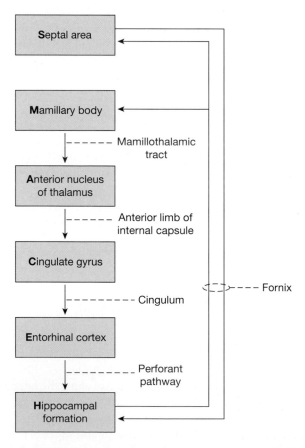

FIGURE 6-18. **Papez circuit.** The Papez circuit was originally proposed as a circuit for memory and emotional processing. Although it is not a true circuit, structures of the "circuit" contribute to memory and emotional processing and constitute the limbic system.

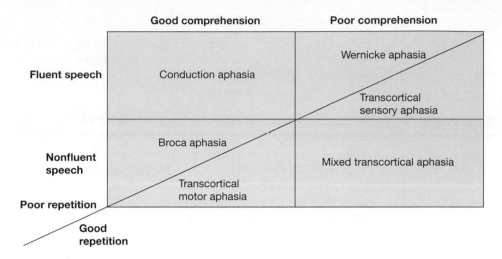

FIGURE 6-19.   **Aphasia square.** The six most commonly tested aphasias.

- Wernicke aphasia: Inability to comprehend both verbal and written language, produce coherent speech, or repeat sentences.
- Conduction aphasia: Inability to repeat after hearing a sentence.
- Mixed transcortical aphasia: Inability to spontaneously produce words or coherent speech; however, repetition is intact.
- Global aphasia: All language function is impaired.

DEEP BRAIN STRUCTURES

Basal Ganglia

LOCATION

Lateral to the internal capsule bilaterally.

STRUCTURES

Striatum (caudate + putamen), globus pallidus internus and externus, and the substantia nigra (Figure 6-20).

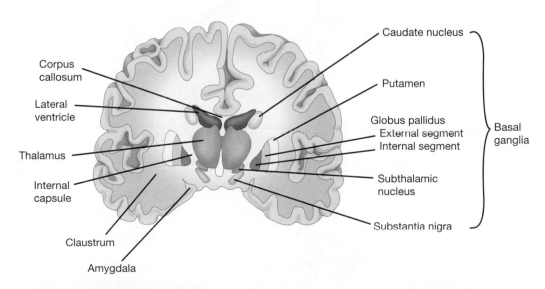

FIGURE 6-20.   **Major structures of the basal ganglia.**

FUNCTIONS

- Initiation of purposeful movement (Figure 6-21) via the direct and indirect pathways.
  - Dopamine (DA) is released into the caudate/putamen from neurons that originate in the substantia nigra pars compacta.
  - Direct pathway (promotes movement):
    - Cortex → caudate/putamen → globus pallidus internus → thalamus → spinal cord.
    - DA activates this pathway via D_1 receptors (G_s), promoting movement.
  - Indirect pathway (inhibits movement):
    - Cortex → caudate/putamen → **globus pallidus externus → subthalamic nucleus** → globus pallidus internus → thalamus → spinal cord.
    - DA inhibits this pathway via D_2 receptors (G_i), promoting movement.
- **Lesions and corresponding deficits:**
  - Substantia nigra DA neurons: lesion results in **Parkinson disease.**
  - Small and medium spiny GABAergic neurons of the caudate and putamen: lesion associated with **Huntington disease.**
  - Subthalamic nucleus: lesion results in **hemiballismus.**

Thalamus

LOCATION

Surrounding the third ventricle, just above the midbrain.

STRUCTURES

Eleven nuclei (Table 6-5 and Figure 6-22).

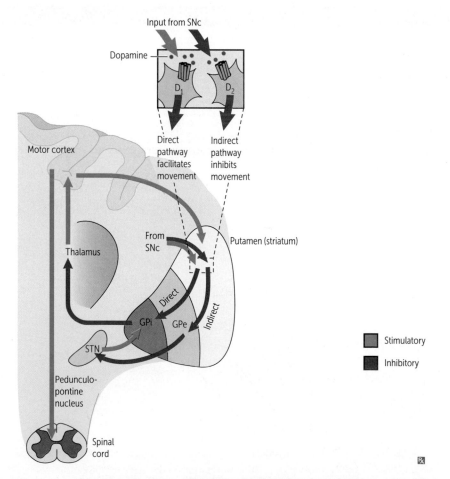

FIGURE 6-21.   Basal ganglia direct and indirect pathways. D_1, dopamine D_1 receptor; D_2, dopamine D_2 receptor; GPe, globus pallidus externus; GPi, globus pallidus internus; SNc, substantia nigra pars compacta; STN, subthalamic nucleus.

TABLE 6-5.   Nuclei and Functions of the Thalamus

NUCLEUS	FUNCTION	INPUTS	OUTPUTS
Ventral posterolateral	Relay somatic sensory information from the trunk and limbs	Spinothalamic tract, dorsal columns (via medial lemniscus)	Primary sensory cortex
Ventral posteromedial	Relay somatic sensory information from the head	Trigeminal tract	Primary sensory cortex
Ventral lateral	Relay motor information	Cerebellum, globus pallidus	Primary motor cortex and supplementary motor area
Ventral anterior	Relay motor planning information	Cerebellum, globus pallidus	Prefrontal cortex
Anterior nuclei	Relay emotion/memory information; part of Papez circuit	Mamillary bodies	Cingulate gyrus
Medial dorsal	Relay cognitive/memory information	Prefrontal cortex, olfactory, and limbic systems	Prefrontal association cortex

FUNCTIONS

- **Sensory relay station:**
    - The thalamus receives sensory input of all sensory modalities.
    - Sensory input is "filtered."
    - The thalamus sends processed signals to other areas of the cortex.
- **Emotion and memory:** The thalamus is part of the Papez circuit, which is involved in emotion and memory.

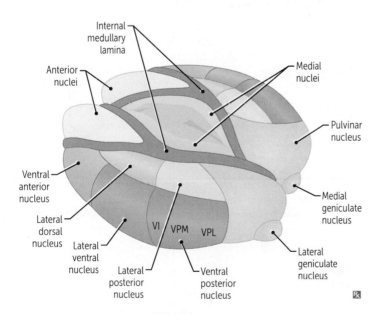

FIGURE 6-22.   Thalamic nuclei. The thalamus has two lobes, one on each side of the third ventricle. The geniculate bodies include the medial and lateral geniculate bodies/nuclei that relay auditory and visual sensory information, respectively. VI, ventral intermediate nucleus; VPM, ventral posteromedial; VPL, ventral posterolateral.

- **Motor relay station:** The thalamus receives input from the motor cortex and basal ganglia and sends signals to the descending motor tracts.
- **Lesion associated with motor and sensory deficits:** Involving multiple areas of the body, and **thalamic pain syndrome** (Dejerine-Roussy syndrome), which is pain perceived without an appropriate stimulus.

BLOOD SUPPLY

Posterior communicating artery, anterior choroidal artery (a branch of the internal carotid artery; see Figure 6-12).

Internal Capsule

The internal capsule is the site of convergence of all ascending and descending white matter tracts to and from the cortex.

LOCATION

White matter lateral to the thalamus and caudate, and medial to the lenticular nucleus (globus pallidus and putamen) as illustrated in Figure 6-23.

DIVISIONS

Anterior limb, posterior limb, genu (the bend or "elbow" between the anterior and posterior limbs), retrolenticular limb, and sublenticular limb.

- Anterior limb: Frontopontine fibers (between frontal cortex and pons), thalamocortical fibers (between medial/anterior nuclei of thalamus and frontal lobes).
- Posterior limb: Descending corticospinal tract, ascending sensory fibers (medial lemniscus, anterolateral/spinothalamic tract).

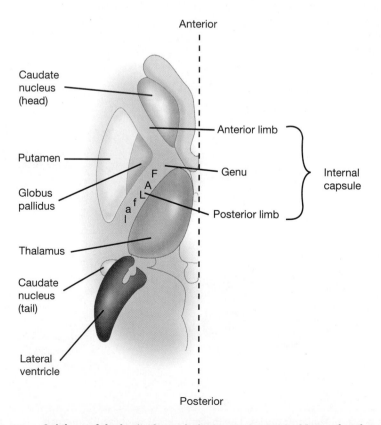

FIGURE 6-23. **Axial cut of the brain through the internal capsule.** Notice that descending motor fibers for the face, arm, and leg (F, A, and L) run anterior to the ascending sensory fibers (f, a, and l) in the posterior limb of the internal capsule.

- Genu: Descending corticobulbar tract (between cortex and brain stem).
- Retrolenticular limb: Optic radiation (between lateral geniculate nucleus and primary visual cortex).
- Sublenticular limb: Auditory radiation (between medial geniculate nucleus and primary auditory cortex).

Lesion causes motor (genu, posterior limb) and sensory (posterior limb) deficits involving multiple areas of the body.

Blood Supply

Medial striate branches from the ACA and lenticulostriate branches from the MCA.

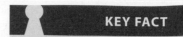

Hypothalamus

The hypothalamus is involved in homeostasis and instinctive actions, such as eating, drinking, sleeping, and sex. Like the thalamus, it is divided into several nuclei controlling various functions (Figure 6-24 and Table 6-6).

Diseases of the Hypothalamus

- **Central diabetes insipidus:**
  - Lesion of the antidiuretic hormone (ADH) pathways to the posterior lobe of the pituitary gland leads to inappropriately low ADH secretion.
  - Polyuria and polydipsia with hypernatremia.
- **Syndrome of inappropriate ADH (SIADH):**
  - May be due to direct injury to the hypothalamus.
  - Can also be due to lung tumors that secrete ADH-like hormone (small-cell lung carcinoma) or drugs that increase ADH secretion (carbamazepine, chlorpromazine).
  - Manifests as fluid retention with hyponatremia.

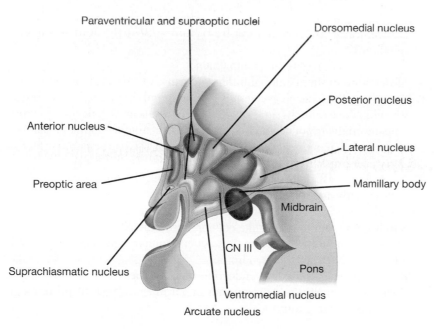

FIGURE 6-24.   Hypothalamic nuclei.

TABLE 6-6. Hypothalamic Nuclei and Major Functions

NUCLEUS	FUNCTION
Supraoptic and paraventricular nuclei	Synthesizes ADH, oxytocin, CRH. Neurophysins serve as carrier peptides for ADH and oxytocin transport to the posterior pituitary for release. Regulates water balance via ADH. Lesion → **diabetes insipidus**
Anterior nucleus	Temperature regulation (heat dissipation). Lesion → **hyperthermia.** Stimulates parasympathetic nervous system
Preoptic nucleus	Releases gonadotropic hormones. Sexual dimorphic nucleus. Lesion → arrested sexual development, impotence, amenorrhea
Suprachiasmatic nucleus	Regulates circadian rhythms (eg, cyclic release of CRH, melatonin). Input from retina, output to pineal gland
Dorsomedial nucleus	Stimulation → obesity, disinhibition
Posterior nucleus	Temperature regulation (heat conservation). Lesion → **poikilothermia** (poor thermoregulation). Stimulates sympathetic nervous system
Lateral nucleus	Feeding center: Stimulation → increased eating (lateral nucleus causes you to grow laterally). Lesion → starvation
Mamillary body	Damaged in Wernicke encephalopathy/Korsakoff psychosis (confabulation, amnesia, and ataxia). Hippocampus → fornix → mamillary body → anterior nucleus of thalamus (part of Papez circuit)
Ventromedial nucleus	Satiety center: Stimulation → decreased eating (ventromedial nucleus causes you to shrink medially), lesion → obesity, hyperphagia, "savage" behavior
Arcuate nucleus	Produces hypothalamic releasing and inhibiting factors that act on the anterior pituitary. Inhibits prolactin release via dopamine (prolactin-inhibiting factor)

ADH, antidiuretic hormone; CRH, corticotropin-releasing hormone.

MNEMONIC

Lesions of the **L**ateral nucleus make you **L**ose weight

MNEMONIC

Lesions of the ventro**M**edial nucleus give you **M**ad hunger.

KEY FACT

The pituitary gland, or adenohypophysis, is formed from an outpouching of the ectodermal diverticulum of the primitive mouth cavity, the **Rathke pouch.** The pouch ascends until it is adjacent to the neurohypophysis, forming the adenohypophysis/neurohypophysis complex that rests in the **sella turcica.** Remnants of the Rathke pouch may give rise to a **craniopharyngioma.**

- Craniopharyngioma:
  - Congenital tumor originating from remnants of the Rathke pouch (oral ectoderm).
  - Often calcified, resembling tooth enamel.
  - Most common supratentorial tumor and cause of hypopituitarism in children.
  - Pressure on the optic chiasm results in **bitemporal hemianopia;** pressure on CN VI within the cavernous sinus can lead to abducens nerve palsy (see Figure 6-14).
  - Pressure on the hypothalamus results in hypothalamic syndrome (loss of function of the hypothalamus).
- Pituitary adenomas:
  - Although not officially part of the hypothalamus, the pituitary is closely related both spatially and functionally.
  - Location of 15% of clinically symptomatic intracranial tumors.
  - Rarely seen in children (unlike craniopharyngiomas).
  - Produces symptoms similar to those of craniopharyngioma (bitemporal hemianopia and hypothalamic syndrome).
  - If endocrine-active, produce endocrine abnormalities (eg, amenorrhea, galactorrhea from prolactin-secreting tumor or acromegaly/gigantism from a growth hormone-secreting tumor).

CEREBELLUM

The cerebellum extends dorsally from the level of the pons at the base of the brain. Important structures include the **vermis,** situated medially, and the hemispheres on either side. The cerebellum is divided into three lobes: the **anterior, posterior,** and **flocculonodular** (Figure 6-25). Major functions include coordination of movement and posture. The hemispheres primarily control purposeful limb movements, and the vermis primarily controls axial posture. Lesions of the cerebellum can result in dysdi-adochokinesia (inability to alternate contraction between antagonistic muscle groups), action tremor, dysmetria, nystagmus, scanning speech, and ataxia.

Anatomy

- **Peduncles** (see Figure 6-26):
  - **Superior cerebellar peduncle (SCP):** Contains major output from the cerebellum, including the dentatorubrothalamic tract, and an afferent pathway, the ventral spinocerebellar tract.
  - **Middle cerebellar peduncle (MCP):** Contains incoming pontocerebellar fibers.
  - **Inferior cerebellar peduncle:** Contains three major afferent tracts: the dorsal spinocerebellar tract, the cuneocerebellar tract, and the olivocerebellar tract from the contralateral inferior olivary nucleus.
- **Layers** (Figure 6-27):
  - **Molecular layer:** Outer layer containing stellate cells, basket cells, the dendritic arbor of Purkinje cells, and parallel fibers of granule cells.
  - **Purkinje cell layer:** Contains cell bodies of Purkinje cells.
  - **Granule layer:** Innermost layer containing granule cell bodies, Golgi cells, and cerebellar glomeruli.
  - **Cerebellar glomeruli:** Consists of a mossy fiber rosette, granule cell dendrites, and a Golgi cell axon.
- **Neurons and fibers** (Table 6-7).

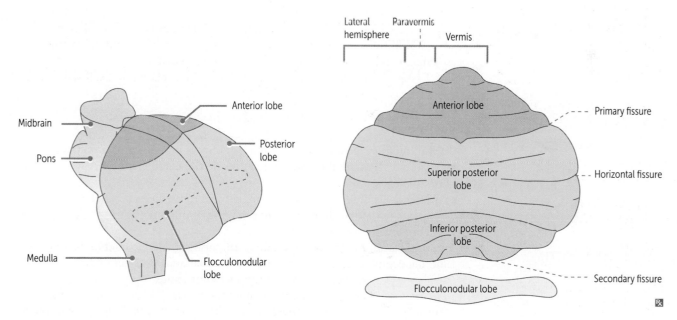

FIGURE 6-25. **Regional anatomy of the cerebellum.** The cerebellum is divided into anterior and posterior segments in the sagittal plane **A** and into the midline vermis and lateral hemispheres in the axial plane **B**.

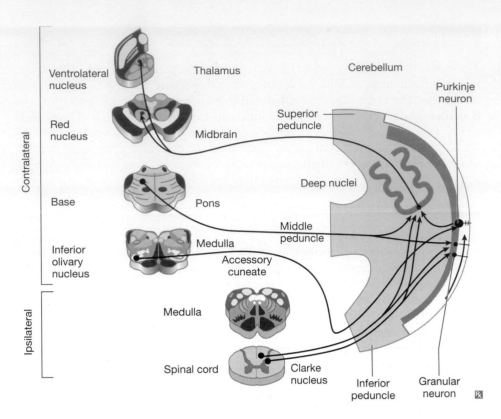

FIGURE 6-26. Cerebellar pathways. Major cerebellar pathways traversing the three peduncles.

- **Deep nuclei:** The deep cerebellar nuclei process input from the cerebellar hemispheres and transmit output signals through the superior cerebellar peduncle (Figure 6-26).
  - **Dentate nucleus:** Receives input from Purkinje cells in the lateral cerebellar hemispheres and transmits output through the dentatorubrothalamic tract.
  - **Emboliform and globose nuclei:** Transmits cerebellar output relating to the upper and lower limbs after a movement has been initiated.
  - **Fastigial nucleus:** Transmits cerebellar output relating to axial stability, especially during standing or walking.

Major Pathways

- Climbing fibers arising from the inferior olivary nucleus project via the olivocerebellar tract through the inferior peduncle to the cerebellar cortex and synapse on Purkinje cells.
- Purkinje cells of the cerebellar cortex project to the deep cerebellar nuclei, especially the dentate nucleus, and form the only inhibitory (GABA-ergic) synapses in the cerebellar circuitry.
- Dentate nucleus cells project via the dentatorubrothalamic tract to the red nucleus and the ventral lateral motor nucleus of the thalamus (see Figure 6-26).
- Thalamic neurons project to the primary motor cortex.
- The motor cortex projects to the pontine nuclei via the corticopontine tract.
- Pontine nuclei project via the pontocerebellar tract (MCP) to the contralateral cerebellar cortex (mossy fibers), completing the cerebrocerebellar circuit.

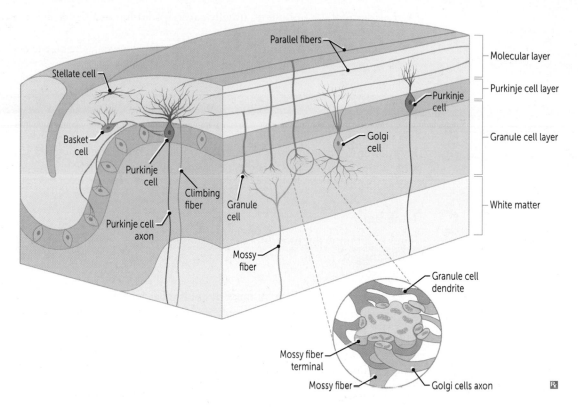

FIGURE 6-27. **Histologic organization of the cerebellum.** Purkinje cells have trees of dendrites that spread along a plane perpendicular to the parallel fibers, forming a matrix for information processing.

Cerebellar Dysfunction and Syndromes

- Signs of cerebellar dysfunction frequently include:
  - **Disequilibrium** (loss of balance, truncal and gait ataxia).
  - **Dyssynergia** (loss of coordination) includes dysmetria, intention tremor, dysdiadochokinesia, and coarse nystagmus more prominent when gazing toward the side of the lesion.
  - **Hypotonia.**

TABLE 6-7. **Neurons and Fibers of the Cerebellum**

CELL/FIBER	LOCATION	PATHWAY	NEUROTRANSMITTER
Purkinje cells	Cell body in Purkinje cell layer; dendritic tree in molecular layer	Only output from cerebellar cortex Receive input from parallel fibers (granule cells) and climbing fibers (inferior olivary nucleus) Project to deep cerebellar nuclei	GABA
Granule cells	Cell body in granule cell layer; axons (parallel fibers) in molecular layer	Receive input from Golgi cells and mossy fibers from spinal cord, medulla, and pons Project to Purkinje, basket, stellate, and Golgi cells through parallel fibers	Glutamate
Parallel fibers	Molecular layer	Axons of granule cells	Glutamate
Mossy fibers	Cell bodies in spinal cord, pons, and vestibular nuclei; terminate in granule cell layer	Originate in spinocerebellar, pontocerebellar, and vestibulocerebellar tracts Terminate as mossy fibers on granule cell dendrites	Glutamate
Climbing fibers	Cell bodies in inferior olivary nucleus; terminate on Purkinje cell dendrites	Carry information from olivocerebellar tract to cerebellar nuclei and Purkinje cells	Aspartate

GABA, γ aminobutyric acid.

- Lesions of the hemispheres usually cause **ipsilateral** cerebellar signs with ataxia of the extremities.
- Lesions of the vermis usually cause gait or truncal ataxia. The classic cerebellar gait is wide-based.

BRAIN STEM

The brain stem lies between the thalamus and the spinal cord. It consists of three main components, from superior to inferior: midbrain, pons, and medulla (Figure 6-28). It develops from the mesencephalon (midbrain), the metencephalon (pons), and the myelencephalon (medulla).

Midbrain

The midbrain is the most superior aspect of the brain stem. Strokes or lesions in the midbrain give rise to several well-known syndromes (see Figures 6-28 and 6-29 and Table 6-8).

- Blood supply: PCA, SCA, branches of the basilar artery (BA).
- Consists of a dorsal tectum (roof), an intermediate tegmentum (floor), and a base.

Pons

The pons is the region of the brain stem shown in Figure 6-30.

- Blood supply: Paramedian branches of the basilar artery and AICA.
- Contents and lesions (Tables 6-9 and 6-10).

KEY FACT

Brain stem lesions often produce **alternating hemiplegia:** Ipsilateral loss of some functions and contralateral loss of other functions. Many of the tracts that travel to and from the brain and spinal cord synapse and cross the midline within the brain stem.

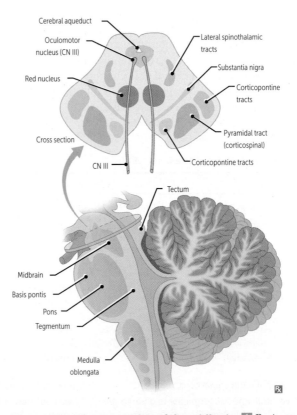

FIGURE 6-28. **Brain stem and cross-section of the midbrain.** A Basic parts of the brain stem include the midbrain, pons, and medulla. Tegmentum = "floor"; tectum = "roof." B The tectum is above the aqueduct, the tegmentum below.

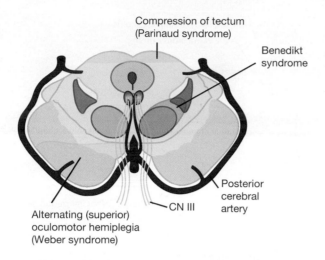

FIGURE 6-29. **Lesions of the midbrain.** Parinaud (loss of upward gaze due to compression of superior colliculus frequently by a pineal gland tumor), Benedikt (paramedian midbrain syndrome that can be caused by occlusion of the posterior cerebral artery), and Weber syndromes (CN III palsy with contralateral hemiparesis).

TABLE 6-8. **Lesions of the Midbrain**

LESION	STRUCTURE	DEFICIT
Perinaud syndrome: lesion of the dorsal tectum	Superior colliculus and pretectal area	Paralysis of upward (less frequently downward) gaze, pupillary disturbances, absence of convergence
	Cerebral aqueduct	Obstruction leads to noncommunicating hydrocephalus (bilateral papilledema)
	Pineal gland	If the underlying cause of **Parinaud syndrome** is a pineal tumor, inadequate *melatonin* production may result in insomnia. Pineal cysts are often asymptomatic
Benedikt syndrome: lesion of the tegmentum	CN III nucleus/root	Ptosis (paralysis of the levator palpebrae muscle), fixed and dilated ipsilateral pupil, complete ipsilateral oculomotor paralysis, causing the eye to be "down and out" due to unopposed actions of the lateral rectus (CN VI) and superior oblique (CN IV) muscles
	Dentatothalamic fibers	Contralateral cerebellar ataxia with intention tremor
	Medial lemniscus	Contralateral loss of light touch and position sensation from the extremities
Weber syndrome: lesion of the base of midbrain	CN III nucleus/root	See Benedikt syndrome above
	Corticospinal tracts	Contralateral spastic paralysis of extremities
	Corticobulbar fibers	Contralateral weakness of the lower face (CN VII), tongue (CN XII), and palate (CN X); the uvula points away from the lesion, but the protruded tongue points toward the lesion

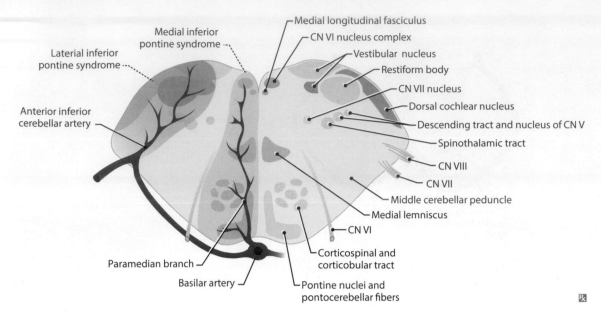

FIGURE 6-30. **Cross-section through the pons.** Note the regions of the lateral inferior pontine syndrome and medial inferior pontine syndrome due to occlusions of the anterior inferior cerebellar artery and the paramedian branches of the basilar artery, respectively.

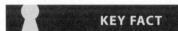

KEY FACT

Charcot triad of MS includes:
1. Scanning speech
2. Intention tremor
3. Nystagmus (MLF syndrome/ internuclear ophthalmoplegia; see discussion)

The pons contains an important structure for conjugate gaze, known as the **medial longitudinal fasciculus (MLF).** The MLF connects the CN VI nucleus with the contralateral CN III nucleus to achieve lateral conjugate gaze. A lesion of the MLF produces **MLF syndrome (internuclear ophthalmoplegia):**

- Medial rectus palsy on attempted lateral conjugate gaze and nystagmus in the abducting eye.
- Often seen in **multiple sclerosis (MS).**

Caloric nystagmus is used to test brain stem function. Nystagmus has two phases: a slow phase in one direction (tracking movement), followed by a fast phase (resetting movement) in the opposite direction. The direction of nystagmus is determined by the direction of the fast phase (Figure 6-31).

- Conscious:
  - Cold water irrigation of the external auditory meatus → reduction of signaling through ipsilateral vestibular afferents (simulating contralateral head turn)

TABLE 6-9. **Contents and Lesions of the Medial Pons (Result from Occlusion of Paramedian Branches of the Basilar Artery)**

STRUCTURE	DEFICIT
Medial longitudinal fasciculus (MLF)	MLF syndrome (internuclear ophthalmoplegia, see previous discussion)
Abducens nucleus (CN VI)	Lateral gaze palsy
CN VII (lower motor neuron)	Ipsilateral Bell palsy without forehead sparing
Medial lemniscus	Loss of contralateral light touch and proprioceptive sensation
Corticospinal tract	Contralateral hemiparesis

TABLE 6-10.   Lateral Inferior Pontine Syndrome (AICA Occlusion)

RELEVANT CEREBRAL ARTERY	ASSOCIATED NEUROLOGIC DEFICIT
Lateral spinothalamic tract	Loss of contralateral pain and body temperature sensation
CN VIII nuclei	Vertigo, hearing loss, tinnitus, nystagmus
CN VII	Bell palsy without forehead sparing
Middle cerebellar peduncle	Ipsilateral ataxia
Spinal trigeminal nucleus/tract	Ipsilateral pain/temperature sensation loss (face)
Descending sympathetics	Ipsilateral Horner syndrome

AICA, anterior inferior cerebellar artery.

→ ipsilateral gaze deviation with nystagmus toward contralateral side (ie, cold water in left ear causes left gaze deviation with right beating nystagmus).

■ Warm water irrigation of the external auditory meatus → increased signaling through ipsilateral vestibular afferents (simulating ipsilateral head turn) → contralateral gaze deviation with nystagmus toward the ipsilateral side (ie, warm water in left ear causes right gaze deviation with left beating nystagmus).

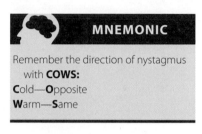

Lesion	Basal eye position	Rotate head left cold calorics right ear	Rotate head right cold calorics left ear
A Normal response			
B Right MLF			
C Left MLF			
D Right frontal			
E Left PPRF			
F Left frontal			
G Right PPRF			

FIGURE 6-31.   Responses to cold caloric testing in brain stem injury. **A** Normally, cold calorics in the right ear simulates a left head turn and induces a right lateral gaze. Calorics in the left ear induces a left lateral gaze. **B** In right MLF syndrome, the right medial rectus does not contract on left lateral gaze, and the right eye remains fixed in midline. **C** In left MLF syndrome, the left medial rectus does not contract on right lateral gaze, and the left eye remains fixed in midline. **D** A right frontal eye field lesion leads to fixed right lateral gaze at rest but does not inhibit left lateral gaze in response to calorics. **E** A left PPRF lesion leaves the eyes fixed in right lateral gaze. **F** A left frontal eye field lesion leads to fixed left lateral gaze at rest but does not inhibit right lateral gaze in response to calorics. **G** A right PPRF lesion leaves the eyes fixed in left lateral gaze. MLF, medial longitudinal fasciculus; PPRF, paramedian pontine reticular formation.

- Unconscious with brain stem intact: Cold water irrigation leads to deviation of the eyes toward the ipsilateral side.
- Bilateral MLF lesion: Cold water irrigation leads to deviation of only the ipsilateral (abducting) eye toward the same side.
- Low brain stem lesion: No response.
- Other important clinical correlations:
  - **Vestibular schwannoma (acoustic neuroma):** Benign tumor of the Schwann cells of CN VIII that arises in the area of the internal auditory meatus and cerebellopontine angle. If bilateral, frequently associated with **neurofibromatosis type 2** (NF2). May impinge on several cranial nerves that pass near the cerebellopontine angle:
    - CN VIII leads to tinnitus, unilateral sensorineural deafness, vertigo, nystagmus, nausea, vomiting, unsteady gait.
    - CN VII results in ipsilateral facial weakness and loss of corneal reflex (efferent limb).
    - CN V is associated with paresthesias, anesthesia of the ipsilateral face, loss of corneal reflex (afferent limb).
  - **"Locked-in" syndrome:** Lesion of the base of the pons from infarction, trauma, tumor, or demyelination.
    - Affects bilateral corticospinal and corticobulbar tracts, and is associated with complete paralysis from head to toe.
    - Spares the oculomotor and trochlear nerves; the patient is only able to communicate with vertical eye movements and blinking.
    - Patient is awake and aware.
  - **Osmotic demyelination syndrome (ODS):** Formerly known as central pontine myelinolysis. ODS is demyelination of the base of the pons due to overly rapid correction of chronic (more than 2 days) hyponatremia. The exact pathogenesis of ODS is not clear. However, brain cells respond to chronic hyponatremia by losing solutes to the extracellular fluid (ECF). Rapid correction via a hypertonic solution results in cell shrinkage and demyelination. Affects the corticospinal and corticobulbar tracts and results in spastic quadriparesis, pseudobulbar palsy, mental changes; may progress to "locked-in" syndrome.

Medulla

- Blood supply: Vertebral artery (VA), anterior spinal artery (ASA), PICA.
- Contents are shown in Figure 6-32.
- Lesions result in important clinical syndromes (Tables 6-11 and 6-12). **Wallenberg syndrome** is particularly common as a result of occlusion in PICA.

Other functions of the medulla include:

- **Vomiting center (chemoreceptor trigger zone):** Neurons at the base of the fourth ventricle (**area postrema**) sample CSF and send inputs to the nucleus of the solitary tract and other autonomic control centers in the brain stem.
- **Respiratory regulation:** At low blood pH, receptors in the medulla activate the **reticular formation** (a diffuse group of neurons controlling vital functions) within the medulla. The phrenic nerve is then activated via CN IX and X, stimulating contraction of the diaphragm and inspiration. Lesion causes respiratory depression, decreased response to hypercapnia.
- **Consciousness:** Disruption of the reticular formation secondary to lesions or alterations in neurotransmitters may lead to changes in consciousness (eg, coma) and even death. Injuries to the reticular formation may result from neck trauma, tumor, and herniation.
- **Blood pressure (BP) regulation:** Receptors in the medulla, the carotid bodies, and the aorta sense stretching of the vessel and send signals to the medulla to increase or decrease BP as needed. Lesion results in hypotension, orthopnea.

KEY FACT

The most common brain tumor found at the cerebellopontine angle is **vestibular schwannoma.**

KEY FACT

Neurofibromatosis 2 (NF2) is often associated with **bilateral** vestibular schwannomas in adults. In children, the vast majority of vestibular schwannomas, even unilateral, are associated with NF2.

KEY FACT

The medulla is the level at which the corticospinal tract crosses the midline (decussates). The crossing fibers of the corticospinal tract constitute the **pyramidal decussation.**

KEY FACT

Horner syndrome:
- Ptosis
- Miosis
- Hemianhidrosis (lack of sweating)
- Apparent enophthalmos (sunken eyeball)

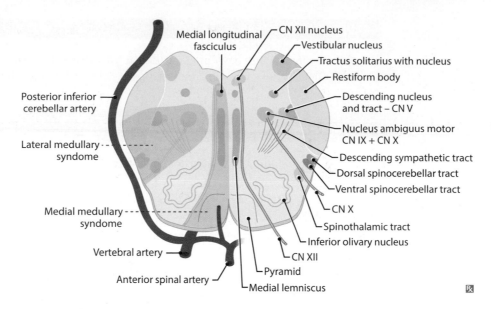

Medial longitudinal fasciculus
CN XII nucleus
Vestibular nucleus
Tractus solitarius with nucleus
Restiform body
Descending nucleus and tract – CN V
Nucleus ambiguus motor CN IX + CN X
Descending sympathetic tract
Dorsal spinocerebellar tract
Ventral spinocerebellar tract
CN X
Spinothalamic tract
Inferior olivary nucleus
CN XII
Pyramid
Medial lemniscus
Posterior inferior cerebellar artery
Lateral medullary syndome
Medial medullary syndome
Vertebral artery
Anterior spinal artery

FIGURE 6-32. Cross-section through the medulla. Note the regions involved in the lateral medullary (Wallenberg) syndrome and medial medullary syndrome due to occlusion of the posterior inferior cerebellar artery and anterior spinal artery, respectively.

TABLE 6-11. Medial Medullary Syndrome (Vertebral or Basilar Artery Occlusion)

STRUCTURE	DEFICIT
Corticospinal tract	Contralateral spastic hemiparesis
Medial lemniscus	Contralateral loss of tactile, vibrational, and proprioceptive sense from trunk and extremities
CN XII nucleus/fibers	Ipsilateral flaccid hemiparalysis of the tongue (tongue points to side of lesion)

TABLE 6-12. Lateral Medullary/Wallenberg/Posterior Inferior Cerebellar Artery Syndrome

STRUCTURE	DEFICIT
Vestibular nuclei	Nystagmus, vertigo
Inferior cerebellar peduncle	Ipsilateral cerebellar signs
Nucleus ambiguus	Dysarthria, hoarseness, dysphagia, loss of gag reflex
Spinothalamic tracts/spinal trigeminal nucleus and tract	*Contralateral* loss of pain and temperature sensation from trunk and extremities, with *ipsilateral* loss of pain and temperature sensation in the face
Descending sympathetic tract	Ipsilateral Horner syndrome

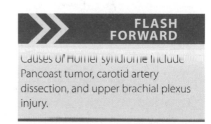

FLASH FORWARD

Causes of Horner syndrome include Pancoast tumor, carotid artery dissection, and upper brachial plexus injury.

CLINICAL CORRELATION

Maintaining balance requires at least two of the three functions: proprioception, vestibular function, and vision. Having a patient stand with feet together and eyes closed isolates vestibular function and proprioception. If the patient loses balance, the Romberg sign is positive, meaning a proprioception defect is likely.

NEUROTRANSMITTERS

Several neurotransmitters have important diffuse functions in the brain. They are present in high concentrations within certain groups of cells that control their release (Table 6-13).

SPINAL CORD

The spinal cord continues caudally from the brain stem as a long cordlike structure that gives off branches along the length of the spine.

Blood Supply

Anterior (ASA) and posterior spinal arteries (PSAs).

Function

The spinal cord carries information from the brain and brain stem to different parts of the body.

Levels of the Spinal Cord

Cervical spinal nerves C1–C7 share the same number as the vertebral segment **below** them. Spinal nerve C8 exits below the C7 vertebrae, and all spinal nerves below C8

TABLE 6-13. Neurotransmitters

	LOCATION IN BRAIN	FUNCTION	ANXIETY	DEPRESSION	SCHIZOPHRENIA	ALZHEIMER DISEASE	HUNTINGTON DISEASE	PARKINSON DISEASE
Acetylcholine	Basal nucleus of Meynert, caudate, putamen	PNS, NMJ, preganglionic sympathetic fibers, postganglionic sympathetic fibers of sweat glands and blood vessels				↓	↓	↑
Dopamine	Substantia nigra pars compacta, ventral tegmentum, arcuate nucleus	Reward pathway, inhibits prolactin release	↓	↑			↑	↓
GABA	Nucleus accumbens		↓				↓	
Norepinephrine	Locus ceruleus	Excess in anxiety, panic attacks, low in mood disorders	↑	↓				
Serotonin	Raphe nuclei	Low in MDD, mediates pain during migraines	↓	↓				↑

GABA, γ-aminobutyric acid; MDD, major depressive disorder; NMJ, neuromuscular junction; PNS, peripheral nervous system.

share the same number as the spinal segment **above** it. Each spinal segment receives sensory input from dermatomal regions of the body and sends motor output to myotomal regions (Figure 6-33).

- Cervical (C1–C8)
- Thoracic (T1–T12)
- Lumbar (L1–L5)
- Sacral (S1–S5)
- Coccygeal

Unique Structures

- **Conus medullaris:** Terminal end of the spinal cord at L3 in newborns and at the lower border of L1 in adults (Figure 6-34).
- **Cauda equina ("tail of the horse"):** At its caudal end (conus medullaris), the spinal cord splits into multiple separate motor and sensory roots, which exit the vertebral canal through the lumbar intervertebral and sacral foramina.

Myotatic Reflex

The myotatic reflexes are monosynaptic, ipsilateral **muscle stretch reflexes,** also known as deep tendon reflexes. Interruption of either the afferent or efferent limb results in **areflexia.** The pathway of the myotatic reflex is as follows (Figure 6-35):

KEY FACT

During growth, the spinal column elongates much more than the spinal cord within it. Thus, the spinal cord terminates at a more cranial level in adults than in newborns.

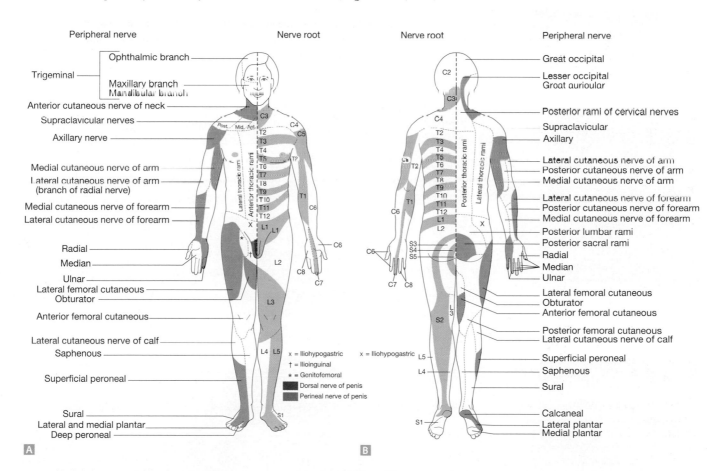

FIGURE 6-33. **Cutaneous innervation (anterior and posterior views).** **A** Cutaneous innervation (anterior view). The segmental or radicular (nerve root) distribution is shown on the left side of the body, and the peripheral nerve distribution on the right side of the body. **B** Cutaneous innervation (posterior view). The segmental or radicular (nerve root) distribution is shown on the left side of the body, and the peripheral nerve distribution on the right side of the body.

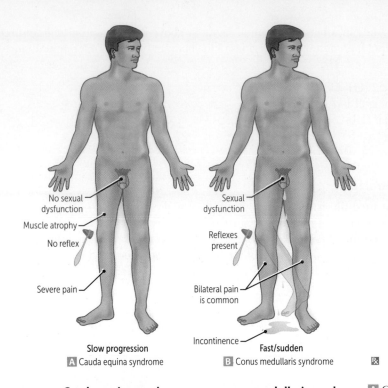

Slow progression
A Cauda equina syndrome

Fast/sudden
B Conus medullaris syndrome

No sexual dysfunction
Muscle atrophy
No reflex
Severe pain

Sexual dysfunction
Reflexes present
Bilateral pain is common
Incontinence

FIGURE 6-34. **Cauda equina syndrome versus conus medullaris syndrome.** **A** Cauda equina syndrome is characterized by preservation of sexual function, muscle atrophy, unilateral pain and areflexia, and a slow progression. **B** Conus medullaris syndrome is characterized by sexual dysfunction, bilateral mild pain, incontinence, and preservation of reflexes.

- Afferent limb: Muscle spindle (receptor) → Ia fiber → dorsal root ganglion neuron.
- Efferent limb: Ventral horn motor neuron → striated muscle (effector).

Reflexes and Corresponding Levels

Reflexes are used to test the integrity of the spinal cord at their corresponding levels (Table 6-14).

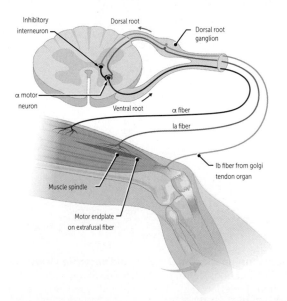

Inhibitory interneuron
Dorsal root
Dorsal root ganglion
α motor neuron
Ventral root
α fiber
Ia fiber
Ib fiber from golgi tendon organ
Muscle spindle
Motor endplate on extrafusal fiber

FIGURE 6-35. **Myotatic reflex pathway.** Diagram of the myotatic/stretch reflex. The Ia fibers transmit information on muscle length, and the Ib Golgi tendon organ fiber transmits information about tension in the tendon.

KEY FACT

Anterior spinal artery (ASA) infarction (ASAs are more susceptible than posterior spinal arteries due to sparse collaterals) presents with:
- Bilateral loss of pain and temperature (spinothalamic tract [STT]).
- Bilateral spastic paresis (corticospinal tract [CST]).
- S2–S4: loss of bladder control.
- Above T2: Horner syndrome.
- The dorsal columns and tract of Lissauer (tract in which the STT travels superior and inferior) are spared.
- Flaccid paralysis (LMN).

KEY FACT

Romberg sign is a test for proprioception, not cerebellar dysfunction. The patient stands with her feet together and closes her eyes. The sign is positive if the patient falls or loses balance.

TABLE 6-14. Deep Tendon Reflexes

MUSCLE STRETCH REFLEX	CORD SEGMENT	MUSCLE
Ankle jerk	S1	Gastrocnemius
Knee jerk	L2–L4	Quadriceps
Biceps jerk	C5–C6	Biceps
Forearm jerk	C5–C6	Brachioradialis
Triceps jerk	C7–C8	Triceps

Cross-Section of the Spinal Cord

- Gray matter: Central "butterfly" that contains the cell bodies of neurons that send projections either to the periphery or up through the spinal cord tracts.
- White matter: Myelinated tracts of the spinal cord.
- White communicating rami: Contain myelinated preganglionic sympathetic fibers. Found only from T1 to L3 in conjunction with the lateral horn and intermediolateral cell column.
- Gray communicating rami: Contain unmyelinated postganglionic sympathetic fibers.

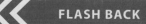

FLASH BACK

The **intermediolateral (IML) cell column** contains neuron cell bodies for the entire sympathetic system. It appears as the **lateral horn** from T1 to L3. Fibers arising from the IML cell column exit the spinal cord via the **white communicating rami** from T1 to L3.

Tracts of the Spinal Cord

The spinal cord is similar to a bundle of electrical wires with various types of information traveling along their respective paths (Figure 6-36).

- **Motor** pathways travel **away** from the brain. The names of motor pathways begin with the brain structure and end with **-spinal** (ie, rubro**spinal** tract).
- **Sensory** pathways travel **toward** the brain. The names of sensory pathways begin with **spino-** and end with the brain structure (ie, **spino**thalamic tract) except the dorsal columns (cuneate and gracile fasciculi).

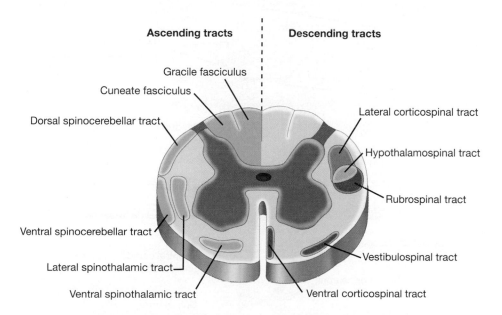

FIGURE 6-36.   Tracts of the spinal cord.

Corticospinal Tracts

The major motor tracts from the cortex. Conduct signals directing purposeful actions (Figure 6-37).

- **Lateral corticospinal tract:** Mediates voluntary skilled motor activity, primarily of the upper limbs.
  - Origin: Cell bodies are the **giant cells of Betz** in layer V of the cortex (see Figure 6-37).
    - Primary motor cortex (Brodmann area 4).
    - Premotor cortex (Brodmann area 6).
    - Supplementary motor cortex (Brodmann area 6).
  - Course:
    - Cortex: The axons of the cells of Betz pass through the posterior limb of the internal capsule, which then forms the crus cerebri as it enters the midbrain.

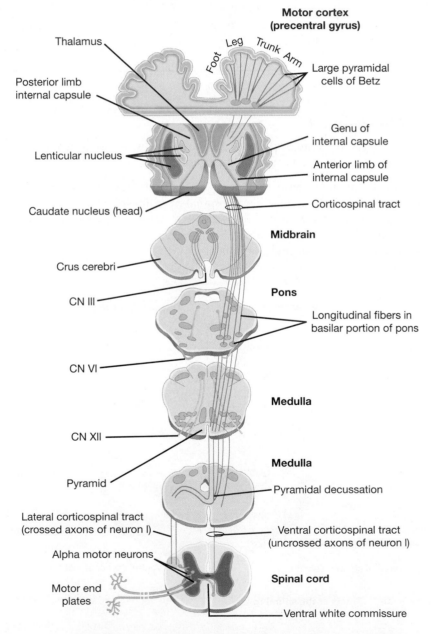

FIGURE 6-37. Lateral and ventral corticospinal tracts. The lateral and ventral tracts deviate from each other at the level of the medulla.

- Brain stem: The fibers continue through the ventral part of the brain stem and decussate in the medulla, forming the medullary "pyramids."
        - Spinal cord: The axons travel along the corticospinal tract in the lateral aspects of the spinal cord.
    - Termination: The fibers synapse onto interneurons within the adjacent gray matter, which then synapse onto alpha motor neurons within the ventral horn of the spinal cord.
    - Transection:
        - Above the decussation, injury results in **contralateral spastic hemiparesis and Babinski sign.**
        - In the spinal cord (below the decussation), transection results in **ipsilateral spastic hemiparesis and Babinski sign.**
- **Ventral corticospinal tract:** Mediates posture and gross movements involving the neck and trunk and lower limbs.
    - Origin: Premotor cortex (Brodmann area 6).
    - Course: Same as that of the lateral corticospinal tract **until the decussation of the pyramids** in the **medulla,** where the ventral corticospinal tract does not decussate and continues ipsilaterally along the ventral white matter of the spinal cord.
    - Termination: The fibers then terminate **bilaterally** near the level of exit of the corresponding alpha motor neurons. Decussating fibers contribute to the **ventral white commissure.** Axons then synapse on alpha motor neurons in the ventral horn of the ipsilateral and contralateral spinal cord. These motor neurons innervate axial muscles used in balance and posture.
    - Transection results in axial/truncal instability (transection in the brain stem and spinal cord have the same manifestation because this tract is uncrossed). Unilateral transection results in more subtle defects because the axial muscles have bilateral innervation.
- **Hypothalamospinal tract:** Carries autonomic information from the hypothalamus.
    - Origin: Hypothalamus.
    - Course: Travels from the hypothalamus through the lateral tegmentum of the brain stem and down through the dorsolateral quadrant of the lateral funiculus.
    - Termination: Ciliospinal center of the intermediolateral cell column at T1–T2.
    - Transection causes **Horner syndrome:** Ipsilateral miosis, ptosis, hemianhidrosis, and apparent enophthalmos.
- **Other motor tracts:** Mediate coordination of movements and balance. The specific functions are beyond the scope of this text.
    - Vestibulospinal tract
    - Rubrospinal tract

Sensory Pathways

- **Dorsal column–medial lemniscus pathway:** Mediates light touch discrimination, vibration sensation, form recognition, and conscious proprioception (joint and muscle position sense; Figure 6-38).
- **Sensory receptors:** Pacinian corpuscles, Meissner corpuscles, Merkel discs, Ruffini corpuscles, joint capsule receptors, muscle spindles, Golgi tendon organs (Table 6-15).
- **First-order neurons:** Cell bodies are located in the dorsal root ganglia. Dendrites terminate as receptors in the periphery. Axons project to the spinal cord and give rise to the following:
    - The **gracile fasciculus** (medial) arises from sensory axons in the lower extremities and ascends the spinal cord and synapses on the gracile nucleus.
    - The **cuneate fasciculus** (lateral) arises from sensory axons in the upper extremity and ascends the spinal cord and synapses on the cuneate nucleus.
    - Spinal reflex collaterals that branch off the main axon and synapse on Ia fibers (see "myotatic reflex," Figure 6-35).

KEY FACT

Before the decussation, the lateral and ventral corticospinal tracts run together. At the pyramids in the medulla, 85–90% of corticospinal fibers decussate and form the **lateral corticospinal tract;** the remaining 10–15% continue as the **ventral corticospinal tract.**

KEY FACT

The lateral corticospinal tract inhibits the **Babinski reflex.** Because myelination of the lateral corticospinal tract is not complete until the second year of life, children < 2 years old often have a positive Babinski sign. Any **upper motor neuron lesion** or lesion of the tract above the alpha motor neuron synapse (ie, spinal cord, cortex) can also result in a positive Babinski sign.

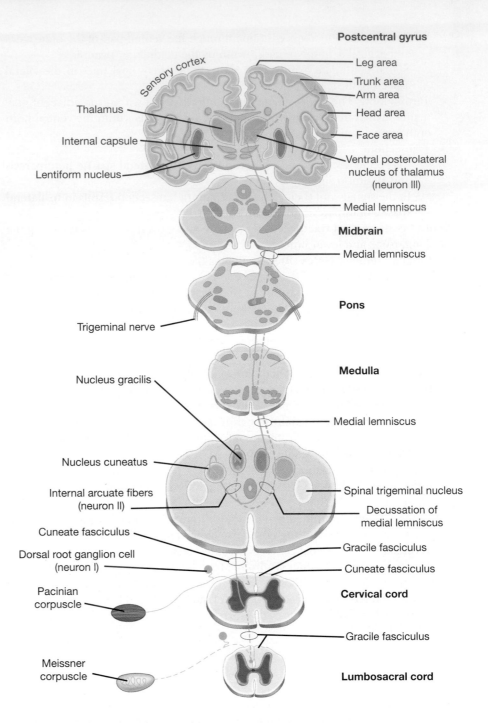

FIGURE 6-38. Dorsal column–medial lemniscus pathway. Impulses from light touch, pressure, and vibration travel along this pathway.

- **Second-order neurons:**
  - Cell bodies: Gracile and cuneate nuclei of the caudal medulla.
  - Axons: Decussate in the medulla as **internal arcuate fibers,** form the **medial lemniscus,** and then ascend in the contralateral brain stem.
  - Termination: Synapse on neurons of the **ventral posterolateral (VPL) nucleus** of the thalamus.
- **Third-order neurons:** Located in the VPL nucleus of the thalamus. Axons project through the posterior limb of the internal capsule to the **primary somatosensory cortex** (Brodmann areas 1, 2, 3) in the postcentral gyrus.

KEY FACT

Since the **cuneate fasciculus** carries sensory axons from the upper extremity to the spinal cord, it does not exist below T2, the most inferior level of nerves supplying the upper extremity.

TABLE 6-15.   Major Sensory Corpuscles

	MEISSNER CORPUSCLE	PACINIAN CORPUSCLE AND RUFFINI CORPUSCLE	MERKEL CORPUSCLE	GOLGI TENDON ORGAN	MUSCLE SPINDLE
Mediates	Light touch, pressure (dynamic)	Deep pressure, vibration, stretching of skin	Light touch, pressure (static)	Muscle tension	Muscle stretch
Description	Small encapsulated	Large encapsulated	Tactile disks associated with peptide-releasing cells		
Location	Between dermal papillae	Dermis	Dermis	Within tendon (in series with muscle fibers)	Within muscle fiber (in parallel with muscle fibers)
Location in the body	Glabrous skin, palms, and soles	Skin, joint capsules, ligaments, serous membranes, and mesenteries	Fingertips, hair follicles, and hard palate	Within tendon	Within muscle fiber

- Transection:
  - **Above the decussation** of the internal arcuate fibers leads to **contralateral** loss of light touch, vibration, and proprioception.
  - In the **spinal cord (below the decussation)** results in **ipsilateral** loss of the above modalities.
- **Lateral spinothalamic tract:** Mediates pain and temperature sensations (Figure 6-39).
  - **Receptors:** Free nerve endings divided into **fast- and slow-conducting pain fibers** (Aδ and C fibers, respectively).
  - First-order neurons: Cell bodies are found in the dorsal root ganglia. Dendrites terminate as free nerve endings. Axons project to the spinal cord and ascend or descend a few levels within the **tract of Lissauer** (lateral root entry zone) before synapsing ipsilaterally on second-order neurons in the dorsal horn (**substantia gelatinosa**).
  - Second-order neurons: Cell bodies are found in the dorsal horn (substantia gelatinosa). Axons decussate in the **ventral white commissure** and ascend in the contralateral **lateral funiculus**. Axons terminate in the VPL nucleus of the thalamus.
  - Third-order neurons: Like those of the dorsal column-medial lemniscus tract, third-order neurons are located in the VPL nucleus of the thalamus. Axons project through the posterior limb of the internal capsule to the **primary somatosensory cortex** (Brodmann areas 1, 2, 3) in the postcentral gyrus.
  - Transection causes ipsilateral loss of pain and temperature sensation for a few levels above and below the lesion along the Lissauer tract and **contralateral** loss of pain and temperature sensation for all levels **below** the decussation.

Brown-Séquard Syndrome

Hemisection of the spinal cord or the brain stem results in Brown-Séquard syndrome. Brown-Séquard syndrome is characterized by its striking clinical manifestation of **ipsilateral** hemiparesis, **ipsilateral** loss of vibratory and tactile sensation, and **contralateral** loss of pain and temperature (Figure 6-40). Additionally, it also involves **ipsilateral** loss of pain and temperature sensation within two levels of the lesion because the first-order neurons of the lateral spinothalamic tract traverse within the **Lissauer tract** a few levels up or down the spinal cord before synapsing on second-order neurons in the substantia gelatinosa, which then cross the midline via the ventral white commissure. A hemisection at or above the level of T1 also causes ipsilateral Horner syndrome.

KEY FACT

Both the dorsal column–medial lemniscus and the spinothalamic tract follow the same rule: Primary afferents synapse ipsilaterally; secondary afferents synapse, then cross. However, the decussations occur at different levels: brain stem for the former and spinal cord for the latter.

KEY FACT

Fasciculations are coordinated spontaneous depolarizations of a group of muscle fibers innervated by one motor neuron. Manifest as twitches.

Fibrillations are small spontaneous depolarizations of a single muscle fiber that has been denervated.

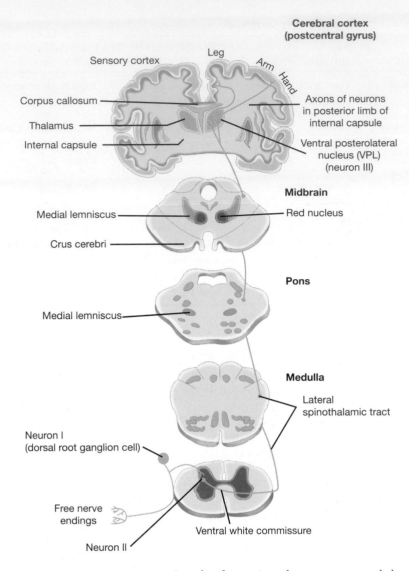

FIGURE 6-39.   Spinothalamic tract. Impulses from pain and temperature travel along this pathway.

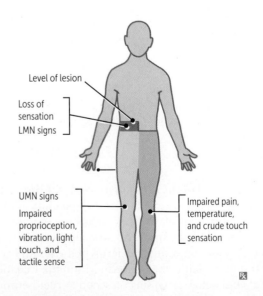

FIGURE 6-40.   Brown-Séquard syndrome.

Lesions of the Spinal Cord

These result in various symptoms, depending upon which tracts are affected (Table 6-16 and Figures 6-41 and 6-42).

TABLE 6-16. Lesions of the Spinal Cord

CATEGORY	LESION	MECHANISM	CLINICAL MANIFESTATION	EXAMPLES/OTHER FACTS
Motor pathway lesions	Upper motor neuron (UMN)	Transection of or damage to the corticospinal tract or cortical motor neurons	Spastic paresis with a positive Babinski sign	Stroke, ischemic/traumatic injury to brain stem or spinal cord
	Lower motor neuron (LMN) (see Figure 6-41A)	Damage to alpha motor neurons	Flaccid paralysis, areflexia, atrophy, fasciculations, and fibrillations of the muscle fibers	Poliomyelitis, Werdnig-Hoffman disease ("floppy baby")
	Combined UMN and LMN (see Figure 6-41C)	Damage to both corticospinal tracts and alpha motor neurons	Both UMN and LMN symptoms	ALS
Sensory pathway lesions	Dorsal column (see Figure 6-41E)	Destruction of the dorsal column	Loss of tactile discrimination and position and vibration sensation; shooting pain and paresthesias; **Romberg sign**	Tabes dorsalis in **tertiary syphilis**
Combined motor and sensory lesions	Spinal cord hemisection (Brown-Séquard syndrome, see Figure 6-41F)	Damage to: ■ Dorsal columns ■ Lateral corticospinal tract ■ Lateral spinothalamic tract ■ Ventral (anterior) horn	Gives rise to: ■ Ipsilateral loss of tactile discrimination, position, vibration ■ Ipsilateral loss of pain and temperature sensation (within 2 segments of lesion) ■ Ipsilateral spastic paresis (below lesion) ■ Contralateral loss of pain and temperature sensation (below lesion) ■ Ipsilateral Horner (lesion T1 or above) ■ Ipsilateral flaccid paralysis (at segment of the lesion)	Trauma
	Anterior spinal artery occlusion (see Figure 6-41D)	Infarction of anterior two-thirds of spinal cord; damage may be unilateral or bilateral; characteristically spares dorsal columns and Lissauer tract	**Preserved** tactile, position, and vibration sense; **loss** of pain and temperature sense; paresis; urinary and stool incontinence; Horner syndrome (lesion T1 or above)	Embolus, aortic dissection
	Subacute combined degeneration (see Figure 6-41G)	Damage to: ■ Dorsal columns ■ Lateral corticospinal tract ■ Spinocerebellar tracts	■ Bilateral loss of tactile discrimination, position, vibration sense ■ Bilateral spastic paresis ■ Bilateral upper and lower ataxia	**Vitamin B₁₂ deficiency,** (eg, pernicious anemia), Vitamin E deficiency, **Friedreich ataxia** (autosomal recessive, no treatment, 40-year life span)

(continues)

TABLE 6-16. Lesions of the Spinal Cord (*continued*)

CATEGORY	LESION	MECHANISM	CLINICAL MANIFESTATION	EXAMPLES/OTHER FACTS
Combined motor and sensory lesions (*continued*)	Syringomyelia (see Figures 6-41F, 6-42)	Central cavitation of the **cervical** cord (C8–T1) of unknown cause; damage to: ■ Ventral white commissure ■ Ventral horns	Results in: ■ Bilateral loss of pain and temperature sensation of upper extremities ■ Bilateral flaccid paralysis of intrinsic muscles of the hands	Commonly seen with Arnold-Chiari syndrome type II; referred to as the sensation of wearing a "cape over the shoulders"
	Multiple sclerosis (see Figure 6-41B)	Random, asymmetrical autoimmune-mediated demyelination of cervical segments of the spinal cord and brain; pathology shows destruction of **oligodendrocytes** and **reactive gliosis**	**Charcot triad:** ■ Scanning speech ■ Nystagmus (internuclear ophthalmoplegia due to MLF lesion) ■ Intention tremor Also spastic paresis and sensory loss	See text discussion
PNS lesions	Guillain–Barré syndrome	Demyelination and edema of motor fibers of ventral roots and peripheral nerves	Facial diplegia, papilledema from elevated protein levels, ascending lower extremity weakness, LMN symptoms, **paresthesias,** life-threatening **respiratory paralysis**	See text discussion
Intervertebral disk herniation	90% L4–S1 10% C5–C7	Prolapse, herniation of the **nucleus pulposus** through defective annulus fibrosus and into vertebral canal, impinging on spinal roots	Paresthesias, pain, sensory loss, hyporeflexia, muscle weakness	Other clues: History of heavy lifting, positive leg-raise test, no relief with sitting
Terminal cord syndromes	Cauda equina syndrome (see Figure 6-34)	Tumor impingement, spinal stenosis, or inflammation at L3–Co	Results in: ■ **Gradual** and **unilateral** onset ■ Radicular **unilateral** pain ■ Loss of sensation in unilateral saddle-shaped area ■ Unilateral muscle atrophy and **absent** patellar (L4) and ankle (S1) jerks ■ **Mild** incontinence and sexual dysfunction	Treat with emergency surgery
	Conus medullaris syndrome (see Figure 6-34)	Impingement of S3–Co from intramedullary tumor (ependymoma)	Results in: ■ **Sudden** and **bilateral** onset ■ **Bilateral** mild pain ■ Loss of sensation in **bilateral** saddle-shaped area ■ **Mild** muscle weakness, **preserved** reflexes ■ **Severe** incontinence and sexual dysfunction	Nonurgent treatment with corticosteroid injection or radiation

ALS, amyotrophic lateral sclerosis; MLF, medial longitudinal fasciculus.

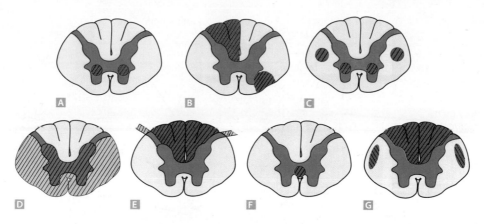

FIGURE 6-41. **Patterns of spinal cord lesions.** Shaded areas demarcate areas commonly lesioned in specific diseases. **A** Poliomyelitis and Werdnig-Hoffmann disease: Lower motor neuron (LMN) lesions only due to destruction of anterior horns; flaccid paralysis. **B** Multiple sclerosis: Mostly white matter of cervical region; random and asymmetrical lesions, due to demyelination; scanning speech, intention tremor, nystagmus. **C** Amyotrophic lateral sclerosis: Combined lower and upper motor neuron (UMN) deficits with no sensory deficit. **D** Complete occlusion of anterior spinal artery; spares dorsal columns and tract of Lissauer. **E** Tabes dorsalis (tertiary syphilis): Degeneration of dorsal roots and dorsal columns; impaired proprioception, locomotor ataxia. **F** Syringomyelia: Crossing fibers of lateral spinothalamic tract in ventral white commissure usually damaged first; results in bilateral loss of pain and temperature sensation in upper extremities ("capelike" distribution) with sparing of fine touch, vibration, and position sense; syrinx expansion can damage anterior horn cells; results in LMN signs. **G** Subacute combined degeneration (eg, vitamin B_{12} neuropathy, vitamin E deficiency, Friedreich ataxia): Demyelination of dorsal columns, lateral corticospinal tracts, and spinocerebellar tracts; ataxic gait, hyperreflexia, impaired position and vibration sense.

CRANIAL NERVES

Twelve cranial nerves innervate the head and neck. Symptoms of lesions of the cranial nerves are important in localizing pathology within the complex anatomy of the head and neck (Figures 6-43 and 6-44 and Tables 6-17 and 6-18).

Cranial Nerve Lesions

Although most lesions are straightforward, some are frequently tested for peculiarities (Table 6-19).

Facial nerve lesions are divided into upper motor neuron (UMN) lesions and lower motor neuron (LMN) lesions:

- UMN lesion (Figure 6-45):
    - Lesion in the motor cortex or connection between the cortex and the facial nucleus.
    - The portion of the facial nerve nucleus innervating the upper face and forehead receives bilateral input from the motor cortex of both cerebral hemispheres.
    - Leads to paralysis of the **contralateral lower face only,** sparing the upper face and forehead.
- LMN lesion (see Figure 6-45):
    - Lesion of the facial nucleus or facial nerve.
    - The portion of the facial nerve nucleus innervating the lower face receives mainly input from the motor cortex of the contralateral cerebral hemisphere.
    - Leads to paralysis of the ipsilateral **upper and lower face.**
    - Idiopathic facial nerve palsy is referred to as **Bell palsy.**

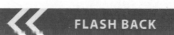

The **nucleus pulposus** is the remnant of the notochord.

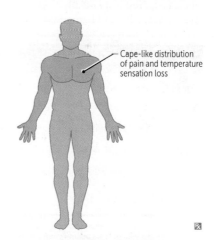

Cape-like distribution of pain and temperature sensation loss

FIGURE 6-42. **Loss of pain and temperature sensation in syringomyelia.** Involves enlargement of the central canal of the spinal cord, damaging fibers of the spinothalamic tract. Sensory loss is often described as feeling like one is wearing a cape over one's shoulders because it is most commonly found in C8–T1. Often seen in Arnold-Chiari malformation.

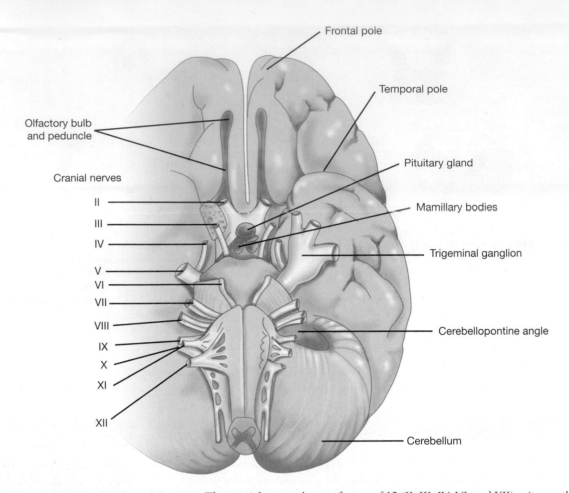

FIGURE 6-43. **Anatomic exits of cranial nerves.** The cranial nerves that are factors of 12 (II, III, IV, VI, and XII) exit near the midline, whereas the rest exit laterally. Of these that exit near the midline, III and IV exit at the level of the midbrain, VI at the level of the pons, and XII at the level of the medulla. Of note, CN IV exits posteriorly and wraps around to the anterior surface.

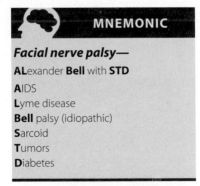

MNEMONIC

Facial nerve palsy—

ALexander **Bell** with **STD**

AIDS
Lyme disease
Bell palsy (idiopathic)
Sarcoid
Tumors
Diabetes

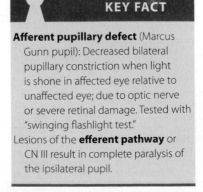

KEY FACT

Afferent pupillary defect (Marcus Gunn pupil): Decreased bilateral pupillary constriction when light is shone in affected eye relative to unaffected eye; due to optic nerve or severe retinal damage. Tested with "swinging flashlight test."

Lesions of the **efferent pathway** or CN III result in complete paralysis of the ipsilateral pupil.

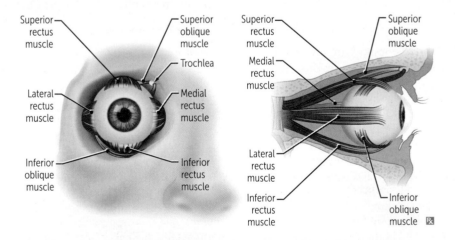

FIGURE 6-44. **Extraocular muscles and their corresponding eye motions.** All muscles are innervated by cranial nerve III with the exception of superior oblique (CN IV) and lateral rectus (CN VI).

TABLE 6-17. Cranial Nerves

NERVE	CN	FUNCTION	TYPE	MNEMONIC
Olfactory	I	Smell	Sensory	Some
Optic	II	Sight	Sensory	Say
Oculomotor	III	Eye movement, pupil constriction, accommodation, eyelid opening	Motor	Marry
Trochlear	IV	Eye movement (superior oblique)	Motor	Money
Trigeminal	V	Muscles of mastication, facial sensation	Both	But
Abducens	VI	Eye movement (lateral rectus)	Motor	My
Facial	VII	Facial movement, taste from anterior 2/3 of tongue, lacrimation, salivation (submandibular and sublingual glands), eyelid closing	Both	Brother
Vestibulocochlear	VIII	Hearing, balance	Sensory	Says
Glossopharyngeal	IX	Taste from posterior 1/3 of tongue, swallowing, salivation (parotid gland), monitoring carotid body and sinus chemo- and baroreceptors	Both	Big
Vagus	X	Taste from epiglottic region, swallowing, palate elevation, talking, thoracoabdominal viscera, monitoring aortic arch chemo- and baroreceptors	Both	Brains
Accessory	XI	Head turning, shoulder shrugging	Motor	Matter
Hypoglossal	XII	Tongue movement	Motor	Most

SENSORY PATHWAYS

Visual System

The visual system performs several important functions, including vision, pupillary reflex, near and far accommodation, and coordination of eye movements or gaze (see Figure 6-44).

Visual Pathway

- **Photoreceptors** of the retina: **Rods** mediate black and white vision; **cones** mediate color vision.
- **Ganglion cells** of the retina: Receive input from the rods and cones via other intermediary cells and send information down axons that form the **optic nerve** (CN II). Ganglion cells from the **nasal** hemiretina project to the **contralateral** lateral

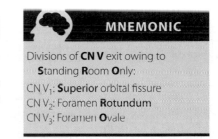

MNEMONIC

Divisions of **CN V** exit owing to **S**tanding **R**oom **O**nly:

CN V$_1$: **Superior** orbital fissure
CN V$_2$: Foramen **Rotundum**
CN V$_3$: Foramen **O**vale

TABLE 6-18. Cranial Nerve and Vessel Exits from the Skull

Cribriform plate (CN I)	
Middle cranial fossa (CN II–VI) through sphenoid bone	1. Optic canal (CN II, ophthalmic artery, central retinal vein) 2. Superior orbital fissure (CN III, IV, V$_1$, VI, ophthalmic vein) 3. Foramen rotundum (CN V$_2$) 4. Foramen ovale (CN V$_3$) 5. Foramen spinosum (middle meningeal artery)
Posterior cranial fossa (CN VII–XII) through temporal or occipital bone	1. Internal auditory meatus (CN VII, VIII) 2. Jugular foramen (CN IX, X, XI, internal jugular vein) 3. Hypoglossal canal (CN XII) 4. Foramen magnum (spinal roots of CN XI, brain stem, vertebral arteries)

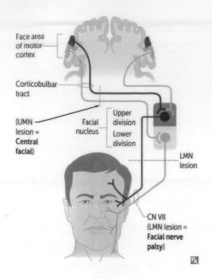

FIGURE 6-45. Facial lesions.
Notice how the upper face receives input from the cortex on both sides, thus a unilateral upper motor neuron (UMN) lesion spares the upper face due to sparing of the contralateral fibers that are innervating the ipsilateral facial nucleus. However, a unilateral lower motor neuron (LMN) lesion disrupts all fibers from the facial nucleus, producing complete paralysis of one side of the face.

TABLE 6-19. Frequently Tested for Cranial Nerve Lesions

CRANIAL NERVE	NOTE ON LESION
III	Triad of ptosis, blown pupil, and "down and out" eyes
VII	Paralysis of **both** the upper and lower face (eg, Bell palsy)
VIII	Sensorineural hearing loss. Weber test: normal > affected. Rinne test: air > bone (see Auditory System section)
X	Uvula deviates **away** from the side of lesion
XI	Weakness turning head to **contralateral** side of lesion
XII	Tongue deviates **toward** the side of lesion ("lick your wounds")

geniculate nucleus (LGN), and those from the **temporal** hemiretina project to the **ipsilateral** LGN. Thus, vision from the right visual field of both eyes is projected to the left LGN and vice versa (Figure 6-46).

■ The **optic nerve** projects from the optic cup at the posterior aspect of the eye through the optic canal to the optic chiasm, where the fibers split.

■ **Papilledema:** Results from congestion of the optic disc and pressure on the root of the optic nerve from increased intracranial pressure (ICP). Results in **enlarged blind spots** with **preserved visual acuity.** Commonly due to mass-occupying lesions in the brain, severe hypertension, or noncommunicating hydrocephalus.

The visual pathway begins at the retina. The **optic tract** is formed from fibers from the ipsilateral temporal hemiretina and contralateral nasal hemiretina. These nerve fibers travel from the optic chiasm to the ipsilateral **LGN, pretectal nuclei,** and **superior colliculus.** Fibers from the LGN then project to the primary visual cortex (Brodmann area 17) through the **geniculocalcarine tract** or **visual radiation.** The **geniculocalcarine tract (visual radiation)** projects through two divisions: the **upper division** and the **lower division (Meyer loop).** The upper division passes through the parietal lobe,

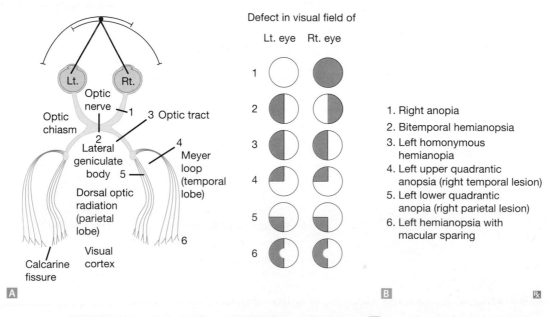

FIGURE 6-46. Visual pathways and associated lesions with clinical manifestations. **A** Visual pathway leading from retina to visual cortex. **B** Lesions along the pathway and corresponding clinical manifestations. Note that lesions proximal to the chiasm can be associated with monocular and ipsilateral defects, and lesions distal to the chiasm lead to contralateral and binocular defects.

and Meyer loop passes through the temporal lobe. Both converge at the **visual cortex.** The posterior area of the visual cortex receives **macular input,** or central vision, the intermediate area receives **perimacular input,** or peripheral vision, and the anterior area receives **monocular input.** Lesions at the various locations of the pathway create different visual defects (Table 6-20).

The **pupillary light reflex pathway** is mediated by the parasympathetic nervous system. It relies on an afferent pathway through CN II and an efferent pathway through CN III (Figure 6-47).

The **pupillary dilation pathway** is mediated by the sympathetic nervous system. Lesions result in ipsilateral **Horner syndrome.**

The **near reflex and accommodation pathway** allows pupils to constrict and focus on near objects.

Auditory System

The auditory system can detect frequencies of **20–20,000 Hz.** The afferent of the auditory system is the cochlear division of CN VIII, the vestibulocochlear nerve (Figure 6-48).

Auditory Pathway

Hair cells of the **organ of Corti** transmit to the:

- Bipolar cells of the **spiral ganglion,** that in turn stimulate the
- Cochlear nerve (enters the brain stem at the **cerebellopontine angle**) ascends to the cochlear nuclei, which sends off fibers that
- Decussate via the **trapezoid body,** and travel to the
- **Superior olivary nucleus** bilaterally,
- Ascends via the **lateral lemniscus** to the

KEY FACT

Argyll Robertson pupil (pupillary light-near dissociation) is the lack of pupillary constriction in response to light, with preservation of pupillary constriction by accommodation to near stimulus. It was formerly referred to as **"prostitute's pupil"** because it "accommodates, but doesn't react." Seen in tertiary **syphilis** and **diabetes.**

KEY FACT

Adie tonic pupil is a large pupil caused by damage to the parasympathetic ciliary ganglion; similar to the **Argyll Robertson pupil,** it has impaired reaction to light, retains accommodation to near vision, but reacts very slowly. Seen in women with diminished knee and ankle reflexes.

TABLE 6-20.   **Lesions of the Visual Pathway**

SITE	LESION	COMMENT
Optic nerve (see Figure 6-46, lesion 1)	Optic nerve	Ipsilateral monocular loss of vision. Loss of ipsilateral (direct) pupillary reflex (light in ipsilateral eye does not induce pupillary constriction of either eye). Contralateral (indirect) pupillary light reflex remains intact (light in contralateral eye induces pupillary constriction in both eyes)
Optic chiasm (see Figure 6-46, lesion 2)	Midsagittal	Bitemporal hemianopia, usually from an enlarging pituitary tumor in adults and a craniopharyngioma in children
	Bilateral lateral	Binasal hemianopia, usually from calcified internal carotid arteries
	Unilateral lateral	Contralateral nasal hemianopia, usually from a calcified internal carotid artery
Optic tract (see Figure 6-46, lesion 3)	Optic tract	Contralateral homonymous hemianopia
Geniculocalcarine tract	Lower division: Meyer loop (see Figure 6-46, lesion 4)	Contralateral upper quadrantanopia, "pie in the sky." If bilateral, it is called upper altitudinopia
	Upper division (see Figure 6-46, lesion 5)	Contralateral lower quadrantanopia. If bilateral, it is called lower altitudinopia
Visual cortex	Perimacular (see Figure 6-46, lesion 6)	Contralateral homonymous hemianopia with macular sparing
	Macular	Central scotoma

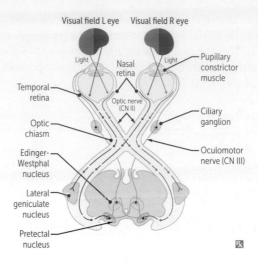

FIGURE 6-47.   Pupillary light reflex pathway. Retinal ganglion cells → CN II (afferent pathway) → pretectal nucleus of the midbrain → bilateral Edinger-Westphal nucleus of CN III (preganglionic parasympathetic fibers) → CN III (efferent pathway) → ciliary ganglion (postganglionic parasympathetic fibers) → sphincter muscle of the iris.

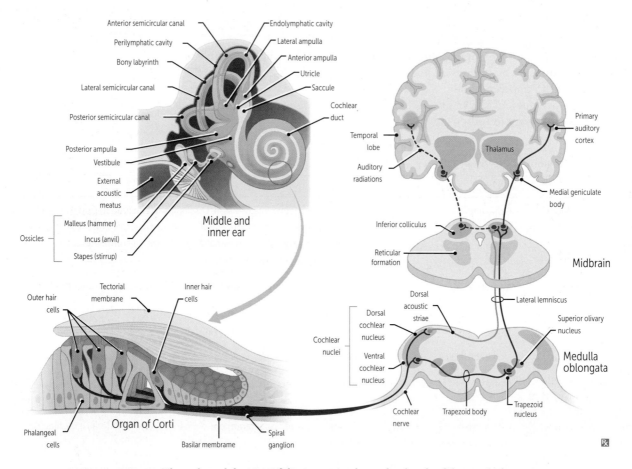

FIGURE 6-48.   Auditory pathway. The enlarged drawing of the inner ear shows the details of the vestibular system.

- **Nucleus of the inferior colliculus,** which projects to the
- **Medial geniculate nucleus (MGN)** via the **brachium of inferior colliculus,** which radiates by way of the **sublenticular part of the internal capsule** to the
- **Transverse temporal gyri of Heschl/primary auditory cortex** (Brodmann areas 41 and 42).

Hearing Defects

- **Conduction deafness:** Caused by anything that prevents sound waves from reaching the organ of Corti. The defect is in the **external** or **middle** ear. May be due to **obstruction** (ie, wax), **otosclerosis,** or **otitis media.**
- **Sensorineural deafness:** Caused by disease of the cochlea, cochlear nerve, or central auditory pathways. Usually due to degeneration of the organ of Corti. May also be due to tumors that disrupt the cochlear nerve (eg, **acoustic neuroma**).
- Two major tests of hearing can be done at the bedside to differentiate between conduction and nerve deafness:
    - **Weber test:** Place a vibrating tuning fork on the top of the skull. Ask the patient which side sounds louder. A normal patient hears the sound equally in both ears.
    - **Rinne test:** Place a vibrating tuning fork on the mastoid process behind the ear until the patient can no longer hear the sound. The patient is using **bone conduction** during this phase of the test. Once the patient no longer hears the sound, the tuning fork is held in front of the ear. Normally, the patient still hears the sound using **air conduction.** Therefore, air conduction > bone conduction in a normal patient.
        - In **conduction deafness,** the sound is louder on the affected side in the Weber test. Bone conduction is greater than air conduction in the Rinne test (abnormal).
        - In **sensorineural deafness,** the sound is louder on the unaffected side in the Weber test. Air conduction is greater than bone conduction in the Rinne test (normal).

Vestibular System

The vestibular system maintains balance and coordinates head and eye movements. **Vertigo** results from disruption of the vestibular system (see Figure 6-48).

Labyrinth

- **Kinetic labyrinth:** Consists of three semicircular canals (superior, lateral/horizontal, and posterior) that are filled with a fluid called **endolymph.** Provides information on **angular acceleration and deceleration** of the head. **Hair cells** lie in the **ampulla** and are activated by endolymph flow.
- **Static labyrinth:** Consists of the **utricle** and **saccule** and responds to **linear acceleration** of the head, including **gravity** (head position). **Hair cells** reside on the otolithic membrane, and bending toward the longest cilium (**kinocilium**) results in activation.

Vestibular Pathways

Hair cells of labyrinth structures → vestibular ganglion → vestibular nuclei in brain stem → cerebellum, MLF, spinal cord, thalamus.

Olfactory System

The olfactory system mediates the sense of smell and involves CN I, the olfactory nerve. It is the only sensory modality that is not relayed by the thalamus before reaching the cortex. Thus, it is thought to be one of the most primal sensory systems.

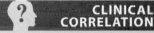

CLINICAL CORRELATION

Olfactory groove meningioma can compress the olfactory and optic nerves, producing the following constellation of symptoms:
- Ipsilateral anosmia (inability to detect smells)
- Ipsilateral optic atrophy
- Contralateral papilledema

KEY FACT

Bilateral acoustic neuroma is a typical manifestation in NF2. In these patients, the Rinne test is normal because the lesion causes nerve deafness. However, the Weber test may be normal also if the nerve deafness affects both ears equally.

Olfactory Pathway

Olfactory receptor cells → mitral cells of the olfactory bulb → olfactory tract/nerve → primary olfactory cortex (piriform cortex) and amygdala.

Gustatory System

The gustatory system mediates taste and is carried by two major nerves: the special sensory division of CN VII (facial nerve), which supplies the anterior two-thirds of the tongue, and CN IX (glossopharyngeal nerve), which supplies the posterior one-third of the tongue.

Gustatory Pathway

- Taste buds of the anterior two-thirds of the tongue → intermediate nerve (CN VII) and chorda tympani (CN VII) travel with the lingual nerve (branch of CN V_3) → geniculate ganglion (cell bodies of the taste buds) → solitary tract and nucleus → ventral posteromedial nucleus of the thalamus → gustatory cortex (parietal operculum, insular cortex).
- Taste buds of the posterior one-third of the tongue → glossopharyngeal nerve (CN IX) → petrosal (inferior) ganglion → solitary tract and nucleus → ventral posteromedial nucleus of the thalamus → gustatory cortex (parietal operculum, insular cortex).

Histology

CELLS OF THE NERVOUS SYSTEM

Neurons

The basic subunits of the CNS and PNS. Several variants (sensory, motor, and interneuron) of these cells all share similar basic components (Figure 6-49):

- Cell body (**soma**): Contains the nucleus, organelles, and prominent clusters of rough endoplasmic reticulum, the latter visualized as **Nissl bodies.**
- Dendrites: Afferent single or multiple extensions of the cell membrane that receive signals from other neurons or the environment of the neuron. They also contain Nissl bodies. In some instances, dendrites can also transmit efferent signals.
- Axons: Efferent extensions of the cell membrane that send signals **away** from the cell body to other neurons or end organs. They may be myelinated or unmyelinated.

Neurons may have any number of dendrites and axons, which can be used for classification purposes:

- **Unipolar** neurons have one dendrite or one axon.
- **Pseudounipolar** neurons have one process that branches into a dendrite and an axon.
- **Bipolar** neurons have one dendrite and one axon.
- **Multipolar** neurons have many dendrites and axons.

Neuronal axons contain both areas that are myelinated and those that are unmyelinated.

- **Myelin:** Multiple layers of membranous phospholipid that form a sheath around an axon. Myelination permits fast transmission of action potentials (APs) along the axon.

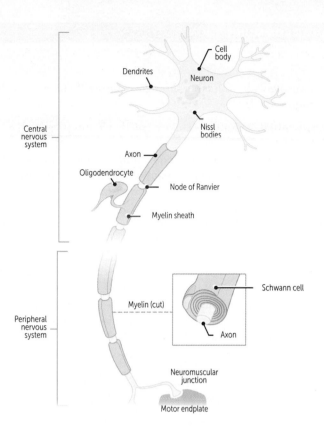

FIGURE 6-45. Central and peripheral neurons. Basic structure of neurons. Note that in the PNS, axons are myelinated by Schwann cells, whereas in the CNS, axons are myelinated by oligodendrocytes.

- **Nodes of Ranvier**: Areas of naked axon in between areas encased by myelin. Contain a high density of ion channels such as voltage-gated Na+ channels that allow current to flow across the axon membrane. Allows rapid saltatory conduction of APs along the axon.

Neuroglia

Neurons are maintained by supportive cells known as neuroglia. Neuroglia come in several forms:

- Astrocytes: Cells that repair and provide nutritional support to neurons, maintain the BBB, and regulate the composition of CSF. They contain the intermediate filament glial fibrillary acidic protein (**GFAP**); stains for GFAP are used to assist in the differential diagnosis of neurologic lesions.
- Ependymal cells: Form a single layer of cells lining the ventricles and produce CSF.
- Microglia: Phagocytes of mesodermal origin with irregular nuclei and little cytoplasm. They proliferate around injured nerve tissue and transform into large ameboid phagocytic cells in response to tissue damage.
- Oligodendroglia: Each cell may myelinate up to 30 neurons in the CNS. Destroyed in central demyelinating diseases such as MS.
- Schwann cells: Each cell myelinates one PNS axon. Gaps between Schwann cells constitute the nodes of Ranvier. They assist in axonal regeneration by creating a pathway for axon growth and secreting growth factors. Mutation of the tumor suppressor gene NF2 may give rise to **schwannomas,** commonly located in the internal acoustic meatus (**acoustic neuroma**). Destroyed in peripheral demyelinating diseases such as **Guillain-Barré syndrome.**

KEY FACT

Wallerian degeneration occurs in a segment of axon after it has been disconnected from the cell body. In the periphery, degradation and phagocytosis of the axon and myelin are followed by proliferation of Schwann cells.

Chromatolysis occurs in a cell body when an axon has been cut off. It is characterized by:
- Disruption and dispersion of Nissl bodies
- Rearrangement of the cytoskeleton with neuronal swelling
- Marked accumulation of intermediate filaments

KEY FACT

HIV-infected microglia form multinucleated giant cells. Characteristic of **HIV encephalitis.**

INTERCELLULAR COMMUNICATION

Synapses

Neurons communicate with each other through **synapses.** Synapses involve the following structures (Figure 6-50):

- Presynaptic membrane: Contains voltage-gated calcium (Ca^{2+}) channels that open in response to APs.
- Secretory vesicles: Contain the neurotransmitter and rest in the cytoplasm, until Ca^{2+} influx recruits them to the presynaptic axon terminal for exocytosis.
- Synaptic cleft: Site where exocytosed neurotransmitter molecules diffuse across to the postsynaptic membrane.
- Postsynaptic membrane: Contains receptors for various neurotransmitters.
- Receptors: Bind the neurotransmitters and facilitate depolarization of the postsynaptic membrane by activating Na^+ channels.
- Ion channels: Include Na^+, potassium (K^+), and Ca^{2+} channels. Sodium channels are responsible for depolarization (AP); K^+ channels are responsible for repolarization (termination of the AP) and maintenance of the resting potential; and Ca^{2+} channels are responsible for permitting increased intracellular calcium concentration that allows for muscle contraction in the PNS.

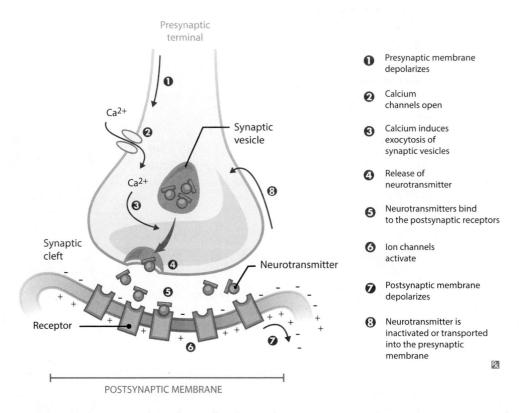

FIGURE 6-50. Steps of synaptic transmission. The small spikes on the postsynaptic membrane represent receptors for neurotransmitters. SER, smooth endoplasmic reticulum.

Neuromuscular Junction

Neurons communicate with muscle fibers through the neuromuscular junction (NMJ), which resembles a synapse except that the postsynaptic membrane is the membrane of a muscle fiber, also known as an **endplate.** The neurotransmitter is always acetylcholine (ACh). The following lists the sequence of events that takes place during activation of the NMJ (Figure 6-51):

- A wave of depolarization propagates down the axon toward the axon terminal, promoting exocytosis of ACh (similar to the process in the synapse, described earlier).
- Nicotinic ACh receptors (ligand-gated ion channels) lie on the postsynaptic membrane and permit Na^+, K^+, and $Ca^{?+}$ (certain subtypes) to traverse the sarcolemma when activated by ACh.
- Calcium channels on the surface of the sarcolemma (dihydropyridine-type) interact with voltage-gated Ca^{2+} channels (ryanodine-type) on the surface of the sarcoplasmic reticulum (SR). The interaction causes a surge of calcium from the SR into the cytosol in a process called **calcium-induced calcium release.**
- Calcium binds troponin C, which moves tropomyosin off myosin-binding sites on actin, allowing myosin heads to bind to actin and generate muscle contraction.
- Meanwhile, acetylcholinesterase (AChE) degrades any ACh that remains in the synaptic cleft.

Diseases of the Neuromuscular Junction

Myasthenia gravis is an autoimmune disease in which antibodies attack the nicotinic ACh receptors, decreasing their numbers partly through the endocytic pathway (Table 6-21). If left untreated, myasthenia gravis can lead to respiratory failure. Diagnosis is via the **Tensilon test:** Administration of **edrophonium,** a short-acting AChE inhibitor rapidly improves symptoms in myasthenia gravis but not in Lambert-Eaton syndrome.

Lambert-Eaton syndrome is an autoimmune disease in which antibodies attack presynaptic voltage-gated Ca^{2+} channels of the neuromuscular junction (see Table 6-21).

> **KEY FACT**
>
> In **neuroleptic malignant syndrome** and **malignant hyperthermia,** muscles of the body involuntarily contract, causing a dangerous elevation of body temperature and damage to muscle fibers. **Dantrolene** can be used to treat these conditions (blocks the ryanodine receptors, inhibiting calcium-induced calcium release).

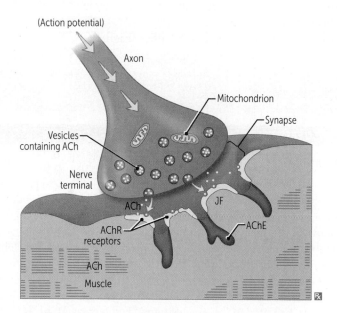

FIGURE 6-51. **Neuromuscular junction.** The "nerve terminal" is the presynaptic bouton. ACh, acetylcholine; AChE, acetylcholinesterase; AChR, acetylcholine receptor; JF, junctional fold.

TABLE 6-21. **Diseases of the Neuromuscular Junction**

MYASTHENIA GRAVIS (MG)	LAMBERT-EATON SYNDROME
Antibodies attack postsynaptic **ACh receptors**	Antibodies attack presynaptic **Ca²⁺ channels**
Associated with **thymoma**	Associated with **small-cell lung cancer**
Muscles are **weaker with repetition**	Muscles are **stronger with repetition**
Manifests with ptosis, diplopia, muscle weakness **at the end of the day**	Manifests with difficulty rising from a chair and weakness of large muscles especially **in the morning**. Respiratory and ocular muscle involvement not as severe as in MG

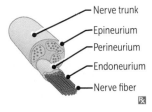

FIGURE 6-52. **Layers of the nerve fiber.**

Sensory Corpuscles

Neurons receive sensory signals through the skin via specialized sensory organs: Meissner, Pacinian, Merkel, and Ruffini corpuscles, muscle spindles, and Golgi tendon organs. Other sensory organs include joint receptors, stretch receptors, baroreceptors, and hair cells of the inner ear (see Table 6-15).

- Pacinian corpuscles: Mediate discrimination of coarse spatial differences.
- Meissner and Merkel corpuscles: Mediate discrimination of fine spatial differences.
- Joint capsule receptors: Sense flexion/extension of the joints.
- Muscle spindles (in parallel with muscle fibers): Sense muscle length.
- Golgi tendon organs (in series with muscle fibers): Sense tension of tendons and muscles.

Organization of Peripheral Nerves

Nerve fibers consist of axons and their myelin sheaths and are bundled together into peripheral nerves. From outermost to innermost, the three layers of a nerve are:

- **Epineurium** (dense connective tissue) surrounds the entire nerve.
- **Perineurium** (permeability barrier) surrounds a fascicle of fibers; must be rejoined in limb attachment surgery.
- **Endoneurium** surrounds a single nerve fiber (Figure 6-52).

Pathology

NEURAL TUBE DEFECTS

Congenital failure of the neural folds and coverings to fuse in the midline leads to deformities in the developing nervous system (Figure 6-3). Clinical presentation varies in severity depending on which layer is defective (see Table 6-1). The development of these defects is associated with low maternal folic acid levels early in pregnancy. Therefore, babies of mothers taking folate supplements prior to conception have a decreased risk of neural tube (NT) defects. Elevated α-fetoprotein (AFP) and acetylcholinesterase (AChE) in amniotic fluid and maternal serum are usually seen. Although there are many causes of elevated AFP in maternal serum, the simultaneous elevation of AFP and AChE in amniotic fluid is diagnostic of an NT defect, even if not visible on ultrasound examination. Elevated AChE suggests an NT defect, as AChE is normally found in fetal CSF. In utero ultrasound can confirm the presence of a deformity.

VENTRICULAR SYSTEM MALFORMATIONS

Disruption in the flow of CSF in the cerebral ventricles and subarachnoid space may lead to hydrocephalus and an increase in ICP (Figure 6-53). Malformations may occur

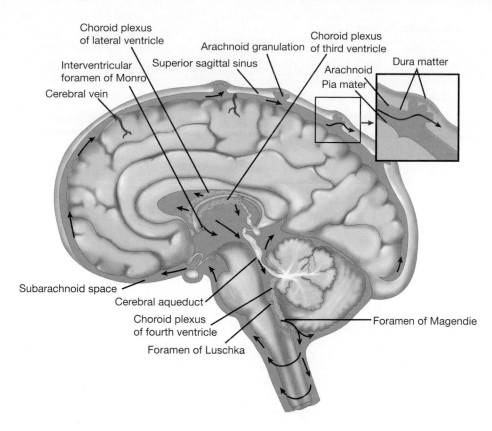

FIGURE 6-53. **Cerebrospinal fluid flow (arrows) through the ventricles.**

anywhere along the pathway and result in a decrease in CSF flow from either **direct blockage of the foramina** or **decreased resorption by the arachnoid granulations.**

PRESENTATION

Hydrocephalus can often manifest with an enlarged calvarium if the cranial bones have not yet fused (ie, the fontanelles are still present). Patients with increased ICP present with the cardinal signs of headache, vomiting, and papilledema.

DIAGNOSIS

- Made by imaging studies (ultrasound, CT, or MRI) showing abnormalities in CSF flow and ventricle dilation.
- Malformations leading to hydrocephalus can be categorized according to whether they are communicating or noncommunicating.
  - **Communicating:** No anatomic block of CSF flow between the ventricles and the subarachnoid space. Examples include meningitis and subarachnoid hemorrhage.
  - **Noncommunicating:** Blockage of CSF flow from the ventricles to the subarachnoid space at any point in the ventricular system.

TREATMENT

Focused on shunting CSF from the ventricular system: Ventricular-peritoneal shunt (most commonly), ventricular-atrial shunt, and third ventriculostomy.

NONCOMMUNICATING HYDROCEPHALUS

Blockage of CSF flow can lead to increased ICP, which causes dilation of the ventricles proximal to the blockage.

KEY FACT

A quad screen is typically done at 15–18 weeks' gestation and measures the levels of AFP, human chorionic gonadotropin (hCG), inhibin-A, and estriol. Elevated hCG and inhibin-A coupled with decreased AFP and estriol indicates an increased risk of having a child with Down syndrome.

KEY FACT

Always get a CT scan of the head prior to performing a lumbar puncture in a patient with signs and symptoms of increased ICP because of the danger of precipitating tonsillar herniation due to a sudden drop in pressure.

Dandy-Walker Malformation

Dandy-Walker malformation is congenital hypoplasia or complete agenesis of the cerebellar vermis resulting in severe cystic dilation of the fourth ventricle and enlargement of the posterior fossa. It is commonly associated with hydrocephalus and spina bifida (see Dandy-Walker syndrome in the section on Congenital Malformations under Brain Development earlier in this chapter).

Congenital Aqueduct of Sylvius Stenosis

The most common cause of hydrocephalus in newborns is obstruction of CSF flow between the third and fourth ventricles. This results in dilation of the ventricles proximal to this obstruction, namely, the third and lateral ventricles.

PRESENTATION

Dilation of the third and lateral ventricles, typically leading to an enlarging head circumference if the cranial suture lines have not yet fused.

DIAGNOSIS

MRI or CT showing enlarged third and lateral ventricles; signs of increased ICP or an enlarging head circumference can be seen on exam.

TREATMENT

Shunt, cerebral aqueductoplasty.

PROGNOSIS

Simple aqueduct stenosis is associated with a very good outcome, with more than half of patients expected to complete normal schooling.

Chiari Malformation

Caudal extension of the medulla and cerebellar vermis through the foramen magnum leads to noncommunicating hydrocephalus (Figure 6-54). This malformation is strongly associated with **cervical syringomyelia** (bilateral loss of pain and temperature sensation in a cape-like distribution) and lumbosacral **meningomyelocele.** A more thorough review of Chiari malformation is provided in the section on Congenital Malformations under Brain Development earlier in this chapter.

COMMUNICATING HYDROCEPHALUS

Communicating (nonobstructive) hydrocephalus has normal CSF flow but **abnormal CSF absorption** by the arachnoid granulations into the dural sinuses, leading to **dilation of all ventricles.** Arachnoid scarring following meningitis is one cause.

Meningitis

Inflammation of the meninges in the CNS (brain and spinal cord) results from bacterial, viral, fungal, or parasitic infection. The consequent postmeningeal scarring and interstitial edema lead to decreased resorption of CSF at the arachnoid granulations and an increase in ICP. The elderly (> 60 years), the very young (< 3 years), and those living in close quarters (military barracks, dorms) are at increased risk.

PRESENTATION

Meningismus: Nuchal rigidity (patient cannot touch chin to chest), headache, and fever.

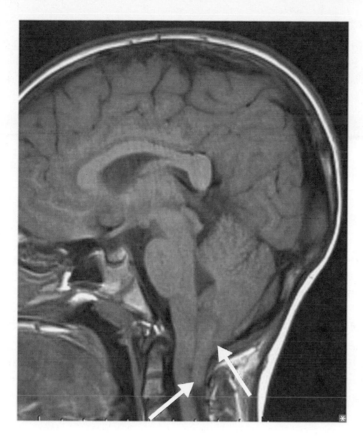

FIGURE 6-54. **Chiari malformation.** MRI showing herniated cerebellar tonsils (arrows).

DIAGNOSIS

CT prior to lumbar puncture if focal neurologic deficits are present (risk of tonsillar herniation if ICP is elevated), CSF profile.

TREATMENT

Empiric antibiotic therapy.

PROGNOSIS

Viral < 1% mortality rate except in neonates; bacterial 25% mortality rate.

Subarachnoid Hemorrhage

Blood in the subarachnoid space (same space as the CSF) may derive from a ruptured intracranial aneurysm or arteriovenous malformation. This results in communicating hydrocephalus because the blood clogs the arachnoid granulations, thereby preventing proper CSF resorption. Five percent of the U.S. population has berry aneurysms (Figure 6-55).

PRESENTATION

Sudden-onset "worst headache of my life," bloody/xanthochromic spinal tap (yellow discoloration from degradation of RBCs), isolated CN III palsy, as well as decreased level of consciousness preceding signs of hydrocephalus.

KEY FACT

Berry (saccular) aneurysms are the number one cause of subarachnoid hemorrhage. Berry aneurysms are a product of uncontrolled hypertension and weakened vasculature. They occur most commonly at vessel branch points due to lack of tunica media in this location.

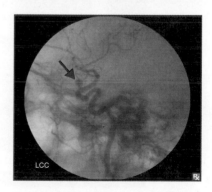

FIGURE 6-55. **Berry aneurysm.** CT angiogram shows an intact berry (saccular) aneurysm (arrow).

FLASH FORWARD

Berry aneurysms are associated with autosomal dominant polycystic kidney disease, Ehlers-Danlos syndrome, and Marfan syndrome. Additional risk factors include old age, hypertension, smoking, and race (higher rates in African Americans).

MNEMONIC

Normal-pressure hydrocephalus manifests with a "wet, wacky, and wobbly" triad: incontinence, dementia, and ataxia.

DIAGNOSIS

Xanthochromic CSF is highly sensitive but usually not present until 2–4 hours after the bleed. CT scan showing blood covering the surface of the brain (through the subarachnoid space) and angiogram to determine whether it is of spontaneous or traumatic origin.

TREATMENT

Surgical clipping of the aneurysm or filling with metal coil.

PROGNOSIS

Forty-five percent die within 1 month following hospitalization.

Normal Pressure Hydrocephalus

Decreased resorption of CSF at the arachnoid granulations leads to a progressive dilation of the ventricles with subsequent stretching of the corona radiata fibers. Most cases are idiopathic. When the etiology is identified, intraventricular hemorrhage, subarachnoid hemorrhage, and meningitis are the most common underlying causes.

PRESENTATION

Classic triad of bladder incontinence, dementia, and slowly developing ataxia. Note that no papilledema or headaches occur because ICP is not increased. The gait is described as a "magnetic gait" in which the patient attempts to initiate each step several times before taking a small step.

DIAGNOSIS

Clinical signs, with CT/MRI showing ventriculomegaly without proportional sulcal atrophy (parenchymal loss) or increased CSF (Figure 6-56).

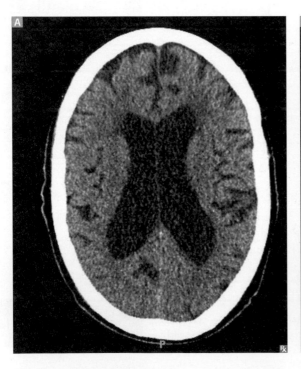
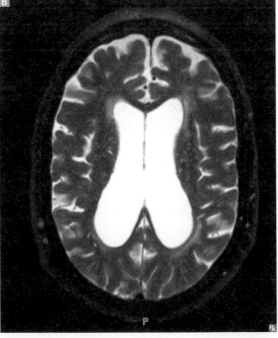

FIGURE 6-56. **Normal pressure hydrocephalus.** **A** CT and **B** T2-weighted MRI of the head showing dilatation of the lateral ventricles out of proportion to the level of diffuse brain atrophy.

TREATMENT

In the acute setting, large-volume lumbar puncture is both therapeutic and diagnostic, with a rapid improvement in symptoms following CSF drainage. Long-term treatment is CSF drainage with a ventriculoperitoneal (VP) shunt.

PROGNOSIS

Normalization of ventricle size is typically associated with reversal of symptoms. Correctly identifying normal pressure hydrocephalus (NPH) early is critical, because NPH is a potentially reversible cause of dementia.

HYDROCEPHALUS MIMICS

Ex Vacuo Ventriculomegaly

PRESENTATION

Often a disease of the elderly. Presents with ventricular dilation and appearance of increased CSF due to a significant decrease in brain tissue (neuronal atrophy). CSF pressure is normal, and the signs and symptoms of hydrocephalus/increased ICP are not present. Causes include Alzheimer disease, stroke, Pick disease, and advanced HIV. Associated with dementia and deficits in cognition, which are actually due to underlying disease process.

DIAGNOSIS

Imaging studies (MRI, CT) showing significant neuronal loss.

TREATMENT

Shunts are not helpful, as the underlying defect is loss of brain parenchyma.

CEREBROVASCULAR DISORDERS

Cerebrovascular disorders arise from any pathologic disorder in the blood vessels supplying the brain (Figure 6-57), such as occlusion by thrombus or embolus, increased vascular permeability, and vessel rupture. The pathologic processes underlying these conditions manifest themselves clinically as ischemia (with or without infarction) or hemorrhage. Strokes are the fifth leading cause of death behind myocardial infarctions and cancer.

PRESENTATION

Depends on the location of the cerebral lesion; see following discussion of the different types.

DIAGNOSIS

CT to detect hemorrhage/blood, diffusion-weighted MRI to detect infarction.

Thrombotic Stroke (Pale Infarction)

The most common type of stroke results from a platelet thrombus that forms over an inflammatory plaque in the middle cerebral artery (MCA) or internal carotid artery (ICA). This causes liquefactive necrosis that usually remains pale due to a lack of reperfusion. The brain exhibits a wedge-shaped area of infarction that develops at the periphery of the cerebral cortex; 1–2 days after infarction, edema develops with loss of demarcation between the gray and white matter; myelin breakdown also occurs.

KEY FACT

Red neurons (eosinophilic change in neuron cytoplasm) are a classic histologic finding in the early stages (12 hours) of stroke.

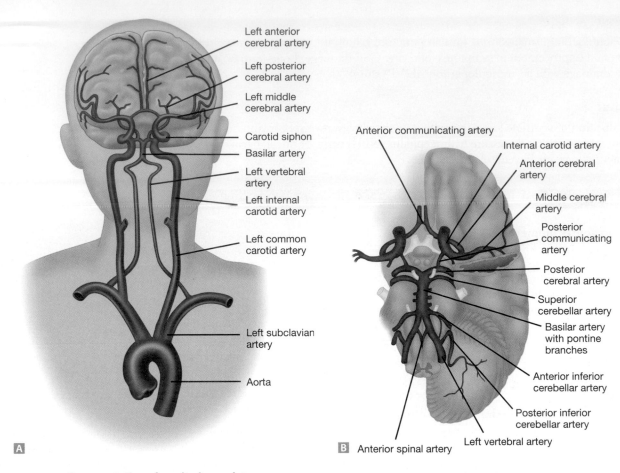

FIGURE 6-57. Representation of cerebral vasculature.

PRESENTATION

Sudden-onset focal neurologic deficits such as unilateral weakness (face, upper extremities, lower extremities), slurring of speech, trouble walking, or visual disturbances, followed by slow improvement over time. Alternatively, patients may wake up in the morning with these symptoms. Transient ischemic attacks, or TIAs (similar symptoms that last < 24 hours), may precede the stroke.

DIAGNOSIS

Symptoms consistent with an infarct in a specific vascular territory (MCA, ACA, PCA, etc). Noncontrast head CT is almost universally obtained in cases with signs suggestive of stroke to look for any signs of cerebral hemorrhage.

TREATMENT

Intravenous (IV) tissue plasminogen activator (tPA) within 4.5 hours of the onset of symptoms to dissolve the thrombus and enable reperfusion of the ischemic region. Most important side effect is bleeding. Contraindications to TPA include intracerebral hemorrhage, recent major surgery, active internal bleeding, systolic blood pressure > 185, diastolic blood pressure > 105, and known bleeding diathesis.

Long-term management with aspirin, statin, and rehabilitation therapy.

Embolic Stroke (Hemorrhagic Infarction)

Hemorrhagic infarction is thought to result from lysis of embolic material following arterial occlusion and ischemic necrosis that leads to partial restoration of blood flow, which causes blood extravasation through the damaged vessel (reperfusion injury). Emboli originate most often from the heart or proximal atherosclerotic plaques in the carotid arteries.

PRESENTATION

Grossly hemorrhagic infarcts extend to the periphery of the cerebral cortex in the distribution of the arterial supply. Clinically indistinguishable from a thrombotic stroke.

DIAGNOSIS

CT or MRI.

TREATMENT

Treat underlying conditions predisposing to emboli: atrial fibrillation, bacterial/nonbacterial endocarditis, or rheumatic heart disease. Anticoagulants (eg, warfarin) are preventive. Rehabilitation therapy.

Intracranial Hemorrhage

These types of hemorrhage are best understood by their anatomic location and typical clinical presentation (Table 6-22, Figure 6-58).

KEY FACT

MRI is the imaging modality of choice for detection of ischemic brain injury, whereas CT is optimal for detecting hemorrhage rapidly.

KEY FACT

Vomiting at the onset of intracerebral hemorrhage occurs much more frequently than with infarction and suggests bleeding as the cause of acute hemiparesis.

TABLE 6-22. Types of Intracranial Hemorrhage

HEMORRHAGE	ETIOLOGY	PRESENTATION	TREATMENT/PROGNOSIS
Epidural (Figure 6-58A)	Rupture of MMA following blunt trauma at pterion (temporoparietal junction). High-pressure hemorrhage with rapid expansion	Characteristic loss of consciousness followed by lucid interval, which can last minutes to hours	Without urgent hematoma clot evacuation and cauterization of the MMA, death can result from increased ICP, uncal herniation, and respiratory arrest
		Bradycardia with increased systolic pressure (Cushing effect)	Permanent brain damage prior to surgical intervention correlates with higher mortality rate
		Noncontrast CT is diagnostic and shows a bright **convex** hematoma between dura and bone; **does not cross suture lines** (Figure 6-58A)	
		Pressure on CN III parasympathetic portion results in blown pupil	
Subdural (Figure 6-58B)	Rupture of bridging (emissary) veins between dural sinuses and arachnoid	Venous bleeding with a delayed onset of symptoms; low-pressure venous system causes slow expansion and delayed onset of symptoms (days to weeks)	Removal of the hematoma by craniotomy is the treatment of choice
	Seen in brain atrophy (eg, alcoholics, the elderly) or abrupt deceleration (eg, shaken baby syndrome, whiplash)	Fluctuating level of consciousness that develops slowly, **crescent-shaped** hemorrhage that covers convexity of brain and **crosses suture lines**	Without treatment, severe cerebral compression and displacement with temporal lobe–tentorial herniation can result in death

(continues)

TABLE 6-22. **Types of Intracranial Hemorrhage** *(continued)*

HEMORRHAGE	ETIOLOGY	PRESENTATION	TREATMENT/PROGNOSIS
Subarachnoid (Figure 6-58C, D)	Trauma is the most common cause. Spontaneous causes include rupture of aneurysm (usually saccular/berry aneurysm) or an arteriovenous malformation that results in blood moving into the same spaces as the CSF	"Worst headache of my life," sudden-onset severe occipital headache	Hemorrhage tends to recur at same site
		Isolated CN III palsy with aneurysm at the junction of the PCA and PComA	Hemorrhage can be prevented with surgical clipping of aneurysm or fill with metal coil prior to rupture
			Level of consciousness at time of arteriography best index of prognosis
		Bloody/xanthochromic spinal tap	Vasospasm resulting in additional cerebral ischemia may occur 3–14 days following original hemorrhage. Vasospasm is diagnosed with transcranial Doppler (TCD) sonography and a CT that is negative for bleeding. Nimodipine, a calcium channel blocker, has been shown to prevent vasospasm and improve outcomes
		Impaired CSF resorption at the arachnoid granules resulting in communicating hydrocephalus (Figure 6-58C, D)	
		Carotid and vertebral angiography only means of demonstrating aneurysm	
Intraparenchymal (Figure 6-58E, F)	Hypertension (most common), amyloid angiopathy, diabetes mellitus, vasculitis, and tumors	Lateral striate artery hemorrhage secondary to hypertension affects the basal ganglia (putamen), thalamus, and internal capsule (Figure 6-58F), leading to hemiplegia, contralateral sensory loss; also affects pons/cerebellum, causing vomiting, inability to sit/stand/walk	44% patients die within 30 days
	Hypertension leads to stress on penetrating vessels (lenticulostriate vessels), causing Charcot-Bouchard microaneurysm with vessel wall thickening; most frequently affects the deep cerebral structures (eg, basal ganglia, thalamus, internal capsule)		Location largely affects the prognosis along with the size of the hemorrhage
			Maintain adequate ventilation, monitor ICP
	Ruptured aneurysms lead to intracerebral hemorrhage, which creates a clot that pushes the brain parenchyma aside		With sustained mean BP > 110 mm Hg, give β-blockers, ACE-inhibitors
			Surgical evacuation of cerebellar hematomas

ACE, angiotensin-converting enzyme; BP, blood pressure; CN, cranial nerve; ICP, intracranial pressure; MMA, middle meningeal artery; PCA, posterior cerebral artery; PComA, posterior communicating artery.

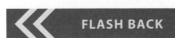

FLASH BACK

All afferent sensory stimuli, except for olfaction, go through the thalamus prior to being relayed to the cortex.

Lacunar Infarcts

Cystic areas of microinfarction result from hyaline arteriolosclerosis (small vessels) secondary to hypertension or diabetes mellitus (DM). Lacunar infarcts often occur in the distal end of small cerebral vessels, causing a number of classic clinical presentations.

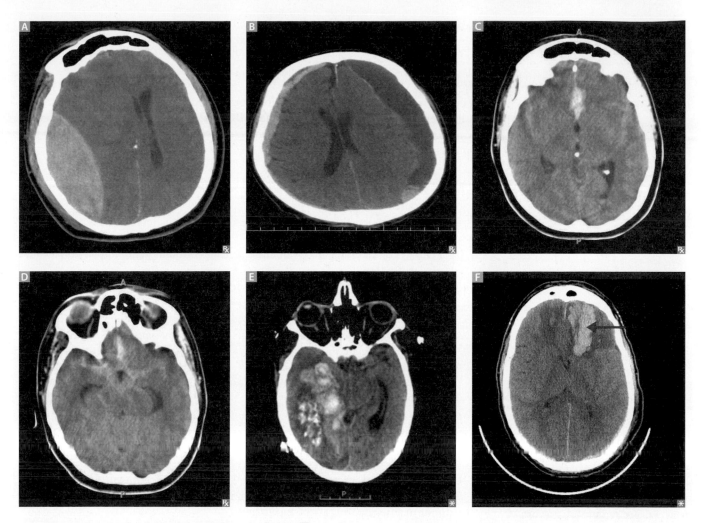

FIGURE 6-58. **CT scans of intracranial hemorrhages.** **A** Epidural hemorrhage with convex lens appearance (does not cross suture lines). **B** Subdural hemorrhage with crescent shape (crosses suture lines). **C D** Subarachnoid hemorrhage. **E** Intraparenchymal hemorrhage draining into left lateral ventricle. **F** Intraparenchymal hemorrhage of left frontal region (arrow).

PRESENTATION

- Pure sensory stroke when the infarct is in the thalamus; characterized by numbness, tingling, pain, or burning sensation without motor symptoms.
- Pure motor hemiparesis from an infarct in the posterior limb of the internal capsule or basis pontis; the face, arm, and leg are almost always involved as opposed to occlusion of the MCA (face and arm worse than the leg) or ACA (leg worse than the face and arm).
- Ataxic hemiparesis from an infarct in the base of the pons; characterized by a combination of cerebellar and motor symptoms.
- Dysarthria and a clumsy hand or arm due to infarction in the base of the pons or in the genu of the internal capsule.
- Pure motor hemiparesis with "motor (Broca) aphasia" due to thrombotic occlusion of a lenticulostriate branch supplying the genu and the anterior limb of the internal capsule and adjacent white matter of the corona radiata.

DIAGNOSIS

Clinical signs and symptoms, imaging studies to exclude hemorrhage, X-ray cerebral angiography.

Q   QUESTION

A 53-year-old woman develops confusion and left-sided weakness 6 days after experiencing a subarachnoid hemorrhage. A rebleed is not evident on CT scan. What medication is the treatment of choice to prevent this complication?

TREATMENT

Modification of risk factors (reduction in BP, control of DM, statins, and aspirin).

PROGNOSIS

Generally fair to good. Depends on the location and extent of damage (as determined by positron emission tomography [PET] scan, MR diffusion with MR perfusion to identify the ischemic penumbra—the area of ischemic tissue on the periphery of the infarct that contains tissue that is still viable).

Stroke Presentation According to Cerebral Location of Occlusion

- **Middle cerebral artery:**
  - Primary sensory cortex involvement results in contralateral hemianesthesia (face and arm worse than leg).
  - Primary motor cortex involvement results in contralateral hemiplegia (face and arm worse than leg).
  - Involvement of Meyer loop in the temporal lobe results in homonymous quadrantanopia.
  - If the **dominant hemisphere** is affected (usually left), aphasia will also develop.
  - If the **nondominant hemisphere** is affected (usually right), sensory neglect and apraxia may develop.
- **Anterior cerebral artery:**
  - Primary sensory cortex involvement results in contralateral hemianesthesia (leg worse than face and arm).
  - Primary motor cortex involvement results in contralateral hemiplegia (leg worse than face and arm).
  - Medial frontal (midline) causes urinary incontinence, reemergence of the grasp reflex.
- **Posterior cerebral artery:** Occipital lobe lesion causes homonymous hemianopia with macular sparing (vs optic tract lesion, which causes homonymous hemianopia without macular sparing).
- **Anterior inferior cerebellar artery (lateral pontine syndrome):**
  - **Ipsilateral:** Paralysis of facial movement (CN VII), facial pain/temperature loss (spinal trigeminal nucleus/tract), Horner syndrome (descending sympathetics), hearing loss/vertigo/nausea and vomiting/nystagmus away from lesion (CN VIII/cochlear nucleus), dystaxia (inferior/middle cerebellar peduncle), which is difficulty controlling voluntary movements.
  - **Contralateral:** Loss of pain and temperature sensation in the body (spinothalamic tract).
- **Posterior inferior cerebellar artery (Wallenberg syndrome/lateral medullary syndrome):**
  - **Ipsilateral:** Limb ataxia and intention tremor (inferior cerebellar peduncle), vertigo/nausea and vomiting/nystagmus away from lesion (vestibular nuclei), paralysis of larynx/pharynx/palate (nucleus ambiguus), facial pain/temperature loss (spinal V), Horner syndrome (descending hypothalamics).
  - **Contralateral:** Loss of pain and temperature sensation in the body (spinothalamic tract).

DYSKINESIAS

Disorders of movement involve disturbance of voluntary movement or the presence of involuntary movements, commonly referred to as **extrapyramidal** diseases because there is no muscle weakness (as is the case in UMN lesions). May arise from basal ganglia lesions and manifest as resting tremor, chorea, or athetosis. Other regions involved are the cerebellar hemisphere, cerebellar vermis, and subthalamic nucleus. Dyskinesias are symptoms that may be part of a syndrome or disease.

Chorea

Chorea is characterized by involuntary, jerky, purposeless movements that arise from basal ganglia lesions.

Diseases Characterized by Chorea

- **Inherited disorders:**
    - Huntington disease
    - Neuroacanthocytosis
    - Wilson disease
- **Infectious:** Streptococcal infection (rheumatic fever)
- **Drug-induced chorea:**
    - Neuroleptics (phenothiazines, haloperidol)
    - Phenytoin
    - Oral contraceptives in women with systemic lupus erythematosus (SLE) and antiphospholipid antibodies
    - Excessive dosage of L-dopa and dopamine agonists
    - Cocaine

Athetosis

An inability to maintain a body part in one position that usually manifests as slow, writhing movements (especially in the fingers) that alternate between extension and flexion. **Characteristic of basal ganglia lesions and antipsychotics** (eg, haloperidol).

Hemiballismus

Sudden, uncontrolled flailing of one limb results from a lesion in the **contralateral subthalamic nucleus.**

PRESENTATION

A lesion in the subthalamic nucleus interrupts the inhibitory indirect pathway (see Figure 6-21) and releases the thalamus from inhibition by the globus pallidus internus results in sudden uncontrolled flailing of the contralateral limb (continuous/intermittent).

DIAGNOSIS

MRI showing signal changes in the contralateral subthalamic nucleus.

TREATMENT

Haloperidol, phenothiazine.

PROGNOSIS

Hemiballismus that persists for weeks without treatment may result in exhaustion and death.

APHASIAS

The muscles involved in generating speech, chewing, and swallowing are intact. Therefore, patients with aphasia do not have a peripheral motor problem, but rather a language problem arising from a cortical lesion (Table 6-23). Speech therapy is recommended for all patients with aphasia (see Figure 6-19 for six most commonly tested aphasias).

KEY FACT

Athetos = not fixed (think snake-like writhing).

KEY FACT

Wernicke aphasia is distinct from Wernicke-Korsakoff syndrome, a disease arising from thiamine deficiency (typically due to chronic alcohol abuse) that manifests with encephalopathy, amnesia, confabulation, ophthalmoplegia, and ataxia.

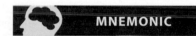

MNEMONIC

Broca's **Bro**ken **Bo**ca (Boca is Spanish for "mouth")
Wernicke is **W**ordy.

KEY FACT

Vascular dementia may be caused by:
- Multiple infarcts: Large-artery atherosclerosis in the circle of Willis (see Figure 6-12) and carotids.
- Binswanger leukoencephalopathy: Loss of white matter secondary to hypertension-related atherosclerosis.
- Lacunar infarcts: Small < 1-cm infarcts of the striatum and thalamus related to arteriolosclerosis.

TABLE 6-23. **Perisylvian Types of Aphasias**

LOCATION	PRESENTATION	PROGNOSIS/TREATMENT
Broca area (inferior frontal gyrus, Brodmann area 44)	■ Motor/nonfluent/expressive aphasia with good comprehension, thus patients are aware of problem, and therefore can be extremely frustrated, cannot say or write what they are thinking, and use mainly short monosyllabic words ■ Often accompanied by contralateral weakness (hemiparesis often on the right side) of the lower face and arm	■ May improve over time, excellent potential for functional recovery ■ Prognosis depends on the size of the lesion, the age of the patient, and the status of the contralateral hemisphere
Wernicke area (superior temporal gyrus, Brodmann area 22)	■ Sensory/fluent/auditory aphasia with impaired comprehension, neologisms, paraphasic errors, and impaired repetition ■ Speech is fluent but nonsensical ("word salad") ■ Unaware of defect ■ Often with contralateral visual defects (right upper quadrant loss because optic radiations from Meyer loop are affected), alexia	■ May improve over time ■ Prognosis depends on the size of the lesion, the age of the patient, and the status of the contralateral hemisphere ■ Patient less likely than those with injury to Broca area to return to normal social life because of severe comprehension defect
Arcuate fasciculus	■ Conduction aphasia because this structure connects Wernicke and Broca areas; poor repetition with intact comprehension and fluent speech ■ Cannot name objects	■ Prognosis depends on the size of the lesion, the age of the patient, and the status of the contralateral hemisphere
Global	■ Both speech and comprehension affected due to large perisylvian or separate frontal and temporal lesions ■ Often accompanied by right hemiplegia, hemianesthesia, and homonymous hemianopia	■ May regain degree of comprehension ■ Clinical picture may resemble Broca aphasia over time

DEGENERATIVE DISEASES

Degenerative diseases, as with other CNS disorders, are best understood by recognizing the functions associated with the specific region(s) in which the lesion develops. Lesions along the corticospinal tract cause motor deficits (Table 6-24).

Generally, symptoms associated with diseases affecting the cerebral cortex include personality changes, memory loss, seizures, and cognitive dysfunction (Table 6-25).

Basal ganglial injuries generally manifest as movement disorders (Table 6-26).

Spinocerebellar lesions affect the spinocerebellar tracts or the cerebellum (or both) and manifest with ataxia (Table 6-27).

Progressive Supranuclear Palsy

Disease is characterized by widespread neuronal loss and subcortical gliosis that notably spares the cerebral and cerebellar cortices.

PRESENTATION

Onset in the sixth decade presenting with difficulty in vertical movement of gaze, pseudobulbar palsy (dysarthria, dysphagia, hyperactive jaw jerk and gag reflexes, and uncontrollable laughing or crying unrelated to emotional state), axial dystonia with repeated falls, and bradykinesia without resting tremor ("atypical Parkinsonism"). Memory and intellect intact.

TABLE 6-24. **Motor Neuron Lesions**

TYPES	PRESENTATION	PATHOLOGY	PROGNOSIS/TREATMENT
Amyotrophic lateral sclerosis (ALS)	Associated with both LMN and UMN signs with sparing of sensation; onset at 40–60 years of age; most common motor neuron disease; rare inherited form in 40- to 60-year-olds (chromosome 21, *SOD1* mutation)	UMN signs (hyperreflexia, spasticity, positive Babinski sign)	Most often fatal within 5 years of disease onset Riluzole delays the onset of ventilator-dependence or tracheostomy and may increase survival by 3–5 months. Its mechanism of action includes blockade of TTX-sensitive Na+ channels (associated with damaged neurons) and both glutamate release and glutamate receptor blockade (reduced excitotoxicity)
	Thenar atrophy first sign (LMN lesion, alpha motor neurons in anterior horns), fasciculations, hyperreflexia (UMN lesion, lateral corticospinal tract)	LMN signs (weakness, fasciculations, hyporeflexia, atrophy)	
Werdnig-Hoffman disease (infantile spinal muscular atrophy type)	Autosomal recessive inheritance that manifests at birth as floppy baby syndrome, tongue fasciculations, LMN disease	Degeneration of anterior horns; no UMN/corticospinal tract degeneration. Defect in gene that normally "turns off" perinatal programmed cell death	Median age of death 7 months, rapidly fatal
Poliomyelitis	Follows infection (fecal-oral) with poliovirus; first replicates in oropharnyx and small intestine before hematologic spread to CNS, presenting with LMN signs	Degeneration of anterior horns of spinal cord	Hospitalize with strict bed rest to reduce rate of paralysis. Ventilation to treat respiratory muscle weakness May develop new muscle weakness after recovery from acute paralytic poliomyelitis
	CSF with lymphocytic pleocytosis and slight elevation of protein		
	Virus recovered from stool or throat		

CNS, central nervous system; LMN, lower motor neuron; TTX, tetrodotoxin; UMN, upper motor neuron.

DIAGNOSIS

Exclusion of other causes, prominent neurofibrillary tangles.

TREATMENT

No definitive treatment. Treatment with L-dopa yields poor results because dopaminergic neurons and receptors are lost.

PROGNOSIS

Death within 6–10 years.

DEMYELINATING DISEASES

Disease is characterized by the destruction of normal myelin (eg, MS) or the production of abnormal myelin (eg, leukodystrophy).

Multiple Sclerosis

MS is an inflammatory autoimmune disorder characterized by demyelination of axons in the brain and spinal cord. There is an increased prevalence in people who lived at higher latitudes north of the Equator for the first decades of their lives. It most often affects Caucasian women 20–30 years of age and is associated with HLA-DR2.

FLASH FORWARD

Wilson disease (hepatolenticular degeneration) results from an autosomal recessive mutation in a membrane-bound copper transporter (*ATP7B* gene) that overwhelms copper capacity because of an inability to excrete copper into bile. Copper is deposited in many tissues, including the brain (basal ganglia and cortex), liver, cornea, and kidney (see Table 6-26).

KEY FACT

Cerebellar lesions (unilateral) present with ipsilateral ataxia, intention/movement tremor (difficulty smoothing out movements), and dysarthria (loss of complex movements of speech if lesions in the lateral hemispheres).

TABLE 6-25. Cerebral Cortex Lesions

TYPES	PRESENTATION	PATHOLOGY	PROGNOSIS/TREATMENT
Alzheimer disease	Slow, progressive mental deterioration with loss of short-term memory, anosmia, difficulties with language and planning skills, decline in executive function. The most common cause of dementia in elderly	Senile plaques (β-amyloid core surrounded by dystrophic neuritis in extracellular space); neurofibrillary tangles (intracellular, abnormally phosphorylated tau protein). The number of neurofibrillary tangles correlates with the severity of the disease	AChE inhibitors that penetrate the BBB (eg, donepezil) increase ACh levels in the brain and alleviate symptoms, but have no effect on disease progression NMDA receptor antagonists (eg, memantine) reduce glutamate-mediated excitotoxicity (also not disease-modifying)
	Generalized cerebral atrophy beginning in the temporal lobe and hippocampus leads to widened sulci and enlarged ventricles (hydrocephalus ex vacuo). Spares primary sensory and motor areas	β-Amyloid is toxic when deposited in neurons and cerebral blood vessel walls (cerebral amyloid angiopathy), leading to weakening of vessel walls and intracranial hemorrhage Decreased ACh due to loss of cholinergic nuclei in the forebrain (nucleus basalis of Meynert)	
	Familial form (10%) associated with onset at < 40 years. Known genetic causes include mutations in presenilin 1 and 2 on chromosomes 1 and 14, respectively (leads to hyperphosphorylated tau and neurofibrillary tangles), *APOE4* allele on chromosome 19, and p-*APP* on chromosome 21. *APOE2* allele decreases risk of developing the disease		
	p-*APP* increases amount of amyloid precursor protein. Trisomy 21 (Down syndrome) is associated with early-onset Alzheimer (near 100% prevalence at age 30–40 years)		
Frontotemporal dementia (Pick disease)	Type of dementia characterized by early personality changes (eg, disinhibition and impaired judgment) due to neuronal loss in the frontal lobe with accompanying language deficits (eg, progressive aphasia) due to neuronal loss in the temporal lobe	Swollen neurons with Pick bodies (intracellular aggregated tau protein); straight filaments observed with silver staining	Limited treatment options targeting neurotransmitters, similar to Alzheimer
	Aspects of Alzheimer (memory loss) except with earlier age of onset (< 50 years)	Loss of white matter underlying atrophic cortex with gliosis, specific for frontal-temporal lobes	

(continues)

TABLE 6-25.   **Cerebral Cortex Lesions** *(continued)*

TYPES	PRESENTATION	PATHOLOGY	PROGNOSIS/TREATMENT
Dementia with Lewy bodies (DLB)	Dementia and visual hallucinations present early in the disease course, followed by parkinsonian symptoms. Extrapyramidal parkinsonian features are due to loss of dopaminergic neurons. Parkinson disease and DLB have overlapping features, but the following are more characteristic of DLB: **episodic delirium** (visual/auditory hallucinations), visuospatial impairment, varying attention, and **undulating** clinical course	Widespread formation of Lewy bodies (α-synuclein aggregates) in substantia nigra, limbic system, nucleus basalis of Meynert, and cerebral cortex	Selegiline and other MAO inhibitors may be helpful with symptoms
Prion diseases (spongiform encephalopathies): Creutzfeldt-Jakob disease (CJD), variant Creutzfeldt-Jakob disease (vCJD), Kuru, fatal familial insomnia (FFI)	CJD—May be inherited or spontaneous. Most common prion disease. Rapidly progressive (weeks to months) dementia with myoclonus ("startle myoclonus"), ataxia (cerebellar involvement), and visual disturbances. Usually sporadic but can be due to iatrogenic exposure (eg, neurosurgical instruments, corneal transplant, HGH) vCJD acquired; exposure to bovine spongiform encephalopathy ("mad cow disease") Kuru acquired; due to practicing cannibalism in some tribal populations FFI—Inherited; severe insomnia and startle myoclonus 14-3-3 protein in CSF; bi- or triphasic spike-wave complexes on EEG; putamen and caudate abnormalities on MRI	Spongiform cortex; prion diseases are due to the conversion of a normal (predominantly α-helical) protein termed prion protein (PrPc) to a β-pleated sheet form (PrPsc), which is resistant to proteases, standard sterilizing procedures, and standard autoclaving Usually sporadic but can be inherited (familial) or transmitted Neuron loss and glial cell proliferation, without an inflammatory response; small vacuoles within neuropil produces spongiform appearance	No treatment; irreversible and uniformly fatal, usually within 1 year of diagnosis
Multi-infarct (vascular) dementia	Second most common cause of dementia A progressive, *stepwise* decline in functioning, which differentiates it from the gradual course of Alzheimer	Secondary to atherosclerosis, arteriolosclerosis, and hypertension	Vascular prophylaxis and stroke prevention

ACh, acetylcholine; AChE, acetylcholine esterase; BBB, blood-brain barrier; CSF, cerebrospinal fluid; EEG, electroencephalography; GABA, γ-aminobutyric acid; HGH, human growth hormone; MAO, monoamine oxidase; NMDA, *N*-methyl-D-aspartate.

PRESENTATION

Multiple neurologic deficits separated in time and space. Classic triad of scanning speech, intention tremor, and nystagmus, as well as UMN lesion signs (hyperreflexia, positive Babinski sign). Also common are optic neuritis (sudden loss of vision), MLF syndrome/internuclear ophthalmoplegia (see discussion on MLF), bowel/bladder incontinence, sexual dysfunction, paraplegia, hemiparesis, and hemisensory paresthesias. MS is often relapsing-remitting.

DIAGNOSIS

The diagnosis is made on the basis of the history and physical exam and must show evidence of multiple lesions occurring or worsening over numerous episodes. Labs may show increased polyclonal IgG (oligoclonal bands on electrophoresis), myelin basic protein, and leukocytes in the CSF. MRI shows multifocal plaques of periventricular demyelination in the white matter and correlates with future disease severity (Figure 6-59). The acute lesion shows perivenular cuffing with activated T cells (mostly CD4+ and some CD8+) and macrophages. The chronic lesion is characterized by gliosis (scarring).

TABLE 6-26.   Basal Ganglia Lesions

TYPES	PRESENTATION	PATHOLOGY	PROGNOSIS/TREATMENT
Huntington disease	Autosomal dominant with complete penetrance and development of progressive athetoid chorea in all four limbs (writhing), dementia, and emotional disturbances. Onset at 20–50 years with anticipation	Atrophy of striatum leads to loss of medium spiny (GABAergic) neurons	Symptomatic treatment with haloperidol effective in suppressing movement disorder (care must be taken not to superimpose tardive dyskinesia; prescribe only for chorea that is functionally disabling)
	Atrophy of the caudate (head) and putamen may make lateral ventricles appear enlarged when imaging ("bat-wing" frontal horns). Hydrocephalus ex vacuo	Expansion of **CAG** triplet repeats (polyglutamine) in *huntingtin* gene on **chromosome 4** results in aggregation of mutant *huntingtin* protein (toxic to neurons)	Incurable; steadily progressive course and death 15–20 years after onset with ↑ rate of suicide; requires supportive therapy and genetic counseling
	Spared memory, increased blinking, impaired initiation, and slowness of both pursuit and volitional saccadic movements and an inability to make a volitional saccade without movement of the head	Associated with decreased levels of ACh and GABA in the brain, along with an increase in dopamine	The number of CAG repeats determines the age of onset and severity. Expansion of repeats typically occurs during spermatogenesis, leading to earlier disease onset in subsequent generations (anticipation). Anticipation occurs more often following paternal transmission
Parkinson disease (PD)	Clinically defined by **TRAPS: T**remor at rest (eg, pill-rolling), cogwheel **R**igidity, **A**kinesia/bradykinesia, **P**ostural instability, **S**huffling gait, flat affect	Lewy body inclusions (eosinophilic with halo, aggregate of α-synuclein representing damaged neurofilaments) diffusely in cortical neurons with few tangles or plaques	Disease course 10–25 years
	Rarely, linked to MPTP exposure (meperidine derivative [synthetic heroin])	Depigmentation of the substantia nigra pars compacta (secondary to loss of dopaminergic neurons)	Dopamine agonists, eg, levodopa, carry risk of drug-related dyskinesias
	Arises from any insult that damages basal ganglia, including antipsychotics that are dopamine antagonists, ischemia, chronic carbon monoxide poisoning, Wilson disease, encephalitis		Deep brain stimulation (DBS) of the STN is effective at improving symptoms in patients with advanced Parkinson disease refractory to drug treatment. Surgical ablation of the STN, while effective, is now rare
			Dementia is a late complication of Parkinson disease (versus dementia with Lewy bodies, in which dementia occurs earlier in the disease with associated parkinsonian symptoms)

(continues)

TABLE 6-26.   Basal Ganglia Lesions *(continued)*

TYPES	PRESENTATION	PATHOLOGY	PROGNOSIS/TREATMENT
Wilson disease	Autosomal recessive defect on chromosome 13; both sexes affected equally. Onset is usually late childhood	Defective hepatocyte transport of copper (Cu) results in (1) decreased Cu incorporation into ceruloplasmin (Cu transport protein in blood); (2) decreased Cu excretion into bile. Eventually, hepatocytes accumulate Cu → Cu leaks into bloodstream → free Cu deposits in tissues (predominantly liver, basal ganglia, and cornea). Free Cu in tissue is toxic; end organ damage is mediated by production of **hydroxyl free radicals** via the Fenton reaction	Deep brain stimulation of the STN is effective at improving symptoms in patients with advanced Parkinson disease refractory to drug treatment. Surgical ablation of the STN, while effective, is now rare Lifetime treatment consisting of two stages: (1) Remove tissue Cu by D-penicillamine (Cu chelator); (2) prevent Cu reaccumulation with zinc (inhibits intestinal absorption of Cu) and a low-Cu diet
	Signs and symptoms include (1) Hepatic dysfunction: acute hepatitis, cirrhosis, and portal hypertension; possible increased risk of developing HCC later in life; (2) Neurologic dysfunction: parkinsonian symptoms, hemiballismus, hepatosplenomegaly, behavior changes, and dementia; (3) Kayser-Fleischer rings: greenish-brown pigmentation around iris due to corneal deposits of Cu+ in Descemet membrane	Laboratory findings: ↑ free serum Cu, ↓ total serum Cu, ↓ **serum ceruloplasmin, ↑ urinary Cu.** Liver biopsy: ↑ Cu and fibrosis. Diagnosis can be made by clinical symptoms plus laboratory values consistent with Wilson disease. Liver biopsy is usually reserved for indeterminate cases	Prognosis is excellent when treated, with the exceptions of acute liver failure and those presenting with advanced disease. Liver transplantation may be considered for acute liver failure, hepatic decompensation not responsive to treatment, and intractable neurologic impairment

ACh, acetylcholine; GABA, γ-aminobutyric acid; HCC, hepatocellular carcinoma; MPTP, 1-methyl-4-phenyl-1,2,3,6-tetrahydropyridine; STN, subthalamic nucleus..

TABLE 6-27.   Spinocerebellar Lesions

TYPES	PRESENTATION	PATHOLOGY	PROGNOSIS/TREATMENT
Olivopontocerebellar atrophy	Ataxia (broad-based gait), dysarthria, intention tremor, generalized rigidity, and dementia	Loss of cerebellar Purkinje cells (GABAergic in cerebellar cortex) MRI shows flattening of pons, enlarged fourth ventricle	Progressive neurodegeneration with no definitive treatment Falls and aspiration pneumonia contribute to morbidity and mortality
Friedreich ataxia	Most common hereditary ataxia (AR inheritance); trinucleotide repeat disease **(GAA)** involving *frataxin* gene, with onset of symptoms in the first decade of life. Loss of proprioception, decreased DTRs, positive Babinski sign Associated with myocarditis, hypertrophic cardiomyopathy, scoliosis, hearing/vision impairment, and high plantar arches (pes cavus)	"Atrophy of spinal cord," diffuse damage to dorsal columns, spinocerebellar tracts, and lateral corticospinal tracts. Pathology mimics SCD of the spinal column (see Figure 6-41G)	Poor prognosis, no definitive treatment

AR, autosomal recessive; DTRs, deep tendon reflexes; SCD, subacute combined degeneration.

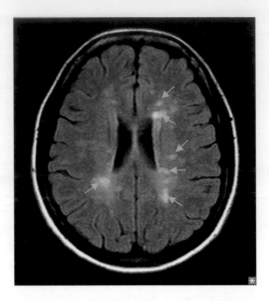

FIGURE 6-59. **Multiple sclerosis.** Axial first-echo image from T2-weighted sequence demonstrates multiple bright signal abnormalities in white matter, typical for MS. These demyelinating lesions may sometimes mimic brain tumors because of the associated edema and inflammation.

TREATMENT

Acute flares are treated with IV steroids. Long-term treatment with disease-modifying agents, such as natalizumab (monoclonal antibody against α4-integrin, preventing cytotoxic T cells from crossing the BBB), glatiramer, and β-interferon, slows disease progression.

PROGNOSIS

Untreated patients typically develop severe physical disability within 20–25 years of onset. Early treatment may help counteract progressive brain atrophy.

Progressive Multifocal Leukoencephalopathy

Progressive multifocal leukoencephalophy (PML) is a fatal, rapidly progressive demyelinating disease resulting from reactivation of latent JC virus infection of B lymphocytes (especially in AIDS patients) that passes through the BBB and cause eventual infection of oligodendrocytes. This leads to widespread destruction of white matter. Increased risk in patients taking natalizumab and rituximab.

PRESENTATION

Weakness (hemiparesis), speech disturbance (aphasia), cortical blindness, and conjugate gaze abnormalities. No change in mental status.

DIAGNOSIS

MRI for white matter lesions. Eosinophilic intranuclear inclusions in abnormal giant oligodendrocytes.

PROGNOSIS

Severe dementia, often progressing to death within 6 months to 1 year. Prognosis may be better in patients with higher CD4+ lymphocyte counts.

Acute Disseminated (Postinfectious) Encephalomyelitis

Demyelinating disease follows infection with measles, mumps, rubella, or chickenpox, with a notable febrile prodrome. Distinct from **subacute sclerosing panencephalitis (SSPE)** by the timing of symptom onset. Specifically, the onset of acute postinfectious encephalomyelitis is much sooner (weeks) than the onset of the SSPE (years).

PRESENTATION

Seen in children and adolescents with a history of recent infection or immunization presenting with abrupt onset of irritability and lethargy, mental status changes, and seizures.

DIAGNOSIS

MRI, CSF to exclude other diagnoses; history of recent vaccination or exanthematous illness.

TREATMENT

High-dose corticosteroids. Plasmapheresis or IV immunoglobulin therapy may be used in resistant cases.

PROGNOSIS

Complete recovery without apparent pathologic sequelae; degree of recovery is unrelated to severity of illness.

Acute Inflammatory Demyelinating Polyradiculopathy

Acute inflammatory demyelinating polyradiculopathy (Guillain-Barré syndrome or GBS) is inflammatory autoimmune destruction of Schwann cells, causing demyelination of peripheral motor ventral roots and cranial nerves often associated with infections. GBS is associated with previous inoculation or infection (1–3 weeks earlier) by herpesvirus, *Campylobacter jejuni*, *Mycoplasma pneumoniae*, and possibly with flu vaccination. Notably, men and women are equally at risk. The autoimmune reaction is presumed to result from an immune response to nonself-antigens that become misdirected against host nerve tissue.

PRESENTATION

Presents with symmetric and ascending, rapidly progressive muscle weakness that begins in the distal lower extremities, with or without paresthesias. Lower-extremity deep tendon reflexes are diminished. A history of antecedent respiratory or gastrointestinal (GI) infection 2–4 weeks prior is common. Significant risk of respiratory muscle paralysis over time. May have autonomic dysfunction, resulting in cardiac dysrhythmias, hypertension, hypotension. Facial diplegia (bilateral facial paralysis in 50% of cases). Deep, aching pain in weakened muscles.

DIAGNOSIS

Clinical presentation, albuminocytologic dissociation (elevated CSF protein with normal cell count), papilledema. Abnormalities of nerve conduction by electromyography.

TREATMENT

Close respiratory monitoring and support are critical, as the disease often ascends to involve the diaphragm. Treatment also includes plasmapheresis and IV immunoglobulins once the diagnosis is made.

KEY FACT

PML only affects white matter. **Rabies** only affects gray matter. **Subacute sclerosing panencephalitis** affects both white and gray matter.

KEY FACT

Viral infection of oligodendrocytes is the key feature of subacute sclerosing panencephalitis (measles paramyxovirus) and progressive multifocal leukoencephalopathy (JC virus).

FLASH BACK

Metachromatic leukodystrophy is an autosomal recessive lysosomal storage disease (arylsulfatase A deficiency; accumulation of sulfatides) that is fatal in the first decade and manifests with progressive paralysis, dementia, and ataxia.

FLASH BACK

Krabbe disease (globoid cell leukodystrophy) is an autosomal recessive disorder associated with defective galactocerebrosidase that leads to an accumulation of galactocerebroside in large, multinucleated histiocytic cells in the CNS. This results in optic atrophy and a classic manifestation of blindness and peripheral neuropathy.

QUESTION

A 37-year-old woman presents with uncontrollable writhing movements of her arms and recent emotional disturbances. Her father died at age 55 after experiencing similar symptoms. On what chromosome is the affected gene?

PROGNOSIS

Death (< 5%) secondary to pulmonary complications within days; therefore, respiratory support is important. Most patients make a full recovery with supportive care. Prognosis is worse if axonal damage is evident.

Osmotic Demyelination Syndrome (Central Pontine Myelinolysis)

Osmotic demyelination syndrome (central pontine myelinolysis [CPM]) is demyelination of neurons due to overly rapid correction of chronic (more than 2 days) hyponatremia. During prolonged hyponatremia, neurons compensate by reducing intracellular osmolytes to prevent cellular swelling. Upon rapid correction, the neurons are hypotonic relative to the suddenly normal serum osmolality. Fluid moves out of neurons into the extracellular compartment, leading to demyelination.

PRESENTATION

Locked-in syndrome: Rapid-onset quadriplegia, dysarthria, dysphagia, and diplopia. Consciousness, alertness, and cognition remain intact; vertical eye movement and blinking may remain intact.

DIAGNOSIS

MRI shows a diamond-shaped, or "bat wing," region of demyelination in the basis pontis that spares neurons and axons. Lack of inflammation distinguishes CPM from MS.

TREATMENT

Avoid by **slow** correction of hyponatremia (to avoid absolute and relative hypernatremia).

PROGNOSIS

Maximum recovery within months; death is common.

SEIZURES

Seizures are characterized by focal or global neuronal hyperactivity, which often causes a sudden change in behavior, but may also be subclinical. This change manifests differently depending on the region of the brain affected (Table 6-28).

CEREBRAL EDEMA

Causes an increase in intracranial pressure (ICP) and commonly occurs 2–4 days post infarction. Edema may be:

- **Cytotoxic:** Secondary to hypoxia and hyponatremia.
- **Vasogenic:** Increased vascular permeability secondary to inflammation, metastasis, trauma, respiratory acidosis → space-occupying lesions that cause mass effect on underlying brain tissue.

PRESENTATION

Classic signs of increased ICP: papilledema (swelling of the optic disc), projectile vomiting, sinus bradycardia, hypertension, and decreased level of consciousness.

TREATMENT

Address the underlying cause if possible and manage ICP (raise the head of the bed, mannitol, hypertonic saline, hyperventilation, sedatives, paralytics, external ventricular drainage, and shunts).

PROGNOSIS

Potential for herniation, which carries a poor prognosis.

TABLE 6-28. **Types of Seizures**

TYPE	PRESENTATION	TREATMENT/PROGNOSIS	ETIOLOGY BY AGE
Partial (one area of the brain)	**Simple:** Consciousness intact with motor, sensory, autonomic, and psychic components	Rx: Carbamazepine, valproic acid, gabapentin, lamotrigine, topiramate, phenobarbital, tiagabine, vigabatrin, levetiracetam Can secondarily generalize	**Children:** Genetic, infection, trauma, congenital, metabolic **Adults:** Tumors, trauma, stroke, infection **Elderly:** Stroke, tumors, trauma, metabolic, infection
	Complex: Components of simple but with alteration of consciousness	Rx: Same drugs as for simple seizures, especially oxcarbazepine	
Generalized	**Absence** (petit mal). 3 Hz, 2 years old to puberty with blank stare. No postictal confusion	Rx absence: Ethosuximide, valproic acid Rx myoclonic: Valproic acid Rx Tonic-clonic: Phenobarbital, phenytoin, carbamazepine (only for secondary generalized, but not primary), valproic acid, topiramate, lamotrigine, gabapentin Note: Do not treat absence seizures with Na^+ channel blockers, as they worsen the seizure. Valproic acid should be avoided in pregnancy as it inhibits folate absorption, increasing the risk of neural tube defects	
	Myoclonic. Quick, repetitive jerks		
	Tonic-clonic (grand mal) Tonic phase characterized by limb stiffening followed by Clonic phase characterized by rhythmic jerking Postictal phase characterized by lethargy and disorientation		
	Tonic Stiffening (usually in children)		
	Atonic "Drop" seizures		

CEREBRAL CONTUSION

Permanent damage to small blood vessels and the parenchyma of the brain, typically due to acceleration-deceleration injuries.

PRESENTATION

Coup (at the site of impact) and contrecoup (opposite the site of impact, usually at the tips of the frontal and temporal lobes) injuries. Contrecoup injuries are typically more devastating because of the increased forces necessary to transmit energy across the brain, resulting in diffuse axonal damage as well.

DIAGNOSIS

CT or MRI.

TREATMENT

Treatment is directed at managing sequelae or lowering elevated ICP. Specific measures to lower ICP include

- Elevating head of bed to 30-degree incline.
- Optimize venous drainage: Head midline, neck neutral, ensure neck brace is not constricting.
- Hyperosmolar agents: Mannitol and hypertonic saline.
- Hyperventilation: Reduces partial pressure of carbon dioxide in arterial blood ($Paco_2$), resulting in cerebral vasoconstriction and reduced ICP.

KEY FACT

Patients with head trauma are often temporarily hyperventilated to produce **respiratory alkalosis,** which causes cerebral vessel constriction by decreasing partial pressure of carbon dioxide (Pco_2). This decreases cerebral blood volume and vessel permeability, thereby reducing the risk of cerebral edema. Note that respiratory *acidosis* causes vasodilation and increased vessel permeability, which enhances cerebral edema.

KEY FACT

Cushing triad: Bradycardia + respiratory depression + hypertension secondary to increased ICP. Also called **Cushing reflex** or **Cushing response.** Both arms of the autonomic system are activated: The sympathetic nervous system drives more blood centrally with concomitant activation of baroreceptors (parasympathetic) to reflexively decrease the heart rate.

Surgical treatment is rare, with the exception of severe cases.

PROGNOSIS

May progress to herniation as edema develops.

PRIMARY BRAIN NEOPLASMS

Neoplasms may result in mass effect, which presents as seizures, dementia, focal lesions, increased ICP (headache worse in the morning, nausea, vomiting, and bradycardia with hypertension). Primary brain tumors seldom undergo metastasis. Most adult primary tumors are supratentorial, whereas the majority of childhood primary tumors are infratentorial (Figure 6-60 and Table 6-29). Half of adult brain tumors are metastases from, in order of decreasing prevalence: lung, breast, skin (melanoma), kidney, GI tract, and thyroid cancers. Metastatic brain lesions present as multiple spherical lesions at the gray-white junction that frequently bleed.

Pituitary Adenomas

Benign neoplasms that arise from one of the five anterior pituitary cell types, and are generally monoclonal. Prolactin-secreting adenoma (prolactinoma) is the most common form.

PRESENTATION

See Table 6-30.

DIAGNOSIS

MRI, endocrine studies. Transsphenoidal surgery confirms the results of clinical and lab studies (determine local levels of relevant pituitary hormones).

TREATMENT

Transsphenoidal surgery, normalization of excess pituitary secretion (dopamine agonists bromocriptine or cabergoline for prolactinomas). Hormone replacement may be necessary depending on patient's age, sex, and presentation.

PROGNOSIS

If the lesion is resectable with preservation of pituitary function, then the prognosis is good.

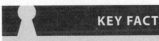

KEY FACT

Astrocytomas account for 70% of neuroglial tumors and are typically located in the frontal lobe of adults and the cerebellum of children.

KEY FACT

Astrocytes can be visualized by staining for glial fibrillary acidic protein (GFAP), an intermediate filament.

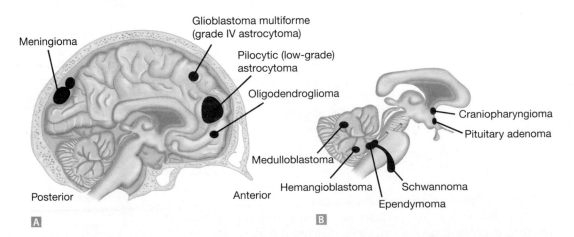

FIGURE 6-60.   **Location of adult and childhood primary brain neoplasms.** A Supratentorial and B infratentorial tumors.

TABLE 6-29. **Primary Brain Neoplasms**

	TYPE	PRESENTATION AND PATHOLOGY	PROGNOSIS/TREATMENT
Adult peak incidence	Glioblastoma multiforme	"Pseudopalisading" tumor cells border central areas of **necrosis** and **hemorrhage,** with ring-enhancing appearance in imaging; found in cerebral hemispheres (frontal lobes most commonly) and may cross corpus callosum ("butterfly glioma"); ill-defined mass; **most common primary brain tumor;** high-grade astrocytoma that stains positive for GFAP	< 1 year life expectancy, poor prognosis; combination of surgical resection, chemotherapy, and radiation
	Hemangioblastoma	Associated with **von Hippel-Lindau syndrome** when found with retinal angiomas; foamy cells and high vascularity are characteristic; may produce erythropoietin, causing secondary polycythemia; mesodermal origin	Resection
	Meningioma	Extra-axial tumor (external to brain parenchyma) arising from meningial arachnoid cells that occurs in convexities of hemispheres and parasagittal region; often asymptomatic but may present with seizures or focal neurologic deficits; symptoms arise from mass effect rather than infiltration of brain parenchyma; spindle cells concentrically arranged in whorled pattern, **psammoma bodies** (laminated calcifications); **most common benign primary CNS tumor in adults;** common cause of new-onset focal seizures	Surgical resection
	Oligodendroglioma	**Slow-growing tumor** most often in white matter of **frontal lobes; "fried egg" cells** with round nuclei and clear cytoplasm; chicken-wire capillary pattern; often calcified	Surgical resection
	Pinealoma	Fifty percent are germinomas that occur more often in males < 30 years old with symptoms similar to pure pineal gland tumor without melatonin abnormalities; pineal gland tumors compress the superior colliculus (**Parinaud syndrome:** vertical gaze palsy, most prominently of upward direction), pretectal area, and cerebral aqueduct (obstructive hydrocephalus); also interrupt melatonin production, leading to disruption of circadian rhythm and insomnia; may calcify with age; precocious puberty	Surgical resection
	Schwannoma-neurofibroma	Third most common primary brain tumor, benign; Schwann cell origin (stain positive for S100) most commonly localized to CN VIII at the cerebellopontine angle (vestibular schwannoma); may arise from any spinal root or CN except I and II (myelinated by oligodendrocytes); densely, uniformly enhancing on MRI; manifest with progressive unilateral tinnitus, hearing loss, ataxia with positive Romberg sign (because localized at cerebellopontine angle); commonly occurs in *NF2*	Surgical resection; may preserve hearing if small and prevent compression of cerebellum, pons, and facial nerve; patient usually deaf at presentation
Childhood peak incidence	Craniopharyngioma	Most common childhood supratentorial tumor, benign; derived from remnants of **Rathke pouch** (ectoderm resembling tooth enamel [ameloblasts]); distinguish from pituitary adenoma by histology (nests of uniform granular cells); present with growth failure, papilledema; compression of pituitary stalk leads to hypopituitarism, whereas compression of optic chiasm leads to bitemporal hemianopsia	Resection, though recurrence is common

(continues)

TABLE 6-29. **Primary Brain Neoplasms** *(continued)*

	TYPE	PRESENTATION AND PATHOLOGY	PROGNOSIS/TREATMENT
Childhood peak incidence *(continued)*	Ependymoma	Ependymal cell tumors most commonly found in fourth ventricle; characteristic perivascular pseudorosettes (ependymal cells around small vessels); rod-shaped blepharoplasts (basal ciliary bodies) found near nucleus; can cause hydrocephalus (nausea, vomiting, nuchal rigidity, increased ICP)	Poor prognosis
	Medulloblastoma	Highly malignant tumor with rosettes or perivascular pseudorosette pattern of cells; arises in cerebellar vermis; small round blue cells; presents with ataxia, projectile vomiting, nuchal rigidity; can compress fourth ventricle, leading to hydrocephalus and increased ICP. Classically responsible for "drop metastasis" to the spinal cord	Radiosensitive, may progress to cerebellar herniation without surgery
	Pilocytic astrocytoma	Diffusely infiltrating benign glioma most often seen in posterior fossa (cerebellar); **Rosenthal fibers** (eosinophilic corkscrew fibers resulting from accumulation of intermediate filament proteins specific to astrocytes); cyst with mural nodule. Cells stain positive for **GFAP**	Good prognosis
	Retinoblastoma	Malignant retinal tumor of childhood; causes leukocoria (abnormal "white pupil" with loss of red pupillary reflex); strabismus and decreased vision are common findings; sporadic cases are generally unilateral, whereas bilateral cases suggests *Rb* gene deletion; two-hit hypothesis prototype	Radiotherapy, cryotherapy, chemotherapy, or enucleation

CN, cranial nerve; CNS, central nervous system; CSF, cerebrospinal fluid; GFAP, glial fibrillary acidic protein; ICP, intracranial pressure.

NEUROCUTANEOUS DISORDERS

Neurocutaneous disorders (phakomatoses) are usually genetic and syndromic in origin. They can present with multiple neurologic and/or cutaneous signs and symptoms, which are outlined in Table 6-31.

TABLE 6-30. **Clinical Features of Pituitary Adenomas**

CATEGORY	HORMONE	PRESENTATION	TREATMENT
Hypersecretion	Prolactin	Men: Hypogonadism, infertility, impotence, ↓ libido, galactorrhea, gynecomastia Women: If premenopausal → menstrual irregularities, oligomenorrhea or amenorrhea, ↓ libido, dyspareunia, vaginal dryness, galactorrhea, anovulation, and infertility Potential mass effects (eg, bitemporal hemianopia, headaches) in both men and women	Dopamine agonists (eg, bromocriptine or cabergoline); surgical resection
	GH	Acromegaly; gigantism if prior to epiphyseal plate closure in a child	Surgical resection
	ACTH	Classic symptoms of Cushing disease (see Chapter 2)	Surgical resection, radiation therapy
	TSH	Classic symptoms of hyperthyroidism (see Chapter 2)	Surgical resection
Hypopituitarism		Compression of hypothalamic-pituitary stalk, leading to decreased production of other pituitary hormones; GH deficiency (lag in growth), hypogonadotropic hypogonadism, etc	Surgical resection followed by hormone replacement

ACTH, adrenocorticotropic hormone; GH, growth hormone; TSH, thyroid-stimulating hormone.

TABLE 6-31. Neurocutaneous Disorders

TYPES	CLINICAL MANIFESTATIONS	ETIOLOGY
Ataxia-telangiectasia (AT, Louis-Bar syndrome)	■ Characterized by progressive cerebellar ataxia, oculocutaneous telangiectasias (dilated vessels in skin and eyes), immune deficiency (IgA deficiency), and thymic hypoplasia ■ Cerebellar atrophy due to Purkinje cell death ■ Associated with increased malignancy (eg, adenocarcinomas, lymphoma, leukemia), increased sensitivity to ionizing radiation, and insulin-resistant diabetes mellitus ■ Increased AFP and CEA	■ AR mutation on chromosome (C.) 11 ■ Mutation of *ATM* (AT mutated) gene results in **failure to repair DNA** double strand breaks and subsequent cell cycle arrest ■ In the absence of ATM, cells collect somatic mutations, leading to malignant transformation
Sturge-Weber syndrome (SWS)	■ Rare vascular disorder; small vessels commonly affected leading to a characteristic facial capillary malformation (**port-wine stain,** nevus flammeus), a benign "birthmark" in the **ophthalmic (V1) and/or maxillary (V2) distribution** of the trigeminal nerve on one side of the face ■ Intellectual disability and seizures (epilepsy) ■ Ipsilateral (same side as facial lesion) leptomeningeal capillary-venous malformation (angioma), usually of parietal and occipital lobes, which can lead to SAH; venous stasis causes tissue ischemia resulting in intraparenchymal calcification ■ Early-onset glaucoma due to episcleral hemangioma blocking outflow of aqueous humor	■ An anomaly of neural crest derivatives secondary to a somatic mosaic mutation of the *GNAQ* gene ■ Congenital, but **nonhereditary (somatic),** thus recurrence is unlikely
Tuberous sclerosis complex (TSC)	■ Characterized by **multiple hamartomas** of the skin and CNS, infantile spasms, subependymal nodular (astrocytic proliferation), and subependymal giant cell tumors in periventricular area of brain ■ Dermatologic features include **ash-leaf spots** (hypopigmented macules), **Shagreen patches** (connective tissue nevi, commonly on lower trunk), ungual fibromas, and facial angiofibromas (adenoma sebaceum, flesh-colored papules in malar region or nasolabial fold) ■ Associated tumors include cardiac rhabdomyoma (very specific, causes mitral regurgitation) and renal angiomyolipoma ■ Intellectual disability and **epilepsy;** seizures are the most common presenting feature and often refractory to medication	■ AD, incomplete penetrance ■ Marked difference in phenotype among family members is due to **variable expressivity** ■ Mutation of either *TSC1* gene (encodes protein hamartin) on C. 9 or the *TSC2* gene (encodes protein tuberin) on C. 16
Neurofibromatosis type 1 (NF1, von Recklinghausen disease)	■ Cutaneous manifestations include **café-au-lait macules** (hyperpigmented macules, typically six or more, occur in 100% of affected individuals before 2 years of age), **Lisch nodules** (pigmented iris hamartomas), and freckling in the axillary or inguinal region (Crowe sign) ■ Skin tumors of NF1 are derived from **neural crest cells;** plexiform neurofibromas (not present in NF2) may undergo malignant transform into MPNSTs (neurofibrosarcoma) involving large nerves ■ Associated with optic pathway glioma and pheochromocytoma	■ AD, 100% penetrance, variable expressivity; half of cases are sporadic ■ Mutation of *NF1* gene encoding neurofibromin (Ras GTPase activating protein) on C. 17
Neurofibromatosis type 2 (NF2)	■ Central form of NF characterized by **vestibular schwannomas,** juvenile cataracts, meningiomas, ependymomas, and spinal cord schwannomas/neurilemmomas of the dorsal roots ■ Often presents as unilateral sensorineural hearing loss and tinnitus in teens or after puberty ■ Unilateral vestibular schwannomas can occur sporadically, but bilateral is a disease defining condition for *NF2*	■ AD, variable expressivity ■ Mutation of *NF2* gene, TSG encoding the protein merlin (schwannomin) on C. 22

(continues)

TABLE 6-31. Neurocutaneous Disorders *(continued)*

TYPES	CLINICAL MANIFESTATIONS	ETIOLOGY
von Hippel-Lindau (VHL) syndrome	<ul><li>Characterized by angiomatosis (eg, cavernous hemangiomas in skin, mucosa, and other organs)</li><li>Variety of benign and malignant tumors, including multiple hemangioblastomas (most common manifestation) of retina, brain stem, cerebellum and spine</li><li>Associated with clear-cell RCC (often bilateral), pheochromocytoma, and endolymphatic sac tumors of the middle ear</li></ul>	<ul><li>AD</li><li>Deletion of TSG, VHL, on C. 3</li><li>*VHL* gene product inhibits HIF1α and HIF2α</li><li>Results in constitutive expression of the TF HIF and activation of angiogenic growth factors</li></ul>

AD, autosomal dominant; AFP, serum alpha-fetal protein; AR, autosomal recessive; CEA, carcinoembryonic antigen; CNS, central nervous system; HIF, hypoxia inducible factor; MPNST, malignant peripheral nerve sheath tumors; RCC, renal cell carcinoma; SAH, subarachnoid hemorrhage; TF, transcription factor; TSG, tumor suppressor gene.

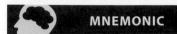

MNEMONIC

PSa**MM**oma bodies are associated with:

Papillary adenocarcinoma (thyroid)
Papillary **S**erous cystadenocarcinoma (ovary)
Meningioma
Mesothelioma

KEY FACT

Meningiomas are associated with neurofibromatosis. Bilateral schwannomas are almost always caused by NF2

KEY FACT

Ependymoma arises in the cauda equina in adults.

SPINAL CORD AND PERIPHERAL NERVE LESIONS

See Tables 6-32, 6-33, and 6-34 and Figure 6-61.

Brown-Séquard Syndrome

Brown-Séquard syndrome results from hemisection of the spinal cord that interrupts conduction through the lateral corticospinal tract (CST, motor), lateral spinothalamic tracts (STT, pain and temperature sensation), and dorsal columns (DC, proprioception and tactile sensation).

Nerves that run from the motor cortex to the spinal cord are referred to as UMNs; nerves that run from the anterior horn of the spinal cord to the periphery are referred to as LMNs.

PRESENTATION

- **Ipsilateral** UMN signs below the lesion (CST).
- **Ipsilateral** loss of tactile, vibration, and proprioception (DC) at and below the lesion.
- **Contralateral** loss of pain and temperature below the lesion (because of crossing fibers, STT).
- **Ipsilateral** loss of pain and temperature a few levels above and below the lesion.
- LMN signs at the level of the lesion.
- If the lesion is above T1, patient may present with Horner syndrome.

DIAGNOSIS

History and physical exam.

TABLE 6-32. Comparison of Lower and Upper Motor Neuron Lesions

MOTOR NEURON SIGNS	UPPER MOTOR NEURON	LOWER MOTOR NEURON
Weakness	+	+
Atrophy	–	+
Fasciculation	–	+
Reflexes	↑	↓
Tone	↑	↓
Babinski	+	–

TABLE 6-33.   Upper Extremity Nerve Injury

NERVE	SITE OF INJURY/DEFICIT IN MOTION	DEFICITS IN SENSATION/COURSE
Radial (C5–C8)	**Shaft of humerus,** leading to loss of triceps brachii, brachioradialis, and extensor carpi radialis; decreased grip strength due to loss of wrist extensors	Posterior brachial cutaneous branch: loss of sensation over posterior arm/forearm and dorsal hand
Median (C5–T1)	**Supracondylar region of humerus,** leaving arm muscle function intact with impaired forearm pronation, wrist flexion (with ulnar deviation), finger flexion, thumb abduction and opposition. Thenar atrophy	Loss of sensation over the lateral palm, thumb and lateral 2.5 fingers, and thumbnail bed
	Carpal tunnel syndrome (repetitive use injury)	Passes through pronator teres, under flexor retinaculum in carpal tunnel
	Slashing the wrist causes loss of thenar muscle innervation, so all thumb movement is lost except for adduction (ulnar)	*Tinel sign* (shock-like pain when lightly tapped on palmar side of wrist) and *Phalen sign* (wrist in flexion reproduces painful symptoms)
Ulnar (C8–T1)	**Medial epicondyle,** causing impaired wrist flexion (radial deviation) and adduction, thumb adduction (adductor pollicis), flexion of the medial two fingers (claw-hand deformity), and wasting of hypothenar eminence and PAD/DAB interosseous muscles	Loss of sensation over medial palm and medial 1.5 fingers
		Passes through carpi ulnaris, at elbow; passes between medial epicondyle and two heads of flexor carpi ulnaris
Axillary (C5 and C6)	**Surgical neck of humerus** or **anterior shoulder dislocation** causes loss of deltoid action (failure to abduct arm > 15 degrees)	Loss of sensation over deltoid muscle; on physical exam, palpable depression under acromion
Musculocutaneous (C5–C6)	Loss of function of coracobrachialis, biceps, and brachialis muscles, along with decreased supination	Passes through coracobrachialis and continues as lateral cutaneous nerve of forearm below elbow

PAD/DAB mnemonic: Palmar adducts/Dorsal abducts.

TABLE 6-34.   Lower Extremity Nerve Injury

NERVE	SITE OF INJURY/ DEFICIT IN MOTION	DEFICITS IN SENSATION/COURSE
Common peroneal (L4–S2) (divides into superficial and deep *branches at the neck of fibula*)	Deep peroneal: Innervates muscles of anterior leg compartment. Loss of foot dorsiflexion, causing foot drop and "steppage" gait	**Anterior compartment syndrome** results from increased pressure that causes compression of the deep peroneal nerve and vasculature, causing foot drop and weak dorsalis pedis pulse
		Deep peroneal: First web space
	Superficial peroneal: Innervates lateral leg compartment muscles. Loss of foot eversion	Superficial peroneal: Dorsal surface of foot except first web space
Tibial (L4–S3) (courses posterior to the medial malleolus)	Tibial nerve: Innervates the posterior compartment of the thigh and leg; Baker cyst (proximal lesion) or tarsal tunnel syndrome (distal lesion); loss of foot plantar flexion	Plantar surface of foot
Femoral (L2–L4)	Loss of knee extension/knee jerk	Paresthesias of anterior/medial thigh and medial leg
Obturator (L2–L4) (exits through the obturator canal to enter the thigh)	Loss of hip adduction	

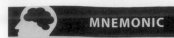

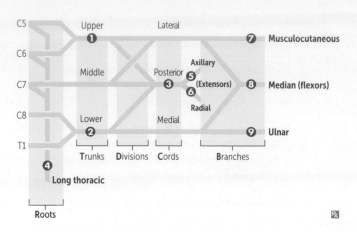

FIGURE 6-61. Diagram of the brachial plexus and associated presentation of lesions. Rad, radial nerve; Ax, axillary nerve; LT, long thoracic nerve; MC, musculocutaneous nerve; Med, median nerve; Uln, ulnar nerve. ❶ Waiter tip (Erb palsy); ❷ Claw hand (Klumpke palsy); ❸ Wrist drop; ❹ Winged scapula; ❺ Deltoid paralysis; ❻ Saturday night palsy (wrist drop); ❼ Difficulty flexing elbow, variable sensory loss; ❽ Decreased thumb function, Pope blessing; ❾ Intrinsic muscles of hand, claw hand.

TREATMENT

Early treatment with high-dose steroids has shown benefit, as have physical therapy and surgery.

PROGNOSIS

Poor; depends on the cause of the syndrome (trauma, infection, disk herniation).

Poliomyelitis

Destruction of the anterior horn of the spinal cord occurs secondary to fecal-oral infection by poliovirus (a picornavirus), leading to LMN destruction (see Figure 6-42, Table 6-24). Poliovirus replicates in the oropharynx and small intestine before spreading through the bloodstream to the CNS.

PRESENTATION

Malaise, headache, fever, nausea, abdominal pain, and sore throat characterize the acute infection. **Signs of LMN lesion** include muscle atrophy, flaccid paralysis, and hyporeflexia, with preserved sensation.

DIAGNOSIS

CSF with lymphocytic pleocytosis and slight elevation of protein. Virus is recovered from stool or the throat.

TREATMENT

Prevention with vaccine (Salk inactive parenteral vaccine). Oral (Sabin) vaccine carries small risk of disease but confers mucosal immunity in contrast to inactive vaccine. Bed rest decreases the incidence of paralysis; intensive care is needed if respiratory muscle weakness occurs.

PROGNOSIS

High mortality rate if bulbar involvement; persistent muscle weakness may develop years after acute infection.

Tabes Dorsalis (Tertiary Syphilis)

Degeneration of the dorsal roots and columns (mainly lumbosacral) that develops 15–20 years after the onset of *Treponema pallidum* infection. Primarily affects the fasciculi gracilis bilaterally.

PRESENTATION

Bilaterally impaired proprioception (positive Romberg sign) and sensation leading to progressive sensory ataxia, paresthesias (shooting pains), Argyll Robertson pupils (accommodate, but do not react to light), and absence of deep tendon reflexes. Purely sensory deficit; muscular power is retained. Associated with Charcot joints (insensitivity to pain in the joint, leading to increased susceptibility to joint injury).

DIAGNOSIS

Clinical and CSF analysis (pleocytosis [> 5 WBC/mm³], increased protein concentration [> 45 mg/dL], and/or VDRL reactivity). Note that the Venereal Disease Research Laboratory (VDRL) test may be positive in autoimmune diseases, mononucleosis, or hepatitis; so follow with specific treponemal tests, such as fluorescent treponemal antibody absorption (FTA-Abs) or microhemagglutination serology to confirm.

TREATMENT

Penicillin; treat symptoms.

PROGNOSIS

If untreated, may progress to paralysis, blindness, and dementia. Residual symptoms may persist after treatment.

Subacute Combined Degeneration (Vitamin B₁₂ Deficiency)

Most commonly results from pernicious anemia (vitamin B_{12} deficiency due to lack of intrinsic factor), which leads to a functional B_{12} deficiency and results in build up of methylmalonyl–coenzyme A (CoA) and its precursor, propionyl-CoA. Propionyl-CoA displaces succinyl-CoA in fatty acid synthesis, resulting in anomalous insertion of odd-chain fatty acids into lipids, such as myelin. Demyelination of the dorsal columns and lateral CST may occur with patients presenting with proprioceptive and motor symptoms.

PRESENTATION

Dementia, ataxic gait (demyelinated spinocerebellar tract), symmetrical spastic paresis (demyelinated CST leads to UMN loss) and impaired position and vibration sense (bilateral demyelination of dorsal columns).

DIAGNOSIS

- Serum B_{12} (cobalamin, Cbl).
- MRI.
- Schilling test:
  1. Give patient oral radiolabeled B_{12} [rB_{12}] plus intramuscular injection of unlabeled B_{12} and measure urine rB_{12} (should be high).
  2. If the first test is abnormal, give rB_{12} and intrinsic factor (to determine if a malabsorption problem exists), and then measure urine rB_{12}.
  3. If still no rB_{12} in urine, give rB_{12} and antibiotics (to rule out bacteria overgrowth) and measure urine rB_{12}.
  4. If still no rB_{12} in urine, then give rB_{12} and pancreatic enzymes (to rule out pancreatitis) and then measure urine rB_{12}.

MNEMONIC

Lower motor neuron lesion = everything **lowered** (↓ muscle mass, ↓ tone, ↓ reflexes, downgoing toes = negative Babinski sign).
Upper motor neuron lesion = everything **up** (↑ tone, ↑ reflexes, and upgoing toes = positive Babinski sign).

KEY FACT

Diabetic polyradiculopathy mimics tabes dorsalis.

KEY FACT

The sciatic nerve (L4–S3) emerges at the midpoint between the greater trochanter and the ischial tuberosity, then branches into the tibial and common peroneal nerves at the short head of the biceps femoris. All gluteal injections should target the superolateral quadrant to avoid damage to the gluteal nerves and sciatic nerve (superomedial quadrant).

KEY FACT

Vitamin B_{12} deficiency may also be caused by **pernicious anemia,** an autoimmune disorder that involves antibodies against *intrinsic factor* or gastric parietal cells (or both). In addition to subacute combined degeneration, vitamin B_{12} deficiency can result in megaloblastic anemia (large, abnormal RBCs).

FLASH BACK

Methylated B_{12} (methylcobalamin) is an essential cofactor for the conversion of homocysteine to methionine, so deficiency results in impairment of DNA synthesis. A high level of homocysteine is a risk factor for cardiovascular disease.

QUESTION

A 63-year-old man with chronic alcoholism presents with increased forgetfulness and confusion, and a serum sodium level of 115 mEq/L. After starting IV hypertonic saline to correct hyponatremia, he develops flaccid quadriplegia. What is responsible?

TREATMENT

Vitamin B$_{12}$ supplements (oral, intramuscular).

PROGNOSIS

Best prognosis is in those with gait disturbance < 3 months prior to commencement of treatment.

Syringomyelia

Enlargement of the central canal of the spinal cord leads to damage of the STT fibers as they cross in the anterior commissure. May also erode the anterior horn, resulting in LMN defects. Often presents in patients with Arnold-Chiari type II malformation (herniation of the cerebellar vermis through the foramen magnum, causing hydrocephalus, meningomyelocele, and syringomyelia).

PRESENTATION

Bilateral loss of pain and temperature sensation in the upper extremities (most often at C8–T1 ["cape and shawl" distribution; see Figure 6-42]) with preservation of touch sensation. LMN signs of flaccid paralysis if the anterior horn cells are affected, causing combined sensory and motor defects. Atrophy of hand interossei (ulnar nerve). Note that amyotrophic lateral sclerosis (ALS, thenar atrophy) can be distinguished from syringomyelia by clinical presentation: ALS patients have motor, but not sensory deficits.

DIAGNOSIS

MRI is diagnostic.

TREATMENT

With Arnold-Chiari malformation, place shunt to treat hydrocephalus before correction of syrinx (posterior fossa decompression).

PROGNOSIS

Highly variable.

Thoracic Outlet Syndrome (Klumpke Palsy)

An embryologic defect in the cervical rib can result in compression of the subclavian artery and the inferior trunk of the brachial plexus (C8, T1). Also seen in Pancoast tumors (apical lung tumor), weightlifters (hypertrophy of the anterior scalene muscle compresses the neurovascular bundle that runs between the anterior and middle scalene muscles), or hyperabduction of the arm (as in falling, breech birth).

PRESENTATION

Thenar and hypothenar eminence (median and ulnar nerves) atrophy, atrophy of the interosseous muscles (ulnar nerve), and sensory deficits on the medial side of the forearm and hand (ulnar nerve, medial cutaneous nerve of the forearm). Disappearance of the radial pulse when the head is rotated toward the opposite side due to compression of the subclavian artery.

DIAGNOSIS

History, physical exam, and radiographic imaging demonstrating cervical rib or apical lung mass.

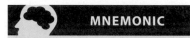

TREATMENT

Anterior scalenectomy (careful to avoid the phrenic nerve that runs on the anterior scalene deep to the prevertebral fascia); surgical removal of cervical rib if present and implicated; physical therapy.

PROGNOSIS

Symptoms may return following treatment secondary to scarring and fibrosis around the nerve roots.

PERIPHERAL NEUROPATHY

Two types occur:

- Demyelination often presents segmentally with sensory changes (discrete sensory loss following the distribution of one or more nerves).
- Axonal degeneration of motor nerves presents as muscle fasciculations and atrophy. Axonal degeneration of sensory nerves occurs first (small fibers are more prone to damage) and presents with a **"stocking-and-glove"** distribution (longer fibers are more prone to damage).

Hereditary Motor and Sensory Neuropathy

Hereditary motor and sensory neuropathy (Charcot-Marie-Tooth disease) is the most common hereditary neuropathy (autosomal dominant). Primarily affects the peroneal nerve. Onset is typically in the first or second decade.

PRESENTATION

Peroneal nerve neuropathy leading to atrophy of the lower leg muscles. This results in an "inverted bottle" appearance of the legs. Associated with scoliosis and foot deformities.

DIAGNOSIS

History and physical exam.

TREATMENT

No therapy to prevent onset or delay progression; patients may benefit from physical therapy and surgery for contractures.

PROGNOSIS

No cure; progressive peripheral neuropathy.

CRANIAL NERVE PALSY

Cranial nerves arise from their nuclei in the brain stem and course toward their targets, primarily in the face. Muscles of facial expression, mastication, autonomic functions, and sensory fibers are supplied by these nerves. Defects result either when the nucleus or the fibers are damaged and may be bilateral or unilateral; unilateral defects commonly present with lesions closer to the periphery (Table 6-35).

KEY FACT

Patients with diabetes mellitus (DM) may develop peripheral neuropathy secondary to osmotic damage to Schwann cells. This is the most common cause of peripheral sensory and motor axonopathy; for this reason, it is extremely important to check the feet of diabetic patients!

KEY FACT

Toxin-associated peripheral neuropathy results from alcohol abuse, exposure to heavy metals, or diphtheria.

KEY FACT

Lyme disease is the most common cause of bilateral facial nerve paralysis in endemic areas.

TABLE 6-35. **Cranial Nerve Palsies**

TYPE/LOCATION	PRESENTATION	ETIOLOGY/NOTES
CN III	Oculomotor paralysis (eg, in transtentorial herniation) leads to denervation of the levator palpebrae muscle, causing ptosis; denervation of the extraocular muscles innervated by CN III, causing "down and out" orientation of eyes; and interruption of ophthalmic parasympathetic innervations, leading to internal ophthalmoplegia (dilated, fixed pupil and impairment in accommodation [cycloplegia])	Transtentorial herniation, posterior communicating artery aneurysm, diabetes, Weber syndrome, brain tumors
CN IV	Extorsion of the eye, weakness of downward gaze, vertical diplopia (worse when looking down), and characteristic compensatory head tilting (pseudotorticollis)	
CN V motor lesion	Jaw deviates toward side of lesion	If lesion is at trigeminal motor nucleus, then ipsilateral loss
		If lesion is higher up in cortex, then contralateral signs
CN VII	Drooping corner of mouth with drooling; loss of buccinator muscle function	Seen in AIDS, Lyme disease, sarcoidosis, tumors, and diabetes
	Difficulty speaking, inability to close eye	
	Loss of taste in anterior two-thirds of tongue (chorda tympani)	
	Loss of lacrimation and salivation	
	Peripheral lesions: paralysis of upper and lower face; Central lesions: paralysis of lower face only (see Figure 6-45)	
CN X lesion	Uvula deviates away from side of lesion	Brain stem infarct
CN XI lesion	Weakness turning head to side contralateral to lesion; shoulder droop on side of lesion	Sternocleidomastoid (SCM) contraction normally moves head to contralateral side
		Loss of SCM and trapezius innervation accounts for presentation
CN XII lesion (LMN)	Tongue deviates toward side of lesion ("lick your wounds")	Anterior spinal artery infarct

KEY FACT

Fibers to the upper facial muscles receive bilateral corticobulbar innervation, which explains why UMN lesions of CN VII present only with lower facial paralysis. Fibers to the lower facial muscles are only innervated by the contralateral cortex.

Defects in Eye Movement

CN III Lesion

PRESENTATION

Lesion causes the eye to point "down and out" (only the lateral rectus and superior oblique muscles are functional), dilation of pupil (loss of parasympathetic fibers), and severe ptosis (as opposed to Horner syndrome, which is characterized by mild ptosis).

ETIOLOGY

- Posterior communicating artery aneurysm compresses the nerve, which causes a fixed, dilated pupil because parasympathetic fibers run along the periphery of the nerve bundle.
- Weber syndrome: Midbrain tegmentum lesion causing ipsilateral CN III palsy and contralateral body hemiplegia.
- Diabetic CN III palsy involves the oculomotor muscles but spares the pupil because it is an ischemic rather than a compressive lesion. Parasympathetic fibers run on

the surface of the nerve, so they are the first to be involved in compression and the last to be involved in ischemia. Oculomotor muscle fibers run along the interior of CN III.

- Mass effect (eg, brain tumor, epidural hematoma), leading to herniation of brain tissue with compression of CN III.

DIAGNOSIS

Physical exam.

TREATMENT

Treatment of underlying etiology (eg, surgical clipping of an aneurysm).

PROGNOSIS

Dependent on etiology.

CN IV Lesion

Eye rotated superior and lateral because of unopposed action of the inferior oblique.

ETIOLOGY

Commonly due to head trauma, brain tumors, or increased ICP resulting in nerve compression.

DIAGNOSIS

Physical exam, imaging to detect underlying cause.

TREATMENT

Treatment is directed at underlying etiology when possible.

PROGNOSIS

Dependent on etiology.

CN VI Lesion

Affected eye fails to abduct; unaffected eye develops nystagmus when the patient tries to abduct the affected eye.

ETIOLOGY

Lesion within the cavernous sinus (ICA aneurysm—CN VI is most susceptible to injury, as it runs directly next to the ICA) or pontomedullary junction; increased ICP, causing a downward shift in the posterior fossa.

DIAGNOSIS

Physical exam and imaging.

TREATMENT

Watchful waiting or treat underlying cause if known.

PROGNOSIS

Most cases resolve within 6 months.

KEY FACT

Trigeminal neuralgia (tic douloureux) presents as severe stabbing pain in the sensory distribution of CN V.

KEY FACT

CN IV (trochlear nerve) is the only cranial nerve to exit the brain stem dorsally and cross the midline; therefore, a lesion at the nucleus results in the contralateral eye deviating superiorly and laterally.

KEY FACT

Cavernous sinus syndrome results from internal carotid aneurysm (mass effect) that presents as ophthalmoplegia and ophthalmic and maxillary sensory loss (CN V_1 and V_2).

KEY FACT

Signs suggestive of brain stem lesions: vertigo (CN VIII), diplopia (CN III, IV, VI), ataxia (cerebellar), perioral numbness (CN V), loss of consciousness (reticular activating system).

KEY FACT

Argyll Robertson pupil, seen in tertiary syphilis, SLE, and DM: accommodation to near objects is intact, but the pupil does not react to light by constricting.

KEY FACT

Marcus Gunn pupil results from a deficit in the afferent light reflex pathway (eg, CN II lesion, retinal detachment). The affected pupil appears to expand when light is switched from the unaffected eye to the affected eye (pupil is actually returning to baseline from a constricted state). Diagnosed by swinging a light from pupil to pupil; usually seen in the context of MS.

KEY FACT

Xerophthalmia (dry eyes) may be caused by vitamin A deficiency (desquamation of conjunctival cells) or Sjögren syndrome (keratoconjunctivitis sicca).

KEY FACT

Macular degeneration occurs secondary to disruption of the retinal membrane, leading to slow-onset loss of central vision with preserved peripheral vision. Most common cause of premature vision loss in the elderly.

KEY FACT

Cataracts (opacification of lens) are seen in the elderly and in those with DM, rubella, and corticosteroid use.

Facial Lesions

UMN Lesion

Lesion of the motor cortex or the connection between the cortex and the facial nucleus results in contralateral paralysis of the lower face only (see Figure 6-45).

LMN Lesion

Ipsilateral paralysis of the upper and lower face.

Visual Field Defects

Lesions occurring anywhere from the retina to the visual cortex result in defects in the visual field (see Figure 6-46). The specific intervention depends on the underlying cause and whether the lesion is a severed tract or a parenchymal injury.

Uveitis

The uveal tract or uvea is the darkly pigmented and vascular, middle layer of the eye. The uvea is composed of three layers (from anterior to posterior): iris, ciliary body, and choroid (Figure 6-62). Uveitis is inflammation of the uvea. Specifically, anterior uveitis or iritis is inflammation of the anterior uvea (composed of iris and ciliary body). Iridocyclitis is anterior uveitis plus inflammation of the adjacent ciliary body. Posterior uveitis (choroiditis and/or retinitis) is inflammation of the posterior uvea (composed of choroid). The retina, while possibly involved, is not part of the uvea.

PRESENTATION

Blurry vision (resulting from inflammation of the iris, ciliary body, and choroids) and may present with retinal detachment and/or acute glaucoma. May have hypopyon (accumulation of pus in the anterior chamber) and/or conjunctival injection.

Associated with:

- **Autoinflammatory disease:** Ankylosing spondylitis, Reiter syndrome, sarcoidosis, ulcerative colitis.
- **Infection:** Toxoplasmosis, cytomegalovirus, toxocariasis (ocular larval migrans), histoplasmosis, tuberculosis (TB), syphilis.

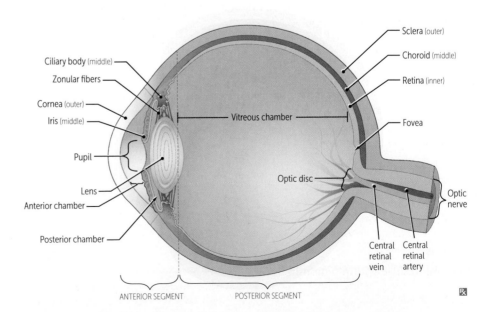

FIGURE 6-62. **Structures of the eye.**

Internuclear Ophthalmoplegia (Medial Longitudinal Fasciculus Syndrome)

Lesion of the medial longitudinal fasciculus (MLF) results in ipsilateral medial rectus palsy on attempted lateral gaze. This lesion is distinguished from CN III palsy by preserved convergence, in contrast to the "down and out" appearance of CN III palsy. Most common cause is MS.

PRESENTATION

When the affected eye is adducting, nystagmus is seen in the abducting opposite eye (Figure 6-63). Normal convergence ("finger to nose" eye test), but loss of conjugate gaze (Figure 6-64). In patients with MS, internuclear ophthalmoplegia (INO) results from demyelination of the MLF.

DIAGNOSIS

Clinical; if bilateral, high suspicion that MS is the cause. Need to exclude myasthenia gravis in patients with isolated medial rectus palsy.

TREATMENT

Underlying condition needs to be managed for MLF syndrome to resolve.

CENTRAL NERVOUS SYSTEM INFECTIONS

Infections that arise in the CNS can be divided into those that affect immunocompetent individuals and those that affect immunocompromised patients, with some specific exceptions. AIDS-defining lesions (fungal, JC viral infection, and *Mycobacterium tuberculosis*) typically occur in immunocompromised patients. Table 6-36 details the types of patients affected and the typical disease course of various CNS infections.

Meningitis

Inflammation of the pia mater covering the brain may be bacterial, viral, or fungal in origin. Usually occurs secondary to hematogenous spread.

HERNIATION SYNDROMES

Under increased intracranial pressure, portions of the brain are displaced through openings of dura partitions or into openings of the skull (eg, foramen magnum) (Figure 6-65). Therefore, treatment is aimed at removing the insult that generated the increased

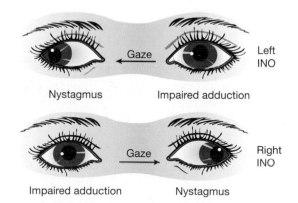

FIGURE 6-63. A clinical exam for medial longitudinal fasciculus (MLF) syndrome. When looking left, the left nucleus of CN VI fires, which contracts the left lateral rectus and stimulates the contralateral nucleus of CN III via the right MLF to contract the right medial rectus. INO, internuclear ophthalmoplegia.

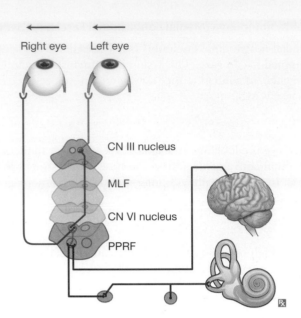

FIGURE 6-64. **Pathway of conjugate horizontal gaze.** CN, cranial nerve; MLF, medial longitudinal fasciculus; PPRF, paramedian pontine reticular formation.

pressure (eg, shunt for hydrocephalus, control of intracranial hemorrhage). Treat with hyperosmotic therapy such as mannitol or hypertonic saline; can use dexamethasone to mitigate cerebral edema (reduce ICP) if that is the underlying cause.

Cingulate/Subfalcine

The cingulate cortex herniates under the falx cerebri and may compress the anterior cerebral artery, leading to symptoms detailed earlier in the cerebrovascular section. The falx cerebri normally separates the two cerebral hemispheres along the midline of the skull (see A in Figure 6-65).

Uncal

DEFINITION AND EPIDEMIOLOGY

The uncus of the medial temporal lobe compresses the crus cerebri by herniating through the tentorium cerebri. Results from a mass lesion that forces the medial aspect of the temporal lobe under the tentorium cerebri (see C in Figure 6-65).

PRESENTATION

- Stretching/compression CN III leads to ipsilateral dilated pupil, ptosis, oculomotor muscle dysfunction (loss of pupillary light reflex proceeds to loss of motor function).
- Compression of the ipsilateral posterior cerebral artery leads to contralateral homonymous hemianopia secondary to hemorrhagic infarct of the occipital lobe.
- Compression of the ipsilateral crus cerebri (lateral CST) leads to contralateral paresis.
- Compression of the contralateral crus cerebri (lateral CST, Kernohan notch) leads to ipsilateral paresis (a "false localizing" sign).
- Caudal displacement of the brain stem (compression of the midbrain) leads to Duret hemorrhages, paramedian artery rupture, and midbrain hemorrhage.

Cerebellar Tonsillar

Herniation of the cerebellar tonsil into the foramen magnum results in cardiorespiratory arrest and/or coma by compression of the medulla (see D in Figure 6-65).

TABLE 6-36.   Central Nervous System Infections According to Type of Microbe

TYPE	PRESENTATION	CAUSATIVE MICROBE
Viral	Acute	Enterovirus is most common cause of aseptic meningitis
	Acute or subacute	Herpes encephalitis
	Subacute to chronic	Progressive multifocal leukoencephalopathy (JC virus), subacute sclerosing panencephalitis (measles)
Bacterial (meningitis)	< 1 month	Group B streptococci, *Escherichia coli, Listeria monocytogenes*
	1 month to 18 years	*Neisseria meningitidis* (*Haemophilus influenzae* is now rare because of vaccine)
	> 18 years	*Streptococcus pneumoniae*
	Immunocompromised	*Mycobacterium tuberculosis* (complication of primary TB)
	Liver/renal disease, aseptic meningitis (Weil syndrome)	*Leptospira interrogans*
Fungal	Immunocompromised (subacute meningitis)	*Cryptococcus neoformans*
	DKA, leukemia	Mucormycosis (*Mucor, Rhizopus*)
Parasitic	Rapidly fatal (immune-competent)	*Naegleria fowleri*
	Rapidly fatal (immunocompromised)	*Acanthamoeba*
	Neurocysticercosis	*Taenia solium*
	AIDS	*Toxoplasma gondii*
	Malaria with CNS infection	*Plasmodium falciparum*
Brain abscess	Bacterial	Streptococci, *Staphylococcus aureus*, Enterobacteriaceae, *Bacillus fragilis, Peptostreptococcus*
	Helminthic	*Taenia solium, Schistosoma*, hydatid cyst (*Echinococcus granulosus*)

CNS, central nervous system; DKA, diabetic ketoacidosis.

Transtentorial

Transtentorial (central) herniation can result in coma and death due to brain stem ischemia from compression of the brain stem and shearing of the basilar artery perforators, leading to brain stem hemorrhages (Duret hemorrhages) (see B in Figure 6-65).

HEADACHE SYNDROMES

A patient presenting with headache (HA) as the primary complaint has a broad differential. Common HA syndromes are presented below. Migraine, tension-type, and cluster HAs are primarily clinical diagnoses based on history and physical exam. However, secondary causes of HA should be considered, including subarachnoid hemorrhage, meningitis, neoplasia, hydrocephalus, and giant cell (temporal) arteritis.

Migraines

PRESENTATION

Migraine HA is usually recurrent in nature and commonly presents as a unilateral, pulsatile/throbbing pain associated with nausea, vomiting, photophobia, and phono-

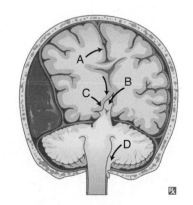

FIGURE 6-65.   Types of cerebral herniation. (A) Cingulate subfalcine herniation; (B) central transtentorial herniation; (C) uncal herniation; (D) cerebellar tonsillar herniation.

phobia. May be precipitated by a trigger (eg, stress, menstruation, visual stimuli, or other factors). Episodes typically last 4–72 hours and may be aggravated by routine physical activity. Classic migraines include an aura, whereas common migraines are not associated with an aura. These HAs are thought to be due to irritation of the trigeminal nerve, meninges, or blood vessels (release of vasoactive peptides, substance P, and/or calcitonin gene–related peptide).

TREATMENT

Abortive pharmacotherapy should be taken only if a person is actively experiencing a migraine and includes nonsteroidal anti-inflammatory drugs (NSAIDs), acetaminophen, and triptans (5-hydroxytryptamine [5-HT]1B/1D agonists). Better results are usually achieved when medications are started as soon as symptoms appear. Prophylaxis for migraine HA includes

- β-Blockers: metoprolol, **propranolol**, timolol
- Antidepressants: **amitriptyline**
- Anticonvulsants: topiramate, valproate
- Ca^{2+} channel blockers: flunarizine, verapamil

Tension-Type Headaches

PRESENTATION

Tension-type HA is the most common HA in the general population. They present as a constant, bilateral pain, often in a "band-like" distribution. Unlike migraine HAs, they are not associated with photophobia, phonophobia, or an aura. They last at least 30 minutes but typically resolve in 4–6 hours.

TREATMENT

Treatment is analgesics, primarily **NSAIDs** or acetaminophen. Amitriptyline can be used as preventive treatment.

Cluster Headaches

PRESENTATION

Cluster HA presents as unilateral, severe periorbital pain, associated with unilateral autonomic manifestations, such as lacrimation, rhinorrhea, conjunctival injection, and a partial Horner syndrome (ptosis and miosis). They usually occur in males and are more common in young smokers. They often occur daily for a period of weeks, followed by a period of remission (hence the term *cluster*).

TREATMENT

One hundred percent supplemental O_2 should be the first abortive therapy attempted. Sumatriptan is first-line pharmacotherapy for abortive therapy. Verapamil is first-line pharmacotherapy for prevention.

Trigeminal Neuralgia

PRESENTATION

Trigeminal neuralgia (TN) presents as a repetitive, unilateral shooting pain in the distribution of one or more branches of the trigeminal nerve (V1, V2, or V3). Pain usually lasts a few seconds per episode (vs cluster HA) and is often described as "electric," "shock-like," or "stabbing." TN is much more common in women. Most cases are believed to be caused by compression of the trigeminal nerve root by an aberrant loop of an artery or vein (classic TN). Causes of secondary TN include herpes zoster (acute or postherpetic), MS, and space-occupying lesions.

DIAGNOSIS

Clinical diagnosis based on history and physical exam. Neuroimaging (MRI or CT) is commonly performed to distinguish between classical and secondary TN.

TREATMENT

The first-line medical treatment for classical TN is carbamazepine. In cases refractory to medical management, surgery is often warranted.

Pharmacology

CENTRAL NERVOUS SYSTEM NEUROTRANSMITTERS

An increase or decrease of certain neurotransmitters or their receptors has been implicated in many neurologic disorders. Certain therapies therefore target neurotransmitters or their receptors. There are multiple subtypes of dopamine, serotonin (5-HT), and noradrenergic receptors throughout the CNS and the rest of the body. Because no two medications in a class of drugs (eg, antidepressants, atypical antipsychotics) have the same action on the same combination of receptors, patents experience differences in the clinical effect and side effects. A very basic example of a synaptic neurotransmission site is shown in Figure 6-66.

Acetylcholine

Acetylcholine (ACh) is a neurotransmitter of both the peripheral (PNS) and central (CNS) nervous systems. This molecule has two classes of receptors: nicotinic and muscarinic. It is formed in the nerve terminal by *choline acetyltransferase* (Figure 6-67). A decrease in levels of ACh is implicated in Alzheimer dementia and Huntington disease, whereas Parkinson disease is associated with a relative increase in ACh. Like histamine receptors, muscarinic receptors are subject to off-target blockade by **antipsychotics** and **tricyclic antidepressants (TCAs)**, resulting in dry mouth, blurred vision, and urinary hesitancy.

Dopamine

A neurotransmitter synthesized from tyrosine, dopamine serves as a precursor to norepinephrine (NE) and epinephrine (Epi; Figure 6-68). Dopamine is implicated in psychosis (increased levels), mania (increased levels), schizophrenia (increased levels), Huntington disease (increased levels), and Parkinson disease (decreased levels).

KEY FACT

The **nucleus basalis of Meynert** is an important site for the production of ACh in the brain.

KEY FACT

The **substantia nigra pars compacta** and the **ventral tegmental area** are important sites of dopaminergic neurons in the brain.

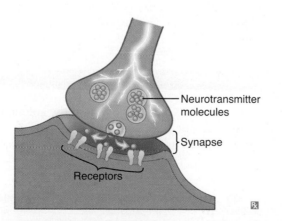

FIGURE 6-66. **Synaptic neurotransmission site.**

$$\text{Acetyl-CoA + Choline} \xrightarrow{\text{Choline acetyltransferase}} \text{Acetylcholine} \xrightarrow{\text{Acetylcholinesterase}} \text{Acetate + Choline}$$

FIGURE 6-67. **Acetylcholine synthesis and degradation.** Acetyl–coenzyme A (CoA) and choline are combined by the enzyme choline acetyltransferase to form acetylcholine. Acetylcholinesterase metabolizes acetylcholine into acetate and choline.

γ-Aminobutyric Acid (GABA)

The major inhibitory neurotransmitter in the CNS, GABA is associated with anxiety (decreased levels) Huntington disease (decreased levels), and epilepsy (decreased levels). Anxiolytics (eg, alcohol, benzodiazepines, and barbiturates) are agonists of the $GABA_A$ receptor (see sections on anxiolytics and hypnotics for further explanation of benzodiazepines and barbiturates).

Glutamate

The major excitatory neurotransmitter in the CNS, glutamate is implicated in epilepsy (increased levels), schizophrenia (increased levels), and Alzheimer disease (increased levels).

Glycine

Glycine is an inhibitory neurotransmitter that controls/modulates glutamate activity in the brain and spinal cord.

Histamine

Histamine is a ubiquitous chemical that, in the CNS, is responsible for sleep modulation and satiety. Antipsychotics and tricyclic antidepressants can cause histamine (H_1)-receptor blockade, leading to side effects such as sedation and increased appetite, leading to weight gain.

Norepinephrine

A catecholamine (precursor to epinephrine), NE is found at sympathetic postganglionic terminals (see Figure 6-68). It is implicated in major depressive disorder (MDD) (decreased levels) and anxiety (increased levels).

Serotonin (5-Hydroxytryptamine)

Serotonin is a monoamine neurotransmitter that regulates mood, body temperature, sexuality, satiety, and sleep. It is converted from tryptophan in a series of reactions (Figure 6-69) and is degraded by the enzyme monoamine oxidase. It is implicated in MDD (decreased), bipolar disorder (decreased), anxiety disorder (decreased), and schizophrenia (increased).

AUTONOMIC DRUGS

Autonomic drugs are chemical agents that act within the autonomic nervous system at sympathetic and parasympathetic nerve terminals (Figure 6-70). These drugs interact with preexisting neurotransmitters in order to achieve desired effects at the junction of the CNS and the PNS.

KEY FACT

Histaminergic neurons are located in the **ventral posterior hypothalamus (tuberomammillary nucleus).**

KEY FACT

The **locus ceruleus,** found in the upper pons, is the primary site of NE synthesis in the brain.

KEY FACT

The **raphe nucleus** in the brain stem releases serotonin to projections throughout the brain.

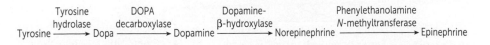

$$\text{Tyrosine} \xrightarrow{\substack{\text{Tyrosine} \\ \text{hydrolase}}} \text{Dopa} \xrightarrow{\substack{\text{DOPA} \\ \text{decarboxylase}}} \text{Dopamine} \xrightarrow{\substack{\text{Dopamine-} \\ \beta\text{-hydroxylase}}} \text{Norepinephrine} \xrightarrow{\substack{\text{Phenylethanolamine} \\ N\text{-methyltransferase}}} \text{Epinephrine}$$

FIGURE 6-68. **Dopa, dopamine, norepinephrine, and epinephrine are all synthesized from the amino acid tyrosine.**

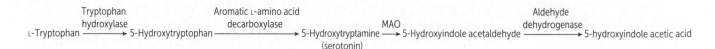

FIGURE 6-69. **Synthesis of serotonin.** MAO, monoamine oxidase.

Neuromuscular Junction Blocking Agents

Neuromuscular junction (NMJ)-blocking agents are drugs used for skeletal muscle relaxation. These agents work at the NMJ, as opposed to inhaled anesthetics or regional nerve blocks, which act at different sites (see Figure 6-51). Because they work only at the NMJ, these agents do not cause analgesia or unconsciousness, **only paralysis.** They are similar in structure to ACh, allowing them to bind to ACh receptors on the muscle membrane. The two classes of NMJ-blocking agents work differently at the ACh receptor; **depolarizing** agents behave as ACh receptor **agonists,** and **nondepolarizing** agents behave as ACh receptor **competitive antagonists.**

Depolarizing Agents

DRUG NAME

Succinylcholine (short-acting).

MECHANISM

In general, depolarizing agents, such as succinylcholine, work as **ACh receptor agonists.** They achieve their desired effect in two distinct phases. In phase I, the drug binds aggressively to the ACh receptor and triggers depolarization of the motor endplate. However, it is resistant to AChE and remains bound to the ACh receptor. Sodium channels found at the motor endplate that initially closed after depolarization remain closed since the drug remains bound to the receptor and prevents repolarization of the motor endplate. Phase II block occurs after the drug remains bound to the ACh receptor over

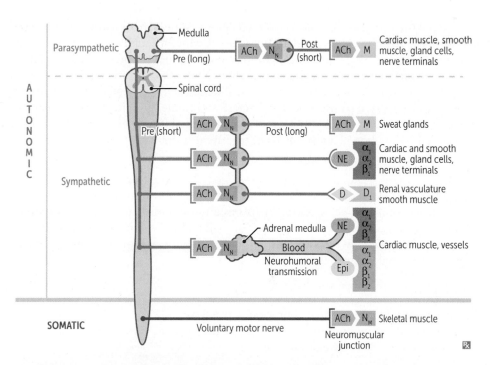

FIGURE 6-70. **The autonomic and somatic nervous systems.** ACh, acetylcholine; D, dopamine; Epi, epinephrine; N, nicotinic receptor; NE, norepinephrine; M, muscarinic receptor; α, alpha-adrenergic receptor; β, beta-adrenergic receptor.

time, inducing a conformational change at the NMJ. This leads to a nondepolarizing neuromuscular block that cannot be reversed. The effects of succinylcholine are evident within 30 seconds and last for 10 minutes (duration of action is limited by diffusion away from the NMJ). **Pseudocholinesterase** metabolizes succinylcholine before the drug reaches the site of action.

USES

Succinylcholine is the only depolarizing agent approved for clinical use in the United States. It is used to effect temporary muscle paralysis (eg, surgery, intubation).

SIDE EFFECTS

- Cardiovascular:
  - Low dose: Negative chronotropic and inotropic effects.
  - High dose: Positive chronotropic and inotropic effects; raises catecholamine levels.
- Fasciculations (visible motor unit contractions in phase I).
- Myalgia.
- Hyperkalemia (can increase serum K^+ levels by 0.5 mEq/L, which is a concern in the setting of **burns,** trauma, spinal cord injury, cardiac disease, and/or metabolic abnormalities).
- Malignant hyperthermia (treat with dantrolene).
- Hypercalcemia.

Nondepolarizing Agents

DRUG NAMES

Mivacurium (short-acting), vecuronium (intermediate-acting), rocuronium (intermediate-acting), atracurium (intermediate-acting), pancuronium (long-acting), doxacurium (long-acting).

MECHANISMS

Nondepolarizing agents operate as ACh receptor **competitive antagonists.** The drug binds to the ACh receptor, but does not cause the motor endplate to depolarize. By binding to the receptor, it prevents ACh from binding, thereby preventing depolarization of the motor endplate and causing paralysis. Most nondepolarizing agents depend on hepatic or renal elimination to terminate their effect. An exception is mivacurium, which is metabolized by pseudocholinesterase and is safe for patients with hepatic or renal dysfunction. Reversal of nondepolarizing block depends on metabolism of the drug or administration of a reversal agent (eg, AChE inhibitor).

USES

Nondepolarizing agents are similar to depolarizing agents in causing muscle paralysis and can substitute for depolarizing agents as a muscle relaxant. Such uses include intubation, prevention of fasciculations (especially important in patients who may be sensitive to variations in serum K^+ levels), decreasing the amount of required inhalational agents, and maintenance of paralysis.

SIDE EFFECTS

- Respiratory failure due to diaphragmatic paralysis.
- Tachycardia (pancuronium).
- Histamine release (mivacurium).

Cholinomimetic Agents

DRUG NAMES

Bethanechol, carbachol, methacholine, and pilocarpine.

USES

These drugs are direct agonists of the ACh receptor. Bethanechol is commonly used in postop and neurogenic ileus, as well as for urinary retention. Carbachol is a pupillary constrictor used in glaucoma. Pilocarpine is used in both open-angle and closed-angle glaucoma for its effects of pupillary constriction and ciliary muscle constriction. Methacholine is a short-acting cholinomimetic used in the diagnosis of asthma.

SIDE EFFECTS

- Bronchospasm
- Bradycardia
- Sweating
- Lacrimation
- Diarrhea

Cholinesterase Inhibitors

DRUG NAMES

Neostigmine, pyridostigmine, edrophonium, physostigmine, cevimeline.

MECHANISMS

These drugs inactivate AChE by electrostatic or covalent binding. They are used to reverse the effects of a nondepolarizing neuromuscular drug. They prevent degradation of ACh at the NMJ and therefore increase the available ACh to compete for ACh receptors, causing the nondepolarizing agent to "wash out." Reversal agents are contraindicated when depolarizing agents are used because they inhibit cholinesterase and pseudocholinesterase, thereby prolonging the phase 1 block.

USES

They are used to reverse nondepolarizing neuromuscular drugs (eg, pancuronium) during surgery; they can also be used to diagnose (edrophonium) and treat myasthenia gravis (eg, pyridostigmine), as well as to treat atropine overdose (physostigmine) and treat dry mouth associated with Sjögren syndrome (cevimeline).

SIDE EFFECTS

- Bradycardia
- Bronchospasm
- Excitation (physostigmine)
- Intestinal spasm
- Increased bladder tone
- Pupillary constriction
- Exacerbation of chronic obstructive pulmonary disease (COPD), asthma, and peptic ulcers (ACh increases gastric acid release)
- Cholinesterase inhibitor poisoning: Caused by cholinesterase inhibitors that irreversibly inhibit AChE (eg, organophosphates found in insecticides). Prolonged activity of ACh leads to an increase in parasympathetic activity (diarrhea, urination, lacrimation, miosis, bradycardia, sweating, and salivation), as well as an excitation of skeletal muscle. Treatment is with atropine (competitive inhibition) and pralidoxime (regenerates AChE).

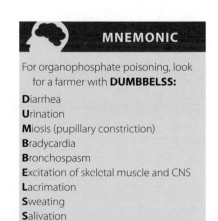

MNEMONIC

For organophosphate poisoning, look for a farmer with **DUMBBELSS:**

Diarrhea
Urination
Miosis (pupillary constriction)
Bradycardia
Bronchospasm
Excitation of skeletal muscle and CNS
Lacrimation
Sweating
Salivation

Anticholinergic (Muscarinic) Drugs

DRUG NAMES

Atropine, scopolamine, benztropine, glycopyrrolate, hyoscyamine, ipratopium, tiotropium, oxybutynin, solifenacin, tolterodine.

MECHANISMS

These drugs competitively block muscarinic ACh receptors and therefore prevent the endogenous neurotransmitter from acting (similar to the way nondepolarizing neuromuscular agents work at the NMJ).

USES

These drugs are primarily used in anesthesiology. However, they have many uses outside of anesthesiology, as they affect many organ systems.

- Glycopyrrolate is commonly used to inhibit oral secretions during intubation in the elderly, or in patients with brain injury, such as cerebral palsy.
- Scopolamine is used to treat motion sickness.
- Benztropine is used in Parkinson disease and acute dystonia.
- Ipratropium and tiotropium act in the respiratory tract and are used to treat COPD and asthma.
- Oxybutynin, solifenacin, and tolterodine act in the genitourinary tract and are used to treat urge incontinence due to cystitis or detrusor instability ("overactive bladder").
- **Atropine** is generally administered for its cardiovascular effects; it is also the first-line treatment for organophosphate poisoning (with pralidoxime):
  - Reversing vagal-stimulated bradycardia.
  - Decreasing respiratory tract secretions.
  - Bronchial smooth muscle relaxation.
  - Reversal of antipsychotic extrapyramidal side effects.

SIDE EFFECTS

- CNS stimulation.
- Cutaneous blood vessel dilation.
- Urinary retention.
- Cycloplegia (paralysis of ciliary muscle of the eye, leading to an inability to accommodate).
- Decreased secretions.
- Constipation.

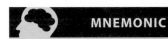

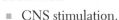

SEAFOOD TOXINS

This section discusses three common seafood toxins. All three are primarily clinical diagnoses based on history and physical exam.

Tetrodotoxin

PATHOGENESIS

Tetrodotoxin is a rapidly acting, highly potent neurotoxin that binds fast voltage-gated Na^+ channels in cardiac and nerve cells, preventing depolarization. Poisoning is most common after eating poorly prepared puffer fish (fugu, a delicacy in Japan) that is contaminated with toxin. Microorganisms associated with puffer fish produce the toxin, which subsequently builds up in the liver and skin of the fish.

CLINICAL MANIFESTATIONS

Symptoms typically begin rapidly after ingestion. GI symptoms include nausea and diarrhea. Neurologic symptoms include weakness, dizziness, hyporeflexia/areflexia, and paresthesias. More severe cases can progress to paralysis, severe hypotension, and death due to respiratory failure.

TREATMENT

Mainly supportive. Gastric lavage and activated charcoal may be used if within 1 hour of ingestion.

Ciguatoxin

PATHOGENESIS

Ciguatoxin is a neurotoxin that opens voltage-gated Na^+ channels, causing depolarization. Poisoning occurs after ingesting contaminated reef fish (eg, amberjack, barracuda, sea bass, grouper, snapper, moray eel). Ciguatoxin is an odorless, tasteless, heat- and acid-stable toxin. Worldwide, it is the most common food poisoning from fish.

CLINICAL MANIFESTATIONS

Symptoms typically begin 3–6 hours after toxin ingestion and mimic cholinergic poisoning. GI symptoms include nausea, vomiting, and diarrhea. Neurologic symptoms include perioral paresthesias, **temperature dysesthesias,** blurry vision, metallic taste in mouth, and a **sense of loose, painful teeth.** Cardiovascular (CV) symptoms include bradycardia, hypotension, and heart block.

TREATMENT

Mainly supportive. Activated charcoal is not warranted, as presentation is usually outside of 1 hour.

Scombroid Poisoning

PATHOGENESIS

Scombroid (histamine) poisoning occurs after ingesting contaminated dark meat fish (eg, tuna, mahi mahi, mackerel, amberjack, and bonito) or Swiss cheese improperly stored at warm temperatures, allowing bacterial overgrowth to occur. Bacterial histidine decarboxylase converts histidine to histamine. Because histamine is the major contributor to symptoms, scombroid poisoning is commonly misdiagnosed as a fish allergy.

CLINICAL MANIFESTATIONS

Patients may complain the fish had a "spicy" or "peppery" taste. Symptoms begin within an hour and mimic an allergic reaction or anaphylaxis. The most common symptoms include urticaria, pruritus, flushing, burning sensation of the mouth, diarrhea, rash, and headache. More severe symptoms (eg, hypotension, bronchospasm, angioedema) are typically in patients with pre-existing asthma or heart disease.

TREATMENT

Mainly supportive, and most cases can be managed with antihistamines. In cases mimicking anaphylaxis, epinephrine is the most important step. Albuterol and glucocorticoids are used if there is respiratory distress.

ANXIOLYTICS AND HYPNOTICS

Both benzodiazepines and barbiturates target $GABA_A$ receptors. Typically, activation of the $GABA_A$ receptor causes a Cl^- ion channel to open, allowing Cl^- to enter and hyperpolarize the cell. With both types of medications, there are concerns about tolerance (decreased responsiveness after repeated doses) and withdrawal (physical dependence; adverse symptoms in absence of medication).

Barbiturates

DRUG NAMES

Phenobarbital, pentobarbital, thiopental, secobarbital.

MECHANISMS

Barbiturates increase the **duration** of Cl⁻ channel opening on $GABA_A$ receptors, resulting in enhanced GABAergic transmission. Barbiturates can block excitatory glutamate receptors in addition to targeting GABA receptors. They also induce CYP-450 microsomal enzymes in the liver so that other drugs that are metabolized by this system are eliminated more quickly.

Phenobarbital is 75% inactivated in the liver and 25% excreted in the urine unchanged.

USES

Barbiturates have many clinical uses. Certain short-acting agents (eg, thiopental, methohexital) are used during anesthesia. Other agents, like phenobarbital, are used as anticonvulsants in the long-term management of tonic-clonic seizures, status epilepticus, and eclampsia. Anxiolytic properties of barbiturates make them applicable for use as mild sedatives that relieve anxiety. Furthermore, clinicians can use barbiturates in the treatment of insomnia but this is typically not recommended because barbiturates suppress REM sleep more than other stages of sleep.

SIDE EFFECTS

- High risk of dependence.
- Synergistic effects with alcohol and benzodiazepines (cross-tolerance).
- Respiratory, cardiovascular, CNS depression sufficient to cause coma and death.
- Induction of cytochrome P450.
- Contraindicated in patients with **acute intermittent porphyria** because barbiturates activate *ALA synthase*, the enzyme that catalyzes the rate-limiting step in heme synthesis.

Treatment of overdose consists of managing symptoms (airway, breathing, circulation [ABCs]) and hemodialysis in severe cases. Alkalinization of urine can aid in the elimination of phenobarbital.

WITHDRAWAL

Barbiturate withdrawal can mimic alcohol withdrawal. The withdrawal syndrome includes:

- Anxiety.
- Irritability.
- Elevated heart rate and respiratory rate.
- Muscle pain.
- Nausea.
- Tremors.
- Hallucinations.
- Confusion.
- Seizures.
- Death is possible if untreated.

Barbiturate withdrawal syndrome is dangerous and must be treated in the hospital. Gradual administration of phenobarbital can be used to treat withdrawal symptoms.

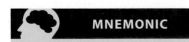

MNEMONIC

Barbi**DURAT**e increases the **DURAT**ion of opening of the $GABA_A$ receptor Cl⁻ channel.

Benzodiazepines

DRUG NAMES

Diazepam, lorazepam, triazolam, temazepam, oxazepam, midazolam, chlordiazepoxide, alprazolam.

MECHANISMS

Increased **frequency** of Cl⁻ channel opening is associated with binding of benzodiazepines on the GABA$_A$ receptor. The entry of Cl⁻ reduces neural excitability by hyperpolarizing the cell, making it more difficult to depolarize. The effects of this class of drugs are terminated through both redistribution and elimination (metabolized by the hepatic microsomal system into active metabolites). Benzodiazepines can cross the placental barrier.

USES

Benzodiazepines have a number of clinical uses. They can be used as anxiolytics (via inhibition of neuronal circuits in the limbic system), as muscle relaxants to treat muscle spasms, as amnesic agents for endoscopic procedures (eg, upper endoscopy, colonoscopy), status epilepticus (lorazepam and diazepam), alcohol withdrawal (lorazepam—important in preventing/treating delirium tremens), night terrors, sleep walking, and as anticonvulsant agents.

SIDE EFFECTS

- Synergistic effects with alcohol and barbiturates (cross-tolerance).
- Respiratory depression and coma (much less than with barbiturates).
- Drowsiness and confusion.
- Tolerance.
- Dependence.

It is possible to reverse the effects of a benzodiazepine with **flumazenil**, a competitive antagonist at the benzodiazepine binding site of the GABA$_A$ receptor. Flumazenil is not effective in treating barbiturate overdose.

WITHDRAWAL

Long-term use of benzodiazepines can lead to tolerance and dependence. Withdrawal is similar to barbiturate withdrawal, but rarely as severe. Signs of benzodiazepine withdrawal include:

- Confusion
- Anxiety
- Agitation
- Restlessness
- Insomnia
- Tension
- Seizures

Opioids

DRUG NAMES

Morphine, hydromorphone, oxymorphone, methadone, meperidine, fentanyl, codeine, hydrocodone, oxycodone, buprenorphine, dextromethorphan, diphenoxylate, loperamide.

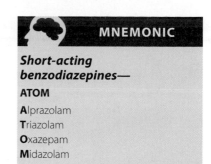

MNEMONIC

Short-acting benzodiazepines—
ATOM
Alprazolam
Triazolam
Oxazepam
Midazolam

KEY FACT

Benzodiazepines decrease latency to sleep onset and increase stage 2 of non-REM sleep. Both REM sleep and slow-wave sleep (stages 3 and 4) are decreased.

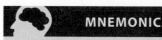

MNEMONIC

Benzodiazepines should be called **FRE**nzodiazepines because they increase the **FRE**quency of Cl⁻ ion entry through the GABA$_A$ receptor.

MECHANISMS

Opioids are analgesics that act on the CNS. Opioids are either endogenous (endorphins, met- and leuenkephalins, and dynorphins) or exogenous (derived from opium or synthetically created). Endogenous endorphins originate from proopiomelanocortin (POMC), which is also the precursor for the formation of adrenocorticotropic hormone (ACTH), melanocyte-stimulating hormone (MSH), and lipotropin (LPH). Synthetic opioids are structurally similar to endogenous opioids, but have been altered to achieve distinct properties. Most opioids provide analgesia by acting as agonists on the μ-opioid receptor, although different formulations have varying strengths (full agonist vs partial or weak agonist). By activating these receptors, the ascending pain pathways are modulated.

USES

Common uses of opioids include local analgesia (eg, regional nerve blocks, epidural nerve blocks, spinal nerve blocks), systemic pain relief (eg, patient-controlled analgesia), and chronic pain management (eg, transdermal patches). They are also used as antitussives (eg, dextromethorphan) and antidiarrheals (eg, loperamide, diphenoxylate). Opioids are frequently substances of abuse for IV drug users (heroin).

SIDE EFFECTS

- Tolerance.
- Dependence (physiologic and psychological).
- Overdose: Treated with the opioid receptor antagonists naloxone or naltrexone.
- Constipation.
- Respiratory and CNS depression.
- Miosis (pupillary constriction).
- Withdrawal: **Piloerection ("goosebumps")**, sweating, fever, rhinorrhea, lacrimation, abdominal cramps, diarrhea, nausea ("flu-like" symptoms), **mydriasis (dilated pupils)**, and **yawning.** Management includes long-term support, as well as methadone and buprenorphine, to prevent full-blown withdrawal in recovering opioid addicts.

Buspirone

MECHANISM

Buspirone is a partial agonist to serotonin 1A (5HT-1A) receptors in the CNS. Because it does not affect GABAergic receptors, it is does not interact with ethanol, nor does it have as profound sedating properties, risk of dependence or tolerance, and associated euphoria as benzodiazepines and barbiturates. Generally takes 1–2 weeks to take effect.

USES

Buspirone is used to treat **generalized anxiety disorder** (see Chapter 7).

SIDE EFFECTS

- May stimulate the locus ceruleus, increasing NE release (causing increased anxiety).
- May not work in patients with a history of benzodiazepine use or severe anxiety.

ANTIDEPRESSANTS

Antidepressants target imbalances in endogenous serotonin, NE, and/or dopamine. Heterocyclic agents (HCAs), selective serotonin reuptake inhibitors (SSRIs), MAO inhibitors, and atypical antidepressants modulate the effects of endogenous neurotransmitters. Extended treatment with antidepressants leads to downregulation of postsynaptic neurotransmitter receptors. There are multiple target receptors; no two antidepressants have the same receptor profile.

Selective Serotonin Reuptake Inhibitors

DRUG NAMES

Citalopram, escitalopram, fluoxetine, paroxetine, sertraline, fluvoxamine.

MECHANISMS

SSRIs are the current first-line treatment for depressive and anxiety disorders. They prevent reuptake of serotonin by the presynaptic terminal, allowing for increased availability of serotonin to the postsynaptic membrane. It can take 3–6 weeks to see a desired effect clinically. Mood is not elevated in nondepressed patients, and mania may be precipitated in patients with bipolar disorder (see Chapter 7). Some SSRIs can be used in pregnant patients and the elderly because they have relatively few side effects.

USES

SSRIs are also used in illnesses other than depressive disorders. They can be used in the specific treatment of panic disorder, generalized anxiety disorder, and obsessive-compulsive disorder. Also, they can be used in the treatment of social anxiety disorder, posttraumatic stress disorder, eating disorders (eg, fluoxetine in bulimia), and trichotillomania (impulsive hair pulling).

SIDE EFFECTS

- Diarrhea.
- Sexual dysfunction (↓ libido, erectile dysfunction, anorgasmia).
- Weight gain.
- Fatigue.
- Discontinuation syndrome (worse with short-acting medications).
- Birth defects (absolute risk is small with all SSRIs, but greatest risk is with paroxetine).
- SIADH in the elderly.
- Serotonin syndrome: Life threatening. Characterized by fever, confusion, myoclonus, hyperthermia, hyperreflexia, flushing, diaphoresis, diarrhea, seizures, and CV collapse. Treat by stopping the serotonergic drugs and giving cyproheptadine (5-HT2 receptor antagonist). Lab values: Increased WBC count, **increased creatine phosphokinase,** decreased serum HCO_3^-. Can develop when used with other drugs that also increase serotonin:
    - SNRIs
    - MAO inhibitors
    - TCAs
    - St. John's Wart
    - Odansetron
    - Fentanyl
    - Meperidine
    - Dextromethorphan

Monoamine Oxidase Inhibitors

DRUG NAMES

Phenelzine, tranylcypromine, isocarboxazid.

MECHANISM

Monoamine oxidase-A (MAO-A) is an enzyme that breaks down NE (see Figure 6-69). Irreversibly inhibiting this breakdown increases the amount of available NE. MAO-A is also responsible for the breakdown of serotonin and tyramine (see Side Effects).

USES

MAO inhibitors are used to treat depressive disorders, including atypical depression (presenting with psychotic, polyphagic, or phobic features). MAO inhibitors are used

KEY FACT

SSRI discontinuation syndrome consists of dizziness, vertigo, nausea, fatigue, headaches, insomnia, shock-like sensations, paresthesias, visual disturbances, muscle pain, chills, irritability, agitation, and suicidal thoughts.

KEY FACT

The most common congenital anomaly associated with SSRI use is ventral septal defect (VSD).

less often since the introduction of SSRIs because of their dangerous interaction with foods containing tyramine (see Side Effects).

SIDE EFFECTS

- Use with tyramine causes potentially fatal side effects and the following symptoms:
    - Hypertensive crisis
    - Diaphoresis
    - Headache
    - Vomiting
- Use with SSRIs can cause **serotonin syndrome.**

Tricyclic Antidepressants

DRUG NAMES

Amitriptyline, imipramine, amoxapine, clomipramine, desipramine, doxepin, nortriptyline, protriptyline.

MECHANISMS

TCAs increase the synaptic concentration of serotonin and NE in the CNS. They achieve this effect by inhibiting serotonin and NE reuptake by the presynaptic terminal, resulting in the availability of more neurotransmitters to bind to postsynaptic neuronal receptors.

USES

TCAs can be used to treat chronic pain, major depression, and anxiety disorders. Historically, TCAs have been used in children for the treatment of enuresis. However, due to the incidence of sudden death, they are not a first-line treatment.

SIDE EFFECTS

- **Constipation**
- **Cardiac arrhythmias**
- **Coma** (overdose potential)
- Sudden death in children (imipramine and desipramine)
- Sedation
- Tremor
- Insomnia
- Orthostatic hypotension
- Psychosis
- Seizures
- Weight gain

Serotonin Norepinephrine Reuptake Inhibitors

DRUG NAMES

Venlafaxine, duloxetine.

MECHANISMS

Both venlafaxine (which is converted to an active metabolite O-desmethylvenlafaxine) and duloxetine work through a similar mechanism to achieve their antidepressant effects. Both medications inhibit the presynaptic reuptake of serotonin > NE.

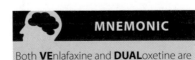

USES

Both drugs are used to treat MDD. Venlafaxine is also used for generalized anxiety disorder, panic disorder, and post-traumatic stress disorder. Duloxetine is used for diabetic peripheral neuropathic pain, chronic musculoskeletal pain, fibromyalgia, and generalized anxiety disorder.

SIDE EFFECTS

- Sedation
- Nausea
- Constipation
- Elevated blood pressure
- Sweating

Nontricyclic Heterocyclic Antidepressants

DRUG NAME

Bupropion.

MECHANISM

Bupropion is a heterocyclic antidepressant that can be used for smoking cessation. Although the mechanism of bupropion is not fully understood, it is generally considered to work by inhibiting the reuptake of dopamine and NE, allowing for increased amounts of both neurotransmitters to bind to their respective receptors in the CNS. This allows the drug to be useful in patients in whom TCAs are not tolerated due to side effects (eg, orthostatic hypotension). Sexual side effects are minimal due to its lack of interaction with serotonin uptake. The mechanism for smoking cessation is also unknown, but it is believed to be mediated by nicotinic ACh receptor antagonism.

USES

Bupropion is a second-line medication used in the treatment of major depression and smoking cessation. They are also used as substitutes in patients who do not tolerate TCAs.

SIDE EFFECTS

- Stimulant effects.
- Tachycardia.
- Insomnia.
- Headaches.
- Seizure risk is greater than with other antidepressant drugs.

Contraindicated in the following conditions:

- Anorexia.
- Bulimia.
- Seizure disorders (lowers seizure threshold).
- MAO inhibitor treatment within the past 2 weeks.

DRUG NAMES

Nefazodone, trazodone, mirtazapine.

MECHANISMS

These medications are serotonin modulators. They block the 5-HT$_2$ receptor and inhibit reuptake of 5-HT and NE. Mirtazapine also antagonizes histaminic H$_1$ receptors and weakly blocks peripheral α_1-adrenergic and muscarinic receptors. Trazodone can antagonize serotonin at low doses and behaves like a serotonin agonist at high doses. In addition to blocking presynaptic serotonin reuptake, trazodone is thought to effect histamine blockade, allowing it to be useful in the treatment of insomnia.

USES

These medications are used to treat major depression and anxiety disorders. In addition, trazodone may be used for insomnia.

SIDE EFFECTS

- Sedation (especially low-dose mirtazapine)
- Increased appetite
- Weight gain
- Dry mouth
- Hepatotoxicity (nefazodone)
- Priapism (trazodone)
- Visual trails (nefazodone)
- Postural hypotension

DRUG NAME

Maprotiline.

MECHANISMS

Maprotiline is a tetracyclic antidepressant that selectively prevents the reuptake of NE. Maprotiline differs from tricyclic antidepressants and other heterocyclic antidepressants in that it does not prevent the reuptake of serotonin.

USES

Maprotiline is used in the treatment of major depression.

SIDE EFFECTS

- Sedation
- Orthostatic hypotension

NEUROLEPTICS

Neuroleptics (classified as first- and second-generation antipsychotics) often block type 2 dopamine receptors (D_2). These drugs are most effective against the positive symptoms of schizophrenia, such as hallucinations and delusions.

First-Generation Antipsychotics

DRUG NAMES

Chlorpromazine and thioridazine (low potency), haloperidol, trifluoperazine, fluphenazine (high potency).

MECHANISMS

First-generation antipsychotics work in the mesolimbic system by blocking postsynaptic D_2 receptors. The low-potency drugs (eg, chlorpromazine, thioridazine) also have an affinity for muscarinic ACh receptors, α-adrenergic receptors, and histaminergic receptors (see side effects). High-potency drugs (eg, haloperidol) have greater affinity for D_2 receptors.

USES

First-generation antipsychotic drugs are useful in the treatment of acute psychosis and schizophrenia as well as in bipolar disorder. Haloperidol can be used in Tourette syndrome (to control tics) and Huntington disease (to combat choreiform movements associated with advanced disease).

SIDE EFFECTS

- Extrapyramidal symptoms, due to dopamine blockade of the nigrostriatal pathway:
- Acute dystonia (hours): Muscle spasm/stiffness; treat with diphenhydramine.

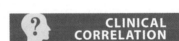

CLINICAL CORRELATION

Antihistamines with significant antimuscarinic effects, such as diphenhydramine, can be used to treat acute dystonic reactions.

- Akathisia (days): Restlessness; treat with β-blockers (eg, propanolol).
- Bradykinesia/parkinsonism (weeks): Treat with benztropine.
- Tardive dyskinesia (months-years): Stereotypic oral-facial movements; irreversible.
- Neuroleptic malignant syndrome: Fever, rigidity, mental status changes, and autonomic instability. Discontinue the drug and treat with dantrolene and dopamine agonists.
- Hyperprolactinemia, due to dopamine blockade in the tuberoinfundibular pathway (dopamine inhibits prolactin release).
- Anticholinergic side effects (low-dose antipsychotics).
- Irreversible retinal pigmentation (thioridazine).
- Corneal and lens deposits (chlorpromazine).
- QT prolongation with possible progression to torsades de pointes.

Second-Generation (Atypical) Antipsychotics

DRUG NAMES

Clozapine, risperidone, olanzapine, quetiapine, ziprasidone, aripiprazole.

MECHANISMS

Atypical antipsychotics have effects on the serotonergic, dopaminergic (with affinity for D_2), and noradrenergic systems. Each medication has a different neuroreceptor profile, accounting for differences in therapeutic action and side effects. Atypical antipsychotics have several advantages over typical antipsychotics. Second-generation antipsychotics are more effective with negative and chronic symptoms of schizophrenia (eg, avolition, alogia, flattened affect). In addition, the risk of tardive dyskinesia, neuroleptic malignant syndrome, and extrapyramidal signs is lower with atypical antipsychotics.

USES

These medications are used to treat schizophrenia, psychosis, bipolar disorder, Tourette syndrome, and for antidepressant augmentation (aripiprazole, quetiapine).

SIDE EFFECTS

- Cardiotoxicity.
- Neuroleptic malignant syndrome.
- Extrapyramidal signs (see previous Side Effects section).
- Agranulocytosis (clozapine): Requires weekly WBC monitoring for the first 6 months.
- Increased chance of seizures.
- Weight gain (clozapine, olanzapine).
- Insulin intolerance, leading to type 2 diabetes (for some second-generation agents, this side effect may be unrelated to weight gain).
- Hyperlipidemia.
- Electrocardiogram abnormalities (prolongation of QT and PR intervals may occur with ziprasidone).
- Increase in prolactin levels (gynecomastia, galactorrhea, and amenorrhea, seen especially with risperidone).

Ziprasidone and aripiprazole have fewer metabolic side effects than do the other second-generation antipsychotics.

MOOD STABILIZERS AND ANTICONVULSANTS

Mood Stabilizers

DRUG NAME

Lithium (Li+).

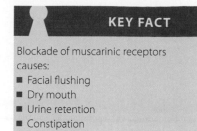

KEY FACT

Blockade of muscarinic receptors causes:
- Facial flushing
- Dry mouth
- Urine retention
- Constipation

Blockade of histamine receptors causes:
- Weight gain
- Sedation
- Orthostatic hypotension
- Tremor
- Sexual dysfunction

KEY FACT

Aripiprazole is a -PRAZOLE that is not a proton pump inhibitor.

MECHANISMS

The exact mechanism of action is unknown. However, Li^+ possibly interferes with the phosphoinositol (IP_3) cascade, depleting CNS inositol, and thus decreasing neurotransmission dependent on inositol.

USES

Lithium is used in the treatment of bipolar disorder and to augment antidepressants in major depressive disorder. The effects of lithium may take 2–3 weeks to manifest, and because of its low therapeutic index, its blood level must be followed and kept to the minimum therapeutic level. Creatinine (renal function), thyroid-stimulating hormone (TSH) (thyroid function), and sodium (hyponatremia increases risk of lithium toxicity) must also be followed regularly.

SIDE EFFECTS

- **Hypothyroidism,** goiter.
- Thirst.
- Tremor.
- Diarrhea.
- Renal dysfunction (**nephrogenic diabetes insipidus** results in increased creatinine and eventual kidney failure).
- Increased appetite and weight gain.
- Cardiac conduction problems.
- Mild cognitive impairment.
- CNS depression (at toxic levels).
- Ebstein anomaly (congenital): Atrialization of the right ventricle (downward displacement of the tricuspid valve).

> **? CLINICAL CORRELATION**
>
> Propranolol is the drug of choice for treating lithium-induced tremor.

Anticonvulsants

Anticonvulsants are agents that suppress uncontrolled neuronal discharge in epileptic seizures. Seizures are characterized as either partial or generalized. Within the category of partial seizures, a patient can have a simple seizure, a complex seizure, or a partial seizure with secondarily generalized tonic-clonic seizure. Within the category of generalized seizures, a patient can have an absence seizure, myoclonic seizure, tonic-clonic seizure, atonic seizure, or status epilepticus. Anticonvulsants inhibit neuronal firing through three different mechanisms to reduce the likelihood that a seizure will occur: (1) increasing GABAergic activity, (2) blocking voltage-activated sodium channels, or (3) blocking voltage-activated calcium channels (see Figures 6-71, 6-72, and 6-73, respectively).

DRUG NAME

Valproic acid.

MECHANISM

Valproic acid, or valproate (its dissociated or ionized form), works via binding to voltage-gated sodium channels and favoring the inactivated state (Figure 6-72). It also has a role in increasing GABA concentration by inhibiting GABA transaminase. Lastly, it decreases Ca^{2+} current in thalamic neurons by acting at T-type Ca^{2+} channels.

USES

Valproic acid is used for the treatment of partial and generalized tonic-clonic seizures, bipolar disorder (mood-stabilizing properties), and intermittent explosive disorder (a behavioral disorder characterized by extreme expression of anger that is disproportionate with inciting cause). Also, it can be used as prophylaxis for migraines and is the second-line treatment for generalized absence seizures after ethosuximide. Use of this drug is decreasing due to the higher number of side effects and its lower efficacy compared with other medications.

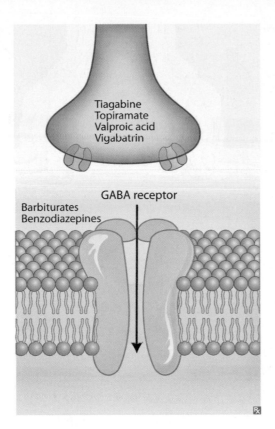

FIGURE 6-71.   **Anticonvulsants that target presynaptic and postsynaptic γ-aminobutyric acid (GABA) and the GABA receptor.** Vigabatrin, valproate, tiagabine, barbiturates, and benzodiazepines all target GABA and its receptor to inhibit central nervous system activity.

Side Effects

- GI upset, with stomach pain, nausea, and diarrhea.
- Increased appetite, leading to weight gain.
- Tremor.
- Sedation.

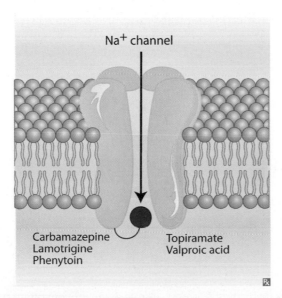

FIGURE 6-72.   **Anticonvulsants that target and extend sodium channel inactivation.** Carbamazepine, phenytoin, topiramate, lamotrigine, valproate, and zonisamide all target voltage-gated sodium channels and aim to prolong their inactivation in the treatment of seizures.

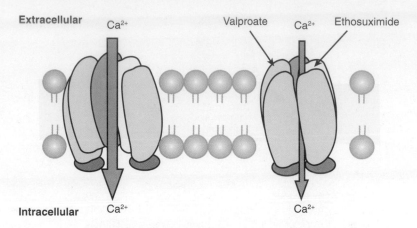

FIGURE 6-73. **Anticonvulsants that target and reduce current through calcium channels.** Only valproate and ethosuximide target and reduce current through T-type calcium channels in the treatment of generalized absence seizures.

- Alopecia.
- Hepatotoxicity.
- Decreased platelet count.
- Possible polycystic ovarian syndrome.
- Congenital neural tube defects (folate antagonist); contraindicated in pregnancy.

DRUG NAME

Ethosuximide.

MECHANISMS

Ethosuximide works by reducing the Ca^{2+} current in thalamic neurons. The thalamus is responsible for the generation of the 3-Hz spike-and-wave rhythms seen in absence seizures. By reducing these T-type currents in the neurons of the thalamus, ethosuximide can stop the rhythmic discharge associated with an absence seizure (see Figure 6-73).

USES

Ethosuximide is the first-line treatment for **absence seizures.**

SIDE EFFECTS

- GI distress
- Lethargy
- Headache
- Urticaria
- Stevens-Johnson syndrome

DRUG NAME

Phenobarbital.

MECHANISMS

A member of the barbiturate drug class, phenobarbital acts on the $GABA_A$ receptor. By doing so, it increases CNS inhibition and raises the seizure threshold (see Figure 6-71).

USES

Phenobarbital has many uses; however, its role as an anticonvulsant includes treatment of partial and generalized tonic-clonic seizures. Side effects limit use in adults. However, it is first-line treatment in neonates for the above-mentioned seizure types.

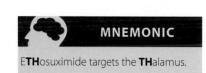

MNEMONIC

ETHosuximide targets the THalamus.

SIDE EFFECTS

- Sedation
- Tolerance
- Dependence
- Induction of cytochrome P450 system

DRUG NAME

Carbamazepine.

MECHANISMS

Carbamazepine reduces the rate of recovery of voltage-activated Na$^+$ channels, blocking the rapid successive firing of action potentials that is classically associated with partial seizures and generalized tonic-clonic seizures (see Figure 6-72).

USES

Carbamazepine is used to treat partial seizures and tonic-clonic seizures (first line) as well as bipolar disorder and **trigeminal neuralgia** (first line).

SIDE EFFECTS

- Aplastic anemia.
- Agranulocytosis.
- SIADH.
- Stevens-Johnson syndrome.
- Hyponatremia.
- Scrotonin syndrome.
- Induces cytochrome P450 enzymes, causing increased metabolism of many drugs, including itself and oral contraceptives.

DRUG NAME

Phenytoin.

MECHANISMS

Like carbamazepine, it acts by slowing the rate of recovery of voltage-activated Na$^+$ channels (see Figure 6-72).

USES

Phenytoin is used to treat all types of partial and generalized seizures (except absence seizures). It is also the first-line treatment for prophylaxis against status epilepticus.

SIDE EFFECTS

Toxicity (at high levels):

- Nystagmus
- Diplopia
- Ataxia
- Sedation
- Gingival hyperplasia
- Megaloblastic anemia
- SLE-like syndrome
- Induction of cytochrome P450
- Fetal hydantoin syndrome: cleft palate, hirsutism, and digital hypoplasia

DRUG NAME

Lamotrigine.

Mechanisms

Lamotrigine blocks voltage-gated Na^+ channels and inhibits glutamate release.

Uses

It is used to treat partial seizures, generalized tonic-clonic seizures, focal epilepsy, Lennox-Gastaut syndrome, and bipolar disorder.

Side Effects

- Skin rash (hypersensitivity reaction).
- Stevens-Johnson syndrome (avoided by increasing the dose very slowly).

Drug Name

Pregabalin.

Mechanisms

Its antinociceptive and antiseizure effects may be due to binding to the α_2-δ subunit of high-voltage-activated Ca^{2+} channels. Pregabalin increases the density of the GABA transporter protein and increases the rate of functional GABA transport. It also decreases presynaptic release of glutamate, NE, and substance P.

Uses

Pregabalin is used to treat neuropathic pain associated with diabetic neuropathy and postherpetic neuralgia and in the adjunctive treatment of partial seizures and fibromyalgia.

Side Effects

- Dizziness
- Somnolence
- Weight gain

Drug Name

Gabapentin.

Mechanisms

Although designed to be a GABA analog, gabapentin does not modulate GABA receptors. It binds avidly to the α_2-δ subunit of high-voltage-activated Ca^{2+} channels, thereby modulating their function. Like pregabalin, gabapentin also acts presynaptically to decrease the release of glutamate.

Uses

Gabapentin is used for sedation as well as to treat partial seizures, pain (including neuropathic), peripheral neuropathy, bipolar disorder, and anxiety.

Side Effects

- Sedation
- Weight gain

TREATMENTS FOR NEURODEGENERATIVE DISEASE

Drugs Used to Treat Alzheimer Disease

The decrease in ACh levels and the increase in the excitatory neurotransmitter glutamate are a notable part of Alzheimer disease. One strategy to manage symptoms of Alzheimer disease is to block the N-methyl-D-aspartate (NMDA) receptors that are activated by excess glutamate. Likewise, since acetylcholinesterase (AChE) breaks down ACh into choline and acetate (see Figure 6-67), blocking the action of AChE may aid in improving cognition. To date, no FDA-approved drug modifies disease progression.

Drug Name

Memantine.

Mechanism

Glutamate is a likely contributor to the development of Alzheimer disease via Ca^{2+} mediated excitotoxicity. At rest, Mg^{2+} is bound to NMDA receptors on neurons, preventing the influx of Ca^{2+}. When glutamate binds the NMDA receptor, the Mg^{2+} is displaced and Ca^{2+} enters the cell. Memantine prevents this influx of Ca^{2+} by noncompetitively inhibiting NMDA receptors. This lowers intracellular Ca^{2+} and spares neurons from further damage.

Uses

Memantine is used to treat moderate to severe Alzheimer disease. It may also have a role in the treatment of vascular dementia.

Side Effects

- Dizziness
- Confusion
- Hallucinations

Drug Names

Donepezil, galantamine, rivastigmine.

Mechanisms

All of these medications are selective inhibitors of AChE in the CNS. By selectively inhibiting AChE in the CNS, levels of ACh increase, which has been shown to improve cognition. The benefits of having centrally acting AChE inhibitors are improved efficacy and decreased peripheral side effects.

Uses

These drugs are generally used in the treatment of Alzheimer disease because they are centrally acting (cross the BBB) unlike other AChE inhibitors used for myasthenia gravis (eg, neostigmine).

Side Effects

- Nausea
- Vomiting
- Diarrhea
- Insomnia
- Urinary incontinence and frequency

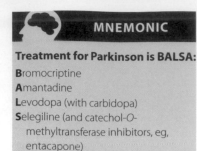

Drugs Used to Treat Parkinson Disease

Parkinson disease is caused by a loss of dopaminergic neurons in the substantia nigra pars compacta, which results in lower levels of dopamine in the CNS. Decreased dopamine manifests clinically with mask-like facies, bradykinesia, resting tremor, muscle rigidity, shuffling gait, and postural instability. Several strategies are used to increase the levels of CNS dopamine: (1) increase endogenous dopamine by preventing its degradation, (2) add an exogenous precursor of dopamine (levodopa) that is converted to dopamine centrally, or (3) give dopamine agonists that directly stimulate D_2 receptors (Figure 6-74).

DRUG NAMES

Bromocriptine, pergolide, ropinirole, pramipexole.

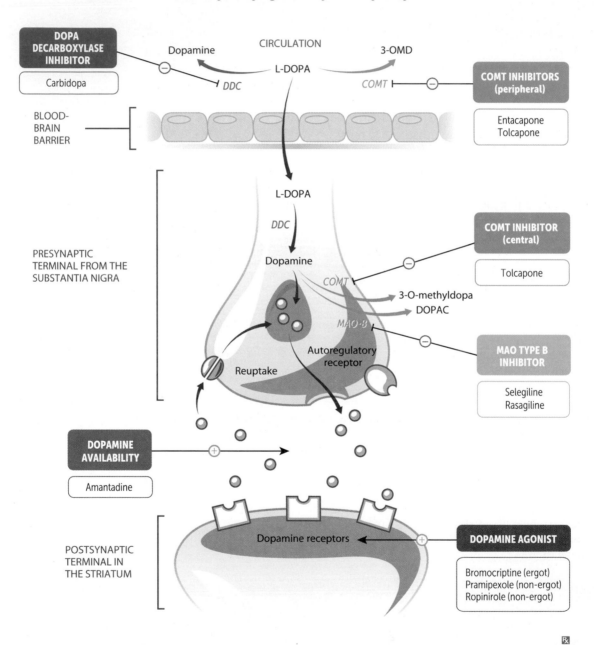

FIGURE 6-74. **Parkinson disease drugs.** 3-OMD, 3-O-methyldopa; COMT, catecholamine O-methyltransferase; DDC, dopa decarboxylase; DOPAC, 3,4-dihydroxyphenylacetic acid.

MECHANISMS

Broadly, these drugs work as dopamine receptor agonists. However, each drug has different effects on the different types of dopamine receptors. For example, pergolide is an agonist of both D_1 and D_2 receptors, ropinirole and pramipexole act only at D_2 receptors, and bromocriptine is a D_2 receptor agonist and D_1 receptor antagonist. Bromocriptine is likely a partial agonist of D_1 receptors in the hypothalamus.

USES

These medications are used to treat Parkinson disease. Bromocriptine can be used to reduce the rate of growth of pituitary adenomas (eg, prolactinoma) and to treat acromegaly. Ropinirole and pramipexole are also used in the treatment of restless leg syndrome. Pergolide is used to treat primary hyperprolactinemia.

SIDE EFFECTS

- Headache.
- Nausea.
- Vomiting.
- Epigastric pain.
- Hypotension/syncope initially, leading to hypertension over time.

DRUG NAME

Levodopa (L-dopa)/carbidopa.

MECHANISMS

Levodopa is a metabolic precursor of dopamine that can cross the BBB. Dopamine itself cannot cross the BBB. Once in the CNS, L-dopa is decarboxylated to dopamine. Levodopa appears in the urine as the metabolites homovanillic acid (HVA) and dihydroxyphenylacetic acid (DOPAC).

USES

First-line medication in the treatment of Parkinson disease. Given with carbidopa (peripheral dopa decarboxylase antagonist) to reduce peripheral conversion of L-dopa to dopamine, which decreases peripheral side effects and increases availability of L-dopa for the CNS.

SIDE EFFECTS

- Nausea and vomiting
- Tachycardia
- Atrial fibrillation
- Dyskinesias
- Depression
- Agitation
- Confusion
- Constipation
- Hallucinations

Levodopa is contraindicated in psychosis and closed-angle glaucoma.

Monoamine Oxidase Inhibitors

Two types of MAO have been distinguished in the nervous system:

- MAO-A) metabolizes NE and serotonin (discussed previously).
- Monoamine oxidase B (MAO-B) metabolizes dopamine.

DRUG NAMES

Selegiline, rasagiline.

MECHANISMS

Selegiline is an irreversible selective inhibitor of MAO-B. MAO-B is found in the striatum and metabolizes dopamine in the brain.

USES

Parkinson disease.

SIDE EFFECTS

Serotonin syndrome (can occur when taken in combination with meperidine, TCAs, or SSRIs).

Catechol-*O*-Methyltransferase Inhibitors

DRUG NAMES

Tolcapone (central and peripheral), entacapone (peripheral).

MECHANISMS

The catechol-O-methyltransferase (COMT) inhibitors tolcapone (central acting) and entacapone (peripheral acting) prolong the action of levodopa by diminishing its central and peripheral metabolism, respectively. Entacapone is preferred to tolcapone (less hepatotoxicity) even though it only has peripheral activity. COMT inhibitors are ineffective if given alone.

USES

Used to increase the levels of levodopa in the treatment of Parkinson disease. Their main indication is in patients with advanced Parkinson disease who prematurely experience motor symptoms due to an end-of-dose effect or "wearing-off" phenomenon.

SIDE EFFECTS

- Dyskinesias
- Nausea
- Confusion

CLINICAL ANESTHETICS AND ANALGESICS

General Anesthetics

General anesthetics are essential to surgery because they cause analgesia, amnesia, and unconsciousness. They also cause muscle relaxation and suppression of reflexes.

Stages of Anesthesia

Four sequential stages:

- Stage 1—Analgesia: "Conscious and conversational."
- Stage 2—Disinhibition: Autonomic variations (changes in blood pressure, heart rate, and respiratory rate).
- Stage 3—Surgical anesthesia: Unconscious with relaxed muscles.
- Stage 4—Medullary depression: Respiratory and vasomotor center depression.

Method of Delivery

Inhaled agents are volatile, halogenated hydrocarbons that were derived from early research and clinical experience with ether and chloroform. On the other hand, IV drugs are typically used for their common property of rapid induction.

Inhaled Anesthetics

Depth of anesthesia can be rapidly altered by changing the inhaled concentration of the drug, making it suitable for maintaining anesthesia. The speed of induction of inhaled anesthetics depends on the alveolar gas and venous blood partial pressures, the solubility of the anesthetic agent in the blood, and the alveolar blood flow. The minimum alveolar concentration, which is very similar to median effective dose (ED_{50}), is equal to the alveolar concentration of an inhaled anesthetic that stops movement in 50% of patients in response to incision.

In order to cross the selectively permeable BBB, drugs must penetrate membrane lipids (lipophilic) or must be actively transported.

DRUG NAMES

Halothane, isoflurane, sevoflurane, desflurane.

MECHANISMS

The mechanism of inhaled anesthetics is poorly understood.

USES

Inhaled anesthetics are used in the maintenance of anesthesia.

SIDE EFFECTS

- Respiratory depression
- Nausea/vomiting
- Hypotension
- Myocardial depression
- Decreased cerebral metabolic demand and O_2 consumption; increased ICP due to increased cerebral blood flow

TOXICITY

- Hepatotoxicity (halothane).
- Nephrotoxicity (methoxyflurane; no longer used in the United States).
- Convulsions (enflurane).
- Expansion of trapped gas in a body cavity (nitrous oxide).
- Malignant hyperthermia: Rare, inherited condition induced by inhaled anesthetics (except nitrous oxide) and succinylcholine; causes fever and severe muscle contractions; treat with dantrolene.

Intravenous Anesthetics

Used to rapidly induce anesthesia, with propofol having the ability to both induce and maintain anesthesia.

TYPES

- Barbiturates
- Benzodiazepines
- Ketamine
- Opiates
- Propofol
- Etomidate

Barbiturates (Thiopental)

Highly lipid-soluble agents that enter the brain rapidly, making them suitable for induction of anesthesia and short surgical procedures. Redistribution from the brain to other

KEY FACT

Drugs with **low** solubility in blood have rapid induction and recovery times. Drugs with **high** solubility in oil or lipids have increased potency. Anesthetics with greater solubility in oil tend to also have greater solubility in blood and vice versa, implying that there is frequently a tradeoff between **potency** and **speed of induction.**

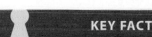

KEY FACT

Dantrolene is used to treat malignant hyperthermia because it interferes with calcium release from the sarcoplasmic reticulum of muscle cells by binding to ryanodine receptors.

tissues causes loss of effects. They are not analgesic and therefore require a supplementary analgesic. IV barbiturates can cause severe hypotension in patients who are hypovolemic or in shock.

Benzodiazepines (Midazolam)

Most common drug used for endoscopy; it is used with inhalational anesthetics and narcotics. Midazolam can cause severe postoperative respiratory depression and amnesia. Treat overdose with flumazenil.

Ketamine (Arylcyclohexylamine)

Acts as a dissociative anesthetic (very high affinity for NMDA receptors). It causes sedation, analgesia, amnesia, immobility, disorientation, bad dreams, and hallucinations. Ketamine is also a cardiovascular stimulant (increases heart rate, BP, and cardiac output) and increases cerebral blood flow.

Opioids (Morphine, Fentanyl, Sufentanil)

Used with other CNS depressants during general anesthesia. Toxicity involves hypotension, respiratory depression, and muscle rigidity.

Propofol

Used for rapid induction of anesthesia and short surgical procedures. An excitatory phase may occur, causing muscle twitching, spontaneous movements, and hiccups. It also can reduce ICP. Propofol is used in the resection of spinal tumors. Since it has much less effect than volatile anesthetics on CNS-evoked potentials, it can be used when assessing spinal cord function.

KEY FACT

Opioids are reversed with naloxone or naltrexone, which antagonize the μ-opioid receptor.

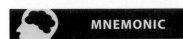

MNEMONIC

B. B. King on **O**piates **PROPO**ses **FO**o**L**ishly:

Barbiturates
Benzodiazepines
Ketamine
Opiates
PROPOFOL

CHAPTER 7

Psychiatry

BASIC DEFINITIONS AND CONCEPTS   534

Defining Psychiatric Illness   534
Classification of Psychiatric Disorders   534
Disorders With Known Biological Causes   536
Transference and Countertransference   536
Psychological Motivators   537
Defense Mechanisms   537
Psychiatric Treatment Approaches   539

PATHOLOGY   539

Cognitive Disorders   539
Schizophrenia and Other Psychotic Disorders   543

Mood Disorders   546
Anxiety Disorders   550
Somatic Symptom and Related Disorders   554
Factitious Disorder and Malingering   557
Dissociative Disorders   558
Personality Disorders   558
Eating Disorders   562
Sleep Disorders   565
Substance Use Disorders   568
Childhood Disorders   577

Basic Definitions and Concepts

The American Psychiatric Association released the *Diagnostic and Statistical Manual of Mental Disorders*, Fifth Edition (DSM-5) in 2013, and this chapter has been updated to reflect DSM-5 changes. However, preclinical students learning the disease processes in psychiatry should not agonize over small differences between DSM versions. The high-yield changes, additions, and deletions in DSM-5 are presented here.

DEFINING PSYCHIATRIC ILLNESS

Mental illness, also called psychiatric illness, is defined by abnormalities in thought, perception, mood, or behavior that deviate from the social norm for an individual's culture and impair social functioning. Although many advances have been made in the diagnosis and treatment of psychiatric illnesses, many patients with psychiatric illness face social stigmatization. This can affect multiple aspects of a patient's life, including relationships, employment, self-perception, and overall quality of life.

As with other areas of medicine, accurate diagnosis of psychiatric illness requires that a patient's subjectively described **symptoms** and objectively observable **signs** be properly identified. Important terms used to describe signs and symptoms of psychiatric illnesses are defined in Table 7-1.

Disordered **thought process, thought content, perception, mood, affect,** and/or **motor activity** are the main hallmarks of psychiatric illness. Refer to Table 7-2 for descriptions and examples of symptoms of disorders within five of these areas. Abnormal mood is discussed in the section on mood disorders.

Observed collections of signs and symptoms that often occur together are grouped into **syndromes.** Specifically recognized syndromes are referred to as **psychiatric disorders. Psychopathology** is the study of mental disorders.

CLASSIFICATION OF PSYCHIATRIC DISORDERS

The DSM-5 is the standard diagnostic text used by American medical and research professionals. Recognizing that our understanding of the etiologies and underlying pathophysiology of many psychiatric disorders is incomplete, the DSM-5 defines mental disorders by a series of inclusion and exclusion criteria.

FLASH FORWARD

Olfactory hallucinations often occur as part of the aura before a seizure.
Visual hallucinations are more commonly associated with medical disorders.
Auditory hallucinations are most consistent with schizophrenia.
Tactile hallucinations are common in delirium tremens (alcohol withdrawal) and in cocaine abusers (during intoxication).

TABLE 7-1. **Important Terminology for Describing Psychiatric Signs and Symptoms**

TERM	DEFINITION
Affect	Outward display of a patient's feelings or emotions, which can be objectively observed. A patient's affect can reflect a normal range of emotions or be flat, blunted, broad, or inappropriate
Mood	Subjective feelings or emotions experienced and expressed by the patient (ie, "How are you feeling today?")
Psychosis	Significant transient or persistent impairment in reality testing (ie, describes transient or persistent distorted perception of reality)
Reality testing	Process of comparing thoughts or ideas to information gathered from the external world
Thought disorder	Abnormal thinking affecting a patient's language, communication, thought content, or thought processes

TABLE 7-2. Definitions and Examples of Symptoms of Disordered Thought, Perception, Affect, Behavior, and Motor Activity

SYMPTOM	DEFINITION	PATIENT EXAMPLE
Disorders of Thought Process		
Thought blocking	Sudden cessation of thought or speech	During an interview, a patient with schizophrenia appears to lose the ability to express thoughts
Short attention span	Inability to complete an act or thought	A man begins to answer a question and rapidly forgets what he is answering
Clang associations	A type of thinking in which the sound of a word, rather than its meaning, provides the impetus for subsequent associations	During a manic episode a woman approaches a man and says, "Hey, man is your name Dan? Plan fans, ban pans!"
Flight of ideas	Rapid succession of thoughts (usually accompanied by rapid and pressured speech); may be difficult to redirect patient back to original topic	While answering a question, a man abruptly and repeatedly switches to unrelated topics
Concrete thinking	One-dimensional thought	A schizophrenic patient interprets a parable in a literal way
Tangential thought	Patient gets lost on an unrelated thought and does not return to the original concept	When asked about his childhood, a man describes riding his bike with friends but soon begins a lengthy recollection of President Kennedy
Circumferential thought	Patient veers from the original idea, but eventually returns to it	When answering a question, a man frequently digresses to related topics before answering the question
Disorders of Thought Content		
Delusions	Fixed, false beliefs that are not shared by the general population. Maintained in spite of proof to the contrary. Can be bizarre (eg, involving supernatural forces) or nonbizarre (eg, fear that organized crime is targeting someone in the family). Specific types of delusion include erotomanic, grandiose, persecutory, referential, and somatic	A man tells his doctor that his landlord is poisoning him with toxic gas
Phobias	Extreme, irrational fear of a situation or an object	A student with agoraphobia becomes extremely anxious when leaving his dorm room
Obsessions	Intrusive and repetitive thoughts	A man believes that his hands remain dirty although he has adequately washed them
Suicidal/homicidal thoughts	Strong desire or preoccupation to kill oneself or others	A patient with schizophrenia plans to kill herself because she fears that she cannot avoid being tortured by her neighbor
Poverty or overabundance of thoughts	Too few or too many ideas	A person does not answer most of a doctor's questions and only speaks one or two words at a time (poverty of thoughts). A person has many different answers to a single question (overabundance of thoughts)

(continues)

TABLE 7-2.   Definitions and Examples of Symptoms of Disordered Thought, Perception, Affect, Behavior, and Motor Activity *(continued)*

SYMPTOM	DEFINITION	PATIENT EXAMPLE
Disorders of Perception		
Illusion	Misperception of real external stimuli	An anxious woman interprets the sound of a door slamming as a shot being fired from a gun
Idea of reference	False belief of being referred to by others	A woman believes that a radio show host is talking about her
Hallucination (visual, auditory, olfactory, tactile, gustatory)	False sensory perception that occurs in absence of actual stimulus	A cocaine abuser feels bugs crawling under his skin (formication, or "cocaine bugs")
Disordered Affect, Behavior, or Motor Activity		
Flat affect	Severe reduction in the range of emotional expression	A patient appears to be staring far into the distance and displays no discernable emotion when describing a traumatic experience
Compulsions	Repetitive behaviors; often associated with temporary relief from obsessive thoughts	After using the bathroom, a man washes his hands five times
Stereotyped movement	Repetitive purposeless movement	A person experiencing amphetamine intoxication repetitively moves her hand in a similar fashion
Hyperactivity (psychomotor agitation)	Increase in activity above a normal level	During a manic episode, a man begins intensely cleaning the entire house
Hypoactivity (psychomotor retardation)	Decreased activity	During a major depressive episode, a woman sits in a chair all day without moving
Catatonia	A syndrome characterized by excited or retarded movement and posturing	A patient with schizophrenia maintains an awkward, rigid pose for hours and ignores all external stimuli

Therefore, DSM-5 provides the field with a consistent classification system and nomenclature that can be used by clinicians and researchers to more effectively communicate patient information and conduct research on mental illness.

All of the disorders described in the DSM-5 are grouped into diagnostic categories, which are organized based on typical age of onset, cause, or common presenting symptoms. Since the DSM-5 is used as the standard for diagnosis of mental disorders in the United States, information about the diagnosis of specific psychopathologic disorders in the following sections is based on the DSM-5 criteria.

DISORDERS WITH KNOWN BIOLOGICAL CAUSES

Many general medical conditions can manifest with signs or symptoms of mental illness. Therefore, to correctly describe a patient's condition it is important to understand the terms **secondary** and **substance-induced** (Table 7-3).

TRANSFERENCE AND COUNTERTRANSFERENCE

During the evaluation and treatment of a psychiatric patient it may be important to understand the concepts of transference and countertransference:

TABLE 7-3. **Classification of Mental Illness With a Known Cause**

TERM	DEFINITION	CLASSIFICATION	EXAMPLE
Secondary	A mental disorder, sign, or symptom that is caused by an identified, specific medical disorder	Classified phenomenologically with related disorders	A mood disorder caused by hypothyroidism is classified in the mood disorders section of the DSM-5
Substance-induced	A sign or symptom of a mental disorder that is primarily the result of substance intoxication or withdrawal	Classified as a substance-related disorder	Psychosis related to LSD intoxication is classified as a substance-related disorder

- **Transference:** A patient unconsciously projects feelings or attitudes from a person or situation in the past onto a person or situation in the present (eg, the patient's physician). For example, a patient may project a parent-like quality onto the doctor and expect that the doctor will provide solutions for all of his problems.
- **Countertransference:** A physician unconsciously projects feelings or attitudes onto the patient. This may be the physician's unconscious response to transference. For example, while treating a patient, a physician may begin to think and act like the patient's parent.

PSYCHOLOGICAL MOTIVATORS

Reporting of symptoms by a patient may be influenced by psychological motivators that can be categorized into primary versus secondary gain. **Primary gain** refers to internal motivations. For example, a patient who is unable to deal with an internal psychological conflict may unconsciously convert the conflict to somatic symptoms (**conversion disorder**). **Secondary gain** refers to external motivators. For example, a patient's disease may allow him/her to garner sympathy or qualify for workers' compensation. The patient may or may not recognize these gains.

DEFENSE MECHANISMS

Defense mechanisms are automatic and unconscious reactions to psychological stress. They function by keeping conflicts out of the conscious mind, thereby helping to alleviate potential anxiety caused by these conflicts. Defense mechanisms can be categorized as immature (includes primitive and neurotic) or mature (Table 7-4). Immature defense

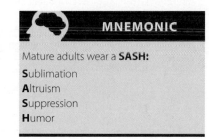

MNEMONIC

Mature adults wear a **SASH:**

Sublimation
Altruism
Suppression
Humor

TABLE 7-4. **Defense Mechanisms**

DEFENSE MECHANISM	CHARACTERISTICS	EXAMPLE
Mature Defense Mechanisms		
Altruism	Negative feelings about oneself are alleviated by helping other people	A Mafia boss makes a large donation to charity
Humor	Focusing on the humorous aspect of an uncomfortable or adverse situation	A nervous patient jokes about an upcoming operation
Sublimation	Replacing a socially unacceptable desire with an action that is similar, but is socially acceptable	A man who has violent thoughts decides to pursue a career as a butcher
Suppression	Voluntarily pushing uncomfortable ideas or feelings out of the conscious mind	A student consciously chooses not to think about upcoming exams until a few days prior to the exams

(continues)

TABLE 7-4. Defense Mechanisms *(continued)*

DEFENSE MECHANISM	CHARACTERISTICS	EXAMPLE
Immature Defense Mechanisms		
Acting out	Unacceptable thoughts or feelings are expressed through attention-seeking actions (ie, bad behavior)	A 16-year-old whose parents are going through a divorce begins to skip classes; a child throwing tantrums
Denial	Refusing to acknowledge the reality of a painful experience or situation	A woman refusing to believe that she was recently diagnosed with cancer
Displacement	Transferring an undesirable or unacceptable idea or feeling for one person onto another person or object	A man who is angry at his boss comes home and yells at his children
Dissociation	Temporary change in memory, personality, or consciousness to avoid emotional stress	A soldier who witnessed the murder of a friend has no memory of the incident
Fixation	Becoming obsessed with and attached to a person, animal, object, or event	An adult avoids obligations by obsessively watching the sports channel
Identification	Unconsciously mimicking the behavior of someone who is often more powerful and/or influential	An abused child grows up to abuse his own children
Intellectualization	Avoiding a distressing situation by focusing on facts and logic rather than emotions	A physician diagnosed with terminal cancer focuses on the pathophysiology of the disease process rather than his emotions
Isolation of affect	Exhibiting a lack of emotion associated with a stressful situation	A woman who witnesses a murder describes the incident in graphic detail with no emotion
Passive aggression	Expressing negativity and performing below expectations as an indirect display of opposition	A disgruntled employee is repeatedly late to work
Projection	Attributing one's own personally unacceptable feeling(s) onto another person	A woman who has desires to cheat on her husband is convinced that her husband is cheating on her
Rationalization	Giving logical reasons for a negative situation in an attempt to convince oneself that the situation is a reasonable one, usually to avoid self blame	A man who did not get the job that he wanted told his friends that it was a good thing because it would have been a very stressful position
Reaction formation	Replacing a personally unacceptable emotion with the opposite attitude	A woman who unconsciously resents her marriage constantly showers her husband with affection and gifts
Regression	Reversion to child-like behaviors. Frequently seen in children during times of stress, such as an illness, punishment, or birth of a new sibling	A 10-year-old boy who recently moved to a new state begins to have enuresis
Repression	A desire is involuntarily excluded from a person's consciousness (versus suppression, which is **intentional** withholding of an idea or desire)	A woman has a phobia of spiders but cannot remember the first time she was afraid of them
Splitting	Labeling people or situations as either purely bad or purely good. Commonly seen in borderline personality disorder	A patient believes that his primary care physician is a terrible person while his therapist is the most wonderful person in the world

mechanisms are developmentally primitive (seen first during early stages of development) and are characterized by the patient reverting back to childlike behavior in response to psychological stress. Although also unconscious reactions, mature defense mechanisms reflect a more developed understanding of the conflict and allow for a healthier approach to reality.

PSYCHIATRIC TREATMENT APPROACHES

Treatment approaches in psychiatry include those that are psychosocial, pharmacologic, or somatic in nature, although several different approaches are often used together to treat a patient's illness. Important examples of specific treatments within these three categories are summarized here and will be mentioned in subsequent sections during the discussion of specific psychiatric disorders.

Psychosocial

Psychosocial treatments include certain forms of psychotherapy, counseling, and social and vocational training. Two important psychosocial treatment approaches are psychodynamic therapy and cognitive behavioral therapy (CBT).

- **Psychodynamic therapy:** A form of psychotherapy that evolved from psychoanalysis. This type of therapy focuses on the unconscious processes that influence a person's thinking and behavior.
- **CBT:** A form of psychotherapy that is based on the idea that a person's thoughts, not the external world, are the basis of his feelings and behaviors. In contrast to psychodynamic therapy, this form of therapy can be shorter in duration and is less centered on the therapeutic relationship between physician and patient.

Pharmacologic

Psychopharmacotherapy involves the use of **psychoactive** medications in the treatment of psychiatric disorders. Important categories of psychiatric drugs include anxiolytics, antipsychotics, antidepressants, and mood stabilizers (Table 7-5).

Somatic

Somatic treatments are a class of psychiatric nonpharmacologic treatment modalities that are centered on a patient's **physical body** rather than her mind. Electroconvulsive therapy (ECT) is a notable example of somatic treatment. In ECT electric currents are passed through the brain. ECT can be effective in treating certain severe psychiatric disorders and is often used for patients who cannot tolerate or have not responded adequately to other treatments.

Pathology

COGNITIVE DISORDERS

Cognitive disorders are categorized into delirium, dementia, and amnestic disorders (Table 7-6). They are the result of central nervous system (CNS) impairment and affect memory, attention, orientation, and judgment. The Mini-Mental State Examination is used to determine the severity of the disorder. This test determines a patient's mental state by testing orientation, registration, attention, recall, language, and calculation.

Delirium

Characterized by a waxing and waning in a patient's level of consciousness **throughout the day.** Patients are easily distracted, disoriented with respect to time and place, have language disturbances, and can experience illusions and hallucinations. Elderly patients often experience symptoms when "sundowning" (delirium worsening at night).

Delirium can be caused by a variety of medical disorders, including infection, trauma, hypoxia, substance withdrawal (eg, alcohol), medications, and toxins (eg, heavy metals). It is commonly seen in **ICUs** and in association with **acute medical illness.**

TABLE 7-5. **Summary of Psychiatric Drugs**

CLASS OF DRUGS	MECHANISM	COMMON/NOTABLE ADVERSE EFFECTS
Anxiolytics		
Benzodiazepines (*short acting:* alprazolam, triazolam, oxazepam, midazolam; *longer acting:* chlordiazepoxide, clonazepam, diazepam, lorazepam)	Potentiate GABA$_A$-mediated inhibition by increasing the **frequency** of Cl$^-$ channel opening	Ataxia, dizziness, somnolence, fatigue, memory difficulties; ↓ **REM sleep; dependence;** additive CNS depression with ETOH. Decreased risk of respiratory depression vs barbiturates. Overdose treated with **flumazenil** (competitive antagonist). Shorter acting have higher addiction potential
Barbiturates (pentobarbital, phenobarbital, secobarbital, thiopental)	Potentiate GABA$_A$-mediated inhibition by increasing the **duration** of Cl$^-$ channel opening	Sedation, **respiratory depression (lethal in overdose),** ataxia, confusion, dependence, dizziness, decreased libido; **contraindicated in porphyria;** additive CNS depression with ETOH; overdose treatment is supportive
Nonbenzodiazepine Hypnotics		
Zolpidem, zaleplon, eszopiclone	Activate BZ1 subtype of GABA receptor	Confusion, ataxia, headaches; moderate amnesia and psychomotor depression. Effects reversed by flumazenil
Nonbenzodiazepine Anxiolytics		
Buspirone	Serotonin 5-HT$_{1A}$ receptor partial agonist	Dizziness, confusion, headache, blurred vision, nervousness; no risk of sedation, addiction, or tolerance; requires 1–2 weeks to take effect; does not interact with ETOH
Antipsychotics		
Typical antipsychotics (**high potency:** haloperidol, fluphenazine, pimozide, trifluoperazine; **low potency:** chlorpromazine, thioridazine)	Antagonize dopamine D$_2$ receptors (increase cAMP)	Parkinsonian symptoms (rigidity, bradykinesia, tremor, masked facies), NMS (hyperthermia, rigidity, autonomic instability, AMS), tardive dyskinesia, anticholinergic symptoms (dry mouth, constipation), hypotension, sedation; can cause QT prolongation
Atypical antipsychotics (risperidone, clozapine, olanzapine, aripiprazole, quetiapine, ziprasidone)	Antagonize dopamine D$_2$, serotonin 5-HT$_{2A}$, α- and H$_1$- receptors	Mild EPS, anticholinergic symptoms, sedation, weight gain, metabolic syndrome, hyperglycemia; can cause QT prolongation; risperidone: most likely atypical to cause EPS; clozapine: agranulocytosis; least likely atypical to cause EPS
Antidepressants		
Selective serotonin reuptake inhibitors (SSRIs: sertraline, paroxetine, fluoxetine, citalopram, escitalopram)	Increase synaptic 5-HT levels by inhibiting presynaptic uptake of 5-HT	Serotonin syndrome (when used concomitantly with an MAO inhibitors, SNRI, or TCA), sexual dysfunction (anorgasmia, decreased libido), GI distress; treatment for serotonin syndrome is **cyproheptadine** (5-HT$_2$ receptor antagonist)
Serotonin-norepinephrine reuptake inhibitors (SNRIs: venlafaxine, duloxetine)	Inhibit 5-HT and NE reuptake at the synapse	**Hypertension,** sweating, weight loss, GI distress, blurred vision, sexual dysfunction (delayed ejaculation, loss of libido, anorgasmia), NMS
Tricyclic antidepressants (TCAs: amitriptyline, nortriptyline, imipramine, desipramine, clomipramine, doxepin, amoxapine)	Inhibit 5-HT and NE reuptake	Heart block (prolongs QT interval), postural hypotension, bloating, constipation, xerostomia, dizziness, somnolence, urinary retention, sedation, tachycardia, dry mouth, **lethal in overdose** Tri-Cs: **C**onvulsions, **C**oma, **C**ardiotoxicity

(continues)

TABLE 7-5. **Summary of Psychiatric Drugs** *(continued)*

CLASS OF DRUGS	MECHANISM	COMMON/NOTABLE ADVERSE EFFECTS
MAO inhibitors (phenelzine, tranylcypromine, isocarboxazid); selegiline (selective MAO-B inhibitor)	Increase 5-HT and NE levels in presynaptic neurons and synapses by inhibiting their breakdown	Hypertensive crisis (with co-ingestion of **tyramine**), serotonin syndrome (with co-ingestion of SSRIs, TCAs, St. John wort, meperidine, or dextromethorphan), dizziness, somnolence, orthostatic hypotension, weight gain
Atypical Antidepressants		
Bupropion	Inhibits presynaptic uptake of NE and dopamine	Tachyarrhythmia, pruritus, sweating, rash, headache, dyspepsia, constipation, dizziness, lowers seizure threshold (contraindicated in anorexia/bulimic patients); no sexual side effects; also used for smoking cessation
Mirtazapine	α_2-Antagonist (increases release of NE and 5-HT) and 5-HT_2 and 5-HT_3 receptor antagonist	Sedation (may be desirable in depressed patients with insomnia), increased appetite, weight gain (may be desirable in elderly or anorexic patients)
Trazodone	5-HT_2 and α_1-adrenergic receptor antagonist	Sedation (commonly used as a sleep aid), nausea, postural hypotension, **priapism**
Mood Stabilizers		
Lithium	Not clearly understood but possible inhibition of phosphoinositol (IP_3) cascade	Acute lithium intoxication (nausea, vomiting, diarrhea, renal failure, ataxia, tremor), bradyarrhythmia, hypotension, hyperkalemia, nephrogenic diabetes insipidus, hypothyroidism, goiter, ECG/EEG abnormalities, leukocytosis, hair loss, psoriasis flares, teratogenic (**Ebstein**), acne, coarse facial features, narrow therapeutic window **First trimester:** Cardiac defects **Second/third trimester:** Goiter, neonatal neuromuscular dysfunction
Lamotrigine	Inhibits neurotransmission by blocking neuronal Na+ channel	**Rash (Stevens-Johnson syndrome,** which can be life threatening, especially in children), ataxia, somnolence, blurred vision
Valproic acid	Affects GABA and NMDA receptors, as well as Na+ and K+ channels	Severe **hepatotoxicity,** nausea, drowsiness, vomiting, pancreatitis; neural tube defects during pregnancy
Stimulants		
Amphetamine, methylphenidate, dextroamphetamine, methamphetamine	Increase catecholamine release from the synaptic terminal, block catecholamine reuptake, weakly inhibit MAO	Hypertension, tachyarrhythmia, restlessness, loss of appetite, addiction potential, dilated pupils, palpitations, diaphoresis, weight loss, psychosis (in overdose)

AMS, altered mental status; cAMP, cyclic adenosine monophosphate; CNS, central nervous system; ECG/EEG, electrocardiogram/electroencephalogram; EPS, extrapyramidal symptoms; ETOH, ethyl alcohol; GABA, γ-aminobutyric acid; HT, hydroxytryptamine; MAO, monoamine oxidase; NE, norepinephrine; NMDA, N-methyl-D-aspartate; NMS, neuroleptic malignant syndrome; QT, ECG interval from beginning of QRS complex to end of T wave.

Symptoms of delirium can last for days or weeks, and if left uncorrected, the condition is associated with a high mortality rate. Correction of the underlying medical disorder resolves the delirium.

DSM-5 Diagnostic Criteria

- Acute change in consciousness.
- Level of consciousness varies throughout the day (ie, waxes and wanes).
- Change in cognition (eg, disorientation, deficits of memory, language disturbance).

KEY FACT

Delirium is more likely to affect the visual system, whereas psychosis is more likely to affect the auditory system.

TABLE 7-6. **Difference Between Delirium and Dementia**

CHARACTERISTIC	DELIRIUM	DEMENTIA
Onset	Acute (from hours to days)	Gradual
Duration	Days to weeks	Months to years (generally irreversible)
Level of consciousness	Fluctuates (varies throughout the day)	Normal (does not change throughout the day)
Symptoms	Fluctuates (worse at night)	Stable but progressive decline over time
Orientation	Impaired	Not impaired in early stages of disease
Memory	Global impairment and dramatic decline in a short period of time	Gradual decline over a longer period of time (recent and remote memory are impaired, but remote memory usually remains more intact than recent memory)
Awareness	Reduced	Normal
Medical status	Usually reversible (after correction of underlying medical disorder)	Most are irreversible (only 15% are reversible if caused by an underlying medical disorder)
Hallucinations	Visual hallucinations common	Hallucinations less common
EEG changes	Present (fast waves/generalized slowing)	None
Causes	Impaired delivery of substrates/blood to the brain, metabolic disturbances, drugs (eg, alcohol, opiates, barbiturates), endocrinopathy (eg, thyroid storm), liver disease, loss of cortical neurons, renal failure, CNS infection, hypoxemia, urinary tract infection, neurosensory disturbance	Alzheimer disease, microvascular disease (vascular dementia), Pick disease/frontotemporal dementia, dementia with Lewy bodies, Huntington disease, Parkinson disease, Creutzfeldt-Jakob disease, normal pressure hydrocephalus

EEG, electroencephalogram.

- Evidence that the change in consciousness is secondary to an underlying medical disorder.

Delirium can be categorized into two groups: quiet and agitated. Patients with quiet delirium may appear depressed.

TREATMENT

- Rule out anticholinergic drug use.
- Correct the underlying medical disorder.
- Pharmacologic therapy: Antipsychotics, benzodiazepines (can also cause delirium; be cautious with their use because they can cause respiratory depression and an increased risk of falls).
- The patient should be placed in a well-lit and quiet environment and in a place where there can be close observation by nurses.
- Constantly reorient patient (eg, tell patient what time it is and where she is).
- Limit the amount of sedation given to the patient (to minimize the amount of napping).

Dementia

Characterized by progressive and usually irreversible impairment of cognitive function and memory. It is a debilitating disorder that affects mainly the elderly. Unlike delirium, the level of consciousness does not vary throughout the day, and the signs and symptoms of dementia generally appear progressively. The incidence increases with age, and 20% of people older than age 80 years suffer from severe dementia. Depression is relatively common in elderly patients and should be ruled out in patients with so-called quiet dementia. The most common causes of dementia include Alzheimer disease (50–60%) and vascular dementia (10–20%).

DIAGNOSIS

The Mini-Mental State Examination is a useful screening test for dementia. A treatable and reversible cause may underlie the symptoms of 15% of patients with dementia. It is important to rule out these treatable causes of dementia. Such causes include depression (pseudodementia), normal pressure hydrocephalus, hypoxia, hypothyroidism, lead toxicity, Lyme disease, meningitis, neurosyphilis, and medications. Malnutrition can cause vitamin B_{12} or thiamine deficiencies, which can manifest with dementia-like symptoms. Folate deficiency is not a malnutrition-related cause of dementia, although emerging evidence suggests that it may be associated with the development of dementia in the elderly. In general, the workup for dementia includes laboratory tests (eg, thyroid-stimulating hormone [TSH] chemistries, HbA_{1c}) and occasionally imaging (eg, head CT without contrast).

TREATMENT

There is no cure for dementia unless it is caused by a treatable medical condition (eg, vitamin B_{12} deficiency, hypothyroidism). Treatment, therefore, usually involves palliative care. Patient and family should be educated, and long-term care should be discussed. In patients with behavioral or emotional symptoms, low-dose antidepressants or neuroleptics can be used. Antipsychotics can be used for paranoia or hallucinations, and benzodiazepines can be used to treat anxiety and agitation.

Amnestic Disorders

These disorders lead to memory impairment without impaired consciousness or other cognitive functions. Like delirium, amnestic disorders are often caused by an underlying medical disorder, including cerebrovascular accident, brain trauma or tumor, hypoxia, hypoglycemia, systemic illnesses, seizures, multiple sclerosis, herpes simplex encephalitis, and substance use (eg, alcohol, medications). Amnestic disorders can be temporary or permanent depending on the underlying cause.

Amnesia can be categorized into two types:

- **Anterograde:** Unable to make new memories and remember things that occur after the CNS insult (eg, alcohol intoxication).
- **Retrograde:** Inability to recall old memories from before the CNS insult. Often seen transiently with electroconvulsive therapy (ECT).

Note that patients may experience a combination of the two types of amnesia. Moreover, a patient may lose only certain classes of memories. For example, a person may be able to remember how to brush his teeth but can't remember his name (procedural vs semantic memory).

TREATMENT

If amnesia is caused by a reversible medical disorder (eg, seizures, hypoglycemia), then the disorder will resolve following treatment of the medical condition. However, when the amnesia is permanent, it is important to discuss the patient's limitations with the patient and his family.

SCHIZOPHRENIA AND OTHER PSYCHOTIC DISORDERS

Psychosis is defined as a distorted perception of reality in which patients experience **delusions, hallucinations,** and **disordered thinking.** Delusions are false beliefs about oneself or others, not shared by other members of society, that persist despite the facts (eg, a patient's thinking aliens are communicating with him or her), and hallucinations are perceptions in the absence of external stimuli (eg, seeing a light that is not actually present). Psychosis can be caused by psychiatric disorders, substance abuse, or medical illness. It is important to note that patients with psychotic symptoms can have intact reality testing despite ongoing hallucinations. For example, a patient might complain of hearing voices but know that it is his psychotic disorder.

Schizophrenia

Largely considered to be one of the most debilitating psychiatric illnesses, schizophrenia is a chronic psychiatric disorder characterized by episodes of psychosis and abnormal behavior lasting **> 6 months.** A specifier was added to DSM-5 to note the presence of catatonia in a patient with schizophrenia. Catatonia can present as profound negativism, motor disturbances with strange posturing, mutism, or incoherent speech; can involve extreme purposeless motion or no motion.

This psychiatric disorder affects about 1% of the population across all ethnic groups and countries studied. Most often, schizophrenia begins to appear in young adults; the age of onset generally ranges from **15 to 25 years in males** and **25 to 35 years in females,** with a slight increase in diagnoses for women during the perimenopausal period. Overall, slightly more men are diagnosed than women (1.4:1). Men with schizophrenia are often less responsive to antipsychotic medications than women and show more social and cognitive deficits.

Genetic factors likely contribute to the development of schizophrenia, as there is an increased rate of diagnosis seen in monozygotic twins relative to dizygotic twins. Three neurologic findings have been associated with some patients:

- Hyperactivity of dopaminergic, serotonergic, and noradrenergic systems; there is also increasing evidence for disordered glutamate utilization.
- Enlargement of the lateral and third ventricles of the brain.
- Abnormalities of the frontal lobes.
- Decreased dendritic branching.

PRESENTATION

Patients demonstrate psychosis and disordered thinking or behavior. These patients generally have normal memory and are oriented to person, place, and time. The symptoms are divided into positive and negative. **Positive symptoms** are thoughts (eg, delusions), sensory perceptions (eg, hallucinations—most often auditory), or behaviors (disorganized speech, disorganized or catatonic behavior) in a person with a psychiatric disorder that are abnormal within the person's culture. **Negative symptoms** are thoughts, sensory perceptions, or behaviors that are present in a normal person but are absent in a patient with mental illness (see following lists of symptoms).

The differences between schizophrenia and type A personality disorders can be subtle and a source of confusion. **Schizotypal personality disorder** is considered part of the spectrum of schizophrenic disorders (Figure 7-1), whereas there is little association between schizophrenia and **schizoid personality disorder.** These disorders are discussed in the personality disorders section. Also, schizophrenia should not be confused with dissociative identity disorder (multiple personality disorder), which is categorized as a dissociative disorder.

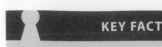

KEY FACT

Diagnostic criteria for psychotic illnesses:
- < 1 month—brief psychotic disorder, usually stress related
- 1–6 months—schizophreniform disorder
- > 6 months—schizophrenia

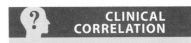

CLINICAL CORRELATION

Frequent cannabis use is associated with psychosis/schizophrenia in teens.

Schizoid	<	Schizotypal	<	Schizophrenia	<	Schizoaffective
Social isolation		Schizoid + odd		Psychotic thinking		Schizophrenia + bipolar or MDD symptoms

Increasing symptoms

FIGURE 7-1. **Keeping "schizo-" straight.** MDD, major depressive disorder.

- **Positive symptoms:**
  - **Delusions:** Can be bizarre (eg, there is an alien living inside the patient's body) or not bizarre (eg, the FBI is secretly investigating his activities). The content of the delusions can be further categorized as ideas of reference, grandiose, paranoid, nihilistic, and erotomanic.
  - **Loose associations:** Patient repeatedly talks about topics completely unrelated to what she was talking about before.
  - **Strange behavior/disorganization.**
  - **Hallucinations:** Typically auditory (40–80%) (eg, hearing voices when no one is really there).
  - Positive symptoms generally respond better than negative symptoms to typical antipsychotics.
- **Negative symptoms:**
  - **Social withdrawal.**
  - **Flat affect:** Patient talks in a monotone voice and does not show any emotion.
  - **Lack of motivation** (avolition).
  - **Thought blocking:** Patient starts talking about a topic but stops in midsentence and is unable to continue with what he was saying.
  - **Poverty of speech** (alogia).
  - Negative symptoms generally respond better to atypical antipsychotics.

DSM-5 Diagnostic Criteria

A diagnosis of schizophrenia requires that **two** or more of the following five symptoms have been present for at least **1 month:**

- Hallucinations
- Delusions
- Disorganized speech
- Disorganized behavior
- Negative symptoms

Furthermore, the following statements must also be true.

- Symptoms cause significant impairment in daily living.
- Symptoms are not due to any other medical condition or substance abuse.

Treatment

Antipsychotic agents (ie, dopamine receptor blockers) and psychosocial interventions (eg, family, individual, and behavioral therapy). Haloperidol decanoate is an example of a long-acting injectable medication that can be useful for noncompliant or poorly compliant psychotic patients. There are long-acting formulations of other antipsychotics as well. The advent of atypical antipsychotics increased the utility of these agents for the treatment of patients with psychotic symptoms because they lack the side effects associated with earlier antipsychotics (Parkinsonism and tardive dyskinesia). Atypical antipsychotics, such as risperidone and clozapine, are combined dopamine and serotonin receptor antagonists.

Prognosis

A continued downward spiral can occur over several years that is associated with frequent treatment noncompliance and recurrent psychotic episodes. Earlier onset of schizophrenia may impair normal brain development and has been shown to indicate a poor prognosis. Better prognosis is highly associated with community support and absence of comorbid substance abuse. Suicide is common, with more than 50% attempting and 10% of those succeeding.

KEY FACT

Schizophrenic patients with predominantly **negative** symptoms have a **poorer** prognosis. Patients with a more rapid onset of illness have a better prognosis.

MNEMONIC

5 A's for negative symptoms of schizophrenia:

flat **A**ffect
Alogia (poverty of speech)
Apathy
Asociality
Attention (impaired concentration)

KEY FACT

Positive symptoms respond well to typical antipsychotics, but negative symptoms respond better to atypical agents.

KEY FACT

If a patient is not oriented or has memory deficits, consider a cognitive disorder (see section on Cognitive Disorders).

Other Psychotic Disorders

Patients presenting with psychosis, delusions, or hallucinations may not meet the diagnostic criteria for schizophrenia, but may in fact be suffering from one of several other psychotic disorders, which include: **brief psychotic disorder, schizophreniform disorder, schizoaffective disorder,** and **substance-induced psychotic disorder** (Table 7-7).

MOOD DISORDERS

Mood is defined as one's internal emotional state, which is affected by internal and external stimuli. Normally, people have some control over their mood, but patients with mood disorders lose this control. Uncontrollable, disruptive emotional states cause significant distress as well as impairment in occupational and social functioning for patients with mood disorders.

There are no ethnic differences in the prevalence of mood disorders. However, due to disparities in health care availability, patients in lower socioeconomic classes often come to the attention of health care providers later and may be misdiagnosed as having schizophrenia. The most common and severe mood disorders are **bipolar disorder** and **major depressive disorder.** The lifetime prevalence for major depressive disorder is about two times higher in women, whereas bipolar disorder is about equal across the sexes.

It is believed that a complex interplay of biological and psychosocial factors leads to the development of a mood disorder. Pathophysiologic changes that are thought to occur in mood disorders include the following:

- Altered neurotransmitter activity.
- Depression is associated with **decreased** levels of serotonin, norepinephrine, and possibly dopamine. Note, however, that simply increasing these neurotransmitter levels in the brain does not show therapeutic utility. Current research suggests that improvements in mood associated with increasing these neurotransmitters pharmacologically or behaviorally result from downstream effects on the cell nucleus and possibly the increased secretion of trophic factors.
- Mania is associated with **increased** norepinephrine levels.
- Limbic-hypothalamic-pituitary-adrenal axis abnormalities.

The major mood disorders are divided into two broad syndromes: bipolar disorder, which is characterized by the presence of at least one manic or hypomanic episode, and major depressive disorder (Table 7-8).

TABLE 7-7.   Characteristics of Other Psychotic Disorders

DISORDER	CHARACTERISTICS
Brief psychotic disorder	Similar symptoms to schizophrenia but lasts **< 1 month** and is often preceded by stressful psychosocial events or factors
Schizophreniform disorder	Same presentation as brief psychotic disorder but psychotic and residual symptoms **last 1–6 months**
Schizoaffective disorder	Schizophrenia with mood disorder symptoms. Lasts **> 2 weeks;** psychotic symptoms with episodic superimposed major depresssion or mania (or both). There must be a period of time in which mood symptoms are absent
Substance-induced psychotic disorder	Related to the use of stimulants, hallucinogens, or withdrawal from sedatives; usually visual or tactile hallucinations and delusions

TABLE 7-8.   Comparison of Mania and Depression

DEPRESSION	MANIA
Sleep disturbances	Decreased need for sleep
Appetite changes	Self-destructive pleasure-seeking activities (eg, sex, drugs, spending, gambling)
Weight changes	Agitation
Reduced libido	Flight of ideas
Fatigue	Pressured speech
Concentration difficulties	Grandiosity
Feeling of worthlessness	Distractible
Suicidal ideation	Increased goal-directed activities

Major Depressive Disorder

With a lifetime prevalence of about 15% (up to 25% in women), major depressive disorder (MDD) is one of the most common and disabling psychiatric illnesses. MDD is two times more common in women during the reproductive years. MDD is characterized by the occurrence of one or more major depressive episodes. It is important to note that a patient who has experienced a manic or hypomanic episode in addition to a major depressive episode should receive a diagnosis of bipolar disorder, not MDD, as treatment with selective serotonin reuptake inhibitor (SSRI) drugs can precipitate mania in a patient with bipolar disorder.

PRESENTATION

Patients with MDD generally present with a history of a sustained, depressed mood with anhedonia (a loss of interest or pleasure in one's typical activities of daily life) and may also exhibit substantial feelings of guilt and worthlessness.

DIAGNOSIS

The diagnosis of MDD is made when a patient has experienced two or more instances of a major depressive episode as specified by the DSM-5 criteria. DSM-5 criteria for a major depressive episode state that a patient must exhibit five or more of the symptoms described in the **"SIG E CAPS"** mnemonic, including either depressed mood or anhedonia for a period longer than ≥ 2 weeks. These symptoms must result in clinically significant distress or impairment in functioning.

In addition to MDD, there are several other distinct depressive disorders with specific features and DSM-5 diagnostic criteria (Table 7-9).

TREATMENT

MDD:

- Pharmacotherapy (ie, SSRIs, tricyclic antidepressants [TCAs], monoamine oxidase [MAO] inhibitors) (Figure 7-2).
- Psychotherapy (ie, CBT).
- ECT can be used when the depression is refractory to other therapies. The patient must be hospitalized if he is at a significant risk for suicide, homicide, or is unable to take care of himself.
  - **Melancholia:** Research suggests that patients with this specific form of MDD may respond well to treatment with antidepressants and ECT.

MNEMONIC

Depressive symptoms are **SIG E CAPS** + depressed mood or anhedonia:

Sleep disturbances (eg, hypersomnia or insomnia; early morning awakenings)
Loss of **I**nterest (ie, anhedonia)
Guilt or feelings of worthlessness
Loss of **E**nergy
Loss of **C**oncentration
Appetite changes/weight changes (usually decreased except in atypical depression)
Psychomotor retardation or agitation (ie, abnormally slow or restless)
Suicidal ideation

KEY FACT

In atypical depression, patients have hypersomnia, weight gain, leaden paralysis (limbs feel weighed down), mood reactivity, and interpersonal rejection sensitivity.

TABLE 7-9.   **Features of Depressive Disorders**

DISORDER	FEATURES
Major depressive disorder (MDD)	Recurrent depressive episodes (two or more), each lasting **> 2 weeks** along with a symptom-free period lasting **at least 2 months**
MDD with melancholic features (melancholia)	Depression with profound anhedonia and dysphoria. Other associated features may include worse mood in the morning, early morning waking, psychomotor abnormality (agitation or retardation), weight loss or decreased appetite, or excessive or inappropriate guilt
MDD with atypical features	Depression that manifests with features that are not considered typical for MDD, including mood reactivity (mood improves in response to positive events), weight gain or increased appetite, hypersomnia, or leaden paralysis. Associated with sensitivity to rejection
Chronic MDD	The criteria for a major depressive episode have been met for **> 2 years**
Postpartum blues	50–85% incidence rate. Characterized by depressed affect, anhedonia, irritability, insomnia, tearfulness, and fatigue starting **2–3 days after delivery** with resolution of symptoms usually within 2 weeks. Treatment is reassurance and support. Follow up is essential, as 20% will progress to depression
Postpartum depression	10–15% incidence rate. Onset is usually within 4 weeks but ranges from **2 weeks to 12 months after delivery.** Characterized by depressed affect, anxiety, feeling inadequate as a mother, poor concentration, decreased libido, suicidal ideation. History of MDD is the biggest risk factor. Diagnostic criteria are the same as for nonpregnant patients. Recurrence rate is high in subsequent deliveries (30–50%). First-line treatment is SSRIs plus CBT
Postpartum psychosis	0.1–0.2% incidence rate. Onset is variable but typically within **4–6 weeks of delivery.** Characterized by mood-congruent delusions, hallucinations, sleep disturbance, emotional lability, and thoughts of harming the baby or self. Risk factors include history of bipolar or psychotic disorder, first pregnancy, family history, recent discontinuation of psychotropic medication. Treatment is hospitalization and initiation of atypical antipsychotic; if insufficient, electroconvulsive therapy (ECT) may be used.
MDD with catatonic features	Patient displays catatonic features similar to those observed in schizophrenia, including posturing, waxy flexibility, catalepsy, negativism, and mutism. Generally observed in patients at the severe and psychotic end of the spectrum of mood disorders
Dysthymic disorder	Mild depression most of the time for **> 2 years** but not meeting the criteria for MDD. These patients cry frequently
Seasonal affective disorder	Depression for at least **2 consecutive years** during the same season and periods of depression are followed by nondepressed seasons

CBT, cognitive behavioral therapy; SSRIs, selective serotonin reuptake inhibitors.

- **MDD with atypical features:** May be difficult to treat and require a combination of medications and psychotherapy. MAO inhibitors have been used successfully for patients with this form of MDD.
- **Chronic MDD:** This condition is generally relatively refractory to existing treatments.
- **Postpartum-onset depression:** Pharmacologic or psychotherapy (or both).
- **Persistent depressive disorder:** The most effective treatment is insight-oriented psychotherapy; however, antidepressants can also be used.
- **Seasonal affective disorder:** Broad-spectrum light therapy, antidepressants, or psychotherapy.

Bipolar Disorder

The second major syndrome of disordered mood is bipolar disorder, which is characterized by the occurrence of at least one manic or hypomanic episode. The lifetime prevalence of bipolar disorder is about 1–3%, and its incidence peaks between the ages of 25

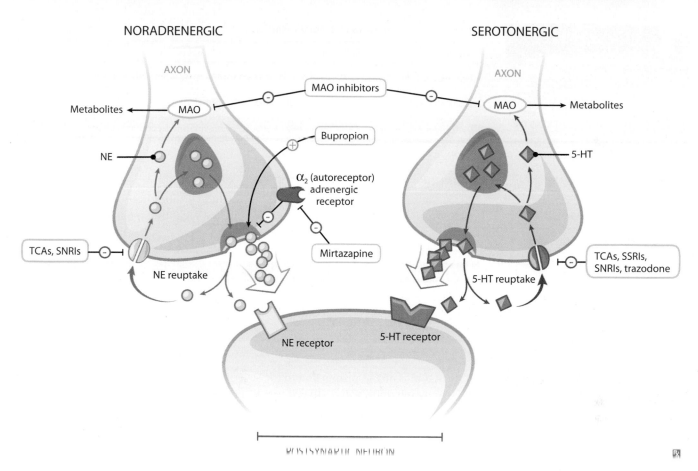

FIGURE 7-2. **Antidepressant and anxlolytic sites of action.** MAO, monoamine oxidase; NE, norepinephrine; SNRIs, serotonin-norepinephrine reuptake inhibitors; SSRIs, selective serotonin reuptake inhibitors; TCAs, tricyclic antidepressants.

and 30. Bipolar disorder affects men and women equally. It is a **strongly** familial disorder—the concordance rate in monozygotic twins is approximately 60%.

PRESENTATION

Patients with bipolar disorder present with a history of a manic or hypomanic episode. A **manic episode** is commonly described as a period during which the patient exhibits an abnormally elevated or irritable mood, rapid speech, hyperactivity, and possibly psychotic symptoms. Note that any episode of increased activity that results in hospitalization is by definition manic. A **hypomanic episode** is similar to a manic episode but is less severe (ie, no hospitalization required), does not cause marked impairment in social or occupational functioning, and is not associated with psychotic symptoms. In either case, the patient typically also experiences periods of depressed mood, although some bipolar patients do not.

DIAGNOSIS

The diagnosis of bipolar disorder is made when a patient has experienced at least one manic (type I) or hypomanic (type II) episode that meets the DSM-5 criteria. The DSM-5 criteria for a manic episode require that a patient experience a period of elevated or irritable mood lasting at least 1 week during which the patient displays three or more of the symptoms described in the "**DIG FAST**" mnemonic. These symptoms must result in clinically significant distress or impairment in functioning.

Features of the bipolar disorders are summarized in Table 7-10.

KEY FACT

ECT can be administered during **pregnancy** in cases of severe depression, catatonia, medication-resistant illness, extremely high suicide risk, or psychosis.

MNEMONIC

Manic symptoms are DIG FAST + excessively elevated or irritable mood:

Distractibility
Insomnia (decreased need for sleep)
Grandiosity
Flight of ideas
Increased **A**ctivity/psychomotor agitation
Pressured **S**peech (nonstop flow of speech)
Thoughtlessness/pleasure seeking/ decreased judgment

TABLE 7-10.   Features of Bipolar Disorders

DISORDER	FEATURES
Bipolar I disorder	Episodes of **mania** and depression. Associated with suicidality
Bipolar II disorder	Episodes of **hypomania** and depression
Cyclothymic disorder	Cyclic mood shifts between dysthymia and hypomania for at least 2 years

TREATMENT

Medications for treatment of these disorders include lithium (a mood stabilizer), anticonvulsants, and antipsychotics (eg, olanzapine). Psychotherapy and ECT have also been shown to be effective in some patients.

ANXIETY DISORDERS

Anxiety is defined as a state of apprehension, terror, and fear in response to an external threat.

Anxiety becomes pathologic when:

- Reaction is **out of proportion** to the severity of the threat.
- Anxiety interferes with daily living.

Collectively, the anxiety disorders—generalized anxiety disorder, posttraumatic stress disorder, panic disorder, phobias, and obsessive-compulsive disorder—are very common (44% combined U.S. lifetime prevalence), although specific phobias and social phobias are roughly twice as prevalent as each of the other anxiety disorders. In general, anxiety disorders are more common in women than in men.

Generalized Anxiety Disorder

Patients with generalized anxiety disorder (GAD) experience excessive anxiety about multiple aspects of their daily lives, unrelated to a specific person, situation, or event, and causes severe impairment of their daily activities. GAD, often described as "free-floating anxiety," has a lifetime prevalence of between 5% and 12%, and affects women more commonly than men (2:1). Two-thirds of patients with GAD have comorbid major depression, and an equally high proportion have an additional anxiety disorder. Typically, symptoms of GAD begin before age 20. Although the cause is not well defined, genetic and psychosocial factors are believed to play a role.

DSM-5 DIAGNOSTIC CRITERIA

- Excessive anxiety about various aspects of life.
- Symptoms have to be present for **more than 6 months** and severely affect daily life.
- The patient is unable to ease the anxiety.
- The anxiety has to be accompanied by at least three of the following:
  - Feeling of being on edge
  - Fatigue
  - Difficulty concentrating
  - Irritability
  - Sleep disturbance (ie, difficulty falling asleep, restless sleep)
  - Muscle tension
  - GI disturbance

TREATMENT

- CBT
- Pharmacotherapy:
    - Benzodiazepines (short-term and low-dose)
    - Buspirone
    - SSRIs
    - Serotonin-norepinephrine reuptake inhibitors (SNRIs): venlafaxine (extended-release)

Patients should be started first on benzodiazepines and then switched to buspirone to avoid dependency; however, the effects of buspirone take 2 weeks to manifest.

Adjustment Disorder

Characterized by emotional or behavioral symptoms that develop in response to a stressor or multiple stressors. Symptoms must **occur within 3 months** of an identifiable stressor and **last no longer than 6 months** after the stressor ends. These symptoms cause significant functional impairment but do not meet the criteria for other DSM-5 psychiatric illnesses. For example, in adjustment disorder with depressed mood, the full criteria for a major depressive episode are not met. The treatment of choice for adjustment disorder is cognitive or psychodynamic psychotherapy.

Posttraumatic Stress Disorder

Posttraumatic stress disorder (PTSD) occurs in individuals who have experienced or witnessed a traumatic situation (eg, war, rape, robbery, serious accident, fire), the memory of which they continue to relive. They commonly avoid anything that reminds them of the experience and may have nightmares or flashbacks. Some patients become emotionally detached and have a restricted affect. PTSD can be preceded by acute stress disorder, which is characterized by anxiety symptoms occurring within 1 month of the trauma and lasting for < 1 month. If the symptoms last **more than 1 month**, then the patient is diagnosed with PTSD. Although almost 90% of patients who have experienced a traumatic event will suffer an acute stress disorder, only about 30% of these patients will go on to manifest PTSD.

KEY FACT

Patients with PTSD are at a greater risk for developing depression and substance abuse.

DSM-5 DIAGNOSTIC CRITERIA

The patient witnessed or experienced a situation in which he felt that his well-being or the well-being of others was threatened, and this experience brought about feelings of extreme fear and helplessness.

- Patient continually relives the experience in one of the following ways:
    - Recurrent and intrusive thoughts.
    - Nightmares.
    - Avoidance of objects or situations that symbolize or resemble an aspect of the traumatic experience.
- The patient goes to great lengths to avoid anything that will trigger the anxiety.
- Emotionally detached/restricted affect.
- Signs of increased arousal (eg, difficulty falling or staying asleep or concentrating; irritability; inappropriate outbursts of anger).
- Daily functioning is severely affected by anxiety.
- Symptoms present for **at least 1 month.**

KEY FACT

If symptoms last between 3 days and 1 month: acute stress disorder.

TREATMENT

- Psychosocial therapy:
    - Exposure therapy (treatment of choice): The patient is gradually exposed to the situation that elicits anxiety and is then taught techniques to ease the anxiety.
    - Relaxation techniques.
    - Support groups.
    - Psychotherapy.

- Pharmacologic therapy:
  - SSRI/SNRI.
  - MAO inhibitor.
  - TCA (imipramine and amitriptyline).
  - Anticonvulsants, prazosin (for nightmares and flashbacks).

Panic Disorder

The defining feature of panic disorder (PD) is unexpected and recurrent episodes (twice or more per week) of panic attacks that develop abruptly and last ~30 minutes (reaching a peak in 10 minutes). There is a strong genetic component; first-degree relatives of patients with PD have a four to eight times greater risk of developing the disorder. Patients with PD have dysregulation of the autonomic nervous system, CNS, and cerebral blood flow. PD is more common in women, with average age of onset of 25 years. The condition is chronic, and attacks can be triggered by psychosocial stressors.

Panic Attacks

PRESENTATION

- Shortness of breath or choking sensation.
- Chest pain/discomfort.
- Palpitations/increased heart rate.
- Sweating, shaking.
- Nausea/abdominal discomfort.
- Feelings of going crazy, losing control, or dying.
- Constantly afraid of having additional attacks.
- Numbness/tingling.
- Chills/hot flashes.
- Light-headedness.
- Depersonalization.

DSM-5 DIAGNOSTIC CRITERIA

Recurrent panic attacks occur in which the trigger is unknown. At least one of the attacks has been followed by **more than 1 month** of at least one of the following:

- Constant worry about having additional attacks.
- Substantial concerns about the implications/consequences of attacks (eg, "going crazy," losing control).
- Impairment of daily functioning due to symptoms. Significant change in behavior related to the attacks, often by avoiding stressors that may precipitate an attack.

The panic attacks must not be due to the direct physiologic effects of a substance or general medical condition (eg, hyperthyroidism or pheochromocytoma) and should not be better accounted for by another mental disorder.

TREATMENT

- **Psychosocial therapy:**
  - Relaxation techniques.
  - CBT (ie, exposure/desensitization therapy).
  - Psychotherapy.
- **Pharmacologic therapy:**
  - Antidepressants: SSRI, TCA, or MAO inhibitor.
  - Benzodiazepines: Short-term use only due to addictive potential and side-effect profile.

Phobias

Social phobia is an extreme fear of social situations in which an individual has to interact with unknown people or is subject to scrutiny by others, thus resulting in embarrassment or humiliation. The lifetime prevalence of social phobia among adults in the United States is 12.1% and occurs with equal incidence in males and females. The most common types of social phobia are public speaking and public washroom use.

Specific phobia is characterized by an extreme and irrational fear of a specific object or situation. Among U.S. adults, specific phobias have the highest 1-year prevalence, although their lifetime prevalence is comparable to or less than that of social phobia, major depressive disorder, and alcohol abuse.

The object or situation that elicits the fear can be placed in one of the following categories:

- Situational (eg, closed spaces)
- Animal/insect/environmental (eg, cats, spiders, heights)
- Other (eg, injections, blood)

Women are twice as likely as men to have specific phobias.

Both social and specific phobias may have a genetic component, as they tend to run in families. Specific phobias may be connected to a traumatic event, and overproduction of adrenergic neurotransmitters may also be a contributing factor.

Agoraphobia is extreme fear of being in a place where escape is difficult. Both PD with and without agoraphobia are more common in women, with average age of onset of 25. The condition is chronic and attacks can be triggered by psychosocial stressors.

> **KEY FACT**
>
> Social phobia is fear of embarrassment in a certain setting, whereas avoidant personality disorder is an overall fear of rejection and sense of inadequacy. Patients can have both disorders concurrently.

DSM-5 Diagnostic Criteria

- **Social phobia:**
  - Intense fear that is triggered by social situations in which the patient might be humiliated or embarrassed.
  - The anxiety response is immediately elicited by the situation.
  - The patient goes to great lengths to avoid the situation.
- **Specific phobia:** Symptoms are similar to those of social phobia, with the exception that intense fear is triggered by a specific object or situation (eg, fear of spiders [arachnophobia]).
- **Agoraphobia:** Great anxiety about being in a situation where escape is difficult in the event of a panic attack. The patient avoids the situation, endures it with great anxiety, or needs someone to accompany him or her. Symptoms cannot be attributed to another mental disorder.

Treatment

- **Social phobia:**
  - SSRI (eg, paroxetine).
  - β-Blockers (for acute situations such as public speaking).
  - CBT.
- **Specific phobia:** CBT (ie, exposure/systematic desensitization).
- **Agoraphobia:** SSRI is first-line treatment.

Obsessive-Compulsive Disorder

Obsessions are persistent and recurrent thoughts that cause great anxiety. The patient realizes that the thoughts are a product of his/her mind and that the response to these thoughts is exaggerated (ie, **ego-dystonic**). Note, that in contrast to obsessive-compulsive disorder (OCD), the symptoms of the cluster C personality disorder known as obsessive-compulsive personality disorder (OCPD) are ego-syntonic. (OCPD is discussed in the section on personality disorders.)

Compulsions are repetitive and inflexible actions that are done by the patient in an attempt to relieve anxiety. The actions are not necessarily logically connected to the anxiety-triggering thoughts (ie, obsessions).

The prevalence of OCD is 2–3%. Females are affected at a slightly higher rate than males in adulthood, although males are more commonly affected in childhood. Studies suggest that OCD is associated with Tourette syndrome and ADHD, and some patients may carry all three diagnoses. Genetics, psychosocial factors, and an imbalance in serotonin levels all contribute to OCD. It is also thought that there is a psychosocial aspect to OCD. In 60% of patients, the symptoms are triggered by a stressful situation. The most common comorbidity in patients with OCD is another anxiety disorder (eg, panic disorder, GAD).

DSM-5 Diagnostic Criteria

- Symptoms of obsession and/or compulsion as defined earlier.
- Symptoms are ego-dystonic.
- Daily living is severely affected by the disorder.

Treatment

- **Cognitive-behavioral therapy:** Exposure and response prevention.
- **Pharmacotherapy:** SSRI (first-line treatment); TCA (clomipramine).

SOMATIC SYMPTOM AND RELATED DISORDERS

These are characterized by physical symptoms that occur in the absence of an identifiable physical pathology and are not being intentionally exhibited by the patient (Table 7-11). These disorders are thought to be unconscious expressions of unacceptable feelings. Although the physical symptoms are brought on by psychosocial factors, patients believe that their symptoms are medical in nature. Primary and secondary gain are associated with the somatic symptoms, but patients are unaware of the gains and do not consciously seek them out. Except for illness anxiety disorder, somatoform disorders are more prevalent in women. It is estimated that 10–30% of primary care visits for somatic complaints may be attributed to somatoform disorders.

TABLE 7-11.   Key Characteristics of Somatic Symptom and Related Disorders

TYPE OF SOMATOFORM DISORDER	KEY CHARACTERISTICS	BUZZWORDS
Somatic symptom disorder	■ Physical symptoms related to multiple organ systems, which cannot be explained by known general medical conditions ■ Numerous visits to the doctor ■ No cure	Multiple organ systems
Conversion disorder	■ Acute onset of neurologic symptoms brought on by a stressor with no identifiable organic cause ■ Patient is not concerned about the condition ■ Tends to recover spontaneously	Neurologic symptoms
Illness anxiety disorder	■ Patient is convinced that he/she has a severe disease ■ Unsatisfied by assurances from her physician ■ Visits many different physicians	Fixed belief that one has severe disease
Body dysmorphic disorder	■ Patient is obsessed about a minor or perceived physical flaw ■ Tries to fix with make-up or repeated plastic surgery, but is usually unsatisfied with the results	Perceived physical imperfection

Somatic Symptom Disorder

Patients have numerous doctor visits complaining of recurrent and multiple physical symptoms that significantly affect their daily lives. Their physical symptoms are related to multiple organ systems but have no underlying organic pathology. It is very important to rule out any medical causes of these complaints while balancing the cost, risk, and possible benefits of diagnostic tests performed. This disorder can be chronic, and potentially lifelong; symptoms can worsen when the patient is exposed to certain stressors.

Females have a 5–20 times greater risk of developing a somatization disorder than males. There is also a greater prevalence of somatization disorder in low socioeconomic groups.

Somatization disorder has a genetic basis, and there is a 30% concordance rate in monozygotic twins. In addition, first-degree female relatives have a greater chance of developing somatization disorder than the general population.

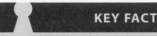

KEY FACT

Half of patients with somatic symptom disorder also suffer from another mental disorder.

DSM-5 Diagnostic Criteria
- At least two GI symptoms.
- At least one neurologic symptom.
- At least one symptom that is sexual or related to the reproductive system.
- At least four pain symptoms.
- Onset before the age of 30 years.
- There is no organic cause of the symptoms.

Treatment

Patients truly believe that there is an organic cause for their symptoms and thus feel the need to see their primary care physician and are resistant to seeing a psychiatrist. As a result, the best way to "treat" such patients is to allow them to see their doctors, but secondary gain should be minimized. Great caution should be used when prescribing medications. Psychotherapy, hypnosis, and relaxation techniques have been shown to be helpful in some patients.

Conversion Disorder

Patients have either sensory or motor symptoms (most often affecting sensory organs of voluntary muscles) that are suggestive of a neurologic deficit but are not consistent with a specific lesion or neurologic disease. Patients may appear to have an inappropriate lack of concern regarding their symptoms (often termed *la belle indifference*). Work-up and physical exam are negative.

Presentation

Neurologic symptoms include:

- Blindness
- Paralysis
- Paresthesias
- Pseudoseizures
- Mutism
- Globus hystericus (ie, feeling of a lump stuck in the throat)
- Seizures
- Speech disturbances

KEY FACT

Levels of serum lactate can be used to differentiate a real seizure from a pseudoseizure: serum lactate is elevated after a seizure but not after a pseudoseizure.

The onset of symptoms is usually brought on by psychological stressors. Unlike somatization disorders, patients with conversion disorder appear to be unconcerned about their condition. Conversion disorder is common, but it affects women two to five times more than men. It is more common in people of low socioeconomic status, uneducated young adults, and in people who "doctor shop." Onset of symptoms can occur at any age but often appear in adolescence or early adulthood.

DSM-5 Diagnostic Criteria

- One or more neurologic symptoms that cannot be explained medically.
- Identifiable psychological stressor that preceded the onset of symptoms.
- Symptoms are not intentional.
- Daily living is severely impaired by symptoms.
- Symptoms are not caused by other mental disorders.

Treatment

Most patients recover without any therapy. However, insight-oriented psychotherapy (ie, education about the diagnosis; first-line therapy), relaxation techniques, and hypnosis have all been shown to be effective in some patients.

Illness Anxiety Disorder

Patients have a constant and exaggerated concern that they have a serious disease. Normal physical findings are misinterpreted by these patients to be signs of severe medical illness. Whereas patients with illness anxiety disorder constantly worry that they *have* a serious illness, some patients with OCD constantly worry that they *will catch* an illness.

Presentation

Patients believe they might be suffering from a serious disease through misinterpretation of normal physical symptoms. They are convinced that they have a serious illness and are not reassured by their doctors. As a result, they visit many different physicians to get different opinions. Symptoms can be exaggerated at times of stress. The average age of onset is 25 years, and both women and men are equally affected.

DSM-5 Diagnostic Criteria

- Constant and exaggerated concern about a serious illness.
- The concern persists despite a normal medical evaluation.
- Symptoms are present for 6 months or more.

Treatment

There is no cure, and patients are often resistant to seeing a psychiatrist. The best way to deal with these patients is to **schedule frequent visits to their primary care doctor.**

Body Dysmorphic Disorder

An obsession with a **perceived** imperfection of a body part. Although the imperfection is minimal or imaginary, patients feel very self-conscious and spend an excessive amount of time trying to correct the perceived imperfection, either through makeup or plastic surgery. Women are more likely than men to develop this disorder. The onset of symptoms usually begins in midadolescence.

DSM-5 Diagnostic Criteria

- Obsession about a perceived flaw of a body part that causes great distress.
- Daily living is severely affected.

Treatment

Although patients use makeup or plastic surgery to correct their perceived imperfection, they are usually not satisfied with the results and continue to be preoccupied with their flaw. Fifty percent of patients respond favorably to SSRIs (fluoxetine).

KEY FACT

Many patients with conversion disorder also suffer from other mental disorders such as depression, anxiety disorders, and schizophrenia.

KEY FACT

Patients with illness anxiety disorder often also suffer from major depression (90%), anxiety disorder (70%), and psychotic disorder (30%).

KEY FACT

- Illness anxiety disorder: patients feel they have a **specific disease.**
- Body dysmorphic disorder: patients feel a **body part** is abnormal.
- Body image disturbance: patients feel their **whole body** is abnormal.

FACTITIOUS DISORDER AND MALINGERING

In DSM-5, these disorders are now grouped as a part of the somatic symptom and related disorders category. In factitious disorder and malingering, a known general medical condition cannot be identified to explain the patient's subjective physical symptoms. However, patients with these disorders consciously mimic physical illnesses for purposes of either primary (factitious disorder) or secondary/external gain (malingering). There are critical distinctions between the somatoform disorders (eg, somatization disorder) and the somatoform-like disorders, which include **factitious disorder, malingering, and specific types of factitious disorders (Munchausen syndrome** and **Munchausen syndrome by proxy)** (Table 7-12).

Factitious Disorder

Patients deliberately (consciously) produce a medical or psychological symptom with the sole purpose of **assuming a sick patient's role** in order to get medical attention. There is **primary (internal) gain** associated with this disorder.

There is a higher incidence in males and in health care workers. The most common symptoms presented include hallucinations, depression, abdominal pain, seizures, and hematuria.

Some patients have a history of child abuse or neglect, which could lead to impaired sexual adjustment and a poor sense of self. As a result, these patients feel the need to play the role of a sick patient to fulfill their need to be in a comforting and safe environment (ie, hospital).

DIAGNOSTIC CRITERIA

Patient presents with a medical or psychological disorder that was deliberately produced with the intention of assuming a sick role. There are no associated monetary or other tangible incentives.

TABLE 7-12. Comparison of Somatoform and Related Disorders

DISORDERS	LEVEL OF AWARENESS	TYPE OF GAIN	CHARACTERISTICS
Somatization	Unaware	Primary and secondary	■ A somatoform disorder. ■ Physical symptoms are brought on by psychosocial factors. ■ Patient truly believes that symptoms have a medical basis.
Factitious	Aware	Primary	■ Not a somatoform disorder. ■ Symptoms are not real. ■ Patient complains of vague symptoms that do not have a medical explanation.
Munchausen syndrome	Aware	Primary	■ A specific type of factitious disorder. ■ Symptoms are not real or are real but intentionally induced. ■ Patients induce symptoms in different ways (eg, take insulin to produce hypoglycemia or add blood to urine).
Munchausen by proxy	Patient is unaware, but the caregiver is aware	Primary	■ A specific type of factious disorder. ■ Symptoms are not real or are real but intentionally induced. ■ Caregivers induce symptoms in different ways (eg, deliberately make a patient sick or appear sick).
Malingering	Aware	Secondary (tangible) gain (eg, monetary)	■ Not a somatoform disorder. ■ Symptoms are not real. ■ Patients pretend to have symptoms (eg, walk around on crutches to mimic an injured leg).

TREATMENT

There is no treatment. Primary care physicians should avoid doing any unnecessary medical procedures and maintain a good relationship with these patients.

Munchausen Syndrome

A chronic form of factitious disorder predominated by physical symptoms. Patients have very specific demands (eg, demanding certain types of medications) and are experienced at producing certain symptoms (eg, taking insulin to achieve a hypoglycemic state; mixing feces in with urine to fake a urinary tract infection). Characterized by a history of multiple hospital admissions and willingness to undergo invasive procedures.

Munchausen Syndrome by Proxy

Another form of factitious disorder in which symptoms are deliberately produced or fabricated in another person (eg, usually a child or elderly person). It is considered to be a form of abuse, though the motivation is often unconscious.

Malingering

Unlike factitious disorders, in which external incentives (eg, monetary gains) are not the primary motivator of the patient's actions, patients who malinger intentionally produce physical or psychological symptoms for secondary (external) gains (eg, avoiding work, obtaining compensation). They often complain of vague symptoms that only improve after they have achieved their desired purpose. Like factitious disorders, it is more common in men than women.

DISSOCIATIVE DISORDERS

Patients have sudden, temporary loss of identity or memory for personal events. These disorders are most commonly seen in women 15–30 years of age. Dissociative disorders are often preceded by a stressful life event. A high proportion of patients with dissociative disorder have a history of trauma or child abuse (Table 7-13).

PERSONALITY DISORDERS

Personality disorders are caused by patterns of enduring, inflexible, and maladaptive personality traits. These disorders cause impaired social or occupational functioning (or both). Patients are often unaware they suffer from a personality disorder (**ego-syntonic**); therefore they do not seek psychiatric help and do not do well in psychotherapy. The pattern of the disorder is usually established by adolescence and is associated with other complications such as violence, depression, psychotic episodes, and suicide. A significant proportion of the general population may meet criteria for one or more personality disorders (10–20%). The prevalence of personality disorders is greater among the psychiatric population; an estimated 50% of inpatients with major depression have a personality disorder. A patient must be > 18 years old to be diagnosed with a personality disorder.

Ten personality disorders are organized into **three personality clusters** (as defined by DSM-5), as summarized in Table 7-14. Note that the cluster B personality disorders generally involve outward expression of traits, whereas patients in cluster A or cluster C have disorders that tend to be inwardly directed. Additional personality disorders that do not fall into one of these traditional clusters are referred to as **personality disorder not otherwise specified (NOS)** and include **passive aggressive personality disorder, sadistic personality disorder,** and **sadomasochistic personality disorder.**

KEY FACT

Malingering is associated with tangible gain (eg, monetary reward), but factitious disorders are associated with psychological gain (ie, feelings that come with being a patient).

MNEMONIC

Schi**zoids avoid** reality, and may daydream or be cold and introverted. Schizo**typals** are odd, magical **types.**

MNEMONIC

Symptoms of borderline personality disorder—
PRAISE

Paranoid ideas
Relationship instability
Abandonment fears, angry outbursts
Impulsiveness
Suicidal gestures
Emptiness

KEY FACT

Patients with antisocial personality disorder commonly have a history of conduct disorder during childhood.

TABLE 7-13. **Key Characteristics of Dissociative Disorders**

DISORDER	DSM-5 CRITERIA	EPIDEMIOLOGY	COURSE	TREATMENT
Dissociative amnesia	■ ≥ 1 episode of inability to recall important personal information regarding a traumatic event ■ Symptoms cause significant impairment in daily living	■ Women > men ■ Adolescents and young adults > the elderly ■ Associated with other mental disorders (eg, major depression) ■ Strongly associated with a history of psychological trauma	■ Most patients regain memory over a period of days ■ Recurrences are uncommon ■ Some patients may present with dissociative fugue, in which they travel to another destination and take on a new identity	■ To prevent recurrence, it is important to help patients recover lost memories ■ Hypnosis and lorazepam are used in the interview to help patients relax and to recover memory ■ Psychotherapy after patient recovers memory
Depersonalization/ derealization disorder	■ Recurrent episodes of feeling detached from body or mind (ie, patients feel like they are observers of their own lives) ■ Patients are aware of symptoms ■ Symptoms cause significant distress	■ Women > men ■ Age of onset: 15–30 years ■ Patients have increased incidence of other mental disorders (eg, major depression)	■ Chronic	■ Treat associated mental disorders (eg, SSRI or antianxiety drugs for major depression or anxiety, respectively)
Dissociative fugue	■ Inability to recall past events, therefore patients are confused about personal identity or assume new identity ■ Patients leave their place of residence and travel to another destination and can take on a new identity (ie, start a new life)	■ Onset preceded by stressful life event ■ Predisposing factors: Substance abuse, mental illness (eg, major depression), head trauma	■ Lasts for a few days to years ■ When patient regains memory of old identity, he or she is unaware of loss of memory	■ A subtype of dissociative amnesia
Dissociative identity disorder (multiple personality disorder)	■ Patient exhibits ≥ 2 distinct identities (with one personality being the dominant one) ■ Identities frequently take control of the patient's life ■ While one personality is in control, patients are unable to recall details of other personalities	■ Women > men ■ Predisposing factors: Childhood abuse, sexual abuse ■ High incidence of other mental disorders (eg, major depression)	■ Patients with earlier age of onset have a poorer prognosis	■ Hypnosis ■ Psychotherapy (insight-oriented)

Cluster A

Patients with cluster A personality disorders avoid social situations and are **unable to develop meaningful relationships.** They do not have psychotic symptoms and are often viewed as weird. Notably, there is a genetic association with schizophrenia. Characteristics of the cluster A personality disorders are presented in Table 7-15.

TABLE 7-14. **Summary of Personality Disorder Clusters**

TYPE	GENERAL CHARACTERISTICS	FAMILIAL ASSOCIATION WITH OTHER DISORDERS	MNEMONIC
Cluster A	"Weird": odd, eccentric	Schizophrenia	**A**ccusatory, **A**loof, **A**wkward
Cluster B	"Wild": dramatic, emotional, erratic	Mood disorders, substance abuse	"**B**ad to the **B**one"
Cluster C	"Worried": anxious, fearful	Anxiety disorders	**C**owardly, **C**ompulsive, **C**lingy

Cluster B

Patients with cluster B personality disorders exhibit emotional lability. They are dramatic, emotional, unstable, and have a higher incidence of substance abuse. They are often seen as "bad" or "wild." Cluster B personality disorders are often familial and have a genetic association with mood disorders. Characteristics of the cluster B personality disorders are presented in Table 7-16.

Cluster C

Patients with cluster C personality disorders appear to be anxious and are fearful. There is a genetic association with anxiety disorders. They are often seen as "worriers." Characteristics of the cluster C personality disorders are presented in Table 7-17.

KEY FACT

Schizoid patients avoid social interaction because they have no desire for such interactions. Avoidant patients desire social interaction, but their extreme fear of social humiliation prevents them from having any kind of social interaction.

TABLE 7-15. **Characteristics of Cluster A Personality Disorders**

TYPE AND EXAMPLE	ETIOLOGY	CLINICAL SYMPTOMS	TREATMENT
Paranoid	▪ Small increased risk in relatives of schizophrenics	▪ Distrustful and suspicious; believe others are plotting to harm or deceive them ▪ Projection is the major defense mechanism ▪ Quick to interpret events or remarks as threatening (sensitive) ▪ Emotionally distant ▪ Differential: Paranoid schizophrenia; paranoid personality disorder patients do not have fixed delusions and are not psychotic	▪ Psychotherapy ▪ Antipsychotics
Schizoid	▪ Increased risk in relatives of patients with schizophrenia and/or cluster A personality disorders ▪ There is a theory that neglectful parenting plays a role	▪ Voluntary social withdrawal—"loners." Does not have nor desire close relationships or sexual encounters. Content with social isolation ▪ Chooses to engage in solitary activities, indifferent to others, avoids personal contact ▪ Flattened affect and emotionally detached ▪ Differential: Paranoid schizophrenia (no fixed delusions in schizoid personality disorder, and no frank psychosis), schizotypal personality disorder (schizoid patients are less eccentric and do not demonstrate magical thinking)	▪ Psychotherapy
Schizotypal	▪ Increased risk in first-degree relatives of schizophrenics	▪ Symptoms similar to schizophrenia but less severe ▪ Odd thought patterns, behavior, and beliefs. Magical thinking (not as severe as schizophrenics), interpersonal awkwardness ▪ Paranoid ideation ▪ Ideas of reference ▪ Inappropriate/constricted affect ▪ Lifetime suicide rate is 10% ▪ Differential: Paranoid schizophrenia (schizotypal patients are not grossly psychotic), schizoid personality disorder (schizotypal patients have more magical thinking and are more eccentric, and schizoid patients avoid people, whereas people avoid schizotypal patients)	▪ Psychotherapy ▪ Low-dose antipsychotics

TABLE 7-16.   Characteristics of Cluster B Personality Disorders

TYPE	ETIOLOGY	CLINICAL SYMPTOMS	TREATMENT
Antisocial	▪ Increased risk in relatives of patients with antisocial personality disorder ▪ Violent, criminal environment leads to greater risk of developing antisocial disorder ▪ Begins in childhood as conduct disorder (eg, fire-setting, animal cruelty, enuresis) ▪ Males > females	▪ Patient must be at least 18 years old to receive diagnosis ▪ Does not conform to societal laws (has criminal behavior) ▪ Disregard for and violation of rights of others ▪ Remorseless, reckless ▪ Deceitful, aggressive, and impulsive ▪ Differential: Drug abuse (important to consider which comes first, because behavior may be attributable to addiction)	▪ Control of behavior (prison or psychiatric hospital) ▪ Psychotherapy ▪ Caution with medications because of high addiction potential in these patients
Borderline	▪ Five times more common in first-degree relatives of borderline patients ▪ Females > males ▪ Increased risk in relatives of alcoholics and patients with mood disorders ▪ Sexual or physical abuse could play a role ▪ Childhood neglect and abuse can be predisposing factors	▪ Forms intense but unstable relationships ▪ Fear of abandonment ▪ Impulsive ▪ Feelings of emptiness or boredom and unstable sense of self ▪ Unable to control anger, impulses ▪ Suicidal gestures (no intent to commit suicide, but may take gestures to dangerous extremes) ▪ Self injury (eg, cutting of arms) ▪ Splitting (ie, alternating between extremes of idealization and devaluation) is the major defense mechanism ▪ Differential: Schizophrenia (borderline patients are not frankly psychotic), mania	▪ Dialectical behavioral therapy ▪ Psychotherapy ▪ Group therapy ▪ CBT ▪ Low-dose antipsychotics or antidepressants (avoid benzodiazepines because of abuse potential) ▪ Medications are more effective in borderline personality disorder than any other personality disorder
Histrionic	▪ Genetic link to antisocial personality and somatic symptom and related disorders	▪ Needs to be the center of attention ▪ Inappropriately seductive and flirtatious (use physical appearance to attract attention) ▪ Considers relationships to be more meaningful than they really are (assumed intimacy) ▪ Unable to maintain intimate relationships ▪ Defense mechanism of regression, an immature defense in which the person returns to an earlier maturational phase in order to avoid conflict ▪ Differential: Borderline personality disorder	▪ Psychotherapy
Narcissistic	▪ Not known	▪ Exaggerated sense of self-worth (grandiosity) and entitlement. Willing to exploit others for personal gain ▪ Arrogant, demands attention ▪ Reacts to criticism with rage ▪ Lack of empathy for others ▪ Low self-esteem underlies outward inflated sense of self ▪ Differential: Antisocial personality disorder (both exploit others, but narcissistic patients want status, whereas antisocial patients want material gain or subjugation of others)	▪ Psychotherapy

TABLE 7-17.   **Characteristics of Cluster C Personality Disorders**

TYPE	ETIOLOGY	CLINICAL SYMPTOMS	TREATMENT
Avoidant	Not known	▪ Extreme fear of humiliation and rejection from others, which leads them to avoid interpersonal contact ▪ Feelings of inadequacy, but desires relationships with others (vs schizoid) ▪ Differential: Schizoid personality disorder (schizoids have no desire for companionship, but avoidants do) ▪ Differential: Social phobia—**situations** are scary because of **embarrassment** vs Avoidant personality disorder—**interpersonal contact** is scary because of **fear of rejection** ▪ Differential: Dependent personality disorder (both cling to relationships; however, avoidant patients are slow to get involved, but dependent patients aggressively seek new relationships)	▪ Psychotherapy ▪ Systematic desensitization ▪ Cognitive therapy ▪ β-Blockers to control anxiety symptoms
Dependent	Not known	▪ Extreme need to be dependent on others for emotional support ▪ Unable to make own decisions (needs advice and assurance from others) ▪ Poor self-confidence ▪ Fear of being deserted or alone ▪ May tolerate abuse by a partner to avoid the situation of being left alone ▪ Differential: Avoidant personality disorder ▪ Differential: Borderline and histrionic personality disorders (all three are dependent on other people, with dependent patients having long-lasting relationships, versus borderline or histrionic patients, who cannot maintain lasting relationships)	▪ Psychotherapy ▪ Assertiveness training ▪ Group therapy ▪ Cognitive therapy
Obsessive-compulsive personality disorder (OCPD)	Not known	▪ Preoccupation with perfectionism and order hinders ability to complete tasks ▪ Devoted to work ▪ Ego-syntonic: Patient views behavior as acceptable to self; as a result, he/she is usually not accepting of change ▪ "Packrat" ▪ Cold and rigid in intimate relationships ▪ Differential: OCD (OCD patients have **recurrent** obsessions or compulsions and are ego-dystonic) ▪ Differential: Narcissistic personality disorder (both are assertive and high achievers, but narcissistic patients are motivated by status, whereas OCPD patients are motivated by work itself)	▪ Psychotherapy ▪ Cognitive therapy

EATING DISORDERS

Patients have a distorted body image and use different methods to try to achieve their perceived ideal body image. The etiology of eating disorders is multifactorial and includes social (eg, cultural/occupational), biological (ie, genetic), and psychosocial (eg, sense of lack of control over aspects of life or history of sexual abuse) factors. Eating disorders are divided into three categories: anorexia nervosa, bulimia nervosa, and binge eating.

Anorexia Nervosa

Characterized by an intense fear of gaining weight and persistent behaviors to prevent weight gain. Patients believe that they are overweight when they are actually dangerously underweight. Anorexic patients restrict their eating or eat in cycles of fasting and binge eating in an attempt to lose weight (Table 7-18).

Anorexic patients are placed into two categories based on their predominant method of achieving weight loss: **restrictive** and **binge eating/purging.** Patients who are restrictive anorexics starve themselves and exercise vigorously. Binge eating/purging anorexic patients binge, then use induced vomiting, laxatives, or diuretics to help them lose

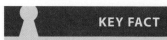
KEY FACT

Anorexic patients have a significantly low body weight, whereas bulimic patients maintain a normal or slightly above normal weight..

TABLE 7-18. **Differences Between Anorexia Nervosa and Bulimia Nervosa**

	ANOREXIA NERVOSA	BULIMIA NERVOSA
Weight	▪ Significantly low body weight	Normal weight or slightly above normal weight
Characteristics	▪ Restrictive type: Starve and exercise vigorously ▪ Binge eating/purging type: Binge then purge or use laxatives/diuretics	▪ Purging type: Similar to binge eating type of anorexia ▪ Nonpurging type: Fast or exercise excessively
Mortality and prognosis	Mortality ~10%	Better prognosis then anorexia nervosa
Ego-dystonic or ego-syntonic	Ego-syntonic	Ego-dystonic

weight. They also exercise excessively. Anorexia nervosa affects 4% of adolescents and young adults, and women are at 10–20 times greater risk than men. Average age of onset is 20 years. Genetics and psychosocial factors both contribute to the development of anorexia nervosa.

DSM-5 Diagnostic Criteria

- Distorted body image.
- Significantly low body weight (< 85% of normal body weight).
- Intense fear of gaining weight.

Associated Mental Disorders

The restrictive type of anorexia nervosa is associated with obsessive-compulsive traits, and many of these patients are socially withdrawn. Major depression and substance abuse are associated with the binge eating/purging type of anorexia nervosa.

Medical Complications

Medical complications that are associated with this disorder include:

- Amenorrhea
- Electrolyte abnormalities (hyperkalemia, hypochloremia, alkalosis)
- Hypercholesterolemia
- Cardiac abnormalities (arrhythmias, cardiac arrest)
- Melanosis coli (due to laxative abuse)
- Leukopenia
- Osteoporosis
- Refeeding syndrome
- Lanugo
- Anemia
- Metatarsal stress fractures

Treatment

If body weight is < 80% of normal body weight, treatment includes inpatient monitoring of weight gain. Behavioral, rehabilitation, and family therapy have also been shown to be beneficial. Anorexia is highly associated with MDD. If anorexia and MDD are both diagnosed in the same patient, antidepressants (usually SSRIs) are also prescribed. Avoid antidepressants, such as bupropion, that lower the seizure threshold (already at risk due to electrolyte abnormalities).

Prognosis

This disorder has a variable course. Some patients have complete recovery, but others have relapses or get progressively worse. Mortality rate is ~10% due to suicide, starvation, or dehydration (resulting in elevated blood urea nitrogen [BUN] and electrolyte imbalances). Additional harmful conditions that can be associated with anorexia include endocrine abnormalities (abnormally low glucose tolerance with fasting hypoglycemia, elevated cortisol levels), osteoporosis, nonspecific ECG abnormalities, and hypothermia.

Bulimia Nervosa

Bulimic patients have a distorted body image but usually maintain normal body weight or may even be slightly overweight. This eating disorder is most common in middle and upper-class white females. Binge episodes are followed by vomiting, excessive exercise, or use of laxatives or diuretics. This behavior occurs weekly for **at least 3 months**. Patients can be categorized into two subtypes: purging and nonpurging. Purging bulimic patients predominantly engage in self-induced vomiting or use of laxatives or diuretics, whereas nonpurging patients exercise excessively or eat little to prevent weight gain. This disorder affects 3% of adolescents and young adults and is more common in women than men. Bulimia nervosa is associated with mood disorders, impulse control disorders, and substance abuse.

PRESENTATION

Medical complications associated with bulimia nervosa include:

- Electrolyte abnormalities (hypokalemic alkalosis and hypochloremia secondary to vomiting).
- Cardiac abnormalities (arrhythmias).
- Dental erosion and reddened knuckles (Russell sign from self-induced vomiting).
- Hypertrophy of parotid salivary gland.

DSM-5 DIAGNOSTIC CRITERIA

- Episodes of binge eating (ie, excessive eating within a 2-hour period associated with a feeling of losing control).
- Binge eating is followed by self-induced vomiting, excessive exercising, or inappropriate use of laxatives or diuretics.
- Symptoms occur at least at least once weekly for 3 months.
- The way in which the patient perceives self is defined by weight.

TREATMENT

Includes psychotherapy (both individual and group), CBT, and antidepressants (SSRI, TCA).

PROGNOSIS

Bulimic patients tend to have better prognoses than anorexic patients. Patients who have onset before age 15 and are able to maintain a healthy body weight for 2 years after onset have better prognoses than patients with later age of onset and those who are hospitalized for their symptoms.

Binge-Eating Disorder

Patients have recurrent episodes of binge eating associated with severe distress. In contrast to anorexia or bulimia, however, these patients do not try to prevent weight gain through excessive exercise, vomiting, or use of laxatives and diuretics. As a result, many patients with this disorder are obese and are thus at risk for obesity-related medical conditions such as hypertension, type 2 diabetes, and cardiac disease.

DSM-5 DIAGNOSTIC CRITERIA

- Recurrent episodes of binge eating that are not associated with other behaviors (eg, excessive exercise).

KEY FACT

Some bulimic patients exhibit the **Russell sign,** which consists of abrasions and scars on the back of the hands due to manual attempts to induce vomiting.

KEY FACT

Bulimic patients are ego-dystonic, unlike anorexic patients, and are thus more likely to want and seek help.

FLASH BACK

Vomiting may lead to hypokalemia, hyponatremia or hypernatremia, and metabolic **alkalosis.** Diarrhea leads to similar electrolyte disturbances as well, but causes metabolic **acidosis.**

KEY FACT

Bupropion is contraindicated in patients with bulimia or anorexia nervosa due to an increased risk of seizures (secondary to electrolyte abnormalities).

- Symptoms are ego-dystonic (eg, patients eat alone because they are ashamed of their eating habits; patients feel guilty and depressed about their behavior).
- Symptoms occur at least once a week for 3 months.
- Three or more of the following symptoms are present:
  - Rapid eating.
  - Eating when not hungry.
  - Consuming an excessive amount of food.
  - Feeling embarrassed or guilty about their behavior; thus, they tend to eat alone.

TREATMENT

- Diet and exercise program
- Psychotherapy
- Psychosocial
  - Behavioral therapy
  - Pharmacologic therapy:
    - Stimulants to suppress appetite
    - Sibutramine to inhibit reuptake of serotonin and norepinephrine

SLEEP DISORDERS

The reticulate-activating system modulates arousal/wakefulness. Sleep disorders are very common and affect approximately one-third of people in the United States. Sleep disorders are classified as either primary or secondary. Secondary sleep disorders are caused by another disorder (eg, mental or medical disorder or substance abuse, see Table 7-19). Primary sleep disorders are not associated with other disorders and are categorized into either dyssomnias or parasomnias.

FLASH BACK

Elevated levels of dopamine or norepinephrine lead to decreased total sleep time.
Melatonin accumulation allows for sleep onset to occur.

TABLE 7-19.   Sleep Disturbances Associated With Psychiatric Disorders*

DISORDER	SLEEP DISTURBANCES
Depression	- Normal sleep onset - Early morning awakenings (ie, waking up before the patient desires) - Decreased REM latency - Increased total REM sleep - Decreased slow-wave sleep - Overall decreased sleep
Bipolar	- Difficulty initiating sleep - Needs less sleep during manic episodes
Anxiety	- Difficulty initiating sleep
Caffeine	- Most common cause of insomnia
Benzodiazepines	- Insomnia (upon discontinuation—withdrawal symptom) - Nightmares and other sleep disturbances, including restless legs syndrome - Nocturnal myoclonus - Hypnagogic hallucinations
Alcohol	- Difficulty initiating sleep; increased arousal and frequent awakenings (associated with withdrawal) - Decrease in sleep quality and associated daytime fatigue (associated with abuse and dependence)

REM, rapid eye movement.

*Including substance abuse disorders.

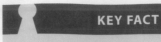
Dyssomnias

Dyssomnias are primary sleep disorders characterized by impairment in the amount, quality, or timing of sleep. Various disorders fall into this category: primary insomnia, primary hypersomnia, narcolepsy, circadian rhythm sleep disorder, and sleep apnea (Table 7-20).

Parasomnias

Parasomnias are also primary sleep disorders characterized by abnormal behavior during the sleep cycle. Disorders that fall into this category include nightmare disorder, sleep terror disorder, and somnambulism (Table 7-21).

TABLE 7-20. Key Characteristics of Dyssomnias

	DIAGNOSIS	EPIDEMIOLOGY/ETIOLOGY	TREATMENT
Primary insomnia	▪ Problems falling asleep and/or staying asleep ▪ Occurs ≥ 3 times/week for at least 1 month	▪ Affects one-third of the population ▪ Anxiety about not getting enough sleep exacerbates the condition	▪ Maintain sleep hygiene (ie, regular sleep schedule, limit caffeine intake, no daytime naps, no alcohol before bed, decrease stimuli in bedroom, avoid light-emitting screens [laptop, television] before bedtime) ▪ Diphenhydramine, zolpidem, zaleplon, trazodone (short term), ramelteon (melatonin agonist), suvorexant (orexin receptor antagonist) ▪ Cognitive behavioral therapy for insomnia (CBT-I)
Primary hypersomnia	▪ Excessive daytime sleepiness or excessive sleep for at least 1 month	▪ Onset often in adolescence	▪ First-line treatment is with amphetamines (stimulants) ▪ SSRIs
Narcolepsy	▪ Primary characteristic is excessive daytime sleepiness ▪ Sudden sleep attacks (repeated) during the day for at least 3 months ▪ Associated with cataplexy (sudden collapse while awake, loss of voluntary muscle tone), short REM latency, sleep paralysis, hypnagogic (while going to sleep) hallucinations are most common, hypnopompic (upon wakening) hallucinations are possible but less common ▪ Immediately go into REM sleep without passing through stages 1–4 ▪ Hypocretin-1 and -2 deficiency on CSF analysis	▪ Uncommon ▪ Onset often during childhood or adolescence ▪ Possible genetic association ▪ Caused by decreased hypocretin (orexin) production in lateral hypothalamus	▪ Scheduled daytime naps ▪ Modafinil is first-line pharmacologic therapy ▪ Amphetamines, methylphenidate (stimulants) ▪ SSRIs or sodium oxalate for cataplexy
Circadian rhythm sleep disorder	▪ Disparity between circadian sleep-wake cycle and environmental sleep demands (eg, jet lag, night shifts)	▪ Seen in frequent travelers, shift workers	▪ Remission, especially in patients suffering from jet lag (in 5–7 days) ▪ Light therapy (for shift workers) ▪ Melatonin (given 5 hours before bedtime)

(continues)

TABLE 7-20. **Key Characteristics of Dyssomnias** *(continued)*

	DIAGNOSIS	EPIDEMIOLOGY/ETIOLOGY	TREATMENT
Sleep apnea	■ Abnormal sleep ventilation (central or obstructive) leading to sleep disruption and subsequently to excessive daytime sleepiness ■ Person stops breathing for at least 10 seconds repeatedly during sleep	■ 10% of population ■ Associated with obesity, pulmonary hypertension, arrhythmias ■ Obstructive sleep apnea (OSA): associated with snoring; seen more commonly in those 40–60 years old; male:female ratio is 8:1 ■ Central sleep apnea: higher incidence in patients with heart failure, alcohol use; more common in the elderly ■ Risk factors for OSA: obesity, tonsillar hypertrophy, hypothyroidism ■ Symptoms: excessive daytime sleepiness, morning headaches, impotence, poor judgment, depression	■ Obstructive: Continuous positive airway pressure (CPAP), surgery (nasal or uvulopalatopharyngoplasty), weight loss ■ Mechanical ventilation

REM, rapid eye movement; SSRIs, selective serotonin reuptake inhibitors.

Other Sleep Disorders

Restless Legs Syndrome

Restless legs syndrome (RLS) is a neurologic disorder characterized by unpleasant sensations in the legs and an uncontrollable urge to move when at rest. The sensations in the legs are often described as burning, creeping, tugging, or like insects crawling inside the legs. The symptoms can begin or worsen during periods of rest or inactivity and are partially or totally relieved by movement. They typically worsen or occur only in the evening or at night and can disturb sleep. Ropinirole, which is used in Parkinson disease, is also approved to treat RLS. There is some evidence to suggest that low iron levels in the brain may play a role.

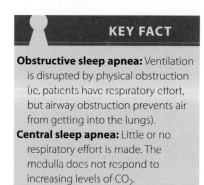

KEY FACT

Obstructive sleep apnea: Ventilation is disrupted by physical obstruction (ie, patients have respiratory effort, but airway obstruction prevents air from getting into the lungs).

Central sleep apnea: Little or no respiratory effort is made. The medulla does not respond to increasing levels of CO_2.

TABLE 7-21. **Key Characteristics of Parasomnias**

	DIAGNOSIS	EPIDEMIOLOGY/ETIOLOGY	TREATMENT
Nightmares	■ Repeatedly being awakened by disturbing dreams and recalling the details of the dream, causing distress ■ Occurs during REM sleep	■ Onset during childhood ■ Increased episodes during times of stress	■ Usually not treated ■ Give TCAs to suppress total REM sleep
Sleep terrors	■ Patients have repeated episodes of extreme frightfulness during sleep ■ Often awaken abruptly with a loud scream, tachycardia, and flushed face ■ Patients have no recollection of these episodes ■ Occurs in stage 3 or 4 of the sleep cycle	■ More frequent in children (boys > girls) ■ Genetic	■ Usually not treated ■ Diazepam at bedtime
Somnambulism (sleepwalking)	■ Patients have repeated episodes of walking during sleep ■ Patients have a blank stare ■ Can be associated with other behaviors (eg, dressing, talking) ■ Patient can be awakened with great difficulty and often is confused when awakened (no recollection of episodes) ■ Episodes occur during stage 3 or 4 of the sleep cycle	■ Onset during childhood (peak at 12 years old) ■ Boys > girls ■ Genetic	■ None

REM, rapid eye movement; TCAs, tricyclic antidepressants.

Nocturnal Myoclonus

Nocturnal myoclonus is also called periodic limb movement disorder. It is a sleep disorder in which the patient moves the limbs involuntarily during sleep and is related to RLS.

This disorder can become worse when taking certain medications such as TCAs and MAO inhibitors. Withdrawal from anticonvulsants, benzodiazepines, and barbiturates can also worsen the symptoms of this disorder. Treatment includes non-ergot-derived dopaminergic drugs.

KEY FACT

Eighty percent of people with restless legs syndrome also have periodic limb movement disorder.

SUBSTANCE USE DISORDERS

DSM-5 no longer uses the terms *substance abuse* and *substance dependence*. Instead, it has replaced these terms with **substance use disorder** (eg, alcohol use disorder, opioid use disorder), which is measured on a continuum from mild to severe based on the number of diagnostic criteria met by an individual.

In general, substance use disorder is diagnosed when the recurrent use of a substance causes clinical and functional impairment, such as health problems, disability, and failure to meet major responsibilities at work, school, or home. According to the DSM-5, a diagnosis of substance use disorder is based on evidence of impaired control, social impairment, risky use, and pharmacologic criteria.

Altered pupillary responses are associated physical signs of substance intoxication or withdrawal and are summarized in Table 7-22.

Substance use disorders are very common and are more prevalent in men than in women.

Depressants

Depressant drugs depress the CNS by increasing the activity of GABA (an inhibitory neurotransmitter). Depressants include **alcohol, barbiturates,** and **benzodiazepines.**

Alcohol Use Disorder

EPIDEMIOLOGY

Approximately two-thirds of U.S. adults consume alcoholic beverages, and it is estimated that up to 10% abuse alcohol. Excessive alcohol use can increase one's risk of developing serious health conditions (eg, hypertension, cardiovascular disease, liver disease, pancreatitis), in addition to those associated with acute intoxication and withdrawal. One study estimated that ethanol intoxication is responsible for over 600,000 emergency department visits each year in the United States.

FLASH BACK

GABA receptors are inhibitory; therefore alcohol, benzodiazepines, and barbiturates have a sedating effect. They also exhibit cross-tolerance (eg, an alcoholic will need a higher dose of benzodiazepines to achieve the same effect as a nonalcoholic).

FLASH BACK

Alcohol → acetaldehyde (via alcohol dehydrogenase).
Acetaldehyde → acetic acid (via aldehyde dehydrogenase—inhibited by disulfiram).
Excess acetaldehyde causes unpleasant "hangover" symptoms, while acetic acid is harmless.

TABLE 7-22.   **Review of Pupillary Response to Substance Intoxication or Withdrawal**

SUBSTANCE	PUPILLARY DILATION	PUPILLARY CONSTRICTION
Amphetamines	Intoxication	Withdrawal
Cocaine	Intoxication	Withdrawal
LSD	Intoxication	
Opioids	Withdrawal	Intoxication **(pinpoint pupils)**
Alcohol	Withdrawal	

PATHOPHYSIOLOGY

Alcohol is primarily absorbed within the stomach of the GI tract and is able to cross the blood-brain barrier to exert its effects on the CNS. Once in the CNS, alcohol potentiates increased Cl^- current through $GABA_A$ channels, which enhances the inhibitory effect of GABA in the brain (Figure 7-3). Alcohol also inhibits glutamate-induced CNS excitation. Long-term alcohol abuse leads to down-regulation of $GABA_A$ receptors (with increased N-methyl-D-aspartate [NMDA] receptors), which can ultimately lead to CNS excitation (withdrawal) upon discontinuation of alcohol.

INTOXICATION

Signs and symptoms of acute alcohol intoxication can include slurred speech, disinhibited behavior, incoordination, unsteady gait, memory impairment, nystagmus, stupor, or coma. Acute alcohol intoxication can also induce multiple metabolic derangements, including hypoglycemia, lactic acidosis, hypokalemia, hypomagnesemia, hypocalcemia, and hypophosphatemia.

DIAGNOSIS

In DSM-5, alcohol use disorder is characterized by a pathologic pattern of alcohol use leading to clinically significant impairment. Alcohol use disorder is believed to arise from a combination of genetic and environmental factors and specific personality traits. It is currently thought that genetic factors are responsible for approximately 50% of the vulnerabilities related to alcohol use disorder.

To be diagnosed with alcohol use disorder, certain DSM-5 diagnostic criteria must be met:

- Recurrent drinking resulting in failure to fulfill role obligations
- Recurrent drinking in dangerous situations
- Continued drinking despite alcohol-related social or interpersonal problems
- Evidence of tolerance
- Evidence of alcohol withdrawal or use of alcohol for relief or to avoid withdrawal
- Drinking in larger amounts or over longer periods than intended
- Persistent desire or unsuccessful attempts to stop or reduce drinking
- Great deal of time spent obtaining, using, or recovering from alcohol
- Important activities given up or reduced because of drinking
- Continued drinking despite knowledge of physical or psychological problems caused by alcohol
- Alcohol craving

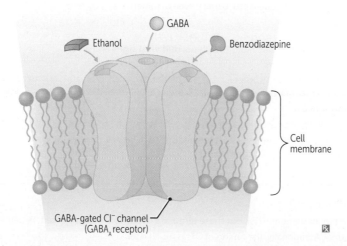

FIGURE 7-3.   **The GABA$_A$ receptor functions as a chloride channel.**

WITHDRAWAL

Signs and symptoms of withdrawal range from tremulousness to hallucinations, seizures, and potentially death. Most symptoms occur between 4 and 72 hours after the last drink or after a reduction in drinking amount and may last up to 5 days (Table 7-23). It's important to keep in mind that alcohol withdrawal is a clinical diagnosis, and its presentation may mimic other life-threatening conditions. As such, it may be necessary to perform extensive testing and imaging to rule out other diagnostic considerations. This is particularly true when the presentation includes altered mental status and fever. Such conditions as infection (eg, meningitis), metabolic derangements, drug overdose, and liver disease can mimic or coexist with alcohol withdrawal.

ALCOHOL WITHDRAWAL TREATMENT

Once the diagnosis of alcohol withdrawal is made, the mainstay of treatment is directed at symptomatic management and correcting metabolic abnormalities:

- Patient should be placed in a **quiet environment;** some may require physical restraints initially.
- **Benzodiazepines** to control psychomotor agitation and prevent withdrawal progression:
  - Intravenous (IV) diazepam, lorazepam, and chlordiazepoxide are frequently used.
  - Patients with advanced cirrhosis or acute alcoholic hepatitis may need shorter-acting benzodiazepines, such as lorazepam or oxazepam.
- **Supportive care:** IV fluids, nutritional supplementation, monitoring vital signs.
  - Thiamine (B_1) and glucose should be given to prevent Wernicke encephalopathy.

Sedative, Hypnotic, Anxiolytic Use Disorder

EPIDEMIOLOGY

Sedatives, hypnotics, and anxiolytics act as CNS depressants. Examples include benzodiazepines (BZDs), barbiturates, and other antianxiety and sleeping medications. At present, BZDs are abused at significantly higher rates than barbiturates.

TABLE 7-23. Alcohol Withdrawal Syndromes

ALCOHOL WITHDRAWAL SYNDROME	SYMPTOMS AND SIGNS	HOURS SINCE LAST DRINK
Mild alcohol withdrawal	Headache, anxiety, tremulousness, insomnia, **autonomic hyperactivity** (sweating, tachycardia, palpitations, variable BP), anorexia, GI upset	6–36
Seizures	Single seizure or multiple generalized tonic-clonic seizures. Usually seen in patients with chronic alcoholism	12–48
Alcoholic hallucinosis	Visual (most common), auditory, and/or tactile hallucinations with **normal vital signs** and **intact sensorium**	12–24
Delirium tremens (DTs)	Generalized tonic-clonic seizures, hyperthermia, hypertension, tachycardia, hyperventilation,* diaphoresis, hallucinations, **disorientation**** Death can result if not properly treated (carries ~5% mortality rate) Hypomagnesemia and hypophosphatemia are common and may predispose to cardiac dysrhythmias and rhabdomyolysis, respectively Symptoms can last up to 5 days	48–96

*Hyperventilation → respiratory alkalosis → decreased cerebral blood flow.

**Many students initially equate alcoholic hallucinosis and delirium tremens (DTs), but these terms are not synonymous. Unlike DTs, sensorium is intact in alcoholic hallucinosis and vital signs are usually normal. Additionally, the timing of DTs is much later.

PATHOPHYSIOLOGY

BZDs are used for sedation and to treat anxiety, seizures, withdrawal states (eg, alcohol), and drug-associated agitation. BZDs exert their effects through binding and modulation of the $GABA_A$ receptor, whereby they potentiate its inhibitory action through increasing Cl^- flux (**membrane hyperpolarization**). BZDs are commonly divided into three groups based on half-life duration: short-acting (half-life < 12 hours), intermediate-acting (half-life 12–24 hours), and long-acting (half-life > 24 hours).

INTOXICATION

Oral BZDs taken in excess without a co-ingestant rarely cause clinically significant toxicity. The classic presentation of a patient with an isolated BZD overdose consists of depressed mental status, slurred speech, and ataxia, with *normal vital signs*. However, severe overdose can cause respiratory depression and stupor/coma. Co-ingestants are common in cases of overdose, the most common being alcohol. Barbiturates have a higher rate of respiratory depression than BZDs.

INTOXICATION TREATMENT

In general, isolated BZD overdose can be treated with symptomatic management and close monitoring. **Flumazenil** is a nonspecific competitive antagonist of the BZD receptor that has been historically used to reverse BZD-induced toxicity. However, administration of flumazenil is not without risks, as it can occasionally precipitate withdrawal seizures. It is also inconsistent in reversing BZD-induced respiratory depression. **Sodium bicarbonate** (weak base) can be given to increase renal excretion of barbiturates (weak acid).

DIAGNOSIS

The new diagnosis requires at least two of the following criteria:

- Continuing to use a substance, in this case a barbiturate, benzodiazepine, or other sedative-hypnotic, despite negative personal consequences
- Repeated inability to carry out major functions at work, school, or home on account of use
- Recurrent use in physically hazardous situations
- Continued use despite recurrent or persistent social or interpersonal problems caused or made worse by use
- Tolerance, as manifested by needing a markedly increased dose to achieve intoxication or desired effect, or by markedly diminished effect with continued use of the same amount
- Withdrawal with the characteristic syndrome, or use of the drug to avoid withdrawal
- Using more of the drug or using for a longer period than intended
- Persistent desire to cut down use, or unsuccessful attempts to control use
- Spending a lot of time obtaining or using the substance, or recovering from use
- Stopping or reducing important occupational, social, or recreational activities owing to use
- Craving or strong desire to use

WITHDRAWAL

Abrupt cessation or drastic reduction in BZD dose in a chronic user can result in clinical withdrawal. The withdrawal syndrome is potentially life threatening, and therefore it is crucial to recognize the signs and symptoms early. Symptoms and signs can include anxiety, tremors, psychomotor agitation, perceptual disturbances, convulsions, dysphoria, and psychosis. Withdrawal can usually be avoided or minimized through the use of BZDs with long half-lives (eg, diazepam, chlordiazepoxide) and/or gradual tapering of the patient's BZD dose over several months. Although many medications have been trialed to treat BZD withdrawal, longer-acting BZDs (eg, diazepam) have proven superior and are the current standard of care.

Stimulants

Stimulants including cocaine, amphetamine, caffeine, and nicotine activate the CNS by increasing the concentration of dopamine. Caffeine and nicotine are the two most commonly abused stimulants.

Cocaine Use Disorder

EPIDEMIOLOGY

Cocaine is an alkaloid extract derived from the leaves of the coca plant and was first used as a local anesthetic in eye surgery. Despite its storied history, cocaine is a common and dangerous drug of abuse that is associated with numerous detrimental health effects.

PATHOPHYSIOLOGY

Cocaine primarily works as an indirect sympathomimetic agent by blocking the reuptake of dopamine, in addition to serotonin, in the synaptic cleft. Cocaine also works by blocking Na^+ channels in neurons, allowing it to serve as a local anesthetic.

DIAGNOSIS

The diagnostic criteria for a substance use disorder were previously described. These criteria apply to cocaine use disorder.

Amphetamines

Stimulants structurally related to catecholamine neurotransmitters can be classified into two groups: classic and substituted (designer). Classic amphetamines (eg, dextroamphetamine, methylphenidate, methamphetamine) stimulate dopamine, NE, and serotonin (5-HT) release at the presynaptic terminal and are used in the treatment of attention deficit/hyperactivity disorder (ADHD) and narcolepsy. Designer amphetamines (methylenedioxymethamphetamine [MDMA, or "ecstasy"] and methylenedioxyethylamphetamine [MDEA, or "Eve"]) have both stimulant and hallucinogenic effects due to the release of dopamine and serotonin, respectively. The clinical presentation and treatment of amphetamine intoxication and withdrawal is similar to that of cocaine (Table 7-24).

Caffeine

DSM-5 classifies caffeine use disorder as a research diagnosis but does not meet the full criteria for abuse or dependence. Caffeine is the most common psychoactive agent used in the United States. It elevates myocardial cAMP by **inhibiting phosphodiesterase** and is an **adenosine antagonist** that also exerts a stimulant effect on the dopaminergic system.

Consumption of 250 mg of caffeine can lead to symptoms of intoxication, which include insomnia, anxiety, restlessness, twitching, rambling speech, flushed face, diuresis, and GI disturbances. If more than 1 g of caffeine (approximately 10 cups of coffee or 20 cups of tea) is ingested, symptoms such as tinnitus, severe agitation, and cardiac arrhythmia can occur. Treatment for caffeine intoxication is symptomatic and supportive.

Caffeine withdrawal also leads to symptoms including headache, anxiety, depression, and drowsiness. Treatment is symptomatic (eg, analgesics for headaches). To avoid subsequent episodes of withdrawal, the patient should slowly taper caffeine consumption.

Nicotine

Stimulates nicotinic acetylcholine receptors. Symptoms of intoxication include insomnia, restlessness, anxiety, and increased GI motility. The definitive treatment for nicotine intoxication is cessation.

Patients suffering from nicotine withdrawal exhibit signs of anxiety, dysphoria, increased appetite, irritability, insomnia, and intense craving. Behavioral counseling, nicotine

TABLE 7-24. Characteristics and Management of Stimulant Intoxication and Withdrawal

SUBSTANCE	INTOXICATION	MANAGEMENT OF INTOXICATION	WITHDRAWAL	MANAGEMENT OF WITHDRAWAL
Cocaine	■ Hypertension, tachycardia, increased myocardial O_2 demand, **chest pain,** arrhythmias, **dilated pupils,** hyperthermia, seizures, psychosis, psychomotor agitation, aggression, anorexia, ischemic or hemorrhagic stroke, formication, increased arousal, euphoria, ischemic bowel, **erythema of turbinates** and **nasal septum** ■ Associated with **placental abruption** in pregnancy	**Agitation:** ■ Benzodiazepines **Cardiac:** ■ ECG, CXR, troponins ■ Aspirin, O_2 ■ Benzodiazepines ■ **Do not administer β-blockers** ■ Nitroglycerin Hypertension: ■ Benzodiazepines; if refractory, consider phentolamine	Irritability, drowsiness, fatigue, hunger, miosis, severe depressed mood ("crash")	■ Supportive treatment ■ No medications shown to be superior ■ If severe agitation or sleep disturbance, may consider BZDs ■ Not life threatening
Amphetamines	■ Diaphoresis, hypertension, tachycardia, arrhythmias, agitation, psychosis, euphoria, increased confidence, talkativeness, **dilated pupils,** abdominal pain, diarrhea	Same as cocaine	Dysphoria, anhedonia, fatigue, increased sleep, vivid dreams, agitation, anxiety, hunger, lethargy	Same as cocaine

BZD, benzodiazepine; CXR, x-ray of the chest; ECG, electrocardiogram.

patch or gum, **varenicline** (partial nicotine receptor agonist), and **bupropion** (antidepressant) have been shown to help reduce nicotine cravings.

Opiate Use Disorder

EPIDEMIOLOGY

Opioid is an inclusive term used to denote the different opiate drugs that currently exist. The most common opiates seen in use in clinical practice are morphine, codeine, methadone, oxycodone, fentanyl, and buprenorphine. Heroin is an opioid often used for illicit purposes. Medically, opioids are most commonly used for **pain relief.** They also have CNS depressant effects, as well as the potential to cause euphoria. Not surprisingly, opioid analgesics are the most commonly abused opioids in the United States, and prescription opioids are the leading cause of opioid-related overdose in the United States. Health consequences of opioid addiction include increased mortality, overdose, infections, endocarditis, and narcotic bowel syndrome.

PATHOPHYSIOLOGY

Opioids activate specific transmembrane receptors (mu, kappa, delta) coupled to G proteins. Activation of endogenous mu opioid receptors results in the prototypic opioid effects of reward and analgesia. Opioid receptors are located in both the central and peripheral nervous systems. Activation of mu receptors in the CNS results in responses such as respiratory depression, analgesia, euphoria, and miosis. Stimulation of peripheral mu opioid receptors, in smooth muscle of the bronchi and intestines, results in cough suppression and opioid-induced constipation. Opiates also affect the dopaminergic system, thus contributing to their addictive and rewarding effects.

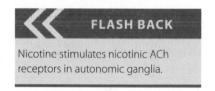

FLASH BACK

Nicotine stimulates nicotinic ACh receptors in autonomic ganglia.

DIAGNOSIS

A problematic pattern of opioid use leading to clinically significant impairment or distress is manifested by two or more of the following within a 12-month period:

- Opioids are often taken in larger amounts or over a longer period than was intended
- A persistent desire or unsuccessful efforts to cut down or control opioid use
- A great deal of time is spent in activities necessary to obtain the opioid, use the opioid, or recover from its effects
- Craving, or a strong desire or urge to use opioids
- Recurrent opioid use, resulting in a failure to fulfill major role obligations at work, school, or home
- Continued opioid use despite having persistent or recurrent social or interpersonal problems caused or exacerbated by the effects of opioids
- Important social, occupational, or recreational activities are given up or reduced because of opioid use
- Recurrent opioid use in situations in which it is physically hazardous
- Continued opioid use despite knowledge of having a persistent or recurrent physical or psychological problem that is likely to have been caused or exacerbated by the substance
- Tolerance
- Withdrawal

INTOXICATION

Patients who are acutely intoxicated can have slurred speech, drowsiness, impaired cognition, hypotension, hypothermia, decreased bowel sounds, and **pinpoint pupils.** If they have injected opioids, then fresh injection sites ("track marks") may be visible on exam.

WITHDRAWAL

Signs of acute opioid withdrawal syndrome include anxiety, restlessness, irritability, depressed mood, lacrimation, pupil dilation, runny nose (rhinorrhea), yawning, muscle twitching, muscle aches, GI symptoms (eg, hyperactive bowel sounds, nausea/vomiting, cramps, diarrhea) and piloerection. Although unpleasant, opiate withdrawal is usually not life threatening.

Methadone and buprenorphine, both of which are synthetic opiates, can be used to treat long-term dependence on heroin (Table 7-25). All three, however, can also lead to physical dependence and tolerance. Methadone and buprenorphine are legally used to substitute for illegal opiates and to prevent withdrawal symptoms. Methadone is a μ-opioid receptor agonist, and buprenorphine is a partial opioid receptor agonist used for long-term maintenance therapy. They block the withdrawal symptoms and euphoric effects of heroin.

> **◀◀ FLASH BACK**
>
> Endogenous opiates include endorphins, dynorphins, and enkephalins.

TABLE 7-25. **Characteristics and Management of Opiate Intoxication and Withdrawal**

SUBSTANCE	INTOXICATION	MANAGEMENT OF INTOXICATION	WITHDRAWAL	MANAGEMENT OF WITHDRAWAL
Opiates	- Drowsiness, CNS depression, nausea/vomiting, constipation, constricted pupils, slurred speech, seizures, respiratory depression (leading to coma/death)	- Overdose is life-threatening - Naloxone or naltrexone for opiate overdose with respiratory depression - Provide ventilatory support if needed	- Not life-threatening - Dysphoria, insomnia, rhinorrhea, yawning, dilated pupils, lacrimation, weakness, sweating, piloerection ("cold turkey"), flulike symptoms (nausea/vomiting, fever, muscle aches)	- Moderate symptoms: Clonidine and/or buprenorphine - Severe symptoms: Methadone (tapered over 7 days)

Hallucinogens (Phencyclidine and Lysergic Acid Diethylamide)

EPIDEMIOLOGY

Hallucinogens are chemicals that alter sensory perception, mood, and thought patterns. Although hallucinogens are used by approximately 1 million Americans each year, the prevalence of abuse is relatively low compared to other illicit drugs. Hallucinogen use frequently begins in adolescence and is more common in males. Lysergic acid diethylamide (LSD) is the prototypical and most historically studied hallucinogen. Phencyclidine (PCP) is another hallucinogen that is known to cause dissociative effects, anesthesia, and aggressive behavior (Table 7-26).

PATHOPHYSIOLOGY

The exact mechanism underlying hallucinations is not known, but a common characteristic of most is their ability to bind 5-hydroxytryptamine$_{2A}$ (5-HT$_{2A}$) receptors. This serotonergic activity may cause serotonin syndrome, which has been associated with LSD and a number of other hallucinogens. PCP is a noncompetitive antagonist of N-methyl-D-aspartate (NMDA) receptors. PCP also inhibits reuptake of dopamine, norepinephrine, and serotonin.

INTOXICATION

Hallucinogens are sought by users for their so-called "psychedelic" effects. These include heightening (or distortion) of sensory stimuli (eg, visual illusions), euphoria, and feelings of blending the senses ("synesthesia"). Unpleasant effects, such as severe anxiety, depression, and paranoia, are also reported. Most hallucinogens also produce sympathomimetic effects, including tachycardia, tremors, hypertension, mydriasis, hyperthermia, and diaphoresis. PCP and LSD intoxication present similarly, but agitation and aggression occur more commonly in patients using PCP. Visual hallucinations and intensified perceptions are hallmarks of LSD intoxication. Further distinguishing features of PCP intoxication and LSD intoxication are outlined in Table 7-26.

DIAGNOSIS

The diagnostic criteria for a substance use disorder were previously described. These criteria apply to hallucinogen-related disorders. Notably, some cultures (eg, Native Americans) may use hallucinogens during religious rituals, and this does not meet diagnostic criteria for substance use disorder.

> **KEY FACT**
>
> The **classic triad** of opiate overdose includes:
> - Respiratory depression
> - Altered mental status
> - Miosis ("pinpoint pupils")

TABLE 7-26.   Characteristics and Treatment of Hallucinogen Intoxication

HALLUCINOGEN	SIGNS AND SYMPTOMS OF INTOXICATION	TREATMENT FOR INTOXICATION
Phencyclidine (PCP)	Impulsiveness, **belligerence, dissociation,** severe agitation, **recklessness,** psychosis, acute brain syndrome, seizures, coma, impaired judgment, ataxia, hypertension, hyperthermia, tachycardia, **multidirectional nystagmus** (rotatory, horizontal, or vertical), **high tolerance to pain, violent behavior** (a common cause of death), other complications*	▪ Place in calm, quiet environment to minimize sensory input ▪ **IV benzodiazepines** (lorazepam, diazepam) for psychomotor agitation; IM injection may be needed if IV access is not attainable; physical restraints may be required for patient and staff safety ▪ Manage complications (hyperthermia, seizures, rhabdomyolysis, and hypertension) ▪ Most cases will resolve with supportive care
LSD	Pupil dilation, tachycardia, **perceptual changes ("synesthesia", time distortion),** ** hallucinations, sweating, palpitations, tremors, impaired coordination	▪ Place in calm, quiet environment to minimize sensory input ▪ **IV benzodiazepines** (lorazepam, diazepam) for acute agitation/dysphoria ▪ If psychotic features persist, may administer IV haloperidol

*Other complications: rhabdomyolysis, seizures, hypoglycemia, prolonged comatose state.

**While intoxicated, most individuals remain oriented and aware that their experiences are drug induced.

Cannabis Use Disorders

EPIDEMIOLOGY

Cannabis (marijuana) is the most commonly used illegal substance worldwide. Recent studies estimate that between 2.5% and 4.0% of the world's population ages 15–64 years use cannabis. Use is particularly high in adolescents, with the highest overall risk for initiating use occurring at age 18 years.

PATHOPHYSIOLOGY

The psychoactive properties of cannabis are primarily attributed to delta-9-tetrahydrocannabinol (THC). The two known cannabinoid receptors, **CB1** and **CB2**, are **G-protein linked** and inhibit adenylyl cyclase to ultimately increase K⁺ conductance across membranes. THC is **lipid soluble,** contributing to its lengthy elimination half-life.

INTOXICATION

The signs and symptoms of cannabis intoxication include tachycardia, increased respiratory rate, hypertension (or, less commonly, orthostatic hypotension), conjunctival injection, dry mouth, increased appetite, slurred speech, nystagmus, impaired reflexes, slowed time perception, impaired short-term memory, impaired motor coordination, and behavioral changes (ie, social withdrawal, euphoria, dysphoria, anxiety). Psychomotor impairment can last up to 12–24 hours due to accumulation of cannabis in adipose tissue. In patients with a history of schizophrenia, cannabis use can increase the risk for psychosis.

DIAGNOSIS

Cannabis use disorder is characterized by the problematic pattern of cannabis use leading to clinically significant impairment, as manifested by two or more of the following within a 12-month period:

- Cannabis taken in larger amounts or over a longer period than was intended
- There is a persistent desire or unsuccessful efforts to cut down or control cannabis use
- A great deal of time is spent in activities necessary to obtain or use cannabis
- Craving, or a strong desire or urge to use cannabis
- Recurrent cannabis use resulting in a failure to fulfill major role obligations at work, school, or home
- Continued cannabis use despite having persistent or recurrent social or interpersonal problems caused or exacerbated by the effects of cannabis
- Important social, occupational, or recreational activities are given up or reduced because of cannabis use
- Recurrent cannabis use in situations in which it is physically hazardous
- Continued cannabis use despite knowledge of having a persistent or recurrent physical or psychological problem that is likely to have been caused or exacerbated by cannabis
- Tolerance

WITHDRAWAL

While cannabis withdrawal can be distressing, it is not life threatening. Symptoms most frequently include fatigue, irritability, yawning, hypersomnia, psychomotor retardation, decreased appetite, anxiety/nervousness, and depressed mood. The withdrawal symptoms typically begin on the first or second day of abstinence and resolve within 1–2 weeks. Only symptomatic and supportive treatment is available for both intoxication and withdrawal syndromes.

KEY FACT

Naloxone = IV route of administration.
Naltrexone = oral (PO) route of administration.
Methylnaltrexone and naloxegol are used to treat opioid-induced constipation.

KEY FACT

Both PCP and LSD alter a person's perception.
PCP intoxication also leads to impulsiveness, beligerence, psychosis, and violent, even homicidal behavior.
LSD intoxication also leads to anxiety or depression.

KEY FACT

Withdrawal from PCP intoxication can lead to sudden onset of random homicidal violence.

CHILDHOOD DISORDERS

Diagnosing psychiatric disorders in children can be more challenging than doing so in adults because the clinical data have to be gathered from various sources. The child, the parents, teachers, and everyone else involved in the child's life should, with appropriate permission, be interviewed. Parents are often excellent sources of information and can give accurate accounts of the child's developmental progress, conduct, school performance, problems with the law, and family history. Teachers and social workers can also give valuable information about academic performance, peer relationships, and the child's social and family environment. Child psychiatric disorders can be categorized into groups depending on the dominant symptoms.

Pervasive Developmental Disorders

Pervasive developmental disorders are characterized by impairments in language and social skills. The disorder is recognized at an early age, and there is a higher incidence in males; the male:female ratio is 3:1 (with the exception of Rett syndrome, which affects females only). Pervasive developmental disorders include autistic disorder, Asperger syndrome, and Rett syndrome. Importantly, language may be normal in breadth in Asperger syndrome.

Autism Spectrum Disorder

Symptoms associated with autism spectrum disorder (ASD) are recognized early in childhood (usually before age 3) due to delayed developmental milestones. There is a high association with mental retardation, fragile X syndrome, and tuberous sclerosis. **Males** have a predilection for autism, and genetics have some role in its inheritance. Children with ASD exhibit impairment in three different areas: social interaction, communication, and restricted and repetitive behaviors. Symptoms must be present from early childhood; both social communication impairment and a restricted, repetitive pattern of behavior must be present to diagnose.

DSM-5 DIAGNOSTIC CRITERIA

According to the DSM-5 criteria, a child has to exhibit six of the following symptoms to be diagnosed with ASD:

- Unable to develop peer relationships
- Unable to express oneself through nonverbal expressions (eg, facial expressions, gestures)
- Does not initiate or reciprocate social interactions
- Does not appropriately reciprocate emotional interactions
- Delayed, impaired speech
- Repetitive use of language
- Repetitive play (eg, continually stacking three blocks in a certain way)
- Exhibit repetitive and rigid rituals
- Obsession with parts of objects

TREATMENT

Treatment of ASD focuses on managing symptoms, which include the following:

- Behavioral management
- Special school curriculum focused on developing social skills
- SSRI (for control of repetitive behaviors)
- Atypical antipsychotics (for treatment of bizarre behaviors, agitation, and tics)
- Stimulants (for hyperactivity)

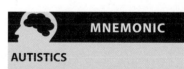

Asperger Disorder

DSM-5 no longer defines Asperger disorder as a separate clinical entity, but rather classifies Asperger disorder as an ASD. Children with Asperger disorder have normal to high intelligence. However, they may suffer deficits in social interaction, narrowed interests, and gross motor clumsiness. Asperger disorder is more prevalent in males, and its cause is not well understood.

DSM-5 DIAGNOSTIC CRITERIA

According to the DSM-5 criteria, patients must exhibit at least two of the following deficits in social interactions:

- Unable to develop peer relationships
- Unable to express oneself through nonverbal expressions (eg, facial expressions, gestures)
- Does not initiate or reciprocate social interactions
- Does not appropriately reciprocate emotional interactions
- Exhibits repetitive behaviors or activities
- Exhibits preoccupation with inflexible routines

TREATMENT

Treatment is geared toward symptom management and is similar to that outlined for autism.

Rett Syndrome

Unlike the other two pervasive developmental disorders, Rett syndrome predominates in females because it is an **X-linked** (ie, *MECP2* gene) **autosomal dominant trait.** It is a very rare disorder, and onset of symptoms often occurs between the ages of 5 and 48 months. Before the onset of symptoms, patients have normal brain development. Following onset of the disease, however, there is a restriction of brain growth and a subsequent regression of development.

KEY FACT

Patients with Rett syndrome exhibit stereotyped hand movements such as clapping and wringing of hands.

DSM-5 DIAGNOSTIC CRITERIA

- Brain development is normal in the first few months of life, followed by a restriction of brain growth (manifested as normal developmental milestones and head circumference initially, but impaired developmental milestones and decreasing head circumference later)
- Regression of development (ie, loss of previously learned skills)
- Exhibits **stereotyped hand movements** (eg, hand clapping and hand wringing)
- Loss of social interaction (could improve over time)
- Impaired gait or truncal ataxia
- Impaired language and psychomotor development

TREATMENT

There is no cure for Rett syndrome; therefore, treatment is supportive with management of symptoms.

Disruptive Behavior Disorders

Disruptive behavior disorders are characterized by behavior that does not conform to societal norms. A disruptive behavior disorder can be categorized as either conduct disorder or oppositional defiant disorder. Both disorders are more prevalent in males.

Conduct Disorder

The presumed etiology of this disorder is multifactorial and includes child-rearing practices (eg, lack of parental discipline), parental or familial factors (eg, parental psychopathology), and family violence. There is an increased incidence of other mental disorders (eg, mood disorder), substance abuse, and criminal behavior in these patients. Many patients diagnosed with conduct disorder will meet the criteria to be diagnosed with antisocial personality disorder after reaching 18 years of age.

DSM-5 Diagnostic Criteria

Patients must exhibit the following behaviors for a period of more than 1 year:

- Persistent behavior that does not conform to societal norms and violates the basic rights of others
- Aggression toward living things
- Destruction of property and stealing
- Behavior causes impairment of daily functioning

Treatment

Children benefit the most from early intervention. Treatment is focused on behavior modification and problem-solving skills. Parents should be involved in the treatment plan and engaged in parenting skills training and family therapy. Antipsychotics or lithium can be used for aggression management, and SSRIs can be used to treat impulsivity, mood lability, and irritability.

Oppositional Defiant Disorder

Unlike conduct disorder, patients with oppositional defiant disorder **do not violate the rights of others.** Onset is in early childhood, but symptoms can regress or progress to conduct disorder. Patients with this disorder have a predilection for substance abuse and have a higher incidence of comorbid mood disorders and ADHD.

DSM-5 Diagnostic Criteria

Patients exhibit at least four of the following symptoms for **at least 6 months:**

- Frequently loses temper
- Disobedient
- Argues with authority figures (ie, teachers and parents)
- Exhibits anger and resentment
- Easily annoyed
- Annoys others on purpose
- Spiteful
- Refuses to take responsibility for his actions

Treatment

Treatment is similar to that for conduct disorder.

Attention Deficit/Hyperactivity Disorder

The prevalence of ADHD among children is 3–5% and is more common in males than females. It is believed that the etiology of ADHD is multifactorial and involves genetic contributors, psychosocial factors, toxin exposure, prenatal trauma, and neurologic factors. The symptoms of most patients remit during adulthood, but 20% of patients ADHD have symptoms that persist into adulthood.

DSM-5 Diagnostic Criteria

Patients must exhibit symptoms for 6 months, symptom onset must occur **before age 12,** and symptoms must be present in **more than one setting** (Table 7-27).

KEY FACT

Children who present with at least one symptom of conduct disorder before 10 years of age are more likely to develop adult antisocial personality disorder than individuals who first display symptoms later in childhood.

MNEMONIC

Children have **C**onduct disorder.
Adults have **A**ntisocial personality disorder.

TABLE 7-27. **Symptoms of Attention Deficit/Hyperactivity Disorder**

HYPERACTIVITY	INATTENTION	IMPULSIVITY
■ Unable to stay seated ■ Unable to play quietly ■ Constantly fidgets ■ Talks excessively ■ Runs around	■ Disorganized ■ Unable to complete task ■ Forgetful ■ Easily distracted ■ Constantly makes careless mistakes ■ Does not listen when spoken to	■ Interrupts or intrudes on others ■ Has difficulty waiting for turn ■ Blurts out answers

TREATMENT

Treatments for ADHD include psychotherapy and pharmacotherapy. Stimulants, such as methylphenidate, are usually first-line pharmacotherapy. Atomoxetine and α_2-adrenergic agonists are also used as pharmacotherapy for those with medical conditions prohibiting stimulant use and/or those wishing to avoid stimulant use in their children. Parents should also go for parenting skills training.

Tourette Disorder

Tourette disorder is a severe tic disorder that involves motor (eg, facial or hand tics) and vocal tics. Tics can be simple (nonpurposeful) or complex (movements or vocalizations that convey meaning). Complex vocal tics can be further categorized into either coprolalia (speaking obscene words) or echolalia (repeating words spoken to the individual). Coprolalia is uncommon in children. The onset of symptoms occurs before age 18, but symptoms can carry on into adulthood. This disorder is more common in males than females. The etiology of Tourette disorder includes genetics and impairment in dopamine regulation. Patients have a high incidence of other psychiatric conditions (eg, OCD and ADHD).

DSM-5 DIAGNOSTIC CRITERIA

Patients exhibit symptoms for **> 1 year** and have an onset prior to age 18:

- Motor and vocal tics
- Symptoms cause significant impairment in daily living

TREATMENT

Treatment includes supportive therapy, α_2-agonists such as guanfacine, benzodiazepines, and, less commonly, antipsychotics such as haloperidol or pimozide. Importantly, patients with Tourette syndrome are not psychotic, but abnormal movement and vocalizations are likely mediated by neurotransmitters that affect the basal ganglia, hence the use of medications that block activity in this region of the brain. For intractable tics, low-dose, high-potency antipsychotics (eg, fluphenazine, pimozide), tetrabenzine, and clonidine may be used.

Separation Anxiety Disorder

This disorder affects 4% of children with an average age of onset of 7 years. It may be preceded by a stressful life event (eg, divorce). Children with this disorder express great fear of being physically separated from their parents and avoid being physically separated (eg, the child may lie about feeling sick to avoid going to school). When they are forced to leave their parents, they express great distress and worry about not seeing their parents again. Treatment includes supportive therapy, family therapy, and low-dose antidepressants for symptom management.

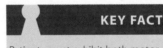

KEY FACT

Patients must exhibit both motor and vocal tics to be diagnosed with Tourette syndrome.

Selective Mutism

This rare disorder occurs more often in women than in men. The onset of symptoms is around 5 years, and it is characterized by **not speaking in specific situations.** Like separation anxiety disorder, it can be preceded by a stressful life event. Treatment includes supportive therapy and behavioral and family therapy.

Intellectual Disability

Intellectual disability (ID, mental retardation) begins in childhood and is defined by limitations in both intelligence and adaptive skills. Formal IQ testing is no longer required to assess severity of ID, but the limitation in intellectual ability usually corresponds to an IQ lower than 65–75 on a scale with a median of 100. ID affects 1% of the population, and the incidence is higher in males than in females. ID has several causes, including genetic (eg, Down syndrome, fragile X syndrome), prenatal infection or toxin exposure, prematurity, anoxia, birth trauma, malnutrition, and hypothyroidism. ID severity is categorized based on the amount of support needed for addressing impaired adaptive functioning in one or more settings (eg, home, work, school). The majority of cases are mild.

Child Abuse

Any physician or medical provider who suspects child abuse is legally required to contact the appropriate authorities (ie, Child Protective Services [CPS]) to file an official report. Should the child be considered in need of urgent medical care, hospitalization is warranted. It is not advisable to confront the parent(s) or caregiver(s) directly, as they may become argumentative or flee the scene with the child. It is preferable to contact CPS immediately once child abuse is suspected. Child abuse tends to be recognized earlier in less affluent families due to more contact with social workers or law enforcement. Child abuse can remain hidden in more affluent families due to lower level of suspicion and the ability of parents to avoid detection and legal consequences.

Once the provider suspects child abuse, the first step is to perform a complete examination. This will require completely removing all of the child's clothes, as the initial focused exam may distract from other long-standing injuries. Injuries such as cigarette burns (circular lesions), multiple fractures in various stages of healing, rib fractures, spiral fractures in children who are not yet walking, or scalding hot water injuries (line of demarcation, absence of splash marks) are very concerning and suggestive of child abuse. Multiple bruises in various stages of healing and orthopedic injuries should prompt a radiologic skeletal survey. Once this comprehensive exam is complete, the physician can determine the appropriate course of action for the patient and whether emergent admission to the hospital is required.

Overall, physicians should have a high index of suspicion for physical/sexual abuse in children with sudden behavioral problems, families with unstable economic backgrounds, or parents with a history of drug/alcohol abuse.

NOTES

CHAPTER 8

Renal

EMBRYOLOGY   584
   Renal Development   584

ANATOMY   587
   Posterior Abdominal Wall   587
   Retroperitoneal Structures   587

HISTOLOGY   590
   Nephron   590
   Juxtaglomerular Apparatus   593
   Renal Calyces, Renal Pelvis, and Ureters   594
   Bladder   594

PHYSIOLOGY   594
   Concepts of Transport   594
   General Renal Physiology   599
   Acid-Base Homeostasis   615

PATHOLOGY   623
   Urinary Casts   623
   Glomerulopathies   623

Nephrotic Syndrome   623
Nephropathies Associated With Systemic Disorders   628
Nephritic Syndrome   630
Renal Stones (Urolithiasis)   636
Urinary Tract Infections   638
Diffuse Cortical Necrosis   639
Renal Papillary Necrosis   640
Acute and Chronic Kidney Injury   640
Cystic Kidney Disease   643
Inherited Renal Syndromes   645
Tumors of the Renal System   647
Electrolyte Abnormalities   650

PHARMACOLOGY   655
Diuretics   655
Antidiuretic Hormone (Vasopressin and Desmopressin)   658
Antidiuretic Hormone Antagonists   658
Angiotensin-Converting Enzyme Inhibitors   659
Angiotensin Receptor Blockers   659
Nephrotoxic Drugs   660

Embryology

RENAL DEVELOPMENT

The urinary system is derived from **intermediate mesoderm** on the posterior wall of the abdominal cavity (Table 8-1). It forms three kidney systems: the pronephros, mesonephros, and metanephros (Figure 8-1):

- **Pronephros:** Rudimentary kidneys that disappear by end of fourth week.
- **Mesonephros:** Another pair of transient kidneys that form after pronephros regression, within which lies a long epithelial duct, the Wolffian duct. This duct then fuses caudally with the cloaca.
- **Wolffian duct (WD):** Paired organ that connects the primitive **mesonephros** to the **cloaca.** The **ureteric bud** is an outgrowth from the caudal WD. The WD coexists with the Müllerian duct, the potential precursor of the female Fallopian tube, uterus, and upper vagina. The presence or absence of hormones secreted from the developing gonads in utero determines which adult analog will form from these ducts. In the male fetus, testosterone from the developing gonads provides stimulus for the development of the epididymus and vas deferens from the WD, while Müllerian inhibitory hormone causes the regression of the Müllerian ducts.
- **Metanephros:** Forms the definitive kidney via reciprocal inductive signaling with the ureteric bud.

Congenital Abnormalities

Potter Sequence

Potter sequence develops as a result of oligohydramnios (decreased amniotic fluid) secondary to any cause of in utero oliguric renal failure (eg, bilateral renal agenesis). During normal fetal development, the fetus continuously swallows amniotic fluid, which is reabsorbed by the gastrointestinal (GI) tract and then reintroduced into the amniotic cavity by the kidneys via urination. Fetuses with bilateral renal agenesis are unable to produce urine, resulting in low amniotic fluid volume. Limb and facial deformities result from compression of the fetus against the walls of the amniotic sac. Infants with this condition have flat facial features (Potter facies). Characteristic features seen at birth include a flat nose, small lower jaw (micrognathia), malformed ears, chest wall abnormalities, club foot (talipes equinovarus), and compression of the skull.

PRESENTATION

The deformities found in Potter sequence can be divided into three groups:

- **Limb deformities:** Clubfoot, flipper hands, hyperextensible joints, and compressed thorax.

KEY FACT

Bilateral renal agenesis is an important cause of oligohydramnios.

KEY FACT

Allantois → urachus → medi**an** umbilical ligament (not the paired medi**al** umbilical ligaments, which are the remnants of the umbilical arteries).
Failure of obliteration of the allantois → **patent urachus** → **urachal fistula** at birth (newborn persistently draining urine from the umbilicus).
Urogenital sinus → urinary bladder and urethra.

MNEMONIC

Babies who can't **P**ee in utero develop **P**otter sequence.

TABLE 8-1.   Renal Development

PORTION OF KIDNEY	EMBRYONIC ORIGIN	ADULT STRUCTURES
Filtration system (nephron)	Derived from **metanephric mesoderm** via reciprocal inductive signaling with the ureteric bud	Glomerulus Bowman capsule Proximal convoluted tubule Loop of Henle Distal convoluted tubule
Collecting system	Derived from the ureteric bud via reciprocal inductive signaling with the metanephric mesoderm	Collecting ducts Major/minor calyces Renal pelvis Ureters (splitting of the ureteric bud can result in double ureters)

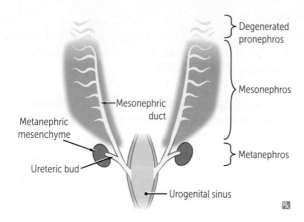

FIGURE 8-1. **Simplified anterior-posterior image depicting early renal system embryology.**

- **Facial deformities:** Sloping forehead, flattened nose, recessed chin, and low floppy ears.
- **Pulmonary hypoplasia:** Fetal lungs mature through swallowing of amnion, which allows the lungs to expand; thus, decreased amniotic fluid causes decreased expansion of the lungs. Physical restriction of the womb preventing full lung expansion also contributes to pulmonary hypoplasia when oligohydramnios is present.

PROGNOSIS

Incompatible with neonatal life.

Renal Ectopy

During development, the embryologic kidneys ascend from the pelvis to their adult position along the posterior abdominal wall. The kidneys must pass under the *umbilical arteries* in this process. If a kidney is unable to pass beneath an umbilical artery, it will remain in the pelvis. Incidence is 1 in 100 births.

PRESENTATION

Obstructive **hydronephrosis** and **vesicoureteric** reflux can be seen in association with renal ectopy. Affected patients may present with pain or infection related to these conditions (eg, pyelonephritis and renal stones).

DIAGNOSIS

Found incidentally on routine antenatal or postnatal imaging or during evaluation for symptoms of associated anomalies.

TREATMENT

Treatment, when required, is generally surgical.

PROGNOSIS

Prognosis is related to the extent of underlying urologic disease.

Horseshoe Kidney

While ascending from their position in the pelvis under the umbilical arteries, the kidneys are sometimes pushed close together, causing the lower poles to fuse **(fusion anomaly)**. The resultant horseshoe-shaped kidney continues to ascend until it is trapped under the **inferior mesenteric artery** (Figure 8-2). It is rare in women and if found should prompt work-up for Turner syndrome (7% of Turner patients have this defect).

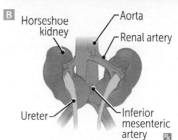

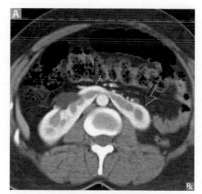

FIGURE 8-2. **Horseshoe kidney.**
Ⓐ Axial CT of abdomen with contrast shows enhancing midline fused kidney (arrows). Ⓑ Diagram of horseshoe kidney.

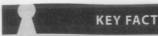

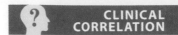

PRESENTATION

Ninety percent are asymptomatic and found incidentally. Most common presentation is **urinary tract infection (UTI)** followed by symptoms of obstruction, hematuria, or abdominal pain. Predisposes to **nephrolithiasis**.

DIAGNOSIS

Most commonly by prenatal ultrasound.

TREATMENT

Usually not necessary unless warranted by symptoms. The renal isthmus can be surgically divided.

Multicystic Dysplastic Kidney

Multicystic dysplastic kidney (MCDK) is a condition that results from the malformation of the kidney during fetal development. It is due to abnormal interaction between the ureteric bud and metanephric mesenchyme and leads to a nonfunctioning kidney consisting of cysts and connective tissue.

PRESENTATION

MCDK is most often asymptomatic and unilateral, with compensatory hypertrophy of the contralateral kidney, due to its maintaining renal function. When MCDK is bilateral, it is often incompatible with life.

DIAGNOSIS

MCDK is often diagnosed during routine prenatal ultrasound.

TREATMENT

For symptomatic cases, including hypertension or malignant transformation, the treatment is surgical removal.

Duplex Collecting System

A developmental defect whereby a ureter is bifid/Y-shaped, with two points of exit at the kidney, or there are two wholly separate ureters entering the bladder, often at inappropriate locations. The upper ureter is almost always the abnormal ureter, owing to the caudal-cranial direction of renal development.

PRESENTATION

Recurring infection is a common presentation in boys and girls. Infections are low in acuity, with low-grade fevers and periodic spikes; urine cultures are often negative, as ectopic ureters often do not drain effectively into the bladder. In boys, epididymitis is more common. Incontinence only occurs as a symptom in girls.

DIAGNOSIS

Often found on prenatal ultrasound, often showing a dilated upper pole with a dilated upper system or a dilated single system.

TREATMENT

Surgical implantation through a common sheath or a ureteroureterostomy.

Posterior Urethral Valve

An abnormality of male embryologic development in which urethral valve leaflets arise from the verumontanum of the prostate (type 1 is most common [95%]). This creates a bladder outlet obstruction, leading to voiding dysfunction, reflux, dilation, and renal dysplasia in utero, as well as consequences of oligohydramnios.

PRESENTATION

In the newborn period, a palpable midline mass representing a hypertrophied bladder can often be identified. Pulmonary hypoplasia and renal dysplasia are often seen early on.

DIAGNOSIS

Ultrasound and physical examination (midline mass).

TREATMENT

Endoscopic valve ablation is the most preferred initial surgical management.

Anatomy

POSTERIOR ABDOMINAL WALL

The posterior abdominal wall is supported by several large muscles attached to the bony thorax, vertebral column, and pelvic bones. The retroperitoneal structures are found atop these muscles and their skeletal insertions. Table 8-2 details these muscles and their innervation, blood supply, and actions.

RETROPERITONEAL STRUCTURES

Much of the urinary system is composed of retroperitoneal organs. Other retroperitoneal organs include the pancreas (except the tail), duodenum (second, third, and fourth parts), ascending colon, descending colon, aorta, inferior vena cava (IVC), rectum, and adrenal glands (Figure 8-3).

Kidney

The kidneys (Figure 8-4) are retroperitoneal organs located at the level of T12–L3 on the left and slightly lower on the right due to the liver. They are embedded in the Gerota fascia (loose connective tissue). The renal arteries and veins, as well as the ureters, adjoin the kidneys at the hilum.

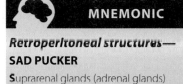

MNEMONIC

Retroperitoneal structures—
SAD PUCKER
Suprarenal glands (adrenal glands)
Aorta/IVC
Duodenum (second through fourth segments)
Pancreas (except tail)
Ureters
Colon (ascending and descending parts)
Kidneys
Esophagus
Rectum

TABLE 8-2. Muscles of the Posterior Abdominal Wall

	ORIGIN/INSERTION	INNERVATION	BLOOD SUPPLY	ACTIONS
Psoas major	Vertebral column (T12–L5) to the lesser trochanter of the femur	Ventral rami of L1–L3	Medial femoral circumflex artery	Flexes thigh and trunk and laterally rotates the hip
Psoas minor	Vertebral column (T12–L1) to the pectineal line	Ventral rami of L1–L2	Various	Flexes the trunk at the hip and stabilizes the thigh
Iliacus	Iliac fossa to the lesser trochanter of the femur	Femoral nerve (L3–L4)	Medial femoral circumflex artery	Powerful hip flexor and lateral rotation
Quadratus lumborum	Transverse processes of L3–L5 to the lower border of the 12th rib and the transverse processes of L1–L3	Ventral branches of T12 and L1–L4	Lumbar arteries	Extends and laterally flexes vertebral column

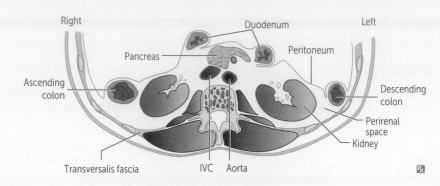

FIGURE 8-3.   **Schematic representation of the retroperitoneum.**

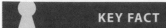

- **Arterial supply:** Renal arteries are branches of the abdominal aorta.
- **Venous return:** Renal veins drain into the IVC.
- **Left renal vein:** Also drains blood from the left gonad and left adrenal gland; is longer than the right renal vein (must cross the aorta to join the IVC).

Lymphatic drainage is to the lumbar nodes, whereas the nerve supply is via the thoracic splanchnic nerves.

The kidney is covered by a capsule of fibrous tissue. Beneath this capsule are the cortex and medulla, which contain the functional components of the kidney. The medulla comprises the early portions of the urinary collecting system:

- Renal pyramids
- Renal papillae
- Minor calyces
- Major calyces

The major calyces join to form the renal pelvis, which then becomes the ureter.

Ureters

The ureters course distally through the retroperitoneum, first crossing posterior (under) to the gonadal arteries, and then entering the pelvis by passing immediately anterior (over) to the external iliac artery where it branches off from the common iliac artery.

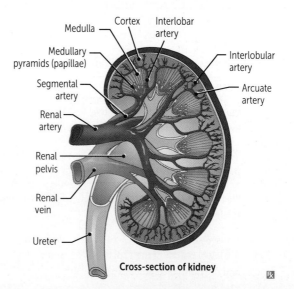

FIGURE 8-4.   **Gross anatomy of the kidney in cross section.**

Prior to entering the bladder, the ureter crosses under the uterine artery or vas deferens (depending on gender) (Figure 8-5).

Bladder

Situated beneath the peritoneum within the bony pelvis. The ureters join the bladder at its posterior-inferior portion, forming two points of the urinary trigone (the third is the urethral orifice). The bladder is an expandable and collapsible organ composed of several layers of smooth muscle (named the detrusor) and transitional epithelium. The bladder muscle has the unique physiologic ability to expand in size without increasing pressures proportionally; it is compliant while retaining the ability to contract forcefully.

Prostate

Surrounds the urethra just below the bladder. Stores and secretes an alkaline fluid constituting over 25% of semen volume. The vas deferens joins the duct of the seminal vesicle to become the ejaculatory duct, which courses through the prostate before emptying into the urethra.

Urethra

The urethra is lined by **transitional epithelium** as it exits the bladder. It then becomes **pseudostratified columnar** epithelium followed by **stratified squamous** cells as it nears the meatus. The urethra differs in men and women.

Male Urethra

Four anatomic divisions, the preprostatic, prostatic, membranous, and penile. Of note:

- **Prostatic:** Passes through the prostate gland, where it receives semen from the ejaculatory ducts (union of vas deferens and duct of the seminal vesicle). The prostate gland itself also contributes prostatic fluid to the ejaculate via several prostatic ducts. Lined by transitional epithelium.
- **Membranous:** Surrounded by striated muscle, which forms the voluntary external urethral sphincter (weakness produces urinary incontinence). Viscous secretions from the bulbourethral glands enter here.

CLINICAL CORRELATION

Ureteral stones are most commonly found at one of three sites: (1) ureter-renal pelvis junction, (2) site where external iliac artery causes a constriction in the ureter, and (3) ureter-bladder junction.

CLINICAL CORRELATION

The detrusor muscle is the target of anticholinergic drugs used to treat incontinence.

KEY FACT

Urachal remnants are most often found at the dome of the bladder. When cancerous, they are most likely adenocarcinoma, rather than urothelial or squamous.

CLINICAL CORRELATION

During hysterectomy the ureter can accidentally be transected.

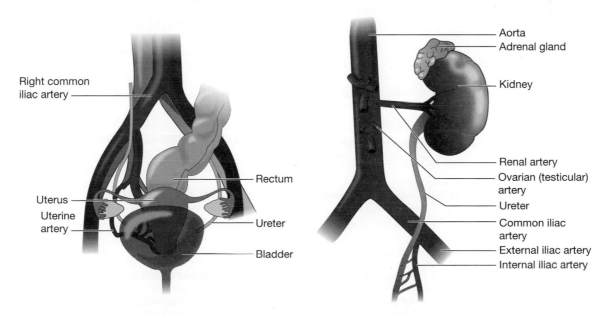

FIGURE 8-5.   Course of ureter with arterial supply.

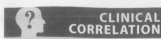
 Penile (including **bulbous** and **pendulous** sections): Longest segment, travels through the corpus spongiosum. Surrounded by Littre glands, which secrete mucus that is incorporated into the semen. Lined by pseudostratified columnar epithelium proximally, stratified squamous epithelium distally.

Female Urethra

Much shorter than the male urethra, which predisposes women to an increased risk of UTIs. It is lined by stratified squamous and pseudostratified columnar epithelium. At its midportion, it is surrounded by the striated muscle of the voluntary external urethral sphincter. The female urethra is also surrounded by Littre glands.

Histology

An overview of the histologic characteristics of the respective structures that form the renal system is provided in Table 8-3.

NEPHRON

The nephron is the primary functional unit of the kidney. It is the body's filtration system, removing substances from the blood and creating urine. It is composed of the **renal corpuscle** and the **tubular system** (Figure 8-6).

Renal Corpuscle

The primary filtering component of the nephron, the renal corpuscle is composed of two distinct functional units: the glomerulus and the Bowman capsule (Figures 8-7 and 8-8). The filtration barrier is composed of (1) fenestrated capillary endothelium, (2) basement membrane, and (3) slit diaphragms between adjacent foot processes of podocytes.

KEY FACT

Glomerulus + Bowman capsule = Renal corpuscle.

TABLE 8-3.   Histologic Characteristics of the Renal System

STRUCTURE	HISTOLOGY
Glomerulus	Fenestrated endothelium
Bowman capsule	Epithelium with two layers: visceral layer and parietal layer
Proximal convoluted tubule	Simple cuboidal epithelium with brush border
Loop of Henle	Thick descending loop; thin descending loop; thin ascending loop; thick ascending loop. Thick segments consist of simple cuboidal epithelium; thin segments consist of simple squamous epithelium
Distal convoluted tubule	Simple cuboidal epithelium without brush border
Collecting tubules	Simple cuboidal epithelium
Collecting ducts	Columnar epithelium
Renal calyces	Transitional epithelium
Renal pelvis	Transitional epithelium
Ureters	Transitional epithelium

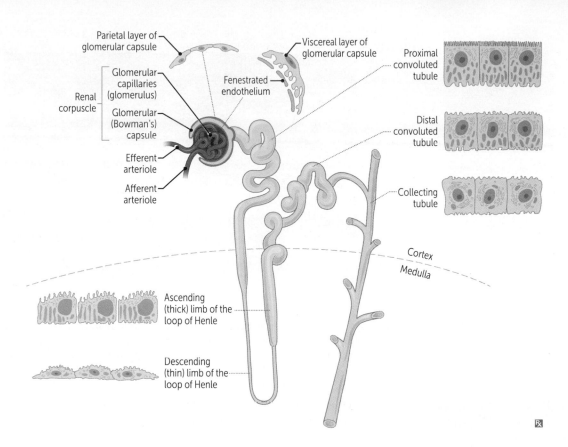

FIGURE 8-6. **Major anatomic divisions of the nephron.**

Glomerulus

A collection of dilated capillaries with fenestrated endothelium, which emerge from the afferent arteriole and drain into the efferent arteriole.

Bowman Capsule

Double-walled epithelial capsule (visceral and parietal) that wraps around the glomerular capillaries. This is where blood is filtered.

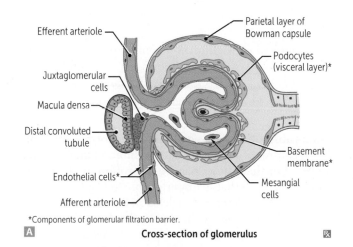

*Components of glomerular filtration barrier.

Cross-section of glomerulus

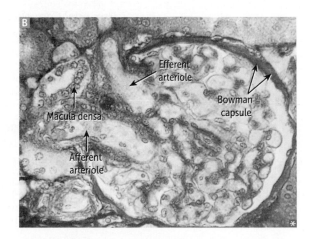

FIGURE 8-7. **Glomerulus.** A Schematic drawing of a cross section of glomerulus. B Normal glomerulus.

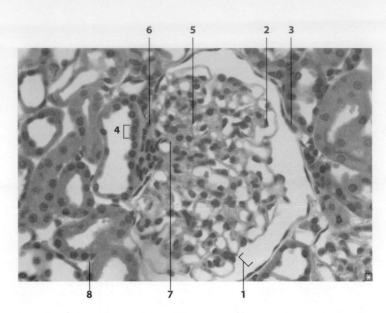

FIGURE 8-8. **Components of the renal corpuscle (hematoxylin and eosin [H&E] stain, normal kidney).** 1, Bowman space; 2, Bowman capsule, visceral layer; 3, Bowman capsule, parietal layer; 4, macula densa; 5, intraglomerular mesangial cell; 6, extraglomerular mesangial cell; 7, arteriole; 8, capillary, peritubular.

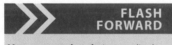

FLASH FORWARD

Heavy proteinuria is a cardinal feature of **nephrotic syndrome.**

- The **visceral layer** is a specialized outer lining on glomerular capillaries that serves as the outermost component of the filtration barrier. The specialized lining is composed of podocytes and their interdigitating foot processes.
- The **parietal layer** does not play a role in filtration. It forms the outer covering of the renal corpuscle and is lined by a simple squamous epithelium. It is continuous with the proximal convoluted tubule (PCT).
- The **urinary space** is found between the visceral and parietal layers. Filtrate collects here after passing through the fenestrated capillary endothelium of the glomerulus, basement membrane, and the visceral layer of the Bowman capsule.

Tubular System

The renal tubular system is divided into several functional units: **proximal convoluted tubule (PCT), loop of Henle, distal convoluted tubule (DCT), collecting tubules,** and **collecting ducts.**

Proximal Convoluted Tubule

The lumen is lined with **simple cuboidal epithelium** containing a **microvillous brush border** (Figure 8-6). This is the "workhorse of the nephron" and reabsorbs all of the glucose and amino acids and most of the Na^+, H_2O, HCO_3^-, Cl^- and PO_4^{3-}.

Loop of Henle

A specialized system that handles absorption and secretion of electrolytes, small molecules, and water (Figure 8-6). It consists of a thick descending limb, a thin descending limb **that is impermeable to Na^+ but that allows passive resorption of H_2O,** a thin ascending limb, and a thick ascending limb **that is impermeable to H_2O but actively pumps out Na^+** (eg, **Na^+ is reabsorbed**). As described in detail in the following sections, these different permeabilities establish the solute gradient critical to the countercurrent mechanism that allows the nephron to excrete a dilute or concentrated urine.

Distal Convoluted Tubule

Lined with **simple cuboidal epithelium** (Figure 8-6). However, it **does not** have a **brush border,** distinguishing it from the PCT. Is considered a "diluting segment" because like the thick ascending limb, the DCT is impermeable to H_2O but actively reabsorbs Na^+.

Collecting Tubules

These units are lined with **simple cuboidal epithelium** (Figure 8-6). They transport the urine from the **functional part** of the **nephron** toward the kidney's **hilum.** Here Na^+ is reabsorbed in exchange for K^+ and H^+ under the influence of aldosterone, and H_2O is reabsorbed under the influence of antidiuretic hormone (ADH).

Collecting Ducts

Lined with **columnar epithelium.** Receive urine from numerous nephrons (Figure 8-6).

Cortical Versus Juxtamedullary Nephrons

Most of the kidney's nephrons are located in the renal cortex. However, the glomerulus of some nephrons is located near the junction of the cortex and medulla. These nephrons are referred to as **juxtamedullary nephrons.**

- **Juxtamedullary nephrons** are central to the filtration, absorption, and secretion of urine. Via exceptionally long loops of Henle, they establish the hypertonic gradient in the kidney, which regulates the production of concentrated urine. The loops **extend deep into the medulla** and consist of a short thick descending limb, a long thin descending limb, a long thin ascending limb, and a short thick ascending limb.
- **Cortical nephrons** have a short thin descending limb and do not have a thin ascending limb. They do not extend into the medulla.

JUXTAGLOMERULAR APPARATUS

The juxtaglomerular apparatus (JGA) consists of **macula densa** cells found in the region of the distal thick ascending limb and early DCT, and **juxtaglomerular cells** found in the walls of the afferent arterioles. The JGA functions to maintain the glomerular filtration rate (GFR) in response to blood pressure (BP) changes in the afferent arterioles.

Macula Densa

A specialized group of epithelial cells in the thick ascending limb/DCT that come in close contact with the afferent and efferent arterioles. The cells of the macula densa are sensitive to sodium concentration and rate of flow through the thick ascending limb/DCT, and regulate GFR through locally active vasoactive peptides, such as angiotensin II, and hormones, such as aldosterone.

Juxtaglomerular (Granular) Cells

Juxtaglomerular (JG) cells are specialized myoepithelial (smooth muscle) cells located in the afferent arterioles. JG cells act as baroreceptors (they sense intrarenal arteriole pressure), which enables them to efficiently monitor BP and maintain normal GFR through the release of renin, the initial enzyme in the renin-angiotensin-aldosterone system (RAAS; see Physiology section for details).

Intraglomerular Mesangial Cells

Specialized pericytes among glomerular capillaries that have the following properties: (1) contract to regulate blood flow of the glomerular capillaries, (2) are a major contributor to extracellular matrix, and (3) phagocytose glomerular basal lamina components and immunoglobulins.

KEY FACT

Despite large fluctuations in arterial BP (75–160 mm Hg), the GFR is maintained within a very narrow range (autoregulation).

FLASH FORWARD

Angiotensin II → cells of efferent arteriole contract → vasoconstriction of efferent arteriole → reduced renal blood flow.

Natriuretic factor → cells of afferent arteriole relax → vasodilation of afferent arteriole → increased renal blood flow.

Extraglomerular Mesangial Cells

Contractile cells with receptors for both angiotensin II and natriuretic factor, enabling them to regulate glomerular flow. Form part of the juxtaglomerular apparatus along with the macula densa and juxtaglomerular (granular) cells of the afferent arteriole.

RENAL CALYCES, RENAL PELVIS, AND URETERS

These structures are lined with **transitional epithelium.** The muscular layer of the calyces, pelvis, and ureters are composed of helically arranged smooth muscle, which becomes more longitudinal as the ureters reach the bladder. The ureters exhibit peristaltic contractions as they pass urine from the kidneys to the bladder.

BLADDER

The wall of the urinary bladder is composed of the following layers (Figure 8-9):

- **Transitional epithelium:** Lines the inner surface. Its thickness depends largely on the bladder's fullness (an empty bladder has much thicker transitional epithelium than its distended counterpart).
- **Smooth muscle:** Three layers of smooth muscle are oriented in various directions and constitute the outer wall of the bladder. The innermost of these layers becomes the involuntary urethral sphincter at the junction between the bladder and the urethra.

Physiology

CONCEPTS OF TRANSPORT

DEFINITIONS

- **Quantity** of a given substance in a solution is expressed in **millimoles (mmol), milliequivalents (mEq),** or **milliosmoles (mOsm).**

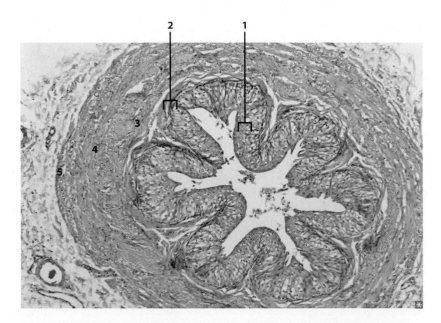

FIGURE 8-9. **Histology of the bladder.** 1, Transitional epithelium; 2, submucosa; 3, inner longitudinal smooth muscle; 4, middle circular smooth muscle; 5, outermost longitudinal smooth muscle.

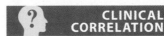

KEY FACT

Surgeons pay special attention to ureteral peristalsis in order to identify and therefore avoid injury to the ureters.

CLINICAL CORRELATION

Micturition is controlled autonomically by the internal sphincter and voluntarily by the external sphincter. Problems with these muscles or the autonomic nervous system can lead to incontinence.

- **Concentration** of a given substance in a solution reflects quantity per given volume. Commonly used units include: **mmol/L, mEq/L,** and **mOsm/L.**

An **equivalent** describes the **quantity of ionized (charged) molecules** in a given solution.

For example, one mole of NaCl in a solution dissociates into one equivalent of Na and one equivalent of Cl. However, one mole of $MgCl_2$ dissociates into two equivalents of Mg (ionized form has two positive charges) and two equivalents of Cl.

An **osmole** defines the number of single particles into which the solute dissociates in solution. Accordingly, **osmolarity** represents the concentration of those particles per given volume (eg, **Osm/L**).

Keeping in mind the previous example, the osmolarity equals molarity for nonionic substances, but they differ for ionic (charged) substances.

Forms of Transport

Concepts of Transport

There are two main types of transport: transcellular and paracellular.

- **Transcellular transport:** Substances are transported across both the apical and basolateral membranes and through the cytoplasm of the cell.
- **Paracellular transport:** The transported substances travel through the tight junctions *between* cells. This form of transport involves **simple diffusion** and/or **carrier-mediated diffusion.**

Substances can be transported via passive or active transport.

Passive Transport

Relies on the concentration gradient across the cell membranes as the driving force (does not require energy).

- **Simple diffusion** involves net transfer of solute down the concentration gradient until the rate of transfer across the membrane becomes equal in both directions (dynamic equilibrium).
- **Facilitated diffusion** is a carrier-mediated process directed down the concentration gradient. The carriers are specific membrane proteins that exhibit a high affinity for the substance. Because the amount of carrier is limited, the transport rate does not increase indefinitely with increasing concentration gradient. Rather, the transport maximum (T_m) for a given substance is achieved when all carrier sites are saturated. Moreover, molecules with structural similarities to the substance may compete for the carrier-binding site, thus reducing the transport rate of the preferred solute; this provides the basis for competitive agonist/antagonist actions.
- **Nonionic diffusion** is a passive process by which impermeant ions derived from the dissociation of weak acids or bases can cross cell membranes. The equation: $[HA] = [H^+] + [A^-]$ depicts the state of equilibrium between the undissociated and dissociated forms of a weak acid. Cell membranes are impermeable to ions, but permeable to the neutral, undissociated free acid form. The system's equilibrium is based on the pH gradient across the membrane.
- **Osmosis** refers to the movement of water across a semipermeable membrane from a region of low solute concentration to a region of high solute concentration. This is the only mechanism by which water is transported across the renal tubular epithelium.

KEY FACT

Equivalents = net charge × molarity (not applicable to neutral molecules)
Osmolarity = number of dissociated particles × molarity

KEY FACT

Osmolarity ≠ molarity for solutes that dissociate into multiple species. For example:
- 10 mmol glucose = 10 mOsm/L glucose
- But, 10 mmol NaCl = 20 mOsm/L NaCl
- (NaCl is ionic and dissociates into Na^+ and Cl^-)

KEY FACT

Examples of substances of physiologic importance that cross the membrane by nonionic diffusion include CO_2 and NH_3. These compounds play important roles in renal regulation of acid-base balance.

- **Osmotic pressure** is the hydrostatic pressure that must be physically applied to the side of a semipermeable membrane containing high-solute concentration (low-water concentration) in order to prevent the osmotic flow of water across the membrane.

Active Transport

Substances transported against their electrochemical gradient require a specific carrier and energy source, the most important of which is ATP.

- **Primary active transport:** Requires a specific ATPase transporter. The **Na^+/K^+-ATPase** and the **Ca^{2+}-ATPase** systems are found on the basolateral membrane of the renal tubules. This allows for Na^+ to be transported in one direction only (from the tubular lumen to the renal interstitial fluid).
- **Secondary active transport:** Two different substances simultaneously bind to the same membrane carrier and are concurrently transported across the membrane; one of the substances moves down its electrochemical concentration gradient while the other moves against it. This process can occur either by co- or countertransport:
- **Cotransport (symport)** occurs when two compounds use the same protein carrier and move in the same direction across the membrane (eg, **Na^+-glucose symporter**).
- **Countertransport (antiport)** occurs when transported substances are moved across the membrane in opposite directions (eg, **Na^+-H^+ antiporter** in the proximal tubule, and the distal tubular **H^+-K^+ antiporter**).

Rate-Limited Transport

The concept of T_m (transport maximum, as described previously) applies to both secretory and reabsorptive epithelial cell transport mechanisms. The different ways in which T_m applies to glucose and *para*-aminohippuric acid (PAH) are discussed later.

Fluid Compartments

Composition of Extracellular Fluid and Intracellular Fluid

The ionic compositions of the extracellular fluid (ECF) and intracellular fluid (ICF) (Figure 8-10) are remarkably different. However, the osmolarities of the compartments are equal, which allows for normal cell homeostasis. These concentration gradients across cell membranes are maintained by transport mechanisms.

The fluid component of the body is divided into several compartments (Figure 8-11). Water accounts for 60% of a person's total weight (known as **total body water,** or **TBW**). Two-thirds of TBW (40% of body weight) is ICF and one-third (20% of total body weight) is ECF.

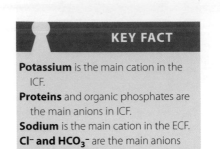

KEY FACT

Potassium is the main cation in the ICF.
Proteins and organic phosphates are the main anions in ICF.
Sodium is the main cation in the ECF.
Cl⁻ and HCO₃⁻ are the main anions in ECF.

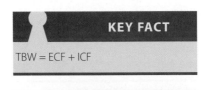

KEY FACT

TBW = ECF + ICF

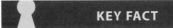

KEY FACT

60-40-20 rule: TBW = 60%, ICF = 40%, and ECF = 20% of body weight.

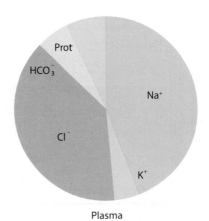
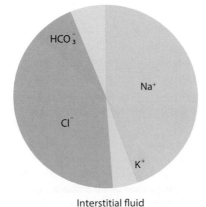
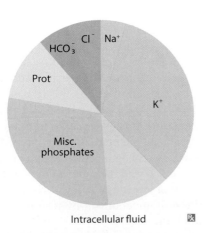

FIGURE 8-10.   **Composition of body fluids.**

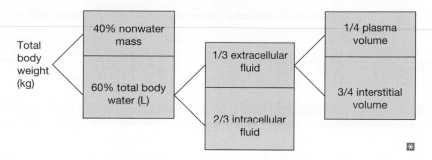

FIGURE 8-11.   Fluid compartments.

In a 70-kg adult, assuming normal hydration, 42 L (60%) of body weight is water, of which 28 L (2⁄3) is in the intracellular space and 14 L (1⁄3) is in the extracellular space.

- TBW varies based on age, sex, and body fat percentage. As body fat increases, the relative percentage of TBW decreases.
- **Infants and children** have higher TBW than adults due to a decreased proportion of fat.
- **Aging** is commonly associated with an increase in body fat (thus decreased TBW).
- **Females,** on average, have more body fat than males, and therefore have lower TBW.

The **ECF compartment** is further divided into interstitial fluid and plasma (Table 8-4).

- **Interstitial fluid** (75% of ECF): Water within the body but outside the cells.
- **Plasma** (25% of ECF): Noncellular fluid of the blood.

Estimating and Measuring Fluid Compartment Volume

Estimating Body Fluid Volumes

The percentage of the fluid compartment multiplied by total body weight (assuming normal hydration).

Measuring Body Fluid Volumes

Accomplished by injecting a known amount of a measurable molecule into the fluid space and allowing it to diffuse. The ideal molecule will enter the compartment(s) of interest and remain there without diffusing into other spaces. Normal physiologic values are depicted in Table 8-5.

The volume of the compartment of interest is calculated by applying the indicator dilution principle in which the distribution volume (V) for the indicator equals the quantity of indicator administered (Q) divided by the measured concentration (C) of indicator after equilibration has occurred.

$$V = Q/C$$

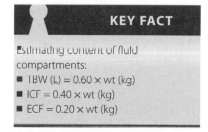

KEY FACT

Estimating content of fluid compartments:
- TBW (L) = 0.60 × wt (kg)
- ICF = 0.40 × wt (kg)
- ECF = 0.20 × wt (kg)

TABLE 8-4.   Composition of Intracellular Versus Extracellular Fluid

FLUID COMPARTMENT	COMPOSITION
ICF	- **Potassium,** magnesium, phosphate ions, organic anions, and protein - Slight negative charge, due to the nature of the cell membrane
ECF	- **Sodium,** chloride, bicarbonate, and calcium - Slight positive charge, due to the nature of the cell membrane

ECF, extracellular fluid; ICF, intracellular fluid.

TABLE 8-5. Normal Values of Fluid Compartments Based on a 70-kg Patient With a Plasma Osmolarity of 280 mOsm/L

COMPARTMENTS	VOLUME (L)	CONCENTRATION (MOSM/L)	TOTAL (MOSM)
TBW	42	280	11,760
ECF	14	280	3,920
ICF	28	280	7,840

ECF, extracellular fluid; ICF, intracellular fluid; TBW, total body water.

The TBW, plasma, and ECF volumes can be determined directly by using the following indicators:

- **TBW indicators:** D_2O (heavy water), ^3H_2O tritium (radioactive water), and $C_{11}H_{12}N_2O$ (antipyrine).
- **Plasma volume (PV) indicators:** Evans blue dye or radioiodinated human serum albumin (^{125}I-albumin).
- **ECF indicators:** Inulin, mannitol, and ^{22}Na.

The ICF, interstitial fluid, and blood volumes can be determined indirectly by using the following relationships:

$$ICF = TBW - ECF$$
$$\text{Interstitial fluid} = ECF - Plasma$$
$$Blood = Plasma / (1 - hematocrit)$$

KEY FACT

Osmolarity of ECF and ICF:
- ECF osmolarity = ICF osmolarity.
- ECF volume changes to maintain this balance.

Intercompartmental Water Dynamics

Under steady-state conditions, the osmolarity of the ECF is equal to that of ICF.

- Under normal physiologic conditions, substances such as mannitol, NaCl, and $NaHCO_3$ are confined to the ECF and do not readily cross the cell membrane.
- Under certain pathophysiologic conditions, this steady state is interrupted.

Volume changes take place in the ECF; ICF changes subsequently occur to equalize osmolarity between these compartments. These compartmental disturbances can be divided into two major groups:

- **Volume contraction** refers to loss of water from the ECF.
- **Volume expansion** refers to increase in the ECF volume.

KEY FACT

Osmolarity = Concentration of osmotically active particles per unit volume.
Normal measured value for body fluid osmolarity (BFO) is 290 mOsm/L (for practical purposes, we can round this to 300 mOsm/L).
Calculated plasma osmolarity $(P_{osm}) = 2 \times [Na^+] + [glucose]/18 + BUN/2.8$.

Furthermore, this can be subdivided based on the osmolarity of the ECF into **iso-osmotic, hypo-osmotic,** and **hyperosmotic** disturbances (all depicted in Figure 8-12, the Darrow-Yannet diagram), followed by practical calculations (Table 8-6).

ECF Pathophysiology Key Facts

- **Iso-osmotic volume contraction:** Prolonged watery diarrhea → hypovolemia and low flow state → activation of the RAAS → lowered urinary output (to retain Na^+ and H_2O).
- **Hypo-osmotic volume expansion:** Distinguish between **psychogenic polydipsia/ water intoxication** and the **syndrome of inappropriate antidiuretic hormone secretion (SIADH).** If psychogenic polydipsia is present, urine will be dilute but will concentrate normally once fluid intake stops. SIADH patients constantly concentrate their urine and thus retain water regardless of water intake.

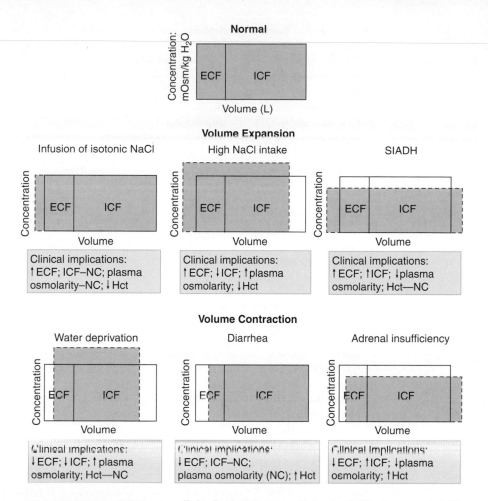

FIGURE 8-12. Darrow-Yannet diagram. ECF, extracellular fluid; ICF, intracellular fluid; Hct, hematocrit; NC, no change; SIADH, syndrome of inappropriate antidiuretic hormone secretion.

GENERAL RENAL PHYSIOLOGY

Renal Clearance: General Concepts

Renal Clearance (C_x)

Volume of plasma cleared of a given substance by the kidney per unit time:

$$C_x = [U_x] \times (V/[P_x])$$

where C_x is the clearance of substance X (mL/min), $[U_x]$ is the urine concentration of substance X (mg/mL), V is the urine flow rate (mL/min), and $[P_x]$ is the plasma concentration of substance X (mg/mL).

It can be determined how a specific substance is handled by the renal tubules by comparing the clearance rate of a substance with the GFR (Table 8-7).

Inulin, a fructose polymer, is freely filtered and neither reabsorbed nor secreted, and as such can be used to determine the clearance of any substance by comparing it with the inulin clearance, expressed through the **clearance ratio.**

$$\text{Clearance ratio} = C_x/C_{inulin}$$

$C_x/C_{inulin} = 1.0$ indicates that the clearance of substance X is equal to that of inulin; the substance is neither secreted nor reabsorbed. Substances with these properties are called **glomerular markers.**

TABLE 8-6.   Sample Calculations

Normal physiologic conditions, normal hydration:

TBW = $0.6 \times$ (70 kg) = 42 L

ICF volume = $0.4 \times$ (70 kg) = 28 L

ECF volume = $0.2 \times$ (70 kg) = 14 L

Body fluid osmolarity (BFO) = 300 mOsm/kg

Total body osmoles = (TBW) $\times$ (BFO) = (42 L) (300 mOsm/kg H_2O) = 12,600 mOsm

ICF osmoles = (ICF) $\times$ (BFO) = (28 L) (300 mOsm/kg H_2O) = 8400 mOsm

ECF osmoles = (ECF) $\times$ (BFO) = (14 L) (300 mOsm/kg H_2O) = 4200 mOsm

Example for SIADH = water intoxication = hypo-osmotic volume expansion:

Assume an extra 6 L of H_2O reabsorption:

Redistribution of H_2O, secondary to volume overload with H_2O

TBW (L) = $0.6 \times$ (70 kg) = 42 L + 6 L = 48 L

ICF (L) = $0.4 \times$ (70 kg) = 28 L + 4 L (⅔ of 6 L) = 32 L

ECF (L) = $0.2 \times$ (70 kg) = 14 L + 2 L (⅓ of 6 L) = 16 L

Comparison of normal versus SIADH:

Normal osmolarity: 12,600 mOsm/42 L TBW = 300 mOsm/kg

SIADH osmolarity: 12,600 mOsm/48 L TBW = 262.5 mOsm/kg

SIADH ICF volume: (ICF osm)/(SIADH osmolarity) = 8400 mOsm/262.5 mOsm/kg = 32 L

SIADH ECF volume: (ECF osm)/(SIADH osmolarity) = 4200 mOsm/262.5 mOsm/kg = 16 L

Final picture of SIADH compared to normal:

Increase in both ECF and ICF volumes

Decrease in body osmolarity (plasma protein dilution)

Hematocrit does not change: decrease in concentration of RBCs is offset by increase in RBC volume (H_2O shifts into the cells)

ECF, extracellular fluid; ICF, intracellular fluid; RBC, red blood cell; SIADH, syndrome of inappropriate antidiuretic hormone secretion; TBW, total body weight.

$C_x/C_{inulin} < 1.0$ indicates that the clearance of substance X is lower than that of inulin, suggesting two possibilities:

- The substance is **not freely filtered** (eg, albumin).
- The substance **is filtered,** but is subsequently **reabsorbed** (eg, glucose, amino acids, urea, phosphate, Na⁺, Cl⁻, and HCO_3^-).

$C_x/C_{inulin} > 1.0$ indicates that substance X is filtered with net secretion.

Glomerular Filtration Barrier

Glomerular filtration is closely regulated by the barrier (Figure 8-13) that separates the blood from the Bowman space and is composed of three main layers.

- **Fenestrated capillary endothelium** originates from the afferent arteriole and ends with the beginning of the efferent arteriole.

TABLE 8-7.   Interpreting C_x

$C_x > GFR$	Substance filtered and secreted
$C_x < GFR$	Substance filtered and partially reabsorbed
$C_x = GFR$	Substance filtered and excreted with no net reabsorption or secretion

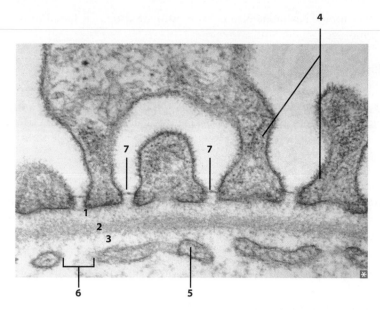

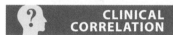

FIGURE 8-13. **Electron photomicrograph of the glomerular filtration barrier.** 1, Lamina rara externae; 2, lamina densa; 3, lamina rara interna; 4, podocytes; 5, capillary endothelium; 6, endothelial pore; 7, filtration slit membrane.

- **Glomerular basement membrane (GBM)** is composed of types IV and V collagen, laminin (glycoprotein), and heparan sulfate (proteoglycan). Laminin and heparan sulfate account for the GBM's **negative charge**, thus keeping plasma proteins, which also have a slight negative charge, from entering the Bowman space. The basement membrane is composed of **three layers**: lamina rara interna, lamina densa, and lamina rara externa.
- **Podocytes** line the outside of the GBM and form part of the visceral layer of the Bowman capsule. They form a network of interdigitating foot processes with intervening filtration slit diaphragms that regulate filtration into the urinary space, preventing large, negatively charged plasma proteins from passing through.

Glomerular Filtrate

Material filtered through the glomerular filtration barrier, normally created at a rate of approximately **120 mL/min**. The glomerular filtration barrier is relatively impermeable to proteins; thus, the filtrate contains little protein. Certain molecules, such as calcium and fatty acids, which are bound to plasma proteins, have a lower-than-expected concentration within the filtrate. Several other factors determine whether a substance will pass through the filtration barrier:

- Molecular size (limited by fenestrated capillary endothelium)
- Shape
- Charge (negative charge of heparan sulfate repels negatively charged proteins)
- Hemodynamic conditions

Glomerular Filtration Rate

Represents renal clearance of a substance that is **neither reabsorbed nor secreted** by the nephron.

- **Inulin** is the gold standard when measuring GFR because it is freely filtered and neither reabsorbed nor secreted (glomerular marker).
- **Creatinine** is more commonly used for GFR calculations. Creatinine is an end product of muscle metabolism and constantly released into the blood. The level of creatinine in the blood primarily depends on production by the muscle and filtration by the kidney. Creatinine clearance is an estimation of GFR and can be measured based on creatinine concentrations in the urine and blood and the urine flow (vol-

CLINICAL CORRELATION

The GBM charge barrier is lost in **nephrotic syndrome,** thereby allowing proteins to leak out of the capillaries, and leading to **albuminuria, hypoproteinemia, and generalized edema. Hyperlipidemia** is also seen in nephrotic syndrome, probably due to the stimulating effect that decreased plasma oncotic pressure has on hepatic lipoprotein synthesis. Hypercoagulability is present as well, due to loss of antithrombin III in the urine.

FLASH FORWARD

The α_3 chain of collagen type IV, the target antigen in **Goodpasture syndrome,** is a component of both the GBM and the alveolar basement membrane.

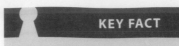

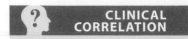

ume over time). Formulae also exist to estimate the GFR based only on serum creatinine, age, gender, and ethnicity.

Renal Blood Flow

The blood flow to the kidneys represents approximately 25% of the total cardiac output. Based on an average cardiac output of 5 L/min, the kidneys receive 1.25 L/min, or 1800 L/day. Because the kidneys handle the entire blood volume many times over each day, they play a crucial role in systemic blood circulation, as well as maintaining normal body fluid volume and composition.

The kidney contains numerous nephrons with vasculature connected in series. Blood flow to the nephrons is supplied by afferent arterioles branching off interlobular arteries within the kidney. Plasma is filtered in the glomerular capillary bed, and the filtered blood flows out into the interlobular veins via the efferent arterioles.

- The average pressure of the **afferent arteriole is 85 mm Hg.**
- The average pressure of the **efferent arteriole is 60 mm Hg.**

Regulation Mechanisms

Systemic BP and perfusion dramatically affect renal function. Physiologic changes in Starling forces and renal vascular resistance allow for regulation of renal blood flow (RBF) and function (Table 8-8, Figure 8-14).

Influencing Factors

The sympathetic nervous system, hormones, and various drugs influence renal function (Figure 8-14).

- **Sympathetic nervous system:** Exerts its action via the catecholamines **epinephrine and norepinephrine,** via activation of α_1 **receptors,** causing vasoconstriction of the renal arterioles (afferent > efferent), and a decrease in RBF and GFR; and via β_1 receptor-mediated renin release. Moderate sympathetic stimulation does not result in a change in GFR.

TABLE 8-8. Modulation of Renal Blood Flow and Filtration

EFFECT	GFR	RENAL PLASMA FLOW (RPF)	FILTRATION FRACTION (GFR/RPF)
Afferent arteriole constriction (as with norepinephrine)	↓ due to ↓ P_{GC}	↓	No change
Afferent arteriole dilation (as with PGE_2 or PGI_2)	↑ due to ↑ P_{GC}	↑	No change
Efferent arteriole constriction (as with angiotensin II)	↑ due to ↑ P_{GC}	↓	⇑
Increased plasma protein concentration (as with multiple myeloma)	↓ due to ↑ π_{GC}	No change	⇓
Decreased plasma protein concentration (as with nephrotic syndrome)	↑ due to ↓ π_{GC}	No change	⇑
Constriction of ureter or urinary tract obstruction	↓ due to ↑ P_{BS}	No change	⇓

P_{GC}, glomerular capillary hydrostatic pressure; P_{BS}, Bowman space hydrostatic pressure; π_{GC}, glomerular capillary plasma colloid osmotic pressure; π_{BS}, Bowman space interstitial colloid osmotic pressure.

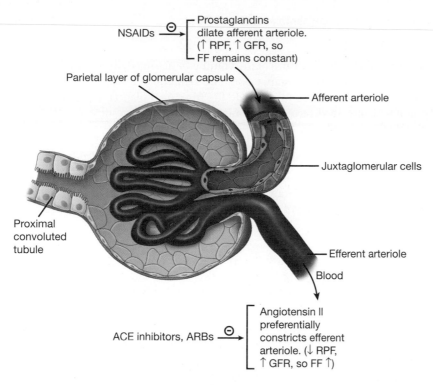

FIGURE 8-14.   **Effects of medications and hormones on renal plasma flow.** ACE, angiotensin-converting enzyme; ARB, angiotensin receptor blocker; FF, filtration fraction; GFR, glomerular filtration rate; RPF, renal plasma flow.

- **Prostaglandins/bradykinin:** PGE_2 and PGI_2 (both produced in the kidneys) cause dilatation of afferent > efferent arterioles, thereby increasing RBF and GFR.
- **Angiotensin II:** A potent vasoconstrictor produced in response to decreased afferent arteriolar pressure from decreased renal blood flow. Angiotensin II constricts both afferent and efferent arterioles, but preferentially constricts the efferent arteriole, thus increasing or maintaining the pressure on the glomerulus. Angiotensin II maintains the GFR even in the face of decreased overall renal blood flow.
- **Dopamine** (precursor of norepinephrine) dilates the renal vessels and suppresses sodium reabsorption in the proximal tubule by inhibiting the action of the basolateral Na^+/K^+-ATPase pump. Dopamine is released directly by the proximal tubule in response to a rise in BP, resulting in increased RBF and GFR.

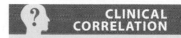

CLINICAL CORRELATION

NSAIDs inhibit prostaglandin synthesis and interfere with the renal protective effects of prostaglandins (GFR and RBF are reduced).

Autoregulation Mechanisms

Autoregulation is the process by which an organ maintains relatively constant blood flow despite variations in BP. These mechanisms typically have limits outside of which they are ineffective (eg, at systolic blood pressures < 80 mm Hg and > 200 mm Hg).

The kidney has two proposed autoregulatory mechanisms: **stretch (myogenic)** and **tubuloglomerular feedback.**

- **Stretch mechanism:** When BP increases, arterioles in the kidney are stretched. This leads to vasoconstriction of the afferent arteriole, which maintains constant RBF and GFR.
- **Tubuloglomerular feedback mechanism:** Increased arterial pressure leads to increased RBF and GFR, and increased flow to the distal tubule, which is sensed by the macula densa. Through a variety of mechanisms, the macula densa causes vasoconstriction of the afferent arteriole, thereby attenuating RBF and GFR and closing the negative feedback loop.

Measurement of Renal Plasma and Blood Flow

Renal Plasma Flow

Renal plasma flow is the measure of the volume of plasma delivered to the kidney in a given amount of time. If a substance could be cleared completely from the plasma, its clearance rate could be used to calculate the true renal plasma flow (RPF). However, RPF cannot be directly determined because there is no known substance that is cleared completely from the plasma.

para-Aminohippuric acid (**PAH**) is an endogenous substance that is 90% excreted from plasma through the kidneys via both filtration and secretion. The amount of PAH in the plasma of the renal artery is approximately equal to the amount of PAH in the urine. Therefore, the clearance rate of PAH can be used to calculate the effective renal plasma flow (**ERPF**).

$$\text{ERPF} = (U_{\text{PAH}} \times V)/P_{\text{PAH}} = C_{\text{PAH}}$$

where U_{PAH} is the urine concentration of PAH, V is the urine flow rate, P_{PAH} is the plasma concentration of PAH, and C_{PAH} is the clearance rate of PAH. ERPF can be used to calculate the value of true RPF and RBF.

True Renal Plasma Flow

The ERPF is an approximation of the true RPF. Because only 90% of PAH is cleared in a single pass through the kidney, the true value of RPF is underestimated by 10%. Therefore, true RPF can be calculated as:

$$\text{True RPF} = \text{ERPF}/0.9$$

Renal Blood Flow

Renal plasma flow can be used to determine RBF, which represents the volume of blood delivered to the kidney in a given period of time. RBF can be determined using the equation:

$$\text{RBF} = (\text{RPF})/(1 - \text{hematocrit})$$

Filtration Fraction

Filtration fraction (FF) is the fraction of plasma filtered across the glomerular filtration barrier. It can be calculated if the GFR and the RPF are known:

$$\text{FF} = \text{GFR}/\text{RPF}$$

Normally, the FF is approximately 0.20. Therefore, about 20% of the RPF enters the renal tubules, while the remaining 80% leaves the glomerulus via the efferent arteriole and becomes the peritubular capillary circulation.

Changes in Filtration Fraction

Changes in the FF alter the plasma protein concentration, and thereby the osmolarity within the peritubular capillaries. For example, an increase in FF reduces the amount and increases the osmolarity of the plasma flowing into the peritubular capillaries. The FF can be modulated by changes in either RPF or GFR.

- **Renal vascular resistance** and the **hydrostatic pressure differential** between the renal artery and vein affect the flow of blood throughout the nephrons (see Table 8-8).
- Increased vascular resistance → decreased RPF, increased hydrostatic pressure differential.

KEY FACT

PAH is filtered and secreted but is NOT reabsorbed. It estimates RPF.

KEY FACT

PAH is freely filtered. Thus, filtration cannot be saturated. An increase in plasma PAH concentration will be matched proportionally by filtration.

KEY FACT

PAH secretion is dependent on the number of transporters present in the membrane. Thus, PAH secretion can be saturated as PAH plasma concentration rises.

■ Decreased vascular resistance → increased RPF, decreased hydrostatic pressure differential.

Changes in renal arterial and venous pressures can affect the FF; however, the autoregulatory mechanisms of the kidney ordinarily maintain the RBF and GFR within a relatively constant and narrow range.

Additionally, the rate of filtration across the glomerular capillaries is dictated by **Starling forces** (Figure 8-15). GFR can be calculated by applying the **Starling equation:**

$$GFR = K_f[(P_{GC} - P_{BS}) - (\pi_{GC} - \pi_{BS})]$$

where K_f is the filtration coefficient, P_{GC} is the glomerular capillary hydrostatic pressure, P_{BS} is the Bowman space hydrostatic pressure, π_{GC} is the glomerular capillary plasma colloid osmotic pressure, and π_{BS} is the Bowman space interstitial colloid osmotic pressure (usually π_{BS} is zero because very little protein is filtered).

Concepts of Reabsorption and Secretion

Glucose

Completely reabsorbed in the **proximal tubules.** However, when serum glucose levels reach about 200 mg/dL, the reabsorption mechanism becomes overwhelmed and glucose may be excreted in the urine (this phenomenon is known as **splay,** or the excretion of a substance in small amounts before the **transport maximum [T_m]** is reached). Splay is caused by heterogeneity of nephrons and relatively low affinity of the Na+-glucose carriers. At serum glucose levels exceeding 350 mg/dL, the transport mechanism becomes completely saturated, resulting in clinical **glucosuria** (Figure 8-16).

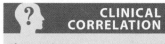

Amino Acids

Reabsorbed by secondary active transport in the **proximal tubules.** The transport mechanism is T_m-limited, and saturation may result in the excretion of amino acids in the urine.

In general, amino acids are not found in the urine unless the individual has a genetic transport deficiency. For example, cystinuria may be observed in patients with defects in the proximal tubule protein mediating cystine reabsorption, possibly leading to formation of cystine stones.

Hartnup disease is an autosomal recessive disorder caused by defective neutral amino acid (ie, tryptophan) transporters in the proximal renal tubule and on enterocytes. Neutral amino acids are lost via the urine (neutral aminoaciduria), and there is decreased absorption of neutral amino acids via the GI tract. Low levels of tryptophan lead to

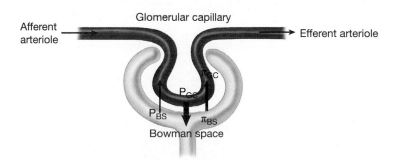

FIGURE 8-15. **Starling forces.** Example of Starling forces acting on glomerular capillaries of a single nephron provided net pressure = 0 mm Hg and filtration equilibrium. Average values: P_{GC}, 45 mm Hg; P_{BS}, 10 mm Hg; π_{BS}, 0 mm Hg; π_{GC}, 27 mm Hg.

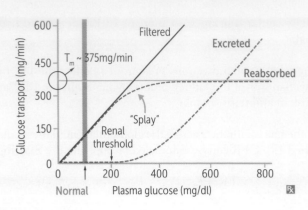

FIGURE 8-16.   Glucose titration curve.

decreased production of niacin. Pellagra-like symptoms of diarrhea, dermatitis, and dementia develop.

Urea

A waste product from the metabolism of amino acids, urea is excreted in large amounts in the urine, and minimally reabsorbed. Urea contributes to the formation of **hyperosmolar urine** through its unique recirculation pathway, which helps to maintain the corticomedullary osmotic gradient (see Figure 8-21, depicting the countercurrent multiplier system [CCMS]).

Para-Aminohippuric Acid

A substance that is both freely filtered through the glomerulus and secreted from the peritubular capillaries into the tubular lumen. PAH is not reabsorbed. As a result, PAH is almost completely cleared from the plasma and is used to estimate RPF (see earlier discussion).

Free Water

Also referred to as solute-free water, it is produced in the thick ascending limb and the early distal tubule. In these diluting segments, NaCl is reabsorbed and the free water remains in the tubules to be excreted in the urine. As urine is produced, water and solutes are excreted in a somewhat independent manner. Excreted solutes can be calculated using osmolar clearance (C_{osm}):

$$C_{osm} = \frac{(U_{osm} \times V)}{P_{osm}}$$

where U_{osm} is the urine osmolarity and P_{osm} is the plasma osmolarity. Free water clearance is equal to the difference between the urine flow rate and osmolar clearance:

$$C_{H_2O} = V - C_{osm}$$

Urine Osmolarity

The clearance of free water can be used to estimate the kidneys' ability to concentrate or dilute urine.

- When C_{H_2O} **is positive**, excess water is excreted and urine is dilute.
- When C_{H_2O} **is negative**, excess solutes are excreted, water is retained, and urine is concentrated.
- When C_{H_2O} **is zero**, urine is iso-osmotic to plasma.

In order to concentrate urine, high levels of ADH (vasopressin) are needed to increase the permeability of the distal tubule and the collecting ducts to water, and an adequate corticomedullary osmotic gradient is required to provide the osmotic drive for water reabsorption.

- In the **presence of ADH,** urine is **concentrated** (conserving water).
- In the **absence of ADH,** urine is **dilute.**

Nephron Physiology and the Tubular System

The **nephron unit** is composed of the **glomerulus,** through which fluid is filtered from the blood, and the **tubular system,** where the filtered fluid is modified through reabsorption and secretion of various solutes to produce urine.

Glomerulus

A network of glomerular capillaries encased in the **Bowman capsule.** Blood flows from the **afferent arteriole** into the glomerular capillaries, where it is either filtered into the Bowman space or continues to flow through the **efferent arteriole** and the peritubular capillary system.

The fluid that is filtered into Bowman space flows into the tubular portion of the nephron. The tubule can be divided into several segments with different characteristics and functions. Each segment relies on the **basolateral Na^+/K^+-ATPase pump** to maintain low intracellular Na^+ concentration, establishing a Na^+ gradient for Na^+ movement from the lumen into the cells.

Proximal Tubule

The major site of reabsorption (Figure 8-17). The cellular mechanism of reabsorption is based on the **transmembrane Na^+ gradient,** which provides energy for numerous **secondary active transport** mechanisms. Solutes and water are reabsorbed passively and proportionally; therefore tubular fluid leaving the proximal tubule is isosmotic to plasma.

- Reabsorbs **all filtered glucose** and **amino acids,** 60–70% of the filtered electrolytes and water, and 50% of filtered urea from the tubular fluid.
- Na^+ is reabsorbed via **cotransport** with amino acids, glucose, lactate, and phosphate, and via **countertransport** with H^+ through the Na^+–H^+ exchanger, which is linked directly to the reabsorption of filtered HCO_3^- through the action of brush border carbonic anhydrase.

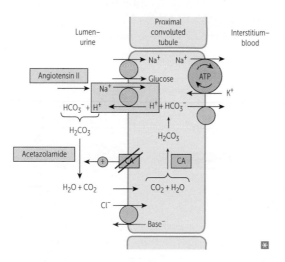

FIGURE 8-17. **Early proximal convoluted tubule, "workhorse of the nephron."** Reabsorbs all of the glucose and amino acids and most of the bicarbonate (HCO_3^-), sodium (Na^+), and water (H_2O). Secretes ammonia, which acts as a buffer for secreted H^+. Pink circles indicate transporters. ATP, adenosine triphosphate; CA, carbonic anhydrase.

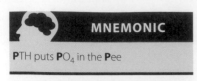
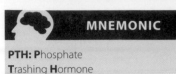
- Ammonia secretion buffers the secreted H$^+$.
- **Na$^+$ is primarily reabsorbed with Cl$^-$ in the late proximal tubule** as follows: Reabsorption of H$_2$O without significant Cl$^-$ reabsorption in the early proximal tubule establishes a high Cl$^-$ chemical gradient that drives Cl$^-$ reabsorption through the cell and into the interstitium; Na$^+$ follows to restore the electroneutrality of the interstitium.
- Angiotensin II and also the sympathetic nervous system (eg, norepinephrine) act on the proximal tubule at the Na$^+$–H$^+$ exchanger to stimulate Na$^+$ reabsorption, whereas atrial natriuretic peptide (ANP) released from stretched atria blocks Na$^+$ reabsorption.
- **Parathyroid hormone (PTH)** decreases phosphate reabsorption by activating adenylate cyclase to increase production of cAMP, which inhibits Na$^+$–phosphate cotransport.

Loop of Henle

Consists of three portions: (1) thin descending; (2) thin ascending; and (3) thick ascending limbs. The majority of action occurs in the thick ascending limb of the loop.

- **Thin descending limb** reabsorbs about 20% of the filtered water, but no solute reabsorption occurs in this segment.
- **Thin ascending limb** is impermeable to water and has no significant reabsorption.
- **Thick ascending limb** is a **diluting segment** of the tubular system (Figure 8-18). It is impermeable to water, yet reabsorbs solutes. This segment actively reabsorbs Na$^+$, K$^+$, and Cl$^-$ via the **Na$^+$–K$^+$–2Cl$^-$ symporter.** Reabsorbed K$^+$ leaks back into the lumen through renal output medullary potassium (ROMK) channels, creating a slight positive charge in the lumen fluid. This positive charge indirectly induces paracellular diffusion of Mg^{2+} and Ca^{2+} into the interstitial fluid.
- The distal thick ascending limb contains the **macula densa** of the juxtaglomerular complex, which provides **tubuloglomerular feedback** for autoregulation of RBF.

Early Distal Convoluted Tubule

- Cortical **diluting segment** of the tubular system (Figure 8-19).
- The distal tubule transport mechanism relies on the Na$^+$–Cl$^-$ cotransporter (situated on the luminal membrane), which provides the basis for Na$^+$, Cl$^-$, K$^+$, Ca^{2+}, and Mg^{2+} trafficking into and out of the lumen. This segment is impermeable to water and urea.
- **Angiotensin II** acts on the early distal tubule to stimulate Na$^+$ reabsorption, while **atrial natriuretic peptide (ANP)** blocks Na$^+$ reabsorption.
- **PTH** acts to increase active Ca^{2+} reabsorption.

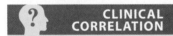
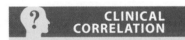
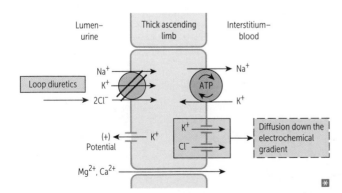

FIGURE 8-18. **Thick ascending limb of Henle.** This structure actively reabsorbs Na$^+$, K$^+$, and Cl$^-$, and indirectly induces the reabsorption of Mg^{2+} and Ca^{2+}. It is impermeable to water. Pink circle indicates transporter.

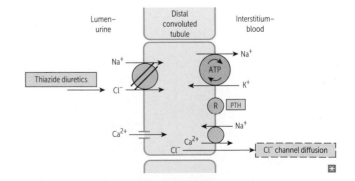

FIGURE 8-19. **Early distal convoluted tubule.** Actively reabsorbs Na$^+$ and Cl$^-$. Reabsorption of Ca^{2+} is under the control of parathyroid hormone. Pink circles indicate transporters.

Late Distal Tubule and Collecting Ducts

Composed of two cell types, principal and intercalated cells (Figure 8-20).

- **Principal cells** reabsorb Na^+ and water and secrete K^+ via the basolateral Na^+–K^+-ATPase pump and apical ROMK channels.
- **α-Intercalated cells** are key players in acid–base regulation of body fluids, as they secrete H^+ and reabsorb K^+ and HCO_3^-. Carbonic acid can be formed in these cells via the catalytic action of carbonic anhydrase on H_2O and CO_2. The carbonic acid then dissociates into H^+ and HCO_3^-. H^+ is secreted into the tubular lumen via the H^+–ATPase and H^+–K^+ exchanger. (*Note:* There are also β-intercalated cells that secrete HCO_3^- and reabsorb H^+.)
- **Aldosterone** stimulates Na^+ reabsorption and K^+ secretion in the principal cells, as well as H^+ secretion in the intercalated cells.
- In the presence of ADH (vasopressin), water channels called aquaporins are inserted into the luminal membrane of principal cells, making them more permeable to water. In the absence of ADH, the late distal and collecting ducts are less permeable to water. The level of ADH therefore controls the concentration of urine.
- **Urea** reabsorption only occurs in the inner medullary collecting ducts (the late distal tubules, the cortical collecting ducts, and the outer medullary collecting ducts are impermeable to urea). ADH increases urea permeability in the inner medullary collecting ducts.

Countercurrent Multiplier System

The countercurrent multiplier system (CCMS) is a U-shaped structure that is an integral part of the nephron known as the **loop of Henle**. The CCMS comprises three loop regions (**thin descending limb, thin ascending limb, and the thick ascending limb**),

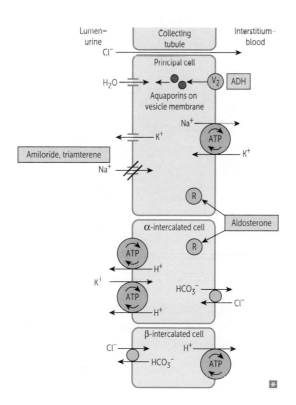

FIGURE 8-20. **Collecting tubules reabsorb Na^+ in exchange for secreting K^+ or H^+ (regulated by aldosterone).** Reabsorption of water is regulated by ADH (vasopressin). Osmolarity of the medulla can reach 1200 mOsm. Pink circles indicate transporters.

which are responsible for establishing the renal medullary interstitial fluid osmotic gradient through a multistep process (see Figure 8-21). The term **countercurrent** describes the fluid movement in opposite directions in adjacent tubes.

Countercurrent Exchanger (Vasa Recta)

How does the water reclaimed from the filtrate make it back to the circulation? The vasa recta are U-shaped capillaries that are freely permeable to water and all solutes except protein. They are situated in close proximity to the loop of Henle, allowing them to equilibrate readily with the surrounding interstitial fluid. The high oncotic pressure in the vasa recta resulting from loss of protein-free filtrate in the glomerulus leads to avid water reabsorption.

The U shape of the vasa recta allows for the preservation of the corticomedullary osmolar gradient (Figure 8-21). As the capillaries run down into the salty medulla, they lose water and gain solute. As they run back toward the cortex, they gain water and lose solute. As such, the vasa recta absorb water and excess solute without dissipating the gradient.

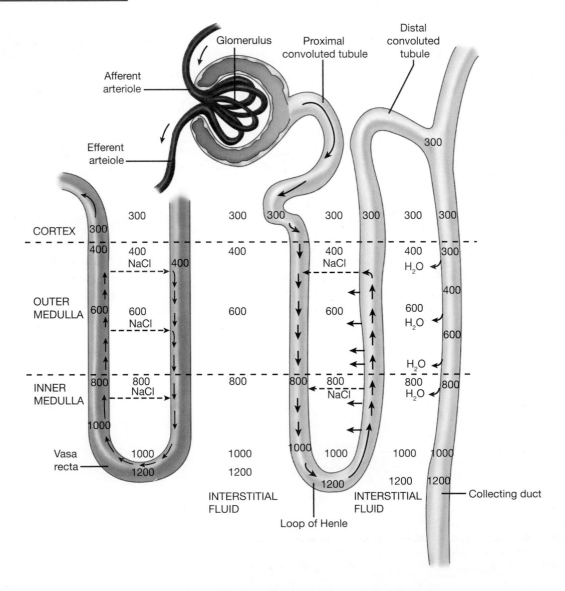

FIGURE 8-21. **Countercurrent multiplier system and vasa recta, the countercurrent exchanger.**

Kidney Endocrine Functions

The kidney performs four major endocrine functions:

- Secretion of erythropoietin (EPO).
- Formation of 1,25-dihydroxycholecalciferol.
- Production of renin (discussed in detail in the later section on the Renin-Angiotensin-Aldosterone System).
- Production of prostaglandins.

Erythropoietin

EPO is a glycoprotein hormone released in response to hypoxia that stimulates RBC production by the bone marrow. In healthy individuals, approximately 90% of all EPO is synthesized in the kidneys. EPO exerts its action through **EPO receptors** on the surface of **proerythroblasts** in the bone marrow. This accelerates the **maturation of proerythroblasts** (to their erythroblastic stage). In the absence of EPO, few RBCs are formed by the bone marrow. Therefore, individuals with insufficient concentrations of EPO (eg, patients with severe kidney disease/failure) may become anemic because they cannot appropriately respond to hypoxia by increasing EPO and RBC production.

Vitamin D: Formation of 1,25-Dihydroxycholecalciferol in the Kidneys

Vitamin D and **PTH** are critical for regulating Ca^{2+} and phosphate metabolism. Vitamin D is a fat-soluble vitamin that is mainly produced in the skin by UV-B light conversion of 7-dehydrocholesterol or ingested in the diet or dietary supplements. Vitamin D is stored in the liver in its inactive form, 25-OH-cholecalciferol; its activation depends on the plasma Ca^{2+} concentration.

Decreased plasma Ca^{2+} levels stimulate PTH secretion, which activates 1α-hydroxylase in the kidneys. This in turn enables the hydroxylation of 25-OH-cholecalciferol (C1 position) into 1,25-$(OH)_2$-cholecalciferol (physiologically active form), which increases intestinal absorption of Ca^{2+} and decreases renal Ca^{2+} and phosphate excretion.

The syndrome of **vitamin D resistance** develops if the kidneys are unable to produce its active metabolite, 1,25-$(OH)_2$-cholecalciferol, despite normal vitamin D intake and availability. This condition can be either inherited (1α-hydroxylase deficiency) or acquired (chronic kidney disease, end-stage renal failure). An extremely rare form of rickets can also result from mutations in the vitamin D receptor gene.

Prostaglandins

Prostaglandins PGE_2 and PGI_2, and **bradykinin** dilate the afferent arterioles to increase RBF and GFR. The use of NSAIDs inhibits prostaglandin production and their effects.

Hormones Acting on the Kidney

Just as the kidney produces several hormones, several others affect kidney function: ANF, PTH, aldosterone, angiotensin II, and ADH (Table 8-9).

Atrial Natriuretic Peptide

The cardiac atria release ANP in response to increased stretching of the muscle fibers (secondary to volume overload or heart failure). ANP causes vasodilation of the afferent arterioles, vasoconstriction of efferent arterioles, and decreased sodium reabsorption in the late distal tubules and collecting ducts.

CLINICAL CORRELATION

Systemic deficiency of EPO and consequent anemia often ensue as a result of chronic kidney disease (CKD), renal malignancy, or as an adverse effect of chemotherapy.

KEY FACT

Human recombinant EPO is available as supportive treatment for patients with advanced chronic kidney disease, end-stage renal disease, HIV-associated anemia, and other similar conditions.

Remember: Patients must also receive proper iron supplementation.

KEY FACT

The action of 1,25-$(OH)_2$-cholecalciferol in the kidney differs from that of PTH:

- **1,25-$(OH)_2$-cholecalciferol** stimulates reabsorption of both Ca^{2+} and phosphate.
- **PTH** stimulates Ca^{2+} reabsorption, but inhibits phosphate reabsorption.

CLINICAL CORRELATION

A related peptide, brain natriuretic peptide (BNP) is released by distended ventricular myocardium under conditions of high volume and/or pressure and as such is often measured to evaluate dyspnea. High values suggest congestive heart failure (CHF) as the etiology.

TABLE 8-9. Summary of Hormones Acting on the Kidney and Their Sites of Action

HORMONE	STIMULUS	MECHANISM AND SITE OF ACTION
ADH	■ Increased plasma osmolarity ■ Decreased blood volume ■ Nausea, pain ■ Stress (ie, surgery)	■ Increases H_2O permeability of principal cells in collecting ducts ■ Increases urea reabsorption in collecting ducts ■ Increases Na^+–K^+–$2Cl^-$ symporter activity in the thick ascending limb
Aldosterone	■ Decreased blood volume (via angiotensin II) ■ Hyperkalemia	Late distal tubule and collecting ducts: ■ Increases Na^+ reabsorption ■ Increases K^+ excretion ■ Increases H^+ excretion
Angiotensin II	■ Decreased blood volume (via renin)	■ Constriction of efferent arteriole resulting in increased GFR ■ Stimulation of Na^+–H^+ exchange in the PCT ■ Stimulation of aldosterone synthesis by the adrenal glands
ANP	■ Increased atrial pressure	■ Decreases Na^+ reabsorption; increases GFR
PTH	■ Decreased plasma Ca^{2+} ■ Increased plasma PO_4^-	■ Increases Ca^{2+} reabsorption ■ Decreases PO_4^- reabsorption ■ Increases 1,25-$(OH)_2$-vitamin D production

ADH, antidiuretic hormone; ANP, atrial natriuretic peptide; GFR, glomerular filtration rate; PCT, proximal convoluted tubule; PTH, parathyroid hormone.

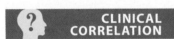
CLINICAL CORRELATION

Renal osteodystrophy results from hyperphosphatemia and hypocalcemia, both the result of little to no phosphate excretion by damaged kidneys, low vitamin D levels, and/or tertiary hyperparathyroidism. Tertiary hyperparathyroidism refers to the situation in which hyperparathyroidism, usually in the context of end-stage renal disease, becomes refractory to normal physiologic regulation and medical therapy.

Parathyroid Hormone

PTH exerts three main actions on the kidneys:

■ Inhibition of phosphate reabsorption in the PCT. This is accomplished by inhibition of the Na^+–phosphate cotransporter. **Phosphaturia** is followed by increased cAMP excretion (**urinary cAMP**). This action of PTH on the kidney is important for the overall Ca^{2+} availability in the ECF. Excess phosphate, resulting from decreased phosphate secretion, leads to "trapping" (complexing) of the free Ca^{2+}, thereby reducing its availability in the plasma.

■ Stimulation of 1α-hydroxylase in the PCT to generate the active form of vitamin D: 1,25-$(OH)_2$-cholecalciferol.

■ Stimulation of Ca^{2+} reabsorption (**hypocalciuric action**) in the DCT. This occurs via the basolateral PTH receptors, which employ a second-messenger system (eg, conversion of ATP to cAMP). This further increases the availability of free Ca^{2+} in plasma.

Renin-Angiotensin-Aldosterone System

The RAAS functions to allow the kidneys to regulate BP (Figure 8-22). Renin is an enzyme synthesized and stored as an inactive compound, prorenin, in the juxtaglomerular cells of the kidneys (located in the walls of the afferent arterioles proximal to the glomeruli).

Several factors affect the **release of renin** into the bloodstream:

■ Fall in arterial BP (hypotension), which results in decreased renal perfusion. This is perceived as a decreased stretch signal by the juxtaglomerular cells, which respond by excreting renin.

■ Increased renal sympathetic activity.

■ β₁-Adrenergic stimulation.

■ Decreased Na^+ delivery to the macula densa.

These conditions initiate the conversion of prorenin to renin in the juxtaglomerular cells, and its subsequent release into the bloodstream, where renin enzymatically cleaves

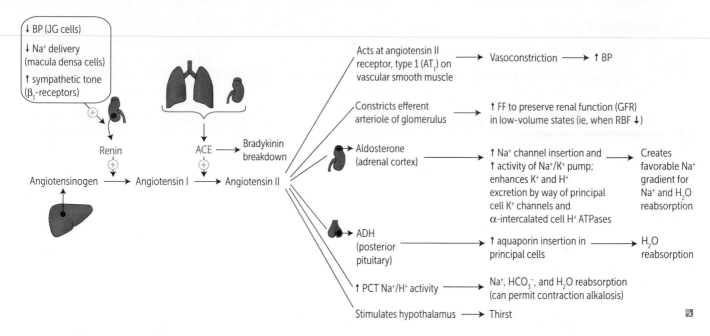

FIGURE 8-22. **The renin–angiotensin–aldosterone system.** ACE, angiotensin-converting enzyme; ADH, antidiuretic hormone; AT, angiotensin; BP, blood pressure; FF, filtration fraction; GFR, glomerular filtration rate; JG, juxtaglomerular; PCT, proximal convoluted tubule; RBF, renal blood flow.

angiotensinogen to release angiotensin I. **Angiotensin I** is then cleaved by angiotensin-converting enzyme (ACE), found in the endothelium of the lung vasculature and kidneys, to form **angiotensin II**.

There are at least three mechanisms by which circulating angiotensin II elevates arterial BP:

- **Direct vasoconstriction (fast response):** Constriction of the arterioles increases total peripheral resistance (TPR), and constriction of the veins promotes increased venous return of blood to the heart, both of which increase BP. The **efferent arterioles** of the kidney are especially affected.
- **Decreased excretion** of salt and water via stimulation of **aldosterone** synthesis in the adrenal glands (**slow response**). Aldosterone promotes Na^+ reabsorption in the distal tubules and collecting ducts, which leads to increases in the ECF and blood volumes.
- **Direct action on the kidneys:** This action is independent of its actions via the aldosterone pathway. In this case, angiotensin II stimulates $Na^+–H^+$ exchange at the level of the proximal tubule, thereby increasing the reabsorption of Na^+ and HCO_3^-.

Angiotensin II only persists in the blood for 1–2 minutes before it is inactivated by angiotensinase. For this reason, the angiotensin II stimulation of aldosterone production is more influential in restoring arterial BP than its direct vasoconstrictive actions.

Aldosterone

A mineralocorticoid synthesized in the zona glomerulosa of the adrenal cortex. Whereas adrenocorticotropic hormone (ACTH) is the primary regulator of the corticosteroid hormones, aldosterone's synthesis and secretion are mainly regulated by changes in ECF volume via the RAAS and changes in serum K^+ levels.

- **Late distal tubule:** Aldosterone exerts its action via stimulation of the mineralocorticoid receptors (MRs) on **principal cells.** This action increases the permeability of their apical (luminal) membrane to Na^+ and K^+ by adding newly synthesized pro-

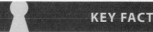

CLINICAL CORRELATION

Na^+ and Ca^{2+} reabsorption are not coupled at the level of the distal tubule as they are in the thick ascending limb. Therefore, **thiazide diuretics** can be used in cases of **idiopathic calciuria** because, though they inhibit Na^+ reabsorption, they also act to increase Ca^{2+} reabsorption.

FLASH BACK

β_1-Agonists (eg, isoproterenol) stimulate renin secretion.
β_1-Antagonists (eg, propranolol) inhibit renin secretion.

KEY FACT

Overall, angiotensin II serves to ↑ intravascular volume and ↑ BP.

KEY FACT

Excess aldosterone causes hypokalemia.

CLINICAL CORRELATION

Potassium-sparing diuretics such as spironolactone inhibit the actions of aldosterone in the distal nephron.

KEY FACT

Mineralocorticoid escape is the ability of the glomerulotubular autoregulatory mechanism to override the action of aldosterone in cases of increased ECF (volume expansion). It is likely that increased ANP secondary to hypervolemia, decreased expression of thiazide-sensitive NaCl cotransporters in the distal tubule, and "pressure natriuresis" resulting from increased blood pressure all may contribute to this escape.

CLINICAL CORRELATION

Syndrome of inappropriate ADH secretion (SIADH) → excessively concentrated urine and inappropriately dilute serum → hyponatremia.
SIADH is most commonly caused by central nervous system (CNS) or pulmonary disease, or as a paraneoplastic syndrome.

teins (epithelial sodium channels [ENaC], ROMK channels) as well as basolateral Na^+–K^+-ATPases and enzymes of the citric acid cycle, which stimulate ATP hydrolysis, reabsorption of Na^+ and water into the blood, and K^+ secretion into the urine.

- **Collecting duct:** Aldosterone also stimulates H^+ secretion by **α-intercalated cells,** thereby regulating plasma HCO_3^- levels and acid-base balance.

Antidiuretic Hormone

Also known as **vasopressin,** ADH plays a major role in determining whether the kidney produces and excretes concentrated or dilute urine (Figure 8-23). It originates in the hypothalamus/posterior pituitary gland, and is produced in response to high serum osmolarity or significantly diminished blood volume. It is also produced in response to angiotensin II as part of the RAAS, which acts to increase blood volume and BP.

- ADH acts on **V2 receptors** of **principal cells** in the **late DCT/collecting ducts.** It causes an increase in the number of functioning water channels (**aquaporins**), thereby increasing the permeability of the collecting ducts to water.
- **Presence of ADH** leads to the passive reabsorption of large amounts of water in the collecting ducts, thereby decreasing urine volume and increasing urine osmolarity (**hyperosmotic** urine).
- In the **absence of ADH,** the collecting ducts are virtually impermeable to water, and large amounts of very dilute (**hyposmotic**) urine are excreted.
- In **high levels, ADH** also acts on **V1 receptors** on arterioles to cause vasoconstriction. This is particularly important in the setting of **hemorrhage, in which ADH helps maintain systemic BP.**
- Decreased pressure leads to activation of the RAAS (Figure 8-22), which raises total peripheral resistance and venous return and stimulates ADH release.
- Systemic baroreceptors (eg, carotid sinus) sense decreased BP, which causes ADH release from the posterior pituitary gland. ADH acts on the kidneys to retain volume, and acts on systemic arterioles to maintain pressure.

The combined efforts of the RAAS and ADH conserve fluid and maintain systemic pressure in the setting of hemorrhagic hypotension (Figure 8-24).

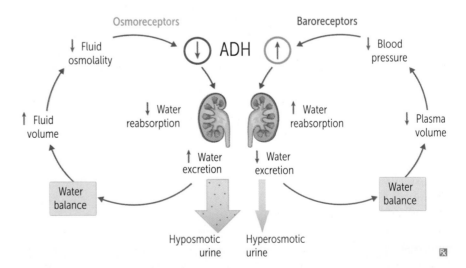

FIGURE 8-23. **Regulation of water balance.** The two major pathways for altering total body water: On the right, changes in antidiuretic hormone (ADH) release from the posterior pituitary are triggered by changes in blood volume. On the left, decreased osmolality causes swelling of osmoreceptor cells in the anterior hypothalamus, which inhibits their firing and inhibits adjacent superoptic nuclei cells, thereby reducing ADH secretion from their axonal extensions in the posterior pituitary.

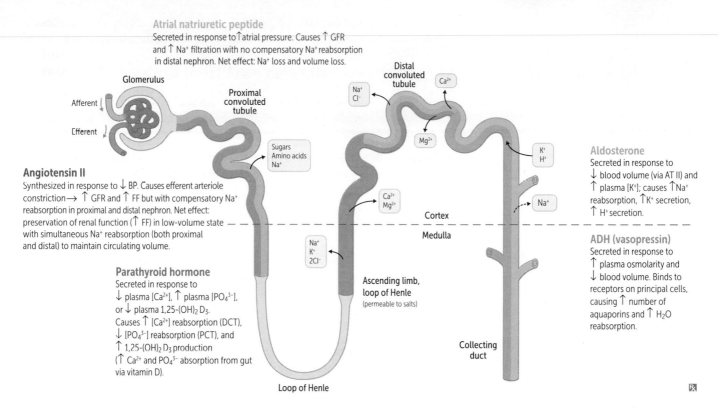

FIGURE 8-24.   **Hormonal action in the kidney.**

ACID-BASE HOMEOSTASIS

Acids and Bases

The body maintains serum pH within a tight range (approximately 7.40 ± 0.05) via a complex system that regulates acid production by metabolic processes. Importantly, most enzymes in the body function optimally within a very small pH range.

Acids

Molecules capable of releasing hydrogen ions into solution are known as acids.

- **Strong acids** rapidly dissociate into their ionic components in solution (eg, HCl → H^+ + Cl^-).
- **Weak acids** are less likely to dissociate into their ionic components, and therefore less readily release H^+. Carbonic acid (H_2CO_3) is an example of a weak acid.

Bases

Any ion or molecule that can accept a hydrogen ion. They often have a net negative charge in solution.

- **Strong bases** readily and strongly accept hydrogen ions in solution, rapidly reducing the hydrogen ion concentration. For example, the hydroxide ion (OH^-) is a strong base.
- **Weak bases** less readily accept hydrogen ions. Bicarbonate (HCO_3^-) is an example of a weak base.

Buffers

Ionic compounds that resist changes in pH when acid or base is either added or removed. Buffers function along a titration curve and are most effective along the linear portion of the curve (±1.0 pH unit from the pK_a value for that particular buffer). The pH of a buffer solution can be calculated using the **Henderson-Hasselbalch equation.**

$$pH = pK_a + \log [A^-]/[HA]$$

where A^- is the base form of the buffer and HA is the acid form of the buffer.

Acid Production

Acid production within the body is of two types: **volatile** and **nonvolatile.** Most of the acids in the body are weak acids, with the exception of hydrochloric acid (HCl^-), which is secreted in the form of gastric acid.

Volatile Acid

Produced in the form of CO_2 via cellular metabolism. The CO_2 produced then reacts with H_2O via the enzyme carbonic anhydrase to produce carbonic acid as shown:

$$CO_2 + H_2O \leftrightarrow H_2CO_3 \leftrightarrow H^+ + HCO_3^-$$

Nonvolatile Acid

Protein catabolism generates sulfuric acid, and phospholipid catabolism creates phosphoric acid. Other nonvolatile acids produced by the body include salicylic acid, lactic acid, and ketones.

Physiologic Buffers

Several molecules act as a buffer system. These are categorized based on their location in relation to the cellular membrane: **intracellular** and **extracellular.**

Intracellular Buffers

Consist of proteins and organic phosphates.

- **Proteins:** Certain chemical moieties in amino acids, such as α-amino groups and imidazole groups, have pK_a values within the physiologic pH range and are therefore able to act as buffers. Hemoglobin is also an intracellular buffer. In the physiologic pH range, deoxyhemoglobin is a better buffer than oxyhemoglobin.
- **Organic phosphates:** These include metabolic substrates such as AMP, ADP, ATP, and 2,3-bisphosphoglycerate (2,3-BPG).

Extracellular Buffers

Consist of HCO_3^- and phosphates.

- **Major:** HCO_3^- is the major extracellular buffer ($pK_a = 6.1$). It is produced via a reaction catalyzed by carbonic anhydrase (see previous formula).
- **Minor:** Phosphate is the minor extracellular buffer ($pK_a = 6.8$). Its most important function is as a buffer of urine. $H_2PO_4^-$ is referred to as a **titratable acid.**

Acid-Base Homeostasis

The body uses chemical buffer systems to regulate acid-base homeostasis.

Buffer Systems

Consist of a pair of substances: a **weak acid** and **weak base** that undergo a reversible chemical reaction. The weak acid yields free H^+ as the hydrogen ion concentration $[H^+]$ starts to fall, and the weak base can bind free H^+ when $[H^+]$ starts to rise.

The **Henderson-Hasselbalch equation** describes the relationship between $[H^+]$ and the members of a buffer pair. This equation fits the titration curve for all weak acids.

$$pH = -\log [H^+]\, pK_a + \log \frac{\text{proton acceptor}}{\text{proton donor}} = pK_a + \log \frac{[A^-]}{[HA]}$$

Inserting the values that describe the **blood bicarbonate buffer,** where $(0.03\ \text{P}_{CO_2})$ is essentially equal to $[H_2CO_3]$:

$$pH = 6.1 + \log \frac{[HCO_3^-]}{0.03\ \text{P}_{CO_2}}$$

The major chemical buffer system that the body uses to regulate extracellular acid-base balance is the carbonic acid/bicarbonate buffer system catalyzed by carbonic anhydrase:

$$CO_2 + H_2O \leftrightarrow H_2CO_3 \leftrightarrow H^+ + HCO_3^-$$

This is a reversible equilibrium reaction. The body regulates hydrogen ion concentration via CO_2 and HCO_3^- concentrations in the blood. The kidneys and lungs are the principal organs responsible for regulation of acid–base homeostasis.

Physiologic pH

Normal blood pH is 7.4, but it may fluctuate from 7.35 to 7.45. Values outside the range of 6.8–8.0 are typically incompatible with life due to changes in enzymatic function and protein denaturation.

- **Acidemia** versus **acidosis:**
    - **Acidemia** is a nonspecific term describing an increase in $[H^+]$ in the blood and is applicable when pH falls below normal (< 7.35).
    - **Acidosis** describes the specific physiologic derangement responsible for a lower than normal pH (eg, metabolic acidosis).
- **Alkalemia** versus **alkalosis:**
    - **Alkalemia** is a decrease in $[H^+]$ or increase in $[HCO_3^-]$ that increases the pH above normal levels (> 7.45).
    - **Alkalosis** describes the specific physiologic derangement responsible for a higher than normal pH.

Acid-Base Homeostasis: The Kidney

Through a variety of mechanisms, the kidney is the primary regulator of $[H^+]$ and $[HCO_3^-]$ in the serum over the long term. Since renal compensation occurs through chemical buffers under hormonal control, renal-mediated changes in serum pH develop relatively slowly (eg, over hours to days).

- **Renal production of H^+ and HCO_3^-:** Proximal and distal tubule cells contain intracellular carbonic anhydrase that produces H^+ and HCO_3^- from CO_2 and H_2O via the intermediate H_2CO_3.
- **Secretion of H^+:** The H^+ may be secreted as either titratable acid ($H_2PO_4^-$) or ammonium (NH_4^+).
- **Secretion as $H_2PO_4^-$:** Excretion of H^+ as titratable acid depends on the amount of urinary buffer (phosphate) present, as well as the pK_a of that buffer. HPO_4^{2-} is relatively abundant and has a favorable pK_a (6.80), making it the major urinary buffer. Once H^+ is secreted, it combines with HPO_4^{2-}, resulting in a net secretion of H^+. This accounts for the minimum pH of urine being lower than that of serum, approximately 4.5.
- **Secretion as NH_4^+:** This mechanism is a function of the amount of ammonia synthesized (from glutamine) by renal tubular cells. Secretion of NH_3 depends largely

on urine pH. The lower the pH, the greater the excretion of H^+ as NH_4^+. In states of **acidemia,** there is a compensatory increase in this process in order to increase H^+ excretion.

■ **Reabsorption of HCO_3^-:** Reabsorption of bicarbonate is regulated by P_{CO_2} and ECF volume. Decreased ECF volume stimulates the RAAS to produce angiotensin II, which stimulates the Na^+–H^+ exchange pump in the PCT. This in turn leads to an increase in HCO_3^- reabsorption and eventual **contraction alkalosis.** On the other hand, increased ECF volume causes decreased HCO_3^- reabsorption and **dilutional acidosis.**

Acid-Base Homeostasis: The Lungs

The lung is also a primary regulator of acid-base homeostasis. Although altered ventilatory states may be responsible for primary derangements, they may also compensate for primary metabolic derangements. Variations in ventilatory rate can change the serum pH within minutes. Therefore, the respiratory system is responsible for acid-base homeostasis in the acute setting.

■ **Compensation states:** Metabolic derangements resulting in an abnormal $[HCO_3^-]$ are followed by a compensatory change in respiratory rate, which affects the carbon dioxide concentration.
  ■ Metabolic alkalosis ($\uparrow HCO_3^-$) → **decreased respiratory rate,** promoting retention of CO_2 and a decrease in pH toward the normal range.
  ■ Metabolic acidosis ($\downarrow HCO_3^-$) → **increased respiratory rate,** decreased CO_2, and an increase in pH toward the normal range.
■ **Derangement states:** The lungs may also be the primary cause of either a respiratory alkalosis or acidosis.

Metabolic Acidosis/Alkalosis

Metabolic Acidosis

Occurs secondary to either a loss of HCO_3^- or an excess of H^+. Conditions that lead to metabolic acidosis can be differentiated based on the **anion gap,** defined as:

$$\text{Unmeasured serum anions} = [Na^+] - ([HCO_3^-] + [Cl^-])$$
$$(\text{normal} = 10\text{–}12 \text{ mEq/L})$$

An anion gap greater than the normal range indicates the presence of an unexpected, unmeasured serum anion (eg, lactate in lactic acidosis). In elevated anion-gap acidosis, the concentration of an unmeasured anion is increased to replace lost HCO_3^-. In contrast, in normal anion-gap (hyperchloremic) acidosis, the concentration of Cl^- is increased to replace lost HCO_3^-. See mnemonic in the margin for typical causes of metabolic acidosis. A brief explanation of some of the less obvious causes follows:

■ Hyperalimentation in this context refers to total parenteral (eg, IV) nutrition (TPN). Acidosis can occur in patients receiving TPN for a variety of reasons, including insufficient thiamine in the formulation or, more commonly, coexisting renal, pulmonary, and or gastrointestinal disease.

KEY FACT

Winter's formula gives the expected P_{CO_2} based on a measured HCO_3^- and is used to determine if the respiratory compensation for a metabolic acidosis is appropriate:

$$P_{CO_2} = [(1.5 \times HCO_3^-) + 8] \pm 2$$

If the expected P_{CO_2} corresponds with the measured P_{CO_2}, then the respiratory compensation is adequate.

MNEMONIC

Anion-gap acidosis vs normal anion gap, or hyperchloremic acidosis—

$\uparrow$ Anion gap: MUDPILES:	Normal anion gap: HARDUP:
Methanol	**H**yperalimentation
Uremia	**A**cetazolamide
Diabetic ketoacidosis	**R**enal tubular acidosis (Table 8-10)
Phenformin,	
Paraldehyde	**D**iarrhea
Isoniazid,	**U**reteroenteric shunt
Infection, **I**ron	
Lactic acidosis	**P**ancreatic fistula
Ethylene glycol, **E**thanol	
Salicylates	

TABLE 8-10. Characteristics of the Different Renal Tubular Acidosis

	TYPE 1	TYPE 2	TYPE 4
Defect	$\downarrow$ Distal acid secretion by α-intercalated cells	$\downarrow$ Proximal tubular cell HCO_3^- reabsorption	$\downarrow$ Aldosterone effect
Plasma K^+	$\downarrow$	Variable	High (cardinal feature)
Urine pH	> 5.5	< 5.5	< 5.5

- Ureteroenteric shunts divert urine from the urinary system to the bowel. Contact between the intestinal mucosa and urine can result in reabsorption of urinary ammonium and chloride and HCO_3^- secretion.
- Pancreatic fistulas result in loss of the bicarbonate-rich pancreatic fluid.
- Severe infections can result in shock, leading to lactic acidosis.
- Iron poisoning, though exceedingly rare, can also lead to shock. Moreover, hydration of ferric ions (Fe^{3+}) generates protons ($Fe^{3+} + 3\ H_2O \rightarrow Fe(OH)_3 + 3\ H^+$).

Metabolic Alkalosis

Occurs secondary to either a loss of acid or excess of base:

- Emesis (loss of H^+ leaves HCO_3^- behind in blood; hypokalemia).
- Hyperaldosteronism ($\uparrow H^+$ secretion and new HCO_3^- formation by DCT/CD).
- Diuretics (loop and thiazide) → "contraction alkalosis" ($\downarrow$ ECF volume → $\uparrow$ renin → $\uparrow$ angiotensin II → $\uparrow Na^+$–H^+ exchange and HCO_3^- reabsorption in PCT).
- Laxative abuse. (Because intestinal secretions ordinarily contain relatively high HCO_3^- concentration, diarrhea normally results in a metabolic acidosis. The alkalosis seen in laxative abuse is not well explained, but may result from hypokalemia.)
- Hypercalcemia/milk-alkali syndrome (repeated ingestion of calcium and absorbable alkali).
- Hypokalemia ($\uparrow NH_3$ synthesis → $\uparrow H^+$ excretion as NH_4^+; transcellular H^+–K^+ exchange: H^+ into cells, K^+ out of cells).

Respiratory Acidosis/Alkalosis

Respiratory Acidosis

Occurs secondary to retention of CO_2. This can result from conditions that inhibit the medullary respiratory center ($\downarrow$ respiratory drive), weakening or paralysis of the muscles of respiration, or decreased CO_2 exchange (Table 8-11).

Respiratory Alkalosis

Occurs due to low plasma concentrations of CO_2. This can result from conditions that affect the CNS, the respiratory system, or from iatrogenic causes (Table 8-12).

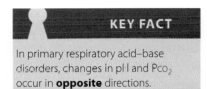

KEY FACT

In primary respiratory acid–base disorders, changes in pH and P_{CO_2} occur in **opposite** directions.

TABLE 8-11.   Causes of Respiratory Acidosis

MECHANISM	CAUSES
Inhibition of medullary respiratory center	- Drugs (opiates, sedatives, anesthetics) - CNS tumors/trauma - CNS hypoxia - Hypoventilation of obesity (Pickwickian syndrome)
Weakening or paralysis of muscles of respiration	- Guillain-Barré syndrome, polio, ALS, MS - Myasthenia gravis - Toxins (botulinum toxin, organophosphates) - Muscle relaxants - Scoliosis, certain myopathies, muscular dystrophy
Decreased CO_2 exchange	- COPD - ARDS
Airway obstruction	

ALS, amyotrophic lateral sclerosis; ARDS, acute respiratory distress syndrome; CNS, central nervous system; COPD, chronic obstructive pulmonary disease; MS, multiple sclerosis.

TABLE 8-12. **Causes of Respiratory Alkalosis**

MECHANISM	CAUSES
Central	■ Head trauma ■ Stroke ■ Anxiety, stress, hyperventilation ■ Drugs (salicylate intoxication) ■ Certain endogenous compounds (eg, progesterone in pregnancy)
Pulmonary	■ Pulmonary embolism ■ Asthma ■ Pneumonia ■ High altitude
Iatrogenic	■ Increased respiratory rate while on controlled ventilation

Acid-Base Clinical Implications

The key points when approaching a clinical scenario involving an acid-base disturbance (Table 8-13) are the following:

■ The lungs regulate the concentration of P_{CO_2}.
■ The kidneys regulate the concentration of HCO_3^-.
■ Compensation is never complete (eg, pH never returns to 7.40 unless there is a second acid-base disturbance).

TABLE 8-13. **Summary of Primary Acid–Base Disturbances**

DISORDER	PCO_2	+	H_2O	$\leftrightarrow$	H^+	+	HCO_3^-	RESPIRATORY COMPENSATION	RENAL COMPENSATION
Metabolic acidosis	↓				↑		⇓	Hyperventilation	↑ [H$^+$] excretion ↑ [HCO$_3^-$] reabsorption ↓ 1.2 mm Hg in P_{CO_2} for every ↓ 1 mEq/L in [HCO$_3^-$]
Metabolic alkalosis	↑				↓		⇑	Hypoventilation	↓ [H$^+$] excretion ↓ [HCO$_3^-$] reabsorption ↑ 0.7 mm Hg in P_{CO_2} for every ↑ 1 mEq/L in [HCO$_3^-$]
Respiratory acidosis	⇑				↑		↑[a]	None	↑ [H$^+$] excretion ↑ [HCO$_3^-$] reabsorption ↑ 1 mEq/L in [HCO$_3^-$] for every ↑ 10 mm Hg in P_{CO_2} (acute—ICF buffering) ↑ 3.5 mEq/L in [HCO$_3^-$] for every ↑ 10 mm Hg in P_{CO_2} (chronic—renal compensation)
Respiratory alkalosis	⇓				↓		↓	None	↓ [H$^+$] excretion ↓ [HCO$_3^-$] reabsorption ↓ 2 mEq/L in [HCO$_3^-$] for every ↓ 10 mm Hg in P_{CO_2} (acute – ICF buffering) ↓ 5 mEq/L in [HCO$_3^-$] for every ↓ 10 mm Hg in P_{CO_2} (chronic—renal compensation)

⇑ or ⇓ = Primary disturbance.

↑ or ↓ = Effect of primary disturbance or compensation.

[a]May be unchanged or slightly lower according to the Henderson-Hasselbalch equation:

$pH = 6.1 + \log [HCO_3^-]/[CO_2]$ Normal $[HCO_3^-]/[CO_2] = 20$.

Respiratory compensation for metabolic acid-base disturbances is essentially instantaneous. In contrast, it takes time for the kidney to compensate for a primary respiratory disorder by excreting or retaining HCO_3^-. Thus, for primary respiratory derangements, the next step in analysis is to determine whether the disturbance is an acute (ICF buffering only) or chronic (ICF buffering + renal compensation) process:

- For respiratory acidosis, we expect:
    - ↑ 1 mEq/L in $[HCO_3^-]$ for every ↑ 10 mm Hg in P_{CO_2} (acute—ICF buffering).
    - ↑ 3.5 mEq/L in $[HCO_3^-]$ for every ↑ 10 mm Hg in P_{CO_2} (chronic—renal compensation).
- For respiratory alkalosis, we expect:
    - ↓ 2 mEq/L in $[HCO_3^-]$ for every ↓ 10 mm Hg in P_{CO_2} (acute—ICF buffering).
    - ↓ 5 mEq/L in $[HCO_3^-]$ for every ↓ 10 mm Hg in P_{CO_2} (chronic—renal compensation).
- If the compensation is not appropriate, there must be another process occurring simultaneously. That is, a **mixed acid-base disorder** exists.

Signs of mixed disorders include:

- In general, suspect mixed disorders when the values observed differ substantially from those expected.
- Marked change in P_{CO_2} and $[HCO_3^-]$ with little change in pH, implying offsetting abnormalities.

If a **mixed disorder** that includes an **elevated anion gap metabolic acidosis** is suspected, calculate the deviation of the anion gap from normal and the deviation of the $[HCO_3^-]$ from normal. Use these two computed values to perform **delta-delta analysis** as shown:

$$\Delta \text{ Anion gap (AG)} = \text{Calculated AG} - 12$$
$$\Delta [HCO_3^-] = 24 - \text{Measured } [HCO_3^-]$$

The delta-delta ratio is defined as

$$\Delta/\Delta = \Delta \text{ AG} / \Delta [HCO_3^-]$$

and can be interpreted using the following criteria:

- $\Delta/\Delta < 1 \rightarrow$ elevated-AG metabolic acidosis + non-AG metabolic acidosis.
- $1 < \Delta/\Delta < 2 \rightarrow$ elevated-AG metabolic acidosis **only.**
- $\Delta/\Delta > 2 \rightarrow$ elevated-AG metabolic acidosis + metabolic alkalosis.

An overview for approaching acid-base disturbances is provided in Table 8-13 and Figure 8-25.

Acid-Base Nomogram

The acid-base nomogram is a quick reference tool that can be used during clinical rotations (Figure 8-25).

Although the acid-base nomogram is an indispensable clinical tool, it is practically impossible to memorize for test purposes. Figure 8-25 provides a simplified version depicting the center of the nomogram. Knowing this basic setup enables you to answer the simple acid-base problems very quickly. It also helps to narrow down the possibilities if dealing with a complicated mixed disorder.

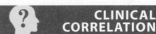

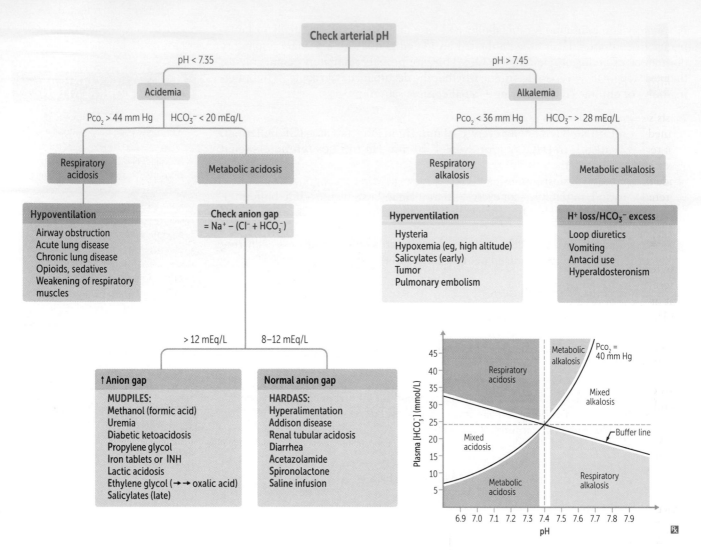

FIGURE 8-25. **Algorithm depicting acidemia and alkalemia analysis and simplified acid-base (Davenport) nomogram (bottom right).**

Acid-Base Problem Solving

Another approach to acid-base problem solving involves performing the same six steps for every problem:

1. Clinical scenario: What might you expect from the clinical information? (eg, loss of HCO_3^- in diarrhea vs loss of H^+ in vomiting).
2. pH: above or below 7.4?
3. What is primary acid-base disturbance? Compare patterns of HCO_3^- above/below 24 and P_{CO_2} above/below 40 (eg, pH 7.25, HCO_3^- 18, P_{CO_2} 28 is a pattern consistent with metabolic acidosis).
4. Is there compensation for the primary disturbance? (eg, in metabolic acidosis, expected $P_{CO_2} = 1.5 \times HCO_3^- + 8 +/- 2 = 1.5(18) + 8 +/- 2 = 33-37$). Expected P_{CO_2} of 33–37 is higher than actual P_{CO_2} of 28, thus a respiratory alkalosis is also present.
5. Anion gap: If over 20, then a high anion gap metabolic acidosis is present; consider etiologies.
6. $\Delta/\Delta = \Delta\,AG\,/\,\Delta\,[HCO_3^-]$: Look for additional metabolic alkalosis or nongap metabolic acidosis.

Pathology

URINARY CASTS

Casts seen on urinalysis can be an indication of tubular pathology. **Cellular casts** are formed within the tubular lumen; hence, their presence indicates that the disease process is of renal origin. **Hyaline casts,** on the other hand, are of little diagnostic significance. They can be seen in normal individuals and in volume-depleted states. All casts are made of a protein matrix primarily composed of **Tamm-Horsfall mucoprotein** secreted by renal tubular cells (Table 8-14).

GLOMERULOPATHIES

The term **glomerulopathies** applies to a group of conditions that affect the glomeruli. These entities are divided into two major groups, nephrotic and nephritic syndromes, that are broken down based on their pathogenesis and clinical manifestations (Table 8-15). Table 8-16 explains the nomenclature of glomerular disorders.

NEPHROTIC SYNDROME

This condition results from an **increased permeability** of the **glomerular basement membrane (GBM),** secondary to cytokines released by mononuclear cells. These cytokines induce fusion of podocytes and obliterate the negative charge of the GBM. Thus, there is **loss of plasma proteins** (predominantly low-molecular-weight, negatively charged **albumin**) in the urine, which is often described as "frothy."

TABLE 8-14.   Urinary Casts

CASTS	CAUSES	FINDINGS
Epithelial cell casts	▪ ATN, ethylene glycol toxicity, heavy-metal poisoning, acute rejection of transplant graft	▪ Desquamated tubular cells in a protein matrix
RBC casts	▪ Glomerulonephritis: IgA nephropathy, poststreptococcal glomerulonephritis, and Goodpasture syndrome ▪ Malignant hypertension ▪ Vasculitis ▪ Renal ischemia	▪ Clumps of dysmorphic RBCs with blebs and buds indicate RBCs are of glomerular origin versus bladder origin (eg, bladder cancer)
WBC casts	▪ Pyelonephritis ▪ Interstitial nephritis ▪ Lupus nephritis	▪ WBC casts indicate inflammation in renal interstitium, tubules, and/or glomeruli ▪ WBCs in urine indicate lower UTI
Hyaline casts	▪ Often seen in normal urine ▪ Pyelonephritis	▪ Glassy looking ▪ Composed of Tamm-Horsfall protein
Granular casts	▪ ATN ▪ Chronic renal failure ▪ Nephrotic syndrome	▪ Derived from the breakdown of cellular casts, especially epithelial cell casts
Fatty casts	▪ Nephrotic syndrome	▪ Fat droplets in hyaline matrix ▪ **Maltese-cross configuration** due to presence of cholesterol (when viewed under polarized light)

ATN, acute tubular necrosis; UTI, urinary tract infection.

TABLE 8-15. General Division of Glomerular Diseases

CONDITIONS THAT MANIFEST WITH NEPHROTIC SYNDROME (INCREASED FILTRATION BARRIER PERMEABILITY)	CONDITIONS THAT MANIFEST WITH NEPHRITIC SYNDROME (INFLAMMATORY DAMAGE TO THE GLOMERULI)
Minimal change disease	Acute proliferative glomerulonephritis (poststreptoccocal/infectious)
Focal segmental glomerulosclerosis	Rapidly progressive glomerulonephritis (crescentic)
Membranous glomerulopathy	Anti-GBM disease Goodpasture syndrome
Membranoproliferative glomerulonephritis (MPGN[a])	MPGN[a]
Diabetic nephropathy associated with systemic disease	IgA nephropathy (Berger disease)
Renal amyloidosis associated with systemic disease	Hereditary nephritis (Alport syndrome)
Lupus nephritis[a]	Lupus nephritis[a]

[a]MPGN and lupus nephritis can present as either nephrotic or nephritic syndrome.

GBM, glomerular basement membrane.

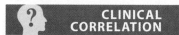

KEY FACT

High ratio of low- to high-molecular-weight proteins (eg, albumin to immunoglobulin) in the urine indicates **highly selective proteinuria.**

KEY FACT

Proteinuria (> 3.5 g/24 h), hypoalbuminemia, edema, hyperlipidemia, urinary fatty casts, and hypercoagulation are the hallmarks of **nephrotic syndrome.**

Key findings in nephrotic syndrome:

- **Massive proteinuria** (> 3.5 g/24 h).
- **Hypoalbuminemia** (plasma albumin level < 3 g/dL) develops in part due to losses in urine. Albumin accounts for ~60% of total human plasma proteins and is the main mediator of the serum oncotic pressure. In the setting of massive proteinuria, the liver cannot keep up with albumin synthesis, leading to reduced serum oncotic pressure and edema. In addition, decreased total albumin leads to decreased total serum calcium because much of the serum calcium (positively charged) is bound to albumin (negatively charged). However, the serum ionized calcium does not change.
- **Edema** develops due to lowered oncotic pressure, which leads to loss of fluid from the circulation into the interstitial space. Decreased intravascular volume leads to activation of the renin–angiotensin–aldosterone system (RAAS), increased sympathetic activity, release of vasopressin, and decreased atrial natriuretic peptide (ANP)

TABLE 8-16. Description of Glomerular Disorders

TERM	DESCRIPTION
Focal glomerulonephritis	Only a few glomeruli are affected
Diffuse glomerulonephritis	All glomeruli are affected
Proliferative glomerulonephritis	> 100 nuclei in affected glomeruli (hypercellular glomeruli)
Membranous glomerulopathy	Thick GBM but no proliferation
Membranoproliferative glomerulonephritis	Thick GBM with hypercellular glomeruli
Focal segmental glomerulosclerosis	Fibrosis of only a segment of the affected glomeruli
Crescentic glomerulonephritis	Proliferation of the parietal epithelial cell lining of Bowman capsule (forms a crescent)

GBM, glomerular basement membrane.

release. All of these changes result in increased renal electrolyte and water retention, thereby exacerbating the edema.

- **Hyperlipidemia** and concomitant **lipiduria** result from an increased production of lipoproteins by the liver in an attempt to maintain the falling oncotic pressure. However, the liver is not able to synthesize sufficient quantities of lipoproteins to successfully counteract the edema. Furthermore, hypoalbuminemia triggers an increase in cholesterol synthesis by the liver through a poorly understood mechanism.
- **Hypercoagulability** secondary to loss of antithrombin III through the damaged glomeruli. There is an increased risk for renal vein thrombosis and other venous thromboses.

Many different pathologies result in a clinical presentation of nephrotic syndrome. The definitive diagnosis can only be made with a **renal biopsy.** However, each of the following disorders has characteristic symptoms and time courses that help to guide diagnosis and treatment.

Minimal Change Disease

Minimal change disease is the **most frequent cause** of nephrotic syndrome in **children** (> 80% of cases seen in those aged 2–3 years). It is so named due to the normal appearance of the glomeruli observed under **light microscopy.** However, **electron microscopy** shows fusion **(effacement)** of the visceral epithelial foot processes, thereby causing increased glomerular permeability. Minimal change disease is **often preceded by respiratory infection or routine immunization.**

Proximal tubules are often heavily laden with lipids secondary to increased tubular reabsorption of lipoproteins that passed through the injured glomeruli, hence, another name for this disease is "**lipoid nephrosis.**"

PRESENTATION

Children between the ages of 2 and 3 years most frequently suffer from this disorder. Symptoms manifest as an insidious onset of nephrotic syndrome without any other obvious clinical disease (eg, no hypertension). The **proteinuria** is termed "selective" because primarily albumin (low-molecular-weight) is lost. Renal function is normally maintained, with only a slight decline in glomerular filtration rate (GFR) in 10–30% of patients.

DIAGNOSIS

As with all glomerulopathies, diagnosis depends on renal biopsy.

- **Light microscopy** (Figure 8-26): No obvious morphologic changes are seen in the glomeruli. Note the lipoid appearance of the cells in the proximal tubules **(lipoid nephrosis).**
- **Electron microscopy: Effacement** of visceral epithelial foot processes and increased lipoproteins in the proximal convoluted tubules **(PCTs).**

Definitive diagnosis of minimal change disease can only be made when nephrotic syndrome is accompanied by diffuse effacement of foot processes on electron microscopy.

TREATMENT

Initial therapy includes **high-dose oral glucocorticoids** (eg, **prednisone**) for up to 8 weeks. For those that fail to achieve lasting remission (defined as either relapse during steroid therapy, or recurrence more than three times per year after the steroid taper), **alkylating agents** such as cyclophosphamide or chlorambucil have been shown to be effective.

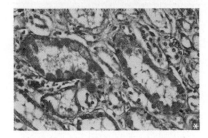

FIGURE 8-26. Histology of minimal change disease (lipoid nephrosis). Light micrograph. Note the foamy (or granular) appearance of the cells of the proximal tubules due to reabsorption of lipoproteins leaking through diseased glomeruli.

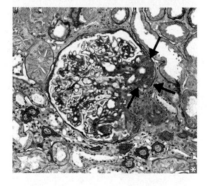

FIGURE 8-27. Histology of focal sclerosing glomerulosclerosis. Light micrograph showing segmental sclerosis and hyalinosis of the glomerulus (arrows).

ANSWER

Steroids are commonly the first-line treatment for minimal change disease, which is the likely diagnosis in this patient.

PROGNOSIS

In children, prognosis is excellent, with 90% of cases responding to treatment. In adults, prognosis is not as good, with only 50% responding to treatment.

Focal Segmental Glomerulosclerosis

Focal segmental glomerulosclerosis (FSGS) is considered to be a more severe form of minimal change disease due to the similar fusion of visceral epithelial foot processes. The pathologic lesion is sclerosis of < 50% of glomeruli (hence the name **focal**), with the sclerosis involving only distinct portions of the affected glomeruli (hence the name **segmental**). The cause is still unknown. This disease accounts for about 33% of nephrotic syndrome in adults and 50% of cases in African Americans.

PRESENTATION

Patients present with nephrotic syndrome. Unlike in minimal change disease, patients have **nonselective proteinuria** as well as **hypertension,** mild hematuria, and possibly decreased renal function. This disorder is associated with HIV, heroin use, and sickle cell disease.

DIAGNOSIS

Definitive diagnosis is based on renal biopsy.

Light microscopy: Two distinct features are notable: **focal** accumulation of hyaline material and **segmental** sclerosis (Figure 8-27). Proper tissue biopsy is important because the prognosis of this disorder is worse than that of minimal change disease.

TREATMENT

Unlike with minimal change disease, only 20–40% of patients experience remission when treated with **oral glucocorticoids.** If there is no remission of proteinuria with steroids, **cyclophosphamide** and **cyclosporine** can be used at doses similar to those for minimal change disease.

PROGNOSIS

Generally poor, with approximately 50% of patients with this disorder developing end-stage renal disease (ESRD) within 10 years. Even following renal transplantation, there is a great risk of disease recurrence.

Diffuse Membranous Glomerulopathy

The pathogenesis of membranous glomerulopathy is not clearly established. However, immunofluorescence studies have led to a hypothesis of immune complex deposition, which is supported by its association with certain infections and systemic diseases. It is the **leading cause** of **nephrotic syndrome** in **adults,** accounting for 30–40% of cases in adults but less than 5% of cases in children. Peak incidence is from ages 30–50, and it is seen predominantly in men (2:1 ratio).

PRESENTATION

Insidious onset of **nephrotic syndrome** with **nonselective proteinuria** in otherwise healthy patients. Membranous glomerulopathy occurs in association with

- systemic diseases, such as systemic lupus erythematous (SLE) and rheumatoid arthritis (RA)
- sexually transmitted infections, such as hepatitis B, hepatitis C, and syphilis
- less-common infections, such as schistosomiasis, malaria, and leprosy
- drugs, such as penicillamine and gold-containing compounds

DIAGNOSIS

Based on renal biopsy.

- **Light microscopy:** Diffuse GBM thickening due to **subepithelial deposits** nestled against the GBM (Figure 8-28).
- **Electron microscopy:** Subepithelial deposits in a **"spike"** (extensions of GBM around deposits) and **"dome"** (deposits in the GBM) pattern. The deposits have been shown to be IgG and C3 using immunofluorescent staining.

TREATMENT

Given the high rate of spontaneous remission, only patients with severe disease should be treated with immunosuppressive therapy. Cyclophosphamide and cyclosporine when combined with glucocorticoids reduce proteinuria and slow the decline of GFR. Transplantation has been shown to be effective for patients that progress to ESRD.

PROGNOSIS

Remission is spontaneous in 40% of patients. Among those who received cyclophosphamide and glucocorticoid therapy, 40% undergo complete remission, 50% develop a chronic clinical picture with frequent relapses, and the remaining 10% go on to develop ESRD in 10–15 years.

Membranoproliferative Glomerulonephritis

Membranoproliferative glomerulonephritis (MPGN) can occur idiopathically or, more commonly, secondary to monoclonal immunoglobulin deposition diseases, autoimmune diseases such as SLE, chronic thrombotic microangiopathies, or chronic infections. There are two distinct types.

- **Type I (two-thirds** of cases): Due to deposition of immune complexes (type III hypersensitivity). Associated with hepatitis B, hepatitis C, and cryoglobulinemia. Some cases have a **nephritic presentation.**
- **Type II (one-third** of cases): Often associated with the **C3 nephritic factor (C3NeF).** It is also called **dense deposit disease,** due to the deposition of an electron-dense material between the lamina densa and subendothelial space of the GBM. Although C3 is present, there are **no IgG** deposits.

PRESENTATION

Patients with **type I** disease tend to present with **nephrotic** syndrome, whereas those with **type II** can present with **either** nephrotic or nephritic syndrome, or a mix of the two.

DIAGNOSIS

Diagnosis is based on clinical presentation and renal biopsy. The disorder is characterized on tissue section by thickening of the GBM and proliferation of mesangial cells.

Electron microscopy: Generally the GBM appears to be divided by an electron-dense material.

- **Type I** shows **subendothelial,** electron-dense deposits of IgG and C3. Ingrowth of the mesangium splits the GBM, creating a **tram-track appearance.**
- **Type II** shows **intramembranous** deposits and increased size of glomeruli, as well as increased cellularity of the mesangial cells. The capillary wall often shows a double contour, or **tram-track appearance,** as a result of GBM splitting.

TREATMENT

There is no effective therapy for this disease, although plasma exchange with albumin has been shown to slow disease progression in some patients with circulating C3NeF.

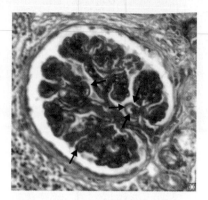

FIGURE 8-28. Histologic image of membranous glomerulopathy. Note capillary and glomerular basement membrane thickening occurs throughout entire glomerulus (arrows).

KEY FACT

C3NeF is a C3-convertase-specific autoantibody, which prevents its degradation. Sustained C3 activation results in low C3 levels, which is an important diagnostic feature.

KEY FACT

MPGN = Tram-track appearance on electron microscopy and subendothelial humps (type I) or intramembranous deposits (type II).

QUESTION

A 22-year-old black man presents with several weeks of lower-extremity and periorbital edema. Urinalysis reveals 4+ protein without RBCs or signs of infection. He has a history of multiple hospital admissions since early childhood. What chronic medical condition does he most likely have?

Prognosis

Differs between types I and II.

- **Type I** has a less aggressive course than type II, but most patients still progress to ESRD within 20 years.
- **Type II** tends to have a worse prognosis, with GFR declining more quickly than type I. A majority of patients progress to ESRD after 5–10 years.

NEPHROPATHIES ASSOCIATED WITH SYSTEMIC DISORDERS

Many systemic disorders ultimately affect the kidneys. Specific diseases associated with nephrotic syndrome include **diabetic nephropathy, renal amyloidosis,** and **lupus nephritis.**

Diabetic Nephropathy

Diabetic nephropathy is the **leading cause of ESRD in Western society,** secondary to glomerular hypertension and hyperfiltration. These glomerular changes are caused by hyaline arteriolosclerosis secondary to nonenzymatic glycation of the vascular basement membrane, which is also the cause of all microvascular pathologies associated with diabetes mellitus.

The **first sign** of injury to the glomerulus is **microalbuminuria,** which occurs about 5–10 years before other symptoms develop. If untreated, microalbuminuria slowly progresses to nephrotic-range proteinuria. Nephropathy is generally more common in type 1 diabetes mellitus (DM-1) than DM-2, occurring in ~30% of cases.

Presentation

Typically, chronic renal failure (CRF) aggravated by glomerulosclerosis leads to fluid filtration abnormalities and a full spectrum of other disorders of kidney function. Cardinal symptoms include **hypertension** and **edema** (as a result of fluid retention). Other complications may include **arteriosclerosis** of the **renal artery** and the **efferent arterioles.** If left untreated, **nephrotic-range proteinuria** ultimately develops.

During its early course, diabetic nephropathy has virtually no symptoms. Late-stage diabetic nephropathy manifests as full-blown CKD.

Diagnosis

Usually diagnosed on **clinical grounds** without the need for a renal biopsy. Should be suspected in patients with either DM-1 or DM-2 who have already developed evidence of end-organ damage from DM, such as retinopathy and neuropathy, and have dipstick-positive proteinuria.

Light microscopy: Thickening of the GBM and expansion of the mesangium. Classic **Kimmelstiel-Wilson lesions,** areas of nodular glomerulosclerosis, may be found (Figure 8-29).

Treatment

Treatment should be started for patients long before their symptoms have progressed to overt nephrotic syndrome.

- Patients who develop microalbuminuria should be started on **angiotensin-converting enzyme (ACE) inhibitors** or **angiotensin receptor blockers (ARBs)** (to counteract hyperfiltration), which have been shown to delay the progression of nephropathy in diabetic patients.

KEY FACT

The first sign of diabetic nephropathy is microalbuminuria secondary to glomerular hyperfiltration.

KEY FACT

Hyaline arteriolosclerosis is a hallmark of DM; efferent arterioles are affected before afferent arterioles.

KEY FACT

Kimmelstiel-Wilson, or "wire-loop," lesions are pathognomonic for diabetic nephropathy.

A **ANSWER**

Sickle cell anemia is a common cause of focal sclerosis glomerulosclerosis, a severe nephrotic syndrome.

■ **Good glucose control** with diet, exercise, and hypoglycemic agents has also been shown to delay the development and progression of symptoms.

PROGNOSIS

Without adequate treatment, ESRD typically arises within 5–10 years following the development of nephrotic-range proteinuria (Figure 8-30).

Renal Amyloidosis

Amyloidosis is characterized by the deposition of fibrous, insoluble proteins in a β-pleated sheet conformation in the extracellular space of organs (eg, renal glomeruli). It is a **multisystem disorder of protein folding** and can be acquired or hereditary.

The two types that affect the kidneys are **amyloid L (AL)** and **amyloid A (AA)** (see Table 8-17 for more information about amyloid). When immunoglobulin light chains lacking the β-pleated configuration deposit in the kidney, the disease is called **light-chain deposition disease.**

PRESENTATION

Nephrotic-range proteinuria, severe edema, and renal insufficiency are common in renal amyloidosis. If amyloidosis is caused by a secondary disease (eg, multiple myeloma, tuberculosis, rheumatoid arthritis, etc.), the patient will also show signs and symptoms of the primary disease.

DIAGNOSIS

Definitive diagnosis is based on renal, abdominal fat pad, or rectal biopsy.

Light microscopy: Tissue stained with **Congo red** has deposits of amyloid that show **apple-green birefringence** under polarized light. In addition, mesangial expansion is present with amorphous hyaline material (amyloid) and thickening of the GBM.

TREATMENT

Some improvement has been shown with a combination of **melphalan** and **prednisone.** Treatment for **AA amyloidosis** is based on the underlying cause of the condition. Transplantation is an option for patients with both AA and AL amyloidosis, although extrarenal organ involvement may be a contraindication.

PROGNOSIS

Prognosis for renal involvement by **AL** is uniformly poor.

Lupus Nephritis

A part of the pathophysiologic spectrum of SLE.

PRESENTATION

During the early course of SLE, patients may or may not have symptoms of kidney disease. However, as the disease progresses, kidneys are almost uniformly affected, and patients present with either nephrotic or nephritic syndrome, or both, ultimately leading to ESRD. Most common symptoms resulting from glomerular pathology include weight gain, high BP, darker foamy urine, and swelling around the eyes, legs, ankles, or fingers.

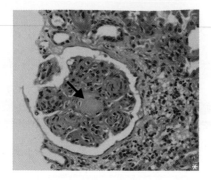

FIGURE 8-29. **Diabetic nephropathy.** Note Kimmelstiel-Wilson nodules (arrow), which are pathognomonic for this disease.

KEY FACT

Congo red stain → Apple-green birefringence = amyloidosis.

QUESTION

A 43-year-old obese man with a 10-year history of type 2 diabetes mellitus comes to your office for his annual checkup. He was recently diagnosed with nonproliferative diabetic retinopathy. Urine studies reveal microalbuminuria. What anomalies are mostly likely to be appreciated on renal biopsy?

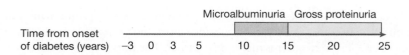

FIGURE 8-30. **Time course of development of diabetic nephropathy.**

TABLE 8-17. **Description of the Common Types of Amyloid**

AMYLOID TYPE	DESCRIPTION
AL	Derived from immunoglobulin light chains, eg, Bence Jones protein in the blood or urine is associated with multiple myeloma
AA	Associated with chronic inflammation, eg, RA, TB
$A\beta$	Main constituent of amyloid plaques in Alzheimer disease
ATTR	Found in familial amyloid polyneuropathy (caused by a genetic mutation) and senile cardiac amyloidosis (caused by wild-type ATTR accumulation)
$A\beta_2M$	Derived from β_2-microglobulin, associated with long-term hemodialysis
IAPP (amylin)	Found in type 2 DM
PrP	Misfolded prion protein found in Creutzfeldt-Jakob disease

DM, diabetes mellitus; RA, rheumatoid arthritis; TB, tuberculosis.

DIAGNOSIS

A diagnosis of SLE is enough to suspect lupus nephritis. The gold standard to confirm lupus nephritis is renal biopsy. There are six classes of lupus nephritis that progress from normal histology (class I) to advanced sclerosis lupus nephritis (class VI). **Diffuse proliferative nephritis** (class IV) is the most common type seen in SLE.

TREATMENT

The treatment is based on the level of renal involvement. It progresses from general SLE treatment to increasing doses of corticosteroids and, finally, to immunosuppressant drugs. Class VI is usually resistant to all drug therapies, so treatment should mainly focus on management of the general symptoms.

PROGNOSIS

Chiefly depends on age of onset and the overall systemic involvement and response to therapy. Lupus nephritis may ultimately lead to ESRD.

NEPHRITIC SYNDROME

The pathology of this condition is the result of **inflammation of the glomerulus** and **neutrophil-related injury.** Nephritic syndrome is characterized by a distinct set of symptoms:

- **Hematuria** secondary to destruction of glomerular capillaries and loss of RBCs into the Bowman space, resulting in dysmorphic RBCs and RBC casts on urinalysis.
- **Oliguria** and **azotemia** (increased blood urea nitrogen and creatinine) secondary to glomerular injury as a result of infiltration of inflammatory cells and immune complex deposition. This infiltration leads to obstruction of the glomerular capillary lumen, thereby decreasing the GFR.
- **Hypertension** secondary to the increased fluid retention by the kidney due to the decreased GFR. Mild **proteinuria** may be observed as a result of the glomerular capillary injury.

As with nephrotic syndrome, there are many different types of nephritic syndrome. Also like nephrotic syndrome, each type has specific causes and presentations while maintaining the core nephritic symptoms mentioned earlier. The presumptive diagnosis is made

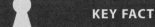

KEY FACT

Hematuria, oliguria, azotemia, and hypertension are the hallmarks of **nephritic syndrome.** In addition, **RBC casts** are often found in the urine.

ANSWER

Kimmelstiel-Wilson nodules.

through clinical suspicion, but the definitive diagnosis can only be made with **renal biopsy.** The cause of this condition is important, since as with nephrotic syndrome, it has implications for both treatment and prognosis.

Important **serologic markers** to obtain when nephritic syndrome is suspected include **C3 levels, anti-GBM titer,** and **antineutrophil cytoplasmic antibody (ANCA) titer.** The corresponding patterns of these laboratory findings may obviate the need for renal biopsy in some cases.

Acute Proliferative Glomerulonephritis (Poststreptoccocal/Infectious)

This form of nephritic syndrome most frequently develops following an infection with certain strains of **group A β-hemolytic streptococci** (GABHS). Pathogenesis is secondary to immune-complex deposition in the glomerulus with resulting complement activation and inflammation. Patients are typically children between the ages of 2 and 6 years due to the effective immunity one develops after infection, although adults occasionally develop this disease as well.

PRESENTATION

Classic presentation is **nephritic syndrome,** usually 10 days after pharyngeal infection or 2–3 weeks after skin infection with GABHS.

DIAGNOSIS

Effective diagnosis can be made based on history and clinical findings reflecting common nephritic symptoms.

- **Serum chemistry:** Antistreptolysin-O (ASO) titers or other streptococcal antibodies (anti-DNAase B) are elevated in > 90% of patients. C3 levels tend to be low; ANCA and anti-GBM antibodies are negative.
- **Urinalysis:** "Smoky brown" colored urine, RBCs and RBC casts, and in some instances proteins.
- **Pathology:** Renal biopsy if needed.
- **Light microscopy** (Figure 8-31): Hypercellular and enlarged glomeruli.
- **Electron microscopy:** Characteristic subepithelial electron-dense deposits (**humps**).
- **Immunofluorescence:** IgG and C3 coarse granular deposits, with a "**lumpy–bumpy**" appearance.

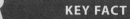

KEY FACT

Poststreptococcal glomerulonephritis can follow either pharyngeal or skin infections, even if the initial infection is treated. In contrast, **poststreptococcal rheumatic fever** can only follow pharyngeal infection, and treatment of the initial infection can effectively prevent its development.

FLASH BACK

One key difference between poststreptococcal glomerulonephritis (PSGN) and IgA nephropathy is the onset. PSGN usually occurs weeks after an upper respiratory infection, whereas IgA nephropathy occurs within a few days.

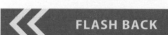
QUESTION

An 83-year-old man presents with six months of back pain and lower extremity edema. Skeletal survey reveals multiple lytic bone lesions in the axial skeleton. What should be used to diagnose this patient's renal problems? What would it show?

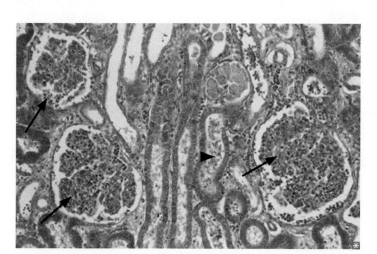

FIGURE 8-31. **Light microscopy of acute proliferative glomerulonephritis.** This low-power view shows three enlarged, hypercellular glomeruli (hypercellularity caused by proliferation of mesangial cells, endothelial cells, and global leukocytic infiltration in all lobules of the glomerulus) (arrows). Several tubules contain red cells and proteinaceous material (arrowhead). Mild interstitial edema is also evident.

TREATMENT

Conservative therapy aimed at maintaining proper water and electrolyte balance. **Diuretics** and other **antihypertensive** drugs are used to control the hypertension and edema that may develop. Penicillin may be administered to eradicate GABHS. Although it does not prevent subsequent development of poststreptococcal glomerulonephritis, it does prevent progression to rheumatic fever.

PROGNOSIS

Excellent in **children,** with complete recovery when adequately treated. In **adults,** complete recovery can also be achieved, although the risk of developing RPGN is greater, as is progression to ESRD due to residual renal impairment.

Rapidly Progressive Glomerulonephritis

Rapidly progressive glomerulonephritis (crescentic RPGN) is not a disease, per se, but rather is an aggressive form of nephritic syndrome, in which progressive loss of kidney function occurs within weeks or months following the primary insult. The disorder is most common in adults aged 30–60 years and is slightly more common in men.

PRESENTATION

Classic nephritic syndrome; varies based on the underlying cause. There are **three distinct types of RPGN** (Table 8-18).

DIAGNOSIS

Effective diagnosis can be made based on history and histologic findings.

- **Serum chemistry:**
    - BUN and creatinine may rise rapidly.
    - Anti-GBM-antibody positive in association with Goodpasture syndrome.
    - ANCA presence varies based on the underlying cause.
    - Complement levels may be decreased in some cases.
- **Urinalysis:** Blood (RBCs), protein, WBC (monocytes), and casts.
- **Pathology:** Renal biopsy.
- **Light microscopy** confirms crescent formation (Figure 8-32). Crescents largely consist of proliferated glomerular parietal cells; Bowman space is filled with monocytes and macrophages. Large amounts of **fibrin** accumulate within the cellular layers of the crescents.

TREATMENT

Depends on the underlying cause.

TABLE 8-18. **Types of Rapidly Progressive Glomerulonephritis**

TYPE	DISEASES	IMMUNOFLUORESCENCE FINDINGS
I	Goodpasture syndrome	**ANCA-negative,** linear IgG and C3 deposits along the GBM
II	Poststreptoccocal GN, SLE, IgA nephropathy, Henoch-Schönlein purpura	**ANCA-negative,** granular "lumpy-bumpy" deposits
III	Granulomatosis with polyangiitis or idiopathic	**ANCA-positive,** no deposits on the GBM

ANCA, antineutrophil cytoplasmic antibody; GBM, glomerular basement membrane; GN, glomerulonephritis; SLE, systemic lupus erythematosus.

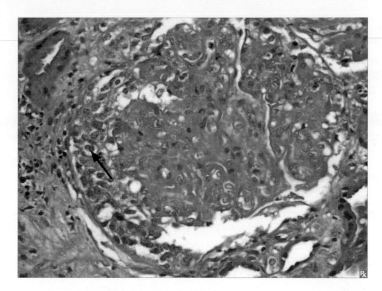

FIGURE 8-32. **Light microscopy of crescent formation.** Note the hypercellular glomerulus with a crescent of epithelial cells filling Bowman space (arrow), characteristic of RPGN.

Antiglomerular Basement Membrane Disease (Goodpasture Syndrome)

Disease characterized by **antibodies against proteins in the GBM.** Symptoms can be isolated to the kidney or may also be seen in the lung due to cross-reactivity of antigens (eg, α_3 chain of collagen type IV) that are common to both alveolar and GBMs. The underlying pathogenesis is based on a type II hypersensitivity reaction. This disease accounts for < 1% of glomerulopathies.

- **Goodpasture syndrome** (Figure 8-33): Both alveolar and glomerular symptoms occur.
- **Idiopathic anti-GBM disease:** Symptoms are isolated to the kidney.

PRESENTATION

Hematuria and other nephritic symptoms, subnephrotic range proteinuria, and RPGN over the course of a few weeks is common. Pulmonary hemorrhage presenting with **hemoptysis** and dyspnea occurs in those patients with both glomerular and alveolar injury.

DIAGNOSIS

Gold standard is renal biopsy with immunofluorescence. Chest plain film shows bibasilar shadows in cases with pulmonary involvement.

- **Serum chemistry: Anti-GBM antibodies** are **positive** in > 90% of patients. ANCA levels are typically negative, but are occasionally mildly elevated. C3 levels are normal.
- **Urinalysis:** RBCs, RBC casts, and mild proteinuria.
- **Pathology:** Renal biopsy is the gold standard for proper diagnosis.
- **Light microscopy:** Cellular accumulation in the Bowman space; crescent formation.
- **Immunofluorescence: Linear, ribbon-like** deposits of IgG along the GBM as opposed to granular deposits characteristic of the immune complex causes detailed earlier.

TREATMENT

Emergency **plasmapheresis** is performed daily until anti-GBM titers become negative.

- **Prednisone** and either **cyclophosphamide** or **azathioprine** are started simultaneously to suppress formation of new GBM antibodies.

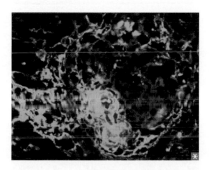

FIGURE 8-33. **Light micrograph with immunofluorescence staining of Goodpasture syndrome.** Note the characteristic linear pattern that is diagnostic of Goodpasture syndrome.

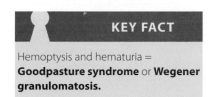

KEY FACT

Hemoptysis and hematuria = **Goodpasture syndrome** or **Wegener granulomatosis.**

■ Patients are monitored frequently for rising titers of anti-GBM antibodies and receive plasmapheresis as needed.

PROGNOSIS

Without treatment, patients tend to develop ESRD within 1 year. When aggressive, immunosuppressive regimens are started early, > 90% of patients maintain renal function after 1 year. Although this disease is rare, the diagnosis must be made early to ensure appropriate treatment and good prognosis.

IgA Nephropathy (Berger Disease)

IgA nephropathy usually affects **children** and **young adults.** It is suspected to arise in individuals with an abnormality in IgA production and clearance (increased production of IgA in ~50% of individuals with this disease), leading to **deposition of the antibodies in the mesangial matrix** (Figure 8-34), which leads to glomerular injury and nephritic symptoms. It is the **most common** glomerulopathy worldwide.

IgA nephropathy can present as disease limited to the kidneys or as a component of **Henoch-Schönlein purpura.**

PRESENTATION

Episode of gross hematuria 24–48 hours after a nonspecific upper respiratory tract infection or GI infection. **Hematuria** typically lasts for several days and then spontaneously resolves, only to recur every few months. Hypertension is unusual at presentation.

DIAGNOSIS

Suspected in patients with new-onset hematuria within 1–2 days of either an upper respiratory or GI infection.

■ **Serum chemistry:** ANCA- and anti-GBM-negative, C3 levels are normal.
■ **Urinalysis:** Painless spontaneous hematuria.
■ **Pathology:** Renal biopsy.
■ **Light microscopy** (Figure 8-34): May range from normal to overt focal crescentic proliferative glomerulopathy.
■ **Immunofluorescence** (Figure 8-35): Granular IgA deposits with specific distribution in mesangial cells.

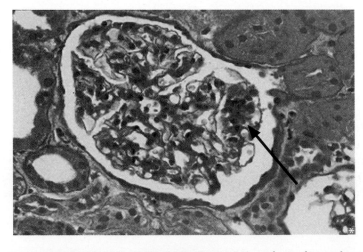

FIGURE 8-34. **Light microscopy of IgA nephropathy.** IgA nephropathy can have variable histologic findings, ranging from normal to overt crescentic glomerulonephritis. The glomerulus in this high-power view (periodic acid-Schiff [PAS] stain) shows mild changes consisting of segmental proliferation of mesangial cells and mesangial widening by matrix accumulation (arrow).

TREATMENT

Glucocorticoids have been shown to be effective in cases of modest proteinuria. Patients with severe disease can be treated with plasma exchange and immunosuppression (controversial) or with high-dose immunoglobulins. Angiotensin-converting enzyme (ACE) inhibitors may retard disease progression to ESRD.

PROGNOSIS

Most patients have recurring episodes every few months or during mucosal infections. Between 20% and 50% of patients suffer ESRD after 20 years unless HTN is controlled and persistent proteinuria does not develop.

Hereditary Nephritis (Alport Syndrome)

Alport syndrome is a **hereditary form of glomerular injury** that is typically **X-linked recessive,** most commonly caused by an error in the synthesis of the **α5 chain of type IV collagen.** This form of collagen is a major component of the GBM, and defects lead to renal dysfunction. Type IV collagen is also found in many other tissues, and therefore patients with this genetic defect tend to develop **sensorineural deafness, lens dislocation,** and early development of **cataracts.**

PRESENTATION

Patients are typically between 5 and 20 years old. Initially, Alport syndrome is asymptomatic, though patients may complain of painless gross hematuria, and there may be family history of nephritic syndrome and deafness in males. Later stages are characterized by chronic glomerulonephritis and systematic glomerular destruction, leading to hematuria and diminished GFR, and ultimately to ESRD.

DIAGNOSIS

Based on the following findings:

- **Serum chemistry:** ANCA- and anti-GBM-negative, C3 levels are normal.
- **Urinalysis:** Gross hematuria, mild proteinuria.
- **Pathology:** Renal biopsy.
- **Light microscopy:** Glomerular and mesangial proliferation. **Foam cells** may be present, which are interstitial cells with accumulation of lipids.
- **EM:** Splitting of the lamina densa (component of GBM).

TREATMENT

No specific therapy, though ACEIs/ARBs are often used to slow disease progression. Dialysis is used for patients who progress to ESRD. Renal transplantation is an option for those patients in renal failure, as allografts do not have similar genetic mutations so relapse does not occur. Because Alport syndrome is X-linked, this disorder is more severe in males than in females, who often have a benign course and serve as genetic carriers of the disease.

PROGNOSIS

Prognosis depends on the kind of mutation. Around 90% of patients develop ESRD by age 40. Patients with a deletion or loss-of-function mutation of the α_5 chain of type IV collagen have a significantly higher chance of developing ESRD than do those with minor mutations.

Granulomatosis with Polyangiitis

Granulomatosis with polyangiitis (GPA), formerly Wegener granulomatosis, is a systemic disease that presents as focal necrotizing vasculitis and necrotizing granulomas in both the upper and lower respiratory tract (lungs), in association with necrotizing glomerulonephritis. Renal injury occurs in up to 80% of patients with this disorder.

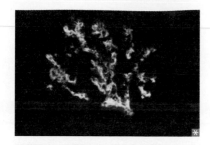

FIGURE 8-35. Immuno-fluorescence of IgA nephropathy. Immunofluorescent stain shows deposits of IgA primarily in mesangial regions.

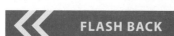

FLASH BACK

Henoch-Schönlein purpura's *extrarenal* symptoms include:
- **Skin:** Purpural lesions found on the extensor surfaces of the lower extremities, buttocks, and arms.
- **GI:** Abdominal pain, intestinal bleeding.
- **Musculoskeletal:** Joint pain.

KEY FACT

Male patients exhibit full spectrum of this disease: deafness, cataracts, and renal failure.
Female patients are carriers; symptoms are limited to mild hematuria.

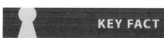

KEY FACT

Confirmation of renal involvement is necessary to make a definitive diagnosis of **granulomatosis with polyangiitis.**

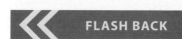

FLASH BACK

Chronic sinusitis, hemoptysis, and hematuria → granulomatosis with polyangiitis.

PRESENTATION

Patients typically present with **nonspecific symptoms,** such as fever, arthralgias, lethargy, and malaise. Renal involvement presents with **nephritic** symptoms and an occasional **mild proteinuria.**

DIAGNOSIS

Cytoplasmic staining ANCA (c-ANCA)–positive in 80% of patients with renal involvement.

Biopsy is required and demonstrates focal, segmental necrotizing glomerulonephritis with occasional crescent formation. Unlike in respiratory tract biopsies, granulomas are only rarely seen. There is a lack of immunoglobulin or complement on immunofluorescence, **anti-GBM** is **negative,** and **complement levels** are **normal.**

TREATMENT

Glucocorticoids and cyclophosphamide. For patients who present with pulmonary hemorrhage or severe renal injury, plasma exchange can be life saving. Dialysis and renal transplantation are good options for those patients who progress to ESRD with little recurrence of the disorder in the allograft.

PROGNOSIS

Most patients respond well to treatment, although flare-ups occur in 25–40% of cases. A majority of patients suffer from long-term complications, such as chronic renal failure and hearing loss.

RENAL STONES (UROLITHIASIS)

Stone formation can take place anywhere in the urinary collecting system (most commonly in the collecting duct) and largely depends on sex, age, diet, climate, and genetic makeup. Their size can vary from crystals to large stones. They occur more commonly in men and in the summer due to insufficient fluid intake. There are several different types:

- **Calcium oxalate stones** are the most common. They can form from a high concentration of calcium in the urine that is caused by excess GI absorption, excess renal excretion, and/or excess bone resorption. They can also form with hyperoxaluria (eg, hereditary primary hyperoxaluria, high vitamin C intake, inflammatory bowel disease, or as a result of ethylene glycol [antifreeze] ingestion).
- **Calcium phosphate stones** are the next most common and often occur in the setting of immobilization or bone-mineral disease. Examples are hypercalcemia secondary to hyperparathyroidism, vitamin D intoxication, and sarcoidosis.
- **Struvite (magnesium ammonium phosphate) stones** occur in patients with persistently alkaline urine from urinary tract infections (UTIs) caused by **urease-positive** organisms, such as *Proteus vulgaris*, staphylococci, *Klebisella*, and *Pseudomonas* (but **not** *Escherichia coli*). The urine pH is alkaline. When the stone creates a cast of the renal pelvis and calyceal system, it is referred to as a **staghorn kidney stone.**
- **Uric acid stones** are associated with **gout** or diseases that cause rapid cell turnover (**leukemia,** myeloproliferative diseases). They are more likely to form in **acidic urine.**
- **Cystine stones** are seen in patients with genetic defects in the PCT resorption of cystine, ornithine, lysine, or arginine. They are more likely to form in **acidic urine.**

PRESENTATION

Kidney stones classically present with severe flank pain that **radiates to the groin** and is colicky in nature. **Hydronephrosis** and **infection** proximal to the site of obstruction can occur as a result of prolonged impediment of the urine outflow.

DIAGNOSIS

- **Colicky pain in flank radiating to the groin,** nausea, vomiting, patient constantly moves to relieve pain.
- An **abdominal radiograph** (Figure 8-36) is helpful in cases of calcium oxalate, calcium phosphate, and struvite stones (which are **radiopaque**) but is of no value for uric acid and cystine stones, which are **radiolucent** and cannot be visualized on a radiograph. Thus, **noncontrast CT** is valuable in diagnosing such cases.
- **Urinalysis** is likely to show hematuria.

TREATMENT

Mainly depends on the type and size of stones (see Table 8-19). **Increased fluid intake** and appropriate **pain management** while waiting for the stone to pass is sufficient for stones smaller than 5 mm. Stones from 5 to 9 mm in diameter usually require medical management with alpha blockers (tamsulosin) to facilitate stone passage. Larger stones (> 9 mm in diameter) may require extracorporeal shockwave **lithotripsy** (ESWL) or surgical treatment (**nephrolithotomy**). Prevention strategies include drinking more water, and other dietary and medication therapies depending on the type of stone (see Table 8-19). Alkalization of the urine can be useful for treating uric acid and cystine stones, but this may cause the formation of calcium phosphate stones. Decreasing calcium intake is not advised, since doing so may lead to greater oxalate absorption.

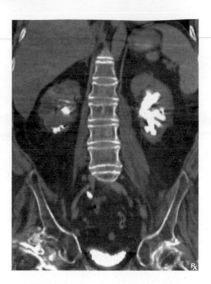

FIGURE 8-36. Staghorn calculi. Noncontrast CT scan shows staghorn calculi in the left and right kidneys, and innumerable stones in the bladder.

TABLE 8-19. Common Types of Kidney Stones

STONE TYPE	FREQUENCY	CAUSES	RADIOLOGY	APPEARANCE	TREATMENT
Calcium oxalate	Most common in adults and in children	Idiopathic hypercalciuria, hyperoxaluria, hypocitraturia	Radiopaque	Envelope or octahedron	Low sodium diet to reduce hypercalciuria, sufficient citrate in diet; low-oxalate diet (no chocolate or nuts); and if necessary, thiazide diuretics to reduce hypercalciuria
Calcium phosphate	Common in individuals with bone-mineral disease or immobilization	Immobilization, cancer, ↑ PTH; ↑ vitamin D, milk-alkali syndrome	Radiopaque	Usually amorphous	Treat underlying disorder, low-sodium diet and thiazide diuretics can reduce hypercalciuria
Struvite (ammonium magnesium phosphate)	Second most common	■ UTI with urease-positive bacteria (*P vulgaris, Staphylococcus,* or *Klebsiella*)	Radiopaque; stone creates a cast of the renal pelvis and calyceal system	Rectangular prism, like coffin lids	Surgical removal Antibiotics to eliminate bacteria, prevent UTI
Uric acid	Less common	■ Hyperuricemia: gout ■ High cell turnover: leukemia and myeloproliferative diseases	Radiolucent	Yellow or red-brown, diamond or rhombus	Allopurinol Alkalinize urine Limit purines in diet
Cystine	Least common	■ Cystinuria: genetic defects in PCT resorption of cystine, ornithine, lysine, and arginine	Faintly opaque, ground glass	Flat, yellow, hexagonal	Increase fluid intake Alkalinize urine Low-sodium diet Low-protein diet

PTH, parathyroid hormone; UTI, urinary tract infection.

URINARY TRACT INFECTIONS

UTIs are infections, usually bacterial, of the **lower urinary tract.** Common bacteria that cause UTIs include *E coli* and *Staphylococcus saprophyticus.* UTIs are extremely common in several different populations and settings:

- **Outpatient:** Especially common among young sexually active females and are thought to be due to the short female urethra and the small distance between the urethra and the anus.
- **Inpatient:** Very common, especially with Foley catheter use. *E coli* is the most common causal organism. *Klebsiella, Proteus, Enterobacter,* and *Serratia* are also common offenders. Likely to be asymptomatic. Have a high suspicion for UTI in any febrile inpatient.
- **Pregnancy:** Asymptomatic bacteriuria is common in pregnant women. There is a higher risk for UTIs to develop into pyelonephritis in pregnant women. UTIs also raise the risk for preterm labor and low birth weight. Bacteriuria in a pregnant woman should *always* be treated, whether or not it is symptomatic.
- **Children:** Children with recurrent UTIs should be evaluated for vesicoureteral reflux (VUR) and/or sexual abuse.

PRESENTATION

- Dysuria, frequency, urgency, suprapubic pain, and hematuria.
- In an uncomplicated UTI, there should **not** be fever, nausea, vomiting, or costovertebral angle (CVA) tenderness (as in pyelonephritis).

DIAGNOSIS

Can be made by history alone.

- Clean-catch urinalysis usually shows pyuria (PMNs in the urine), bacteriuria, leukocyte esterase, and nitrites (if caused by member of the Enterobacteriaceae family).
- Urine culture identifies the specific pathogen but is only indicated for children, inpatients, patients for whom antibiotic therapy has failed, or complicated cases of UTI.

TREATMENT

Uncomplicated UTIs can be treated with oral antibiotics such as trimethoprim/sulfamethoxazole (TMP/SMX), ciprofloxacin, or nitrofurantoin. Around 50% of people recover without treatment within a few days to weeks. Ingestion of cranberry juice and urination immediately after sexual intercourse may decrease the incidence of UTIs. Patients with asymptomatic bacteriuria should only be treated if they are **pregnant, require or have had surgical urological intervention, or have had hip arthroplasty.** All other asymptomatic patients should not have their bacteriuria treated. Appropriate treatment during pregnancy includes nitrofurantoin, ampicillin, or cephalexin.

Acute Pyelonephritis

Pyelonephritis is an infection, usually bacterial, of the upper urinary tract including the kidneys. Common bacterial causes include *E coli* and Enterococci species. It typically results from an ascending infection from the lower urinary tract. It affects the same populations as do uncomplicated UTIs but in much smaller numbers overall.

PRESENTATION

Fever, nausea/vomiting, flank pain and CVA tenderness. Can occur in the presence or absence of typical symptoms of lower UTI (dysuria, frequency, urgency).

DIAGNOSIS

Based on history and physical exam, especially vital signs and CVA tenderness.

CLINICAL CORRELATION

Acute UTI is a common cause of acute delirium in elderly patients.

KEY FACT

Escherichia coli is the most common cause of UTIs in women, followed by *Staphylococcus saprophyticus.*

CLINICAL CORRELATION

Sterile pyuria in the setting of a negative urine culture suggests infection by *Neisseria gonorrheae* or *Chlamydia trachomatis.*

CLINICAL CORRELATION

Treatment of acute UTI during pregnancy is complicated by many antibiotics being contraindicated. Nitrofurantoin is normally first-line treatment during pregnancy. Cephalexin, amoxicillin, and amoxicillin-clavulanate can also be used.

CLINICAL CORRELATION

White blood cell casts in the urine are pathognomonic for **acute pyelonephritis.**

- **Urinalysis (UA)** and **urine culture** with **antimicrobial sensitivities** should be performed in all patients with suspected acute pyelonephritis because of the risk of serious sequelae if treatment is inappropriate. Urinalysis demonstrates **pyuria. WBC casts,** if present, are diagnostic of acute pyelonephritis.
- **Microbiology:** The pathogens responsible for pyelonephritis are the same as those responsible for uncomplicated UTIs.

TREATMENT

Oral or IV antibiotics such as TMP/SMX and ciprofloxacin.

Chronic Pyelonephritis

Recurrent or persistent infections of the kidneys ultimately lead to irreversible interstitial scarring.

Underlying factors leading to this condition are almost exclusively structural abnormalities such as **obstructions** of the urinary tract (eg, from stones, benign prostatic hypertrophy [BPH], or congenital ureteropelvic junction obstruction) or **VUR** in children.

PRESENTATION

- May have asymptomatic pyuria.
- May complain of low-grade fevers, flank pain, and nausea/vomiting.
- May have evidence of renal insufficiency such as hypertension, proteinuria, or failure to thrive in children.

DIAGNOSIS

Based on the following findings.

- **Renal ultrasound** to evaluate for renal damage. A **CT scan** may offer additional information for diagnosing the underlying pathology.
- **Voiding cystourethrogram** can help diagnose VUR in children.
- Laboratory data may show **pyuria, proteinuria,** and **azotemia.**
- **Pathologic specimens:**
  - Chronic inflammation and asymmetrical corticomedullary scarring.
  - Deformities in renal pelvis and calyces.
  - **Thyroidization** of kidney (Figure 8-37).

TREATMENT

Antibiotics such as TMP/SMX and nitrofurantoin, and surgical repair.

DIFFUSE CORTICAL NECROSIS

Diffuse cortical necrosis (DCN) develops as a result of diffuse or patchy **infarction of the cortices** of the kidney secondary to ischemia. Often multifactorial and can progress to acute kidney injury (AKI), especially in the third trimester of pregnancy.

PRESENTATION

Signs and symptoms of the systemic process (sepsis, disseminated intravascular coagulation [DIC], obstetric complications) resulting in cortical necrosis. Anuria, evidence of AKI, flank pain, and fever.

DIAGNOSIS

Based on the following findings:

- **Serum chemistry:** Azotemia, DIC (eg, low platelets, increased fibrin split products).
- **UA:** Proteinuria, hematuria, red blood cell casts, granular casts (derived from dead renal tubule cells).
- **Pathology:** Cortical necrosis, microthrombi of small vessels.

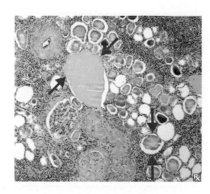

FIGURE 8-37. Chronic pyelonephritis. Light micrograph of a renal biopsy of a patient with chronic pyelonephritis. Note the prominent thyroidization (arrows).

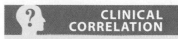

CLINICAL CORRELATION

Conditions associated with **DCN:**
- Abruptio placentae
- Eclampsia/preeclampsia
- Septic shock
- Hemolytic-uremic syndrome (in children)

TREATMENT

Treat underlying condition.

PROGNOSIS

Reversible if treatment of underlying process is initiated early. Fatal if untreated.

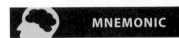

Conditions associated with **renal papillary necrosis:**

- DM
- Acute pyelonephritis
- Chronic analgesic use, especially those containing phenacetin
- Sickle cell disease/trait

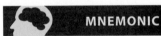

SAAD PAPa with **PAP**illary necrosis:

Sickle cell disease/trait
Acute pyelonephritis
Analgesics (chronic use)
Diabetes mellitus

MNEMONIC

Dialysis is indicated for **AEIOU:**

Acidosis
Electrolyte abnormalities (hyperkalemia)
Intoxicants (eg, ethylene glycol, methanol, and Li)
fluid **O**verload
Uremia

RENAL PAPILLARY NECROSIS

Renal papillary necrosis results from an ischemic insult to the renal papillae.

PRESENTATION

Polyuria, rust-colored urine, AKI, flank pain.

DIAGNOSIS

UA: Sediment, casts, blood, and necrotic renal papillae. Plain radiographs may show a ring of calcification, especially in disease resulting from analgesic use.

TREATMENT

Treat the underlying condition. Stop offending drugs if analgesic nephropathy is suspected.

ACUTE AND CHRONIC KIDNEY INJURY

Many conditions can lead to either AKI or chronic kidney injury (CKI). Definitions of key terms pertinent to kidney injury are provided in Table 8-20. The three main categories of kidney injury are summarized in Table 8-21. The pathophysiologic mechanisms of renal failure are discussed in each section.

Acute Kidney Injury

Abrupt-onset decrease in renal function as measured by GFR (not necessarily urine output). Leads to reduced ability to maintain serum electrolytes and excrete nitrogenous waste. AKI is classified as shown in Figure 8-38.

TREATMENT

- Maintain fluid and electrolyte balance and avoid nephrotoxic medications.
- Treat obstruction if indicated.

TABLE 8-20. **Key Definitions in Acute and Chronic Kidney Injury**

TERM	DEFINITION
Glomerular filtration rate (GFR)	The volume of filtrate that crosses the glomerular capillary membrane into Bowman capsule per unit time. Normal is 90–120 mL/min
Azotemia	Elevated BUN and serum creatinine levels; may have causes other than renal dysfunction
Uremia	Syndrome caused by biochemical derangement from severe metabolic waste product accumulation. Findings include encephalopathy, platelet dysfunction/bleeding, pericarditis, anorexia, and vomiting. Uremic symptoms are most often seen in the setting of renal symptoms secondary to AKI/CKI
Oliguria	Urine output < 500 mL/24 hours
Anuria	Urine output < 100 mL/24 hours
Polyuria	Urine output > 3 L/24 hours

AKI, acute kidney injury; BUN, blood urea nitrogen; CKI, chronic kidney injury.

TABLE 8-21.   Types of Kidney Injury

VARIABLE	PRERENAL	RENAL	POSTRENAL
Urine osmolality (mOsm/kg)	> 500	< 350	< 350
Urine Na (mEq/L)	< 20	> 40	Variable
FE_{Na}	< 1%	> 2%	> 4%
BUN/Cr ratio	> 20	< 15	> 15

BUN, blood urea nitrogen; Cr, creatinine; FE_{Na}, fractional excretion of sodium.

■ **Dialysis** is indicated for severe uremia (including uremic pericarditis), hyperkalemia unresponsive to medication, metabolic acidosis, refractory fluid overload (usually presents as pulmonary edema), etc.

Acute Tubular Necrosis

A disease state of the kidney clinically manifested as AKI and pathologically by destruction of tubular epithelial cells. Acute tubular necrosis (ATN) is an intrinsic renal disease and is the **most common cause of AKI** (Figure 8-39). It can be either ischemic or nephrotoxic in origin (Table 8-22).

> **CLINICAL CORRELATION**
>
> Associated with **ATN:**
> ■ Muddy brown casts
> ■ Rhabdomyolysis
> ■ Crush injury

PRESENTATION

There are three stages of ATN: inciting event, oliguric phase, and polyuric phase. Most patients present with oliguria and azotemia, though some patients are asymptomatic.

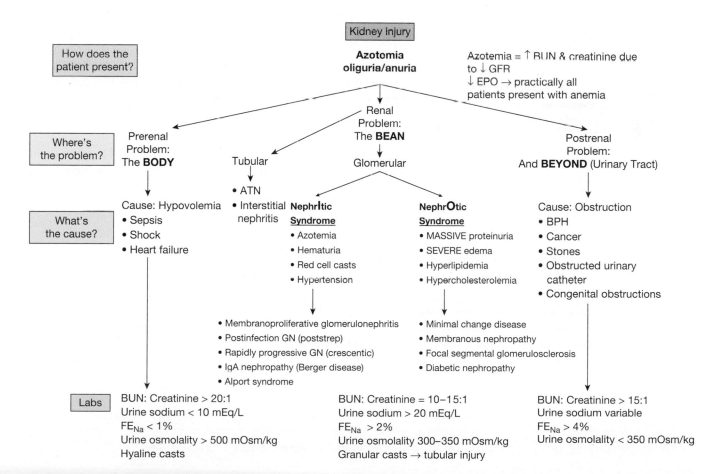

FIGURE 8-38.   Pathophysiology of acute kidney injury.

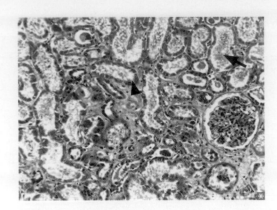

FIGURE 8-39. **Kidney with acute tubular necrosis.** Note the loss of nuclei (arrowhead), dilation of tubules, interstitial edema, sloughing of epithelium (arrows), and glomerular congestion.

The oliguric, or maintenance phase, is dangerous because many patients may become hypovolemic and/or hyperkalemic. If this is left untreated for a significant period of time (longer than two weeks), a polyuric, or recovery phase, can develop. This final phase is most notable for polyuria (up to 3 L per day) and electrolyte wasting due to the re-epithelialization of the nephron while the tubules are still damaged. Hypokalemia is a major risk due to a large loss of dissolved solutes during this phase.

DIAGNOSIS

Azotemia; $FE_{Na} > 1\%$ and **muddy brown casts** on microscopy.

TREATMENT

Address the underlying disease, and remove the offending agent (medication, contrast medium, etc.). When rhabdomyolysis or crush injury is the insulting factor, large volumes of IV fluid are required to maintain adequate perfusion. In addition, IV fluids can dilute nephrotoxic substances such as myoglobin and possibly prevent ATN from occurring in patients with crush injuries or rhabdomyolysis. Look for and treat electrolyte abnormalities.

Chronic Renal Failure

Also called chronic kidney disease (CKD), this disease is characterized by a substantial decrease in renal function, usually less than 20% of normal GFR, developing over a long period of time (usually > 6 months). CKD can be asymptomatic for many years, followed by increasing uremia and associated symptoms as GFR drops below 60 mL/min. Causes of CKD, all of which are chronic disease processes, are shown in Table 8-23.

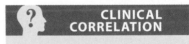

CLINICAL CORRELATION

Contrast nephropathy can result from IV contrast agents used for contrast CT scans. Fluid bolus and n-acetylcysteine can be used prophylactically to prevent contrast nephropathy.

TABLE 8-22. **Common Causes of Acute Tubular Necrosis**

TYPE	ETIOLOGY	DAMAGE
Nephrotoxic	▪ **Drugs:** NSAIDs, radiocontrast, cyclophosphamide, aminoglycosides, diuretics, and heavy metals (eg, lead, mercury) ▪ **Disease:** Rhabdomyolysis, hemolysis, gout, pseudogout, and multiple myeloma	▪ PCT ▪ Tubular basement membranes remain intact
Ischemic	▪ Decreased blood flow to the kidney	▪ Straight segment of PCT ▪ Medullary segment of TAL ▪ Tubular basement membranes are disrupted

NSAIDs, nonsteroidal anti-inflammatory drugs; PCT, proximal convoluted tubule; TAL, thick ascending limb (of loop of Henle).

TABLE 8-23. Causes of Chronic Kidney Disease

	CAUSE
Prerenal	▪ Renal artery stenosis ▪ Embolism (both kidneys)
Parenchymal	▪ DM ▪ SLE ▪ Hypertension ▪ Amyloidosis ▪ Chronic glomerulonephritis ▪ Chronic tubulointerstitial nephritis ▪ Adult polycystic kidney disease ▪ Renal cancer
Postrenal	▪ Chronic urinary tract obstruction

DM, diabetes mellitus; SLE, systemic lupus erythematosus.

TREATMENT

- Dietary management of protein and electrolytes.
- Dialysis (indicated when GFR ≤ 20 mL/min).
- Renal transplantation (cadaveric or living donor) when GFR < 20 mL/min.
- Control of renal osteodystrophy through the use of calcimimetics like cinacalcet or calcitriol replacement therapy.

Consequences of Renal Failure

Renal failure results in multiple systemic consequences (Table 8-24). The primary effects of ARF are electrolyte imbalances and disruption of the kidneys' control of excretion. ARF typically manifests itself as uremic syndrome, hyperkalemia, and metabolic acidosis. CKD has more gradual effects on multiple systems, and the dysregulation of sodium and water can lead to **congestive heart failure (CHF)** and **pulmonary edema.**

CYSTIC KIDNEY DISEASE

Autosomal Dominant Polycystic Kidney Disease

PRESENTATION

Autosomal dominant polycystic kidney disease (ADPCKD) is caused by mutations in **PKD1** or **PKD2** on chromosomes 16 and 4, respectively. It is characterized by multiple cysts in both kidneys that destroy the intervening parenchyma (Figure 8-40). Patients usually present in their 40s with flank pain, intermittent hematuria, a palpable abdominal/flank mass, hypertension, and a positive family history of kidney disease.

DIAGNOSIS

A positive family history and bilateral kidney cysts detected by ultrasound. Liver cysts may also be present.

TREATMENT

Largely supportive, including antihypertensives, diuretics, and a low-salt diet. UTIs should be promptly treated with antibiotics. Treatment of ESRD includes dialysis and renal transplantation.

PROGNOSIS

CRF begins at age 40–60 and is the most common cause of death. Complications include refractory hypertension and urinary infection. There is an association with

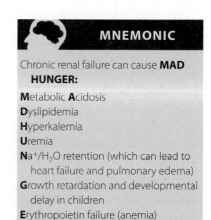

MNEMONIC

Chronic renal failure can cause **MAD HUNGER:**

Metabolic **A**cidosis
Dyslipidemia
Hyperkalemia
Uremia
Na⁺/H₂O retention (which can lead to heart failure and pulmonary edema)
Growth retardation and developmental delay in children
Erythropoietin failure (anemia)
Renal osteodystrophy

TABLE 8-24. **Consequences of Renal Failure**

Uremic syndrome	▪ Occurs as BUN rises; lethargy, seizures, myoclonus, asterixis, pericardial friction rub ▪ Urea typically travels from the liver to the kidney, where it is excreted. The failing kidney cannot excrete urea and therefore the gut enzyme urease converts the extra urea into ammonia, causing **hyperammonemia** ▪ Urinalysis: Isosthenuria (specific gravity of urine becomes fixed around 1.010, regardless of the fluid intake because the kidney cannot concentrate or dilute the urine), proteinuria, abnormal sediment with tubular casts
Hyperkalemia	▪ When GFR significantly decreases, the kidney cannot excrete dietary K+ ▪ Hyperkalemia → look for **peaked T waves on ECG, which can lead to ventricular fibrillation**
Metabolic acidosis	▪ GFR < 50% impairs renal production of HCO_3^- so H+ cannot be excreted. This causes an **elevated AG metabolic acidosis**
Sodium and water retention	▪ **Early CKD** causes **decreased urine concentration,** which causes easy dehydration and sodium wasting ▪ **Late CKD** causes **volume overload** as the kidney is no longer able to excrete sodium. This can lead to **pulmonary edema**
Renal osteodystrophy	▪ Following hydroxylation in the liver by 25-hydroxylase, 25-hydroxycholecalciferol (25-(OH)-D_3) is then converted to its biologically active form, 1,25-dihydroxycholecalciferol (1,25-(OH)$_2$-D_3), in the kidney by 1α-hydroxylase ▪ CKD causes loss of **1-α hydroxylase** activity in the kidney, thereby causing decreased vitamin D activation and increased bone turnover ▪ Decreased phosphate excretion results in hyperphosphatemia. This leads to hypocalcemia, which induces secondary hyperparathyroidism and also increases bone turnover
Anemia	▪ Failure of **EPO production** causes decreased hematocrit
Hypertension	▪ Benign hypertension causes hyaline arteriolosclerosis. Malignant hypertension causes hyperplastic arteriolosclerosis, fibrinoid necrosis of the arterioles and small arteries, and intravascular thrombosis ▪ Long-standing damage and scarring of the kidney from reflux nephropathy causes hypertension as one of the first indications of renal disease ▪ Can be caused by APKD
Fanconi syndrome	▪ Damage to proximal tubules compromises reabsorption of glucose, amino acids, phosphate, and bicarbonate

AG, anion gap; APKD, adult polycystic kidney disease; CKD, chronic kidney disease; ECG, electrocardiogram; EPO, erythropoietin; GFR, glomerular filtration rate.

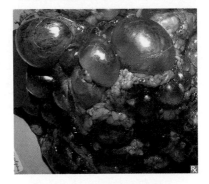

FIGURE 8-40. Autosomal dominant polycystic kidney disease (ADPKD). Photograph of a resected kidney demonstrating the multitude of cysts that can form over time in patients with ADPKD.

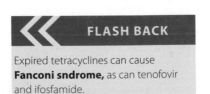

FLASH BACK

Expired tetracyclines can cause **Fanconi sndrome,** as can tenofovir and ifosfamide.

saccular aneurysms affecting the circle of Willis, leading to a high incidence of **subarachnoid hemorrhage.**

Autosomal Recessive (Childhood) Polycystic Kidney Disease

PRESENTATION

Autosomal recessive polycystic kidney disease (ARPCKD) is a rare, autosomal recessive, developmental disease due to mutations in PKHD1. Neonates present with enlarged kidneys at birth. Maternal oligohydramnios leads to Potter facies and pulmonary hypoplasia in newborns.

DIAGNOSIS

Ultrasound and other imaging studies reveal enlarged kidneys (Figure 8-41). Disease can be diagnosed after 24 weeks in gestation in severe cases. Neither parent has renal cysts, which distinguishes ARPCKD from ADPCKD.

TREATMENT

No specific treatment. Mechanical ventilation, dialysis and blood pressure management may improve survival.

PROGNOSIS

Fifty percent of affected neonates die, and one-third of those who survive develop ESRD in 10 years. Patients who survive develop cysts in the liver and ultimately develop congenital hepatic cirrhosis.

INHERITED RENAL SYNDROMES

Fanconi Syndrome

Fanconi syndrome results from loss of function of the PCT and involves all, or nearly all, PCT transporters. Hereditary causes include Wilson disease, tyrosinemia, cystinosis, and glycogen storage diseases. Expired tetracyclines, ifosfamide, tenofovir, lead poisoning, ischemia, and multiple myeloma can also lead to the development of Fanconi syndrome.

PRESENTATION

Patients often present with symptoms of acidosis (type II RTA, specifically) due to defective reuptake of bicarbonate in the proximal tubule. Patients may also present with polyuria and polydipsia due to defective reuptake of Na and H_2O. Patients may also have incidentally found renal glycosuria, which occurs with normal serum glucose levels due to dysfunction of the Na^+/glucose cotransporters. Lastly, children may often present with failure to thrive and/or rickets, the latter because of hypophosphatemia and urinary phosphate losses related to dysfunction of the Na^+/PO_4^{3-} co-transporter.

DIAGNOSIS

Diagnosis is made through discovery of loss of multiple PCT transport functions. The underlying cause of the disorder is specific to each case.

TREATMENT

These patients require replacement of the electrolytes lost in the urine, as well as treatment of any underlying etiologies. The prognosis depends on the underlying disorder.

Bartter Syndrome

Rare autosomal recessive disorder due to mutations in any of the transporters of the thick ascending limb of Henle. Symptoms similar to those seen in patients taking loop diuretics.

PRESENTATION

Presents in early life, often in neonatal period or prenatally with polyuria (or polyhydramnios) and postnatal volume depletion. There can be growth delays and electrolyte abnormalities including hypokalemia, hypochloremic metabolic alkalosis, and hypercalciuria.

DIAGNOSIS

Normally a clinical diagnosis. Patients have polyuria in the setting of volume depletion and multiple electrolyte abnormalities. High renin, high aldosterone. Rule out vomiting and diuretic abuse. Genetic tests available.

TREATMENT

The mainstay of treatment is NSAIDs. These help by decreasing RBF, GFR, and urinary sodium wasting. Potassium supplements are generally needed along with a high sodium, high potassium, high fluid diet. Caution is needed with use of diuretics as these block essential compensatory mechanisms for the sodium wasting. Similar caution is needed if RAAS blockade is introduced.

PROGNOSIS

With early identification and treatment, prognosis is good. However, because treatment is supportive and only mitigates symptoms, patients often have short stature and ongoing need for high fluid intake, high sodium intake, and high potassium intake. Patients with significant hypercalciuria can develop interstitial calcium deposition (nephrocalcinosis), which can lead to tubulointerstitial scarring and eventual CKD and ESRD.

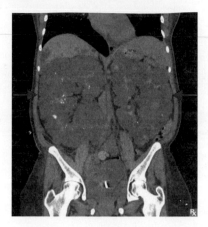

FIGURE 8-41. **Autosomal recessive polycystic kidney disease (ARPCKD).** CT scan revealing grossly enlarged kidneys (arrows) in a child with ARPKD.

Gitelman Syndrome

Rare autosomal recessive disorder due to defects in the thiazide-sensitive Na^+–Cl^- cotransporter in the DCT. Symptoms are similar to those seen in patients using thiazide diuretics. It is a more benign condition than Bartter syndrome and is often not diagnosed until late childhood or early adulthood.

PRESENTATION

Cramps and severe fatigue. Electrolyte abnormalities include **hypochloremic metabolic alkalosis, hypokalemia,** and **hypocalciuria.** Hypomagnesemia secondary to hypermagnesuria is present in most cases. **No hypertension.**

DIAGNOSIS

It is a clinical diagnosis as described previously, along with the associated fluid and electrolyte abnormalities with volume depletion, hypokalemia, hypochloremic metabolic alkalosis, and hypocalciuria. Hypocalciuria versus hypercalciuria helps to differentiate Gitelman syndrome from Bartter syndrome. Despite volume depletion, there is polyuria and an elevated urine sodium and FE_{Na}. Renin and aldosterone levels are elevated but measurement is not typically necessary. Rule out vomiting and diuretic abuse. Genetic testing is available.

TREATMENT

NSAIDs can be used to decrease RBF, GFR, and urinary sodium wasting. Potassium supplements are generally needed along with a high sodium, high potassium, and high fluid diet. Caution is needed with use of diuretics as these block essential compensatory mechanisms for sodium wasting. Similar caution is needed if RAAS blockade is introduced.

PROGNOSIS

Prognosis is excellent. Unlike patients with Barrter syndrome, patients with Gitelman syndrome do not have hypercalciuria, so there is no risk of tubulointerstitial scarring and ESRD.

Liddle Syndrome

An autosomal dominant disorder characterized by severe hypertension due to gain of function mutation in the collecting duct epithelial sodium channel (ENaC). Excess sodium reabsorption increases ECF volume and causes hypertension and hypokalemia.

PRESENTATION

Children are frequently asymptomatic. Adults can present with weakness, fatigue, and palpitations. Findings include **hypokalemia** and **metabolic alkalosis** with **hypertension.** Presentation is similar to hyperaldosteronism, but is independent of mineralocorticoids.

DIAGNOSIS

Persistent hypertension, hypokalemia, and metabolic alkalosis. Genetic testing is available.

TREATMENT

ENaC antagonists, such as amiloride or triamterene. Spironolactone and eplerenone are not effective in treating Liddle syndrome, as they regulate the actions of aldosterone, and the mutation in Liddle syndrome occurs downstream of aldosterone.

PROGNOSIS

Once diagnosed, prognosis is excellent with blood pressure–lowering ENaC antagonists. Since it is so rare, there is often a delay in making the diagnosis and starting administration of an ENaC antagonist.

TUMORS OF THE RENAL SYSTEM

As with other neoplasms, tumors of the renal system can be malignant or benign, primary or secondary (metastatic). In this section, we address the most common primary malignancies of the kidneys.

Renal Cell Carcinoma

Renal cell carcinoma is the most common primary tumor of the kidney in the adult population, accounting for ~80% of kidney tumors (affecting men more than women, at an average age of 60–70 years). It arises from the tubular epithelium, most often in the proximal convoluted tubule, and can be sporadic (most common) or hereditary. Risk factors include smoking, exposure to cadmium, petroleum, gasoline, asbestos, and lead, and acquired cystic disease from chronic dialysis. Three common forms exist:

- **Clear-cell carcinomas** (80%) have **clear** or **granular cytoplasm** (Figure 8-42). Both familial and sporadic forms are commonly associated with an underlying genetic defect in the **VHL gene** (a tumor suppressor gene on **chromosome 3**).
- **Papillary renal cell carcinomas** (15%) have a **papillary growth pattern** and affect the proximal tubules. Familial and sporadic forms exist, with the underlying genetic defect being in the **MET gene** (a proto-oncogene on **chromosome 7**). Familial forms frequently exhibit **trisomy of chromosome 7.**
- **Chromophobe renal carcinomas** (< 5%) affect the cortical collecting ducts, stain darkly, and are characterized by **loss of an entire chromosome**, frequently chromosomes 1, 2, 6, 10, 13, 17, and 21.

PRESENTATION

The classic **triad of clinical symptoms** includes:

- Painless hematuria (microscopic or macroscopic).
- Palpable flank mass.
- Flank pain.

But most patients will present without the full triad.

> **? CLINICAL CORRELATION**
>
> **Renal cell carcinoma** can be associated with **von Hippel-Lindau disease (VHL).**

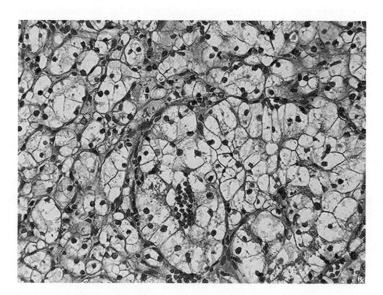

FIGURE 8-42.   Clear-cell carcinoma. Histologically, the clear-cell variant is the most common type. The tumor has an alveolar architecture created by a prominent network of thin-walled vascular septae demarcating collections of tumor cells. Tumor cells have abundant clear cytoplasm. The nuclei are round and fairly uniform in appearance in low-grade tumors (as seen here) or may be highly pleomorphic and vesicular with prominent nucleoli in high-grade tumors.

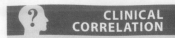
CLINICAL CORRELATION

Paraneoplastic syndromes associated with **renal cell carcinoma:**
- Hypercalcemia due to high levels of PTH-related protein.
- Polycythemia from excess EPO production.

The cancer may spread **hematogenously** via the renal vein and inferior vena cava (IVC) to the bones or lungs, causing bone pain or respiratory symptoms secondary to a lung mass, respectively. Invasion of the left renal vein can cause **left-sided varicocele** due to blockage of left spermatic vein drainage.

DIAGNOSIS

Renal **ultrasound** shows the presence of a mass. **CT** can provide precise information on the size and location of the tumor, as well as detect enlarged lymph nodes and metastases. The most common appearance of clear-cell renal carcinoma is an upper pole mass with cysts and hemorrhage.

TREATMENT

Standard treatment involves **radical nephrectomy** with removal of local lymph nodes.

- Partial nephrectomy/nephron-sparing surgery is commonly performed in cases of **VHL.**
- Additional treatments have included **interleukin-2** in metastatic disease.

PROGNOSIS

Renal cell carcinoma usually metastasizes late and may recur years after the tumor has been removed. The prognosis is poor if the tumor has extended through the renal capsule or into the renal vein, with a 5-year survival rate of 10–15%. The best prognosis is with the chromophobe subtype.

Transitional Cell Carcinomas

Transitional cell carcinomas are twice as common as renal cell carcinomas and affect men more than women, frequently between the ages of 50 and 70 years. They arise in the urinary tract outside of the kidney, predominantly in the bladder, originating from transitional epithelium.

KEY FACT

Schistosomiasis is associated with *squamous* cell carcinoma of the bladder, not transitional cell carcinoma.

MNEMONIC

Associated with problems in your **P**ee **SAC:**

Phenacetin
Smoking and **S**chistosomiasis
Aniline dyes (**A**romatic amines)
Cyclophosphamide

Bladder tumors are more common in people with exposures to β-naphthylamine, cigarette smoking, cyclophosphamide, and phenacetin (analgesic).

PRESENTATION

Painless hematuria with the risk factors mentioned and in the appropriate age range. Other presentations depend on the location of the tumor. If a ureter is involved or outflow of the ureters is blocked, there may be an obstructive presentation with flank pain, suprapubic fullness and pain, increased urinary frequency, and hydronephrosis.

DIAGNOSIS

Cystoscopy reveals the lesion within the bladder, and **urine cytology** shows malignant cells. **Pelvic CT** may help with level of invasion.

TREATMENT

Superficial tumors may be treated with transurethral resection and/or injection of chemotherapeutic agents, such as bacillus Calmette Guérin (BCG), into the bladder. More invasive tumors may require cystectomy with radiation or chemotherapy (or both).

PROGNOSIS

Tend to recur following treatment, but most low-grade recurrences can be treated with repeat conservative excision.

Wilms Tumor (Nephroblastoma)

Wilms tumor is the **most common** primary tumor of the kidney in children between the ages of 2 and 5 years, and is due to **loss of WT1** (a tumor suppressor gene on chromosome 11). **Nephrogenic rests** are precursor lesions associated with bilateral Wilms tumors.

KEY FACT

Wilms tumor is associated with loss of *WT1* on chromosome 11 via a **two-hit mechanism.** Mutation of one copy of *WT1* in the germ-line followed by mutation of the second copy of *WT1* in the kidneys predisposes to tumor development.

PRESENTATION

Large, palpable abdominal mass that may extend into the pelvis. Some patients have hypertension due to excessive renin secretion. Wilms tumor is also associated with other underlying disorders such as Beckwith-Wiedemann syndrome (hemihypertrophy), WAGR (Wilms tumor, aniridia, genitourinary malformations, mental retardation/intellectual disability), and Denys-Drash syndrome. Tumors this size can also cause intestinal obstruction. Other presenting symptoms include abdominal pain, fever, and hematuria.

DIAGNOSIS

Abdominal ultrasound shows an intrarenal mass and any invasion into the IVC. **CT scan** (chest, abdomen, and pelvis) can evaluate for metastatic disease.

- Grossly, these tumors are **tan-gray with areas of hemorrhage and necrosis.**
- Histologically, there is a variable mix of blastemal, stromal, and epithelial cell types.

TREATMENT

Nephrectomy with chemotherapy (vincristine, actinomycin D, and doxorubicin if lung metastases are found). Abdominal radiation may also be used in selected patients.

PROGNOSIS

The aforementioned therapy offers excellent 5-year survival rates (> 90%).

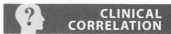

CLINICAL CORRELATION

Syndromes associated with **Wilms tumor** include:
- **WAGR** complex: **W**ilms tumor, **A**niridia, **G**enitourinary malformation, and mental-motor **R**etardation.
- **Denys-Drash syndrome:** Gonadal dysgenesis, renal abnormalities (eg, diffuse mesangial sclerosis), and Wilms tumor.
- **Beckwith-Wiedemann syndrome:** Enlarged organs, hemihypertrophy of extremities, and Wilms tumor.

Neuroblastoma

Neuroblastoma is the most common extracranial solid tumor in children and the most common tumor in the first year of life. It arises via malignant transformation of cells of the sympathetic nervous system of **neural crest cell origin** and is most often found in the **adrenal glands.** For this reason, distinguishing between neuroblastoma and Wilms tumor in a small child can be difficult without assessing the tumor pathology. **A small number of cases are familial and are caused by a mutation in the anaplastic lymphoma kinase (ALK) gene.** Most neuroblastomas have an amplification of the **N-myc** gene. Neuroblastomas are one of the types of malignant tumors that can rarely undergo **spontaneous regression.**

PRESENTATION

Most patients present with a rapidly growing abdominal mass. Other symptoms are mostly constitutional and include fatigue, fever, and loss of appetite. Due to the location of the tumor, hypertension is often present as well due to compression of the renal artery.

DIAGNOSIS

Most patients have an increase in their urine catecholamines and catecholamine degradation products (eg, vanillylmandelic acid [VMA]) that can be used as a screening test. Neuroblastomas can have calcifications on CT scan. They also can be positively identified on metaiodobenzylguanidine (mIBG) scan, as well as scans using radioactive iodine. Definitive diagnosis requires tissue biopsy.

TREATMENT

Patients are stratified into low, intermediate, and high-risk groups. Low-risk patients often can be observed without treatment, whereas some receive surgical resection. Intermediate-risk patients undergo surgical resection. High-risk patients receive a combination of surgery, chemotherapy, radiotherapy, bone marrow transplantation, and antibody therapy with granulocyte-macrophage colony-stimulating factor (GM-CSF) and interleukin-2 (IL-2), depending on the specific biochemical markers presented by the tumor.

PROGNOSIS

Low and intermediate-risk patients fare well, with an overwhelming majority of patients achieving complete remission. Between 20% and 50% of high-risk patients do not respond to treatment, and a majority of those who do respond have recurrence of disease. Many survivors are afflicted by other chronic conditions later in life, and those receiving chemotherapy often have hearing loss as a result of the treatment.

ELECTROLYTE ABNORMALITIES

Electrolyte abnormalities (see Table 8-25) can be diagnosed with a standard laboratory chemistry panel and are frequently the manifestation of some underlying pathology. The common electrolyte abnormalities are discussed in the following sections.

Hypernatremia

Serum sodium level > 145 mEq/L.

PRESENTATION

Excessive thirst, doughy skin, and mental status changes (confusion, seizures, and muscle twitching).

CAUSES

Most commonly, hypernatremia is due to a loss of free water versus a gain of sodium without adequate rehydration (due to impairment of the thirst mechanism or lack of access to water).

Specific causes include iatrogenic from hypertonic saline, medications (diuretics, lithium, or sodium-containing drugs), hyperglycemia in the setting of diabetic ketoacidosis, and central or nephrogenic diabetic insipidus.

TREATMENT

Treatment includes correction of the underlying cause and IV hydration. The amount of IV fluid to give is determined by the following formula:

$$\text{Free water deficit} = \text{Total body water} \times [(\text{Plasma Na}/140) - 1]$$

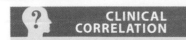

CLINICAL CORRELATION

Neurologic symptoms associated with **hypernatremia:** irritability, delirium, and coma.

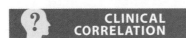

CLINICAL CORRELATION

Correcting hypernatremia too quickly can lead to **cerebral edema** and **herniation.**

TABLE 8-25. Electrolyte Abnormalities

	PRESENTATION	CAUSES
Hypernatremia	Excessive thirst, **doughy skin,** and mental status changes	Hypertonic saline, diuretics, diabetic ketoacidosis, and central or nephrogenic DI
Hyponatremia	Headaches, nausea, muscle cramps, depressed reflexes, and disorientation; beware of **CPM** during correction	Skin or GI losses, **SIADH,** water intoxication, and liver or heart failure
Hyperkalemia	Palpitations, muscle weakness; **peaked T waves,** widened QRS interval, flattened P waves, ventricular fibrillation	Lab error (hemolysis), acute or chronic kidney injury, crush injury, hypoaldosteronism
Hypokalemia	Fatigue, muscle weakness, hyporeflexia; **flattened T waves, U waves, prolonged PR interval,** ST-segment depression	Insulin, diuretics, vomiting, hyperaldosteronism, hypomagnesemia, types I and II RTA
Hypercalcemia	"Renal stones, abdominal groans, painful bones, and psychiatric moans." QT-segment shortening	Malignancy, hyperparathyroidism, granulomatous disease
Hypocalcemia	Muscle cramps, depression, tetany, convulsions; QT-segment prolongation; Chvostek and Trousseau signs	DiGeorge syndrome (in children), hypoparathyroidism (following parathyroidectomy), furosemide, and vitamin D deficiency
Hypomagnesemia	Often asymptomatic; anorexia, nausea, vomiting, lethargy	Dietary deficiency; difficult to correct hypocalcemia or hypokalemia in the setting of hypomagnesemia

CPM, central pontine myelinolysis; DI, diabetes insipidus; RTA, renal tubular acidosis; SIADH, syndrome of inappropriate secretion of antidiuretic hormone.

Hyponatremia

Serum sodium level < 136 mEq/L.

PRESENTATION

The symptoms are largely manifested neurologically: headaches, nausea, muscle cramps, depressed reflexes, and disorientation.

CAUSES

To identify the cause of hyponatremia, it is essential to identify **serum osmolality** and **volume status.** Figure 8-43 offers an approach to identifying the cause of hyponatremia. Low serum sodium and low serum osmolality are most frequently encountered.

TREATMENT

Treatment of hyponatremia depends on the underlying cause, but if the patient is symptomatic, the administration of IV hypertonic saline (3% saline) may be indicated. Care must be taken to slowly correct the sodium level because of the risk that **central pontine myelinolysis (CPM)** may develop.

Hyperkalemia

Serum potassium > 5.0 mEq/L, making the resting membrane potential **less** negative and hence the cell **more** excitable.

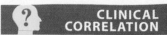

CLINICAL CORRELATION

Central pontine myelinolysis (CPM) develops as a result of severe damage to the myelin sheath of neurons in the pons. Most often caused by rapid correction of **chronic hyponatremia.** If the osmolarity of the external environment is suddenly increased, the neurons rapidly shrink, which causes myelinolysis.

Symptoms of CPM include sudden para- or quadriparesis, dysphagia, dysarthria, double vision, and loss of consciousness.

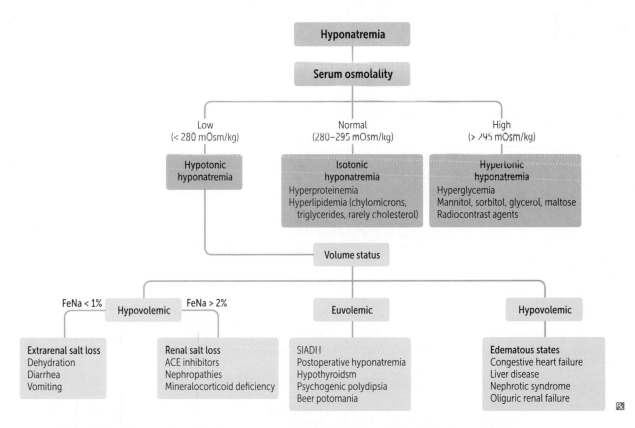

FIGURE 8-43. **Evaulation of hyponatremia using serum osmolality and extracellular fluid volume status.**

PRESENTATION

Clinically, the patient may experience palpitations or muscle weakness. Potassium causes the heart to be more excitable (possibly leading to **ventricular fibrillation**) and the effects on the heart should be investigated with an **electrocardiogram (ECG)** (Figure 8-44):

- Peaked T waves
- Widening of the QRS complex, progressing to a sine wave ECG as K⁺ increases
- Flattening of the P wave

CAUSES

Most common underlying pathology includes renal failure or trauma due to extensive crush injury with release of potassium from muscle cells. Also common in diabetes patients as insulin facilitates potassium entry into cells. Finally, hypoaldosteronism is a less common but important cause of hyperkalemia.

TREATMENT

Treatment focuses on removing potassium from the body and stabilizing the myocardium (monitor the serum K⁺ levels and ECG findings during treatment). The systematic approach to treating hyperkalemia includes:

- **Calcium gluconate** first to stabilize the myocardium.
- **Insulin** with concurrent glucose infusion (insulin ↑ cellular K⁺ uptake).
- **β-Agonists** (drive K⁺ into cells).
- If the patient is acidemic, administer **bicarbonate** to facilitate shifting K back into cells.
- If the patient has residual renal function, **furosemide + IV fluids** is a potent method of removing K⁺.
- **Sodium polystyrene sulfonate** (causes excretion of K⁺ from the GI tract).
- Dialysis.

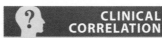
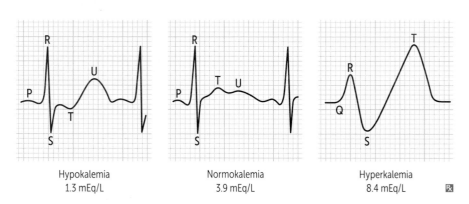

Hypokalemia	Normokalemia	Hyperkalemia
1.3 mEq/L	3.9 mEq/L	8.4 mEq/L

FIGURE 8-44. **Electrocardiographic effects of hyperkalemia and hypokalemia.** Electrocardiographic changes characteristically progress from symmetrically peaked T waves, often with a shortened QT interval, to widening of the QRS complex, prolongation of the PR interval, loss of the P wave, loss of R-wave amplitude, and ST-segment depression (occasionally elevation)—to an ECG that resembles a sine wave—before final progression into ventricular fibrillation or asystole. Note progressive flattening of the T wave, an increasingly prominent U wave, and ST-segment depression.

Hypokalemia

Serum K^+ < 3.6 mEq/L, making the resting membrane potential **more** negative and hence cells are **less** excitable.

PRESENTATION

Patients present with general, nonspecific symptoms of fatigue, muscle weakness, intestinal ileus, and/or hyporeflexia.

Classic ECG findings (Figure 8-44) include:

- Flattened T waves.
- Presence of U waves.
- ST-segment depression.

CAUSES

Insulin, alkalosis, diuretics (loop or thiazide), vomiting (eg, eating disorders), increased aldosterone levels, and hypomagnesemia.

TREATMENT

Treat the underlying cause. Low-serum K^+ is treated with administration of IV or PO K^+. Unless the patient has emergent ECG changes, treating with oral K^+ is always preferred to IV repletion. During treatment, monitor the ECG and plasma levels of K^+. If the hypokalemia is caused by hypomagnesemia, Mg^{2+} must be corrected before the K^+ will appropriately correct.

Hypercalcemia

Serum Ca^{2+} level > 10.2 mg/dL, increasing the threshold potential and thus cells are **less** excitable (acidosis has a similar effect).

PRESENTATION

Many patients are asymptomatic. Levels over 12.0 mg/dL may produce ECG changes (**shortened QT interval;** Figure 8-45), and more dramatic symptoms, such as renal **stones** (nephrolithiasis), abdominal **groans** (nausea, vomiting, constipation), psychiatric **moans** (delirium, psychosis), and painful **bones** (osteitis fibrosa cystica).

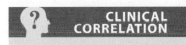

CLINICAL CORRELATION

Renal stones, abdominal groans, painful bones, and psychiatric moans are classic findings for **hypercalcemia.**

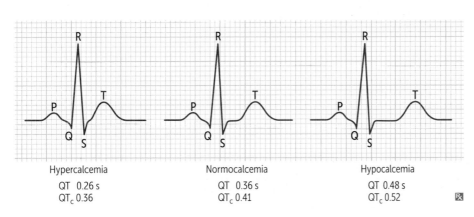

Hypercalcemia	Normocalcemia	Hypocalcemia
QT 0.26 s	QT 0.36 s	QT 0.48 s
QT_c 0.36	QT_c 0.41	QT_c 0.52

FIGURE 8-45.   Electrocardiographic effects of hypocalcemia and hypercalcemia.
Prolongation of the QT interval (ST-segment portion) is typical of hypocalcemia. Hypercalcemia may cause abbreviation of the ST segment and shortening of the QT interval. QT_c is the QT interval corrected for heart rate.

CAUSES

The most common cause in the inpatient setting is **malignancy** (metastases to bone or ectopic production of PTH-related protein), but the most common cause in the outpatient setting is primary **hyperparathyroidism** (adenoma > hyperplasia > carcinoma). Other common causes include hyperthyroidism, thiazide diuretic use, granulomatous disease (sarcoidosis), renal failure, and **milk-alkali syndrome.**

TREATMENT

Treat the underlying cause. If patients is symptomatic, hydrate with **IV normal saline** and give **furosemide** with consideration given to the addition of **bisphosphonates to inhibit bone resorption by osteoclasts.** In severe refractory cases, hemodialysis may be indicated.

Hypocalcemia

Serum calcium level < 8.5 mg/dL, decreasing the threshold potential and thus cells are **more** excitable (alkalosis has a similar effect).

PRESENTATION

Frequently asymptomatic. More severe symptoms occur at very low serum levels: muscle cramps, perioral paresthesias, **tetany,** and convulsions. **QT segment prolongation** is seen on ECG (see Figure 8-45).

- **Chvostek sign:** Tapping the facial nerve results in twitching of facial muscles.
- **Trousseau sign:** Carpopedal spasm resulting from inflation of a BP cuff on the forearm.

CAUSES

In newborns and infants, consider **DiGeorge syndrome.** Hypoparathyroidism (secondary to treatment of hyperparathyroidism), pseudohypoparathyroidism, vitamin D deficiency, osteomalacia, rickets, and diuretics (furosemide).

TREATMENT

If the patient is symptomatic, calcium can be replaced via **IV calcium gluconate** while monitoring ECG. Less severe cases can be treated with **PO calcium** and **vitamin D.**

Hypomagnesemia

Serum Mg^{2+} level < 1.5 mEq/L.

PRESENTATION

Anorexia, nausea, vomiting, lethargy, and personality changes. Also look for hypocalcemia and hypokalemia in the setting of low Mg^{2+} levels because low magnesium decreases PTH release and increases efflux of intracellular K^+, which is then excreted.

CAUSES

Dietary deficiency complicated by poor absorption.

TREATMENT

Low Mg^{2+} is treated with magnesium replacement, usually magnesium sulfate.

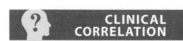

CLINICAL CORRELATION

Preeclampsia patients treated with magnesium sulfate need serial neurologic exams to detect hyporeflexia, an early sign of **hypermagnesemia.**

Pharmacology

DIURETICS

Diuretics (Figure 8-46) are drugs that act to **increase urine volume** by altering ion transport in the nephron. A generally safe class, diuretics are **first-line drugs** in the treatment of **hypertension** and **edematous states** such as **CHF, nephrosis,** and **cirrhosis.** Common side effects of diuretics (Table 8-26) are

- Volume depletion.
- Hypokalemia (loop diuretics and thiazides).
- Hyponatremia.
- Hyperglycemia (thiazides; opposite action on pancreatic β-cells as sulfonylurea drugs).
- Metabolic acidosis (acetazolamide and K+-sparing diuretics [eg, spironolactone]).
- Metabolic alkalosis (loop diuretics and thiazides).
- Hypercalciuria (loop diuretics).
- Specific side effects are discussed with each of the following drug classes.

There are **five main classes** of diuretics:

- Osmotic agents: Mannitol and urea (mainly in patients with SIADH).
- Carbonic anhydrase inhibitors: Acetazolamide.
- Loop agents: Furosemide, bumetanide, and ethacrynic acid.
- Thiazides: Hydrochlorothiazide (HCTZ) and metolazone.
- Potassium-sparing agents: Spironolactone, eplerenone, triamterene, and amiloride.

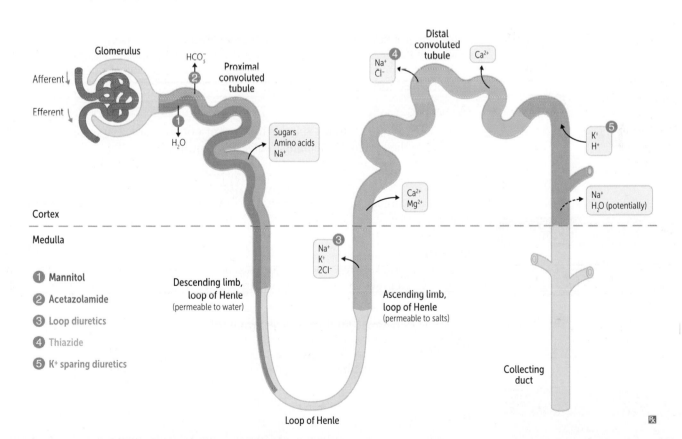

FIGURE 8-46. **Overview of diuretic sites of action.**

TABLE 8-26. Common Electrolyte Changes Seen With Diuretic Use

CLASS	DRUGS	MECHANISM OF ACTION	ELECTROLYTE CHANGES
Carbonic anhydrase inhibitors	Acetazolamide	Inhibits carbonic anhydrase in PCT, blocks Na^+/H^+ exchange	▪ Hyperchloremic metabolic acidosis ($\uparrow Cl^-$, $\uparrow H^+$) ▪ Hypokalemia ($\downarrow K^+$)
Osmotic agents	Mannitol, urea	Increases tubular fluid osmolarity in entire tubule	▪ Hypernatremia ($\uparrow Na^+$)
Loop agents	Furosemide, bumetanide, ethacrynic acid	Inhibits $Na^+-K^+-2Cl^-$ transporter in thick ascending limb of loop of Henle	▪ Hypokalemia ($\downarrow K^+$) ▪ Hyponatremia ($\downarrow Na^+$) ▪ Hyperuricemia ($\uparrow$ urea) ▪ Hypocalcemia ($\downarrow Ca^{2+}$) ▪ Hypomagnesemia ($\downarrow Mg^{2+}$) ▪ Metabolic alkalosis ($\downarrow H^+$)
Thiazide diuretics	HCTZ, metolazone	Blocks Na^+-Cl^- cotransport in DCT	▪ Hyperglycemia ($\uparrow$ glucose) ▪ Hyperlipidemia ($\uparrow$ lipids) ▪ Hyperuricemia ($\uparrow$ urea) ▪ Hypercalcemia ($\uparrow Ca^{2+}$) ▪ Hypokalemia ($\downarrow K^+$) ▪ Hyponatremia ($\downarrow Na^+$) ▪ Metabolic alkalosis ($\downarrow H^+$)
Potassium-sparing agents	Spironolactone, eplerenone, amiloride, triamterene	▪ Spironolactone and eplerenone are competitive aldosterone receptor antagonists in the collecting tubule ▪ Other agents block Na^+ channels (ENaC) in the collecting tubule	▪ Metabolic acidosis ($\uparrow H^+$) ▪ Hyperkalemia ($\uparrow K^+$)

DCT, distal convoluted tubule; ENaC, epithelial sodium channel; HCTZ, hydrochlorothiazide; PCT, proximal convoluted tubule.

Osmotic Agents (Mannitol and Urea)

MECHANISM

Mannitol is filtered into the tubular lumen but not reabsorbed, increasing osmotic pressure in the lumen and retaining water in the urine.

USES

Reduction of intraocular or intracranial pressure, increases excretion of water more than sodium, urinary excretion of metabolic toxins.

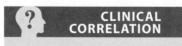

CLINICAL CORRELATION

Pulmonary edema is a contraindication to the use of mannitol.

SIDE EFFECTS

▪ Dehydration without adequate water intake.
▪ Increased ECF volume, leading to **pulmonary edema.**

Carbonic Anhydrase Inhibitors (Acetazolamide)

MECHANISM

Blocks carbonic anhydrase, which in the PCT prevents reabsorption of sodium bicarbonate, leading to diuresis.

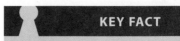

KEY FACT

Since it contains the sulfa group ($R-SO_2-NH_2$), acetazolamide is contraindicated in patients allergic to sulfonamides.

USES

Glaucoma (decreases production of aqueous humor), acute mountain sickness (stimulates ventilation via metabolic acidosis), elimination of acidic toxins (alkalinizes urine, leading to increased excretion of weak acids), pseudotumor cerebri (decreases CSF production), and corrects alkalosis.

SIDE EFFECTS

■ Renal stones (decreases concentration of urine citrate and alkalinizes urine, increasing risk for calcium phosphate stones).
■ Potassium wasting (increased Na^+ delivery to distal nephron increases K^+ excretion).
■ Hyperchloremic metabolic acidosis.

Loop Agents (Furosemide, Bumetanide, and Ethacrynic Acid)

MECHANISM

Inhibit Na^+–K^+–$2Cl^-$ transporter in thick ascending limb. Decreases positive luminal potential, leading to increased excretion of calcium and magnesium.

USES

Treatment of acute pulmonary or other edema, hypercalcemia, hyperkalemia, hypertension, pseudotumor cerebri, and volume overload in AKI.

SIDE EFFECTS

■ Hypokalemic metabolic alkalosis.
■ **Ototoxicity.**
■ Hyperuricemia (thus causing **gout**).
■ Hypomagnesemia.
■ Hypocalcemia.
■ Renal calculi (due to hypercalciuria).
■ Severe dehydration.
■ Allergic reactions (all loop diuretics are sulfonamide derivatives except ethacrynic acid).

> **CLINICAL CORRELATION**
>
> Ethacrynic acid may be used in patients allergic to sulfonamides.

Thiazide Diuretics (Hydrochlorothiazide and Metolazone)

MECHANISM

Inhibit Na^+–Cl^- cotransporter in DCT.

USES

First-line agent for treatment of hypertension, CHF, nephrosis, hypercalciuria, and nephrogenic DI (thiazides reduce ECF volume → activates RAAS → ↑ proximal reabsorption of NaCl and H_2O → ↓ delivery of fluid to distal nephron → ↓ urine output).

SIDE EFFECTS

■ Dehydration.
■ Hypokalemia.
■ Hypercalcemia.
■ Hyperglycemia.
■ Hyperlipidemia.
■ Hyperuricemia.
■ Hyponatremia.
■ Allergic reactions (sulfonamide derivatives).
■ Thiazides increase Li^+ reabsorption in the proximal tubules, possibly causing Li^+ toxicity.

> **CLINICAL CORRELATION**
>
> Thiazides have added benefit in hypercalciuric patients.

Potassium-Sparing Agents (Spironolactone, Eplerenone, Amiloride, and Triamterene)

MECHANISM

Spironolactone and eplerenone directly antagonize the mineralocorticoid receptor (target of aldosterone), thereby reducing Na^+ reuptake in the late DCT and collecting duct. Both drugs prevent the aldosterone-mediated increase in apical membrane permeability to K^+ (ROMK channels) and therefore are considered "potassium-sparing."

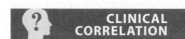
Amiloride and triamterene directly inhibit ENaCs in the late DCT and collecting duct, which also reduces Na+ reabsorption. This renders the charge in the lumen more positive, which is unfavorable for K+ secretion. Hence, these ENaC antagonists are also considered "potassium-sparing."

Uses

- **Spironolactone and eplerenone:** Primary hyperaldosteronism (Conn syndrome) and edematous states caused by secondary hyperaldosteronism (cirrhosis, nephrotic syndrome, and cardiac failure). Antiandrogen activity can be useful for treatment of polycystic ovary syndrome and hirsutism.
- **Amiloride and triamterene:** Counteract K+ loss caused by other diuretics, adjunct therapy to other diuretics to treat edema or hypertension.

Side Effects

Hyperkalemia, hyperchloremic metabolic acidosis, gynecomastia (spironolactone), impotence (males), abnormal menses (females).

ANTIDIURETIC HORMONE (ADH) (VASOPRESSIN AND DESMOPRESSIN)

Mechanism

Upregulates selective water channels (aquaporin 2) in apical membrane of collecting ducts.

Uses

Central DI, enuresis.

Side Effects

- Vasoconstriction
- Headache
- Nausea

ANTIDIURETIC HORMONE ANTAGONISTS

Demeclocycline

Mechanism

Nonselectively inhibits action of ADH in collecting ducts by decreasing cAMP levels. Member of tetracycline family of antibiotics.

Uses

SIADH, decrease intravascular fluid volume in heart or liver failure.

Side Effects

- Nephrogenic DI
- Renal failure

Tolvaptan

Mechanism

Competitively inhibits arginine vasopressin receptor 2, thus promoting excretion of free water.

USES

SIADH, decreases intravascular fluid volume in heart or liver failure.

SIDE EFFECTS

- GI upset
- Polyuria, polydipsia
- Renal failure

ANGIOTENSIN-CONVERTING ENZYME INHIBITORS

Lisinopril, Enalapril, Captopril, and Ramipril

MECHANISM

Inhibit ACE, which catalyzes conversion of angiotensin I to angiotensin II, thereby interrupting the renin–angiotensin–aldosterone axis. Also **increases** levels of **bradykinin** (a potent vasodilator) because ACE normally degrades bradykinin. In the kidney, ACE inhibitors decrease efferent arteriolar resistance, improving renal blood flow and reducing GFR.

USES

Treatment of hypertension. Proven renal protective function in all patients with CKD, for example, diabetic nephropathy (decreases hyperfiltration and proteinuria, slowing down progression of glomerular scarring and renal function loss).

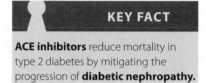

KEY FACT

ACE inhibitors reduce mortality in type 2 diabetes by mitigating the progression of **diabetic nephropathy.**

SIDE EFFECTS

- Dry cough (due to increased levels of bradykinin).
- Teratogenic (do **not** give to pregnant women).
- Hypotension.
- Acute renal failure (patients with **bilateral renal artery stenosis**).
- Hyperkalemia.
- Angioedema (due to increased levels of bradykinin).

ANGIOTENSIN RECEPTOR BLOCKERS

Losartan, Candesartan, Irbesartan, and Valsartan

MECHANISM

Block vasoconstriction and aldosterone-producing effects of angiotensin II at receptor sites in vascular smooth muscle and adrenal glands, thereby interrupting the renin–angiotensin–aldosterone axis. **Unlike ACE inhibitors, ARBs do not affect bradykinin,** and thus are rarely associated with the persistent dry cough and/or angioedema that limit ACE inhibitor therapy.

USES

First-line treatment for hypertension in non-blacks and diabetics. Alternative drug therapy for patients who cannot tolerate ACE inhibitors.

SIDE EFFECTS

- Hypotension.
- Teratogenic (do **not** give to pregnant women).
- Acute renal failure.
- Hyperkalemia.

NEPHROTOXIC DRUGS

The kidneys are critical organs for removal of most drugs from the body. Table 8-27 lists commonly used drugs and frequently encountered toxins that impair renal function.

TABLE 8-27. Common Renal Manifestations of Adverse Drug Reactions and Toxins

DRUG CLASS	COMMON DRUGS	TOXIC RENAL ACTION(S)
Antihypertensives	ACE inhibitors, ARBs	Fetal renal toxicity (teratogenic)
Antibiotics	Aminoglycosides (eg, gentamycin, neomycin), β-lactams (eg, methicillin), sulfonamides (eg, sulfamethoxazole), trimethoprim, rifampin	Range from mild renal impairment to ATN (aminoglycosides) or AIN
Antivirals	Acyclovir, ganciclovir, foscarnet	Formation of urinary crystals (acyclovir) and transient renal dysfunction
Antifungals	Amphotericin B, polymyxin	Dose-related nephrotoxicity (direct acute tubular injury)
Anti-inflammatory	NSAIDs (eg, ibuprofen, indomethacin, naproxen), COX-2 inhibitors (eg, rofecoxib)	▪ AIN, renal papillary necrosis, direct tubular injury due to ischemia ▪ Inhibition of COX isoenzymes inhibits renal PGI_2 production, leading to altered excretion of Na^+, edema, and hypertension
Immunosuppressive drugs	Cyclosporine, tacrolimus (FK506)	Dose-related nephrotoxicity (direct acute tubular injury)
Chemotherapy drugs	Cisplatin, cyclophosphamide, ifosfamide	Dose-related nephrotoxicity (cisplatin and ifosfamide), hemorrhagic cystitis (cyclophosphamide and ifosfamide)
Radiocontrast dyes	Iodinated contrast agents	ATN/contrast-induced nephropathy, usually in patients with underlying CKD (eg, patients with diabetic nephropathy) are at higher risk for CIN
Endogenous toxins	Myoglobin (rhabdomyolysis), hemoglobin (hemolysis)	ATN, oliguria
Other exogenous toxins	Ethylene glycol Heavy metals (eg, arsenic, lead)	Renal failure at high doses ATN, oliguria Precipitation of calcium oxalate stones (ethylene glycol)
Lithium	Lithium	Nephrogenic diabetes insipidus and tubulointerstitial fibrosis

ACE, angiotensin-converting enzyme; AIN, acute interstitial nephritis; ARBs, angiotensin receptor blockers; ATN, acute tubular necrosis; CIN, contrast-induced nephropathy; COX, cyclooxygenase; NSAIDs, nonsteroidal anti-inflammatory drugs; PGI_2, prostaglandin I_2.

CHAPTER 9

Reproductive

EMBRYOLOGY 662
Reproductive Development 662
Review: Male and Female Genital Homologs 674

ANATOMY 674
Lower Abdomen and Perineum 674
Male Reproductive System 675
Female Reproductive System 679

PHYSIOLOGY 681
Gametogenesis 681
Spermatogenesis 682
Oogenesis 684
Menstrual Cycle and Ovulation 686
Gonadal Steroids 687
Sexual Response 689
Fertilization 691
Pregnancy 692
Menopause 698

PATHOLOGY—GENETIC DISEASES 700
Klinefelter Syndrome (47,XXY) 700
Turner Syndrome 700
Double Y Males (XYY Syndrome) 701
Male Pseudohermaphrodite 701

Female Pseudohermaphrodite 702
Ovotesticular Disorder of Sex Development
    (Formerly True Hermaphroditism) 702
Kallmann Syndrome 703
Müllerian Agenesis 703

PATHOLOGY—FEMALE 703
Pregnancy Pathology 703
Vaginal Diseases 712
Cervical Pathology 713
Ovarian Pathology 715
Uterine Pathology 721
Breast Pathology 727
Sexually Transmitted Infections and Other Genital Infections 731

PATHOLOGY—MALE 733
Penile Pathology 733
Diseases of the Testes 734
Prostate Diseases 738
Sexually Transmitted Infections and Other Genital Infections 741

PHARMACOLOGY 741
Drugs That Modulate the Gonadotropin Axis 741
Drugs That Modulate the Male Reproductive System 741
Drugs That Modulate the Female Reproductive System 744

Embryology

REPRODUCTIVE DEVELOPMENT

Determination of Sex

According to the World Health Organization, human sex is defined as the biological and physiological characteristics that define men and women. Gender is the social constructed role, behavior, and activity that society considers appropriate for a man or a woman. Human sex can be defined by three criteria:

- Genetic sex: Presence or absence of a Y chromosome.
- Gonadal sex: Presence of testes or ovaries.
- Phenotypic sex: Appearance of the external genitalia.

Genotypic Sex

Genetic sex, or karyotype, is determined at conception. The oocyte provides an X chromosome, and the sperm carries either an X or Y chromosome. Thus, at fertilization, either an XX female or XY male is created. The **sex-determining region (SRY) gene** on the Y chromosome encodes **testis-determining factor (TDF)**, a transcription factor whose targets induce the male phenotype. In the absence of SRY, a female phenotype develops. Notably, the genes from both X chromosomes are needed for female development, but can be overridden by SRY (ie, XXY). Phenotypic sex is also affected by expression of certain hormones during development (Table 9-1). The **female phenotype is the default** (ie, no Y chromosome equals female phenotype), but the male phenotype requires expression of testosterone by the interstitial Leydig cells and Müllerian-inhibiting factor (MIF) by Sertoli cells.

Early Development

Reproductive organs regardless of the genetic sex undergo an initial common stage of development beginning the fifth week of gestation, known as the **indifferent stage.** The SRY gene is not activated until the **seventh week** of gestation.

Gonads

Primordial germ cells, the precursors to gametes, migrate out to the yolk sac wall during gastrulation. Between the fourth and sixth weeks, they return to the embryo through the gastrointestinal (GI) tract, surrounding peritoneum, and dorsal mesentery while undergoing mitotic divisions (Figure 9-1). The cells **invade the gonadal ridge** (a mass of mesodermal tissue at the back of the abdominal cavity and precursor to the gonads), proliferate, and become embedded medial to the developing mesonephros. Three primary cell types (mesenchymal cells, mesothelial cells, and primordial germ cells) develop in the gonadal ridge (Table 9-2).

TABLE 9-1. **Role of Hormones in Sexual Differentiation During Gestation**

HORMONE	EXPRESSION	INTERNAL STRUCTURES	EXTERNAL GENITALIA
Testosterone	8th week	Stimulates development of the vas deferens, seminal vesicles, and epididymis	
MIF	8th week	Inhibits development of the uterus, fallopian tubes, cervix, and upper vagina	
DHT	9th–12th weeks	Stimulates development of the prostate	Stimulates development of the penis and scrotum

DHT, dihydrotestosterone; MIF, Müllerian-inhibiting factor.

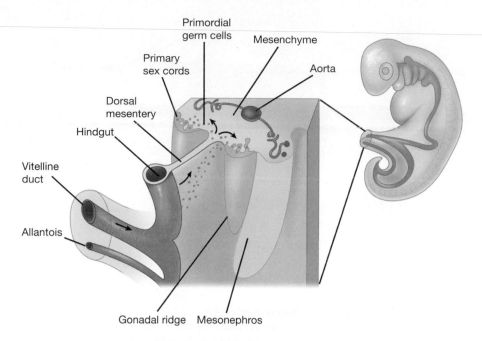

FIGURE 9-1. **Primordial germ cell migration and gonadal ridge formation.** The primordial germ cells (blue specks) migrate from the wall of the yolk sac to the gonadal ridge, where they settle into the primary sex cords.

Genital Ducts

The **mesonephric (Wolffian)** and **paramesonephric (Müllerian)** ducts are mesodermal derivatives that form the male and female genital duct systems, respectively (Figure 9-2).

The mesonephric ducts are derived from intermediate mesoderm. They form as longitudinal solid cords of tissue dorsolateral to the mesonephric tubules in the thoracic region. The solid cords grow caudally and fuse with the ventrolateral walls of the cloaca, the urogenital sinus. Subsequently, each cord detaches from everything except the urogenital sinus and canalizes, forming a lumen. During the sixth to tenth weeks of gestation, each duct **drains urine from the mesonephros,** a temporary kidney.

The paramesonephric duct forms lateral to the mesonephric duct via an invagination of celomic epithelium on the cranial aspect of the mesonephros. The invaginated portion of the paramesonephric duct forms the ostium at the future fimbriated end (infundibulum) of the uterine tube, which opens into the celomic cavity, the future peritoneal cavity. The duct then grows caudally and crosses over the mesonephric duct. The right and left paramesonephric ducts fuse at the midline, forming a canal that will **become the uterus** (see Figures 9-2 and 9-3). The fused tip presses on the urogenital sinus, forming a small protrusion.

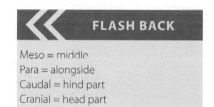

FLASH BACK

Meso = middle
Para = alongside
Caudal = hind part
Cranial = head part

TABLE 9-2. **Gonadal Ridge Cell Types**

CELL TYPE	FATE
Mesenchymal cells	Gonadal ridge medulla: Male = Leydig cells; Female = ovarian support stroma
Mesothelial cells	Gonadal ridge and primary sex cord cortex: Male = seminiferous tubules; Female = ovarian follicles
Primordial germ cells	Enter primary sex cords as future gametes: Male = spermatogonia; Female = oogonia

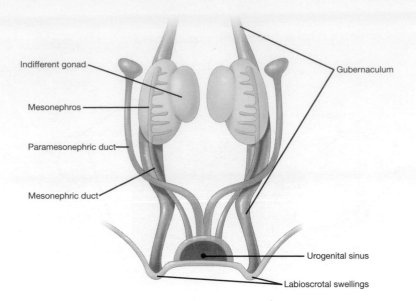

FIGURE 9-2. **Indifferent genital duct formation.** Once it becomes hollow, the mesonephric duct drains urine for the mesonephros. The paramesonephric duct forms lateral to the mesonephric duct and fuses at the midline. This fused tip becomes the uterus.

External Genitalia

In the fourth week of gestation, **five mesenchymal swellings** covered with ectoderm form around the cloacal membrane: one **genital tubercle,** two **urogenital folds,** and two **labioscrotal folds** (Figure 9-4). The cloacal membrane divides in half and ruptures, forming the urogenital orifice and anus. A ligament, the **gubernaculum,** forms between the indifferent gonads and the labioscrotal swellings (see Figure 9-2). In males, the gubernaculum guides the testis inferiorly from the abdominal cavity into the scrotal sac. In females, the gubernaculum becomes the round ligament of the uterus and several ligaments of the ovary.

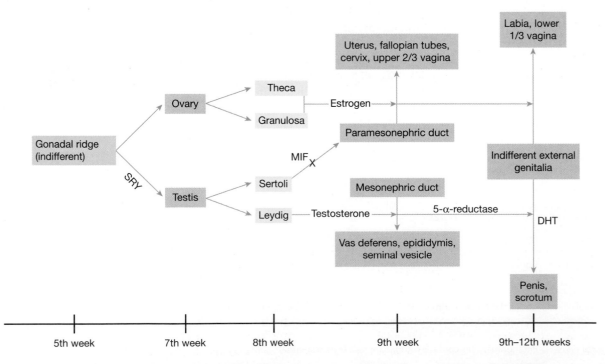

FIGURE 9-3. **Overview of sexual differentiation.** DHT, dihydrotestosterone; MIF, Müllerian-inhibiting factor; SRY, sex-determining region.

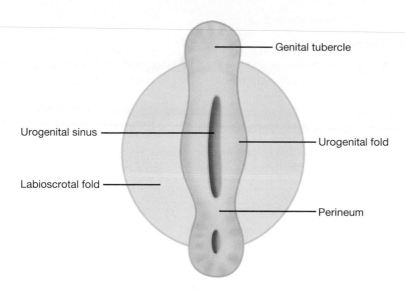

FIGURE 9-4. **Indifferent external genitalia development.** The indifferent external genitalia consist of five mesenchymal swellings: one genital tubercle, two urogenital folds, and two labioscrotal folds.

Differentiation

Gonads

At the seventh week of gestation, if a Y chromosome is present, the SRY gene leads to the development of testes; absence of SRY leads to formation of ovaries. Determination of the gonadal sex (ie, formation of either testes or ovaries) leads to differentiation of the germ cells. In male development, Leydig and Sertoli cells develop by week 8, producing testosterone and MIF, respectively.

For the male, the testes remain high in the abdomen until about the 30th week (seventh month) of gestation. Under the influence of MIF, testosterone, and dihydrotestosterone (DHT), testes undergo transabdominal and transinguinal descent.

Genital Ducts

Testosterone stimulates differentiation of the Wolffian duct, producing the epididymis, vas deferens, and seminal vesicle. MIF reduces aromatase biosynthesis, thereby reducing conversion of androgens to estrogens and suppressing development of the Müllerian duct. In females, the lack of these factors allows the Müllerian duct to develop into the fallopian tubes, uterus, cervix, and upper part of the vagina, whereas the Wolffian duct degenerates. An overview of these pathways is illustrated in Figure 9-3.

External Genitalia

Male and female external genitalia can be differentiated by the 9th week of fetal life and are fully developed by the 12th week.

Masculinization (virilization) or feminization of the external genitalia also depends on the presence or absence of male hormones. Whereas testosterone mainly affects the internal structures, **DHT** affects the development of the prostate, penis, and scrotum. In the female, lack of testes—and thereby vastly reduced levels of androgens—leads to development of the lower vagina and labia. Although estrogens from the mother or exogenous sources can contribute to feminization of the genitalia in either gender, intrinsic fetal estradiol has little to no effect on sexual differentiation. The roles of these hormones in determining gonadal and phenotypic sex are summarized in Table 9-1.

KEY FACT

Aromatase converts androgens to estrogens.

FLASH FORWARD

Anastrozole and exemestane are **aromatase inhibitors.** By inhibiting aromatase, they reduce serum estrogen levels. Clinical trials show that both are effective as primary prevention in reducing the incidence of invasive breast cancer in select high-risk women.

Disorders of Sex Development

Gonadal Agenesis

If primordial germ cells do not form or migrate, gonads do not develop, and the duct systems and external genitalia differentiate along the female development path until birth, regardless of the genetic sex.

Ovotesticular Disorder of Sex Development

In ovotesticular disorder of sex development, which is very rare, the histology of the gonad contains both ovarian follicles and testicular tubular elements. Previously known as true hermaphroditism.

Pseudohermaphroditism

This condition is characterized by gonads and karyotype of one gender, combined with secondary sex characteristics of the other gender.

- Male pseudohermaphroditism (eg, complete androgen insensitivity symdrome):
  - XY, undervirilized male/female phenotype.
  - By definition, testes are present.
  - Most common cause is complete androgen insensitivity syndrome (also called testicular feminization).
  - Complete lack of response to androgens despite high circulating androgen levels. As such, the child is genotypically XY, but due to the lack of androgenic sensitivity, the Wolffian ducts degenerate, and the external genitalia are feminized.
- Female pseudohermaphroditism:
  - Most common cause is congenital adrenal hyperplasia (CAH) due to 21-hydroxylase deficiency; virilization is secondary to increased adrenal androgen production.
  - XX, overvirilized female/male phenotype.
  - By definition, ovaries are present.

Male Development

Testes

The *SRY* gene is transcribed during the seventh week of gestation. Its transcription factor product, TDF, acts on the indifferent gonads (Figure 9-5) causing them to differentiate into:

- Primary sex cords (middle): Coiled, solid **testis cords.**
- Primary sex cords (ends): Stay straight, join near hilum = **rete testes.**
- Rete testes + mesonephric tubule remnants: **efferent ductules.**
- Mesenchyme thickening: **tunica albuginea.**
- Mesothelial cells: **Sertoli cells.**
- Mesothelial cells between testis cords: Interstitial cells (**Leydig cells**).

The testes enlarge and separate from the mesonephros, following the lower gubernacula to reach the scrotum via the inguinal canal (Figure 9-6). At the same time, the upper gubernacula degenerate to allow the testes to descend. As the testes travel, the layers of the abdominal wall travel ahead, forming the layers of the scrotal wall and spermatic cord (see Figure 9-6). A thin fold of peritoneum, the **processus vaginalis,** also descends, but its connection to the abdomen is lost between the future deep ring of the inguinal canal and the upper pole of the testis. However, it remains in the scrotum as the **tunica vaginalis,** which covers the spermatic cord and testes. In a vast majority of cases, the testes finish their descent and are present in the scrotum at birth.

CLINICAL CORRELATION

5α-Reductase type 2 deficiency, one of the milder forms of 46,XY disorder of sex development, leads to deficiency of DHT and thereby to ambiguous external genitalia until puberty, when the external genitalia become more masculine. It is believed that the increase of levels of testosterone at the beginning of puberty produces sufficient levels of DHT either by the action of 5α-reductase type 1 (present in the adult liver, nongenital skin, and some brain areas) or through the expression of low levels of 5α-reductase type 2 in the testes.

CLINICAL CORRELATION

Direct inguinal hernias are acquired hernias that occur when bowel protrudes through a weak point of the abdominal wall: the superficial inguinal ring of the inguinal canal. **Indirect inguinal hernias** are congenital hernias and occur when bowel protrudes through the deep inguinal ring due to **patent processus vaginalis,** an incomplete closure of the inguinal canal. A **hydrocele** is a collection of serous fluid that can accumulate in the tunica vaginalis as a result of patent processus vaginalis.

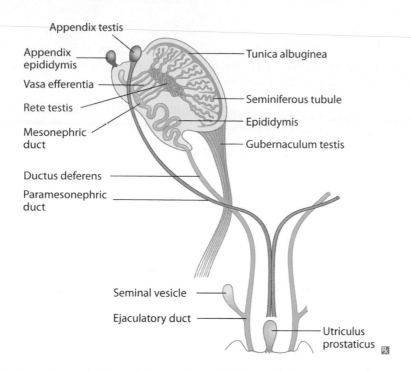

FIGURE 9-5. **Gonadal differentiation in the male (after week 7).**

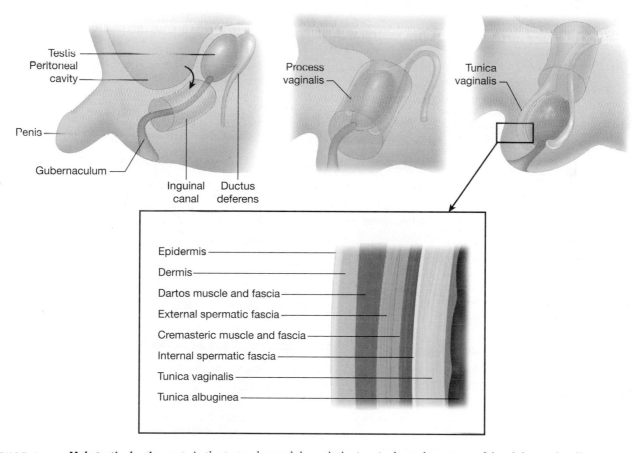

FIGURE 9-6. **Male testicular descent.** As the testes descend through the inguinal canal, portions of the abdominal wall precede them, forming the layers of the scrotal wall and sheath of the spermatic cord.

Internal Genitalia

In the eighth week of gestation, Sertoli cells secrete MIF, which induces **regression of the paramesonephric (Müllerian) ducts.** Leydig cells begin to secrete androgens that stimulate **differentiation of the mesonephric (Wolffian) ducts.** The mesonephric ducts form several structures (Figure 9-7).

- Seminal vesicle: Gland that is lateral to the ductus deferens and ends in the prostatic ejaculatory duct.
- Epididymis: Coiled ducts, form caudally.
- Ejaculatory duct: Connects ductus deferens and seminal vesicle ducts to the prostatic urethra.
- Ductus deferens: Thick smooth muscle coat, ends in prostatic ejaculatory duct.

Another important structure, the **prostate,** forms as an endodermal outgrowth from the urogenital sinus. There are two zones of glandular tissue surrounded by mesenchyme. The outer zone of prostatic glands constitutes the **posterior lobe.** The inner zone of mucous glands, which constitute the **median lobe,** also contains mesoderm from the mesonepheric duct and Müllerian duct remnants. Additionally, the urogenital sinus forms the prostatic urethra.

External Genitalia

Testosterone secreted by Leydig cells also induces changes in the external genitalia (Figure 9-8).

- Phallus enlarges to become the glans (distal end).
- Urogenital folds fuse to form the ventral shaft of the penis.
- Labioscrotal swelling develops into the scrotum.

The fusion of the urogenital folds encloses the endodermally derived urethra. The fusion process leaves a line called the **scrotal/penile raphe.** All structures are covered in ectoderm, but the ectoderm over the glans breaks down to form the **foreskin,** or **prepuce.**

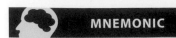

MNEMONIC

Mesonephric duct derivatives—
SEED

Seminal vesicles
Epididymis
Ejaculatory duct
Ductus deferens

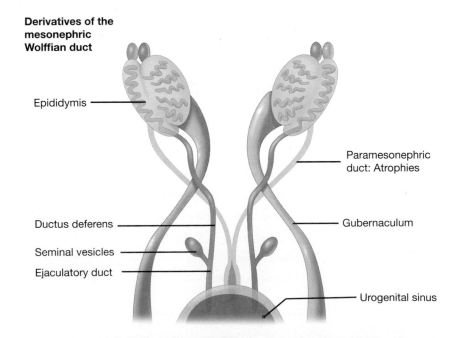

Derivatives of the mesonephric Wolffian duct

Epididymis

Paramesonephric duct: Atrophies

Ductus deferens

Gubernaculum

Seminal vesicles

Ejaculatory duct

Urogenital sinus

FIGURE 9-7. **Male internal genitalia development.** The mesonephric (Wolffian) duct differentiates to form the epididymis, ductus deferens, seminal vesicle, and ejaculatory duct, whereas the paramesonephric (Müllerian) duct atrophies.

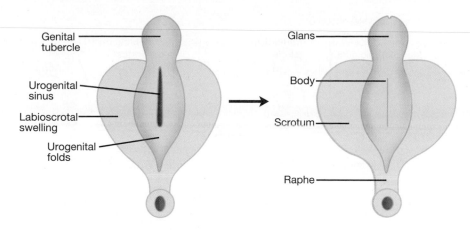

FIGURE 9-8.   Male external genitalia development. During development of the male external genitalia, the phallus enlarges and the urogenital and labioscrotal folds fuse at the midline. This results in formation of the penile glans, penile body, and scrotum, respectively.

Male Congenital Malformations

Cryptorchidism

Failure of the testes to descend can occur secondary to abnormalities in either androgen production or shortening of the gubernaculum. Undescended testes typically migrate to the scrotum within 3–6 months after birth. If testicular descent does not occur, surgery is required to either lower the testes (orchidopexy) or remove the testes. Testes require cooler temperatures for sperm production. Thus, undescended testes are unable to produce mature spermatozoa because of the higher temperature inside the body.

Congenital (Indirect) Inguinal Hernia

Incomplete closure of the processus vaginalis/inguinal canal creates a passage from the abdominal canal to the scrotum through which the intestines can herniate.

Hypospadias

Hypospadias is an abnormal opening of the penile urethra on the ventral side of the penis (Figure 9-9). The opening is secondary to failure of the **urogenital folds** to close. This condition is the most common penile abnormality and must be corrected to prevent urinary tract infections (UTIs). Hypospadias occurs in 10% of patients with cryptorchidism.

Epispadias

Epispadias is an abnormal opening of the penile urethra on the dorsal side of the penis (Figure 9-9). This opening occurs due to malpositioning of the **genital tubercle.** This condition is associated with **exstrophy of the bladder,** a condition in which the bladder is exposed, inside out, and protrudes through the abdominal wall. Epispadias is less common than hypospadias.

Female Development

Ovaries

In the absence of the *SRY* gene, the indifferent gonads follow a female pattern of differentiation (Figure 9-10). They differentiate to form:

- Primary sex cords: Degenerate.
- Cortical sex cords: Break up into a single layer of mesothelial follicular cells surrounding each germ cell (**primordial follicles).**
- Primordial germ cells: Differentiate to **oogonia** and undergo mitosis to increase their numbers.
- Mesenchyme: Connective tissue stroma for follicular support.

Hypospadias

Epispadias

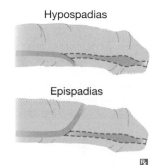

FIGURE 9-9.   Penile urethral abnormalities. In hypospadias, an abnormal opening of the urethra occurs on the ventral side of the penis. In epispadias, an abnormal opening of the urethra occurs on the dorsal side of the penis.

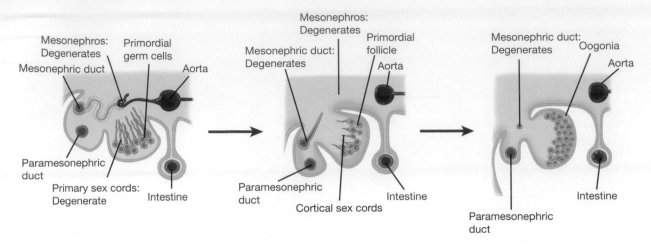

FIGURE 9-10. **Ovarian development.** As the ovaries develop, the mesonephros and primary sex cords degenerate. The primordial germ cells migrate into the cortical sex cords and form primordial follicles. These follicles then differentiate into oogonia.

Before birth, the oogonia enter meiosis I prophase, and no further division is possible. Arrests occur in the diplotene stage of meiosis I, and meiosis II does not begin until the egg is fertilized by the sperm. The ovaries separate from the mesonephros and become suspended in the pelvic mesentery. The peritoneal covering of the ovary is lost. After puberty, the ova are extruded into the peritoneal cavity and gathered into the ostium of the infundibulum by the fimbriae.

Internal Genitalia

The female internal genitalia develop due to the **absence of testosterone** and **MIF.** Without these substances, the mesonephric (Wolffian) duct regresses and the paramesonephric (Müllerian) duct begins to differentiate. The paramesonephric ducts partially fuse at the midline to form several structures (Figure 9-11).

- **Oviduct** (fallopian tubes): Upper, nonfused portion of ducts.
- **Fimbriae:** Elongations of oviducts.
- **Uterus:** Lower, fused portion of ducts.
- **Vagina** (upper two-thirds): Lower, fused portion of ducts.

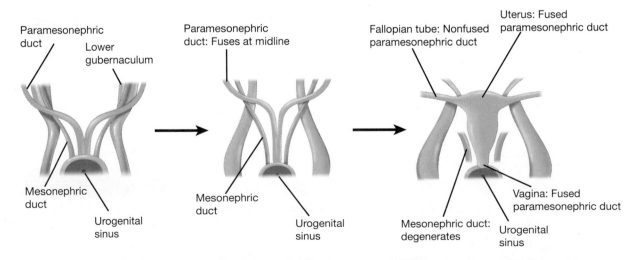

FIGURE 9-11. **Female internal genitalia development.** The lower portion of the paramesonephric duct fuses at the midline, forming the uterus and upper vagina. The upper portion of the paramesonephric duct does not fuse and forms the oviduct (fallopian tube).

The uterus develops a layer of **myometrium** from the surrounding mesenchyme and a layer of peritoneal covering, the **perimetrium** (serosa). The lower third of the vagina is formed from two outgrowths of the urogenital sinus wall, the **sinovaginal bulbs.** The ascending sinovaginal bulbs fuse with the descending paramesonephric system, creating the vaginal plate. The vaginal plate canalizes only with the thin covering of the hymen remaining. The greater (**Bartholin glands**) and the lesser vestibular glands (**Skene glands**) are endodermal outgrowths of the urogenital sinus.

Ligaments

Several peroneal ligaments are formed from the gubernaculum attached to the indifferent gonads (Figures 9-12 and 9-13). The gubernaculum is initially separated into upper and lower portions. As the Müllerian ducts fuse in the midline, the lower ligament is further separated, creating a total of three segments: **suspensory ovarian ligament** (attaches ovary to pelvic wall, carries ovarian vessels), **ovarian round ligament** (attaches ovary to lateral surface of uterus), and **uterine round ligament** (attaches uterus to labia majora via the inguinal canal; supplied by the Sampson artery).

The **broad ligament,** which covers the entire uterus, develops when the paramesonephric ducts descend through the pelvis, pulling a fold of celomic, or body cavity, epithelium and mesenchyme with them (see Figures 9-12 and 9-13). The broad ligament consists of three parts: mesovarium (covers ovaries), mesosalpinx (covers oviducts), and mesometrium (covers uterus). The **cardinal ligament** attaches the cervix to the lateral pelvic wall at the ischial spine and contains the uterine vessels (see Figures 9-12 and 9-13).

The female peroneal ligaments are summarized in Table 9-3.

External Genitalia

Under the influence of estrogen (Figure 9-14):

- The genital tubercle becomes the glans, which then becomes the clitoris.
- Urogenital folds partially fuse to become labia minora.
- Labioscrotal swellings partially fuse to become labia majora.

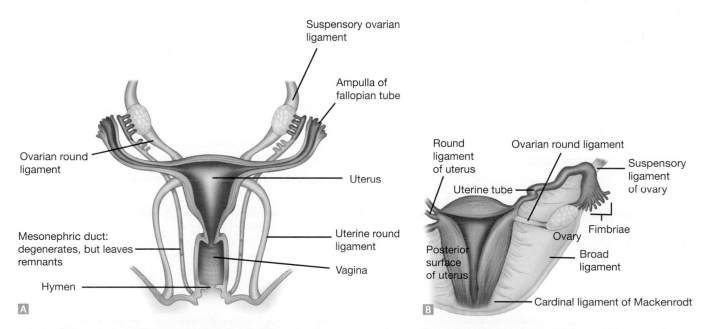

FIGURE 9-12.   Female ligament development. **A** The gubernaculum is separated into three segments that form the suspensory ovarian ligament, ovarian round ligament, and uterine round ligament. **B** The broad ligament covers the entire uterus and forms as the developing uterus descends through the pelvis, pulling epithelium and mesenchyme from the lining of the body cavity.

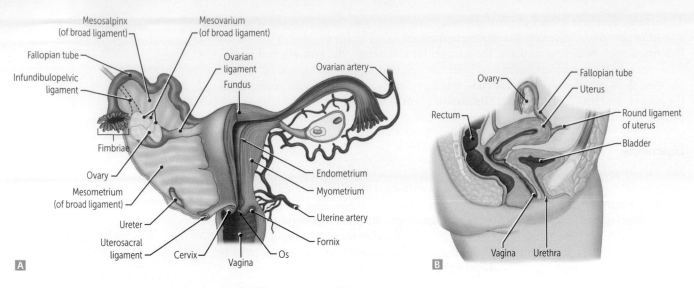

FIGURE 9-13.   Female reproductive anatomy. A Posterior and B sagittal views.

The skin covering the clitoris does not break down as in male development, so there is no foreskin equivalent.

Breast Development

Mammary glands develop from **apocrine sweat glands** in the mesenchymal layer just beneath the skin. Embryologically, breast development is identical in males and females.

- Week 4: The **mammary ridge,** a line of thickened ectoderm, develops from the inguinal region to the axilla.
- Weeks 4–6: The mammary ridge regresses except in the pectoral region.
- Week 6: Single mammary buds form as downgrowths of the mammary ridge.
- Weeks 6–birth:
    - Placental hormones (eg, lactogen) cause lactiferous duct branching.
    - The surrounding mesenchyme develops into fat and connective tissue.
    - The nipple is formed by depression of the skin before birth.
- Postnatal: The skin surrounding the nipple pit grows, raising the nipple.
- Puberty: If estrogen is present, female mammary glands develop.

> **CLINICAL CORRELATION**
>
> If portions of the mammary ridge do not regress, accessory nipples form along the thoracoabdominal region of the milk line. This is the most common congenital abnormality of breast development.

TABLE 9-3.   Female Peroneal Ligaments

LIGAMENT	CONNECTS	STRUCTURES CONTAINED
Infundibulopelvic ligament (suspensory ligament of the ovary)	Ovaries to lateral pelvic wall	Ovarian vessels
Ovarian round ligaments	Ovary to uterus	
Uterine round ligament	Uterus to labia majora via inguinal canal	Sampson artery
Broad ligament	Uterus, fallopian tubes, and ovaries to lateral pelvic wall	Uterus, round ligament of uterus, fallopian tubes, ovaries, ovarian ligaments
Cardinal ligament	Cervix to lateral pelvic wall	Uterine vessels
Uterosacral ligaments	Cervix to sacrum	

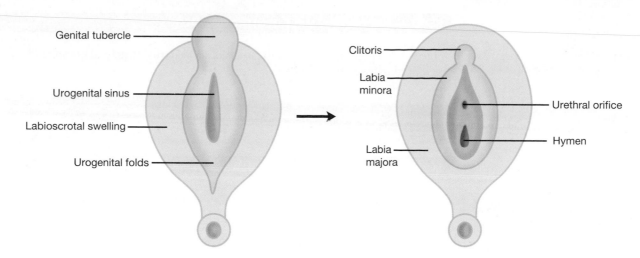

FIGURE 9-14. **Female external genitalia development.** The genital tubercle develops into the clitoris, and the urogenital and labioscrotal folds develop into the labia minora and labia majora, respectively.

Female Congenital Malformations

Uterine Canal Abnormalities

The paramesonephric ducts first fuse to form a Y-shaped tubular structure, which develops into the uterus and upper vagina. Once this Y-shaped structure is formed, fusion occurs followed by resorption/canalization of the intervening septum. Combinations of failed fusion and resorption can cause several different anomalies, including a double uterus, a bicornuate or septate uterus, or a unicornuate uterus (Figure 9-15). Abnormalities of uterine development often lead to infertility.

Atresia of the Uterine Canal

This condition occurs when there is narrowing or complete occlusion of the paramesonephric ducts (uterine atresia) or of just the sinovaginal bulbs (vaginal atresia).

Ovarian Hypoplasia

This underdevelopment of the ovary is seen in patients with Turner syndrome (XO). Primordial germ cells migrate toward the undifferentiated gonad, but follicles do not form. The vulnerable germ cells degenerate and the gonads do not produce hormones after birth, leaving the genitalia in an infantile state.

CLINICAL CORRELATION

A hysterosalpingogram visualizes the internal surface of the female reproductive tract via radiopaque dye and is used to evaluate anatomic causes of infertility.

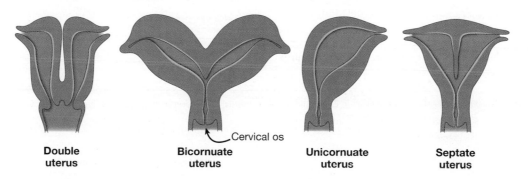

Double uterus   Bicornuate uterus   Unicornuate uterus   Septate uterus

Cervical os

FIGURE 9-15. **Uterine canal abnormalities.** Abnormal fusion of the paramesonephric ducts results in a double uterus (no fusion), a bicornuate uterus (incomplete fusion), or a septate uterus (incomplete resorption). Failure of one paramesonephric duct to develop results in unicornuate uterus.

Table 9-4 and Figure 9-16 review the internal and external structural homologs between the reproductive systems of the two sexes.

Anatomy

LOWER ABDOMEN AND PERINEUM

From superficial to deep, the abdominal wall consists of:

- Skin
- Subcutaneous fat (Camper fascia)
- Scarpa fascia
- External oblique muscle
- Internal oblique muscle
- Transversus abdominis muscle
- Transversalis fascia
- Preperitoneal fat
- Peritoneum

The aponeuroses of the abdominal muscles form the rectus sheath. Above the arcuate line, the sheath has anterior and posterior portions that wrap around the rectus abdominis. Below the arcuate line, however, the rectus sheath only travels anterior to the rectus abdominis. In other words, the posterior rectus sheath is absent inferior to the arcuate line (Figure 9-17).

The inguinal (Poupart) ligament is derived from the inferior border of the external oblique muscle aponeurosis. This ligament serves as the inferolateral border of the Hesselbach triangle and as the superiomedial border of the femoral triangle (Figure 9-18).

The pelvic region contains four named fasciae:

- Camper fascia: Fatty layer of the superficial fascia of the lower abdomen.
- Scarpa fascia: Membranous layer of the superficial fascia of the lower abdomen (deep to Camper fascia).
- Buck fascia: Membranous layer of the deep penile fascia, unique to men.
- Colles fascia: Membranous layer of the superficial fascia of the urogenital region (perineum).

FLASH BACK

Protrusion of peritoneum through the femoral canal results in a **femoral hernia.**

KEY FACT

Scarpa and Colles fasciae are contiguous.

FLASH BACK

The **inguinal (Hesselbach) triangle** is the area defined by the **rectus abdominis muscle** medially, the **inguinal ligament** inferiorly, and the **inferior epigastric vessels** superiorly and laterally. It is in this region that **direct inguinal hernias** protrude through the abdominal wall.

CLINICAL CORRELATION

Germ cell tumors (from testes or ovaries) spread first to the para-aortic lymph nodes.

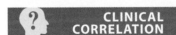
TABLE 9-4. **Derivatives of Embryonic Urogenital Structures**

	MALE	FEMALE
Mesonephric duct	Ureter, renal pelvis, calyces, collecting tubules, ductus (vas) deferens, duct of epididymis, ejaculatory duct, seminal vesicle	Ureter, renal pelvis, calyces, collecting tubules
Paramesonephric duct		Uterus, fallopian tubes, cervix, upper two-thirds of vagina
Urogenital sinus	Urinary bladder, urethra, prostate gland, bulbourethral glands	Urinary bladder, urethra, lower third of vagina, urethral and paraurethral glands, greater vestibular glands
Gubernaculum	"Scrotal ligament"	Ovarian ligaments, round ligament of the uterus

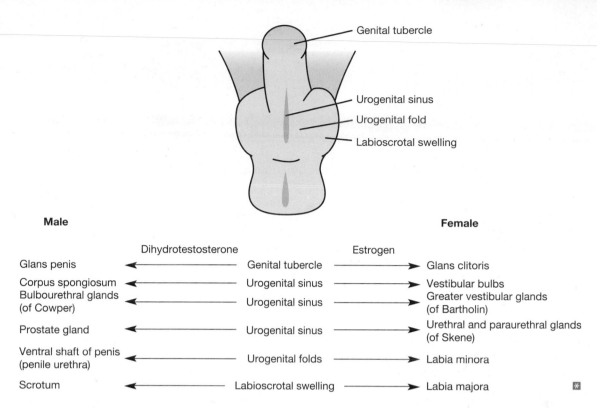

FIGURE 9-16.   **Male and female genital homologs.**

Venous drainage of the gonads differs between the right and left sides. The right gonadal vein drains directly into the interior vena cava (IVC) while the left drains first into the left renal vein, which then connects to the IVC.

Lymphatic drainage of both male and female gonads is to the para-aortic lymph nodes. However, lymphatic drainage of the scrotal skin/labia is to the superficial inguinal nodes.

> **?** **CLINICAL CORRELATION**
>
> Varicoceles are varicose veins of the testicles that cause pain and can lead to testicular atrophy. Varicocele is cited as a major cause of male infertility.

MALE REPRODUCTIVE SYSTEM

Reproductive structures in the male are located both within and outside the pelvis, as shown in Figure 9-19.

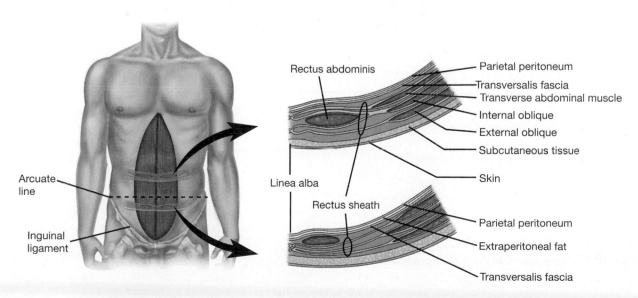

FIGURE 9-17.   **Layers of the abdominal wall.**

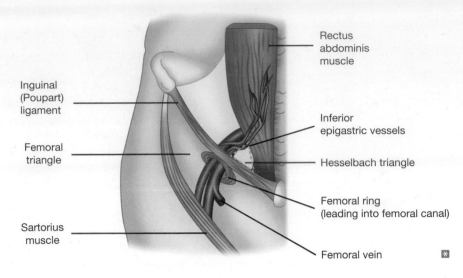

Rectus
abdominis
muscle

Inguinal
(Poupart)
ligament

Inferior
epigastric vessels

Hesselbach triangle

Femoral
triangle

Femoral ring
(leading into femoral canal)

Sartorius
muscle

Femoral vein

FIGURE 9-18. **Anatomic borders formed by the inguinal ligament.**

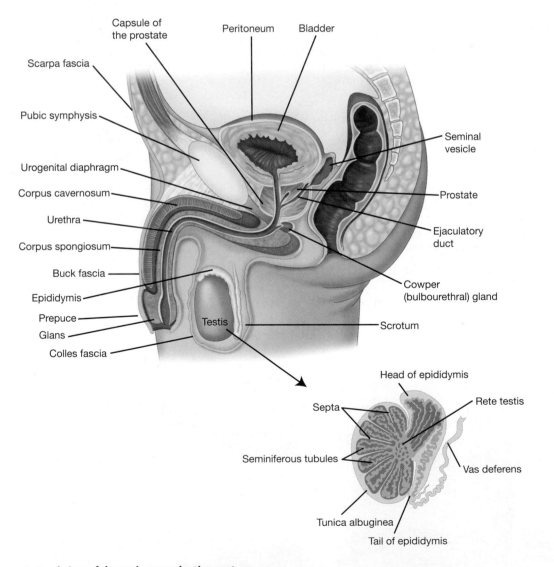

Capsule of
the prostate

Peritoneum

Bladder

Scarpa fascia

Pubic symphysis

Seminal
vesicle

Urogenital diaphragm

Prostate

Corpus cavernosum

Urethra

Ejaculatory
duct

Corpus spongiosum

Buck fascia

Epididymis

Cowper
(bulbourethral) gland

Prepuce

Glans

Testis

Scrotum

Colles fascia

Head of epididymis

Septa

Rete testis

Seminiferous tubules

Vas deferens

Tunica albuginea

Tail of epididymis

FIGURE 9-19. **Lateral view of the male reproductive system.**

The pelvic fasciae are illustrated in Figures 9-19 and 9-20.

Between the testis and inguinal canal, the vas deferens runs within the **spermatic cord.** Cremasteric muscle fibers, the testicular artery, the pampiniform venous plexus, and the genital branch of the genitofemoral nerve are also found within this structure. The ilioinguinal nerve (a branch of the first lumbar nerve) runs atop the spermatic cord. The genitofemoral nerve is responsible for the cremasteric reflex, which describes contraction of the cremasteric muscle (genital branch) when the skin of the medial thigh (femoral branch) is touched. The ilioinguinal nerve supplies sensation to the skin of the medial thigh, mons pubis, and scrotum or labia majora.

In the scrotum, the **tunica dartos,** a thin muscular layer superficial to Colles fascia, allows the scrotal skin to become tense. It also forms the scrotal septum, which keeps the spermatic cords from getting tangled. The **gubernaculum** (sometimes called the "scrotal ligament") further limits movement of the testes by tethering them to the inferior aspect of the scrotum. The left testis often hangs lower than the right.

In conjunction with the **cremaster muscle,** which covers each testis, the tunica dartos allows the testes and scrotum to be drawn up closer to the body in cold environments.

The layers of the scrotum are reviewed in Figure 9-21 and Table 9-5.

The penis is formed from three bodies of erectile tissue. During erection, this tissue stiffens because it is filled with blood from deep arteries of the penis and the arteries of the bulb of the penis. An erection is maintained because the expansion of erectile tissue compresses the dorsal veins of the penis, which keeps blood in the penis. The two dorsal erectile bodies are called corpus cavernosum, and the ventral body is called the corpus spongiosum. The urethra passes through the corpus spongiosum on the ventral side of the penis. At the distal end of the penis, the corpus spongiosum expands to form the glans penis (see Figures 9-19 and 9-20).

Sperm Cells

A sperm cell (Figure 9-22) is composed of a head, a middle piece, and a principal piece (eg, tail). The head contains the nucleus and the acrosome. The front part of the head

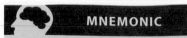

MNEMONIC

The pathway sperm take to exit the body—
SEVEn UP
Seminiferous tubules (site of **S**permatogenesis)
Epididymis
Vas deferens
Ejaculatory ducts
Urethra
Penis

KEY FACT

Loss of cremasteric reflex is common in testicular torsion in younger males. However, this reflex is often absent in older adult males.

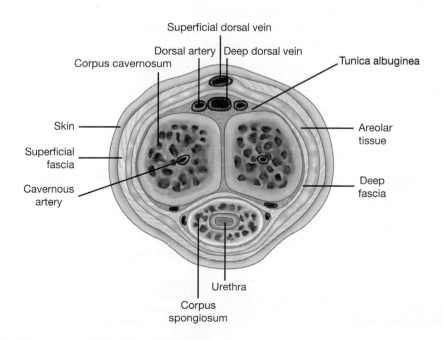

FIGURE 9-20. **Cross section of the penis.**

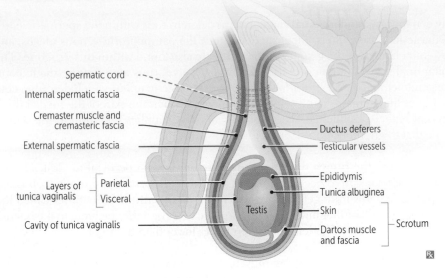

FIGURE 9-21.   **Layers of tissue within the scrotum.**

contains the **acrosome,** a structure derived from the Golgi apparatus that contains enzymes to digest the extracellular matrix (ECM) and zona pellucida of the egg. The postacrosomal region contains a haploid nucleus. The sperm cell membrane in this region also contains receptors for the egg. The spiral midpiece consists of fused mitochondria that use fructose to generate adenosine triphosphate (ATP) to move the **9+2 axoneme** in the proximal portion of the tail (called the flagellum). The sliding of the microtubules generates the whip-like motile force characteristic of sperm cells.

Prostate

About the size and shape of a walnut, the prostate stores and secretes a clear, alkaline fluid found in semen. Prostatic fluid constitutes roughly one third of the volume of the semen. The alkalinity of semen helps neutralize the acidity of the vaginal tract, prolonging the lifespan of sperm. Located at a major anatomic hub with the seminal vesicles and vas deferens, this fluid from the prostate is mixed with seminal fluid and spermatozoa. The ejaculatory ducts, which are located in the middle lobe and lined with transitional epithelium, are found posterior to the urethra. Smooth muscle within the prostate helps expel semen during ejaculation.

Though the gross anatomy of the prostate can be described by lobes, the more common approach is by pathologic zones (Figure 9-23). Table 9-6 lists the approximate equivalencies between the two classification systems.

TABLE 9-5.   **Spermatic Cord Derivatives of Abdominal Layers**

ABDOMINAL STRUCTURE	DERIVATIVE IN SPERMATIC CORD
External oblique muscle aponeurosis	External spermatic fascia
Internal oblique muscle	Cremaster muscle
Transversalis fascia	Internal spermatic fascia
Extraperitoneal fatty tissue	Areolar tissue
Peritoneum	Processus vaginalis

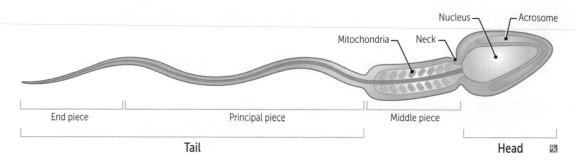

FIGURE 9-22.   Sperm anatomy.

The stroma, which accounts for 5% of the weight of the prostate, contains no glands—only muscle and fibrous tissue.

FEMALE REPRODUCTIVE SYSTEM

The female reproductive organs and accessory structures are illustrated in Figure 9-24. In situ, the uterus is usually anteverted (tilted forward), with its anteroinferior face resting against the bladder. As such, it is the posterior side of the uterus that is visualized when looking down at the pelvic floor.

Once released by the ovary, ova are caught by the fimbriae of the fallopian (uterine) tube and travel toward the uterus. The fallopian tubes, also known as the **oviducts** or **salpinges**, contain four sections: the infundibulum, ampulla, isthmus, and interstitium. The infundibulum contains fimbriae and the ampulla is the usual site of fertilization.

The pelvic fasciae are labeled in Figure 9-25. As in the male, the female urogenital diaphragm is bordered by superior and inferior fascia. Colles fascia is continuous with the posterior aspect of the inferior fascia.

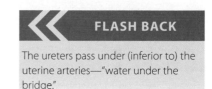

FLASH BACK

The ureters pass under (inferior to) the uterine arteries—"water under the bridge."

The Breasts

Breast tissue, a composite of connective tissue (collagen and elastin), adipose tissue, and glands, changes over time and secondary to hormonal influences. At puberty, as

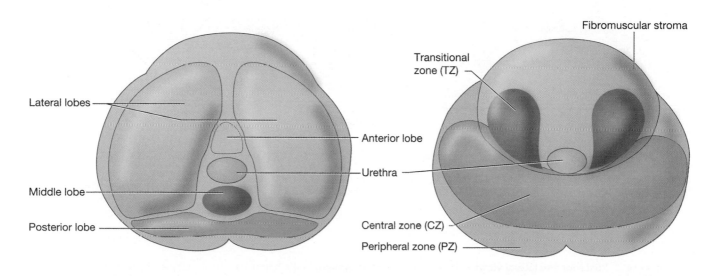

FIGURE 9-23.   Prostatic lobes (left) and prostatic zones (right).

CLINICAL CORRELATION

BPH involves hyperplasia of cells in the periurethral zone (lateral and middle lobes), resulting in urinary symptoms. **Prostatic adenocarcinoma** affects the androgen-sensitive cells of the peripheral zone (posterior lobe), allowing easy metastasis to the spine via the Batson plexus.

▶▶ FLASH FORWARD

Breast cancer in situ: Ductal carcinoma in situ (DCIS) tends to occur unilaterally, whereas lobular carcinoma in situ (LCIS) has a greater chance of affecting both breasts.

KEY FACT

The dermatome at the level of the nipple is T4 in males.

MNEMONIC

T4 at the teat pore.

TABLE 9-6. **Anatomic Lobes and Pathologic Zones of the Prostate**

ANATOMIC LOBE	PATHOLOGIC ZONE
Anterior lobe (isthmus)	Transitional zone (TZ)
Posterior lobe	Peripheral zone (PZ)
Middle lobe (median lobe)	Central zone (CZ)
Lateral lobe	All zones

estrogen increases, the breasts increase in size and softness as the mammary glands develop and more fat is deposited. Growth of breast epithelium is primarily estrogen mediated, while ductal growth is both estrogen and progesterone dependent. After the birth of a child, the number of glands roughly doubles, allowing for the secretion of milk. Overproduction of estrogen, either during menstruation or at the beginning of menopause, can make the breast tissue more tender. The consistency of the breast tissue itself also varies during this period. With time, the **Cooper ligaments**—the suspensory ligaments of the breast—weaken.

A normal breast (Figure 9-26) possesses a nipple surrounded by the **areola**, a pigmented section of skin containing sebaceous glands. The mammary glands within the breast tissue connect to the nipple via lactiferous ducts. The breast itself sits atop the pectoralis major muscle, spanning from approximately the second to the sixth rib, though a thin layer of mammary tissue reaches several ribs above and below. The **"tail of Spence"** extends diagonally from the superior lateral quadrant to the axilla.

The majority of the lymph from the breast drains to the ipsilateral axillary lymph nodes. The parasternal, abdominal, and contralateral axillary lymph nodes may also be involved.

The nipples in both men and women are highly sensitive and highly vascular. Table 9-7 and Figure 9-27 review, respectively, the important nerves and vessels in the breast.

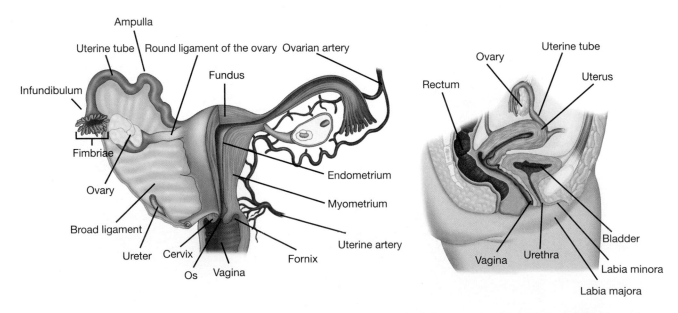

FIGURE 9-24. **Posterior and lateral views of female reproductive system.** In the left image, the ureter runs perpendicular to the plane of the page (the broad ligament).

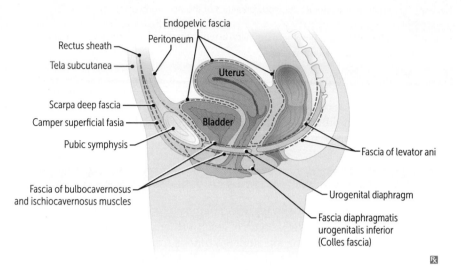

FIGURE 9-25.   **Lateral view of the female perineum illustrating the pelvic fascia.**

Physiology

GAMETOGENESIS

Human sexual reproduction depends on many factors, but formation of healthy gametes is probably the most important. Though the synchronicity and location of spermato-

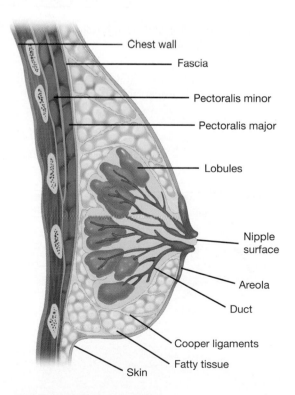

FIGURE 9-26.   **Lateral view of the female breast.**

TABLE 9-7.   Principal Nerves and Vessels of the Breast

Nerves	Anterior and lateral cutaneous branches of thoracic intercostal nerves T3–T5
Arteries	Internal thoracic (internal mammary) artery, lateral thoracic artery, thoracodorsal artery, thoracoacromial artery
Veins	Axillary vein, internal thoracic vein

FLASH BACK

Ploidy = number of homologous sets of chromosomes:
- Diploid (46 chromosomes)
- Haploid (23 chromosomes): parent
- Chromatid = one-half of a replicated chromosome

genesis and oogenesis differ, the cells go through nearly analogous stages (as suggested by their suffixes). Table 9-8 reviews these stages.

SPERMATOGENESIS

Spermatogenesis, which occurs in the seminiferous tubules of the testes, is a stepwise process of mitosis followed by two rounds of meiosis (Figure 9-28). It is important to note two things: (1) Some spermatogonia undergo mitosis (replication) but do not advance further, thus maintaining a constant supply of cells for spermatogenesis, and (2) dividing sperm cells remain connected by threads of cytoplasm so they develop at the same time (Figure 9-29). Upon release from Sertoli cells, mature but nonmotile spermatozoa move from the lumen of the seminiferous tubules to the epididymis, where they become motile. However, it is muscle contraction in the male reproductive tract rather than flagellar movement that moves the sperm cells prior to ejaculation.

Sertoli cells are supportive cells that make numerous contributions to developing sperm cells, including:

- The **blood-testis barrier,** which blocks penetration by cytotoxic agents and white blood cells.
- Secretion of substances that aid in meiosis.
- Phagocytosis of residual cytoplasm during the final stage of spermatogenesis when spermatids become spermatozoa.
- Secretion of other factors, including androgen-binding protein (ABP), inhibin, giant-cell line–derived neutrophilic factor (GDNF), and estradiol.

Leydig cells are interstitial cells that produce testosterone, which diffuses into the seminiferous tubules. A very high local concentration of testosterone in the seminiferous

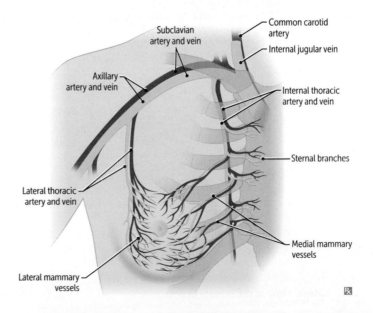

FIGURE 9-27.   **Selected vessels in the female breast.**

TABLE 9-8.   Overview of Gametogenesis in Males and Females

CHROMOSOMES	CELL TYPE (SINGULAR FORM)	CHROMATIDS
Diploid (46)	Spermatogonium/oogonium	2N
	Primary spermatocyte/primary oocyte	4N
Haploid (23)	Secondary spermatocyte/secondary oocyte	2N
	Spermatid/ootid	N
	Spermatozoon/ovum	

tubules is required for spermatogenesis, and this is partly achieved by Sertoli cell–produced **ABP,** which traps androgens in the seminiferous tubules.

Leydig cells are stimulated by luteinizing hormone (LH), and Sertoli cells are stimulated by follicle-stimulating hormone (FSH); both hormones are secreted by the anterior pituitary.

Via standard feedback inhibition, **inhibin** secreted by Sertoli cells and testosterone secreted by Leydig cells inhibit the hypothalamus and anterior pituitary from secreting gonadotropin-releasing hormone (GnRH) and LH/FSH, respectively (Figure 9-30).

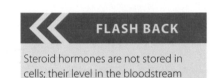

FLASH BACK

Steroid hormones are not stored in cells; their level in the bloodstream depends on their rate of synthesis.

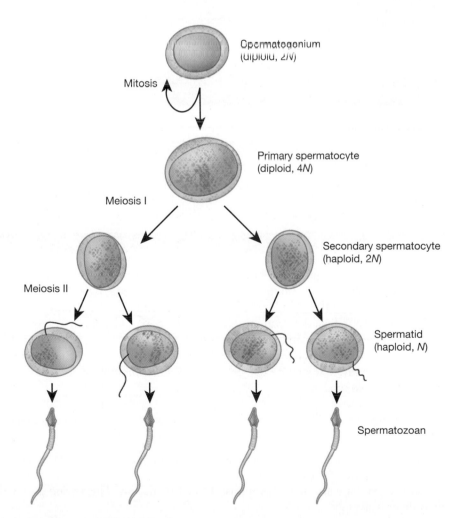

Spermatogonium
(diploid, 2N)

Mitosis

Primary spermatocyte
(diploid, 4N)

Meiosis I

Secondary spermatocyte
(haploid, 2N)

Meiosis II

Spermatid
(haploid, N)

Spermatozoan

FIGURE 9-28.   Spermatogenesis.

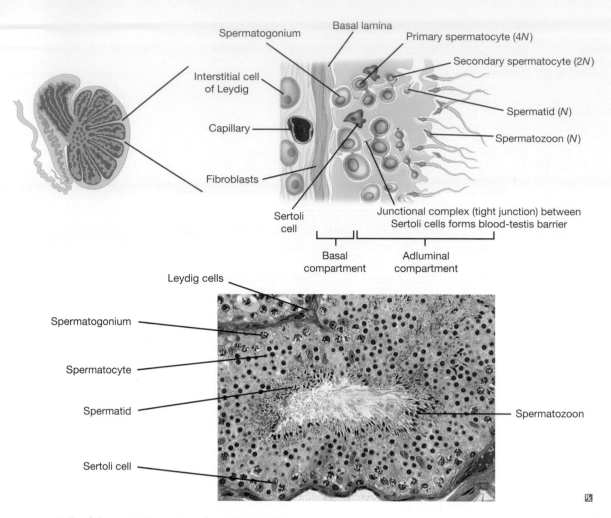

FIGURE 9-29.   Cells of the seminiferous tubule and interstitium.

Spermatogenesis begins at puberty and continues until death, although the quantity and quality of the sperm cells wane somewhat in the later years as plasma testosterone levels fall.

OOGENESIS

The female sex cell, the ovum, is a spherical structure produced within **mature Graafian follicles** in the ovary. The outermost layer, the **corona radiata,** is two to three cells thick and is derived from the granulosa cells on the inner portion of the ovarian follicle. Deep to the corona radiata is the **zona pellucida (striata),** a glycoprotein layer that binds to invading sperm cells and allows the acrosome reaction to occur. Deeper still is the **perivitelline space,** which contains both the mature oocyte and, after fertilization, the second polar body. The mature oocyte possesses a cell membrane, copious cytoplasm, and a haploid nucleus.

Oogenesis occurs in the follicle without the aid of centrosomes. It is analogous to spermatogenesis, although the timing is different:

- Oocytogenesis is completed in the perinatal period, thus providing a newborn female with all the oocytes she will ever have ($\sim 7 \times 10^6$).
- Primary oocytes are arrested in **prophase I until ovulation.** This period is called dictyate or dictyotene.

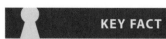

KEY FACT

Upon fertilization, meiosis II is completed, allowing the secondary oocyte (2N) to become an ootid/ovum (N) and avoid multiploidy.

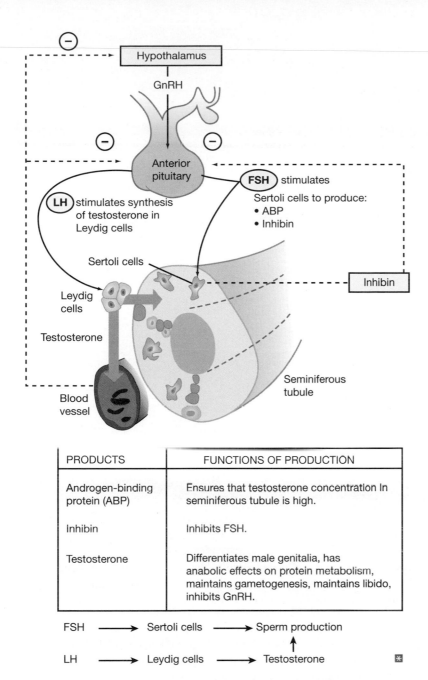

PRODUCTS	FUNCTIONS OF PRODUCTION
Androgen-binding protein (ABP)	Ensures that testosterone concentration in seminiferous tubule is high.
Inhibin	Inhibits FSH.
Testosterone	Differentiates male genitalia, has anabolic effects on protein metabolism, maintains gametogenesis, maintains libido, inhibits GnRH.

FSH ⟶ Sertoli cells ⟶ Sperm production

LH ⟶ Leydig cells ⟶ Testosterone

FIGURE 9-30. **Hormonal regulation of spermatogenesis.** FSH, follicle-stimulating hormone; GnRH, gonadotropin-releasing hormone; LH, luteinizing hormone.

- After ovulation, the oocyte completes meiosis I, forming the first polar body and a secondary oocyte that is arrested in **metaphase II until fertilization.**
- Within minutes of fertilization, the secondary ooctye completes meiosis II and produces an ootid and second polar body. The ootid becomes an ovum, a cell with both paternal and maternal pronuclei. When the pronuclei fuse, the ovum becomes a zygote.

Also in contrast to spermatogenesis, the effort in oogenesis is concentrated on one cell. The two **polar bodies** degenerate (Figure 9-31).

Until ovulation (and possible subsequent fertilization) occurs, maturation of the oocyte takes place within an ovarian follicle (Figure 9-32).

FLASH BACK

Breast budding **(thelarche)** and growth of pubic hair are the first signs of a girl's entry into puberty. Physicians monitor these changes using Tanner staging.

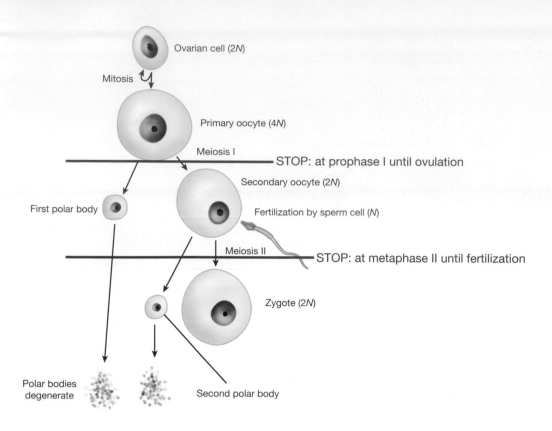

FIGURE 9-31. **Oogenesis and fertilization.**

MENSTRUAL CYCLE AND OVULATION

Menarche, or a woman's first menstrual period, occurs, on average, at 12.5 years of age in American girls. It precedes regular ovulation by several months to a year.

Granulosa cells, the female analog of Sertoli cells, respond to FSH and encourage growth of 15–20 follicles. LH-responsive theca cells stimulate growth of the corpus luteum and produce androgens, which can be converted to estrogen by the granulosa cells.

Estrogen encourages growth of the endometrium and generally provides negative feedback to the anterior pituitary to inhibit the release of FSH and LH (Figure 9-33). High levels of estrogen at the end of the follicular phase actually stimulate gonadotropin release, leading to a midcycle gonadotropin surge.

Approximately 1 week before ovulation, one of the developing follicles becomes dominant and increases its expression of FSH receptors above the other developing follicles (more sensitive to FSH). This follicle secretes inhibin, blocking the production of FSH from the anterior pituitary and thus causing the other follicles to undergo atresia. In anticipation of a preovulatory rise in estrogen levels from the dominant follicle, granulosa cells express both FSH and LH receptors, and theca cells increase their expression of LH receptors. An LH surge results in ovulation.

During ovulation, the wall of the ovary at the location of the dominant follicle degrades and ruptures, releasing the oocyte into the peritoneal space, where it is captured by the fimbriae at the end of the fallopian tube. The granulosa cells surrounding the ruptured follicle are filled with cholesterol esters and become the corpus luteum ("yellow body").

The corpus luteum secretes high levels of progesterone and lower levels of estrogen. Progesterone transforms the proliferating endometrium into secretory endometrium to prepare the uterus for implantation. It also thickens the cervical mucus.

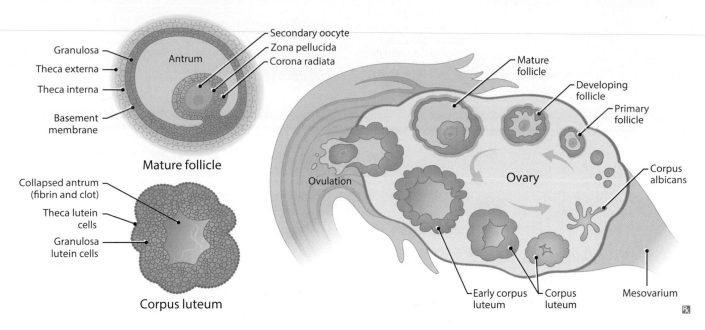

FIGURE 9-32. Follicular development in situ.

If fertilization and implantation occur, the extraembryonic trophoblasts produce **human chorionic gonadotropin (hCG).** This hormone acts like LH and causes the corpus luteum to continue secreting high levels of progesterone, stimulating further development of the endometrium.

If fertilization and implantation do not occur (Figure 9-34), the corpus luteum degenerates into scar tissue called the **corpus albicans** ("white body") after approximately 14 days. Consequently, estrogen and progesterone levels drop, and the functional portion of the endometrium is shed via menstruation. The whole process of follicular recruitment through menstruation takes approximately 28 days.

Figure 9-35 shows the variation of FSH and LH levels with age. These two hormones normally stimulate production of estrogen, but after menopause, there are no more ovarian follicles, so estrogen, progesterone, and inhibin levels drop despite continuing high levels of FSH and LH. A woman's lifetime estrogen exposure is an important risk factor for the development of breast cancer and endometrial cancer. Increased estrogen exposure is associated with early menarche, late menopause, nulliparity, and not breast-feeding.

GONADAL STEROIDS

Steroid hormones, which are derived from cholesterol (Figure 9-36), can be organized into five groups: mineralocorticoids, glucocorticoids, androgens, estrogens, and progestogens. The latter three groups are vital for normal genital development and, later, fertility. Their functions are reviewed in Table 9-9. Dehydroepiandrosterone (DHEA), a weak androgen, and androstenedione are both produced in the adrenal gland (zona reticularis) and the gonads. By comparison, the stronger androgens and estrogens (eg, testosterone, DHT, and estradiol) are primarily produced in the gonads.

CLINICAL CORRELATION

Insulin stimulates the ovaries to produce estrogen. Consequently, type 2 diabetics with insulin resistance and hyperinsulinemia may have a greater risk of breast cancer and endometrial carcinoma.

FLASH BACK

A female fetus has high levels of FSH and LH during the second trimester, owing to development of the genitalia.

KEY FACT

Testosterone and androstenedione are converted to estradiol and estrone, respectively, in adipose tissue by the enzyme **aromatase.**

CLINICAL CORRELATION

Like hyperinsulinemia, obesity can increase the risk of breast cancer. Adipocytes allow peripheral conversion of androgens to estrogens through the action of aromatase.

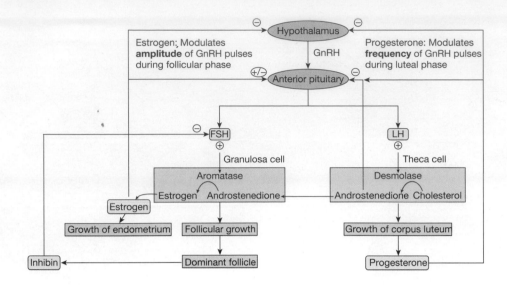

FIGURE 9-33. **Female hormonal axis (follicular phase).** FSH, follicle-stimulating hormone; GnRH, gonadotropin-releasing hormone; LH, luteinizing hormone.

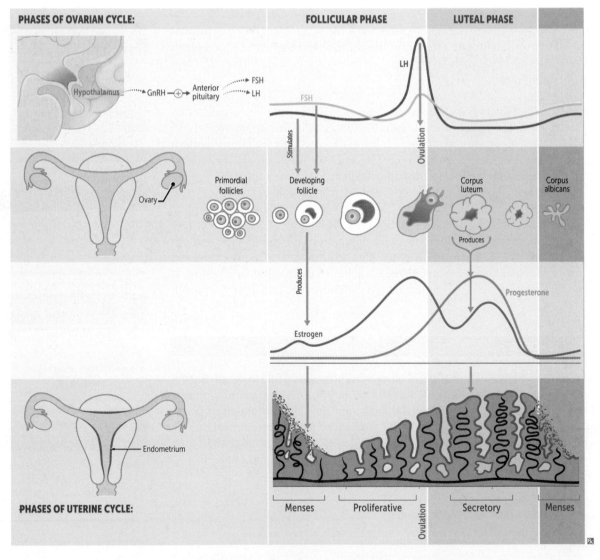

FIGURE 9-34. **Endometrial and hormonal changes in a menstrual cycle.** FSH, follicle-stimulating hormone; LH, luteinizing hormone.

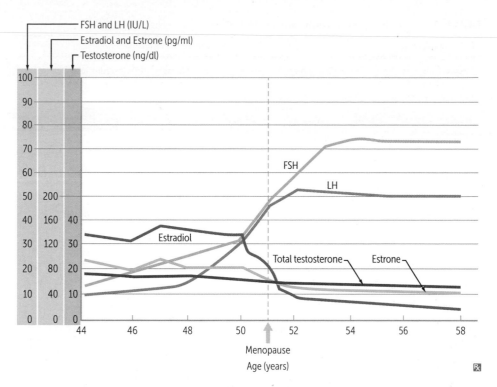

FIGURE 9-35. **Plasma gonadotropin levels throughout a woman's lifetime.** FSH, follicle-stimulating hormone; LH, luteinizing hormone.

SEXUAL RESPONSE

The trajectory of sexual response in both men and women consists of four phases: desire, excitation (parasympathetic), orgasm (sympathetic), and resolution. Men experience increased blood flow into and decreased venous return out of the cavernous spaces of the penis, yielding an **erection**. Women, too, experience similar changes in blood flow to the clitoris and vestibular bulbs. This process is all mediated by the pelvic splanchnic nerves (parasympathetics, S2–S4).

> **KEY FACT**
>
> Progesterone is the only naturally occurring human progestagen. Progestins are synthetic progestagens used for hormonal contraception because they inhibit ovulation by blocking the LH surge.

> **MNEMONIC**
>
> **PRiSM**
>
> **P**rogestins cause **R**elaxation of **S**mooth **M**uscle, which accounts for the observed vasodilation and decreased myometrial excitability and GI motility.

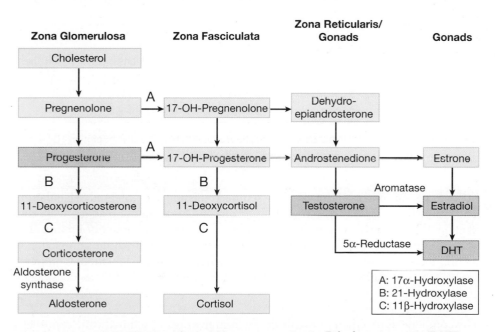

FIGURE 9-36. **Organization of steroid hormone synthesis.** Dihydrotestosterone (DHT) is produced by peripheral conversion. Estradiol can be made directly in the gonads or by peripheral conversion as well.

TABLE 9-9.   Androgens, Estrogens, and Progestins

ANDROGENS

Source	Testis (DHT and testosterone), adrenal glands (androstenedione)
Biological potency	DHT > testosterone > androstenedione
Targets	Skin, prostate, seminal vesicles, epididymis, liver, muscle, brain
Function	1. Differentiation of the Wolffian duct system into internal gonadal structures 2. Secondary sexual characteristics and growth spurt during puberty 3. Required for normal spermatogenesis 4. Anabolic effects (increased muscle size, increased RBC production) 5. Increased libido

ESTROGENS

Source	Ovary (estradiol), placenta (estriol), adipose (estrone, estradiol)
Biological potency	Estradiol > estrone > estriol
Function	1. Growth of follicles 2. Endometrial proliferation 3. Development of genitalia 4. Stromal development of the breast 5. Female fat distribution 6. Hepatic synthesis of carrier proteins 7. Feedback inhibition of FSH 8. LH surge (estrogen feedback on LH and FSH secretion switches from negative to positive just before the LH surge) 9. Increased myometrial excitability 10. Increased HDL, decreased LDL

PROGESTINS

Source	Corpus luteum, placenta
Function	1. Stimulation of endometrial glandular secretions and spiral artery development 2. Uterine smooth muscle relaxation 3. Maintenance of pregnancy 4. Production of thick cervical mucus, which inhibits sperm entry into the uterus 5. Increased body temperature 6. Negative regulation of gonadotropins (LH, FSH)

DHT, dihydrotestosterone; FSH, follicle-stimulating hormone; HDL, high-density lipoprotein; LDL, low-density lipoprotein; LH, luteinizing hormone; RBC, red blood cell.

FLASH BACK

Estrogen promotes proliferation of breast epithelium and is the main driver of breast growth during puberty. Normal breast ductal development requires the coordinated action of both estrogen and progesterone.

KEY FACT

The parasympathetics stimulate the release of nitric oxide (NO), which increases cyclic guanosine monophosphate (cGMP) in vascular smooth muscle and closes Ca^{2+} channels. The arterial smooth muscle relaxes, and the erectile tissue fills with blood.

In men, orgasm consists of two substeps: **seminal emission** and **antegrade ejaculation**. The sympathetic nervous system (T10–L2) controls closure of the bladder neck, contraction of the seminal vesicle, and deposition of semen in the posterior urethra. The somatic and visceral pudendal nerves (S2–S4) then stimulate rhythmic contraction of the ischiocavernosus and bulbocavernosus muscles, allowing ejaculation. Continued sympathetic stimulation ends the erection (**detumescence**) by inducing vasoconstriction of the arteries.

The components of semen primarily derive from five organs: seminal vesicle, prostate, testes, bulbourethral (Cowper) gland, and epididymis. The seminal vesicle secretes fructose, ascorbic acid, prostaglandins, phosphorylcholine, and flavins (60% of semen volume). The prostate secretes zinc, citric acid, phospholipids, acid phosphatase, and profibrolysin (20% of semen volume). The testes produce sperm (15% of semen volume). The bulbourethral gland secretes thick, alkaline mucus to help neutralize the acidity of the vagina (< 5% of semen volume). The epididymis secretes carnitine and acetyl carnitine (< 5% of semen volume).

In women, orgasm involves "tenting" of the vagina (relaxation of the vaginal muscularis) and contractions of the pelvic diaphragm and uterus. Detumescence of the clitoral and vestibular erectile tissue is slower, which allows women to experience multiple orgasms.

FERTILIZATION

Successful fertilization depends on four sequential steps:

- Gamete delivery.
- Binding of the sperm to the egg.
- Activation of the egg.
- Fusion of the sperm and egg.

Ovulation occurs within 24–48 hours of the midcycle surge of LH. Usually, only one egg is released, entering the fallopian tube via ciliary action. The egg can survive only 24 hours in the female tract, so fertilization must occur around the time of ovulation.

By comparison, sperm can survive in the female tract for up to 5 days. In their journey to the fallopian tubes, they are aided by estrogen-induced watery uterine mucus and peristaltic uterine contractions. Before being able to fertilize the egg, sperm must be **capacitated** in the female tract—a set of changes that alter membrane fluidity, membrane potential, and even movement of the tail.

Fertilization takes place in the fallopian tube (ampulla). Capacitated sperm penetrate the corona radiata and bind to the zona pellucida. This species-specific interaction triggers the acrosome reaction and allows the entire sperm cell to burrow deeper into the egg.

The unfertilized egg is metabolically quiescent. After fusing with the sperm cell, the egg undergoes a signal transduction cascade that stimulates the egg to complete meiosis II (formation of the second polar body and a haploid ovum) and release cortical granules to prevent polyspermy (Figure 9-37). Sperm already bound to the zona pellucida are removed, and new sperm are prevented from binding.

The egg's cytoplasm causes the sperm nucleus to decondense and form the male pronucleus. The mitochondria and tail disintegrate, but the sperm cell contributes a centriole for cell division. The male and female centrioles organize an aster, allowing the two pronuclei to slowly come together over the course of 12 hours. During this time, DNA replication occurs. Thus, when the male and female pronuclei finally fuse, the zygote can undergo mitosis to form two diploid cells.

While undergoing cell division, the zygote travels down the oviduct to the uterus, where it implants 5 days after fertilization.

At best, the probability of fertilization following intercourse is 35%, and only two-thirds of fertilized eggs develop successfully. Thus, the probability of a successful pregnancy is about 25%.

CLINICAL CORRELATION

Sildenafil treats erectile dysfunction (ED) by inhibiting the enzyme **phosphodiesterase-5 (PDE-5)**, which normally catabolizes cGMP. Inhibiting PDE-5 increases intracavernous cGMP levels and improves erectile response to sexual stimulation in many men.

MNEMONIC

Distinction for autonomic control of erection vs ejaculation:

Point (**P**arasympathetic) and **S**hoot (**S**ympathetic)

KEY FACT

Fertilization of a single egg with multiple sperm would result in aneuploidy, **not** multiple, viable zygotes.

CLINICAL CORRELATION

Ectopic pregnancy occurs when the zygote implants somewhere other than the uterus. Implantation in the fallopian tube can lead to tubal rupture.

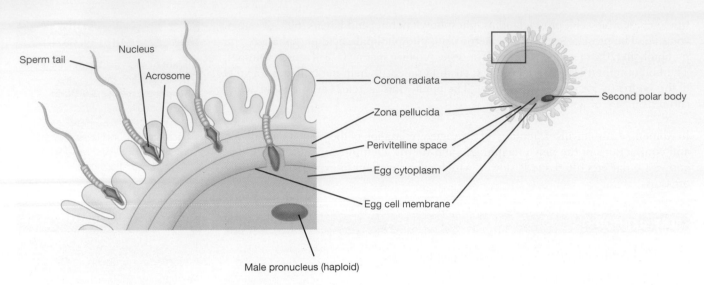

FIGURE 9-37. **Penetration of the ovum by a sperm cell.** The second polar body only appears after fertilization takes place.

PREGNANCY

Designed to optimize the welfare of the fetus, numerous metabolic and physical changes occur in the mother's body during pregnancy.

Osmoregulation

Pregnancy is a state of chronic volume overload and has many features similar to those of congestive heart failure, including edema and polyuria. The fetus, placenta, and amniotic fluid contribute about half of the 6- to 8-L increase in the woman's total body water. As Table 9-10 illustrates, increased glomerular filtration rate (GFR), progesterone, prostaglandins, human chorionic gonadotropin (hCG), atrial natriuretic peptide (ANP), and lying in the left lateral decubitus position favor Na$^+$ excretion. Decreased GFR and increased aldosterone, estrogen, and deoxycorticosterone favor Na$^+$ retention. Despite net Na$^+$ retention, serum concentrations (and plasma osmolality) actually decrease due to dilution. Similarly, hemodilution causes **physiologic anemia** and a compensatory increase in cardiac output.

TABLE 9-10. **Factors That Favor Na$^+$ Excretion and Retention**

SODIUM EXCRETION	SODIUM RETENTION
↑ GFR	↓ GFR
Progesterone	Aldosterone
Prostaglandins	Estrogen
hCG	Deoxycorticosterone
ANP	Lying supine (uterus compresses IVC, which ↓ preload and ↓ CO, thus ↓ renal perfusion)
Left lateral decubitus position ↑ renal perfusion)	

ANP, atrial natruretic peptide; CO, cardiac output; GFR, glomerular filtration rate; hCG, human chorionic gonadotropin; IVC, inferior vena cava.

Urinary System

Positioning of the fetus can lead to decreased bladder capacity and increased urinary frequency and incontinence. An additional effect of progesterone-mediated smooth muscle relaxation is dilation of the ureters. Secondary to fluid overload, the renal pelves/calyces also dilate, literally opening the kidneys up to UTIs and subsequent infection. Volume overload dilutes the serum levels of blood urea nitrogen (BUN), creatinine, and uric acid, and increases the effective renal plasma flow and GFR. The renal tubular absorptive capacity is surpassed, which may result in physiologic glucosuria (but not proteinuria). Similarly, small amounts of blood may also appear in the urine.

Cardiovascular System

Increased heart rate (HR) and stroke volume (SV) result in a 30–50% increase in cardiac output (CO). Nonetheless, blood pressure (BP) actually decreases secondary to progesterone acting on smooth muscle to decrease systemic vascular resistance (SVR). By the third trimester, BP returns to baseline. A low-grade systolic flow murmur and mild left ventricular hypertrophy are other normal physiologic changes seen during pregnancy.

Though the mother's blood volume increases about 50%, plasma expands at a faster rate than RBC mass, hastening the development of physiologic anemia. Platelet count may also progressively decline (gestational thrombocytopenia). Nonetheless, due to increased fibrinogen, decreased protein S, and increased venous stasis in the legs, the mother is actually in a **hypercoagulable state.**

Respiratory System

Pregnancy results in elevation of the diaphragm, which decreases the residual volume. The total lung capacity (TLC) decreases only slightly, however. The net effect is decreased residual volume but increased inspiratory capacity. Notably, on spirometry testing, forced vital capacity (FVC) and forced expiratory volume in 1 second (FEV_1), are unchanged.

These changes have no effect on respiratory muscle function itself. The tidal volume (TV) actually increases to allow for increased minute ventilation (MV) and chronic hyperventilation. Hyperventilation leads to decreased CO_2 partial pressure, which causes chronic (mild) respiratory alkalosis and compensatory metabolic acidosis, facilitating fetal off-loading of acidic wastes and CO_2.

Blood flow to the nasopharynx is increased during pregnancy, causing many women to experience nasal congestion and intermittent epistaxis. On histology, the upper respiratory mucosa shows increases in gland activity, phagocyte activity, mucopolysaccharide production, and hyperemia. These changes are similar in appearance to an allergic reaction, but they are actually due to increased levels of female sex hormones during pregnancy. Of note, the mucosal appearance in pregnant but asymptomatic women often has the same microscopic appearance.

Digestive System

Most changes to the digestive system are side effects of hemodilution, estrogen, and progesterone. Albumin and total protein levels appear decreased due to volume overload. Nonetheless, the body's new set point favors Na^+ and water absorption in the large intestine. Progesterone reduces small-bowel motility, leading to constipation. Estrogen increases 3-hydroxy-3-methylglutaryl coenzyme A (HMG-CoA) reductase activity, and progesterone delays gallbladder emptying, thus promoting supersaturation of bile with cholesterol and the formation of gallstones. Smooth muscle relaxation of the lower esophageal sphincter leads to gastroesophageal reflux disease and nausea. Lastly, portal

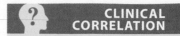

hypertension, spider angiomas, and palmar erythema due to high estrogen levels can mimic liver disease.

Endocrine System

Human placental lactogen induces maternal insulin resistance to ensure continued transport of nutrients from mother to fetus. This leads to fasting hypoglycemia and postprandial hyperglycemia in the mother, in other words, glucose intolerance. With the body's response to insulin numbed, pancreatic β-cell hypertrophy results in **hyperinsulinemia** and an increased risk of gestational diabetes.

Triglycerides (TGs), high- and low-density lipoproteins (HDLs and LDLs), and total cholesterol levels all increase during pregnancy, as they are necessary precursors for steroidogenesis in the maternal adrenal glands. Progesterone, a cortisol antagonist, prevents Cushing-like effects that might otherwise be caused by increased adrenal function and delayed plasma clearance of cortisol.

Effects on the pituitary and thyroid are more subtle. Despite negative feedback by estradiol and progesterone (which decrease FSH and LH), the pituitary gland enlarges and increases its secretion of prolactin. Although hCG mimics the activity of thyroid-stimulating hormone (TSH) in the first trimester (potentially abnormal thyroid function tests), the mother remains euthyroid throughout the pregnancy. Estrogen causes an increase in hepatic synthesis of thyroxine-binding globulin (TBG), but free triiodothyronine (T_3) and thyroxine (T_4) levels remain relatively normal.

Immune System

Changes to immune function during pregnancy are complex. Estrogen and cortisol cause a progressive rise in white blood cell count—mostly polymorphonuclear leukocytes. This preference for granulocytes over lymphocytes and monocytes favors innate immunity over adaptive immunity. Progesterone, on the other hand, reduces the immune response, ostensibly to prevent rejection of the "foreign" fetus. The pregnant uterus is also an immune-privileged site, utilizing a number of sophisticated mechanisms to promote tolerance of the fetus.

Skin and Bones

To maintain her center of gravity, a pregnant woman experiences increased inward curvature of the spine (spinal lordosis). In anticipation of the birthing process, the woman's pubic symphysis also widens. **Relaxin,** the peptide hormone responsible for this process, causes relaxation of other ligaments as well.

Increased levels of active vitamin D [1,25-$(OH)_2$] increase intestinal absorption of Ca^{2+} so it can be transported across the placenta. Calcitonin keeps Ca^{2+} resorption from bone from becoming overactive to protect the maternal skeleton. Parathyroid hormone levels, on the other hand, are not particularly high because increased intestinal absorption keeps Ca^{2+} levels from falling too low. Despite all of these changes, the maternal serum ionized Ca^{2+} and phosphate levels remain normal.

Some of the most obvious changes during pregnancy occur in the skin. Estrogen-induced angiogenesis accounts for facial flushing, and estrogen also plays a role in the tearing of collagen that leads to stretch marks. Hyperinsulinemia may contribute to **linea nigra** (a hyperpigmented band down the midline) and hirsutism.

Table 9-11 reviews the key physiologic changes during pregnancy in these organ systems.

Other important aspects of pregnancy are related to the health of the fetus.

TABLE 9-11.   Maternal Adaptations to Pregnancy

SYSTEM	PARAMETER	ALTERATION
Blood	Volume	Increases by 50% in second trimester
	Hematocrit	Decreases slightly
	Fibrinogen	Increases
	Systemic coagulation	Hypercoagulable state
Cardiovascular	Heart rate	Gradually increases 10–15%; increased incidence of arrhythmias
	Blood pressure	Gradually decreases 10% by 34 weeks, then increases to prepregnancy values
	Stroke volume	Increases to maximum at 19 weeks, then plateaus; ejection fraction unchanged
	Cardiac output	Rises rapidly by 20%, then gradually increases an additional 10% by 28 weeks
	Peripheral venous distention	Progressive increase to term
	Peripheral vascular resistance	Progressive decrease to term
Gastrointestinal	Sphincter tone	Decreases
	Gastric emptying time	Unchanged; increases only with opioid administration and during painful labor
	Intestinal motility	Gallbladder, small and large intestine decreased
Pulmonary	Respiratory rate	Unchanged
	Tidal volume	Increases by 30–40%
	Expiratory reserve	Gradual decrease
	Vital capacity	Unchanged
	Respiratory minute volume	Increases by 40%
Renal	Renal plasma flow	Increases early by 50–80%, then declines to term
	Glomular filtration rate	Increases 40–50% by early second trimester, then declines slightly to term
	Solute and electrolyte values	Decreased creatinine and blood urea nitrogen, slight decrease in plasma osmolarity and sodium
Weight	Uterine weight	Increases from about 60–70 g to about 900–1200 g
	Body weight	Average 11-kg (25-lb) increase

Prenatal Testing

Standard prenatal screening tests include routine blood work, urinalysis, and ultrasound examinations. Other tests may be offered based on the mother's risk factors, such as age, race, and comorbidities.

Maternal serum α-fetoprotein (AFP) was one of the first screening tests developed. High levels suggest an open neural tube defect such as cephalocele or spina bifida, whereas

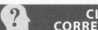

CLINICAL CORRELATION

hCG levels are elevated in women with hydatidiform mole (HM) and choriocarcinoma. hCG can activate TSH receptors, as hCG and TSH share an identical alpha subunit. Thus, HM and choriocarcinoma can present with signs and symptoms of thyrotoxicosis (anxiety, tachycardia, tremor, warm skin) due to very high hCG levels.

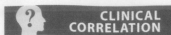
CLINICAL CORRELATION

Though ABO blood type incompatibility occurs in approximately 20% of pregnancies, only a minority of these cases result in hemolytic anemia. This is because, unlike Rh incompatibility, which generates IgG antibodies that readily cross the placenta, ABO incompatibility generates IgM antibodies that do not. Thus, fetal hemolysis is uncommon in ABO incompatibility. Nonetheless, ABO blood type incompatibility is the most common cause of neonatal jaundice in the developed world.

CLINICAL CORRELATION

Preeclampsia (hypertension, edema, and proteinuria) is a disease of the placenta. It is due to defective spiral artery remodeling and trophoblast invasion. The resulting placental hypoperfusion and ischemia cause the release of antiangiogenic factors into the maternal circulation, which alters vascular endothelial cell function.

FLASH BACK

Fetal Circulation:
Oxygenated blood flows into the IVC → RA → foramen ovale → LA → LV → aorta → head.
Deoxygenated blood flows into the SVC → RV.
Mixed blood flows from the RV → pulmonary artery → ductus arteriosus → aorta → lower body.

KEY FACT

After birth, inspiration increases Po_2 and causes release of bradykinin, two factors that close the ductus arteriosus. Indomethacin, a nonsteroidal anti-inflammatory drug, can also be used to close the shunt in hypoxic newborns by inhibiting prostaglandin production, specifically PGE2, which helps to keep the ductus open.

low levels suggest Down syndrome. The **quad test,** which makes use of multiple markers (AFP, estriol, hCG, and inhibin-A) is even more accurate (low false-positive rate).

Chorionic villus sampling (CVS) and amniocentesis are two common means of testing for chromosomal abnormalities. They are compared in Table 9-12.

The Placenta

Trophoblasts, cells forming the outer layer of the blastocyst, are the first cells to differentiate from the fertilized egg. They go on to develop into two layers: the inner cytotrophoblasts and outer syncytiotrophoblasts. The latter cells secrete hCG and attach to the uterine wall (endometrial stroma).

In the second trimester, the placenta takes over production of estrogen and progesterone, causing the corpus luteum to degrade into a corpus albicans.

The placenta is illustrated in Figure 9-38. Each gram of placenta can support 7 g of fetal tissue.

Fetal Circulation

The fetal circulatory system (see Figure 9-38) is different from that of the adult. It must both make use of the maternal blood supply via the placenta and avoid overperfusing the lungs while no gas exchange is occurring there (Figure 9-39). The three fetal shunts that allow this to occur are described in Table 9-13 (see also Figure 1-9).

Furthermore, fetal hemoglobin (HbF) is more concentrated in fetal blood and has a greater affinity for O_2 than does maternal HbA. In other words, at any given oxygen partial pressure (Po_2), HbF has a greater O_2 saturation than HbA. This is the case because the γ-subunit of HbF has a weaker positive charge than the adult β-subunit, so 2,3-bisphosphoglycerate (2,3-BPG) has less of an effect on lowering its O_2 affinity.

For an adult, these circulatory modifications are unnecessary. Thus, three key changes allow for the transition from fetal to normal adult circulation:

- Pulmonary vascular resistance (PVR) decreases.
- SVR increases.
- The fetal shunts close so the pulmonary and systemic circulations operate in parallel.

At birth, the sphincter in the ductus venosus constricts and closes the ductus venosus; cutting off the placental blood supply causes portal blood to enter the hepatic sinusoids, resulting in a drop in BP in the IVC and right atrium (RA). Inspiration by the newborn increases Po_2 and causes release of bradykinin, which induces vasoconstriction and closure of the ductus arteriosus. Accompanied by reduced PVR from lung expansion,

TABLE 9-12. **Diagnostic Testing for Chromosomal Abnormalities**

	CVS	AMNIOCENTESIS
What is it?	Biopsy of rapidly dividing cells in the placenta	Amniotic fluid retrieval of amniocytes
When can it be done?	Early pregnancy (10–12 wk)	Midpregnancy (15–19 wk)
Risk of pregnancy loss?	1%	0.5%

CVS, chorionic villus sampling.

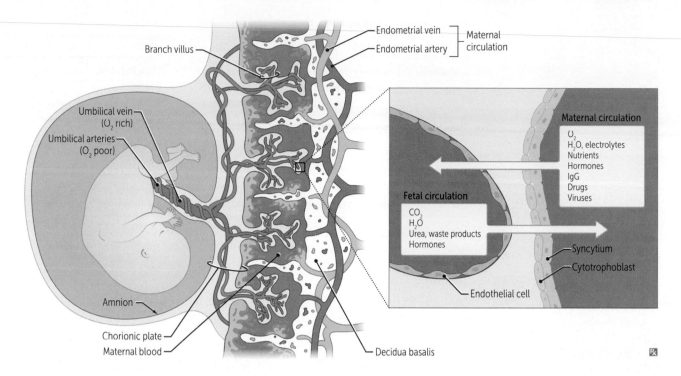

FIGURE 9-38. **The placenta in cross-section.**

this results in increased pulmonary blood flow. The left atrial (LA) pressure rises and the RA pressure decreases, closing the foramen ovale, and thus functionally setting up the normal adult systemic circulation. Anatomic closure occurs with the formation of fibrous tissue.

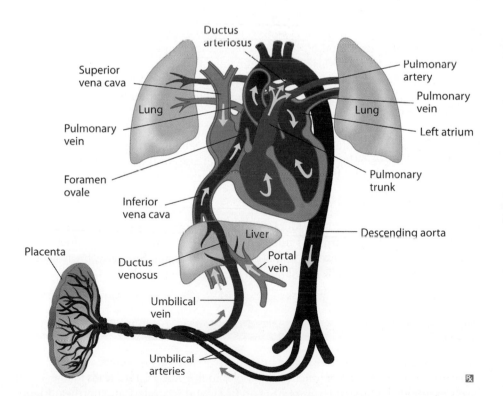

FIGURE 9-39. **Overview of fetal circulation.** Path of fetal blood flow from the umbilical veins through the physiological fetal shunts and out through the umbilical arteries.

> **KEY FACT**
>
> There is no direct contact between maternal and fetal blood.

> **CLINICAL CORRELATION**
>
> Maintaining a patent ductus arteriosus (PDA) with prostaglandins may actually be necessary in anatomic abnormalities such as **coarctation of the aorta, transposition of the great arteries,** and **tetralogy of Fallot.**

> **KEY FACT**
>
> Monozygotic twins are always of the same sex (except in cases of meiotic nondisjunction, eg, XO).
> Dizygotic twins can be the same or different sex.

TABLE 9-13. **Shunts in the Fetal Circulation**

SHUNT	LOCATION	FUNCTION	FLOW	OXYGENATION
Ductus arteriosus	Between the aorta and pulmonary trunk (artery)	Decreases pulmonary blood flow	High PVR, low pulmonary blood flow	Mixed blood
Foramen ovale	Between the RA and LA	Decreases pulmonary blood flow	High PVR, low pulmonary blood flow	Mixed blood
Ductus venosus	Connects umbilical vein to the IVC (bypasses liver)	Imports maternal blood	Regulated by a sphincter	Oxygen-rich blood

IVC, inferior vena cava; LA, left atrium; PVR, pulmonary vascular resistance; RA, right atrium.

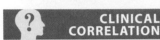
CLINICAL CORRELATION

Chorionicity in monozygotic twins can usually be determined by ultrasound. Some dichorionic, diamniotic gestations, however, feature a fused placenta, which falsely gives the appearance of a monochorionic, diamniotic pregnancy.

KEY FACT

Twinning can only occur within the first 15 days following fertilization.

KEY FACT

Having monozygotic twins is primarily based on chance (1:250 pregnancies) and not greatly affected by newer reproductive technology. The likelihood of having dizygotic twins can be influenced by many factors such as fertility drugs, in vitro fertilization, and increased maternal age at conception (due to higher levels of FSH). Thus, dizygotic twins may run in families, but monozygotic twins do not.

KEY FACT

Breast milk contains antimicrobial, immunomodulating, and anti-inflammatory agents not found in formula.

Twinning

Multiple fetal gestation, though not a true pathologic state, is a natural cause of premature birth. The average gestational age for twins is 35 weeks, and for triplets it is 33 weeks.

Fraternal (dizygotic) twins, which result from two fertilized ova (two sperm, two eggs), always have their own chorion and amniotic sac. Identical (monozygotic) twins, derived from a single ovum (one sperm, one egg), usually share a chorion but have separate amniotic sacs. About one-third of monozygotic twins do have unique chorions and amniotic sacs, however, depending on when the ovum splits. Figure 9-40 illustrates this timeline.

Breast-Feeding

During pregnancy, estrogen and progesterone levels are high. These hormones ready the breasts for milk production. However, estrogen antagonizes **prolactin,** preventing lactation. After expulsion of the placenta, estrogen and progesterone levels drop, removing the blockade of prolactin. The suckling of an infant on the breast stimulates prolactin secretion from the anterior pituitary and subsequent milk production. The posterior pituitary secretes **oxytocin,** which expels the milk into the lactiferous ducts (the milk "letdown" reflex).

Breast milk is a dynamic fluid that changes both throughout the day and over the course of lactation. For example, though the volume decreases over a single feeding, the fat content increases. Similarly, breast milk is particularly rich in immunoglobulins (IgA) within the first 5 days after delivery.

It is believed that breast-feeding reduces a child's chances of acquiring acute infections (eg, respiratory syncytial virus, GI infections, and otitis media), chronic illnesses (eg, leukemia, irritable bowel disease, and obesity), and allergies. Similarly, breast-feeding seems to reduce the mother's risk of ovarian and premenopausal breast cancer, as well as that of osteoporosis and anemia.

MENOPAUSE

The cessation of menstruation, called menopause, occurs at an average age of 52 years and results from depletion of functional follicles in the ovaries. This leads to low serum levels of estradiol, elevated levels of FSH and LH, and secondary amenorrhea. Figure

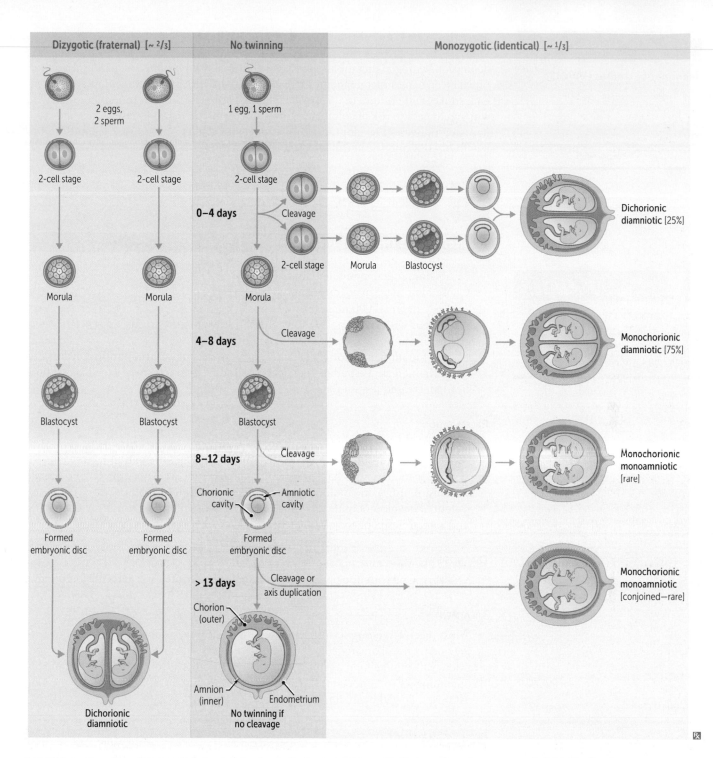

FIGURE 9-40. **Development of single fetus (no twinning) and dizygotic (fraternal) and monozygotic (identical) twins.**

9-35 shows the variation of FSH and LH levels with age. Recall that these two hormones normally stimulate production of estrogen, but after menopause, estrogen and inhibin levels drop due to ovarian failure. Lack of feedback inhibition generates very high levels of FSH and LH. A woman's lifetime estrogen exposure is an important risk factor for the development of breast and endometrial cancers. Increased estrogen exposure is associated with early menarche, late menopause, nulliparity, and not breast-feeding.

Some women experience symptoms such as palpitations, joint pain, decreased libido, vaginal dryness, and poor sleep (leading to forgetfulness and irritability) during meno-

KEY FACT

Hormonal changes in menopause lead to reduced estrogen, higher FSH, higher LH (no surges), and higher GnRH.

pause. Estrogen hormone replacement therapy (HRT) counteracts many of these symptoms, positively affecting the central nervous system to improve cognition and reducing depression. Estrogen therapy also preserves bone mass and inhibits hot flashes. However, unbalanced oral estrogen therapy increases a woman's risk of thromboembolic phenomena, stroke, and endometrial cancer. Similarly, estrogen-progesterone therapy (EPT), which reduces the risk of colorectal cancer, increases the risk of breast cancer and coronary heart disease. Development of these negative effects, of course, depends on the length of HRT and the age at which it is given.

Pathology—Genetic Diseases

KLINEFELTER SYNDROME (47,XXY)

- Most common congenital abnormality.
- Cause of primary hypogonadism.
- Affects 1 in 500–1000 male births.
- Associated with maternal meiotic nondisjunction and advanced maternal age, though it can be maternal or paternal in origin.
- Loss of functional Sertoli cells and increased aromatase function in Leydig cells results in increased estradiol, increased LH and FSH (due to loss of feedback inhibition), decreased testosterone, and decreased inhibin.

PRESENTATION

- Hypogonadism: Small and firm testes; **infertility** due to azoospermia.
- **Tall, eunuchoid body shape with disproportionately long extremities.**
- Female secondary sex characteristics at puberty, such as gynecomastia and female hair distribution, due to decreased testosterone:estradiol ratio.
- Potential developmental delay, inability to sustain attention, impulsive behavior, and sometimes poor social interaction.

DIAGNOSIS

47,XXY karyotype with one of the X chromosomes inactivated in each cell (Barr body).

TREATMENT

- Most receive lifelong testosterone therapy to induce puberty and maintain male secondary sex characteristics.
- Men with Klinefelter may still father children through advanced fertility techniques, including sperm retrieval via testicular biopsy and intracytoplasmic sperm injection (ICSI), followed by in vitro fertilization (IVF).

TURNER SYNDROME

Primary hypogonadism in phenotypic females resulting from partial or complete monosomy (45,X). Short stature is related to loss of regions on the short arm of the X chromosome. Loss of regions of the long arm of the X chromosome is associated with amenorrhea and premature loss of ovarian follicles but not with short stature. If there is any Y chromosome mosaicism, there is increased risk for gonadoblastoma (germ cell tumor) and removal of ovaries is required. Patients typically have either primary ovarian failure (primary amenorrhea) or premature ovarian failure (premature menopause).

PRESENTATION

- Newborns may have **webbed neck** (cystic hygroma), edema of the hands and feet, **coarctation of the aorta,** characteristic triangular facies, pulmonary stenosis, and **bicuspid aortic valve.**
- Children and adolescents classically are described as being **short in stature** and having a "shield chest" with widely spaced nipples, streak ovaries, and **amenorrhea.** These girls often maintain prepubescent genitalia with little pubic hair and fail to develop secondary sex characteristics.

DIAGNOSIS

Karyotyping (no Barr body) is the definitive diagnostic test. High FSH:LH ratio due to decreased estrogen.

TREATMENT

Teenage patients need counseling regarding stigmata of their condition and treatment with hormone therapy. Estrogen is given for development of secondary sexual characteristics, normal menstruation, and osteoporosis prevention. Growth hormone may be given to increase the height of affected patients.

PROGNOSIS

Patients with 45,X (most common) or 45,X mosaicism have a low fertility rate. Those who become pregnant have increased rates of spontaneous abortion (30%), stillbirths (6–10%), and maternal death (2%).

DOUBLE Y MALES (XYY SYNDROME)

- Affects 1 in 1000 male births and results from paternal nondisjunction in meiosis II, resulting in a sperm with an extra Y chromosome.
- Tall males, severe cystic acne, lower mean IQ, and more behavioral problems than unaffected males.
- Mild delay in motor and language development. Increased incidence of autism spectrum disorder and attention-deficit hyperactivity disorder (ADHD).
- Increased tendency to be convicted of a criminal offense due to poor judgment and low socioeconomic status, not aggressiveness as previously thought.

MALE PSEUDOHERMAPHRODITE

Genetic male (46,XY) with ambiguous or female external genitalia (eg, vagina with blind pouch). Testes are present. However, there is either an **absolute** or **functional testosterone** deficiency, possibly due to any of the following causes:

- Defective testicular differentiation.
- Impaired secretion/production of testosterone.
- Failure of conversion of testosterone to DHT (**5α-reductase deficiency**).
- Defect of androgen receptors (most common is **androgen insensitivity syndrome**).

5α-Reductase Type 2 Deficiency

- 5α-Reductase catalyzes the conversion of testosterone to DHT, a potent androgen required for the development of male external genitalia and secondary sexual characteristics.
- Affected males have female or ambiguous external genitalia at birth due to defective virilization in utero, though testes are functional and possess normal internal male genitalia.

- Since functioning testes produce testosterone and MIF, **internal genitalia** develop in a male pattern.
- Increased testosterone production at **puberty** generates sufficient levels of DHT either via 5α-reductase type 1 activity in the liver, skin, and brain or low-level expression of 5α-reductase type 2 in the testes. This causes **masculinization** and increased growth of external genitalia.

Androgen Insensitivity

- X-linked disorder. Genetically male (46,XY) but phenotypically female. Most common cause of male pseudohermaphroditism.
- Mutation of androgen receptor. Decreased or absent response to androgens, though androgen production is normal.
- Complete (CAIS) and partial androgen insensitivity (PAIS) forms exist. Degree of androgen receptor function determines phenotype.
- CAIS phenotype: Normal female external genitalia, short blind-ending vagina. Functional testes found in labia majora, inguinal canal, or abdominal cavity. At puberty, breast development, sparse to absent pubic hair, and primary amenorrhea are seen.
- CAIS internal sex organs: Testes produce MIF and testosterone. MIF inhibits development of paramesonephric structures (uterus, cervix, fallopian tubes, and upper two-thirds of vagina). Male mesonephric structures (ductus deferens, prostate gland, epididymis, and seminal vesicles) cannot respond to testosterone and are absent.
- CAIS diagnosis: Karyotype is essential. Most hormone levels are normal. After puberty, slightly elevated testosterone, DHT, LH, and estradiol levels may be seen.
- PAIS: Less severe. External genitalia may appear female, male, or ambiguous. Phenotype varies from female, with mild virilization, partially fused labioscrotal folds, and clitoromegaly, to fertile but poorly virilized men. Testes can be inguinal to scrotal.
- PAIS is often called "penis at 12" syndrome. Increased androgen production during puberty raises DHT levels sufficiently to cause appreciable penile growth.
- In CAIS, and if testes are cryptorchid in PAIS, there is an increased risk of developing germ cell tumors and gonadoblastoma. Orchiectomy is recommended in these cases.

FEMALE PSEUDOHERMAPHRODITE

- Genetic females (XX) with virilized or ambiguous external genitalia due to excessive and inappropriate exposure to androgens during the 8th to 13th weeks of gestation.
- Commonly seen in congenital adrenal hyperplasia.

OVOTESTICULAR DISORDER OF SEX DEVELOPMENT (FORMERLY TRUE HERMAPHRODITISM)

- Presence of both ovaries and testes in the same individual, which may be due to XX/XY mosaicism or abnormal crossover of a region of the Y chromosome containing the SRY region with the X chromosome in an XX individual.
- The external genitalia may be normal male, ambiguous (most common), or normal female.
- Cryptorchidism and hypospadias are common.
- The gonads are most often ovotestes, followed by ovaries, and, least commonly, testes.
- The development of the genital ducts follows that of the ipsilateral gonad.
- Germ cell tumors, inguinal hernias, and obstructed genital tracts frequently occur in true hermaphrodites.

KEY FACT

Mosaicism is the presence of two or more genetically distinct cell lines in one individual.

KALLMANN SYNDROME

- Autosomal dominant. A form of secondary hypogonadotropic hypogonadism.
- Presents as failure to complete puberty in both males and females. Secondary sex characteristics are absent or severely reduced.
- Due to defective neuron migration of GnRH producing cells.
- Decreased hypothalamic GnRH production, with a subsequent decrease in FSH, LH, and testosterone production, and infertility.
- Low sperm count in males; amenorrhea in females.
- Patients also fail to form an olfactory bulb, resulting in the characteristic finding of anosmia (lack of sense of smell).

MÜLLERIAN AGENESIS

Characterized by the congenital absence of the vagina with variable uterine development. It is the second most common cause of primary amenorrhea.

The incidence rate is 1 in 4000–5000 live female births. Affected individuals have normal ovaries and normal secondary sexual characteristics. The exact cause is unknown.

PRESENTATION

- Primary amenorrhea in the presence of normal secondary sexual characteristics.
- The vagina may be absent or shortened.
- The labia majora, labia minora, and clitoris are normal.
- Ectopic kidneys are common. Some patients may present with voiding difficulties, recurrent UTIs, and urinary incontinence.

DIAGNOSIS

- Ultrasound or MRI can often be diagnostic.
- Laparoscopy is performed if there is an unclear diagnosis or pain from functioning obstructed Müllerian remnants, possibly with a higher rate of endometriosis.
- After administration of IV contrast medium and subsequent excretion by the kidneys, a pyelogram is performed to assess for frequently associated urinary tract abnormalities.

TREATMENT

- Progressive dilation or reconstructive surgery on the foreshortened vagina can be performed to make the vagina more functional, and this may establish sexual functioning. Sometimes intercourse itself can serve this same purpose.
- Rudimentary uterine horns may need to be excised to prevent pain if they have functioning endometrium.

FLASH BACK

Fused lower ends of the Müllerian (paramesonephric) ducts form the uterus, fallopian tubes, cervix, and upper two-thirds of the vagina.

KEY FACT

The stratified squamous epithelium of the anus and vagina are derived from the cloaca and have somatic innervation from the pudendal nerve. The structures superior have columnar epithelium and visceral innervation.

KEY FACT

Renal abnormalities are found in 20–30% of women with Müllerian duct abnormalities.

Pathology—Female

PREGNANCY PATHOLOGY

Teratogens

The fetus is most susceptible to damage by teratogens during organogenesis (weeks 3–8 of gestation). Exposure before 3 weeks is likely to result in loss of the pregnancy. Exposure later in pregnancy usually affects fetal growth and maturation of fetal organs (Table 9-14).

TABLE 9-14. Teratogens

TERATOGEN	EFFECT(S) ON FETUS	NOTES
Medications (common uses)		
Angiotensin-converting enzyme (ACE) inhibitors (hypertension, renal protection in type 2 diabetes)	Renal agenesis/dysfunction, leading to subsequent congenital malformations (ie, Potter sequence)	
Alkylating agents (chemotherapy)	Absence of digits	
Aminoglycosides (antibiotics)	Ototoxicity	Aminoglycosides can also cause ototoxicity in adults when given in high enough doses
Carbamazepine (anticonvulsant, neuropathic pain)	Facial dysmorphism, developmental delay, neural tube defects, phalanx/fingernail hypoplasia	
Diethylstilbestrol (DES; prevention of miscarriage)	Vaginal clear cell adenocarcinoma, congenital Müllerian anomalies	DES is a synthetic estrogen that is no longer manufactured due to its known teratogenic effects. Patients who may have been exposed in utero were born in the 1940s–1970s
Folate antagonists, eg, methotrexate and trimethoprim (chemotherapy, immunosuppression, antimicrobial/antiparasitics)	Neural tube defects	
Isotretinoin (treatment of acne)	Multiple severe birth defects	Females are required by the federal government to be on two forms of contraception. All patients are barred from donating blood due to fear it may be transfused into a pregnant woman
Lithium (bipolar disorder)	Ebstein anomaly (atrialized right ventricle)	
Methimazole (hyperthyroidism)	Aplasia cutis congenita	
Phenytoin (anticonvulsant)	Fetal hydantoin syndrome (cleft palate, cardiac defects, phalanx/fingernail hypoplasia)	
Tetracyclines (antibiotic)	Discolored teeth	
Thalidomide (antinausea)	Limb defects	Now strictly contraindicated for use in pregnancy but still used as an immunomodulator in many diseases, including leprosy and multiple myeloma
Valproate (anticonvulsant)	Neural tube defects due to inhibition of maternal folate absorption	
Warfarin (anticoagulant)	Bone deformities, fetal hemorrhage, abortion, eye abnormalities	Heparin is the anticoagulant of choice in pregnancy because it does not cross the placenta
Environmental exposures		
Alcohol	Fetal alcohol syndrome, which includes developmental delay, heart defects, and characteristic head/face abnormalities (microcephaly, smooth philtrum, hypertelorism)	**Most common cause of intellectual disability in the United States**

(continues)

TABLE 9-14. Teratogens *(continued)*

TERATOGEN	EFFECT(S) ON FETUS	NOTES
Cocaine	Intrauterine growth restriction (IUGR), usually secondary to decreased placental blood flow, placental abruption	Most of cocaine's effects are mediated by its action as a powerful vasoconstrictor
Smoking	IUGR/low birth weight, preterm labor, placental insufficiency	The nicotine found in tobacco is a vasoconstrictor, which reduces placental blood flow. CO found in tobacco smoke binds hemoglobin more avidly than O_2, resulting in decreased oxygen delivery to the fetus
X-rays	Microcephaly, intellectual disability	
Nutritional		
Folate (B_9) deficiency	Neural tube defects	Nutritional folate deficiency is exceedingly rare in industrialized countries due to the addition of folate to food products (eg, flours, cereals) and use of prenatal vitamins
Iodine deficiency or excess	Thyroid issues (cretinism or congenital goiter)	
Maternal diabetes	Caudal regression syndrome, congenital heart defects, neural tube defects	Maternal diabetes may be preexisting or brought on by gestation
Vitamin A excess	Extremely high risk for spontaneous abortions and birth defects	Vitamin A excess is rare and usually due to massive oversupplementation (or consumption of liver)

Placental Disorders

Placental Abruption

Separation of normally implanted placenta due to hemorrhage in the decidua basalis of the endometrium before the delivery of the fetus (Figure 9-41A). Severe abruptions have a 25% rate of perinatal mortality.

PRESENTATION

Painful **vaginal bleeding** in third trimester, **tender uterus,** fetal distress, hypertonus, and/or stillbirth. Sometimes, the bleeding may be severe, leading to shock, and it can also lead to disseminated intravascular coagulation (DIC). The bleeding is often painful. Risk factors include hypertension, previous placental abruption, and **cocaine use.**

DIAGNOSIS

Mainly clinical. A retroplacental clot on ultrasound is specific for abruption.

TREATMENT

Prompt delivery of the fetus via cesarean section if mother is hemodynamically unstable or fetus is showing signs of distress. Vaginal delivery is preferred if the fetus is deceased and the mother is stable.

Placenta Accreta

Defect in the decidua basalis leading to abnormal implantation of the placenta (Figure 9-41B). When the Nitabuch membrane is deficient, the trophoblastic tissue attaches directly to the myometrium. Incomplete separation of the placenta during delivery leads to profuse hemorrhage.

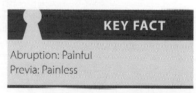

KEY FACT

Abruption: Painful
Previa: Painless

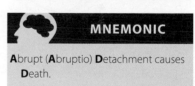

MNEMONIC

Abrupt (**A**bruptio) **D**etachment causes **D**eath.

PRESENTATION

Profuse placental hemorrhage during delivery.

DIAGNOSIS

Sonography may help diagnosis in the antepartum period.

TREATMENT

Hysterectomy.

Placenta Previa

Implantation of the placenta over or near the internal cervical os (Figure 9-41C). The incidence of placenta previa is 1 in 300 deliveries in the United States. Risk factors include multiparity, previous placenta previa, and prior cesarean section.

PRESENTATION

Painless vaginal bleeding at the end of the second trimester or later. The uterus is soft and nontender.

DIAGNOSIS

Sonography is the initial investigation of choice for localization of the placenta.

> **CLINICAL CORRELATION**
>
> **Do not** perform vaginal examination in any woman who is > 20 weeks pregnant with vaginal bleeding. The digital examination may rupture the previa or worsen placental abruption.

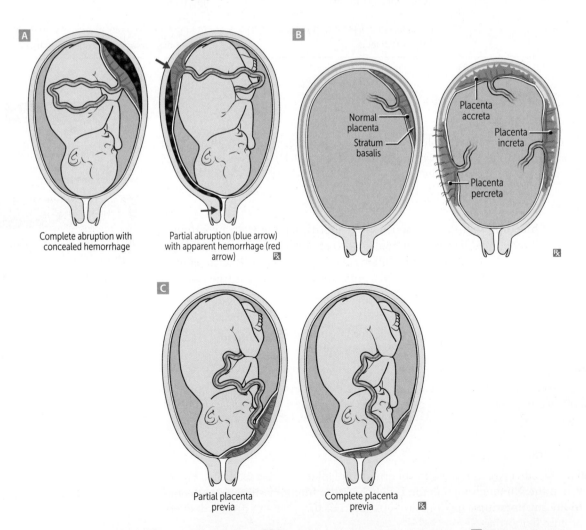

A Complete abruption with concealed hemorrhage

Partial abruption (blue arrow) with apparent hemorrhage (red arrow)

B Normal placenta / Stratum basalis / Placenta accreta / Placenta increta / Placenta percreta

C Partial placenta previa

Complete placenta previa

FIGURE 9-41. **Placental disorders.** **A** Placental abruption. **B** Placenta accreta, increta, and percreta. **C** Placenta previa.

TREATMENT

The choice of treatment depends on gestational age, maternal and fetal conditions, and the amount of bleeding. Delivery is via cesarian section.

EXPECTANT MANAGEMENT

If fetal lung maturity is not achieved, the pregnancy may be prolonged using tocolytics and dexamethasone.

COMPLICATIONS

- **Maternal:** Hemorrhage, shock, and death.
- **Fetal:** Prematurity and perinatal mortality.

Ectopic Pregnancy

Implantation of blastocysts outside the uterine cavity. The most common location for ectopic pregnancy is the **ampulla of the fallopian tube.** The rate of ectopic pregnancy is 2% of all pregnancies in the United States, with African Americans at increased risk. Risk factors include **previous tubal or abdominal surgery, previous ectopic pregnancy, IUD use, pelvic inflammatory disease (PID)**, infertility, and current smoking. A pregnancy in a patient with an IUD is more likely to be ectopic because the chances of an intrauterine pregnancy are greatly reduced.

PRESENTATION

Patient classically presents with amenorrhea, abdominal pain, vaginal bleeding, fainting, or dizziness. On examination, abdominal tenderness and cervical motion tenderness may be present, and an adnexal mass can be palpated.

DIAGNOSIS

Urine pregnancy test, sonogram, and measurement of β-hCG are extremely sensitive diagnostic tests. Transvaginal sonography is more sensitive for a gestational sac.

TREATMENT

- **Medical:** Methotrexate (MTX) is the drug of choice for medical management. MTX is a folate antagonist that is able to kill rapidly dividing trophoblastic cells.
- **Surgical:** Laparoscopic salpingostomy or salpingectomy. A laparotomy approach can be used in unstable patients.

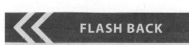

FLASH BACK

MTX inhibits dihydrofolate reductase, resulting in a decrease in deoxythymidine monophosphate, purine nucleotides, and amino acids and a consequent decrease in DNA and protein synthesis.

Amniotic Fluid Abnormalities

Amniotic fluid is produced by the fetus, aids in normal growth and development, and helps protect the fetus. Too much (polyhydramnios) or too little (oligohydramnios) amniotic fluid can lead to abnormalities in the developing fetus.

Polyhydramnios

- May result from inability to swallow amniotic fluid.
- Associated with fetal intestinal atresia, esophageal/duodenal atresia, anencephaly, maternal diabetes, neural tube defects, and multiple gestations.
- Amniotic fluid index (AFI) > 24 cm or amniotic fluid volume > 1.5–2 L.

Oligohydramnios

- Associated with ruptured membranes, Potter syndrome, placental insufficiency, and agenesis of posterior urethral valves (in males) and resultant inability to excrete urine.
- AFI < 5 cm or amniotic fluid volume < 0.5 L.

Hypertension in Pregnancy

Gestational Hypertension

Elevated BP without proteinuria after 20 weeks of gestation and followed by disappearance within 12 weeks of delivery.

Preeclampsia

Defined as new-onset **hypertension** and **proteinuria** after 20 weeks of gestation. It has an incidence of 23.6 per 1000 deliveries in the United States. Placental dysfunction causes release of excess soluble fms-like tyrosine kinase-1 (sFlt-1), which binds growth factors vascular endothelial growth factor and **placental growth factor,** rendering them unavailable. This leads to vascular endothelial damage, vasoconstriction, hypertension, renal glomerular endothelial cell damage, and coagulation abnormalities. Intense vasospasm is induced by the release of various mediators like endothelin and thromboxane A_2. The degree of preeclampsia depends on the level of trophoblastic invasion by the placenta.

The criteria for preeclampsia:

- Systolic blood pressure (BP) > 140 mm Hg or diastolic BP > 90 mm Hg after 20 weeks of gestation, on two readings taken 4 hours apart while the patient is on bed rest.
- Proteinuria: 0.3 g or more per 24 hours, or protein/creatinine ratio ≥ 0.3.
- With or without edema (caused by loss of albumin in the urine).

Severe Preeclampsia

Preeclampsia is considered severe if there is severe end-organ dysfunction as manifested by one or more of the following criteria:

- Systolic BP > 160 mm Hg or diastolic BP > 110 mm Hg after 20 weeks of gestation measured on two readings taken 4 hours apart while the patient is on bed rest.
- Proteinuria: > 3 g on two random samples collected 4 hours apart.
- Oliguria (< 500 mL/24 h).
- **Severe headache.**
- Cerebral or visual disturbances.
- Pulmonary edema or cyanosis.
- **Epigastric or right upper quadrant tenderness.**
- Elevated liver enzymes.
- Low platelets (< 100,000/mm³).
- Intrauterine growth restriction.
- Death resulting from **cerebral hemorrhage** and **acute respiratory distress syndrome.**

Eclampsia

New-onset grand mal seizure in the setting of preeclampsia.

PRESENTATION

High BP with proteinuria or signs of severe preeclampsia with convulsive seizures, as discussed earlier. May lead to DIC.

TREATMENT

Delivery of the fetus is the definitive cure for preeclampsia. During labor and delivery, **magnesium sulfate** may prevent severe preeclampsia and eclampsia. Hydralazine and labetalol can be used to lower the BP. Vaginal delivery should be attempted whenever possible, weighing possible risks and benefits.

FLASH BACK

Prostacyclins and nitric oxide (potent) are vasodilators, and endothelin (potent), thromboxane A_2, and angiotensin II are vasoconstrictors.

KEY FACT

When symptoms of preeclampsia are present at < 20 weeks' gestation, suspect an underlying disorder such as lupus, a gestational trophoblastic neoplasm, or preexisting hypertension.

KEY FACT

Eclamptic seizures may occur as long as 48 hours after delivery.

Preeclampsia Superimposed on Chronic Hypertension

Sudden new-onset proteinuria, acute increase in hypertension, and/or development of HELLP syndrome.

HELLP Syndrome

- **H**emolysis, **E**levated **L**iver enzymes, and **L**ow **P**latelets in a pregnant woman.
- Mortality rate of 7–35%.
- Can occur during antepartum period and up to 1 week postpartum with or without superimposed preeclampsia or eclampsia.
- A positive feedback loop of endothelial damage and platelet activation, leading to release of thromboxane A_2 and serotonin, causing vasoconstriction and platelet aggregation.

PRESENTATION

- May present with vague complaints of malaise, epigastric pain, nausea and vomiting, and headache.
- The diagnosis is often delayed in the absence of superimposed eclampsia.
- Physical examination may reveal epigastric or right hypochondriac tenderness, edema, and hypertension with or without proteinuria.

DIAGNOSIS

- Hemolytic anemia (microangiopathic).
- Elevated liver enzymes and low platelets.

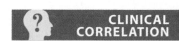

CLINICAL CORRELATION

Complete blood count and liver function tests should be done in any pregnant woman in the third trimester presenting with malaise. Suspect HELLP syndrome in a pregnant woman with a low platelet count.

TREATMENT

The best treatment for HELLP syndrome is termination of the pregnancy. **Corticosteroids** should be given to all patients with HELLP syndrome. Severe HELLP syndrome requires immediate delivery.

Sheehan Syndrome

Sheehan syndrome (postpartum hypopituitarism) is ischemic necrosis (infarction) of the pituitary gland due to postpartum hemorrhage. During pregnancy, the pituitary gland enlarges, and sudden massive obstetrical bleeding or hypovolemia may cause hypoxia, leading to pituitary necrosis. The anterior pituitary is more often involved than the posterior pituitary.

PRESENTATION

- Difficulty in lactation or failure to lactate (lack of prolactin) is the most common initial presentation.
- Other features include oligomenorrhea or amenorrhea.
- If diagnosis is missed at an earlier stage, may present with features of panhypopituitarism, such as hypothyroidism, secondary adrenal insufficiency, or adrenal crisis.

DIAGNOSIS

- Diagnosis made by features of hypopituitarism seen in a patient with a history of postpartum hemorrhage.
- Decreased levels of pituitary hormones, such as adrenocorticotropic hormone (ACTH), thyroid-stimulating hormone (TSH), FSH, LH, and growth hormone (GH), followed by a decreased level of target hormones, such as thyroxine, cortisol, estrogen, and progesterone.

TREATMENT

Replacement of target hormones, such as hydrocortisone, thyroxine, estrogen, and progesterone.

Amniotic Fluid Embolism Syndrome

- Embolism of amniotic fluid during labor and delivery.
- High mortality rate of 80–90%.
- Exact mechanism is unknown, but inflammatory cytokines and mediators are probably involved.

PRESENTATION

- Sudden-onset dyspnea, tachypnea, and cyanosis during or after labor and delivery.
- May also present with cardiogenic shock, hypoxemia, seizures, DIC, and bleeding.

DIAGNOSIS

- Arterial blood gas shows severe hypoxemia.
- Prolonged bleeding times, clotting times, hypofibrinogenemia, and increased fibrin degradation products can occur in the setting of DIC.
- Electrocardiogram may reveal sinus tachycardia, right ventricular strain pattern, and nonspecific ST segment changes.

TREATMENT

Supportive.

Erythroblastosis Fetalis

- Alloimmunization because of previous maternal exposure to foreign fetal RBCs leads to destruction of fetal RBCs by maternal antibodies directed against them.
- There are several types of RBC alloimmunization, but the most common is Rh incompatibility (especially RhD).
- An Rh-negative mother is sensitized with Rh-positive fetal RBCs and produces antibodies.
- During a subsequent pregnancy, Rh-specific IgG crosses the placenta into the fetus and coats Rh-positive fetal RBCs, causing hemolysis, hydrops, and hemolytic disease of the newborn.

PRESENTATION

- Anemia, hepatosplenomegaly, and jaundice.
- May present with edema, ascites, and pericardial/pleural effusion.
- Respiratory distress due to deficiency of surfactant and pulmonary hypoplasia.

DIAGNOSIS

Blood typing, Rh factor, and antibody screening of all pregnant patients, with paternal testing if maternal antibodies are found.

TREATMENT

- Rh immunoglobulin (RhoGAM) consisting of IgG anti-RhD antibodies (passive immunization) is given to the mother at 28 weeks of gestation, and again within 72 hours after delivery as prophylaxis.
- This solution of immunoglobulins binds and leads to the destruction of fetal RhD-positive red blood cells that have passed from the fetal circulation into the mother's circulation, and hence, does not allow for the mother to mount an immune response to RhD antigens.

KEY FACT

Passive immunization: Transfer of active presynthesized antibodies.
Active immunization: Transfer of an immunogen that stimulates the host's humoral immune system.

- RhoGAM is also routinely given to Rh-negative mothers after abortion, D&C, amniocentesis, chorionic villus sampling, abruptio placentae, placenta previa, and ectopic pregnancy, or after any bleeding during pregnancy.

Gestational Neoplasms

Hydatidiform Mole

Benign tumor of the chorionic villus resulting from abnormal fertilization of an ovum and characterized by abnormal proliferation of trophoblastic cells. The incidence is 7–10 times higher in Southeast Asian countries than in the Western world. Occurs in 1 of 1500 pregnancies in the United States. Increased maternal age is only a risk factor for complete mole and *not* incomplete mole.

Hydatidiform moles are classified into two different types (Table 9-15):

- **Complete mole:** Results from fertilization of an empty ovum by two sperm or a haploid sperm that divides its nuclear material and forms diploid chromosomes (46,XX or 46,XY). Therefore, the **complete** mole is **completely** paternal in origin. Fetal parts are **completely** absent, and the placenta is **completely** neoplastic.
- **Partial mole:** Results from fertilization of a normal ovum by two sperm cells or duplication of one sperm. It has **triploid chromosomes (69,XXY, 69,XXX, or 69,XYY)**. Partial mole is both maternal and paternal in origin and **partially** consists of identifiable fetal parts (see Table 9-15). Not all placental villi are neoplastic.

PRESENTATION

- **Complete mole:** First-trimester vaginal bleeding is the most common presentation. Additional features include excessive elevations in hCG, theca lutein cysts > 5 cm in diameter, excessive uterine size, hyperemesis gravidarum, **symptoms of preeclampsia in the first trimester,** and hyperthyroidism.
- **Partial mole:** Vaginal bleeding or the features of missed or incomplete abortion are the most common presentations of partial mole. The uterus is usually small for date.

TABLE 9-15.   **Classification of Hydatidiform Moles**

	COMPLETE MOLE	INCOMPLETE MOLE
Karyotype	46,XX (most common) or 46,XY	69,XXY or 69,XXX or 69,XXY
Components	Empty egg + 1 duplicated sperm or empty egg + 2 sperm	1 egg + 1 duplicated sperm or 1 egg + 2 sperm
Fetal parts	No	Yes
Histologic features	- Generalized swelling of chorionic villi - Diffuse trophoblastic hyperplasia - Marked trophoblastic atypia	- Focal swelling of chorionic villi - Focal trophoblastic hyperplasia - Mild trophoblastic atypia
hCG levels	Excessively elevated	Sometimes elevated
Progress to choriocarcinoma	2%	Rare
Risk of complications	15–20% malignant trophoblastic disease	Low risk of malignancy (< 5%)

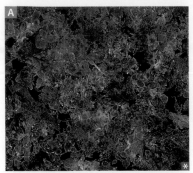

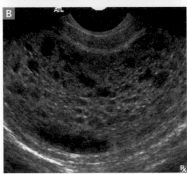

FIGURE 9-42. Hydatidiform mole. A Complete hydatidiform mole. Note the grape-like, fluid-filled clusters of chorionic villi. B "Snowstorm" ultrasound characteristic of complete mole.

DIAGNOSIS

- **Complete mole:** hCG is excessively elevated. Sonography is sensitive and specific, revealing a "snowstorm" pattern. "Honeycombed" uterus, appearance like a cluster of grapes on imaging, and swollen villi without fetal RBCs are other important features (Figure 9-42).
- **Partial mole:** hCG is rarely elevated above levels that are normal for pregnancy. Sonography shows focal cystic changes in the placenta and a ratio of transverse to anteroposterior diameter > 1.5.

TREATMENT

- **Suction curettage** is the method of choice for evacuation of the uterine cavity. It should be followed by curettage with a sharp curette to confirm complete evacuation of the products of conception.
- **Follow-up:** Postevacuation molar pregnancy should be followed up with weekly hCG measurements until three consecutive tests are negative.

PROGNOSIS

With complete mole, there is a 15–20% chance of development of postmolar gestation trophoblastic neoplasia (invasive mole and choriocarcinoma). With partial mole, the risk is only 2–4%.

Choriocarcinoma

Aggressive, malignant tumors composed of cytotrophoblasts and syncytiotrophoblasts arising from gestational chorionic epithelium. They usually follow evacuation of a mole with 2% of complete moles becoming choriocarcinoma.

PRESENTATION

- Recurrent vaginal bleeding after evacuation of a mole or following delivery, ectopic pregnancy, or abortion. hCG levels continue to rise after evacuation. Histologically, the cancer appears as hemorrhagic, necrotic masses within the uterus. **Chorionic villi are not present.**
- Metastases spread hematogenously and seed the lung (50%), vagina (35%), liver, and brain. Chemotherapy (methotrexate) is often curative.

VAGINAL DISEASES

Vaginismus

The involuntary contraction of the muscles of the pelvic floor, which causes pain and prevents vaginal penetration, including sexual intercourse and insertion of a speculum in gynecologic examinations. The exact cause is unknown, but it is important to investigate both physiologic and psychological causes. Treatment should be individualized based on the patient's condition.

Condyloma Acuminata (Genital Warts)

Occurs on the female genitalia, perineum, perianal area, and rectum. Genital warts result from human papillomavirus (HPV) infection acquired during sexual intercourse. Genital warts appear as soft, tan, cauliflower-like warts. Histologically, genital warts have epidermal hyperplasia with cytoplasmic vacuolization (**koilocytic change**) (Figure 9-43).

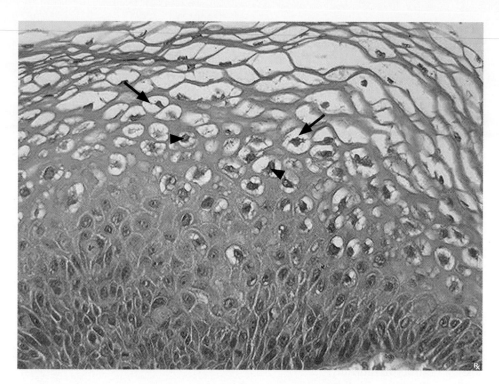

FIGURE 9-43.   Koilocytic change caused by human papillomavirus. Cytoplasmic vacuolization (arrows) is found around pyknotic nuclei (arrowheads).

Vaginal Tumors

Squamous Cell Carcinoma

Most common form of vaginal cancer with a mean age at presentation of 60 years. Squamous cell carcinoma may present with painless vaginal bleeding and discharge, commonly after intercourse. Commonly, it is an extension of a cervical squamous carcinoma with the primary lesion associated with high-risk HPV (eg, types 16, 18).

Clear Cell Adenocarcinoma

Correlated with girls in their late teens whose mothers took **diethylstilbestrol** (DES), an estrogen once believed to prevent miscarriage, during pregnancy. In one-third of the at-risk population, small glandular or microcystic inclusions appear in the vaginal mucosa (vaginal adenosis). Microscopically, malignant cells appear with clear cytoplasm.

Sarcoma Botryoides (Embryonal Rhabdomyosarcoma Variant)

Rare. Encountered in children < 5 years who present with vaginal bleeding and soft polypoid grape-like masses that protrude from the vagina. Histologically, sarcoma botryoides appears as a small, round, blue-cell tumor with skeletal muscle differentiation. It also expresses muscle-specific proteins including **desmin**.

CERVICAL PATHOLOGY

Dysplasia and Carcinoma in Situ

Abnormal organization of cells in cervical epithelium starting from the basal layer. It has a tendency to progress from mild to severe dysplasia, and finally to invasive carcinoma. Ninety-nine percent of cervical intraepithelial neoplasia (CIN) is associated with HPV infection. On biopsy, CIN is histologically classified as:

FLASH FORWARD

HPV types 16 and 18 cause 70% of cervical cancers. HPV expresses E6 and E7 oncoproteins that interact with p53 and Rb, respectively, leading to malignant transformation.

KEY FACT

The most common cancer of the vagina is squamous cell carcinoma, followed by adenocarcinoma. Malignant melanoma is the third most common cause of vaginal cancer.

The most common cancer of the vulva is also squamous cell carcinoma. However, melanoma ranks second for vulvar cancer.

KEY FACT

HPV attaches to and infects the basal layer of stratified squamous epithelium. This layer is most exposed, and therefore most likely to be infected, at the squamocolumnar junction (SCJ) between the endo- and ectocervix. In fact, it is the basal layer that is targeted in Pap tests.

- CIN I (mild dysplasia): Involves the basal third of the epithelium.
- CIN II (moderate dysplasia): Involves the basal two-thirds of the epithelium.
- CIN III (severe dysplasia): Involves more than two-thirds of the epithelium.
- Carcinoma in situ: Involves the entire thickness of the epithelium.

According to the Bethesda system for cytologic Papanicolaou (Pap) smear examinations, atypical squamous cells are classified into those of undetermined significance (ASCUS), low-grade squamous intraepithelial lesion (LGSIL), and high-grade squamous intraepithelial lesion (HGSIL) (Figure 9-44).

Invasive Carcinoma

Early cervical cancer is often asymptomatic. Risk factors for development include **early age at first intercourse, multiple partners, cigarette smoking,** and **high-risk HPV infection** (most important risk factor). Progression from HPV infection to invasive carcinoma requires approximately 10 years (Figure 9-45). Cervical cancer can invade directly into the uterus, vagina, peritoneal cavity, bladder, or rectum, and by lymphatic or hematogenous dissemination.

PRESENTATION

Postcoital vaginal bleeding, abnormal vaginal bleeding, or a mucinous discharge. In late-stage disease, the patient may present with foul-smelling vaginal discharge, weight loss, or obstructive uropathy.

High-Risk HPV (Types 16, 18, 31, 33, 35, and 39)

HPV 16 and 18 account for 70% of cases of cervical cancer and precancerous cervical lesions. High-risk HPVs integrate into the host's DNA and express the proteins E6 and E7, which inactivate p53 and Rb, respectively, allowing uncontrolled cellular proliferation.

DIAGNOSIS

Pap smear is a screening test that screens for abnormal cervical cells while the patient is asymptomatic. Increased detection of abnormal cells with Pap smears has reduced the number of cervical cancer cases in developed countries. Women with abnormal cytology should undergo colposcopy. Rectal examinations may reveal nodularity when carcinoma invades the parametrium. Biopsy alone is sufficient for diagnosis.

PREVENTION

Vaccination against HPV-16 and -18 reduces the risk of developing cervical neoplasia and cervical cancer.

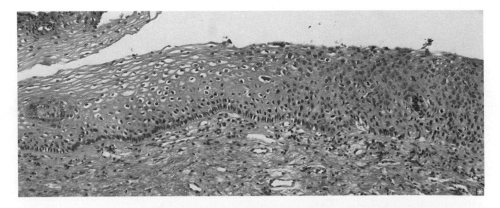

FIGURE 9-44. **Spectrum of squamous intraepithelial lesion (SIL) and cervical dysplasia.** This LEEP cone biopsy shows the spectrum from normal, to borderline koilocytosis, to low-grade SIL, to high-grade SIL, all in one field.

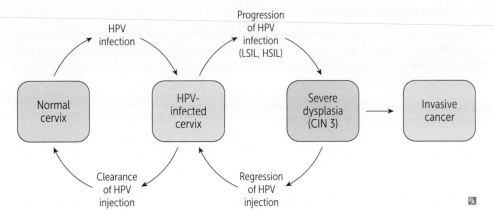

FIGURE 9-45. **Potential outcomes of genital human papillomavirus infection.** Subclinical infection and spontaneous resolution are the most common outcomes. Progression to invasive cancer usually develops over a period of approximately 10 years.

TREATMENT

Cervical conization, simple hysterectomy, radical hysterectomy, or radiation therapy and chemotherapy, depending on the stage.

PROGNOSIS

Five-year survival is > 80% with early-stage disease. Five-year survival is < 10% with late-stage disease.

Acute Cervicitis

PRESENTATION

Foul-smelling, purulent vaginal discharge, abnormal bleeding, or dyspareunia (pain during sexual intercourse). Classic physical exam finding is cervical motion tenderness.

TREATMENT

Cervicitis is often due to sexually transmitted infections. Treatment is usually antibiotics targeted to the causative organism(s). May also be associated with bacterial vaginosis. Untreated cervicitis secondary to chlamydia or gonorrhea may progress to PID. PID is discussed in detail later in the text.

PROGNOSIS

Acute cervicitis generally resolves with appropriate antibiotic treatment. However, a single episode of PID can decrease female fertility in the future.

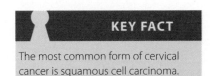

KEY FACT

The most common form of cervical cancer is squamous cell carcinoma.

OVARIAN PATHOLOGY

Primary Ovarian Insufficiency (Formerly Premature Ovarian Failure)

Primary ovarian insufficiency, once called premature ovarian failure, is defined as primary hypogonadism in a female younger than 40 years. Due to atresia of ovarian follicles. Characteristics include infertility and loss of oocytes, folliculogenesis, and ovarian estrogen production. Etiology is usually not known, but some causes include fragile X syndrome, Turner syndrome, certain drugs, and radiation. Low serum estradiol and very high FSH are common.

Polycystic Ovarian Syndrome

Characterized by chronic anovulation, hirsutism, obesity, and enlarged polycystic ovaries. The most important features of polycystic ovarian syndrome (PCOS) are anovulation and signs of hyperandrogenism. Ovaries are enlarged with multiple small cysts and the cortex is thickened.

PATHOGENESIS

Most women with PCOS have elevated LH secretion, which stimulates the ovarian theca and stroma to secrete excessive quantities of androgens, including androstenedione and testosterone. In addition, many women with PCOS are insulin resistant with chronic hyperinsulinemia, which further stimulates the ovaries to secrete androgens. Elevated androgens stunt follicle growth, which results in failure to trigger an LH surge and anovulation (Figure 9-46).

PRESENTATION

Patients with PCOS present with hirsutism, obesity, chronic anovulation, insulin resistance, infertility, and anemia. Symptoms typically begin around menarche. Patients are also at increased risk for endometrial hyperplasia and carcinoma due to prolonged unopposed estrogen exposure.

DIAGNOSIS

There are three major diagnostic criteria (two of three should be met for diagnosis):

- Any form of hyperandrogenism: clinical (eg, acne, hirsutism) or endocrine (high levels of androgens).
- Oligomenorrhea or amenorrhea indicating ovarian dysfunction.
- Sonogram showing enlarged ovaries, with multiple (> 12) small cysts (2–9 mm in diameter) in a "string of pearls" configuration.
- Other endocrinopathies must be ruled out, such as hypothyroidism, hyperprolactinemia, or late-onset congenital adrenal hyperplasia.
- Laboratory studies show increased LH production (leading cause of anovulation) and hyperandrogenism due to inappropriate increased synthesis of androgens by theca cells.

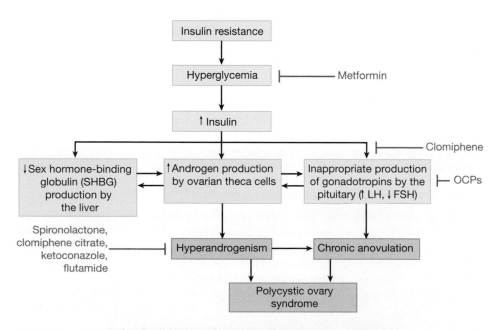

FIGURE 9-46.   **Pathophysiologic pathways in polycystic ovary syndrome.**

TREATMENT

Weight loss, oral contraceptive pills (OCPs), GnRH agonists, metformin, ketoconazole, spironolactone, clomiphene citrate, and pergonal (menotropins) have been used with varying degrees of success.

Follicular Cysts

When the LH surge does not occur and the Graafian follicle does not extrude the ovum, it grows and results in a follicular cyst that does not usually require treatment. It goes away on its own after two or three menstrual cycles. Sometimes an OCP can be used.

Corpus Luteum Cysts

Hemorrhage into a persistent corpus luteum. Normally after the LH surge, the ovum is extruded. The follicle then turns into a corpus luteum. However, the corpus luteum can sometimes accumulate fluid, thus becoming a corpus luteum cyst. It can grow up to 6 cm in diameter and has a potential to rupture or cause ovarian torsion. Corpus luteum cysts are also called *hemorrhagic cysts*. The cysts usually regress spontaneously. There is an association of corpus luteum cysts with the use of ovulation-inducing medication such as clomiphene citrate.

KEY FACT

Hemorrhagic (corpus luteum) cysts are a common gynecologic cause of ovarian torsion and acute abdomen in a young female.

Theca Lutein Cysts

Lined with theca interna cells, theca lutein cysts are usually bilateral and often regress spontaneously. They may grow to a large size and rupture. The cysts are associated with molar pregnancy, choriocarcinoma, twin pregnancy, Rh isoimmunization, and ovulation-inducing agents such as clomiphene citrate.

Ovarian Neoplasms

Asymptomatic until growing tumor becomes large enough to produce symptoms of abdominal distention or fullness, or a dragging sensation due to mass effect. A tumor mass also predisposes to ovarian torsion, causing intermittent intense and sharp pain. Constitutional symptoms of fever, chills, and unintentional weight loss may also be present. Ovarian neoplasms are broadly divided into the following categories, depending on their origin:

CLINICAL CORRELATION

Individuals who are carriers of a *BRCA* mutation are recommended to pursue elective prophylactic bilateral salpingo-oophorectomy after childbearing is complete to reduce risk of developing ovarian cancer.

- Epithelial cell tumors
- Germ cell tumors
- Sex cord/stromal cell tumors
- Metastatic tumors

Epithelial Cell Tumors

Typically arise from the epithelial lining of the fallopian tubes rather than from the ovaries themselves. It usually appears at the fifth or sixth decade of life and accounts for 75–80% of all ovarian cancer. CA-125 is a surface-derived ovarian cancer marker that is used to follow tumor burden during treatment and to detect recurrence; however, it is not diagnostic of ovarian cancer because it can be elevated in other conditions.

Risk factors include family history, low parity, infertility, early menarche, and late menopause. Genetic predisposition is the most significant risk factor. Incidence of epithelial cell derived tumors is increased in patients with *BRCA-1* and *-2* mutations, hereditary nonpolyposis colorectal cancer, and Turner syndrome. Oral contraceptive use at any point during a woman's lifetime decreases the risk of developing epithelial carcinoma of the ovary. The ability of OCPs to decrease the number of ovulatory cycles is the underlying mechanism providing protection, as the development of ovarian epithelial carcinoma is related to the number of ovulatory cycles.

CLINICAL CORRELATION

CA-125 is used to assess treatment efficacy and detect recurrence but is never diagnostic!

Types include:

- Serous
- Mucinous
- Brenner
- Endometrioid

Serous

- **Serous cystadenoma:**
  - Benign.
  - Smooth-walled cyst filled with pale yellow serous fluid.
  - Bilateral in 10–25% of cases.
  - Treatment is either unilateral salpingo-oophorectomy or ovarian cystectomy.
- **Serous cystadenocarcinoma:**
  - Malignant.
  - Characterized by ingrowths of papillary and glandular structures with stromal invasion.
  - **Psammoma bodies** are present in 80% of cases.
  - **Poorly differentiated** cancer may present as solid sheets of cells.

MNEMONIC

PSa**MM**oma bodies are round collections of calcium seen in:
Papillary carcinoma of the thyroid
Serous cystadenocarcinoma
Meningioma
Mesothelioma

Mucinous

- **Mucinous cystadenoma:**
  - Benign.
  - Filled with sticky mucin; tends to be **multiloculated.**
  - Bilateral in < 5% of cases.
  - Can present very large.
  - Treatment is either unilateral salpingo-oophorectomy or ovarian cystectomy.
- **Mucinous cystadenocarcinoma:**
  - Malignant.
  - Characterized by multiple loculi lined with mucin-secreting epithelium and stromal invasion.
  - Bilateral in 8–10% of cases.
  - **Pseudomyxoma peritonei** is excessive mucus production in the abdominal cavity. The primary tumor is most commonly a mucinous adenocarcinoma of the **appendix,** with metastasis to the ovary and seeding of the peritoneal surface. If not treated, mucin accumulates and compresses structures in the abdominal cavity.

Brenner Tumor

- Usually benign.
- Characterized by **transitional (bladder) epithelium** with stromal invasion.

Endometrioid Carcinoma

- Characterized by similar adenomatous pattern seen in endometrial carcinoma of the uterus.
- Often arises out of endometriosis deposits in the ovaries.
- Often present with abdominal distention, pelvic or abdominal pain, and **abnormal vaginal bleeding.**
- Presents at early stage; therefore, has relatively good prognosis.

Germ Cell Tumors

Derived from primordial germ cells of ovaries and constitute 20% of all ovarian tumors. They are similar to testicular germ cell tumors (see previous discussion).

PRESENTATION

Can occur at any age, but peak incidence is in the early 20s.

- About one-third of germ cell tumors diagnosed in children and adolescents are malignant, but most diagnosed in adults are benign (primarily mature cystic teratomas).
- Often present at early stages, unlike epithelial ovarian tumors, which are slow growing and often present at late stages.
- Pelvic pain.
- Menstrual irregularities.
- Rapidly growing pelvic mass with pressure symptoms on the bladder and rectum.
- Adnexal mass, ascites, and pleural effusion may be present.

DIAGNOSIS

- **Sonogram** may reveal adnexal mass measuring > 2 cm with cystic or solid components.
- Karyotyping may be necessary because germ cell tumors tend to occur in dysgenetic gonads (can be seen in 46,XY females).

TYPES

- Dysgerminoma
- Endodermal sinus tumor
- Embryonal carcinoma
- Choriocarcinoma
- Teratomas

Dysgerminoma

The most common malignant germ cell tumor in females. Analogous to seminoma of the testes. Associated with elevated **placental alkaline phosphatase (PLAP), lactate dehydrogenase (LDH),** and **human chorionic gonadotropin (hCG)** (Table 9-16).

- Typically unilateral; bilateral in **10–15% of cases.**
- The capsule appears thin, and the cut surface is spongy and gray-brown in color. Histologically, dysgerminomas exhibit large, round cells with clear cytoplasm and large nuclei with prominent nucleoli.
- Increased risk in Turner syndrome and pseudohermaphrodites (46,XY females).
- Highly sensitive to radiation and chemotherapy.

TABLE 9-16. Germ Cell Tumors, Tumor Markers, and Characteristic Features

GERM CELL TUMORS	TUMOR MARKERS	CHARACTERISTIC FEATURES
Dysgerminoma	PLAP, LDH, and hCG	Large round cells with clear cytoplasm
Endodermal sinus tumor	AFP	Blood vessels with cancer cells resembling primitive glomeruli (Schiller-Duval bodies)
Embryonal carcinoma	hCG and AFP	Large cells, basophilic cytoplasm with indistinct borders
Choriocarcinoma	hCG	Syncytiotrophoblast and cytotrophoblast
Teratoma	AFP and hCG	Differentiated somatic cells from endoderm, ectoderm, and mesoderm

AFP, α-fetoprotein; hCG, human chorionic gonadotropin; LDH, lactate dehydrogenase; PLAP, placental-like alkaline phosphatase.

Yolk Sac Tumor

Also known as endodermal sinus tumor in both males and females.

- Second most common germ cell tumor of the ovary; occurs in those < 30 years of age.
- Associated with elevated AFP levels (see Table 9-16).
- Shows glandular and papillary structures.
- Papillary structures resemble primitive glomeruli (Schiller-Duval bodies).
- Radioresistant but chemosensitive.

Embryonal Carcinoma

- **hCG** and **AFP** are usually elevated.
- Appears as an ill-defined invasive mass containing foci of hemorrhage and necrosis.
- The cells are large and primitive looking, with basophilic cytoplasm, indistinct cell borders, and large nuclei with prominent nucleoli.
- May secrete estrogens, leading to precocious puberty.
- Responds to combination chemotherapy.

Choriocarcinoma

Grossly, primary tumors are small, nonpalpable lesions. Microscopically, **cytotrophoblasts** and **syncytiotrophoblasts** are seen.

- **hCG** is **elevated** (see Table 9-16).
- Increased frequency of theca-lutein cysts.
- Responds well to chemotherapy; therefore, good prognosis.

Teratoma

Differentiated neoplastic germ cells along somatic cell lines. They contain differentiated somatic cells from multiple germ layers (ectoderm, mesoderm, and endoderm). Teratomas are firm masses that, on cut surface, often contain cysts and recognizable areas of cartilage. AFP and hCG are associated tumor markers. Histologically, there are three major variants:

- **Mature dermoid cyst:** "Dermoid" because this tumor has hair and keratin (Figure 9-47). Most frequent benign ovarian tumor.
  - **Benign.**
  - **Bilateral in 10–15%.**
  - **Most common during reproductive years.**
  - Cyst lined by epidermis and adnexal structure.
  - Contains **well-differentiated** bone, cartilage, hair, muscle, and/or thyroid follicles.
- **Immature dermoid cyst:**
  - **Malignant.**
  - Common in younger age groups.
  - Solid tumor with areas of hemorrhage and necrosis.
  - Contains **poorly differentiated** elements of bone, cartilage, hair, muscle, and/or thyroid tissues.
  - Immature areas are always immature neuroepithelium.
- **Specialized teratoma:** Primarily monodermal in origin. An example is **struma ovarii,** which contains mostly mature thyroid tissues. Sometimes can cause **hyperthyroidism** (rare).

Sex Cord Stromal Tumors

Fibroma

Benign tumor of fibroblasts. Key feature is Meigs syndrome: pleural effusions and ascites.

KEY FACT

hCG is a product of the trophoblast (cells that form the villi of the placenta).

KEY FACT

AFP is a product of yolk sac cells.

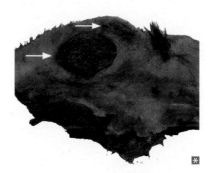

FIGURE 9-47. Mature cystic teratoma of the ovary. White arrows indicate two subcutaneous cysts.

Granulosa Cell Tumor

Estrogen-secreting tumor. Granulosa cells secrete estrogen, which can be used as a tumor marker.

- In prepubertal girls, often associated with pseudoprecocious puberty.
- In reproductive age group, associated with menstrual irregularities, endometrial carcinoma (5%), and endometrial hyperplasia (50%).
- Some secrete inhibin, which can be used as a tumor marker.
- Grossly, smooth with lobulated surfaces; size can range from few millimeters to 20 cm.
- Cells often arrange themselves around a central cavity like a primordial follicle **(Call-Exner bodies).**
- Coffee bean (grooved) nuclei are common.
- Bilateral in < 2% of cases.

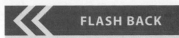

FLASH BACK

Granulosa cells convert androstenedione and testosterone into estrone and estradiol, respectively, via aromatase.

Sertoli-Leydig Cell Tumor

Androgen-producing tumor and may contain **Reinke crystals.**

- Occurs between 30 and 40 years of age.
- Because of the type of hormone produced, commonly presents with signs of virilization such as amenorrhea, breast atrophy, acne, hirsutism, deepening of the voice, and receding hairline.
- Elevated testosterone and androstenedione with normal dehydroepiandrosterone sulfate (DHEA-S).
- Bilateral in < 1% of cases.

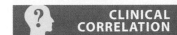

CLINICAL CORRELATION

Unexplained pleural effusion and ascites (Meigs syndrome) may be due to an occult ovarian fibroma. Excision of the tumor is curative.

Metastatic Tumors

- **Krukenberg tumor:** Metastatic tumor to ovaries commonly from the stomach and less commonly from other sites such as the colon, breast, or biliary tract.
- Occurs in ovarian stroma.
- Cells are typically mucin-filled, with **"signet ring" appearance.**
- Usually bilateral (evidence for hemometastasis).

UTERINE PATHOLOGY

Clues to uterine pathology include lower abdominal pain, changes in the menstrual cycle (more or less frequent, heavier or lighter), or a range of constitutional symptoms (fever, chills, and unintentional weight loss). To determine the specific underlying cause, pay attention to the age of the patient and the characteristics of the menstrual cycle with regard to symptoms.

Pelvic Inflammatory Disease

PID is infection and inflammation of the upper genital tract. Causative organisms include:

- *Neisseria gonorrhoeae.*
- *Chlamydia trachomatis.*
- *Gardnerella vaginalis.*
- Anaerobic bacteria.
- Less commonly *Haemophilus influenzae*, enteric gram-negative rods, and streptococci.
- In regions where tuberculosis is endemic, PID is commonly caused by *Mycobacterium tuberculosis.*

PID commonly occurs in young, sexually active, nulliparous women. Progestin-containing OCPs and barrier methods may have a protective effect against PID. Risk factors include smoking, douching, and nonwhite race.

PRESENTATION

Patients present with lower abdominal pain, fever with chills, and purulent cervical discharge. On examination, cervical motion tenderness (**chandelier sign**) and adnexal tenderness may be noted. However, many patients with PID may exhibit subtle signs and symptoms, making it difficult to diagnose. Because the sequelae are grave, PID criteria are defined broadly with low sensitivity in order to catch all cases.

TREATMENT

Azithromycin and ceftriaxone are used to cover *C trachomatis* and *N gonorrhoeae*, respectively.

COMPLICATIONS

Even with treatment, 25% of patients with acute PID develop recurrent PID, chronic pelvic pain, dyspareunia, **ectopic pregnancy,** or **infertility.** May also progress to Fitz-Hugh-Curtis syndrome.

Endometritis

Infection of the endometrium. Frequently preceded by parturition or miscarriage and is related to retained products of conception. Presents with fever and abdominal pain in the postpartum period. Chronic endometritis can occur in association with chronic gonorrheal disease, miliary tuberculosis, intrauterine devices, or spontaneously. Histologically, there is irregular proliferation of the glands with infiltration of chronic inflammatory cells, specifically plasma cells.

Endometriosis

Presence of functional endometrial tissue outside the uterus. The most common sites of implantation are the pelvic viscera (ovaries are most common, rectosigmoid pouch of Douglas is second most common) and the peritoneum (Figure 9-48). Other sites of

KEY FACT

PID with right upper quadrant tenderness suggests associated perihepatitis (infection of the liver capsule) from bacterial transmigration across the peritoneum. This condition is known as **Fitz-Hugh-Curtis syndrome.**

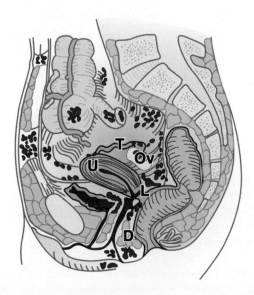

FIGURE 9-48. **Common locations of endometriosis.** The most common sites of endometrial implants are the uterus (U), uterine tubes (T), ovaries (Ov), uterine ligaments (L), and the rectosigmoid pouch of Douglas (D).

implantation include laparotomy scars, lungs, pleura, diaphragm, kidneys, nasal mucosa, spinal canal, stomach, and breast. Endometriosis is believed to occur in 6–8% of women of reproductive age in the United States.

PATHOPHYSIOLOGY

The exact cause of endometriosis is unknown; however, several theories have been proposed to explain its occurrence, including the retrograde menstrual flow theory, celomic metaplasia, and multifactorial genetic predisposition.

- **Regurgitant flow theory (retrograde menstruation, or Sampson's theory):** Menstrual regurgitation occurs in 80–90% of women during normal menstruation. The endometrial cells get implanted elsewhere and function as if they were in the uterine cavity.
- **Celomic metaplasia:** Conversion of one normal cell type to another (eg, hemoptysis and epistaxis concurrent with each menstrual period suggest upper respiratory endometriosis).
- **Induction theory:** Some believe that under the influence of immunologic and hormonal factors, undifferentiated peritoneal cells get transformed into endometrial cells.
- **Genetic factors:** A relative risk of 7 has been shown in women who have first-degree relatives affected with endometriosis. Twin studies support the role of genetic influences.

PRESENTATION

There are a variety of manifestations, ranging from no complaints to the following:

- Cyclic bleeding with **dysmenorrhea** (severe menstrual pain).
- **Subfertility or infertility.**
- Dyspareunia.
- Chronic pelvic pain.
- **Pain on defecation** (due to involvement of rectovaginal pouch of Douglas).
- Pain on urination.
- GI symptoms like nausea, vomiting, bloating, distention, and altered bowel habits.

The physical examination may be normal in the majority of women. However, the following findings may be present:

- Pelvic tenderness.
- Adnexal tenderness.
- Tenderness and **nodularity** over the uterosacral ligaments or in the posterior cul-de-sac.
- Unilateral ovarian enlargement.
- Retroverted uterus.

DIAGNOSIS

- A transvaginal sonogram has excellent specificity and sensitivity in detecting ovarian endometriotic cysts.
- Findings on laparoscopy include "powder-burn" lesions, serous or clear vesicles, and scarring. On biopsy, these areas show endometrial glands, endometrial stroma, and hemosiderin-laden macrophages.

TREATMENT

- Progestins and progestin-dominant, estrogen-progestin contraceptives stop proliferation of endometrial cells by shutting down the hypothalamic-pituitary-ovarian axis, resulting in endometrial atrophy.

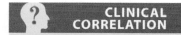

CLINICAL CORRELATION

Suspect **endometriosis** in women with new-onset cyclic dysmenorrhea.

KEY FACT

Endometrioma is a pseudocyst formed by accumulation of menstrual debris from shedding and bleeding of a small endometrial implant over the ovarian cortex. These are also called **chocolate cysts** because of the color of the fluid.

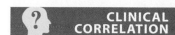

CLINICAL CORRELATION

Combination estrogen-progestin OCPs do not worsen endometriosis. Rather, combination OCPs are one means of treatment.

- Danazol is useful in endometriosis because of its antigonadotropin activity. Danazol directly acts on the pituitary to decrease the level of gonadotropins.
- A GnRH analog given in a continuous fashion (vs pulsatile) also acts by decreasing the levels of LH and FSH, thereby decreasing the estrogen level.
- The goal of **surgical management** is to preserve fertility and decrease symptomatology. The least expensive and least invasive procedures should be the preferred choices.

Adenomyosis

Presence of endometrial glands and stroma in the myometrium of the uterus. The proliferating stratum basalis is nonfunctional, and it may occur focally or diffusely.

PRESENTATION

- Menorrhagia and dysmenorrhea.
- Asymptomatic in one-third of cases.
- Pelvic examination may reveal **a symmetrically enlarged, soft,** bulky uterus, a uterine mass, or uterine tenderness.

DIAGNOSIS

- Transvaginal sonography is the initial imaging technique of choice.
- MRI is the most accurate diagnostic test for adenomyosis.

TREATMENT

Hysterectomy is the only definitive treatment.

COMPLICATION

Anemia due to menorrhagia.

Neoplasms

Endometrial Hyperplasia

Proliferation of endometrial glands and stroma in a greater-than-normal gland:stroma ratio. **Endometrial hyperplasia usually occurs due to prolonged unopposed action of estrogen on endometrial tissue.** Causes include early menarche, late menopause, nulliparity, PCOS, and any other condition associated with anovulation (unopposed estrogen), granulosa cell tumor (secretes estrogen), tamoxifen (an endometrial estrogen-receptor agonist, despite being a breast estrogen-receptor antagonist), or unopposed estrogen therapy without concomitant use of a progestin.

The different types of endometrial hyperplasia are described in Table 9-17.

PRESENTATION

Patients with endometrial hyperplasia present with abnormal uterine bleeding, such as menorrhagia, metrorrhagia, or postmenopausal bleeding. Amenorrhea may also be a presenting symptom, especially in anovulatory patients.

DIAGNOSIS

The diagnosis is based on histologic examination of specimens obtained either from dilatation and curettage (D&C) or endometrial biopsy in an office setting.

TREATMENT

Progesterone therapy is quite effective for hyperplasia without atypia. However, complex hyperplasia with atypia may require hysterectomy because 25% of patients with atypical

TABLE 9-17. Types of Endometrial Hyperplasia, Cytologic Features, and Progression to Endometrial Carcinoma

TYPE	CYTOLOGIC FEATURES	PROGRESSION TO ENDOMETRIAL CANCER (%)
Simple	Cystic hyperplasia without atypia 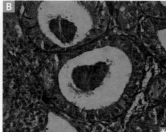	1
Complex	Adenomatous hyperplasia without atypia 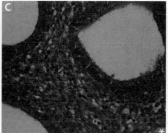	3–5
Simple with atypia	Cystic hyperplasia with atypia	8–10
Complex with atypia	Adenomatous hyperplasia with atypia	29

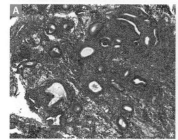
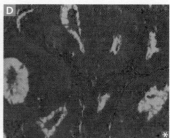

hyperplasia detected on endometrial biopsy or curettage specimens are found to have well-differentiated endometrial carcinoma. Women who have not completed childbearing can be treated with progestins and followed closely to preserve fertility.

Endometrial Carcinoma

Cancer arising from the endometrium of the uterus. It is the **most common gynecologic malignancy,** and 2–3% of women develop endometrial carcinoma in their lifetime. Seventy-five percent of endometrial cancer occurs in women > 50 years of age. It ranks as the fourth most common malignancy in women after breast, lung, and colon cancers. Increased estrogen exposure throughout a woman's lifetime is the most important risk factor for endometrial cancer. The most common risk factors for endometrial carcinoma include:

- Nulliparity
- Late menopause
- Early menarche
- Obesity
- Diabetes mellitus
- Estrogen replacement therapy
- Atypical endometrial hyperplasia
- Tamoxifen therapy for breast cancer

Endometrial carcinoma can arise in two different pathologic settings:

- **Endometrioid:** Carcinomas frequently arise on a backdrop of endometrial hyperplasia. These tumors are termed endometrioid because they appear similar to normal endometrial glands. They originate in the mucosa and may infiltrate the myometrium and enter the vascular spaces, with metastases to regional lymph nodes.
- **Papillary serous and clear cell:** Poorly differentiated cancers that arise from atrophic endometrium rather than endometrial hyperplasia and are much more aggressive tumors. Not associated with unopposed estrogen exposure.

Most patients present at their perimenopausal or postmenopausal period with complaints of vaginal bleeding or discharge. The peak age of incidence is in the sixth and seventh decades of life.

KEY FACT

Any factor that causes the endometrium to undergo unopposed estrogen exposure increases the risk of **endometrial carcinoma.**

KEY FACT

There is no appropriate screening test for endometrial carcinoma.

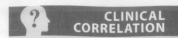
CLINICAL CORRELATION

Postmenopausal vaginal bleeding is endometrial carcinoma until proven otherwise.

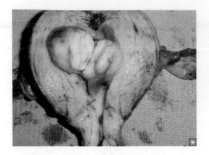

FIGURE 9-49.   Submucosal leiomyoma.

DIAGNOSIS

Endometrial aspiration biopsy is the best initial investigation of choice.

TREATMENT

Total abdominal hysterectomy plus bilateral salpingo-oophorectomy with peritoneal sampling is routinely done.

Leiomyoma (Fibroid)

Leiomyoma (uterine fibroid) is a benign tumor arising from smooth muscle and connective tissue of the uterus. **Most common of all tumors in females.** Leiomyomas are clonal and arise from a single myometrial cell. Leiomyomas occur in 20–50% of women of reproductive age and may be:

- **Intramural:** Tumors embedded within the myometrium.
- **Submucosal:** Tumors directly beneath the endometrium (Figure 9-49).
- **Subserosal:** Tumors directly beneath the serosa.

Sometimes leiomyomas are found in the peritoneal cavity, broad ligament, and cervix. The exact cause is unknown. Grossly, leiomyomas are sharply circumscribed, firm, gray-white masses with a **characteristic whorled cut surface.** Microscopically, the cells appear to have uniform size and shape with scarce mitotic figures. Malignant transformation is very rare.

PRESENTATION

Peak incidence is 20–40 years of age. The clinical features of leiomyoma depend on the location, size, and number of tumors. Symptoms include the following:

- Menorrhagia, which may lead to iron deficiency anemia.
- Pain symptoms such as dysmenorrhea, dyspareunia, or pelvic pressure. Acute pain may result from torsion of a pedunculated fibroid.
- Pressure symptoms such as frequency, urgency, incontinence, constipation, or venous stasis of the lower extremities.
- Reduced fertility and recurrent abortions.
- Ascites.
- Polycythemia.

DIAGNOSIS

Pelvic examination may reveal an asymmetrically enlarged uterus or an adnexal or pelvic mass. Sonography shows a concentric, solid hypoechoic mass. The diagnosis is confirmed by histopathology, which shows uniform-sized cells with few mitotic figures.

TREATMENT

- **Medical:** Continuous administration of GnRH agonists decreases the levels of FSH, LH, and estrogen. Long-term use of GnRH agonists is limited by their side effects (eg, hot flashes).
- **Surgical:** Hysterectomy, myomectomy, or embolization.

COMPLICATIONS

Calcification, ossification, mucinous or cystic degeneration, and **red degeneration;** anemia and venous stasis in the lower extremities are common complications of leiomyoma. Leiomyomas are estrogen-sensitive and therefore may enlarge during pregnancy.

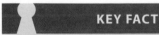
KEY FACT

Red degeneration is a form of coagulative necrosis in a hemorrhagic, meaty, cut surface.

Leiomyosarcoma

- Arises from mesenchymal cells of the myometrium, *not* from preexisting leiomyomas.
- Appears similar to leiomyomas but diagnostic features include **pleomorphic spindle cells with relatively frequent mitoses.**

- Older females are affected, and pathology reveals at least 10 mitotic figures per high-power field, atypia, and necrosis.
- Treat with surgical resection.

BREAST PATHOLOGY

Benign Breast Disease

The female breast progresses through normal anatomic changes during pre-, peri-, and postmenopausal years. Differentiating normal from pathologic anatomic changes is important in clinical practice and in answering test questions. Keys to identifying the underlying disease process are the patient's age, history, changes related to the menstrual cycle, nipple discharge, and findings on ultrasound, mammogram, or biopsy (Table 9-18). The presence of a myoepithelial cell layer around glands is an important distinguishing factor between benign and malignant breast disease. This layer is normally absent in invasive breast cancer.

Fibroadenoma

Most common benign tumor of the female breast, and the most common tumor in women < 25 years of age. It is thought to be caused by an increase in estrogen activity. Grossly, fibroadenomas are firm, with a uniform tan-white color on cut section, punctuated by softer yellow-pink specks. Clinically, they present as a **solitary, discrete, movable mass** in a young woman and rarely become malignant.

Fibrocystic Changes

Fibrocystic changes are common, benign changes involving the tissues of the breast that manifest as palpable lumps. They are the consequence of an exaggeration and distortion of the cyclic breast changes that occur normally in the menstrual cycle. Fibrocystic changes are divided into two categories: nonproliferative and proliferative.

- **Nonproliferative (cysts and fibrosis):** The most common fibrocystic change, it is characterized by an increase in fibrous stroma associated with dilation of ducts and formation of cysts of various sizes without epithelial cell hyperplasia. The secretions within the cysts can calcify and appear radiodense on mammograms. Types of nonproliferative change include blue dome cysts (filled with serous, turbid fluid) and apocrine metaplasia (cysts lined by large, polygonal cells that have abundant granular, eosinophilic cytoplasm with small, round deeply chromatic nuclei).
- **Proliferative (hyperplasia and sclerosing adenosis):** The terms *epithelial hyperplasia* and *proliferative fibrocystic change* encompass a range of lesions within the ductules, terminal ducts, and sometimes lobules of the ducts. Atypical hyperplasia is associated with the development of carcinoma and is estrogen sensitive.

TABLE 9-18.   Classification of Benign and Malignant Breast Diseases

BENIGN BREAST DISEASES	MALIGNANT BREAST DISEASES
- Fibrocystic changes	Carcinoma in situ
- Intraductal papilloma	- Ductal
- Fibroadenoma	- Lobular
- Phyllodes tumor (benign or malignant)	Invasive carcinoma
- Traumatic fat necrosis	- Ductal
- Acute mastitis	- Medullary
- Gynecomastia	- Tubular
	- Mucinous (colloid)
	- Papillary
	- Inflammatory
	- Lobular

Intraductal Papilloma

A neoplastic papillary growth (double-layered epithelial cells overlying a myoepithelial layer) within a lactiferous duct or sinus. Presentation includes **serous or bloody nipple discharge,** subareolar tumors, or, rarely, nipple retraction. A single papillary growth with a myoepithelial layer is likely to be benign, whereas multiple growths lacking a myoepithelial layer are more likely to be carcinoma.

Phyllodes Tumor

Arises from the intralobular stroma and rarely from a preexisting fibroadenoma. These lesions may clinically mimic a fibroadenoma but tend to occur in older women. Most grow to a **massive size,** distending the breast. On gross section, they exhibit leaf-like clefts and slits (*phyllon* is Greek for leaf). Only about 15% are malignant, and < 20% metastasize. **There is no ductal invasion and, therefore, no bleeding.**

Fat Necrosis

An uncommon and innocuous lesion significant only because it produces a mass, usually after some antecedent trauma to the breast. The lesion consists of a central focus of necrotic fat cells surrounded by polymorphonuclear neutrophils; it later becomes enclosed by fibrous tissue, and then scars. **The necrotic fat is phagocytosed by macrophages, which then become lipid-laden.** Can progress and cause skin retraction.

Acute Mastitis

Inflammation of the breast tissue caused by infection. Acute mastitis in the setting of breastfeeding (lactation mastitis) is normally **unilateral** and occurs the first few weeks after birth. It typically presents as a **tender,** swollen, firm, and red area of the breast with associated **fever.** Flu-like symptoms (eg, myalgia, chills, and malaise) are common. Bacteria are the most common pathogen; fungi are rare. *Staphylococcus aureus* is the most common pathogen isolated and can lead to abscess formation. Treatment includes antibiotics (cephalosporins, dicloxacillin), cold compresses, nonsteroidal antiinflammatory agents, and emptying of the breast by continuing breastfeeding, pumping, or hand expression. Cessation of lactation is not necessary.

Gynecomastia

Gynecomastia is defined as benign proliferation of glandular tissue of the breast in men. Proliferation and enlargement of breast tissue in males is due to increased estrogen levels, increased estrogen precursors, or decreased androgen levels. Physiologic enlargement may be present at birth, during puberty, or in old age. Pathologic enlargement is usually due to cirrhosis, testicular tumors, Klinefelter syndrome, specific drugs (spironolactone, digoxin, cimetidine, alcohol, ketoconazole), or obesity.

Malignant Breast Tumors

In the United States, breast cancer is the most frequently diagnosed cancer and the most common breast mass in women older than 50 years. Breast cancer is the second most common cause of death related to cancer in women in the United States. However, the morbidity and mortality associated with breast cancer are decreasing due to earlier detection and treatment.

PRESENTATION

The initial chief complaint may be a palpable breast mass. Some patients may present with abnormal mammographic findings such as irregular masses and calcifications. The key to identifying the underlying pathology involves breast examination and tissue biopsy of the mass.

Risk factors include family history, early menarche, late menopause, late first pregnancy (after 30 years), nulliparity, never having breast-fed, previous history of breast cancer, and family history of first-degree relative with breast cancer at a young age. Women having mutations in *BRCA1* and *BRCA2* genes have a 60–80% chance of developing breast cancer in their lifetimes. *BRCA1* and *BRCA2* gene mutations are transmitted in an autosomal dominant fashion.

TREATMENT

Treatment of breast cancer is specialized based on the location of the primary lesion, lymph node involvement, and the expression of hormone receptors or the HER2 protein.

- **Estrogen/progesterone receptors:** It is believed that estrogen and progesterone receptors normally present in breast epithelium, and often present in breast cancer cells, may interact with various growth promoters to create an autocrine mechanism of tumor development. Assessment of these receptors' expression is critical as there are targeted therapies such as tamoxifen (a breast estrogen receptor antagonist) and aromatase inhibitors.
- ***ERBB2:*** The *ERBB2* (formerly *HER2/neu*) protooncogene has been found to be amplified in up to 30% of sporadic breast cancers. It is a member of the epidermal growth factor receptor family and is associated with a poor prognosis. The importance of evaluating *ERBB2* expression is to predict responsiveness to the monoclonal antibody trastuzumab, which targets the *ERBB2* receptor. It is one of the first antitumor antibody therapies based on specific genetic abnormalities.
- **Sentinel node biopsy:** This has been introduced as an alternative, less morbid procedure to replace a full axillary nodal dissection. The first one to two draining nodes are identified with a dye or radiolabel. A negative sentinel node is highly predictive of no metastatic cancer in the remaining nodes. However, the significance of finding micrometastases is unknown.

Carcinoma in Situ

- **Ductal carcinoma in situ (DCIS):** Usually arises from the major ducts. Nonpalpable. Commonly contains microcalcifications. Comedocarcinoma is a distinct variant of DCIS characterized by central necrosis. One-third of DCIS cases eventually invade. Treated with lumpectomy.
- **Lobular carcinoma in situ (LCIS):** Involves the terminal duct lobular unit. Nonpalpable. Signet ring cells are common. Usually estrogen and progesterone receptor-positive and e-cadherin negative. One-third of cases eventually invade. Fifty percent to 75% increased incidence of cancer in the opposite breast.

Paget Disease of the Breast

Caused by the extension of DCIS into the lactiferous ducts and the skin of the nipple. Common complaints of itching, pain, and burning may occur before disease is clinically apparent. Clinically, there is a unilateral crusting and exudate over the nipple and areolar skin (Figure 9-50). Nipple retraction is rare, but may occur in advanced disease. Paget cells have an abundant clear cytoplasm. Palpable mass in only 50% of cases.

Invasive Carcinoma

Ductal

Term used for all nonlobular carcinomas that cannot be subclassified into one of the specialized types listed here; they account for most breast cancers (70–80%). It is usually associated with DCIS. Invasion of lymphovascular spaces or nerves may be seen. Roughly two-thirds express estrogen-progestin receptors and about one-third overexpress ERBB2. Types of frank ductal carcinoma include the following (Table 9-19):

KEY FACT

Tamoxifen acts as an estrogen receptor antagonist in breast tissue and an agonist in endometrium and bone tissue. **Raloxifene** acts as an estrogen receptor antagonist in breast tissue and an agonist in bone tissue. It has no effect on the endometrium.

FLASH BACK

Paget disease has a similar histologic appearance to pagetoid spread of melanoma.

KEY FACT

Paget disease of the breast is associated with underlying DCIS/invasive carcinoma in > 95% of cases.

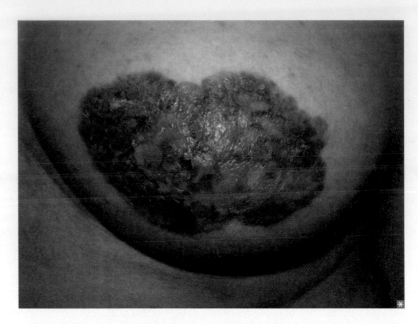

FIGURE 9-50. **Paget disease of the nipple.** Scaly and erythematous plaque involving the nipple and areola.

- **Medullary:** 1–5% of all breast cancers. Associated with *BRCA1* mutations. Occur at younger age. Bulky, soft tumor with large cells and infiltrate of leukocytes. Although they lack estrogen and progesterone receptors, they have a better prognosis.
- **Tubular:** Presents as irregular mammographic densities. The carcinoma consists of well-formed tubules with low-grade nuclei. Affects young females. Metastases are rare, prognosis is good, and hormone receptors are normally expressed.
- **Mucinous (colloid):** Cancer cells produce mucus and grow into a jelly-like tumor; associated with a better prognosis. Usually affect the elderly.
- **Papillary:** Papillary architecture and fibrovascular cores. Often expresses progesterone and estrogen receptors.
- **Inflammatory:** Presents as an enlarged, swollen, erythematous breast, usually without a palpable mass. The blockage of numerous dermal lymphatic spaces by carcinoma

CLINICAL CORRELATION

The skin dimpling seen in inflammatory ductal carcinoma is due to Cooper ligaments that focally anchor the skin to the chest wall. The surrounding areas of skin swell due to dermal lymphatic invasion.

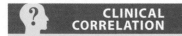

TABLE 9-19. **Characteristics of Different Subtypes of Invasive Ductal Carcinoma**

TYPE	AGE	PATHOLOGIC FINDINGS	PROGNOSIS
Medullary	Young	▪ Sheet-like growth with absent ducts or alveolar pattern ▪ Estrogen/progesterone receptor absent	Better
Tubular	Young	▪ Well-formed tubules with low-grade nuclei ▪ Estrogen/progesterone receptor present	Better
Mucinous	Elderly	▪ Neoplastic cells surrounded by mucin ▪ Estrogen/progesterone receptor present	Better
Papillary	Elderly	▪ Papillary architecture with fibrovascular cores ▪ Estrogen/progesterone receptor present	Better
Inflammatory	Young	▪ Swollen, erythematous base with invasion to dermal lymphatics and dimpling of the skin (peau d'orange) ▪ Estrogen/progesterone receptor present in < 50%	Poor

results in dimpling like an orange peel—"peau d'orange". Most of these have distant metastases and an extremely poor prognosis.

Lobular

Often bilateral but less common than infiltrating ductal carcinoma. The cells invade single-file into stroma and are often aligned in strands or chains. Lobular carcinomas, more often than ductal carcinomas, metastasize to cerebrospinal fluid and elsewhere. Nearly all of these tumors express hormone receptors.

SEXUALLY TRANSMITTED INFECTIONS AND OTHER GENITAL INFECTIONS

Sexually transmitted infections (STIs) are a significant cause of morbidity with short- and long-term consequences. Table 9-20 summarizes the common STIs and other genital infections.

TABLE 9-20.   **Sexually Transmitted Infections and Other Genital Infections**

DISEASE (PATHOGEN)	PRESENTATION	DIAGNOSIS	TREATMENT
Syphilis (*Treponema pallidum*)	**Primary:** Small papule that turns into a painless ulcer (chancre) with well-defined borders **Secondary:** Lymphadenopathy, rash on the palms and soles of the feet, condylomata lata, meningitis, hepatitis **Tertiary:** Thoracic aneurysm, tabes dorsalis, gummas, Argyll Robertson pupils **Congenital:** Stillbirth, hepatomegaly, snuffles, rash, bone abnormalities (eg, saber shins, mulberry molars, saddle nose, Hutchinson triad [notched central incisors, interstitial keratitis, 8th nerve palsy])	▪ Darkfield microscopy ▪ VDRL/RPR (nonspecific): Measure cardiolipin antibody; titers fall after treatment ▪ FTA-Abs (specific): Remains positive after treatment	Penicillin G, azithromycin, ceftriaxone, or erythromycin
Gonorrhea (*Neisseria gonorrhoeae*)	▪ Attaches to the mucosal epithelium of the urethra via pili. May ascend to infect the prostate, epididymis, and testes in men or cause PID in women ▪ Purulent urethral discharge ▪ Swelling around the meatus ▪ Pain with urination	Culture of discharge shows gram-negative diplococci	Ceftriaxone (also treat for *C trachomatis* with azithromycin or doxycycline)
Nongonococcal urethritis (*Chlamydia trachomatis*, serotypes D-K or *Ureaplasma urealyticum*)	▪ Most common STI ▪ Purulent urethral discharge ▪ Pain with urination ▪ May ascend to infect the prostate, epididymis, and testes in men or cause PID in women	▪ Gram-negative intracellular organism ▪ Serologic testing ▪ **Reiter syndrome:** Uveitis, arthritis, urethritis ("can't see, can't pee, can't climb a tree")	Azithromycin or doxycycline (also treat for *N gonorrhoeae* with ceftriaxone)
Lymphogranuloma venereum (*C trachomatis*, serotypes L1-L3)	▪ Ulcerative genital lesion ▪ Regional lymphadenopathy (buboes): Granulomatous inflammatory reaction with irregularly shaped foci of necrosis and neutrophilic infiltrate; potential formation of draining sinuses ▪ Proctitis, rectal strictures	▪ Gram-negative intracellular organism ▪ Serologic testing	Tetracycline, doxycycline, erythromycin, or cotrimoxazole
Chancroid (*Haemophilus ducreyi*)	▪ Tender, erythematous papule that ulcerates ▪ Lesions are painful ▪ Base of ulcer covered by yellow-gray exudate	Based on clinical criteria. Very difficult to culture	Azithromycin, ceftriaxone, or erythromycin

(continues)

TABLE 9-20. Sexually Transmitted Infections and Other Genital Infections (continued)

DISEASE (PATHOGEN)	PRESENTATION	DIAGNOSIS	TREATMENT
Granuloma inguinale (donovanosis, caused by *Klebsiella granulomatis*)	▪ Sharply demarcated ulcer with beefy-red granulation tissue ▪ Lymph nodes are spared ▪ Lesion is painless	Based on clinical criteria. Very difficult to culture	Erythromycin, tetracycline, ampicillin, or TMP-SMX
Condylomata acuminata (HPV types 6 and 11)	▪ Squamous cell proliferation (genital warts) ▪ Small sessile lesions to large papillary lesions	**Koilocytosis:** Hyperchromatic nuclei surrounded by a perinuclear halo	Chemical destruction (podophyllin, trichloroacetic acid, or 5-FU/epinephrine gel) or surgical excision
Genital herpes (HSV types 1 and 2)	▪ Usually caused by HSV-2 ▪ Prodrome of burning and tingling ▪ Active lesions are painful vesicles	Microscopy: **Cowdry type A inclusion bodies** (viral inclusions that appear as light purple intranuclear structures surrounded by a clear halo)	Acyclovir, famciclovir, valacyclovir
Bacterial vaginosis (*Gardnerella vaginalis*)	▪ **Fishy-smelling** discharge after unprotected intercourse ▪ No inflammatory signs on examination	▪ Microscopy: **Clue cells** (epithelial cells covered with adherent *Gardnerella vaginalis*; Figure 9-51) ▪ pH > 4.5 (abnormal) ▪ Whiff test (addition of KOH to vaginal discharge generates fishy, amine-like odor) may be positive	Metronidazole or clindamycin
Trichomoniasis (*Trichomonas vaginalis*)	▪ Purulent, thin, greenish frothy vaginal discharge associated with pruritus, dysuria, and dyspareunia ▪ Erythema of the vulva and vagina ▪ Punctate hemorrhages on the vagina and cervix ("strawberry cervix")	▪ Microscopy: Motile trichomonads and leukocytes ▪ **Whiff test** (addition of KOH to vaginal discharge generates fishy amine-like odor) may be positive	Metronidazole
Candidiasis (*Candida albicans*)	▪ Thin to homogeneously thick vaginal discharge ▪ Vaginal soreness, pruritus, dyspareunia, and vulvar burning ▪ Curdy white patches on the vulva and vagina ▪ May have had recent antibiotic use, pregnancy, or diabetes as these conditions decrease lactobacilli and allow overgrowth of fungi	▪ pH < 4.5 (normal) ▪ Mycelia on KOH preparation	Topical azoles or oral fluconazole

FTA-Abs, fluorescent treponemal antibody absorption; 5-FU, 5-flurouracil; HPV, human papillomavirus; HSV, herpes simplex virus; PID, pelvic inflammatory disease; STI, sexually transmitted infection; TMP/SMX, trimethoprim-sulfamethoxazole; VDRL/RPR, Venereal Disease Research Laboratory, rapid plasma reagin.

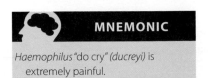

MNEMONIC

Haemophilus "do cry" (*ducreyi*) is extremely painful.

The pH of the normal vagina is < 4.5 and is maintained by the production of lactic acid. Estrogen-stimulated vaginal epithelial cells are rich in glycogen, which is broken down into glucose. The vaginal cells and lactobacilli convert glucose into lactic acid. Frequent sexual intercourse or the use of douches causes the vaginal pH to be alkaline, which predisposes to bacterial vaginosis (Figure 9-51).

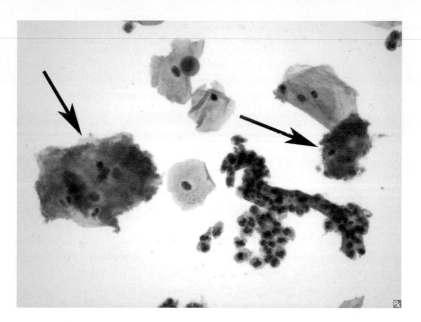

FIGURE 9-51. **Clue cells.** Clue cells can be seen on Pap smears of patients with bacterial vaginosis caused by overgrowth of *Gardnerella*. The image shows the organisms coating squamous cells forming a purple, velvety coat (*arrows*).

Pathology—Male

PENILE PATHOLOGY

Anatomic/Structural

Peyronie Disease

A dense, subcutaneous fibrous plaque forms on the tunica albuginea on the penis, which causes the penis to curve laterally when erect. It mainly affects older men; however, the cause is unknown. If the curvature of the penis interferes with normal sexual intercourse, surgical correction is recommended. If erectile dysfunction or infertility occurs, then a penile implant should be considered.

Priapism

Priapism is a persistent painful erection in the absence of sexual desire or stimulation. Etiologies include sickle cell disease or trait, spinal cord trauma, antidepressants (trazodone), antipsychotics (chlorpromazine), penile vascular injury (trauma), and erectile dysfunction drugs (sildenafil).

Inflammatory

Balanitis

Inflammation of the glans penis. It is called **balanoposthitis** when the foreskin and prepuce are also inflamed. Balanitis is commonly seen in unhygienic uncircumcised men. The collection of smegma, which is carcinogenic, and the lack of aeration causes irritation and inflammation, accounting for the increased rates of penile cancer seen in uncircumcised males. Balanitis can be complicated by phimosis and meatal stenosis leading to urinary retention. Treatment includes cleaning of the area and antibiotics.

KEY FACT

Trazodone is an antidepressant that can cause **priapism.**

Phimosis

Extremely tight foreskin that is too small to be retracted over the glans penis. Tight foreskin is normal very early in life but considered pathologic after age 3 years. Often occurs in uncircumcised males that experience chronic infections and inflammation of the glans penis (**balanitis**), sometimes due to poor hygiene of the area. Circumcision can be used as a treatment after the initial infection is treated with broad-spectrum antibiotics.

Premalignant and Neoplastic Diseases

Bowenoid Papulosis

Small, multiple, red, brown, or flesh-colored patches on the skin of the penis. It is a premalignant condition with a 2–3% chance of progression to cancer. Bowenoid papulosis has a close link to high-risk HPV and is described as being between genital warts and Bowen disease of the penis in severity. Many cases of Bowenoid papulosis spontaneously regress, but close follow-up is required as it has malignant potential.

Bowen Disease

Bowen disease is defined as squamous cell carcinoma (SCC) in situ originating anywhere on the skin and is not limited to the penis or scrotum. SCC in situ of the male external genitalia usually presents as a solitary, red or gray well-demarcated and velvety plaque on the penis, scrotum, or inguinal or suprapubic skin. Variations are possible and include the presence of multiple lesions, scaling, ulceration, and keratotic and elevated plaques. The lesions tend to grow slowly over many years. Patients may experience pain, itching, and bleeding.

Bowen disease is associated with previous high-risk HPV infection (eg, HPV-16), lack of circumcision, and chronic inflammation. Surgical excision of lesions is the treatment of choice if possible. It is a precursor to invasive SCC and has a 10% chance of progression if not treated.

Erythroplasia of Queyrat

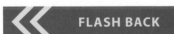

Bowen disease, specifically of the glans penis, is termed erythroplasia of Queyrat. The most common presentation is on the mucosal surface of the glands or prepuce. Lesion appearance, risk factors, and treatment are similar to Bowen disease (see Bowen disease above).

Penile Squamous Cell Carcinoma

Penile cancer is rare in the United States, representing < 1% of cancers in males. It is frequently seen in uncircumcised and unhygienic men with a prior history of genital warts and high-risk HPV (Figure 9-52).

DISEASES OF THE TESTES

Congenital Abnormalities

Cryptorchidism

PRESENTATION

A failure of one or both testes to descend from the abdominal cavity into the scrotum by 4 months of age. The undescended testis can frequently be palpated as a mass in the inguinal canal. Usually spontaneously descends by 3 months of age.

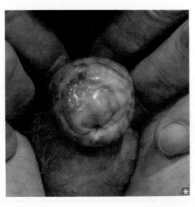

FIGURE 9-52. Squamous cell carcinoma of the penis.

COMPLICATIONS

Ipsilateral inguinal hernia, testicular torsion, trauma, and infertility. An increased risk of germ cell tumors, usually seminomas and embryonal carcinomas, is associated with cryptorchidism, even after surgical intervention, and in both the normal and cryptorchid testis.

TREATMENT

Orchiopexy (testes repositioned into scrotal sac) is done as soon as possible after 6 months of age and no later than 2 years. It helps to fix the testes in place, prevent torsion, and increase fertility, and aids in detection of cancer because the external position of the testis better facilitates examination.

Infectious Diseases

Orchitis

- Inflammation of the testes usually caused by the mumps virus (Paramyxovirus) and usually affects only one testis.
- If **bilateral (uncommon)**, it **may lead to sterility** resulting from atrophy of the seminiferous tubules. In the case of sterility, serum testosterone is decreased but serum FSH and LH are increased. While sterility is more common if infected with the mumps virus after puberty, it is still very rare.

Epididymitis

An infection of the epididymis that can be caused by a variety of bacteria.

- < 35 years old: *Chlamydia trachomatis* and *Neisseria gonorrhoeae*.
- > 35 years old: *Escherichia coli* and *Pseudomonas aeruginosa*.
- Patients often suffer from pain and swelling in the scrotum, tenderness, and a positive **Prehn sign** (a marked decrease in pain in association with elevation of the scrotum).

Structural/Anatomic Abnormalities

Torsion

A twisting of the spermatic cord that compromises blood supply to the testes, potentially resulting in testicular infarction and gangrene (Figure 9-53).

- Possible loss of cremasteric reflex, though this reflex is often absent in older men.
- **Surgical correction** within 6 hours of occurrence usually results in full recovery of the testis.

Varicocele

Dilated and tortuous veins located in the pampiniform plexus of the spermatic cord that most often appears as a **"bag of worms"** on examination.

- The left testis is more likely to have a varicocele because its pampiniform plexus drains into the left renal vein before the inferior vena cava (IVC), causing increased pressure in the venous plexus.
- Any type of **obstruction of the left renal vein,** such as in renal cell carcinoma, can cause a varicocele.
- Varicocele is the most common cause of treatable male **subfertility.**

Hydrocele

A collection of serous fluid that distends the tunica vaginalis. Most commonly caused by a **persistent processus vaginalis** that enables communication between the scrotum and the peritoneal cavity. Also can be due to infection or lymphatic blockage as a result of a tumor.

KEY FACT

Normal descent of the testes:
- Transabdominal phase (mediated by MIF)
- Inguinoscrotal phase (mediated by androgens, hCG)

KEY FACT

Epididymitis is more common in men 19–40 years of age, and **orchitis** is more common in boys (< 10 years).

CLINICAL CORRELATION

Etiology of epididymitis determines empiric treatment. Men younger than 35 years are treated with doxycycline and ceftriaxone. Men older than 35 years are treated with fluoroquinolones.

FLASH BACK

Right testicular vein → IVC
Left testicular vein → left renal vein → IVC

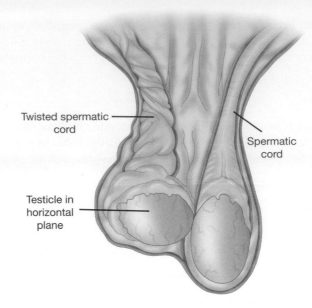

FIGURE 9-53. **Testicular torsion.** Note the unilateral pulling of the testis into the horizontal plane due to the twisting of the spermatic cord.

- The most frequent cause of **enlargement of the scrotum** in young boys.
- Can be distinguished from tumors by transillumination (Figure 9-54). Hydroceles transilluminate; tumors do not.

Hematocele

A collection of blood in the tunica vaginalis. Hematocele often results from testicular trauma and presents with pain, tenderness, and absent transillumination. A hematocele sometimes results from tapping a hydrocele during examination. If a hematocele is not drained, it can form a clot, which requires orchidectomy.

Spermatocele

A retention cyst distended with fluid containing spermatozoa in the epididymis or rete testis. Spermatocele is often present in the head of the epididymis and behind the upper pole of the testis. Small ones can be ignored; larger ones should be aspirated or excised through a scrotal incision.

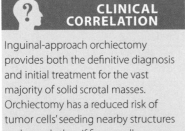

CLINICAL CORRELATION

Inguinal-approach orchiectomy provides both the definitive diagnosis and initial treatment for the vast majority of solid scrotal masses. Orchiectomy has a reduced risk of tumor cells' seeding nearby structures and vessels than if fine needle aspiration or biopsy is performed. Excisional biopsy is rarely performed as well for diagnosis.

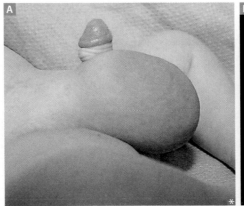
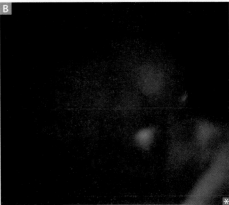

FIGURE 9-54. **Hydrocele and transillumination. A B** Note the translucent appearance when a light is shone through the testis filled with serous fluid.

Testicular Neoplasms

Germ Cell Tumors

Seminoma

Most common germ cell tumor of the testes. Large, soft, well-demarcated, gray-white tumor that bulges from the cut surface of the affected testis. A seminoma is confined beneath an intact tunica albuginea. Microscopically, large cells with distinct cell borders, pale nuclei, and prominent nucleoli ("fried egg" appearance) as well as a lymphocytic infiltrate are seen. **Seminoma** can be associated with an increase in **hCG** and **placental alkaline phosphatase (PLAP)**. It mainly affects males between the ages of 15 and 35 years old. Seminoma metastasizes via the lymphatics and is **exquisitely radiosensitive** with an excellent prognosis (Figure 9-55 and Table 9-21).

Yolk Sac Tumor

Large, may be well demarcated. Microscopically, cells appear as cuboidal to columnar epithelium forming sheets, glands, papillae, and microcysts, and are often associated with **hyaline globules. Schiller-Duval bodies,** which are structures resembling primitive glomeruli, are a distinctive feature of yolk sac tumors. This is the most common primary testicular neoplasm in children < 3 years. α-Fetoprotein **(AFP)** can be demonstrated within the cytoplasm of these neoplastic cells.

Choriocarcinoma

Grossly, primary tumor is small and nonpalpable. Microscopically, choriocarcinoma is composed of sheets of small cuboidal cells irregularly intermingled with or capped by large, eosinophilic syncytial cells containing multiple dark, pleomorphic nuclei; these represent **cytotrophoblastic and syncytiotrophoblastic differentiation,** respectively. **hCG is elevated.** Choriocarcinoma frequently metastasizes to visceral organs, specifically the lungs, via hematogenous spread. Pharmacologic treatment for metastatic disease is methotrexate.

Teratoma

Firm masses that contain cysts, cartilage, and other tissue types. Originating from germ cells, they differentiate into ectoderm, endoderm, and mesoderm. Histologically, there are three major variants: mature, immature, and mixed.

- **Mature:** Fully differentiated tissues from multiple germ cell layers (eg, neural tissue, cartilage, adipose, bone, and epithelium) in a random array.
- **Immature:** Somatic elements reminiscent of developing fetal tissue.

KEY FACT

Cryptorchidism results in an increased risk of **seminomas.**

KEY FACT

Testicular tumors metastasize first to the periaortic lymph nodes.

CLINICAL CORRELATION

hCG, TSH, FSH, and LH share a common alpha subunit. Thus, elevated hCG may present with symptoms of hyperthyroidism or gynecomastia.

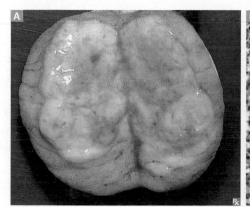
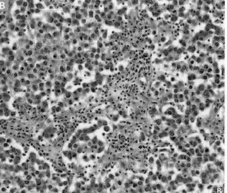

FIGURE 9-55. Testicular seminoma. A Gross specimen shows well-defined borders with involvement of most of the parenchyma. B Histologic specimen shows lymphocyte infiltration of the parenchyma.

TABLE 9-21. Characteristics, Tumor Markers, and Prognosis of Germ Cell Testicular Tumors

MALIGNANCY	CHARACTERISTICS	TUMOR MARKERS	PROGNOSIS
Seminoma	Large, well-demarcated mass	Increased hCG, PLAP	Excellent
Yolk sac tumor	Schiller-Duval bodies	Increased AFP	Good
Embryonal carcinoma	Ill-defined masses with foci of necrosis and hemorrhage	Increased hCG	Poor
Choriocarcinoma	Trophoblastic tissue	Increased hCG	Poor
Teratoma	Derivatives from multiple germ layers (ectoderm, endoderm, mesoderm)	Increased AFP and/or hCG	Good

AFP, α-fetoprotein; hCG, human chorionic gonadotropin; PLAP, placental alkaline phosphatase.

KEY FACT

In males, both immature and mature teratomas are considered malignant. In females, **only** immature teratomas are considered malignant.

- **With malignant transformation:** Development of frank malignancy in preexisting teratomatous elements, usually in the form of a squamous cell carcinoma or adenocarcinoma. Usually occurs in adults.
- **Mixed:** Combinations of any of the germ cell tumors above may occur in mixed tumors, the most common being a combination of teratoma, embryonal carcinoma, and yolk sac tumors. **hCG and AFP are elevated.**

Embryonal Carcinoma

Ill-defined invasive mass containing foci of hemorrhage and necrosis. Metastases are common. Histologically, the cells are large and primitive looking, with basophilic cytoplasm, indistinct cell borders, and large nuclei with prominent nucleoli. The cells may be arranged in undifferentiated, solid sheets or glandular structures. Embryonal carcinoma is associated with **an increase in hCG.**

Sex Cord Stromal Tumors

Leydig Cell Tumor

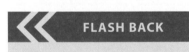

FLASH BACK

Most testicular tumors have an ovarian counterpart.

Arises from Leydig cells that contain rod-shaped **Reinke crystals,** and is usually benign. Golden-brown mass consisting of large, uniform cells with indistinct cell borders. It produces androgens or estrogens, leading to gynecomastia in men and precocious puberty in boys. Treatment is orchidectomy.

Sertoli Cell Tumor

Arises from Sertoli cells. Grossly, it is a gray-white to yellow mass. Microscopically, it shows cord-like structures resembling seminiferous tubules. Secretes a small amount of androgens or estrogens that is typically insufficient to induce gynecomastia, loss of libido, and aspermia. It is usually a benign condition, and orchiectomy is curative.

Malignant Lymphoma

Originates as a diffuse large-cell lymphoma and causes secondary involvement of both testes. The most common testicular cancer in **elderly men.** Prognosis is poor.

PROSTATE DISEASES

Benign Prostatic Hyperplasia

Benign enlargement of the prostate gland due to cellular proliferation (**hyperplasia**), usually at the periurethral central zone (Figure 9-56).

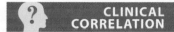

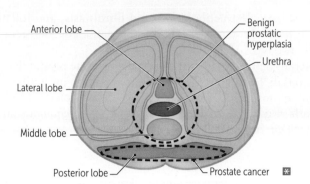

FIGURE 9-56. **Transverse section of prostate showing location of benign prostatic hypertrophy (BPH) and prostatic carcinoma.** The central portion of the prostate is sensitive to estrogen and dihydrotestosterone and is the site for BPH, whereas the peripheral zone is sensitive to androgen and is the site for prostatic carcinoma.

- It is commonly seen in males > 50 years of age.
- Family history (first-degree relative) is a risk factor.
- With age, estrogen levels tend to increase, in turn inducing surface expression of androgen receptors in the central zone of the prostate. Therefore, despite the generally lower androgen levels in older men, their prostate hypertrophies because of increased **sensitivity** to DHT.

PRESENTATION

Patient presents with lower urinary tract symptoms including urgency, frequency, nocturia, dribbling of urine, poor stream, sensation of incomplete voiding, incontinence, urinary retention, and often UTI. This may lead to distention and hypertrophy of the bladder due to incomplete emptying and straining during urination.

DIAGNOSIS

- Firm, smooth, and uniform enlargement of the prostate on digital rectal examination.
- Sonogram shows a diffusely enlarged prostate.
- Prostate-specific antigen (PSA) level is checked to rule out prostate cancer. PSA can be elevated in BPH, but is typically < 10 ng/mL.

TREATMENT

Medical treatment includes nonselective α-blockers (doxazosin, prazosin, and terazosin), selective α-blockers (tamsulosin), and 5α-reductase inhibitors (finasteride). Surgical management involves transurethral resection of the prostate or prostatectomy.

Prostatitis

Inflammation of the prostate gland.

PRESENTATION

- Dysuria, urinary frequency, malaise, lower back pain.
- Poorly localized pelvic pain.
- May be acute or chronic.
  - **Acute:** Caused by *E coli* and other gram-negative rods. Neutrophilic infiltrate, congestion, and edema. Microabscesses may form. The prostate is often **tender and boggy.** Leukocytosis and fever are also seen. In patients < 35 years of age, the pathogens *C trachomatis* and *N gonorrhoeae* are most likely. In patients older than 35 years of age, *E coli*, *P aeruginosa*, and *Klebsiella pneumoniae* are most likely.

CLINICAL CORRELATION

Digital rectal exam (DRE) is one screening test for prostate cancer. The peripheral zone of the prostate is easily palpated during a DRE.

FLASH FORWARD

Prazosin, doxazosin, and terazosin relax the bladder neck and prostate by blocking α-adrenergic receptors located in smooth muscle. They are used to treat urinary retention in BPH.

FLASH FORWARD

The 5α-reductase inhibitor finasteride inhibits conversion of testosterone to DHT. DHT normally causes increased proliferation of smooth muscle in the central zone of the prostate.

■ **Chronic:** Tissue destruction, **increased fibroblasts,** and inflammatory cells characteristic of chronic infections. Can be caused by recurrent UTIs or STIs. There are two types of chronic prostatitis:
  ■ **Bacterial:** Same organisms responsible for acute prostatitis.
  ■ **Abacterial:** The most common form of chronic prostatitis. Leukocytes are found in prostatic secretions but there are no bacteriologic findings. There is no history of recurrent UTI. However, *C trachomatis* and *Ureaplasma urealyticum* have also been implicated.

TREATMENT

For bacterial prostatitis, antibiotic treatment with trimethoprim/sulfamethoxazole or ciprofloxacin is effective. For abacterial prostatitis, no therapies have been shown to be effective. Nonsteroidal anti-inflammatory drugs (NSAIDs) can be used as an adjunctive therapy.

Prostatic Adenocarcinoma

■ Arises mostly from the peripheral zone (70%) of the prostate (Figure 9-56).
■ It occurs in 20–30% of men > 50 years of age and in 90% of men > 70 years of age.
■ Most are very slow growing and never present in the man's lifetime.
■ With advancing age, the androgen level declines. When the androgen level declines, regressive changes occur, mainly in the peripheral zone, and prostatic carcinoma arises in these settings.

PRESENTATION

■ Appears as a hard, irregular mass during digital rectal examination.
■ Since the peripheral zone is typically involved, urinary symptoms are a late manifestation of the disease.

SPREAD

■ Spreads via hematogenous or lymphatic channels and by direct invasion.
■ Spreads to the **lungs** hematogenously and via the vertebral venous plexus to **pelvic bones and lumbosacral spine.**
■ Lymphatic spread occurs to presacral, internal iliac, para-aortic, and supraclavicular nodes, whereas direct spread may invade the bladder, ureter, seminal vesicles, and other pelvic structures.
■ The rectum is rarely involved due to the presence of the rectovesical fascia.

DIAGNOSIS

■ Prostatic biopsy with histologic examination is required for a definitive diagnosis. The Gleason grading system assigns a score of 1–5 to tissue samples based on architecture. Higher Gleason scores portend a worse prognosis.
■ On digital rectal examination, the prostate appears to be **stony hard with obliteration of the median sulcus.**
■ **PSA** (glycoprotein produced by normal and abnormal ductal epithelium) > 10 ng/mL is suggestive, and > 35 ng/mL is diagnostic of advanced cancer.
■ **Alkaline phosphatase** is elevated either due to hepatic or bone metastasis.
■ Radiologic findings in case of metastasis include characteristic sclerotic, osteoblastic metastases in lumbar vertebrae and pelvic bones.

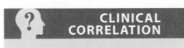

CLINICAL CORRELATION

PSA is often used to monitor tumor recurrence. Digital rectal exams do not increase the false-positive rate of PSA.

TREATMENT

Radical prostatectomy can be done as a curative treatment for early disease, but palliative treatment is the only option for advanced disease. The palliative treatment involves deprivation of androgens via bilateral orchidectomy or by giving antiandrogens such as flutamide. Other treatment options include radiation and gonadotropin-releasing hormone (GnRH) agonists administered in a continuous fashion (suppresses anterior pituitary secretion of FSH and LH).

SEXUALLY TRANSMITTED INFECTIONS AND OTHER GENITAL INFECTIONS

See Table 9-20 in the Pathology—Female section for a summary of common STIs and other genital infections.

Pharmacology

DRUGS THAT MODULATE THE GONADOTROPIN AXIS

Gonadotropin-Releasing Hormone Mixed Agonists/Antagonists (Leuprolide, Buserelin, Nafarelin, Goserelin)

MECHANISM OF ACTION

Decrease secretion of FSH and LH when used in a **continuous** fashion by desensitizing pituitary GnRH receptors, resulting in downregulating of the receptor. Use in a **pulsatile** fashion has GnRH agonist activity, resulting in increased FSH/LH.

USES (FIGURE 9-57)

Pulsatile administration: Infertility.
Continuous administration: Prostate cancer, uterine fibroids, endometriosis, PCOS, precocious puberty.

SIDE EFFECTS

Menopausal symptoms (eg, hot flashes, bone density loss), headache, nausea, vomiting.

Gonadotropin-Releasing Hormone Pure Antagonists (Ganirelix, Cetrorelix)

MECHANISM OF ACTION

Competitively bind GnRH receptor in the pituitary, decreasing secretion of FSH/LH.

USES

Control of ovulation via suppression of premature LH surges in IVF cycles, endometriosis, menorrhagia, gynecomastia.

SIDE EFFECTS

Virilization in females, GI disturbances, weight gain, fluid retention, dizziness, muscle cramps, headache.

DRUGS THAT MODULATE THE MALE REPRODUCTIVE SYSTEM

Androgen Agonists (Testosterone, Methyltestosterone)

MECHANISM OF ACTION

Agonist at androgen receptor, resulting in modification of gene transcription upon conversion to DHT in target cells and decreased release of LH from the anterior pituitary.

USES

Hypogonadism/testicular failure, anemia, stimulation of anabolic activity.

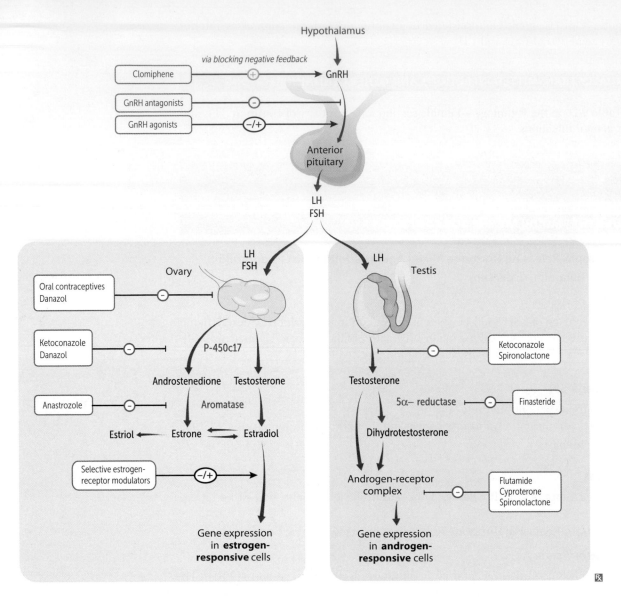

FIGURE 9-57. **Pharmacologic control of reproductive hormones.** FSH, follicle-stimulating hormone; GnRH, gonadotropin-releasing hormone; LH, luteinizing hormone.

SIDE EFFECTS

Decreased release of LH, resulting in decreased testicular production of testosterone and gonadal atrophy, increased low-density lipoprotein (LDL), decreased high-density lipoprotien (HDL), premature closure of epiphyseal plates.

Antiandrogens

Androgen Antagonists (Flutamide)

MECHANISM OF ACTION

Competitive antagonist at androgen receptor.

USES

Prostate cancer, hirsutism in women.

SIDE EFFECTS

Gynecomastia, impotence, decreased libido, decreased volume of ejaculate, hot flashes, diarrhea, nausea, hepatitis.

5α-Reductase Inhibitors (Finasteride)

MECHANISM OF ACTION

Decrease conversion of testosterone to the more potent DHT.

USES

BPH, androgenic alopecia.

SIDE EFFECTS

Loss of libido, erectile dysfunction, breast enlargement/tenderness, testicular pain, GI distress. Pregnant women should avoid exposure due to risk of hypospadias in a male fetus.

Nonhormonal Drugs

Phosphodiesterase 5 (PDE-5) Inhibitors (Sildenafil, Vardenafil, Tadalafil)

MECHANISM OF ACTION

Vasodilate by inhibiting cGMP phosphodiesterase (cGMP increased), resulting in increased blood flow to the corpus cavernosum and penile erection.

USES

Erectile dysfunction.

SIDE EFFECTS

Life-threatening hypotension in patients taking nitrates, headache, changes in blue-green color vision, flushing, dyspepsia.

Tamsulosin

MECHANISM OF ACTION

Inhibits smooth muscle contraction in the prostate by acting as an $\alpha_{1A,D}$ antagonist.

USES

BPH.

SIDE EFFECTS

Retrograde ejaculation, hypotension, poor outcomes for cataract surgery.

Minoxidil

MECHANISM

Direct arteriolar vasodilator.

USES

Androgenic alopecia.

SIDE EFFECTS

Local irritation/burning, unwanted hair growth.

DRUGS THAT MODULATE THE FEMALE REPRODUCTIVE SYSTEM

Labor Modulators

Uterine Contractants (Oxytocin, Ergometrine)

MECHANISM OF ACTION

Bind oxytocin receptor, stimulating the release of intracellular calcium and inducing contraction of smooth muscle in uterus and mammary myoepithelial cells.

USES

Induction of labor, postpartum hemorrhage, stimulation of milk letdown.

SIDE EFFECTS

Generally well tolerated.

Uterine Relaxants (Ritodrine, Salmeterol, Terbutaline)

MECHANISM OF ACTION

β_2-agonists that relax the smooth muscle of the uterus.

USES

Blockade of contractions in preterm labor.

SIDE EFFECTS

Pulmonary edema, tremor, arrhythmia.

Hormone Agonists

Estrogen Agonists (Ethinyl Estradiol, DES, Mestranol)

MECHANISM OF ACTION

Estrogen receptor agonists, resulting in stimulation of endometrial growth and development/maintenance of secondary sex characteristics.

USES

Hormone replacement therapy in women without a history of breast cancer, osteoporosis, contraception.

SIDE EFFECTS

Thrombosis, weight gain, breast tenderness, increased risk of endometrial cancer, migraine, increased risk of clear cell vaginal adenocarcinoma in female offspring (DES).

Progesterone Agonists (Medroxyprogesterone, Norethindrone)

MECHANISM OF ACTION

Stimulate vascularization of endometrium and maintenance of pregnancy.

USES

Abnormal uterine bleeding, endometrial cancer, contraception, appetite stimulation in cachetic patients.

SIDE EFFECTS

Thrombosis, hypertension, acne, fluid retention, weight gain, depression, decreased libido, breast discomfort, irregular periods.

Androgen Agonists (Danazol)

MECHANISM OF ACTION

Synthetic androgen that acts as a partial agonist at androgen and progesterone receptors and displaces testosterone from sex hormone binding globulin, resulting in increased serum testosterone levels.

USES

Can be used for endometriosis because it decreases estrogen levels in females but has largely been replaced by other therapies due to its hyperandrogenic effects. Also used in hereditary angioedema.

SIDE EFFECTS

Masculinization, hirsutism, acne, decreased HDL levels, weight gain, edema, hepatotoxicity.

Hormone Antagonists

Selective Estrogen Receptor Modulators (Clomiphene, Tamoxifen, Raloxifene)

MECHANISM OF ACTION

Clomiphene: Estrogen receptor (ER) antagonist in hypothalamus, resulting in decreased negative feedback and increase gonadotropin release, causing ovulation.

Tamoxifen: Estrogen antagonist in breast tissue, **agonist in endometrium** and bone.

Raloxifene: Estrogen antagonist in breast tissue and endometrium, agonist in bone.

USES

Induction of ovulation (clomiphene), ER-positive breast cancer and osteoporosis (tamoxifen and raloxifene).

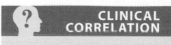

CLINICAL CORRELATION

Oral contraceptives are contraindicated in women older than age 35 who smoke due to risk of venous thromboembolism.

SIDE EFFECTS

Clomiphene: Multiple births, ovarian enlargement, breast tenderness, abdominal pain, hot flashes, visual disturbances.

Tamoxifen: **Endometrial cancer,** thrombosis, hot flashes.

Raloxifene: Thrombosis, hot flashes.

Aromatase Inhibitors (Anastrozole, Exemestane)

MECHANISM OF ACTION

Competitively (anastrozole) and noncompetitively/irreversibly (exemestane) bind aromatase enzyme, preventing the conversion of testosterone to estradiol.

USES

Chemotherapy in postmenopausal women with ER-positive breast cancer.

SIDE EFFECTS

Osteoporosis, infertility.

Progesterone Inhibitors (Mifepristone, aka RU-486)

MECHANISM OF ACTION

Competitive inhibitor of progesterone receptor.

USES

Termination of pregnancy.

SIDE EFFECTS

Heavy bleeding, abdominal pain, GI upset.

Antiandrogens (Ketoconazole, Spironolactone)

MECHANISM OF ACTION

Inhibit steroid synthesis (both) and displace estradiol and DHT from sex hormone binding protein (spironolactone), resulting in increased estradiol to testosterone ratio.

USES

PCOS.

SIDE EFFECTS

Amenorrhea, gynecomastia, liver toxicity.

Oral Contraceptives (Combined Progesterone and Estrogen)

MECHANISM OF ACTION

Inhibition of FSH/LH secretion via negative feedback, resulting in suppression of development of the follicle and ovulation. Progesterone also inhibits endometrial proliferation and thickens cervical mucus.

USES

Contraception.

SIDE EFFECTS

Increased risk of blood clots in older women/smokers, weight gain, nausea, fluid retention, hypertension, depression.

HER2/neu Antagonists (Traztuzumab, Pertuzumab)

MECHANISM OF ACTION

Monoclonal antibody targeting *HER2/neu* receptor, causing selective immune-modulated cytotoxicity.

USES

HER2/neu-positive breast cancer.

SIDE EFFECTS

Cardiotoxicity.

CHAPTER 10

Respiratory

EMBRYOLOGY   748
Respiratory Development   748
Congenital Malformations   751

ANATOMY   753
Airways   754
Lungs   754
Diaphragm   756
External Anatomy   757
Muscles of Respiration   757
Flail Chest   758

HISTOLOGY   758
Respiratory Epithelium   759
Alveoli   759
Olfactory Cells   761

PHYSIOLOGY   761
Lung Volumes and Capacities   761
Ventilation   763
Blood Gases   770

PATHOLOGY   779
Pathology on Physical Examination   779
Nasopharynx   781
Obstructive Lung Diseases   783
Restrictive Lung Diseases   790
Pulmonary Vascular Diseases   798
Respiratory Tract Cancers   803
Pulmonary Infections   808
Pleural Effusion   815
Pneumothorax   815
Allergy   817
Hypersensitivity Pneumonitis   818

PHARMACOLOGY   818
Histamine Blockers   818
Mucoactive Agents   819
Dextromethorphan   819
α-Adrenergic Agonists   820
Pulmonary Hypertension Drugs   820
Asthma Drugs   821

Embryology

RESPIRATORY DEVELOPMENT

The respiratory system allows for blood oxygenation and clearance of carbon dioxide (CO_2), sustains aerobic metabolism, and maintains acid-base balance. The respiratory system develops in the fluid-filled womb, devoid of air. Development occurs in a cranial-to-caudal fashion. The upper respiratory tract (larynx to trachea) develops first, followed by the lower respiratory tract (bronchi and lungs). Lung development is further subdivided into pseudoglandular, canalicular, saccular, and alveolar stages (Figure 10-1).

The respiratory system develops from the laryngotracheal groove on the ventral foregut during gestational weeks 3 and 4 (Figure 10-2). The groove develops into a diverticulum (outpouching) and elongates to form the laryngotracheal tube. The developing respiratory system is partitioned off from the esophagus by the tracheoesophageal septum. The proximal end of this tube becomes the larynx, the middle becomes the trachea, and the distal end forms the lung buds.

Larynx

The larynx is a musculocartilaginous structure in the anterior neck that protects the airway, aids in respiration, and produces sound (vocalization). Located just below the pharynx, it marks the division between the respiratory and digestive systems. It is suspended from the hyoid bone by muscle and ligaments and attached to the trachea inferiorly. The laryngeal cartilage and musculature are derived from the fourth and sixth

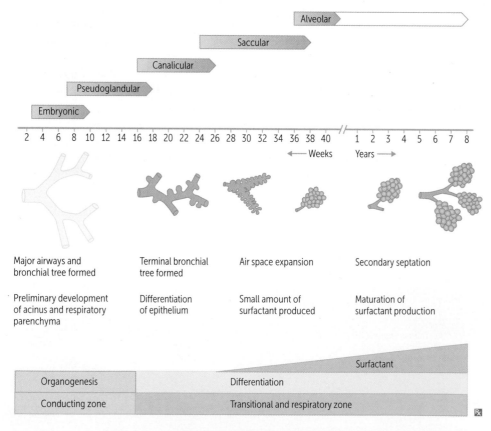

FIGURE 10-1. **Overview of respiratory system development.** After development of the larynx and trachea, the other conducting zones develop through branching. The transitional and respiratory zones develop after the conducting zone.

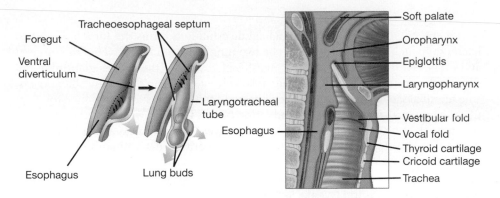

FIGURE 10-2. **Larynx and trachea development.** The larynx begins as the ventral diverticulum. As the diverticulum lengthens, lung buds form at its distal end. This will ultimately give rise to the trachea and lungs.

pharyngeal arches and are innervated by the superior laryngeal nerve (CN X) and recurrent laryngeal nerve (CN X), respectively. As the pharyngeal arches develop, a primitive laryngeal orifice arises below the fourth arch. During week 5, swellings develop lateral to the orifice and eventually form the arytenoid cartilages. An anterior swelling becomes the epiglottis. During week 6, this region develops into a T-shaped orifice (Figure 10-3). Epithelial tissue occluding the orifice breaks down during week 10, with surrounding epithelial folds differentiating into the false and true vocal folds.

Trachea

The trachea is a conducting airway derived from the middle portion of the laryngotracheal tube. The epithelium and glands are derived from the tube endoderm; cartilage, smooth muscle, and connective tissue are derived from splanchnic mesoderm (the ventral part of the lateral mesoderm).

Bronchi and Bronchioles

The lower laryngotracheal tube divides into bronchi, which further divide into bronchioles. The first division is asymmetrical, accompanied by movement of the **smaller left bud** to a **more lateral position** than the **larger right bud.** The second division of the bronchi is also asymmetrical, with three branches on the right and two branches on the left. The tertiary bronchi continue to divide dichotomously until terminal bronchioles with distal alveoli are formed.

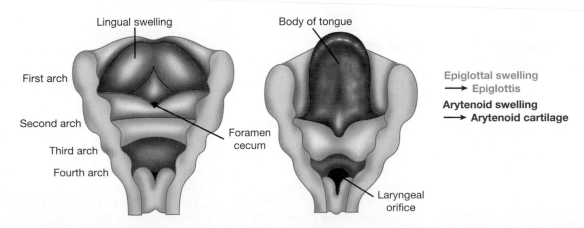

FIGURE 10-3. **Larynx development from pharyngeal arches.** The cartilage and musculature of the larynx are derived from the pharyngeal arches. An epiglottic swelling will give rise to the epiglottis, and an arytenoid swelling will give rise to the arytenoid cartilages. The foramen cecum is a depression along the groove that divides the tongue into two symmetric halves.

Lungs

At the end of week 4, the laryngotracheal diverticulum forms the lung buds as two lateral outpouchings (Figure 10-1). The two lung buds go on to develop the bronchi and bronchial tree between 2 and 7 months of gestation (the **pseudoglandular** and **canalicular** periods). The lungs mature relatively late compared to many other organs. The terminal sacs and eventually alveoli begin to form in week 26 when the bronchial tree is completed, and **surfactant production begins between weeks 25 and 28** with a rise in production over time (the **saccular** and **alveolar** periods). As a result, the developmental maturity of the lungs is one of the most critical determinants of survival in premature neonates.

Pseudoglandular Period (Weeks 5–16)

Branching continues and all major parts of the lung are formed, except for the gas-exchange elements—respiratory bronchioles and alveoli (Figure 10-1).

Canalicular Period (Weeks 16–26)

The **airways increase in diameter and lung vasculature** develops. **Primitive end-respiratory units,** consisting of a respiratory bronchiole, alveolar duct, and terminal sac, are formed (Figure 10-1).

Saccular Period (Week 26–Birth)

Terminal sacs develop, distinguished by their **thin epithelial lining.** Type I squamous epithelial cells form the gas-exchange surface; type II secretory pneumocytes produce surfactant (Figure 10-1).

Alveolar Period (Prenatal–Childhood)

Clusters of primitive alveoli form, allowing "breathing" in utero via aspiration and expulsion of amniotic fluid. The fluid in the lungs keeps the pulmonary vascular resistance high throughout gestation. At birth, the lungs are half-filled with liquid that must be expelled through the mouth or absorbed into the blood and lymph. The replacement of fluid with air results in a decrease in pulmonary vascular resistance at birth. The alveoli continue to mature after birth, growing in number for the first 3 years and then increasing in both number and size for the next 5 years (Figure 10-1).

Pleural Cavities

The lungs invaginate to penetrate part of the intraembryonic coelom, or body cavity, as they grow and branch. This leaves a layer of **visceral pleura** from the splanchnic mesoderm covering the lung, and a layer of **parietal pleura** from the somatic mesoderm directly abutting the body wall (Figure 10-4).

Diaphragm

The diaphragm develops more superiorly than its postnatal location but maintains its innervation from cervical roots C3, **C4,** and C5. It is formed from four embryologic structures that fuse by week 7 (Figure 10-5):

- The **septum transversum** is formed by mesodermal tissue that projects from the ventral body wall to partially separate the thoracic cavity and abdominal cavity. In the adult, the septum transversum forms the **central tendon** of the diaphragm.
- The **pleuroperitoneal folds** extend from the dorsolateral sides of the body wall to form the pleuroperitoneal membranes, which then fuse with the septum transversum.
- The **body wall** also extends from the dorsal and lateral sides (after the pleuroperitoneal folds have closed the thoracic cavity) to form the peripheral, muscular portion of the adult diaphragm.
- The **dorsal mesentery of the esophagus** forms the portion that is dorsal to the esophagus and ventral to the aorta.

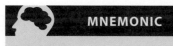

MNEMONIC

C3, 4, 5 keep the diaphragm alive.

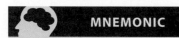

MNEMONIC

Several **P**arts **B**uild a **D**iaphragm:

Septum transversum
Pleuroperitoneal folds
Body wall
Dorsal mesentery of the esophagus

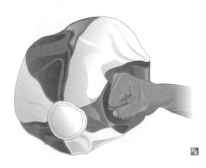

FIGURE 10-4. Pleural cavity development. Imagine pushing on a partially inflated beach ball. As the ball invaginates over your fist, it creates two juxtaposed layers. The surface in contact with your fist is the visceral pleura, and the outer surface is the parietal pleura. The pleural cavity is a potential space that normally contains < 10 mL fluid and lies between the visceral and parietal pleura.

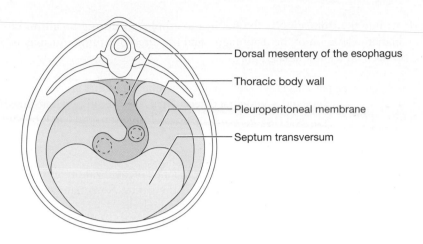

FIGURE 10-5. **Embryonic origins of the diaphragm.**

CONGENITAL MALFORMATIONS

Esophageal Atresia and Tracheoesophageal Fistula

The ventral laryngotracheal diverticulum is separated from the dorsal gut tube (esophagus at this region) by the **tracheoesophageal septum** (mesoderm-derived tissue). Anomalies in the tracheoesophageal septum can lead to **esophageal atresia** (EA) and/or **tracheoesophageal fistula** (TEF) (see also Chapter 3). A fistula is an abnormal communication between two body cavities. Atresia refers to an absence or abnormal narrowing of an opening in the body.

The most common combination of findings is a proximal EA with a distal TEF. However, other variants have been described (Figure 10-6).

Esophageal closure can form as a result of posterior deviation of the tracheoesophageal septum (see Figure 10-6). Embryos in whom there is an EA with no proximal TEF are unable to swallow amniotic fluid, leading to fluid accumulation, polyhydramnios, and an enlarged uterus.

Infants with a TEF have a conduit that allows oral and/or acidic gastric contents to communicate with the lungs, which can cause coughing during feedings. Chemical irritation of the airway mucosa by gastric contents is termed **aspiration pneumonitis.** Infection of the lungs by this process is called **aspiration pneumonia.** In addition, pas-

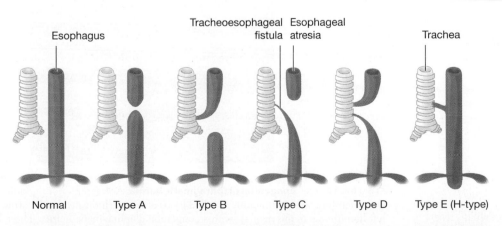

FIGURE 10-6. **Congenital malformations of the trachea and esophagus.** Normal. Type A (8%): esophageal atresia (EA) only. Type B (1%): proximal tracheoesophageal fistula (TEF) and distal EA. Type C (86%): proximal EA and distal TEF. Type D (1%): proximal TEF and distal TEF. Type H (4%): TEF only.

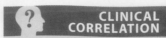
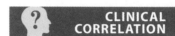
sage of air into the stomach (via the trachea to esophagus during breathing) causes gastric dilation, elevation of the diaphragm, and impaired breathing. Air may be seen in the stomach on a chest radiograph.

TEF and EA may be part of a larger pattern of congenital anomalies known by the acronym **VACTERL,** which includes Vertebral defects, Anal atresia or imperforate anus, Cardiac defects, TEF, Esophageal atresia, Renal agenesis/obstruction, and Limb hypoplasia.

Laryngeal Atresia

Discontinuity of the larynx is thought to be due to failed recanalization during development. Although rare, it is considered a medical emergency. A neonate with laryngeal atresia will asphyxiate unless tracheostomy is performed.

Laryngomalacia

Laryngomalacia is a congenital laxity (weakness) of immature laryngeal cartilages that leads to collapse of the larynx during inspiration, audible as a "wet" inspiratory stridor. It is common in neonates and usually resolves spontaneously without treatment.

Congenital Diaphragmatic Hernia

A **congenital diaphragmatic hernia** (CDH) may result if the components of the developing diaphragm fail to properly fuse. The newborn presents with respiratory distress and bowel sounds in the thoracic cavity. A chest radiograph will show abdominal contents (loops of bowel) within the thoracic cavity (Figure 10-7). CDH is the most common cause of pulmonary hypoplasia.

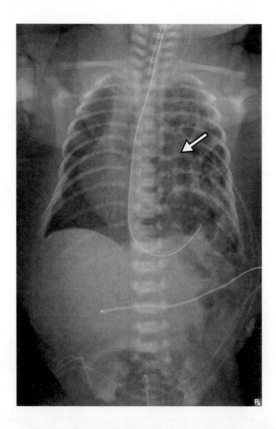

FIGURE 10-7. **Congenital diaphragmatic hernia.** Anteroposterior portable chest and abdomen film shows numerous air-filled loops of bowel (indicated by the arrow) in the left hemithorax in this neonate with a congenital diaphragmatic hernia. There is a shift of mediastinal structures to the right. An orogastric tube lies within the stomach.

Pulmonary Hypoplasia

Failure of the lungs to develop fully may be primary or, more commonly, secondary to another defect such as oligohydramnios, or due to compression by a CDH or tumor (Figure 10-8). The hypoplastic lung lacks respiratory exchange capacity and has overgrowth of smooth muscle elements, which leads to pulmonary hypertension. Unilateral hypoplasia is compatible with life; bilateral usually results in early death. In rare cases, the lungs may fail to develop entirely, termed **pulmonary aplasia.**

Congenital Cysts

Congenital cysts are saccular enlargements of the terminal bronchiole. They are usually solitary and can be associated with chronic infection secondary to poor drainage.

Respiratory Distress Syndrome

During weeks 25–28, type II pneumocytes begin to produce surfactant, a phospholipoprotein fluid that facilitates alveolar opening by reducing surface tension during expiration. Due to the absence of surfactant, a fetus delivered prior to 25 weeks of gestation may not be viable. A baby delivered prematurely during the period between the onset of surfactant secretion and term gestation has some degree of surfactant deficiency (Figure 10-9). The static surface tension of surfactant-deficient alveoli results in collapse of some air spaces and hyperexpansion of others due to LaPlace's law ($P = 2T/r$). The impaired ventilation contributes to vascular congestion and leakage of proteins, resulting in formation of hyaline membranes. Respiratory distress syndrome (RDS) is further discussed under Interstitial Lung Diseases. Clinically, the infant exhibits superficial, rapid breathing **(tachypnea)** and **cyanosis.** The incidence of RDS is inversely related to gestational age at birth. The most important intervention for RDS is to prevent premature birth, if possible. The first-line treatment is administration of antenatal corticosteroids (stimulates fetal surfactant production) to all pregnant women who are at risk of delivery between 23 and 34 weeks' gestation. Initial postnatal treatment includes nasal continuous positive airway pressure (CPAP). Exogenous surfactant replacement, endotracheal intubation, and mechanical ventilation are used for more severe RDS.

Anatomy

The respiratory system consists of the nasal passages and mouth, pharynx, trachea, bronchi, bronchioles, lungs, and the muscles that control respiration, as shown in Figure 10-10.

> **KEY FACT**
>
> The conducting airways are surrounded by a layer of smooth muscle that hypertrophies and undergoes spastic contractions in **asthma,** an obstructive lung disease.

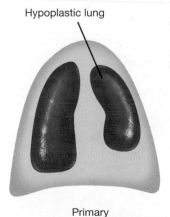

Hypoplastic lung

Primary

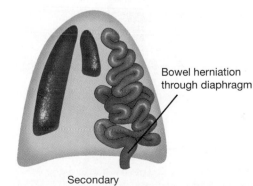

Bowel herniation through diaphragm

Secondary

FIGURE 10-8. **Lung hypoplasia and congenital diaphragmatic hernia (CDH).** Failure of a lung to fully develop may occur as an isolated event (left) or secondary to another defect such as bowel herniation through the diaphragm (right).

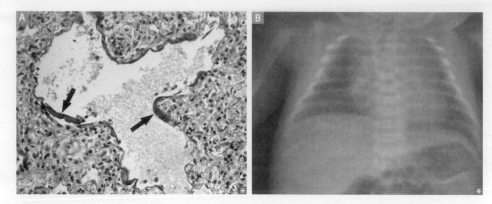

FIGURE 10-9. Indications of surfactant deficiency in a premature infant.
A Photomicrograph shows collapsed alveoli surrounding dilated alveolar ducts lined by smooth homogeneous hyaline membranes (arrows). **B** X-ray of the chest shows diffuse ground-glass opacities and prominent air bronchograms consistent with neonatal respiratory distress syndrome.

AIRWAYS

The passages that transmit air from the environment to the lungs can be divided into conducting and respiratory airways (Table 10-1).

LUNGS

The right and left lungs are structurally distinct (Table 10-2).

Blood Supply of the Lungs

- The right and left **pulmonary arteries** transport relatively deoxygenated blood from the right ventricle to the lungs.
- The **bronchial arteries** branch from the descending aorta to supply the bronchi and pulmonary connective tissues with nourishing, O_2-rich blood. In reality, the perfusion provided by these vessels is not clinically significant. They are not commonly reanastomosed during lung transplantation.
- Branches of the pulmonary and bronchial arteries enter the **bronchopulmonary segments** centrally alongside the **segmental (tertiary) bronchi.**

MNEMONIC

RALS:

Right pulmonary artery is **A**nterior, **L**eft pulmonary artery is **S**uperior to the bronchi.

KEY FACT

An aspirated foreign object is more likely to lodge in the right mainstem bronchus than the left mainstem bronchus due to the smaller angle of entry and wider diameter of the right mainstem bronchus (see Figure 10-10).

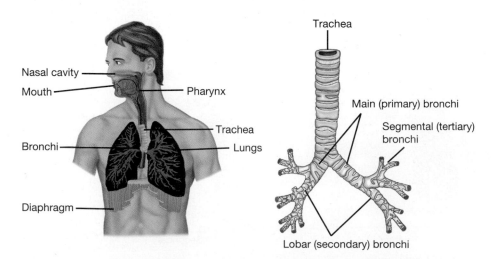

FIGURE 10-10. Gross anatomy of the respiratory system. Overview (left) and conducting airways (right).

TABLE 10-1.   Conducting and Respiratory Airways

	CONDUCTING AIRWAYS	RESPIRATORY AIRWAYS
Function	Warm, humidify, and filter air; no gas exchange (anatomic dead space)	Gas exchange
Structures	Nose/mouth, pharynx Trachea Bronchi Bronchioles Terminal bronchioles	Respiratory bronchioles Alveolar ducts Alveoli

- Small **bronchial veins** unite to form a single vessel in each lung that empties into the **azygos vein** on the right and the **hemiazygos vein** on the left.
- The **pulmonary veins** transport highly oxygenated blood from the alveoli to the left atrium.

The relationship among the conducting airways, respiratory airways, and blood supply to the alveoli is shown in Figure 10-11.

Pleura

The lungs are located within a bilayered pleural sac in the thoracic cavity.

- The **visceral pleura**, or **pulmonary pleura**, adheres tightly to the outer surface of the lungs.
- The **parietal pleura** covers the inside of the thoracic cavity, including the diaphragm, chest wall, and the mediastinum.
- The **pleural reflections** are the angled boundaries between the parietal pleura lining one surface and the parietal pleura lining another. For example, the costal pleura is continuous with the diaphragmatic pleura, forming the costal line of pleural reflection at the boundary between the ribs and the diaphragm, also called the **costophrenic angle.**

Between the visceral and parietal pleura is a potential space, the **pleural cavity**, which normally contains < 10 mL of fluid. In some disease states, fluid accumulates in the pleural cavity, forming a **pleural effusion.** When the patient is erect, the fluid fills the **costodiaphragmatic recess** located at the inferior part of the thoracic cavity. On a chest radiograph, the costophrenic angles are normally sharply demarcated and unoccupied by tissue or fluid, but pleural effusions blunt these angles, as seen in Figure 10-12.

KEY FACT

The visceral pleura lacks sensory innervation. The parietal pleura is innervated by branches of the intercostal and phrenic nerves, and is thus highly sensitive to pain, but the visceral pleura is not.

MNEMONIC

The **P**arietal pleura feels **P**ain.

FLASH BACK

A pleural effusion may be classified as **transudative** or **exudative.**

- **Transudate:** increased capillary pressure or decreased oncotic pressure secondary to congestive heart failure (CHF), cirrhosis, or nephrotic syndrome.
- **Exudate:** increased vascular permeability and inflammation secondary to lung infection, malignancy, or pulmonary embolism (PE), although some PEs produce a transudative pleural effusion.

CLINICAL CORRELATION

A pneumothorax occurs when air fills the pleural cavity due to compromise of one or both of the pleurae (often caused by trauma or ruptured blebs). Positive pleural pressure resulting from air entering the thorax leads to collapse of the ipsilateral lung, as well as dissociation of the lung–chest wall system. These events may manifest as shortness of breath (dyspnea), particularly when the pneumothorax is large.

TABLE 10-2.   Anatomy of the Right and Left Lungs

	RIGHT	LEFT
Lobes	Three (upper, middle, and lower)	Two (upper with lingula, and lower)
Main bronchus entry	Smaller angle (more continuous with trachea)	Sharper angle (greater deviation from trachea)
Main bronchus shape	Shorter and wider	Longer and narrower
Pulmonary artery entry	Anterior to right mainstem bronchus	Superior to left mainstem bronchus

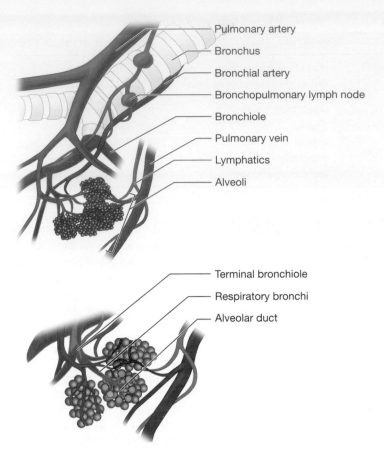

FIGURE 10-11. **Anatomy of the bronchopulmonary segments.** Each lobe of the lung is subdivided into several functional bronchopulmonary segments, each supplied by its own artery and tertiary bronchus. The pulmonary and bronchial arteries approach the alveoli alongside the bronchi, and the pulmonary vein drains blood separately.

DIAPHRAGM

The thoracic diaphragm is a domed, musculotendinous structure that forms the inferior border of the thoracic cavity. During physiologic inspiration, the central part of the diaphragm descends, decreasing intrathoracic pressure and increasing lung volume.

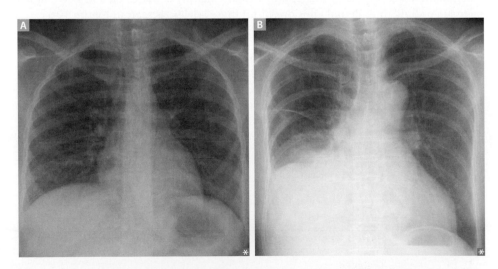

FIGURE 10-12. **Chest radiographs.** **A** Normal chest radiograph. **B** Plain chest radiograph shows pleural effusion in the right hemithorax.

The peripheral parts of the diaphragm are fused to the thoracic wall and are thus immobile. The left and right crura (singular: crus) affix the diaphragm posteriorly to the vertebral column.

The diaphragm is a useful landmark in radiographs, as it has three openings at specific vertebral levels, which allow structures to penetrate: (1) the inferior vena cava (IVC) through the caval opening at T8; (2) the esophagus and vagus nerve through the esophageal hiatus at T10; and (3) the aorta, azygos vein, and thoracic duct through the aortic hiatus at T12 (Figure 10-13).

EXTERNAL ANATOMY

Landmarks outline the location of the lungs and surrounding pleural cavities (Figure 10-14).

- The lung apices are superior to the first rib, extending into the **supraclavicular fossa.** This is of clinical significance in penetrating trauma to the lower neck and upper thoracic regions, as the lung apex can be damaged and a pneumothorax can result.
- At full exhalation, the lower lung borders extend to the sixth rib anteriorly, eighth rib at the midaxillary line, and 10th rib posteriorly.
- The pleural reflection extends to the eighth rib anteriorly, descending to the 10th rib at the midaxillary line, and to the 12th rib posteriorly.

These landmarks are important when performing thoracic procedures. A **thoracentesis** allows for sampling of pleural effusions by introducing a needle into the pleural space. The needle is typically inserted against the superior border of the corresponding rib, because the intercostal vein, artery, and nerve lie at the inferior rib margin (Figure 10-15).

MUSCLES OF RESPIRATION

The diaphragm is the primary muscle of respiration. It is innervated by the **phrenic nerve,** which is formed by branches of the C3, C4, and C5 nerve roots.

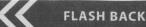

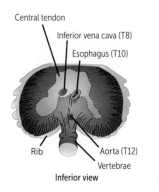

FLASH BACK

The **right crus** of the diaphragm wraps around the esophagus to prevent the formation of a **hiatal hernia,** in which the stomach begins to slide into the thoracic cavity (refer to the Pathology section in Chapter 3 for details).

Central tendon
Inferior vena cava (T8)
Esophagus (T10)
Rib
Aorta (T12)
Vertebrae
Inferior view

FIGURE 10-13. **The diaphragm and penetrating structures.**

MNEMONIC

I 8 10 EGGs AAT 12 ("I ate ten eggs at twelve"):

Inferior vena cava: I**8**
EsophaGus, vaGus nerve: T**10**
Aorta, Azygos vein, Thoracic duct: T**12**

MNEMONIC

The intercostal **V**ein, **A**rtery, and **N**erve travel in a **VAN** inferior to the rib, in a superior-to-inferior direction:
V → A → N.

CLINICAL CORRELATION

A lesion of the phrenic nerve results in ipsilateral paralysis of the diaphragm. On a chest radiograph, this can be seen as elevation of the ipsilateral diaphragm.

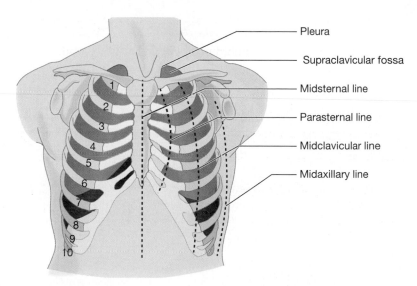

Pleura
Supraclavicular fossa
Midsternal line
Parasternal line
Midclavicular line
Midaxillary line

FIGURE 10-14. **External landmarks of the thoracic cavity.** Note the difference between the extent of the lungs at normal inflation (pink) and at full inspiration (dark red). The floating ribs (11 and 12) are not illustrated.

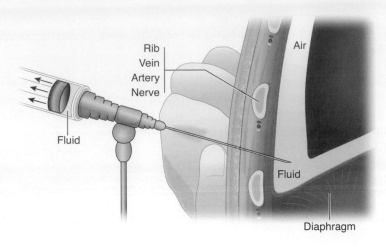

FIGURE 10-15. **Thoracentesis.**

The diaphragm (and to a lesser extent, the external intercostals and scalenes) is involved in **quiet inspiration** (inspiration at rest), while **quiet expiration** is a passive activity. Multiple additional accessory muscles are involved in **forced respiration,** which occurs during heavy activity (Table 10-3).

FLAIL CHEST

Flail chest is usually due to significant blunt trauma and is defined as three or more adjacent ribs with fractures at two or more locations. The result is an unstable chest wall segment with **paradoxical breathing motion.** The flail segment moves inward during inspiration and outward during expiration—opposite from the surrounding uninjured chest wall. Crepitus may be present as well. Pulmonary contusion underlying the flail segment often results in respiratory compromise. Treatment is beyond the scope of this text but may include pain control, incentive spirometry, and mechanical ventilation.

Histology

Within the lungs, there are two distinct functional regions: the **conducting airways,** which partition, humidify, and filter the air, and the **respiratory airways,** which allow for

TABLE 10-3. **Respiratory Muscles**

	QUIET RESPIRATION	FORCED RESPIRATION
Inspiration	Diaphragm External intercostals Internal intercostals (interchondral part)	Diaphragm External intercostals Internal intercostals (interchondral part) Scalenes Sternocleidomastoids
Expiration	None (passive)	Rectus abdominis Internal/external obliques Transversus abdominis Transversus thoracis Internal intercostals (interosseous part)

gas exchange. Specialized epithelial cell layers along these different airways contribute to their distinct functional capacities. The conducting airways are lined by thick pseudostratified columnar epithelium, and the alveoli are lined by exceedingly thin type I pneumocytes and interspersed surfactant-secreting type II pneumocytes.

RESPIRATORY EPITHELIUM

The proximal portion of the upper respiratory tract consists of **stratified squamous epithelium,** which lines the following:

- Oropharynx
- Laryngopharynx
- Anterior epiglottis
- Upper half of posterior epiglottis
- True vocal cords

The remainder of the conducting portion of the respiratory tract is lined mostly by **ciliated pseudostratified columnar epithelium ("respiratory epithelium")** from the nasal cavity to the terminal bronchioles, where the lining transitions to ciliated simple cuboidal (respiratory bronchioles) and then simple squamous (alveolar ducts and alveoli) epithelium.

Cilia of the respiratory epithelium sweep mucus and foreign particles toward the mouth, thereby protecting the lower respiratory tract. **Goblet cells,** which secrete mucus, are interspersed in the respiratory epithelium from the nasopharynx to the primary bronchioles. These cells can be identified by their distinct shape and pale-staining cytoplasm.

Clara cells lack cilia, are located in the terminal bronchioles, and secrete protein to help protect the airway lining from damage. Microscopically, Clara cells can be identified by secretory granules in the apical cytoplasm.

ALVEOLI

The alveoli are composed of multiple cell types. These cells are described in Table 10-4 and illustrated in Figure 10-16.

TABLE 10-4. Types of Alveolar Cells

	TYPE I CELLS	TYPE II CELLS	ENDOTHELIAL CELLS	MACROPHAGES	CLARA CELLS
Prevalence	Cover 95% of alveolar surface area. Comprise 10% of cell population	Cover 5% of alveolar surface area. Comprise 12% of the cell population	40% of the cell population	Variable	11% in terminal bronchioles; 22% in respiratory bronchioles
Structure	Flat and extremely thin (< 500 nm)	Cuboidal	Thin, wrapped into cylinders to form capillaries	Amorphous	Nonciliated; low-columnar/cuboidal with secretory granules
Function(s)	Allow for gas exchange with the adjacent capillaries Nonproliferative	Secrete surfactant Proliferate after lung damage Are source of precursors for new alveolar cells (types I and II)	Allow for gas exchange with the alveolus	Engulf debris ("dust cells")	Secrete component of surfactant; degrade toxins; act as reserve cells

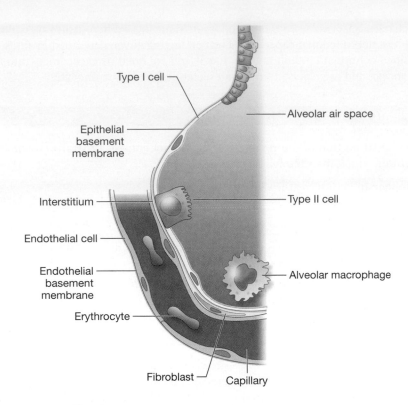

FIGURE 10-16. **Alveolar structure.**

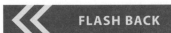
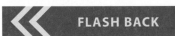
Pulmonary surfactant is a mixture of phospholipids (80%, primarily dipalmitoylphosphatidylcholine [DPPC], which is a type of lecithin), surfactant-associated proteins (12%), and lipids (8%). Surfactant is stored in the whorled cytoplasmic **lamellar bodies** of type II alveolar cells (Figure 10-17).

Pulmonary capillary endothelial cells are joined by tight junctions to form a continuous endothelium without fenestrations. This configuration prevents fluid leakage but still permits gas exchange across the thin cell bodies.

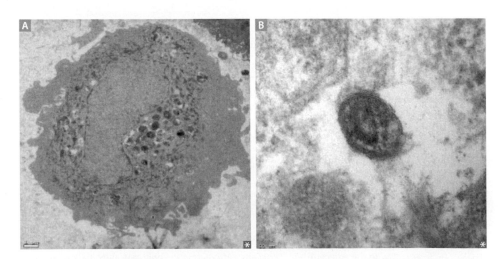

FIGURE 10-17. **Type II pneumocytes.** **A** Electron micrograph of type II pneumocytes. **B** Higher magnification electron micrograph showing lamellar bodies.

OLFACTORY CELLS

In the nasal cavity, the **pseudostratified olfactory epithelium** is found in the superior conchae. Among other supportive cells in this epithelium, **olfactory cells** are bipolar neurons that generate action potentials in response to specific odor molecules. Each olfactory cell has a single dendrite containing a few nonmotile cilia that function to increase the surface area for olfactory receptors.

Physiology

The respiratory system is a means for inspiring air, facilitating gas exchange between the air and blood, and expelling air. As illustrated by the ideal gas law and Boyle's law, air and its component gases are characterized by their quantity, volume, and pressure. Likewise, respiratory physiology may be described as a series of **pressure-driven changes in the volume of gas in the lung** that enables the **regulation of oxygen, carbon dioxide, and pH in the blood.** This section introduces lung volumes and capacities and then discusses in detail (1) the movement of gas into and out of the lungs (**ventilation**) and (2) the regulation of O_2 and CO_2 transport (the **blood gases**).

LUNG VOLUMES AND CAPACITIES

Important lung volumes and capacities are defined in Table 10-5 and depicted graphically in Figure 10-18.

- Forced expiratory volume in 1 second (FEV_1) is normally 70–80% of the forced vital capacity (FVC), or **FEV_1/FVC = 0.7–0.8.**
- In obstructive lung diseases, like **asthma** or **emphysema**, FEV_1 is decreased more than FVC, so **$FEV_1/FVC < 0.7$** (Figure 10-19 and Table 10-6).

FLASH BACK

Increased capillary hydrostatic pressure within the lungs, as occurs in severe left ventricular systolic failure, can cause leakage of fluid into the lungs **(pulmonary edema).**

KEY FACT

Ideal Gas Law
$PV = nRT$
where
P = absolute pressure (pascals)
V = volume (m³)
n = number of gas molecules (moles)
R = universal gas constant
    (8.314 J/[K * mol])
T = temperature (Kelvin)

KEY FACT

Boyle's Law
Special case of the ideal gas law that states: For a fixed amount of an ideal gas at a constant temperature, the pressure and volume of the gas are inversely proportional.
$PV = k$, where k is a constant.

TABLE 10-5. Lung Volumes and Capacities

NAME	DESCRIPTION
Volumes	
Tidal volume (TV or V_T)	Volume of air taken into the lungs during resting inspiration after a resting expiration.
Inspiratory reserve volume (IRV)	Maximal additional volume of air that can be inspired beyond tidal inspiration.
Expiratory reserve volume (ERV)	Maximal volume of air that can be expired beyond resting expiration.
Residual volume (RV)	Volume of air in lungs that cannot be expired regardless of effort.
Capacities (Sums of 2 or more volumes)	
Inspiratory capacity (IC)	Maximal volume of air inhaled after a quiet expiration at rest. IC = IRV + TV
Functional residual capacity (FRC)	Volume of air remaining after tidal expiration. FRC = ERV + RV
Vital capacity (VC) Forced vital capacity (FVC)	Maximum expiratory volume after a maximal inspiration. The FVC is the *measured* VC when the patient exhales forcefully after maximal inspiration. VC = IRV + TV + ERV = TLC – RV
Forced expiratory volume in 1 second (FEV_1)	Volume of air forcefully expired in 1 second following a maximal inspiration.
Total lung capacity (TLC)	Total volume of air contained in the lungs after maximal inspiration.

ᵃFor 70-kg male.

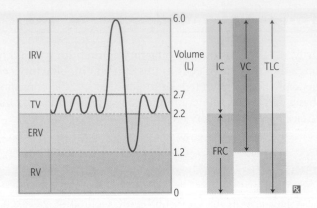

FIGURE 10-18.   **Lung volumes and capacities.** A spirometry tracing showing all of the lung volumes (left) and capacities (right). Values are typical for a 70-kg male. ERV, expiratory reserve volume; FRC, functional residual capacity; IC, inspiratory capacity; IRV, inspiratory reserve volume; RV, residual volume; TLC, total lung capacity; TV, tidal volume; VC, vital capacity.

■ In restrictive lung diseases, like **pulmonary fibrosis,** FEV_1 is decreased to the same extent as, or less than, FVC, so $FEV_1/FVC \geq 0.7.$

Measurement of Lung Volumes and Capacities

Some lung volumes and capacities can be measured simply by having a patient perform various breathing maneuvers into a spirometer. For example, having a patient take a maximal inspiration to total lung capacity (TLC) followed by a maximal expiration to residual volume (RV) generates a volume equivalent to the VC. However, since RV, functional residual capacity (FRC), and TLC cannot, by definition, be measured as expired volumes on spirometry, other methods are used. They include:

■ **Dilution tests:** A known volume and concentration of an inert gas such as helium is inhaled at the end of a tidal expiration. This inert gas is diluted by the air already in the lungs, so the change in concentration of the gas that is expired can be used to calculate the FRC. Specifically, if X is the unknown lung volume of the patient, then

$$X = \frac{V_o \cdot (C_o - C)}{C}$$

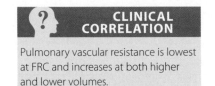

CLINICAL CORRELATION

Pulmonary vascular resistance is lowest at FRC and increases at both higher and lower volumes.

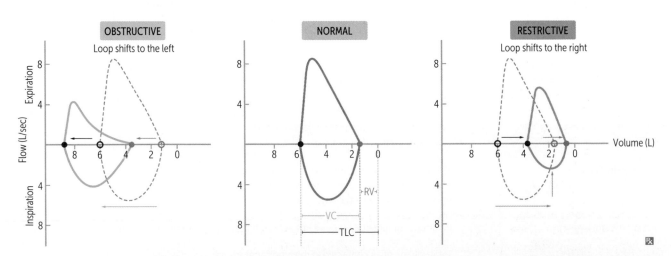

FIGURE 10-19.   **Obstructive versus restrictive lung diseases.** Forced vital capacity (FVC) and forced expiratory volume in 1 second (FEV_1) in normal subjects and patients with lung disease. RV, residual volume; TLC, total lung capacity; VC, vital capacity.

TABLE 10-6. **Lung Volumes in Restrictive Versus Obstructive Disease**

	RV	FRC	TLC	FVC	FEV_1	FEV_1/FVC
Obstructive	↑↑	↑	↑	↓	↓↓	↓
Restrictive	↓	↓	↓	↓↓	↓	↑ or normal

FEV_1, forced expiratory volume in 1 second; FRC, functional residual capacity; FVC, forced vital capacity; RV, residual volume; TLC, total lung capacity.

where V_o and C_o are the original volume and concentration of helium in the spirometer, and C is the final concentration of the helium after equilibration with the patient's lungs.

- **Body plethysmography:** The patient sits in an airtight box with a known pressure and breathes through a mouthpiece. At end expiration, the mouthpiece is closed and the patient attempts to inhale. Chest expansion against the closed system increases the measured pressure within the box. The FRC volume can thus be computed by Boyle's law. In contrast to dilution tests, body plethysmography can detect air that is not in communication with the airways.

Anatomic Dead Space

The volume of air in the conducting airways that does not participate in gas exchange (ie, everything but the respiratory bronchioles, alveolar ducts, and alveoli). It is **normally ~150 mL** and should not change for a given individual under different respiratory conditions.

Physiologic Dead Space (Total Dead Space)

The total volume of inspired air that does not participate in gas exchange, comprised of the **anatomic dead space** and the **alveolar dead space**. The alveolar dead space represents the alveoli that are filled with air but not perfused by blood ($\dot{V}/\dot{Q}$ mismatch, where $\dot{V}$ is ventilation rate and $\dot{Q}$ is blood flow; see Hypoxemia section under Blood Gases). Conceptually, dead space (or more specifically V_D/V_T) is proportional to the fraction of tidal volume that reaches areas that do not contribute expired CO_2 (no gas exchange due to absence of perfusion). Thus, in healthy lungs, the total dead space is essentially equal to the anatomic dead space, while diseased lungs may have elevated physiologic dead space. The Bohr equation computes the physiologic dead space:

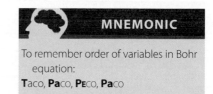

MNEMONIC

To remember order of variables in Bohr equation:

Taco, **Pa**co, **Pe**co, **Pa**co

$$V_D = V_T \cdot \frac{P_{aCO_2} - P_{ECO_2}}{P_{aCO_2}}$$

where V_D is the physiologic dead space (mL); V_T is the tidal volume (mL); P_{aCO_2} is the arterial partial pressure of carbon dioxide (mm Hg); and P_{ECO_2} is the partial pressure of carbon dioxide in expired air (mm Hg).

VENTILATION

Alveolar Function

Gas Exchange

The alveolus enables robust gas exchange, even during rigorous exercise. To accomplish this, the approximately spherical alveolar surface is criss-crossed by a network of narrow capillaries barely wider than a single red blood cell, or about 10 μm. Oxygen and CO_2 must diffuse across a trilaminar barrier: the endothelial cell wall, the basement membrane, and a type I pneumocyte. The total thickness of this barrier is approximately

500 nm in a healthy human lung. At normal respiratory rates, RBCs are fully saturated with O_2 after traversing a quarter of the length of an alveolar capillary. The remaining length provides the capacity to accommodate increased cardiac output during exertion.

Surface Tension

The collapsing pressure of the alveoli is governed by Laplace's law:

$$P = (2T)/r$$

where P is collapsing pressure (the pressure required to hold the alveolus open); T is surface tension; and r is the alveolar radius.

When r is small, greater pressure is required to keep the alveolus open. Thus, alveoli are most likely to collapse on expiration, when their radii are at a minimum; this alveolar collapse is called **atelectasis. Surfactant** reduces the surface tension to protect small alveoli from collapsing.

Surfactant

As described previously (see Alveoli in the Histology section), surfactant is synthesized by **type II alveolar cells** and is composed primarily of **DPPC**.

- Surfactant lines alveoli and acts as a detergent, reducing surface tension during expiration. This helps prevent alveolar collapse.
- Surfactant production in the fetus may begin as early as week 24, and is usually present by week 35. A **lecithin (DPPC):sphingomyelin ratio > 2:1** indicates mature surfactant production.
- **Neonatal respiratory distress syndrome** can occur in premature infants due to a low level of surfactant. These infants have **atelectasis, decreased compliance,** trouble with inspiration, and **hypoxemia** due to $\dot{V}/\dot{Q}$ mismatch and shunting.

Other Lung Products

The lung produces many important substances besides surfactant, including:

- **Prostaglandins:** Various functions, including contraction or relaxation of vascular smooth muscle.
- **Histamine:** Promotes vascular permeability and exudative processes.
- **Kallikrein:** Activates bradykinin.
- **Angiotensin-converting enzyme (ACE):** Converts angiotensin I to angiotensin II (see also Renin-Angiotensin-Aldosterone System in the Physiology section of Chapter 8); inactivates bradykinin.

Ventilation Rate

Minute Ventilation

The total amount of air inspired in 1 minute.

$$\text{Minute ventilation} = (\text{Dead space ventilation} + \text{alveolar ventilation}) \times \text{Breaths/min}$$

Alveolar Ventilation

The total amount of air reaching the alveoli (air that participates in gas exchange) in 1 minute. It is different from minute ventilation due to dead space.

$$\text{Alveolar ventilation} = (V_T - V_D) \times \text{Breaths/min}$$
$$\dot{V}_A = \dot{V}_{CO_2}/F_{A CO_2} = 0.863\, \dot{V}_{CO_2}/Pa_{CO_2}$$

KEY FACT

Decreased or dysfunctional surfactant in acute respiratory distress syndrome (ARDS) and the lack of surfactant in neonatal RDS contribute to decreased lung compliance and atelectasis.

KEY FACT

Angiotensin-converting enzyme (ACE) not only converts angiotensin I to angiotensin II but is also responsible for breaking down bradykinin. Hence, ACE inhibitors increase bradykinin levels, potentially causing cough and angioedema as adverse effects.

where $\dot{V}_A$ is alveolar ventilation (L/min), $\dot{V}_{CO_2}$ is the rate of CO_2 production in the body (mL/min), F_{ACO_2} is the fraction of alveolar CO_2, P_{aCO_2} is the partial pressure of CO_2 in the arterial blood, and 0.863 is the temperature and pressure-adjusted conversion between F_{ACO_2} and P_{aCO_2}.

Increasing alveolar ventilation through increased depth (tidal volume) or rate of breathing results in a proportionate decrease in P_{aCO_2}.

Inspiration

Inspiration is an active process that always requires at least some muscle activity (see also Table 10-3).

- **Diaphragm:** The most important muscle of inspiration. When the diaphragm contracts, the volume of the thoracic cavity increases vertically. This creates negative intrathoracic pressure, thus drawing air into the lungs.
- **External intercostals, scalenes, and sternocleidomastoids:** Normally used only during times of increased work of breathing, such as **exercise,** but may be used **at rest in patients with lung disease.** The actions of these muscles on the upper and lower ribs are different because the upper ribs are firmly attached to the sternum and relatively parallel to the horizontal plane, whereas the lower ribs descend as they curve around the body anteriorly. As a result, movement of the upper ribs is often compared to a pump-handle, where the ribs and sternum move up and out as a unit and increase the anteroposterior (AP) diameter of the chest. In contrast, movement of the lower ribs is more like lifting bucket handles from either side of the thorax, resulting in an increased transverse diameter (Figure 10-20).

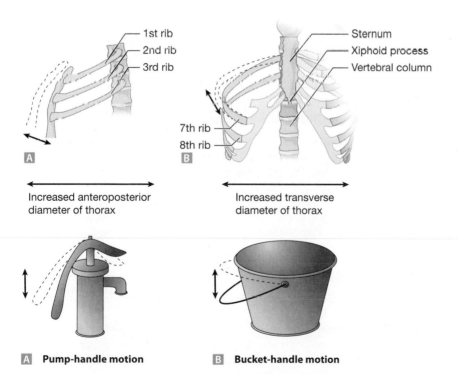

FIGURE 10-20.   Pump-handle versus bucket-handle movement. **A** When accessory muscles lift the upper ribs, which are directly affixed to the sternum, the sternum lifts up and out as if it were a water pump, thereby increasing the anteroposterior diameter of the thorax. **B** When accessory muscles lift the lower ribs, which have a significant downward angle and indirect attachment to the sternum, they primarily lift up like the handle of a bucket, thereby increasing the transverse diameter of the thorax.

Expiration

Expiration is normally passive, secondary to the elastic recoil of the lung–chest wall system. The lung–chest wall system is minimally distended at FRC, so once the active muscle activity of inspiration is removed, the lungs recoil back to FRC.

Expiratory muscles are used during **exercise,** coughing, or when airway resistance is elevated in disease (eg, **asthma**). Such muscles include the interosseous part of the internal intercostals, rectus abdominis, transversus abdominis, and internal/external obliques.

Lung Compliance

Compliance (C) is the distensibility of an object; in other words, the volume change that results per unit of pressure applied. The more compliant the lung, the easier it is to inflate and deflate it. Compliance is the reciprocal of elastance and is therefore inversely proportional to the amount of elastic tissue.

$$\text{Compliance } (C) = \Delta \text{ Volume } (V) \, / \, \Delta \text{ Pressure } (P)$$

where C is in mL/cm H_2O, V is in mL, and P is in cm H_2O (1 cm H_2O = 0.74 mm Hg).

When inspiration and expiration are plotted on a volume-versus-pressure graph (Figure 10-21), the slope of the curve is the compliance (this is a **static** compliance curve, meaning that the points correspond to measurements made after airflow is halted at different stages of inspiration or expiration). Notice that the compliance changes as a function of pressure and according to whether a person is breathing in or out (this path-dependence is termed *hysteresis*).

Compliance of the Lung–Chest Wall System

Since the act of breathing involves both the lungs and the chest wall, the separate compliance curves for both must be summed in order to understand the mechanics of the respiratory cycle (Figure 10-22).

Mechanics of Breathing During the Respiratory Cycle

The respiratory cycle involves the repeating pattern of inspiration → expiration → rest. The volumes and key pressures during a prototypical tidal breath are graphed in Figure 10-23 and described in detail in the following sections.

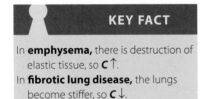

KEY FACT

In **emphysema,** there is destruction of elastic tissue, so **C** ↑.
In **fibrotic lung disease,** the lungs become stiffer, so **C** ↓.

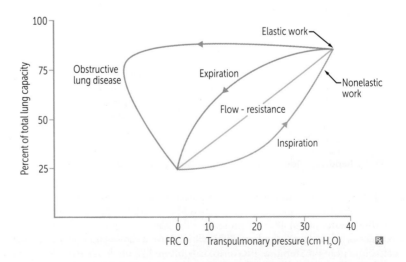

FIGURE 10-21. **Hysteresis curve.** Percent of total lung capacity versus transpulmonary pressure.

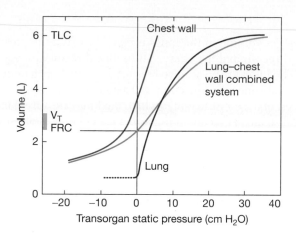

FIGURE 10-22. **Lung–chest wall system.** Pressure and volume tracings for the lung, chest wall, and the combined system. FRC, functional residual capacity; TLC, total lung capacity; V$_T$, tidal volume.

Forces Defined

- **Inward recoil of the lungs:** Inward-directed force created by the elastic tissue in the lungs. In isolation, the lungs always collapse to a minimal volume, regardless of how much air they contain.
- **Outward recoil of the chest wall:** Outward-directed force created by the chest wall's tendency to expand to its resting state (~70% of TLC).
- **Intrapleural pressure:** The pressure within the pleural cavity.
- **Intra-alveolar pressure:** The pressure within the alveoli of the lungs; the major determinant of air flow between the lungs and the environment. Varies from negative during inspiration to positive during expiration.
- **Transpulmonary pressure:** Intra-alveolar pressure minus intrapleural pressure, ie, the pressure difference across the lung wall.
- **Negative pressure:** When the intra-alveolar pressure is lower than the ambient pressure at the airway opening, air flows down the pressure gradient into the lungs.
- **Positive pressure:** When the intra-alveolar pressure is greater than the airway opening pressure, air flows down the pressure gradient out of the lungs.

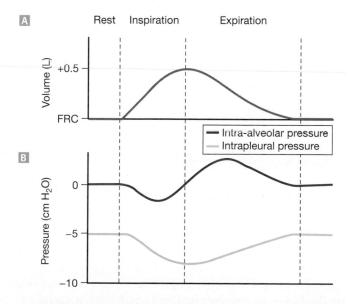

FIGURE 10-23. **Spontaneous respiration.** **A** Volume of the lung relative to functional residual capacity (FRC) during spontaneous respiration. **B** Intrapleural (blue) and intra-alveolar (red) pressures during spontaneous respiration.

At Rest

At rest, when the gas volume in the lungs is equal to FRC, the pressures created by the lungs (inward recoil) and the chest wall (outward recoil) are equal and opposite (Figure 10-22). The lungs create positive pressure because they tend to collapse due to their elasticity. At the same time, the chest wall generates negative pressure because the ribcage and the rest of the thoracic wall to which the lungs are affixed resist deformation from their natural shape. These opposing forces cancel out, establishing a distending pressure (alveolar pressure) of 0 (Figure 10-23). The respiratory muscles are not involved in this process.

$$\text{Intrapleural pressure} = -5 \text{ cm } H_2O$$
$$\text{Intra-alveolar pressure} = 0 \text{ cm } H_2O$$

In **emphysema,** the lungs have a decreased tendency to collapse due to a loss of elasticity (compliance $\uparrow$). As a result, the lung–chest wall system recalibrates to a new, **higher FRC** at which the forces balance. This is why patients with emphysema are **barrel-chested.**

In **lung fibrosis,** the lungs have an increased tendency to collapse (compliance $\downarrow$), so the system equilibrates to a new, **lower FRC** at which the forces balance.

During Inspiration

The muscles of inspiration contract, generating negative pressure. The intra-alveolar pressure is therefore negative. However, inspiration does not continue indefinitely because the pressure exerted by the chest wall becomes positive as it expands beyond its natural shape, thus opposing the muscles of inspiration. Approximate values for a young, healthy subject are given below; note that there can be significant variation based on age, weight, or health:

$$\text{Intrapleural pressure: Decreases from } -5 \text{ to } -8 \text{ cm } H_2O$$
$$\text{Intra-alveolar pressure} < 0 \text{ cm } H_2O, \text{ so air flows into the lungs}$$

At Maximum Inspiration

At TLC, the positive inward pressures due to the distension of the chest wall and lungs have increased to the point where they exactly cancel out the negative outward pressure generated by the muscles of inspiration. Thus, the lungs are held at full capacity, neither expanding nor contracting.

$$\text{Intrapleural pressure} = -8 \text{ cm } H_2O$$
$$\text{Intra-alveolar pressure} = 0 \text{ cm } H_2O, \text{ so no air flows}$$

During Expiration

The muscles of inspiration relax, removing their strong negative outward force and allowing the intra-alveolar pressure to become positive. This allows the lung–chest wall complex to return to its equilibrium at FRC.

$$\text{Intrapleural pressure: Increases from } -8 \text{ to } -5 \text{ cm } H_2O \text{ (may increase into positive}$$
$$\text{range, depending on the patient)}$$
$$\text{Intra-alveolar pressure} > 0 \text{ cm } H_2O, \text{ so air flows out of the lungs}$$

At Maximum Expiration

At RV, there is still some gas left in the lungs. That is, **we can never exhale enough to fully collapse the lungs.** At RV, the chest wall exerts such a strong negative outward pressure (due to its tendency to recoil outward to its resting shape) that the expiratory muscles are unable to create enough positive inward pressure to exhale any further.

$$\text{Intrapleural pressure} = -5 \text{ cm } H_2O$$
$$\text{Intra-alveolar pressure} = 0 \text{ cm } H_2O, \text{ so no air flows}$$

Mechanical Ventilation

Mechanical ventilators allow physicians to manipulate the pressures and volumes that govern inspiration and expiration. A detailed explanation of mechanical ventilation is beyond the scope of this text, but a brief discussion of the most common modes of mechanical ventilation and how they work may be useful.

Positive end-expiratory pressure (PEEP): With this setting, airway pressure at the end of expiration does not fall to 0, but is instead maintained at a fixed value (eg, 10 cm H_2O). This helps to maintain airway patency during expiration and is particularly useful in hypoxemic states such as acute respiratory distress syndrome (ARDS). In a patient who is initiating all breaths, the equivalent of PEEP is continuous positive airway pressure (CPAP), which may be applied by mask or endotracheal tube in order to maintain airway patency. CPAP is commonly used in the treatment of obstructive sleep apnea.

Airways

Flow

Airflow is proportional to the pressure difference between the mouth (or nose) and the alveoli and is inversely proportional to the resistance of the airway.

$$\dot{V} = \Delta P/R$$

where $\dot{V}$ is the ventilation rate (airflow); ΔP is the pressure gradient; and R is resistance.

Note that the dot over the $\dot{V}$ in the ventilation rate indicates that it is the change in volume with respect to time (ie, dV/dt).

Resistance

Governed by Poiseuille's law:

$$R = (8\eta l)/(\pi r^4)$$

where R is resistance, η is the viscosity of the gas, l is airway length, and r is airway radius.

Since airway radius is the major determinant of resistance (r^4), the major source of airway resistance is the **medium-sized bronchi** (the smaller bronchi have greater numbers arranged in parallel, thus offering less net resistance than the medium-sized bronchi).

Factors That Influence Pulmonary Resistance

- Contraction of bronchial smooth muscle:
  - **Sympathetic stimulation:** Airways dilate via β_2-adrenergic receptors, thus decreasing resistance. **Albuterol** is a common β_2 agonist and is used in an inhaled form by patients with asthma or chronic obstructive pulmonary disease (COPD).
  - **Parasympathetic stimulation:** Airways constrict via M_3-cholinergic receptors, thus increasing resistance. This is seen in **asthma** as part of the immune response. **Ipratropium** is a common anticholinergic drug used to counter this parasympathetic bronchoconstriction in asthma or COPD.
- **Secretions:** Increased and/or thickened airway secretions, a hallmark of chronic bronchitis and cystic fibrosis (CF), lead to increased airway obstruction and resistance.

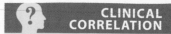

Obstructive sleep apnea occurs when excess body weight, extra pharyngeal tissue, or abnormal anatomy (eg, tonsillar hypertrophy or short mandible) blocks the upper airway passages when the patient is sleeping. This obstruction causes periods of hypoventilation and hypoxia, resulting in nocturnal awakenings, poor sleep, and daytime somnolence. Treatment includes continuous positive airway pressure (CPAP), which is the equivalent in spontaneous breathers of PEEP.

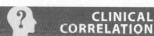

For a mechanically ventilated patient, hypoxia (low O_2) can be corrected by increasing Fio_2 or PEEP, whereas hypercarbia (high CO_2) can be corrected by increasing minute ventilation or tidal volume.

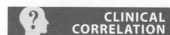

Patients with ARDS are routinely treated with PEEP at low tidal volumes to protect the lungs. CO_2 is lowered by increasing the respiratory rate rather than the tidal volume.

- Lung volumes:
  - **High lung volumes:** The lung tissue surrounding and attached to the airways expands, pulling the airways open, so resistance is decreased.
  - **Low lung volumes:** When the lung volume is low, there is less traction and increased resistance. Airways are more prone to collapse.

BLOOD GASES

Oxygen Transport

Hemoglobin

- **Structure:** Hemoglobin is a globular protein composed of four subunits (two α-family chains and two β-family chains). Each subunit contains a **heme moiety,** which is a porphyrin ring containing a single iron atom at its core. The iron in hemoglobin is in the **ferrous (Fe^{2+}) state and can bind O_2.** If the iron is in the **ferric (Fe^{3+}) state,** it is called **methemoglobin** and **is unable to bind O_2.** Hemoglobin can exist in two forms: **taut,** which has low affinity for O_2, and **relaxed,** which has high affinity for O_2.
- **O_2 saturation (SpO_2):** The percentage of total oxygen-binding sites on hemoglobin that are actually occupied by oxygen, also called the saturation of peripheral oxygen.
- **O_2 content:** The total amount of O_2 in the blood, both dissolved and bound to hemoglobin. Measured in mL of O_2 per deciliter of blood. Depends on hemoglobin concentration, partial pressure of O_2 (PO_2), and the 50% hemoglobin capacity (P_{50}). Calculated by the equation:
  - O_2 content = O_2 bound to hemoglobin + O_2 dissolved in blood
  - O_2 content (mL/dL blood) = (1.34 mL O_2/dL blood × [Hemoglobin] × $\mathbf{SpO_2}$) + (0.0031 mL/mm Hg O_2 × PaO_2)
  - Using typical values of hemoglobin = 14 g/dL, SpO_2 = 1.00 (100%), and partial arterial pressure of oxygen (PaO_2) = 100 mm Hg, one finds that the vast majority (98.5%) of oxygen in the blood is bound to hemoglobin.
- **O_2 capacity:** The maximum amount of O_2 that can be bound to hemoglobin (in mL/dL blood), computed as 1.34 mL O_2/dL blood × [Hemoglobin]. This is approximately equal to the O_2 content of blood at 100% saturation.

Oxygen-Hemoglobin Dissociation Curve

The oxygen-hemoglobin dissociation curve describes how the oxygen saturation of hemoglobin varies with the PO_2 in the blood (Figure 10-24). Its sigmoidal shape reflects positive cooperativity among the four subunits, such that the more oxygen molecules that are bound, the easier it is for an additional oxygen molecule to bind. Factors that decrease the affinity of hemoglobin for oxygen cause the curve to shift right, leading to greater oxygen unloading. On the other hand, a left shift causes more oxygen to become bound in the blood.

- Increases in PCO_2, altitude, 2,3-bisphosphoglycerate (2,3-BPG), or temperature, or a decrease in pH, will cause a rightward shift of the curve.
- Decreases in PCO_2, altitude, 2,3-diphosphoglycerate, or temperature, or an increase in pH, will cause a leftward shift of the curve.
- During exercise, PCO_2 and temperature rise, and pH falls in the active muscle tissue. This promotes a right shift and greater O_2 unloading to the tissues. This is known as the Bohr effect.
- At high altitudes, 2,3-DPG synthesis is increased, facilitating O_2 unloading.
- Fetal hemoglobin ($\alpha_2\gamma_2$) does not bind 2,3-DPG as strongly as adult hemoglobin ($\alpha_2\beta_2$), shifting the curve to the left. This helps the fetus obtain O_2 from the mother's RBCs.

KEY FACT

Fe_2 binds O_2.

MNEMONIC

Hemoglobin:
Taut in **T**issues, **R**elaxed in **R**espiratory tract.

KEY FACT

Methemoglobinemia may result from treatment with nitrites and is thus sometimes induced when amyl nitrite or sodium nitrite is given to treat cyanide poisoning. Methemoglobinemia is treated with **methylene blue,** which reduces the ferric iron reducing agent that converts ferric iron (Fe^{3+}) in methemoglobin to ferrous iron (Fe^{2+}). Remember that only reduced Fe can bind O_2.

MNEMONIC

Causes of a right-shifted hemoglobin dissociation curve—

BAT ACES
BPG (2,3-BPG)
Altitude
Temperature
Acid
CO$_2$
Exercise
Sickle cell

MNEMONIC

A rule of thumb for translating between PO_2 and SpO_2 is the 40-50-60: 70-80-90 rule, where PO_2s of 40, 50, and 60 mm Hg translate to 70%, 80%, and 90% saturation, respectively.

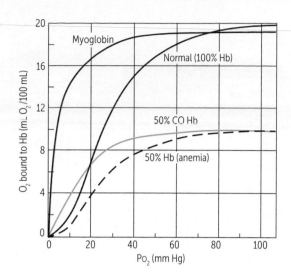

FIGURE 10-24.   **Oxygen dissociation curves.** Normal hemoglobin vs carbon monoxide poisoning (blue line), anemia (dashed line), and myoglobin (red line). Graph illustrates O_2 bound to hemoglobin relative to Po_2. CO, carbon monoxide; Hb, hemoglobin; Po_2, partial pressure of oxygen.

There are several important regions of the oxygen-hemoglobin dissociation curve worth remembering:

- At a **Po_2 of > 70 mm Hg,** hemoglobin is essentially 100% saturated. **Arterial blood** has a Po_2 of around 100 mm Hg.
- At a **Po_2 of 40 mm Hg,** hemoglobin is 70% saturated. **Venous blood** is at this level of oxygenation.
- At a **Po_2 of 25 mm Hg,** hemoglobin is 50% saturated. This is the **P_{50}** (50% saturation point) of hemoglobin.

Carbon Dioxide Transport

CO_2 is produced in the body's tissues and carried to the lungs via the venous blood. It is transported in three forms:

- **HCO_3^- (bicarbonate),** formed by the combination of CO_2 and H_2O by the enzyme **carbonic anhydrase,** is the **major mode** of carbon dioxide transportation, making up 70% of CO_2 in the blood. This reaction reverses in the lungs, where HCO_3^- enters RBCs in exchange for Cl^-, and CO_2 is reformed by carbonic anhydrase and expired (Figure 10-25).
- Dissolved CO_2, 5–9% which is free in the bloodstream.
- Carbaminohemoglobin, 21–25% which is CO_2 bound to hemoglobin. In the lungs, the oxygenation of hemoglobin promotes the dissociation of CO_2 from hemoglobin. This is known as the **Haldane effect** (Figure 10-26).

Respiratory Acid-Base Disturbances

The lungs, kidneys, and molecular buffers are the major determinants of acid-base balance within the body. The kidneys can eliminate and reabsorb both base (HCO_3^-) and acid (H^+ and fixed [nonvolatile] acids) in the urine, whereas the lungs remove volatile acid from the circulation in the form of exhaled CO_2. Molecular buffers are involved with short-term compensation for acidosis.

- **Respiratory acidosis** (Table 10-7): Caused by a **decrease in alveolar ventilation** (hypoventilation) and retention of CO_2 **($Paco_2 > 40$ mm Hg),** leading to an increase in blood $[H^+]$ and $[HCO_3^-]$.
    - **Renal compensation:** Increased excretion of H^+ and NH_4^+ and increased reabsorption of HCO_3^-.

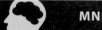

Factors that cause a right shift of the oxygen-hemoglobin dissociation curve—
CADET
↑ Pco_2
Higher **A**ltitude
↑ 2,3-**D**PG
Exercise (buildup of lactic acid and CO_2 → ↓ pH)
↑ **T**emperature

KEY FACT

Carbon monoxide (CO) binds to hemoglobin with 240 times greater affinity than O_2 does, thus creating an allosteric change in the hemoglobin that prevents the unloading of O_2 from other binding sites. This causes a left shift of the curve and results in hypoxemia in CO poisoning. Treatment includes high-flow O_2 to competitively remove the CO from hemoglobin.

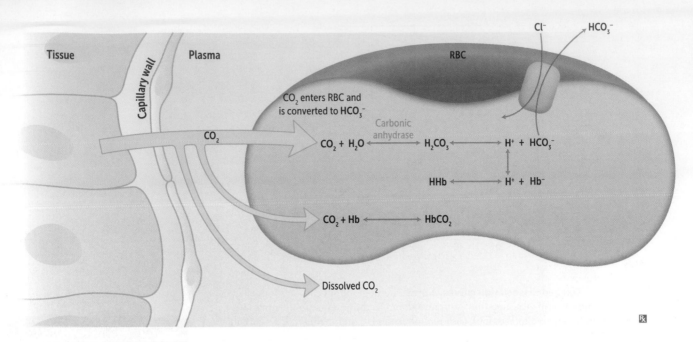

FIGURE 10-25. **Carbon dioxide transport.** CO_2 handling in the RBC. Hb^-, ionized hemoglobin; HHb, deionized hemoglobin.

- **Acute respiratory acidosis:** Renal compensation has not yet occurred (intracellular fluid buffering only). Each 10 mm Hg increase in $Paco_2$ leads to a 1 mEq/L rise in HCO_3^- and a 0.08 decrease in pH.
- **Chronic respiratory acidosis:** Renal compensation has occurred. Each 10 mm Hg increase in $Paco_2$ leads to a 3.5 mEq/L rise in HCO_3^- and a 0.03 decrease in pH.
- Causes of respiratory acidosis include opiates, sedatives, and anesthetics (due to inhibition of the medullary respiratory center), Guillain-Barré syndrome, amyotrophic lateral sclerosis (ALS), and multiple sclerosis (MS) (due to weakening of respiratory muscles), airway obstruction, ARDS, and COPD (due to decreased CO_2 exchange).
- **Respiratory alkalosis** (Table 10-7): Caused by an **increase in alveolar ventilation** (hyperventilation) and a loss of CO_2 (**$Paco_2$ < 40 mm Hg**), leading to a decrease in blood $[H^+]$ and $[HCO_3^-]$.
  - **Renal compensation:** Decreased excretion of H^+ and NH_4^+, decreased reabsorption of HCO_3^-.

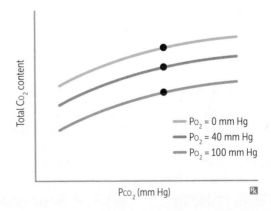

FIGURE 10-26. **Haldane effect.** As RBCs pass through the alveolar capillaries and the partial pressure of oxygen (Po_2) increases from 70% to almost 100%, the CO_2 dissociation curve shifts downward. This promotes the dissociation of CO_2 from the RBCs.

TABLE 10-7.   Acid-Base Disturbances

| | RESPIRATORY | | | |
| | ACIDOSIS | | ALKALOSIS | |
	CHANGE IN HCO₃⁻	CHANGE IN PH	CHANGE IN HCO₃⁻	CHANGE IN PH
Acute	↑ 1 mEq/L	↓ 0.08	↓ 2 mEq/L	↑ 0.08
Chronic	↑ 3.5 mEq/L	↓ 0.03	↓ 5 mEq/L	↑ 0.03

- **Acute respiratory alkalosis:** Renal compensation has not yet occurred (intracellular fluid buffering only). Each 10 mm Hg decrease in $Paco_2$ leads to a 2 mEq/L decrease in HCO_3^- and a 0.08 rise in pH.
- **Chronic respiratory alkalosis:** Renal compensation has occurred. Each 10 mm Hg decrease in $Paco_2$ leads to a 5 mEq/L decrease in HCO_3^- and a 0.03 rise in pH.
- Causes of respiratory alkalosis include pulmonary embolism (PE), high altitude (due to hypoxemia and increased ventilation rate), anxiety, pregnancy, cirrhosis, and salicylate intoxication (due to direct stimulation of the medullary respiratory center).

The lungs play a compensatory role in the cases of metabolic acidosis and alkalosis, which are discussed in greater detail in Chapter 8.

- In **metabolic acidosis,** hyperventilation occurs to blow off excess CO_2 and thus carbonic acid, although this cannot completely compensate for the acidosis.
- Conversely, in **metabolic alkalosis,** hypoventilation occurs to retain CO_2 and thus carbonic acid, although this cannot completely compensate for the alkalosis.

Pulmonary Circulation

Characteristics

The pulmonary vasculature has unique characteristics that set it apart from the rest of the vascular system. These properties relate directly to the physiologic function of the respiratory system (Figure 10-27).

- **Pressures** are much **lower** in the pulmonary circulation than in the systemic circulation (normal pulmonary arterial pressure = 25 mm Hg systolic and 10 mm Hg diastolic).
- **Resistance** is much **lower** than in the systemic circulation.

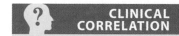

CLINICAL CORRELATION

Treat altitude sickness with acetazolamide, a carbonic anhydrase inhibitor that increases the renal excretion of HCO_3^-.

KEY FACT

Normal pH in the presence of abnormal HCO_3^- or CO_2 suggests a mixed disorder.

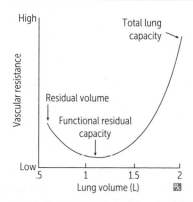

FIGURE 10-27.   Lung volume and pulmonary vascular resistance (PVR). As the lung volume increases from residual volume (RV) to total lung capacity (TLC), PVR changes as shown in the graph. PVR is the sum of the resistance in all pulmonary vessels. PVR is typically lowest at functional residual capacity (FRC).

- Normal pulmonary vascular resistance (PVR) = 20–120 dynes · s · cm⁻⁵. This is ~1/10 of systemic vascular resistance (SVR) (Table 10-8).
- PVR changes with lung volume. At high volumes, the **alveolar vessels** are compressed by stretched alveolar walls and contribute more to PVR. At low volumes, larger extra-alveolar pulmonary vessels are compressed due to decreased elastic traction and increased positive intrathoracic pressure, contributing to an increased PVR.
- Total PVR is at its minimum at FRC.

Distribution of Pulmonary Blood Flow

When a person is supine, blood flow is nearly uniform throughout the entire lung. When standing, however, the lungs are divided into three zones based on blood flow and ventilation as affected by gravity, with zone 1 at the apices, zone 2 in the middle, and zone 3 at the bases. Both blood flow and ventilation are increased as one moves down the lung due to gravity, but blood flow increases to a greater degree than ventilation, resulting in a mismatch between ventilation ($\dot{V}$) and perfusion ($\dot{Q}$). This is known as $\dot{V}/\dot{Q}$ mismatch (Figure 10-28).

- **Zone 1 (apices):** Ventilation exceeds perfusion.
    - Alveolar pressure > arterial pressure > venous pressure.
    - High alveolar pressures compress the capillaries and reduce blood flow.
    - $\dot{Q}$ is reduced relative to $\dot{V}$; therefore, $\dot{V}/\dot{Q}$ is increased. In extreme cases, zone 1 can approximate dead space ($\dot{Q} = 0$, so $\dot{V}/\dot{Q} = \infty$).
    - P_{O_2} is the highest and P_{CO_2} is the lowest in zone 1 due to having greater ventilation relative to blood flow; there is unspent (wasted) ventilation left over even after full oxygenation of the blood.
- **Zone 2 (middle):** Well-matched.
    - Arterial pressure > alveolar pressure > venous pressure.
    - Blood flow here is driven by the difference between arterial and alveolar pressures.
- **Zone 3 (bases):** Perfusion exceeds ventilation.
    - Arterial pressure > venous pressure > alveolar pressure.
    - Blood flow here is driven by the difference between arterial and venous pressures, as in the systemic circulation.
    - $\dot{Q}$ is increased relative to $\dot{V}$, so $\dot{V}/\dot{Q}$ is decreased. In extreme cases, zone 3 can approximate shunt ($\dot{Q} \gg \dot{V}$, so $\dot{V}/\dot{Q} \to 0$).
    - P_{O_2} is the lowest and P_{CO_2} is the highest in zone 3 due to decreased gas exchange and airway closure.

CLINICAL CORRELATION

Reactivated pulmonary TB usually occurs in the lung apices due to the high $\dot{V}/\dot{Q}$ and thus high O_2 concentrations in this region of the lung.

KEY FACT

Pulmonary blood flow can be measured using radioactive isotopes. This method, called **$\dot{V}/\dot{Q}$ scanning,** can detect areas of decreased perfusion and is useful for evaluating for pulmonary embolism (PE) and assessing regional lung function. CT pulmonary angiograms can also be used to identify PEs.

TABLE 10-8. **Calculating Cardiac Output, Pulmonary Vascular Resistance, and Systemic Vascular Resistance**

	CALCULATION	NORMAL VALUE
CO	SV × HR	5–6 L/min
PVR	[(MPAP – MLAP)/(CO)] × 80 **Note:** Units for pressure and CO should be mm Hg and L/min, respectively. The factor of 80 converts the units to dynes · s · cm⁻⁵.	20–120 dynes · s · cm⁻⁵
SVR	[(MAP – MRAP)/(CO)] × 80	770–1500 dynes · s · cm⁻⁵

CO, cardiac output; MAP, mean arterial pressure; MLAP, mean left atrial pressure; MPAP, mean pulmonary artery pressure; MRAP, mean right atrial pressure; PVR, pulmonary vascular resistance; SVR, systemic vascular resistance.

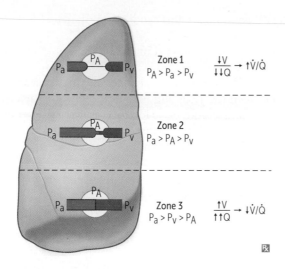

FIGURE 10-28. **Degrees of ventilation and perfusion in the zones of the lung.** Zone 1 (apex) has increased ventilation relative to perfusion due to the negative pleural pressures holding alveoli open and impeding blood flow. Zone 2 (mid lung) has a proportionate amount of ventilation relative to perfusion. Zone 3 (lower lung) has relatively more perfusion due to a less negative pleural pressure from the weight of the lung. P_A, alveolar pressure; P_a, arterial pressure, P_v, venous pressure.

Regulation of Pulmonary Blood Flow

- **Hypoxia:** In the lungs, hypoxia leads to **vasoconstriction.** This phenomenon serves to shunt blood to areas of better ventilation. In chronic hypoxia, pulmonary hypertension can result from prolonged vasoconstriction. This is in contrast to other organs, in which hypoxia leads to vasodilation. Hypoxic vasoconstriction allows blood to be redirected away from poorly ventilated regions and toward well-ventilated areas.
- Several other factors also affect pulmonary blood flow (Table 10-9).

Hypoxemia

Hypoxemia is defined as a below-normal O_2 content in the arterial blood (as opposed to **hypoxia,** which means low O_2 in tissues), usually indicated by a reduced Pa_{O_2}. In a normal individual, the blood leaving the lungs should have an O_2 tension (Pa_{O_2}) approximately equal to the O_2 tension within the alveoli (PA_{O_2}).

$$PA_{O_2} = FI_{O_2}(PB - PH_2O) - (Pa_{CO_2}/R)$$

where FI_{O_2} is the fraction of inspired air that is O_2 (0.21 on room air, 1.00 for pure oxygen); PB is the barometric pressure (760 torr at sea level, where 1 torr = 1 mm Hg = 133 Pa); PH_2O is the vapor pressure of H_2O in the alveoli (47 torr at 37°C); Pa_{CO_2} is the arterial CO_2 tension; and R is the respiratory quotient.

The respiratory quotient, R, which represents the number of molecules of CO_2 produced for every molecule of O_2 consumed, depends on diet. R = 0.7 for fat metabolism, 0.8 for protein metabolism, and 1.0 for carbohydrate metabolism. The typical Western diet is assumed to have an R of about 0.8.

> **? CLINICAL CORRELATION**
>
> Bosentan, a nonselective competitive antagonist of endothelin-1 at the ET-A and ET-B receptors on vascular endothelium, lowers PVR by relaxing blood vessels and is one of the pharmacologic treatments for primary pulmonary hypertension.

TABLE 10-9. **Factors Regulating Pulmonary Blood Flow and Pulmonary Vascular Resistance**

	LOW O_2	LOW PH	HISTAMINE	PROSTAGLANDINS	NITRIC OXIDE	ENDOTHELIN	SYMPATHETIC TONE	PARASYMPATHETIC TONE
Vasoconstriction	X	X				X	X	
Vasodilation			X	X	X			X

For a patient breathing room air, this can be simplified to:

$$P_{AO_2} = 150 - 1.25(Pa_{CO_2})$$

Once P_{AO_2} is calculated, the actual Pa_{O_2} can be measured via arterial blood gas testing. The difference between the P_{AO_2} and Pa_{O_2} is the **alveolar-arterial O_2 gradient** (A-a gradient, or AaD_{O_2}), and should be **< 15 torr,** although this value can increase with normal aging. A good rule of thumb is that the gradient should be less than the patient's age/4 + 4. For example, a 60-year-old should have an A-a gradient no greater than 19 torr. The A-a gradient is important for determining the cause(s) of hypoxemia, discussed in greater detail later and diagrammed in Figure 10-29. In particular, the A-a gradient is increased in the case of shunt, V̇/Q̇ mismatch, and diffusion impairment, but it is unchanged in the case of pure hypoventilation or low F_{IO_2}.

Etiology

There are five main causes of hypoxemia (Figure 10-29). They include:

1. **Hypoventilation:** Hypoventilation is relatively common in lung disease. It is characterized by a reduced Pa_{O_2} and an **increased Pa_{CO_2}.** Since alveolar ventilation is also reduced, there is **no increase in A-a gradient.**
2. **Decreased inspired O_2:** This occurs most commonly at high altitudes, where the P_B is decreased. This causes a reduction in Pa_{O_2} due to the decrease in P_{AO_2}. Thus, there is **no increase in A-a gradient.** There are several physiologic adaptations to high altitude (Table 10-10).
3. **Poor gas exchange (diffusion impairment):** Diffusion impairment occurs due to a failure of P_{O_2} in the pulmonary capillary blood to equilibrate with alveolar gas. This is a rare cause of hypoxemia because most abnormalities in diffusion are too mild to cause hypoxemia unless the patient is exercising. The **A-a gradient is increased.**
   - O_2 is normally a **perfusion-limited** gas. This means that O_2 equilibrates early along the length of the pulmonary capillary (within the first third). This leaves a lot of room for compensation in disease states; thus, a failure in O_2 diffusion is a very rare cause of hypoxemia.
   - O_2 can become a **diffusion-limited** gas under certain circumstances, in which case it does not equilibrate by the end of the pulmonary capillary, resulting in the maintenance of a partial pressure gradient between the alveolus and the capillary. This can occur in **strenuous exercise** (due to increased cardiac output), **pulmonary fibrosis** and ARDS (due to alveolar membrane thickening), and **emphysema** (due to decreased surface area for gas diffusion).
   - Diffusion capacity can be measured using carbon monoxide, resulting in a D_{LCO} (diffusion capacity of the lung for carbon monoxide) value. CO is used in place

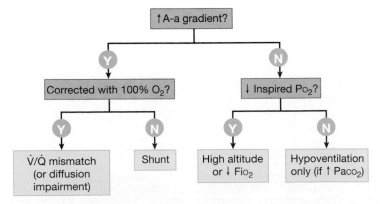

FIGURE 10-29. **Hypoxemia decision tree.** The different causes of hypoxemia can be distinguished as shown. Note, however, that combinations of different mechanisms are common.

TABLE 10-10. **Response to High Altitude**

PARAMETER	RESPONSE
Pa_{O_2}	Decreased (hypoxemia)
PA_{O_2}	Decreased (due to ↓ barometric pressure)
Ventilation rate	Increased (hyperventilation due to hypoxemia)
Arterial pH	Increased (respiratory alkalosis)
Hemoglobin concentration	Increased (polycythemia)
2,3-DPG concentration	Increased
Hemoglobin-O_2 curve	Right shift
PVR	Increased (hypoxic vasoconstriction)

2,3-DPG, 2-3-diphosphoglycerate; PA_{O_2}, partial alveolar pressure of oxygen; Pa_{O_2}, partial arterial pressure of oxygen; PVR, pulmonary vascular resistance.

of oxygen because of the very high affinity of hemoglobin for CO. DLCO is a surrogate for the surface area available for gas exchange.

- DLCO is decreased when useful surface area for gas exchange is lost, such as in emphysema, interstitial lung disease, and pulmonary vascular disease.
- DLCO may be increased in the presence of intraparenchymal hemorrhage, increased blood volume due to CHF, or polycythemia (increased hematocrit).

4. **V̇/Q̇ mismatch:** The V̇/Q̇ ratio is the ratio of ventilation to pulmonary blood flow. Under normal circumstances, V̇/Q̇ ≈ 0.8, although it varies with position in the lungs (see previous discussion of lung zones). When the V̇/Q̇ ratio is altered, hypoxemia can result. There is also an **increased A-a gradient.** Deviation of the V̇/Q̇ ratio from normal indicates the presence of a shunt (Figure 10-30).

- **V̇/Q̇ mismatch in airway obstruction:** If the airway is completely blocked and blood flow remains, then V̇ = 0, so V̇/Q̇ = 0, and there is a **shunt.** Since there is no gas exchange, the values of P_{O_2} and P_{CO_2} for pulmonary capillary blood approach the values of mixed venous blood (Pa_{O_2} = 40 mm Hg, Pa_{CO_2} = 46 mm Hg).
- **V̇/Q̇ mismatch in pulmonary embolism:** If blood flow is completely blocked, then Q̇ = 0, so V̇/Q̇ = ∞ and there is **complete dead space.** This results in increased CO_2 retention, although this is rarely seen since patients with PE often hyperventilate and may even become hypocapnic as a result. Local bron-

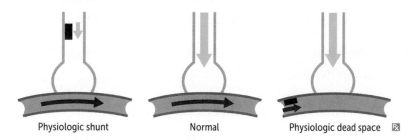

Physiologic shunt   Normal   Physiologic dead space

FIGURE 10-30. **Physiologic dead space.** Under normal circumstances, both ventilation and perfusion are adequate. A physiologic dead space is created when ventilation is greater than perfusion. This may be caused by pulmonary embolism, pulmonary arteritis, necrosis, or fibrosis. A physiologic shunt is created when perfusion is greater than ventilation. In this situation, blood passes through pulmonary vasculature without optimal gas exchange. This may be caused by asthma, COPD, atelectasis, or diseases of the chest wall.

chospasm due to the PE can also contribute to hypoxemia. If the blood flow is low but not zero, the values of P_{O_2} and P_{CO_2} for pulmonary capillary blood approach that of inspired air ($P_{aO_2} = 150$ mm Hg, $P_{aCO_2} = 0$ mm Hg).

- In most cases of $\dot{V}/\dot{Q}$ mismatch, there is neither true shunt nor complete dead space, but simply an **abnormal $\dot{V}/\dot{Q}$ ratio.** Blood from well-ventilated areas is already saturated at baseline, so no amount of effort from well-ventilated areas can compensate for the desaturated blood emerging from areas that are poorly ventilated. Giving the patient **100% O_2 increases the patient's P_{aO_2}.**

5. **Shunt:** As mentioned previously, shunt is an extreme case of $\dot{V}/\dot{Q}$ mismatch that occurs when some blood reaches the systemic circulation without being oxygenated, reducing P_{aO_2}. Since the P_{aO_2} is unaffected, the **A-a gradient is increased.**
    - **Right-to-left shunt:** Occurs when blood from the right side of the heart enters the systemic circulation without passing through the lungs. It is seen in **tetralogy of Fallot** (and other congenital heart conditions causing right-to-left shunts) and always causes a reduction in P_{aO_2}.
    - **Left-to-right shunt:** More common than right-to-left shunt because pressures are higher on the left side of the heart. It is seen with several congenital abnormalities, including patent ductus arteriosus (PDA), atrial septal defect, and ventricular septal defect, as well as with traumatic injury. Left-to-right shunts **do not decrease P_{aO_2}** since oxygenated blood is returning to the right side of the heart, raising the P_{O_2}.
    - True shunt can be differentiated from $\dot{V}/\dot{Q}$ mismatch by giving the hypoxemic patient 100% O_2. This increases P_{aO_2} in the case of $\dot{V}/\dot{Q}$ mismatch but not in the case of a shunt, since in the latter, the blood never communicates with the alveolar gas, regardless of its composition. A patient without a shunt should achieve a P_{aO_2} of at least 400 torr on 100% oxygen.

Hypercapnia

Alveolar ventilation is the main determinant of P_{aCO_2}. Hypercapnia occurs when alveolar ventilation is reduced, which can happen in a number of ways:

- Decreased total minute ventilation without a change in the V_D/V_T ratio.
- Constant minute ventilation with increasing V_D/V_T. This can occur with decreased V_T (eg, a greater percentage of the V_T is taken up by dead space) and increased respiratory rate.
- $\dot{V}/\dot{Q}$ mismatch. Well-perfused areas may be underventilated, whereas underperfused areas may be overventilated. When a large amount of ventilation is "wasted" on underperfused sections of lung, the effect is similar to increasing the dead space: less air is available to exchange gases with the blood, and CO_2 levels in the blood increase.

The response of the body to hypercapnia is often to increase alveolar ventilation by hyperventilating and blowing off more CO_2. Thus, CO_2 retention may not occur even if the preceding criteria are met as long as the body is able to compensate.

Control of Respiration

Central Control of Respiration

- **Medullary respiratory center:** Located in the reticular formation. Damage to or suppression of this region due to stroke, opioid overdose, or other causes can lead to respiratory failure and death.
    - **Dorsal respiratory group:** Responsible for **inspiration** and determines the **rhythm of breathing** (normally 12–20 breaths/minute with an I:E [inspiration-to-expiration] ratio of 1:2). The dorsal respiratory group receives sensory input from peripheral chemoreceptors and lung mechanoreceptors via the vagus and glossopharyngeal nerves. Output travels via the phrenic nerve (C3–C5) and

the intercostal nerves (T1–T11) to the diaphragm and the external intercostal muscles, respectively.
- **Ventral respiratory group:** Responsible for **forced expiration;** not active during ordinary passive expiration. Also involved with increased inspiratory effort (eg, during exercise).
- **Pons:**
  - **Pneumotaxic center:** Located in the upper pons. **Inhibits inspiration,** helping to regulate inspiratory volume and rate.
  - **Apneustic center:** Located in the lower pons. **Stimulates inspiration.**
- **Cerebral cortex:** Exerts voluntary control over breathing.

Chemoreceptors

- **Central chemoreceptors in the medulla:** Respond to the pH of the cerebrospinal fluid (CSF), with decreases in pH causing hyperventilation. CO_2 from arterial blood diffuses into the CSF and combines with H_2O to form H^+ and HCO_3^-.
- **Peripheral chemoreceptors in the carotid and aortic bodies:** Increased Pa_{CO_2} or decreased pH or Pa_{O_2} stimulate these chemoreceptors to increase respiratory rate. Pa_{O_2} must reach low levels (< 60 mm Hg) before breathing is stimulated.

Other Receptors

- **Lung stretch receptors:** Mechanoreceptors located in the airway smooth muscle that are stimulated by distention of the lungs and produce reflex inspiratory time shortening and Hering-Breuer inflation and deflation reflexes. In the Hering-Breuer inflation reflex, excessive stretching of the lungs during a large inspiratory effort leads to inhibition of the dorsal respiratory group and the apneustic center to promote expiration. The deflation reflex acts during expiration to activate the inspiratory control areas.
- **Irritant receptors (nociceptors):** Located between airway epithelial cells and stimulated by noxious substances.
- **Juxtacapillary (J) receptors:** Located close to the capillaries in the alveolar walls. Increases in interstitial fluid, such as during pulmonary edema, PE, or pneumonia, stimulate these receptors, causing rapid, shallow breathing.
- **Joint and muscle receptors:** These are activated by limb movement and help to stimulate breathing early in exercise.

Pathology

Discussion of respiratory pathology will begin with an overview of physical examination findings commonly associated with respiratory dysfunction. Pathologic conditions of the upper airways (eg, nasopharynx, oropharynx, larynx) are then covered, followed by those of the lower airways (eg, tracheobronchial tree, lung parenchyma).

PATHOLOGY ON PHYSICAL EXAMINATION

The pulmonary physical examination has four components: inspection, auscultation, percussion, palpation. This section provides an overview of each component in the context of the USMLE Step 1. The technical aspects of the physical examination are beyond the scope of this text.

Inspection

Signs of respiratory distress include dyspnea (labored breathing), tachypnea (respiratory rate > 20 breaths/min), cyanosis, grunting, nasal flaring, retractions, and using accessory muscles of respiration. Retractions refer to the inward "pulling" of muscles during

KEY FACT

Suspect foreign body aspiration in a child who presents with acute onset wheezing.

inspiration and are commonly seen in the intercostal, subcostal, suprasternal, and abdominal areas. Accessory muscles refer to the muscles primarily involved in forced breathing rather than unlabored diaphragmatic breathing. Increased work of breathing not in the context of exercise or physical exertion is concerning.

Hyperinflated lungs can be a sign of COPD, in particular the "**barrel chest**" seen in emphysema.

Auscultation

On a normal physical examination, breath sounds can be heard differently depending on the auscultated region. Physiologic breath sounds can be described as tracheal (auscultated over the trachea), bronchial (over the manubrium), vesicular (over most of the lung), and bronchovesicular (between the scapulae and in the first and second intercostal spaces anteriorly). Although physiologic breath sounds are usually not directly tested on board exams, it is important to be familiar with the terminology, as it does show up in question stems. On the other hand, adventitious (pathologic) breath sounds are high yield for exams and are described in Table 10-11.

Egophony describes modified voice transmission on lung auscultation. It is classically detected by having the patient produce and hold an "E" sound. In cases of egophony, transmission will be such that the examiner hears an "A" sound through the stethoscope. This finding is highly specific for lung consolidation (ie, lobar pneumonia).

Percussion

Lung percussion provides the examiner with information regarding the nature of the underlying tissue (ie, air-filled, fluid-filled, solid). In general, percussion over solid or fluid-filled cavities tends to generate duller tones, whereas percussion over air-filled cavities produces more resonant or "drum-like" tones. In order of increasing resonance, the five tones generated by percussion are flatness, dullness, resonance, hyperresonance, and tympany (Table 10-12).

> **CLINICAL CORRELATION**
>
> To become more familiar with percussion sounds, you can generate different tones by percussing over certain areas:
> - Flatness—thigh
> - Dullness—liver
> - Resonance—normal lung
> - Tympany—puffed out cheek

TABLE 10-11. **Adventitious Lung Sounds**

SOUND	DESCRIPTION	COMMON ETIOLOGIES
Crackles (rales)	Often equated to the sound of rubbing strands of hair between the fingers or the sound produced by velcro. Due to fluid/consolidation within the lung parenchyma (**wet crackles**) or pulmonary fibrosis (**dry crackles**).	Wet crackles: pneumonia, pulmonary edema (eg, congestive heart failure) Dry crackles: pulmonary fibrosis
Wheezes	Whistling sound. Can be heard during inspiration or expiration. Caused by air passing through **narrowed airways.**	Obstructive diseases: asthma, chronic obstructive pulmonary disease (COPD), bronchitis, foreign body aspiration (FBA)
Rhonchi	Low-pitched **"snoring"** sound. Suggests secretions in large airways.	Asthma, COPD, bronchitis
Stridor	Similar to a wheeze, but louder (often heard without auscultation) and almost entirely inspiratory. High pitch, best heard over trachea, **loudest in the neck.** Indicates partial obstruction of **laryngeal or trachea;** often a medical emergency.	Laryngotracheitis (croup), FBA
Pleural rub	**Scratching** sound when **inflamed parietal and visceral pleura** rub against one another during respiration. Usually heard during both inspiration and expiration. Often localized to a small area of the chest wall.	Connective tissue disorders (systemic lupus erythematosus, rheumatoid arthritis) Infections (viral, bacterial, fungal)

TABLE 10-12. Lung Percussion Findings

SOUND	DESCRIPTION	COMMON ETIOLOGIES
Dullness, flatness	**Fluid** in pleural cavity or lung parenchyma	Pleural effusion, lobar pneumonia
Resonance	Normal lung finding	Normal lung
Hyperresonance, tympany	**Excess air** in pleural cavity or lung parenchyma	Emphysema, pneumothorax

Palpation

The chest wall can be palpated to check for symmetrical chest wall expansion, tenderness, crepitus, as well as tactile fremitus. The patient's neck can also be palpated to check for tracheal deviation. Refer to Table 10-13 for more details.

NASOPHARYNX

Rhinosinusitis

Inflammation of the paranasal sinuses. The paranasal sinuses refer to the hollow, air-filled cavities surrounding the nose, which are lined with mucus and drain into the nasal cavity. They serve to humidify inspired air. The four groups of paranasal sinuses are the frontal, sphenoid, ethmoid, and maxillary sinuses, illustrated in Figure 10-31.

When sinus drainage into the nasal cavity becomes obstructed (typically by mucus), the sinuses can become infected. The vast majority of infectious rhinosinusitis is caused by viral upper respiratory tract infections (URIs). In certain cases, viral URIs can be superimposed by bacterial infections, with the most common organisms being *Streptococcus pneumoniae* (40%), *Haemophilus influenzae* (35%), and *Moraxella catarrhalis* (5%). The widespread use of conjugated pneumococcal vaccination in children is changing the incidence rate of the major pathogens. The percentage of bacterial sinusitis due to *S pneumoniae* is decreasing, while the number of cases caused by nontypeable

TABLE 10-13. Lung Palpation Findings

FEATURE	DESCRIPTION	COMMON ETIOLOGIES
Chest wall expansion	Assessed by placing your hands on each side of the patient's back with thumbs pointed toward the spine and fingers wrapped around each hemithorax. Have the patient take a deep breath and feel for equal movement of your hands away from the midline as the chest expands.	**Asymmetrical expansion:** hemidiaphragmatic paralysis, large pleural effusion, pneumothorax
Tenderness		Trauma, costochondritis
Crepitus	Crackles sensation or "rice krispies" felt under the skin. Indicative of **subcutaneous air.**	Pneumothorax, pneumomediastinum
Tactile fremitus	Vibrations palpated as the patient vocalizes. Detected by placing the ulnar surface of your hands just medial to each of the patient's scapulae and having him/her vocalize.	**Decreased tactile fremitus:** nonspecific (eg, chronic obstructive pulmonary disease, pleural effusion, pneumothorax, atelectasis, thick chest wall) **Increased tactile fremitus:** lobar pneumonia
Tracheal positioning	Palpated along the patient's neck. Tracheal deviation can be ipsilateral or contralateral to the affected lung; can also be confirmed on chest x-ray.	**Ipsilateral deviation:** atelectasis, spontaneous (simple) pneumothorax **Contralateral deviation:** pneumothorax, large pleural effusion

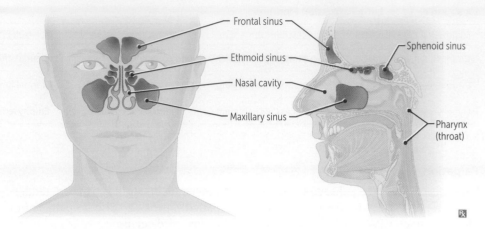

FIGURE 10-31.   Paranasal sinuses

H influenzae is increasing. If indicated, empiric treatment with antibiotics is generally directed toward these agents.

PRESENTATION

- Sinus inflammation presents with tenderness to palpation, a sensation of "fullness" in the affected paranasal regions (may mimic toothache), and, rarely, earache. These symptoms are often associated with viral URI symptoms (eg, rhinorrhea, nonproductive cough).
- When rhinosinusitis is superimposed by bacterial infections, patients present with fever and purulent nasal discharge, in addition to their pre-existing symptoms. Bacterial infections can also be suspected when viral URI symptoms persist or worsen after 1–2 weeks. Antibiotics are generally not indicated for sinusitis, unless symptoms have persisted longer than 10 days, although exceptions exist.

DIAGNOSIS

- Primarily clinical suspicion based on patient history and physical examination.
- CT scan (coronal view) can show air-fluid levels (Figure 10-32). CT is the imaging method of choice but is rarely clinically indicated in uncomplicated sinusitis.
- Nasal swabs for culture are not reliable and almost never indicated.

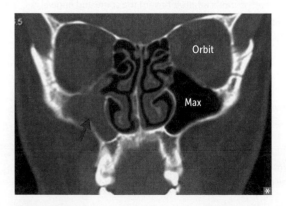

FIGURE 10-32.   Rhinosinusitis. Coronal CT of sinus showing maxillary sinusitis (arrow).

TREATMENT

- Rhinosinusitis due to viral URI is typically self-limiting.
- If complicated by bacterial infections, antibiotics are indicated.
- Amoxicillin-clavulanate is first-line pharmacologic treatment; use doxycycline, ciprofloxacin, or moxifloxacin if patient is allergic to penicillin.

Epistaxis

Epistaxis is a nose bleed; the nasopharynx receives its blood supply from four arteries listed below (origins in parentheses) and illustrated in Figure 10-33:

- Anterior ethmoidal arteries (ophthalmic artery)
- Septal branch of the superior labial artery (facial artery)
- Greater palatine artery (maxillary artery)
- Nasopalatine branch of the sphenopalatine artery (maxillary artery)

The terminal branches of these arteries form an anastomotic network in the anterior segment of the nasopharynx called **Kiesselbach plexus.** Epistaxis most commonly arises from vascular damage within this plexus. Although less common, epistaxis arising from the posterior segment of the nasopharynx (sphenopalatine artery) can be life threatening. If a board question describes a patient who "picks their nose" and presents with persistent large-volume epistaxis, and no other localizing information is given, Kiesselbach plexus or sphenopalatine artery is the likely injured vessel.

OBSTRUCTIVE LUNG DISEASES

The three major obstructive disorders are **COPD** (includes emphysema and chronic bronchitis), **asthma,** and **bronchiectasis.** These diseases are characterized by air outflow obstruction (+/− inflow obstruction) and subsequent air trapping within the lungs. Obstruction can occur from the bronchioles to the mainstem bronchi. Spirometry (pulmonary function tests [PFTs]) shows a markedly decreased FEV_1 and decreased (although possibly normal) FVC. As such, a decreased **FEV_1:FVC ratio** is the hallmark of obstructive disease. RV is increased because of air trapping. Impaired ventilation results in a decreased $\dot{V}/\dot{Q}$ ratio on ventilation-perfusion scan.

FLASH BACK

FEV_1/FVC ratio < 0.7 is characteristic of obstructive lung disease. While FEV_1/FVC is used to diagnose obstructive lung disease, FEV_1 is used to determine the severity of disease.

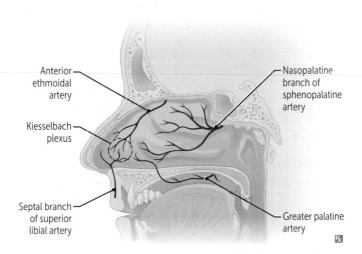

Anterior ethmoidal artery

Nasopalatine branch of sphenopalatine artery

Kiesselbach plexus

Septal branch of superior libial artery

Greater palatine artery

FIGURE 10-33. **Blood supply of nasopharynx.**

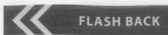
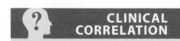
Emphysema

Emphysema is abnormal and permanent airway enlargement distal to the terminal bronchiole, accompanied by progressive destruction of alveolar walls and surrounding interstitium. The result is loss of elastic recoil, **increased lung compliance**, dilation of the terminal air spaces, and air trapping. The loss of elastic recoil in the lung parenchyma shifts the compliance curve of the lung upward and to the left (Figure 10-34).

Normally, alveolar neutrophils and macrophages produce **elastase** in response to air pollutants. Elastase is a proteolytic enzyme that digests elastin (the component responsible for elastic recoil of alveolar walls). α_1-**Antitrypsin** is an anti-proteolytic enzyme (protease inhibitor) that neutralizes elastase, thus maintaining the elastic properties of alveolar walls. **Emphysema develops from either excess elastase or deficient α_1-antitrypsin production.**

Two major causes of emphysema:

- **Smoking:** The most significant risk factor across the population for developing emphysema, so significant that those who do not smoke rarely develop emphysema unless an underlying genetic disorder or uncommon environmental exposure is present. Ash particles in cigarette smoke enter alveoli and attract increased numbers of neutrophils and macrophages, which produce elastase. Over time, excess elastase overwhelms local production of α_1-antitrypsin.
- **Hereditary α_1-antitrypsin deficiency:** Autosomal dominant. Accounts for 1% of emphysema cases. Emphysema develops secondary to unopposed elastase activity. Patients with α_1-antitrypsin deficiency often develop emphysema at a much younger age than smokers, often younger than 45 years.

Air trapping develops in emphysema secondary to **loss of radial traction.** Radial traction is the outward pull on airway walls by lung interstitium. Normally, as the lungs deflate during expiration, the interstitial tissues pull the airways open (ie, increase radial traction), allowing airflow. In emphysema, radial traction is lost (ability to expire is compromised) as the interstitium is destroyed, leading to airway collapse and subsequent air trapping during expiration.

This loss of elastic recoil also explains the **prolonged expiration time** needed to completely empty the lungs. This increases the overall duration of a single respiratory cycle. Because of the ongoing need to ventilate at a high-enough rate to maintain oxygenation, patients often begin inhaling their next breath before exhaling all of the air from the previous breath. This traps nonventilated air in the lungs. As a result, the volume of trapped air increases over the course of several breaths (**dynamic hyperinflation**).

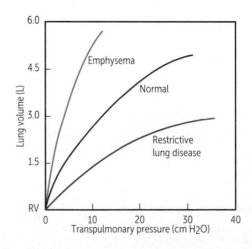

FIGURE 10-34. Lung compliance in pulmonary disease. The lung compliance curve shifts up and to the left in emphysema and down and to the right in restrictive lung disease.

PRESENTATION

- Chronic dyspnea with or without cough. Dyspnea and desaturation are often worsened by exertion and can be exacerbated by respiratory tract infections, air pollutants, bronchospasm, or CHF.
- "Pink puffer": PaO_2 is well preserved, so patients are not cyanotic ("pink"). Although ventilation and perfusion are both decreased, they are often well matched (alveoli and pulmonary capillaries are destroyed equally), so $\dot{V}/\dot{Q}$ mismatch is not severe. Patients require a high minute ventilation to maintain normal levels of PO_2 and PCO_2, so they "puff," working hard to get air in. Although this is the classic presentation, many patients do not fit this description.

DIAGNOSIS

- **Physical exam:**
  - Thin or cachectic.
  - Leaning forward on extended arms ("tripoding"), using accessory muscles of respiration.
  - Signs of hyperinflation: Resonance to percussion; diminished breath sounds bilaterally.
  - Breathing through pursed lips. This increases pressure within the airways and prevents airway collapse during expiration.
  - Prolonged expiration and associated **wheezing** on auscultation.
- **Chest film:** Barrel-shaped chest due to hyperinflated lungs and flattened diaphragm (Figure 10-35). Classic emphysema (smoking related) has decreased vascular markings (arterial deficiency) in the upper lobes with or without bullae. These changes can be seen in the lower lobes in α_1-antitrypsin deficiency.
- **Pulmonary function testing:**
  - **Spirometry:** Decreased FEV_1 and FEV_1:FVC ratio. FVC is often preserved.
  - **Lung volumes:** Increased TLC, FRC, and RV due to hyperinflation and air trapping.
  - **Diffusing capacity (DL_{CO}):** DL_{CO} is directly proportional to the surface area available to participate in gas exchange. Thus, the DL_{CO} is reduced in emphysema due to destruction of alveolar walls and associated capillary beds.
- **Arterial blood gas testing:** Early in the disease, PaO_2 may be mildly decreased or normal but decreases as alveolar damage progresses. More severely affected patients often chronically retain CO_2, resulting in compensated respiratory acidosis (elevated PCO_2, elevated HCO_3, and slightly decreased pH). During an acute exacerbation, PaO_2 drops and $PaCO_2$ increases, resulting in acute respiratory acidosis.
- **Pathology:** Two major subtypes of emphysema.
  - **Panacinar (panlobar) emphysema:** Characterized by dilation of the entire acinus (includes the respiratory bronchioles, alveolar ducts, and alveolar sacs). Primarily affects the lower lobes. **Associated with α_1-antitrypsin deficiency.**
  - **Centriacinar (centrilobular) emphysema (Figure 10-36):** Characterized by dilation of the proximal part of the acinus (the respiratory bronchioles). The pattern of involvement is more irregular and is often localized to the upper parts of the lungs. **Associated with smoking.**

TREATMENT

- **Smoking cessation is most important.**
- Supplemental oxygen is useful in patients with severe hypoxemia.
- Only smoking cessation and supplemental oxygen are proven to reduce mortality. All other treatments, including pharmacotherapy, only reduce symptoms.
- If hospitalization is required for an acute exacerbation, appropriate antibiotics, such as levofloxacin, improve outcome.
- Inhaled bronchodilators can reduce airflow obstruction. These include:
  - β_2-agonists (albuterol, salmeterol, formeterol)
  - Anticholinergics (ipratropium, tiotropium)
- Corticosteroids are used in acute exacerbations (PO/IV) and for long-term control (inhaled).

KEY FACT

Recognizing emphysema on a lateral chest x-ray is high yield. Look for an enlarged retrocardiac clear space (increased distance between sternum and heart) and flattened diaphragm.

KEY FACT

Common nonallergic causes of asthma include aspirin, exercise, occupational exposure, and viral infection.

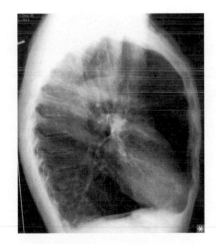

FIGURE 10-35. Lateral chest film of patient with emphysema. Note the increased anteroposterior diameter and "barrel-shape" characteristic of emphysema.

MNEMONIC

Obstructive lung disease—
ABCDE

Asthma
Bronchiectasis
Chronic bronchitis
Decreased FEV_1:FVC ratio
Emphysema

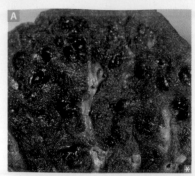

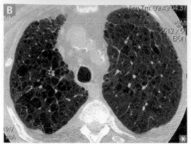

FIGURE 10-36. Centriacinar emphysema. Gross specimen and computed tomography cross-section.

KEY FACT

COPD is a broad term encompassing both emphysema and chronic bronchitis, as these two conditions can coexist.

KEY FACT

The term "blue bloater" is sometimes used to describe the clinical picture of chronic bronchitis. These patients are classically overweight ("bloated") and exhibit varying degrees of cyanosis ("blue") due to hypoxemia.

KEY FACT

Emphysema has decreased DL_{CO}, whereas chronic bronchitis has normal DL_{CO}.

PROGNOSIS

Lifelong and chronic. Often coexists with, or may be complicated by, chronic bronchitis. Spontaneous pneumothorax can occur due to rupture of a surface bleb or tear in the airways.

Chronic Bronchitis

Defined clinically as a **productive cough** occurring for at least 3 months per year over at least 2 consecutive years. Characterized by excessive mucus production in the airways. The mucus itself is typically more viscous than normal.

Smoking causes proliferation and hypertrophy of bronchial mucous glands. It also damages cilia lining the bronchial lumen, impeding mucus clearance. There is also an influx of inflammatory cells, leading to airway inflammation.

The increased mucus production and airway wall thickness decreases the cross-sectional area of the lumen, increasing resistance and inhibiting air flow. The obstruction to airflow in chronic bronchitis is in the terminal bronchioles, which is proximal to the obstruction in emphysema.

PRESENTATION

- Chronic cough **productive with copious mucus and sputum.** Blood-tinged mucus can be seen with rupture of pulmonary microvasculature.
- "Blue bloater": Often hypoxemic and cyanotic ("**blue**") due to decreased ventilation but relatively preserved perfusion; V̇/Q̇ mismatch.
- Often obese ("**bloater**"); can have peripheral edema due to RV.
- Dyspnea, chronic smoking history; large overlap with emphysema.

DIAGNOSIS

- **Physical exam:**
  - Often obese and sometimes cyanotic. The fingertips, lips, and tongue in particular may appear purplish blue.
  - Clubbing of fingertips associated with hypoxemia.
  - Rhonchi and wheezing on auscultation.
- **Chest film:** May show increased airway markings (appearing as a "dirty lung"), and there may be evidence of pulmonary hypertension and cor pulmonale.
- **Pulmonary function testing:**
  - **Spirometry:** Airflow obstruction results in decreased FEV_1 and FEV_1:FVC ratio. FVC is often preserved.
  - **Lung volumes:** In patients with dynamic hyperinflation, TLC, FRC, and RV may be increased.
  - **Diffusing capacity (DL_{CO}):** Typically normal. Despite the airway obstruction due to mucus plugging, the alveolar walls function normally.
- **Arterial blood gas testing:** Pa_{O_2} is often decreased, and Pa_{CO_2} is increased. Bicarbonate is elevated by the kidneys in an attempt to compensate for the decreased pH.
- **Pathology:** Increased number of goblet cells. The **Reid index,** which is the ratio of bronchial mucous gland depth to the total thickness of the bronchial wall, is abnormally high in chronic bronchitis.

TREATMENT

Bronchodilators and corticosteroids are used as in emphysema. Supplemental O_2 can treat hypoxemia, reduce hypoxic vasoconstriction and polycythemia, thereby reducing the incidence of pulmonary hypertension. Supplemental O_2 and cessation of cigarette smoking are the only interventions that have been shown to reduce mortality. Chest physiotherapy (percussion, coughing, and postural changes) can loosen and clear airway secretions, and pulmonary rehabilitation is helpful.

PROGNOSIS

- Chronic hypoxemia increases the risk of developing pulmonary hypertension secondary to pulmonary vasoconstriction. In turn, right-sided heart failure can ensue (**cor pulmonale**).
- In a compensatory effort to increase oxygen delivery to tissues, erythropoietin production is upregulated in the kidneys, resulting in **secondary polycythemia**.

Asthma

Reversible obstructive disease characterized by hyperreactive and hyperresponsive airways that lead to exuberant **bronchoconstriction** with minimal irritation. Prevalence is approximately 9% in the United States, although there is variation between races and sexes. Asthma is frequently seen in patients with a family history of eczema and allergic rhinitis, both of which are also hypersensitivity-mediated conditions. Children exposed to secondhand smoke, as well as infants of mothers who smoke, are at increased risk of developing asthma. Extrinsic and intrinsic subtypes exist, although patients frequently have a combination of the two.

- **Extrinsic asthma:** Mediated by a **type I hypersensitivity** reaction involving IgE and mast cells (see also the section on Allergy at the end of this chapter). Often begins in childhood in patients with a family history of allergies. Common allergens include animal dander (especially cats), pollen, mold, and dust mites.
- **Intrinsic asthma:** Due to nonallergic causes. Precipitating factors include viral URIs, exercise, cold temperatures, air pollutants (eg, cigarette smoke), chronic bronchitis, acid reflux, stress, and medications (especially aspirin).

In both types of asthma, airway inflammation leads to bronchial hyper responsiveness. Implicated in this inflammation are eosinophils, lymphocytes, histamine, leukotrienes, and IgE (see Table 10-14 for specific mediators). As a result of airway smooth muscle contraction, mucosal edema, and secretions within the lumen, the airway narrows, thereby increasing resistance and reducing airflow, especially during expiration. Unlike COPD, the process in asthma is generally reversible, so between attacks, most asthmatics have relatively normal physiology.

TABLE 10-14. **Epithelial-Derived Inflammatory Mediators in Asthma**

MEDIATOR	PHYSIOLOGIC EFFECT(S)
Endothelin-1	Bronchoconstriction
NO PGE$_2$ 15-HETE	Vasodilation
Cytokines: GM-CSF IL-8 RANTES Eotaxin	Inflammation
Growth factors: EGF IGF-1 PDGF	Fibrosis Smooth muscle hyperplasia

EGF, epidermal growth factor; GM-CSF, granulocyte-macrophage colony-stimulating factor; IGF-1, insulin-like growth factor-1; 15-HETE, 15-hydroxyeicosatetraenoic acid; IL-8, interleukin-8; NO, nitric oxide; PDGF, platelet-derived growth factor; PGE$_2$, prostaglandin E$_2$.

FLASH BACK

In contrast to other organs in the body, such as the brain, the pulmonary circulation actually vasodilates in response to high O_2 and vasoconstricts in response to low O_2.

CLINICAL CORRELATION

"Silent chest" is the absence of wheezing and other breath sounds during an asthma attack due to air flow rates too low to generate sound. It is a marker of disease severity and portends a poor prognosis for an acute asthma exacerbation.

KEY FACT

Not all that wheezes is asthma and not all asthma wheezes. Anaphylaxis, foreign body aspiration, COPD, and cardiac wheeze (pulmonary edema due to HF) may present with wheezing. However, a severe asthma exacerbation can result in respiratory muscle failure or so severely obstruct airways that air flow rates are insufficient to produce audible wheezing.

KEY FACT

Some asthmatics may be sensitive to aspirin, which inhibits cyclooxygenase and favors the production of leukotrienes from arachidonic acid. Leukotrienes play a role in airway inflammation and are potent bronchoconstrictors.

CLINICAL CORRELATION

Samter's triad is characterized by aspirin-induced bronchospasm, asthma, and nasal polyps.

FLASH BACK

Pulsus paradoxus is a decrease in systolic blood pressure by 10 mm Hg or more during inspiration. On board exams, it is most commonly tested in the context of cardiac tamponade but can also be seen in asthma, obstructive sleep apnea, and croup.

KEY FACT

Release of major basic protein (MBP) by eosinophils is a major cause of damage to the alveolar lining in asthma.

FLASH BACK

Immune cytokines:
IL-4 is responsible for B-cell class switching to IgE.
IL-5 is responsible for eosinophil recruitment.

CLINICAL CORRELATION

Asthma exacerbations are typically associated with respiratory alkalosis from tachypnea. Signs of acidosis (eg, decreased pH, increased Pa_{CO_2}) suggest impending respiratory failure as the patient's muscles of respiration become fatigued. This is a potential emergency requiring intubation.

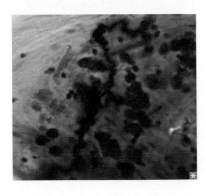

FIGURE 10-37. Curschmann spirals.

PRESENTATION

Acute exacerbation manifests with:

- Sudden-onset dyspnea, wheezing, and tachypnea, usually following an inciting event.
- Patients can also present with coughing, chest tightness, or chest pain.

DIAGNOSIS

- **Physical exam:** Tachypnea. Prolonged expiration and wheezing on auscultation.
- **Methacholine challenge test:** Inhalation of methacholine (direct cholinergic agonist). When performed in asthmatic patients, this precipitates bronchoconstriction at lower doses (hyperreactivity) and increased severity (hyperresponsiveness) compared to normal patients.
- **Pulmonary function testing (PFTs):** During an acute attack, airflow obstruction results in decreased FEV_1 and FEV_1:FVC ratio (FVC is often normal), and dynamic hyperinflation leads to a normal or increased TLC, and an increased FRC and RV. Between attacks, PFTs are often normal, although there may be small changes, such as decreased maximal midexpiratory flow (appearing as a marked concavity on the exhalation curve termed **expiratory coving**) and increased RV (Figure 10-19).
- Patients with asthma can often monitor their own respiratory status with portable peak flow meters.
- **Arterial blood gas testing:** During an attack, Pa_{O_2} is often reduced due to hypoxemia resulting from $\dot{V}/\dot{Q}$ mismatch. Pa_{CO_2} is also reduced due to hyperventilation. Pa_{CO_2} levels that normalize or become elevated during an asthma attack may indicate worsening airway obstruction or a tiring individual who can no longer maintain a high minute ventilation rate.
- **Pathology:**
  - Edema of the bronchial walls with **smooth muscle hypertrophy** and cellular infiltrates (eosinophils and lymphocytes).
  - Denuded epithelium, **enlarged mucous glands,** and increased number of goblet cells.
  - **Curschmann spirals** (whorled mucus plugs) containing shed epithelial cells (Figure 10-37) and eosinophilic crystals (**Charcot-Leyden crystals**) on sputum microscopy.
  - Mucus plugging (Figure 10-38).

TREATMENT

Treatments are listed below. Refer to the Pharmacology section at the end of the chapter for a more detailed discussion of each agent.

- β_2-agonists: albuterol, salmeterol, formoterol
- Corticosteroids: beclomethasone, fluticasone
- Muscarinic antagonists: ipratropium
- Antileukotrienes: montelukast, zafirlukast, zileuton
- Omalizumab
- Magnesium sulfate

PROGNOSIS

May improve with age or be a life-long condition. Avoidance of triggers can avert the worst symptoms. A severe attack that is refractory to bronchodilators (**status asthmaticus**) may require assisted ventilation and can result in death.

Bronchiectasis

Bronchiectasis is irreversible dilation of the airways caused by repeated episodes of infection and/or inflammation with eventual destruction of the bronchi and bronchiole walls. Over time, as the airways lose their elastic recoil, they become unable to expel air. As a result, air is functionally trapped in the lungs. Also, the damaged airways compromise the ability to fight infection. This allows bacterial colonization, pooling of secretions, and additional inflammation, thus perpetuating a vicious cycle. Bronchiectasis (Figure 10-39) has several causes, including the following:

- **Infection:** May be viral, bacterial, or fungal. Examples include tuberculosis, pertussis, and allergic bronchopulmonary aspergillosis.
- **Obstruction** by tumor, foreign body, or mucus plug.
- Defective airway or ciliary clearance:
  - **Smoking:** Irritants from cigarette smoke paralyze cilia and inhibit their ability to clear secretions.
  - **Primary ciliary dyskinesia (Kartagener syndrome):** Genetic dynein arm defect, resulting in immotile cilia. Affected patients also present with **infertility** (due to immotile sperm in males and dysfunctional fallopian tubes in females) and **situs inversus** (dextrocardia on chest x-ray and right-sided point of maximal impulse [PMI]).
- Patients with **cystic fibrosis** develop bronchiectasis due to the production of thick secretions that are difficult to clear as well as chronic infection with multiple pathogens (Figure 10-39). The lungs of these patients are often colonized with *Pseudomonas aeruginosa*, *Staphylococcus aureus*, and *Haemophilus influenzae*; less common organisms include *Burkholderia cepacia*, which almost exclusively appears in patients with cystic fibrosus.

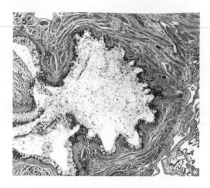

FIGURE 10-38. **Mucus plug.**

> **KEY FACT**
>
> Persistent obstruction of any portion of the respiratory tract (either internal blockage or external compression) can lead to bacterial colonization, inflammation, and eventual destruction of regions distal to the obstruction.

PRESENTATION

Cough; copious mucoid, mucopurulent, or purulent sputum production; dyspnea; rhinosinusitis; hemoptysis.

DIAGNOSIS

- **Physical exam:**
  - Localized crackles or rhonchi may be heard. Some patients also present with wheezing.
  - Clubbing of the fingernails may also be seen in some patients.
- **Chest film:** Often nonspecific abnormal findings, including increased markings, crowded vessels, or "ring" shadows corresponding to the dilated airways.

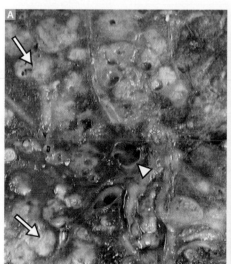
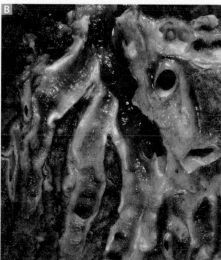
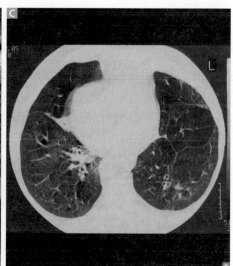

FIGURE 10-39. **Bronchiectasis.** **A** Fibrotic lung parenchyma with numerous areas of pneumonia (arrows) and thick inspissated secretions in areas of bronchiectasis (arrowhead) in a patient with cystic fibrosis. **B** Permanently dilated airways seen with bronchiectasis. **C** Computed tomography scan cross-section showing dextrocardia and bronchiectasis in a patient with Kartagener syndrome.

■ **CT:** Has become the preferred method both to diagnose bronchiectasis and to evaluate location and extent of disease.
■ **PFT:** Often normal, but can also show obstructive pattern.
■ **Arterial blood gas testing:** Usually normal, except in patients with very diffuse disease, who can exhibit hypoxemia and hypercapnia.
■ **Pathology:** Marked dilation of the airways in one of three patterns: cylindrical, varicose, or saccular (Figure 10-39). Increased secretions are also seen. The arteries also enlarge and proliferate. New anastomoses may form, leading to hemoptysis.

TREATMENT

■ Removal of any foreign body or tumor (if possible).
■ Inhaled bronchodilators are useful in patients with coexisting causes of airway obstruction.
■ Antibiotics for both acute and chronic infections.
■ Bronchopulmonary drainage with chest physiotherapy helps to clear secretions from the dilated airways.
■ **DNase** is used to break up thick secretions in CF patients.

PROGNOSIS

In severe cases, cor pulmonale can develop. Colonization with *P aeruginosa* is frequent.

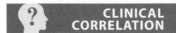

KEY FACT

$FEV_1:FVC$ ratio > 80% is characteristic of restrictive lung disease.

CLINICAL CORRELATION

Restrictive lung disease due to poor muscular effort can also arise from diaphragmatic paralysis, in which one or both phrenic nerves are damaged (eg, trauma) or impinged on (eg, tumor).

RESTRICTIVE LUNG DISEASES

Restrictive lung diseases are characterized by reduced lung expansion (decreased lung volume). **TLC and RV are reduced.** In turn, FEV_1 **and FVC are decreased.** FEV_1 and FVC decrease proportionately, resulting in a **normal $FEV_1:FVC$, or FVC is decreased to a greater degree** than FEV_1, resulting in an **increased $FEV_1:FVC$.** Restrictive lung disease can develop from both pulmonary and extrapulmonary sources (Figure 10-40).

Extrapulmonary Restrictive Disease (Poor Breathing Mechanics)

The restrictive defect is extrinsic to the lung parenchyma. This includes mainly disorders of the chest wall and neuromuscular disease leading to impaired ability to fully expand the lungs. Hypoxemia develops secondary to **hypoventilation.** There are two broad classes: **poor muscular effort** and **poor structural apparatus.**

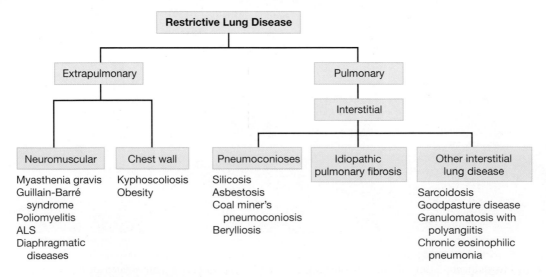

FIGURE 10-40. **Classification of restrictive lung diseases.** ALS, amyotrophic lateral sclerosis.

Poor Muscular Effort

Poor muscular effort is often due to one of several neuromuscular diseases. In each case, hypoventilation develops as the diaphragm and accessory muscles become fatigued. Patients alter their breathing pattern, taking more frequent, shallow breaths. This increases the $V_D:V_T$ ratio, reducing alveolar ventilation and increasing $Paco_2$. Ineffective cough can lead to decreased secretion clearance, atelectasis, and recurrent respiratory infections. Common causes of neuromuscular disease include

- **Poliomyelitis (polio):** Picornavirus infection, which leads to ablation of anterior motor neurons and therefore symptoms of lower motor neuron (LMN) paralysis.
- **Myasthenia gravis:** Autoimmune disorder that causes muscle weakness due to auto-antibodies targeting nicotinic acetylcholine receptors in the neuromuscular junction.
- **Amyotrophic lateral sclerosis (ALS):** Neurodegenerative motor neuron disease affecting both the lateral corticospinal tracts and anterior horns of the spinal cord, leading to signs of upper motor neuron (UMN) and LMN paralysis, respectively.
- **Guillain-Barré syndrome (GBS):** Transient autoimmune destruction of Schwann cells, leading to peripheral demyelination. Classically presents with symmetric ascending paralysis, starting from the lower extremities; symptoms can also include autonomic dysregulation (eg, cardiac arrhythmias, hypertension, or hypotension). Usually follows gastroenteritis (most commonly caused by *Campylobacter jejuni*).

Poor Structural Apparatus

Commonly due to scoliosis and morbid obesity.

- **Kyphoscoliosis:** Lateral curvature of the spine prevents proper chest wall expansion.
- **Morbid obesity:** The excess weight surrounding the chest wall presses down on the wall and inhibits proper expansion. Obesity is also associated with decreased respiratory rate, which also contributes to hypoventilation (see discussion on obesity hypoventilation syndrome below).

PRESENTATION

Dyspnea, especially with exertion. Other possible signs and symptoms are etiology dependent.

DIAGNOSIS

- A-a gradient: **normal,** because gas exchange in alveoli is **not** impaired.
- **Physical exam:**
  - **Neuromuscular disease:** Etiology dependent, nonpulmonary manifestations of specific disease; assess for UMN and LMN lesions (see Chapter 6).
  - **Diaphragmatic disease:** Paradoxical movement of paralyzed regions of the diaphragm upward during supine inspiration.
  - Assess for kyphoscoliosis.
- **Chest film:** Assess for kyphoscoliosis, diaphragmatic paralysis.
- **PFT:** Variable depending on the specific disease and disease severity. In general, FEV_1, FVC, TLC, and RV are usually decreased, but these are neither sensitive nor specific.

TREATMENT

Supplemental O_2 or mechanical ventilation may be needed for patients with severe disease. The underlying disorder must be treated, or irreversible pulmonary sequelae will develop.

PROGNOSIS

Extrapulmonary restrictive diseases resulting in hypoxemia can lead to pulmonary hypertension and cor pulmonale. Progressive disease can lead to chronic respiratory acidosis.

Interstitial Lung Diseases

The restrictive defect is due to abnormalities within the lung parenchyma. It is most commonly due to fibrosis, with the exceptions of ARDS and neonatal respiratory distress syndrome (NRDS), which are discussed below. Because diffusing capacity through the alveolar walls is impaired, **A-a gradient is increased.**

Acute Respiratory Distress Syndrome

Acute respiratory distress syndrome (ARDS) is characterized by acute-onset diffuse alveolar damage and leakage of fluid out of the pulmonary capillaries into the interstitium and alveolar spaces. ARDS is defined by four major criteria, all of which must be met:

1. Reduced arterial oxygen to inspired oxygen ratio Pao_2/Fio_2:
   - Mild ARDS: 200–300.
   - Moderate ARDS: 100–200.
   - Severe ARDS: < 100.
   - A low ratio reflects poor oxygenation despite ample inspired oxygen; normal ratio is 500 mm Hg.
2. Acute onset.
3. Bilateral lung infiltrates (Figure 10-41).
4. Must not be fully explained by left-sided heart failure or fluid overload.

Etiologies include pneumonia, inhalation of irritants, O_2 toxicity, heroin overdose, shock, sepsis, aspiration of gastric contents, trauma, uremia, acute pancreatitis, head trauma, multiple transfusions of blood products (transfusion-related acute lung injury [TRALI]), disseminated intravascular coagulation (DIC), and fat or amniotic fluid embolism. In all of these cases, the initial injury in ARDS affects the type I pneumocytes and/or capillary endothelial cells, resulting in leakage of protein-rich fluid. Alveoli become flooded with fluid, inhibiting gas exchange and oxygenation. This leads to hypoxemia in the forms of shunting and V/Q mismatch, with the latter being exacerbated by altered distribution of pulmonary blood flow due to increased PVR. Additionally, surfactant function and production is altered, resulting in alveolar collapse.

PRESENTATION

Acute-onset dyspnea accompanied by tachypnea and hypoxemia, usually in a critically ill patient.

KEY FACT

Pulmonary edema is an intra-alveolar accumulation of fluid. It can be caused by increased hydrostatic pressure (eg, left ventricular failure), increased capillary permeability (eg, ARDS), or several other mechanisms (eg, high altitude, neurologic injury, or opiate overdose).

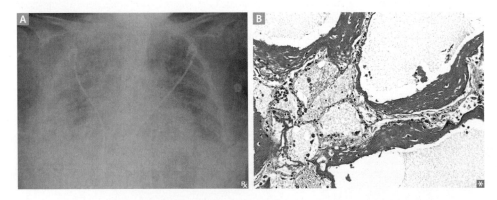

FIGURE 10-41. **Acute respiratory distress syndrome.** A Chest film shows diffuse, bilateral interstitial and alveolar infiltrates with near-complete opacification of lungs with obscured cardiomediastinal silhouette. B Histology: note alveolar fluid (clear, frothy) and thick hyaline membranes (pink).

DIAGNOSIS

- **Physical exam:** Crackles are often heard on auscultation.
- **Chest film:** Diffuse, symmetrical interstitial and alveolar edema (see Figure 10-41; note that this is criterion 3 from the previous diagnostic criteria). Air bronchograms—visualization of distal bronchioles due to the contrasting opacity of infiltrates around the airway—may be present.
- **PFT:** Not usually performed, but would see a restrictive pattern with a reduced D$_{LCO}$.
- **Arterial blood gas testing:** Hypoxemia, with a large A-a gradient. Supplemental O$_2$ may not increase Pao$_2$ significantly due to shunt.

PATHOLOGY

Damage to type I alveolar epithelial cells, with regenerative hyperplasia of type II cells. Interstitial and alveolar fluid is present, with an inflammatory cell infiltrate and areas of alveolar collapse. **Hyaline membranes** (composed of eosinophilic, acellular material), fibrosis, and changes in the pulmonary vasculature can also be seen (Figure 10-42).

TREATMENT

Treat underlying cause; patients are typically intubated and mechanically ventilated using low tidal volume ventilation and high PEEP in an ICU.

PROGNOSIS

High mortality (30–50%), largely due to the underlying cause rather than the pulmonary effects of ARDS.

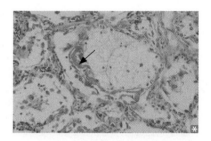

FIGURE 10-42. Alveolar damage In acute respiratory distress syndrome. The alveoli are congested and edematous, and the classic hyaline membrane can be seen (arrow).

Neonatal (Infant) Respiratory Distress Syndrome

Neonatal respiratory distress syndrome (NRDS) is the most common cause of respiratory failure in newborns and the most common cause of death in premature infants. It results from a deficiency of surfactant in immature lungs, leading to atelectasis due to increased surface tension in the air-liquid interface, V/Q mismatch, and shunting.

Predisposing factors include:

- **Prematurity.**
- **Maternal diabetes:** Excess glucose in the mother's blood reaches the fetus through the placenta. Fetal insulin production increases, which suppresses corticosteroids normally involved in surfactant production.
- **C-section delivery:** During a normal vaginal delivery, maternal uterine contractions compress the fetal head, inducing corticosteroid production. This process is bypassed in a C-section, causing the fetus to produce fewer corticosteroids.

Incidence and mortality decrease dramatically with gestational age, with the most severe disease seen prior to the alveolar stage of lung development.

PRESENTATION

Dyspnea and tachypnea in a newborn, with risk factors described above, especially if premature.

DIAGNOSIS

- **Physical exam:** Tachypnea, often with grunting, cyanosis, and retractions; crackles on auscultation.
- Fetal pulmonary maturity can be assessed by measuring the **ratio of surfactant lecithin to sphingomyelin in the amniotic fluid.** A ratio of 2:1 or greater indicates lung maturity.

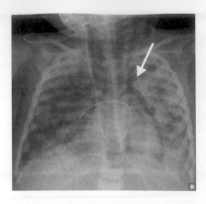

FIGURE 10-43. Neonatal respiratory distress syndrome. X-ray of the chest showing pneumomediastinum (arrow).

CLINICAL CORRELATION

Remember your **ABC**s: **A**irway, **B**reathing, **C**irculation. Assess these three parameters and manage them (if needed) before any other physical examination maneuvers are carried out.

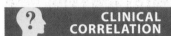

MNEMONIC

Adverse effects associated with supplemental O₂ administration in patients with NRDS—

RIB:

Retinopathy of prematurity
Intraventricular hemorrhage
Bronchopulmonary dysplasia

MNEMONIC

Asbestosis is from the roof (roofers), but affects the base (lower lobes).
Silica and coal are from the base (earth), but affect the roof (upper lobes).

- **Chest film:** Low lung volumes, diffuse ground-glass appearance with air bronchograms (Figure 10-43).
- **Arterial blood gas testing:** Hypoxemia, with a large A-a gradient. Hypoxemia may be refractory to supplemental O_2 due to shunting.
- **Pathology:** Lungs are heavier than normal, with alternating atelectatic areas and dilated alveoli. The pulmonary vessels are engorged, with leakage of fluid into the alveoli. Hyaline membranes are also seen (note that neonatal RDS was formerly called hyaline membrane disease).
- **Differential diagnosis:** Transient tachypnea of the newborn (TTN—self-resolving, relatively benign respiratory distress associated with pulmonary edema), bacterial pneumonia, congenital heart disease.

TREATMENT

Exogenous surfactant administration. Mechanical ventilation with PEEP. Inhaled nitric oxide. Antenatal maternal corticosteroid therapy to promote surfactant production.

PROGNOSIS

Mortality rates have improved dramatically with the use of exogenous surfactant but remain over 10%. NRDS may also be associated with metabolic acidosis, patent ductus arteriosus (PDA), and necrotizing enterocolitis.

Pneumoconiosis

A group of interstitial lung diseases caused by the inhalation of inorganic and organic particulate matter. This produces varying degrees of pulmonary fibrosis, characterized by decreased compliance, reduced lung volumes, and destruction of the alveolar-capillary interface, leading to $\dot{V}/\dot{Q}$ mismatch and hypoxemia. Four common inorganic pneumoconioses are listed in Table 10-15.

PRESENTATION

Dyspnea, especially with exertion.

DIAGNOSIS

- **Physical exam:** Bibasilar crackles heard on auscultation. Clubbing may also be seen.
- **Chest film:** Nodular opacities seen in silicosis, coal worker's pneumoconiosis, and berylliosis. A more linear pattern is seen in asbestosis. Calcified pleural plaques are also seen in asbestosis.
- **PFT:** Decreased TLC, FRC, RV, FEV_1, and FVC, with a normal or increased FEV_1:FVC ratio. D_{LCO} is also decreased.
- **Arterial blood gas testing:** Hypoxemia, often with normo- or hypocapnia.
- **Pathology:** Refer to Table 10-15.

TREATMENT

Avoid further exposure. No curative treatment.

PROGNOSIS

- **Silicosis:** Associated with increased susceptibility to tuberculosis (TB).
- **Coal worker's pneumoconiosis (CWP):** Simple CWP is often inconsequential. If CWP is complicated by progressive massive fibrosis (PMF), it can lead to bronchiectasis, pulmonary hypertension, and death from respiratory failure or right-sided heart failure.

TABLE 10-15. Common Inorganic Pneumoconioses

NAME	EXPOSURE	PATHOLOGY	COMMENTS
Asbestosis	Asbestos fibers (associated with shipbuilding, roofing, plumbing, insulation, construction work)	**"Ivory white" calcified pleural plaques A B** are pathognomonic for asbestos exposure but are not precancerous. **Asbestos (ferruginous) bodies** are golden-brown fusiform rods resembling dumbbells C.	Interstitial fibrosis primarily affects the lower lobes. Associated with an increased incidence of bronchogenic carcinoma and mesothelioma (bronchogenic >> mesothelioma). Concomitant cigarette smoking multiplies the risk of developing lung cancer.
Berylliosis	Beryllium (found in aerospace, electronics, nuclear materials, and manufacturing industries)	Noncaseating granulomas.	Interstitial fibrosis primarily affects the upper lobes. Associated with an increased risk of primary lung cancer. **Can mimic sarcoidosis** (granulomas in multiple organ systems).
Coal workers' pneumoconiosis	Prolonged coal dust exposure (coal miners)	Black lungs; coal dust contains silica and carbon D. Progresses from **anthracosis** (mild, asymptomatic form seen in city dwellers and smokers).	Interstitial fibrosis primarily affects the upper lobes and develops secondary to activation of carbon-laden macrophages. **Not associated with lung cancer.**
Silicosis	Silica (associated with sandblasting; also seen in foundries and mines) quartz and other minerals)	**"Eggshell" calcification** of hilar lymph nodes. Silicotic nodules E.	Interstitial fibrosis primarily affects upper lobes. Silica disrupts phagolysosome in macrophages, **increasing susceptibility to tuberculosis.** Associated with increased risk of bronchogenic carcinoma.

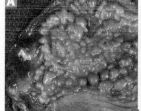 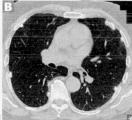 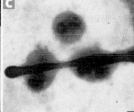 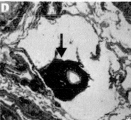 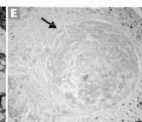

Modified with permission from Le T, et al. *First Aid for the USMLE Step 1 2017.* New York, NY: McGraw Hill Education; 2017.

- **Asbestosis:** Predisposes to bronchogenic carcinoma and, less commonly, malignant mesothelioma of the pleura or peritoneum. Concomitant cigarette smoking multiplies the risk of developing cancer.
- **Berylliosis:** Can mimic sarcoidosis, with granulomas in multiple organ systems.

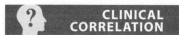

CLINICAL CORRELATION

Caplan syndrome is characterized by rheumatoid arthritis and pneumoconiosis with intrapulmonary nodules.

Sarcoidosis

Inflammatory disease characterized by **noncaseating granulomas,** often involving multiple organ systems. The initial exposure that leads to granuloma formation is unknown.

PRESENTATION

Classic presentation of sarcoidosis is an African-American female in her thirties with progressive dyspnea, often accompanied by a dry or nonproductive cough. More common in women and African Americans. Presents in young adulthood. Often discovered in asymptomatic patients on chest film (Figure 10-44A). Less often, presents with extra-pulmonary symptoms.

DIAGNOSIS

- **Chest film:** Bilateral hilar lymphadenopathy, diffuse (coarse) reticular densities.
- Reduced sensitivity/anergy to skin test antigens.
- **Laboratory findings:** Hypercalcemia (due to increased 1-α-hydroxylase production by activated macrophages leading to increased 1,25-(OH)$_2$-vitamin D), hypercalciuria, hypergammaglobulinemia, increased ACE activity. Hypercalcemia/hypercalciuria may present as nephrolithiasis.
- **Biopsy** showing noncaseating granulomas in the lung with a negative microbiology work-up is highly suggestive. Granulomas are often seen in other organs as well. The granuloma consists of a core of macrophages surrounded by T lymphocytes, as illustrated in Figure 10-44B.
- **Differential diagnosis:** TB, fungal infections (see Table 10-15), other infectious diseases, malignancy, rheumatologic disease.

TREATMENT

Many patients do not need treatment. Criteria for receiving treatment include impaired pulmonary function or worsening radiologic findings, systemic symptoms that interfere with activities of daily living, ocular disease, heart disease, neurologic involvement, and hypercalcemia. Treatment consists of systemic corticosteroids or other immunosuppressive drugs.

PROGNOSIS

Natural history varies widely. In some patients, clinical and radiographic manifestations resolve spontaneously. In others, symptoms persist without progression. In a small minority, the disease progresses to widespread pulmonary fibrosis.

Idiopathic Pulmonary Fibrosis

Idiopathic pulmonary fibrosis (IPF) pathogenesis is believed to be precipitated by an unknown agent that causes cytokine release, resulting in repeated cycles of inflammatory lung injury, followed by wound healing. Collagen deposits accumulate in the lungs with each cycle, eventually leading to fibrosis. IPF accounts for approximately 15% of cases of chronic interstitial lung disease.

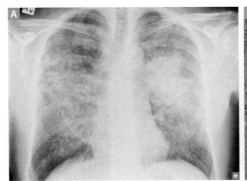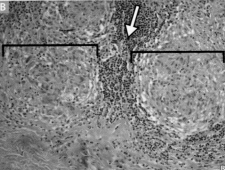

FIGURE 10-44. **Sarcoidosis.** **A** X-ray of the chest shows bilateral hilar adenopathy and coarse reticular opacities. **B** Photomicrograph from a patient with sarcoidosis. Granulomas consist of macrophages and multinucleated giant cells (brackets) surrounded by lymphocytes (arrow).

PRESENTATION

Insidious onset, often between 40 and 70 years of age. Most commonly presents with progressive dyspnea.

DIAGNOSIS

- **Physical exam:** Dry crackles or rales on auscultation, clubbing of fingernails.
- **Chest film and CT:** Diffuse, interstitial pattern bilaterally. Seen more at the bases and peripheral portions of the lung. CT classically shows "honeycombing"—a cavernous network of fibrosis within the lungs (Figure 10-45).
- **Biopsy/pathology:** Provides definitive diagnosis; shows chronic inflammation and fibrosis of the alveolar walls as well as interstitial fibrosis; dilation of bronchioles proximal to fibrotic alveoli produces "honeycomb lung" appearance in UIP.

TREATMENT

Systemic corticosteroids and other immunosuppressive drugs are not effective. Lung transplantation may be an option for younger patients. Two new drugs can now be considered—pirfenidone and nintedanib.

PROGNOSIS

Rapid disease progression with a mean survival of 2–5 years.

Goodpasture Syndrome

Autoimmune disease targeting the lungs and kidneys. Caused by type II hypersensitivity against the α3-chain of type IV collagen, located in the basement membranes of alveoli and glomeruli.

PRESENTATION

Pulmonary hemorrhage with concomitant nephritic syndrome (hematuria, etc; see Chapter 8).

DIAGNOSIS

- **Anti–type IV collagen autoantibodies.**
- **Kidney biopsy:** Immunofluorescence demonstrates linear, ribbon-like deposition of IgG along the glomerular basement membrane. Lung biopsy may be necessary if renal biopsy is not possible.

TREATMENT

Plasmapheresis with or without immunosuppressive therapy to reduce the burden of autoantibodies.

PROGNOSIS

Therapy can often control symptoms. However, immune-mediated damage to the lung parenchyma can result in scarring and eventual fibrosis.

Granulomatosis with Polyangiitis (Formerly Wegener Granulomatosis)

Granulomatosis with polyangiitis is an autoimmune vasculitis affecting primarily the upper respiratory tract, lungs, and kidneys, but also affecting the joints, skin, eyes, or nervous system in certain cases. Characterized by vasculitis of small and medium blood vessels in affected organs, with granulomas surrounding these vessels.

MNEMONIC

Drugs that cause pulmonary fibrosis:

Breathing **A**ir **B**adly [from] **M**edications: **B**leomycin, **A**miodarone, **B**usulfan, **M**ethotrexate

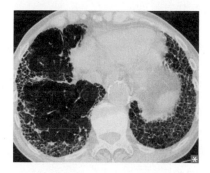

FIGURE 10-45. CT of chest of a patient with idiopathic pulmonary fibrosis. Image demonstrates bibasilar reticular abnormalities with traction bronchiectasis and honeycombing characteristic of usual interstitial pneumonia.

FLASH BACK

Both **Goodpasture syndrome** and **granulomatosis with polyangiitis** are causes of **rapidly progressive glomerulonephritis,** which presents as a nephritic syndrome. Histology will reveal crescent-shaped proliferation of glomerular parietal cells and accumulation of fibrin in glomeruli.

PRESENTATION

Extremely varied. Cough, dyspnea, hemoptysis. Persistent rhinorrhea, bloody/purulent nasal discharge, nasal pain. Nonrespiratory symptoms include nephritic syndrome, eye and ear symptoms, arthritis, and cutaneous vasculitis.

DIAGNOSIS

- **CT:** One or several nodules ("coin lesions") and infiltrates, often with cavitation (Figure 10-46).
- **c-ANCA-positive** (antiproteinase 3 autoantibodies).
- **Biopsy:** Necrotizing granulomatous vasculitis.

TREATMENT

Prednisone used during initial therapy. Cytotoxic agents like cyclophosphamide are also used.

PROGNOSIS

Complete and long-term remission can often be achieved with proper treatment.

Chronic Eosinophilic Pneumonia

PRESENTATION

Presents over weeks to months, with fever, weight loss, dyspnea, and nonproductive cough.

DIAGNOSIS

- **Chest film:** Peripheral pulmonary infiltrates and a pattern suggestive of alveolar filling.
- **Eosinophilia.**
- **Pathology:** Pulmonary interstitium and alveolar spaces infiltrated by eosinophils and macrophages.

TREATMENT

Administration of corticosteroids.

PROGNOSIS

Clinical improvement can be seen within days to weeks after therapy with steroids is initiated.

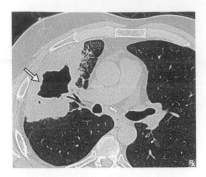

FIGURE 10-46. CT of the lungs of a patient with granulomatosis with polyangiitis. This CT scan shows a large cavitary lesion in the right upper lobe (arrow) (surgically proven).

PULMONARY VASCULAR DISEASES

The pulmonary vasculature receives the entire cardiac output and is susceptible to a number of disease processes. The four major entities discussed here are deep venous thrombosis (DVT), pulmonary embolism (PE), pulmonary hypertension, and sleep apnea.

Deep Venous Thrombosis

DVT refers to the formation of an occlusive blood clot (thrombus) in the deep veins of the lower extremity. The physiologic risk factors that predispose a patient to thrombus formation are described by the **Virchow triad:**

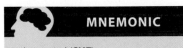

MNEMONIC

Virchow triad (**SHE**):
Stasis
Hypercoagulability
Endothelial damage

- **Stasis:** Occurs in patients who are immobile for prolonged periods (eg, postoperative state, long plane flights, truck drivers).
- **Hypercoagulability:** Due to defects in coagulation cascade proteins. The most common genetic hypercoagulable condition is factor V Leiden. Other causes include malignancy, multiple bone fractures, and use of oral contraceptive pills (OCPs).
- **Endothelial damage:** Exposure of subendothelial collagen activates the clotting cascade (intrinsic pathway).

Most commonly, DVTs form in the **femoral** and **popliteal** veins, as well as the veins in the **calf.**

PRESENTATION

Sudden-onset unilateral lower extremity pain and swelling (Figure 10-47) in a patient with prolonged immobilization or another risk factor mentioned above.

DIAGNOSIS

- Physical exam:
    - Unilateral lower extremity swelling and tenderness to palpation (Figure 10-47). Pitting edema is also seen in the affected leg due to excessive hydrostatic pressure.
    - Calf pain with passive dorsiflexion of the foot (positive **Homan sign**). This finding is not always present.
- **Compression ultrasound** of the lower extremity can be used for confirmation.

TREATMENT

- DVTs are initially managed with **unfractionated heparin** or a low-molecular-weight heparin (LMWH), such as **enoxaparin.** This is followed with oral anticoagulants (eg, warfarin, rivaroxaban) for long-term prophylaxis as outpatient therapy.
- Many hospitalized patients are given heparin (unfractionated or LMWH) prophylactically due to increased risk for developing a DVT secondary to immobilization (stasis).

PROGNOSIS

In some cases, DVTs can break off and become lodged in the pulmonary circulation (PE). The majority of PEs arise from the proximal deep veins of the lower extremity.

Pulmonary Embolism

PE is often missed clinically and is seen in > 60% of autopsies. It occurs when a blood clot from a systemic vein lodges in one or more branches of the pulmonary artery. Most often, a PE arises from a deep vein thrombosis (DVT), but it can also result from embolization of fat, air, bacteria (infectious vegetations), amniotic fluid, and tumor cells (Table 10-16). As mentioned earlier, the majority of PEs arise from DVTs. As such, similar risk factors apply.

Decreased perfusion with continued ventilation causes an increase in dead space following a PE. One may expect this to lead to hypercapnia, but patients often hyperventilate and become hypocapnic. The release of inflammatory mediators can lead to bronchoconstriction, V/Q mismatch, and hypoxemia. Reduced output of the right ventricle can lead to hypotension, syncope, and/or shock.

PRESENTATION

Tachypnea, tachycardia, hypoxia, and **sudden-onset dyspnea** with **pleuritic chest pain** (pain that worsens with breathing) are the classic signs and symptoms, but the presentation is often varied. Can be associated with hemoptysis (secondary to infarcted lung tissue) and syncope. Smaller PEs are often asymptomatic.

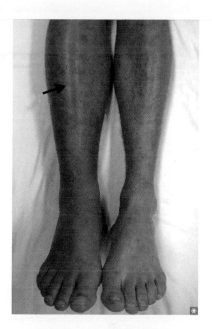

FIGURE 10-47. Deep venous thrombosis in right lower extremity.

> **CLINICAL CORRELATION**
>
> For acute management of DVT, give heparin before transitioning to warfarin. Heparin has a faster onset than warfarin, and this sequence also decreases the risk of warfarin-induced skin necrosis.

> **FLASH BACK**
>
> The differential diagnosis for hypercoagulable states includes primary thrombotic disorders and acquired risk factors. Primary genetic disorders include factor V Leiden, prothrombin G20210A, antithrombin deficiency, protein C or S deficiency, and dysfibrogenemias. Secondary risk factors include antiphospholipid syndrome (APLS), immobility, pregnancy, oral contraceptive use, and obesity.

TABLE 10-16. **Types of Emboli**

TYPE	COMMENTS	EXAMPLE PRESENTATION
Fat	Associated with long-bone fractures and liposuction. Classic triad: Hypoxemia, neurologic abnormalities, and petechial rash on the chest and truck. Pathology: The emboli stain black with osmium tetroxide.	A 24-year-old patient is hospitalized following a motor vehicle accident. The next day, he develops sudden-onset dyspnea and confusion. On physical examination, a petechial rash is seen across his chest.
Air	Develops in divers when nitrogen bubbles precipitate in their blood as they ascend too rapidly.	A 26-year-old patient develops rapid-onset dyspnea and pleuritic chest pain. On further questioning, patient reports symptoms developed while scuba diving.
Thrombus (DVT)	Develops after prolonged immobilization (usually ≥ 3 days).	Five days after abdominal surgery, a 68-year-old woman develops dyspnea and pleuritic chest pain.
Bacteria	Develops in infective endocarditis, when the bacterial vegetations dislodge from the heart valves. Can travel to brain or lungs, resulting in an abscess.	A 36-year-old IV drug user presents with sudden-onset left-sided weakness. His temperature is 101.6°F. Physical examination shows a heart murmur, painless erythematous nodules on his palms, and nail-bed hemorrhages.
Amniotic fluid	Develops when amniotic fluid leaks into the maternal bloodstream, usually postpartum. Can lead to disseminated intravascular coagulation (DIC).	A 27-year-old woman develops sudden-onset dyspnea shortly after giving birth.
Tumor cells	Be suspicious of malignancy when an adult presents with signs of new-onset hypercoagulability.	A 59-year-old man presents with sudden-onset right-sided weakness. He has a 40 pack-year smoking history. Chest x-ray shows a 4-cm lung nodule.

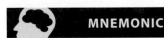

MNEMONIC

Types of emboli:

An embolus moves like a **FAT BAT** (**F**at, **A**ir, **T**hrombus, **B**acteria, **A**mniotic fluid, **T**umor).

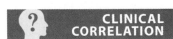

CLINICAL CORRELATION

Lines of Zahn (Figure 10-48B) are interdigitating areas of pink (platelets, fibrin) and red (RBCs) found only in thrombi formed before death. As such, they are used to assess whether a thrombus formed pre- or postmortem.

DIAGNOSIS

- **Physical exam:**
    - Tachycardia and tachypnea.
    - Localized crackles or wheezes; however, the lung exam is often normal.
    - A pleural rub may be present. The pleural rub is produced by a fibrinous exudate that is released from the pleural surface overlying the region of ischemic lung tissue.
    - In the case of a massive PE (Figure 10-48A), the sudden increase in vascular resistance can lead to right ventricular overload (acute cor pulmonale), in which case a right-sided S_4 and loud P_2 may be heard (see Heart Sounds, discussed in Chapter 1). Jugular venous distention (JVD) may also be observed.
    - Lower extremity tenderness, swelling, and a palpable cord suggestive of a DVT may be seen.
- **Laboratory results and imaging:**
    - **CT angiography** can show the filling defect due to the thrombus (Figure 10-48C,D). This is the preferred method of definitive diagnosis.
    - **V̇/Q̇ scan:** Shows an area of V̇/Q̇ mismatch.
    - **Chest film:** Usually nonspecific. Dilation of the pulmonary arteries, **Hampton hump** (wedge-shaped consolidation in the lung periphery adjacent to the pleura), **Westermark sign** (abrupt cutoff of pulmonary vascularity distal to a PE), or a pleural effusion may also be seen.
    - **D-dimer level:** Fibrin degradation product. Elevated levels indicate thrombus formation. Has high sensitivity (hence, used for ruling out PEs).
    - **Arterial blood gas testing:** Decreased Pao_2 due to increased dead space. Decreased $Paco_2$ due to tachypnea. A-a gradient increased due to V̇/Q̇ mismatch.

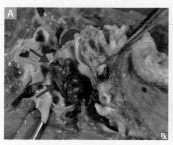 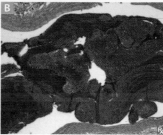 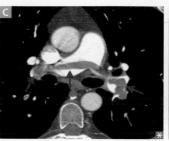 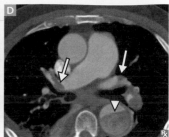

FIGURE 10-48. Pulmonary embolus. A Massive pulmonary embolus. B Lines of Zahn, indicating premortem thrombus formation. C CT angiogram of pulmonary vessels showing a filling defect (arrows). D Bilateral pulmonary emboli (arrows) appear as contrasting regions within the pulmonary vasculature. This axial CT also shows a type B aortic dissection (arrowhead), with the true lumen narrower than the false lumen.

TREATMENT

Supplemental oxygen if hypoxemic. Anticoagulation therapy, usually with IV heparin or low-molecular-weight heparin followed by oral anticoagulation for 3–6 months. Thrombolytic therapy may be useful in a subset of patients with massive PE and hypotension. Placement of a filtering device in the IVC can be used in patients who cannot tolerate anticoagulation due to an elevated bleeding risk.

PROGNOSIS

Variable, ranging from sudden death to asymptomatic resolution.

Pulmonary Hypertension

Pulmonary hypertension is the elevation of intravascular pressure within the pulmonary circulation and includes pulmonary arterial hypertension (PAH) as well as pulmonary venous hypertension. PAH is defined as a mean pulmonary artery pressure > 25 mm Hg at rest or > 35 mm Hg with exertion. Idiopathic (primary) pulmonary arterial hypertension has no known cause and carries a poor prognosis. It occurs in the absence of underlying heart or lung disease and is more common in women than in men. Primary pulmonary hypertension is associated with mutations in genes linked to transforming growth factor beta (TGF-β) signaling and is characterized by vascular hyperreactivity with proliferation of smooth muscle. Congenital idiopathic pulmonary hypertension is associated with abnormally thickened vasculature.

Secondary pulmonary hypertension is more common and is related to lung or heart disease, including:

- Chronic thromboembolic disease.
- Loss of vessels by scarring or destruction of alveolar walls.
- Chronic hypoxemia.
- Increased flow (left-to-right shunt).
- Elevated left atrial pressure, as in CHF or mitral stenosis.
- Chronic respiratory acidosis (eg, chronic bronchitis, obstructive sleep apnea).
- Meconium aspiration at birth, the most common cause of persistent pulmonary hypertension of the newborn.

PRESENTATION

Dyspnea and exertional fatigue. Substernal chest pain, similar to angina pectoris, is sometimes seen. If cardiac output falls enough, syncope can result.

DIAGNOSIS

- **Physical exam:**
  - Lung examination often normal unless pulmonary hypertension is due to concomitant lung disease.
  - Loud P_2, right-sided S_3 and S_4.
  - JVD.
  - Right ventricular heave.
- **CT:** Increased prominence and size of hilar pulmonary arteries, which rapidly taper off. Enlarged cardiac silhouette (particularly RV and RA enlargement). Redistribution of blood flow to the upper lungs (Figure 10-49).
- **PFT:** Spirometry and lung volumes usually normal, with a decreased DLCO.
- **Arterial blood gas testing:** Useful in determining whether hypoxemia or acidosis plays a role in the disease's cause.
- **Echocardiogram:** Elevated right ventricular systolic pressure with possible right ventricular dysfunction or hypertrophy.
- **Pathology:** Intimal hyperplasia and medial hypertrophy of small arteries and arterioles, leading to obliteration of the lumen. Plexogenic (web-like) lesions are typically seen in idiopathic disease. Thickening of the walls of larger arteries is also seen. Right ventricular hypertrophy is also a feature.

TREATMENT

Supplemental O_2 therapy, various vasodilators (eg, sildenafil, bosentan, prostacyclins), inhaled nitric oxide, and possibly anticoagulation therapy. See the Pharmacology section of this chapter for a more detailed discussion.

PROGNOSIS

- Right-sided heart failure can occur due to elevated right-sided pressures.
- Idiopathic (primary) pulmonary hypertension: Poor prognosis, often resulting in death within a few years of diagnosis if untreated.

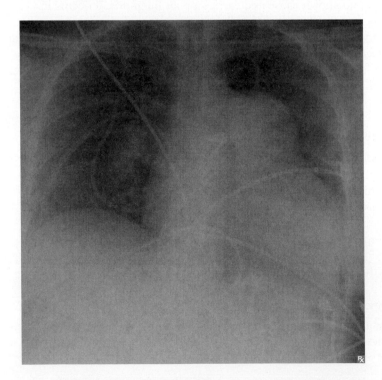

FIGURE 10-49. **Pulmonary arterial hypertension.** Chest x-ray shows characteristic radiologic features.

Sleep Apnea

Sleep apnea is characterized by repeated cessation of breathing for at least 10 seconds during sleep. Apneic episodes disrupt normal sleep cycles, preventing individuals from getting adequate rest. Thus, **daytime somnolence** is a hallmark presentation of sleep apnea.

Etiology of sleep apnea is classified as either obstructive or central. With **obstructive sleep apnea (OSA),** the airways collapse during sleep. This is due to excess weight of the chest wall pressing down on the airways (associated with obesity) and/or decreased vagal tone, which decreases smooth muscle tone and increases the tendency for the airways to collapse on themselves during sleep. **Central sleep apnea (CSA)** is characterized by a lack of respiratory drive during sleep (airways remain patent) and is associated with central nervous system (CNS) injury/toxicity and congestive heart failure.

PRESENTATION

- **OSA:** Daytime sleepiness (most common) or fatigue. Patients are **obese** adults with a history of excessive **snoring** (often reported by the patient's spouse or partner). OSA can also present in children with **tonsillar hypertrophy.**
- **CSA:** Daytime sleepiness and morning headaches. The patient's spouse or partner might report seeing the patient stop breathing during the night, sometimes in the context of **Cheyne-Stokes respirations** (see Key Fact). Look for a previous history of CNS injury.

DIAGNOSIS

- **Physical exam:** If OSA is suspected, look for obesity and/or enlarged tonsils. Physical exam is usually unremarkable in patients with CSA.
- **Polysomnography** (sleep study) is the **gold standard.**
- **Arterial blood gas:** Both OSA and CSA are associated with hypoxemia (decreased Pao_2) and hypercapnia (increased $Paco_2$) during sleep secondary to hypoventilation. If associated with obesity hypoventilation syndrome (see Key Fact), these patients will also have increased $Paco_2$ during the waking hours.
- **Chest radiography:** Right ventricular hypertrophy if sleep apnea is complicated by cor pulmonale.

TREATMENT

The mainstay of treatment for sleep apnea is positive airway pressure (PAP) during sleep.

- Continuous positive airway pressure (**CPAP**): Continuous delivery of positive pressure keeps the airways open in patients with **OSA.**
- Bi-level positive airway pressure (**BiPAP**): Provides a baseline CPAP but also provides additional positive airway pressure whenever the patient initiates a breath. This helps patients with **CSA** take full breaths during sleep. BiPAP can also be programmed to initiate breaths whenever patients fail do so on their own.

PROGNOSIS

If untreated, chronic hypoxemia causes vasoconstriction of pulmonary vessels, leading to pulmonary hypertension and **cor pulmonale.** This is prevented by using PAP during sleep, especially in the case of OSA.

RESPIRATORY TRACT CANCERS

Lung Cancer

Primary lung cancer is the second-most-common cancer by incidence, as well as the leading cause of cancer-related death in both males and females.

KEY FACT

Cheyne-Stokes respirations refer to a cyclic breathing pattern in which a period of apnea is followed by a gradual increase in tidal volume and respiratory rate, then a gradual decrease until the next apneic period. This occurs when damage to the respiratory center causes a delay between the brain stem's detection of changes in blood gas levels (afferent response) and the compensatory adjustments in respiration (efferent response).

KEY FACT

Obesity hypoventilation syndrome (OHS) is a clinical picture in which obese patients have decreased respiratory drive. This condition is characterized by obesity (BMI > 30) and hypercapnia ($Paco_2$ > 45) during the waking hours. Most patients with OHS also have coexisting OSA.

Cigarette smoking is clearly related to certain types of lung cancer. While quitting reduces subsequent risk of developing lung cancer, this risk likely never drops to that of a nonsmoker. Family history and occupational exposures, including arsenic, radon, haloethers, hydrocarbons, and agents associated with pneumoconioses (eg, asbestosis, silicosis), can predispose to lung cancer.

Lung cancer is broadly categorized as small cell or non–small cell subtypes. Non–small cell is further classified as adenocarcinoma, squamous cell carcinoma, large cell carcinoma, and bronchial carcinoid tumors. The five major types of primary lung cancer are discussed below.

Small Cell Lung Cancer

Small cell lung cancer (SCLC), previously known as oat cell carcinoma, is a neuroendocrine tumor arising from **Kulchitsky cells.** It typically arises centrally in the lung from bronchi and is strongly associated with smoking. Commonly associated with upregulation of **c-Kit** and amplification of the **L-myc (MYCL1)** oncogene (gain-of-function transcription factor mutation), SCLC is composed of undifferentiated cells and is very aggressive. A key feature of SCLC is that it is usually **surgically unresectable** due to lymph node invasion and/or distant metastasis at diagnosis. Treatment is therefore chemotherapy and/or radiation, but the prognosis and long-term survival after diagnosis are grim.

Histology shows **small round "blue" cells with sparse cytoplasm,** finely dispersed chromatin, and no distinct nucleoli (Figure 10-50A) that usually stain positive for **synaptophysin, neuron-specific enolase, and chromogranin A.**

SCLC is commonly associated with paraneoplastic syndromes such as Cushing syndrome, syndrome of inappropriate antidiuretic hormone secretion (SIADH), cerebellar ataxia, and **Lambert-Eaton myasthenic syndrome (LEMS).** LEMS is an autoimmune condition involving autoantibodies against presynaptic voltage-gated calcium channels. Inhibition of these channels prevents the release of neurotransmitters. It presents with **proximal muscle weakness** that improves with activity and signs of **autonomic dysfunction,** such as dry mouth and impotence.

Adenocarcinoma

Adenocarcinoma is the most common primary lung cancer (50% of cases) in the overall population, as well as in nonsmokers. It is more common in women than men. There is no clear relationship between adenocarcinoma and smoking. Adenocarcinoma arises from mucin glands located **peripherally** in the lung or old scar sites (usually due to infection or injury and found in a subpleural location). The clinical picture of **hypertrophic osteoarthropathy** is associated with adenocarcinoma of the lung and is characterized by digital clubbing and sudden-onset symmetrical arthropathy, usually involving the wrists and hands.

Adenocarcinoma is associated with activating mutations of *k-ras, EGFR,* and *ALK.* On histology, adenocarcinoma shows a **glandular pattern** that often stains positive for **mucin** (Figure 10-50B). Stains such as periodic acid-Schiff (PAS) or mucicarmine are required to demonstrate intracellular mucin.

Bronchioloalveolar adenocarcinoma (BAC) originally described a subtype of invasive adenocarcinoma of the lung characterized by well-differentiated cytology, peripheral location, and growth along intact alveolar walls ("lepidic" growth pattern). BAC has since been reclassified into new subgroups based on histology. BAC is discussed below; however, a detailed description of each subgroup is beyond the scope of this text.

BAC arises from Clara cells (nonciliated columnar epithelium) and grows along alveolar septa, giving the appearance of **thickened alveolar walls** on histology. Many cases of BAC are asymptomatic and detected after incidental imaging. The classic radiologic presentation of BAC is a solitary pulmonary nodule in the lung periphery, appearing as **ground glass** on chest computed tomography or **hazy infiltrates** on chest radiograph. More extensive disease may present with lobar consolidation, mimicking bacterial pneumonia. BAC rarely invades the basement membrane and has a good prognosis. BAC has been traditionally described as having no relationship to smoking. However, newer studies show a definite and direct relationship between smoking and BAC.

Squamous Cell Carcinoma

Squamous cell carcinoma develops **centrally** in the lung, arising from squamous epithelium of proximal large airways. It can be seen on chest radiographs as a hilar mass (sometimes with **cavitation**) arising from the bronchus (Figure 10-50C). Squamous cell carcinoma is strongly associated with smoking and more common in men than women. Classically, squamous cell carcinoma is associated with the paraneoplastic syndrome **hypercalcemia of malignancy** secondary to production of parathyroid hormone–related peptide (**PTHrP**). On histology, **keratin pearls** (Figure 10-50D) and **intercellular bridges** are characteristic. Staining for **desmoglein** is usually positive.

Large Cell Carcinoma

Large cell carcinoma (LCC) is a highly anaplastic undifferentiated tumor with a poor prognosis. LCC is associated with smoking and arises from epithelial cells, commonly in the lung **periphery,** though central tumors sometimes occur. No glandular or squamous differentiation is present in LCC. Thus, LCC is a diagnosis of exclusion and includes all non–small cell lung carcinomas (NSCLCs) that cannot be further classified. Unlike SCLC, it is less responsive to chemotherapy and is usually **surgically resected.** Histology shows **sheets of pleomorphic giant cells,** polygonal in shape with prominent nucleoli and pale-staining cytoplasm. In some cases, these cells can secrete β-hCG.

Bronchial Neuroendocrine (Carcinoid) Tumors

Bronchial neuroendocrine (carcinoid) tumors (NETs) are a group of lung neoplasms that arise from peptide- and amine-producing neuroendocrine cells. There is no clear association with smoking or genetic predisposition, with rare exceptions (eg, multiple endocrine neoplasia, type 1). Bronchial NETs can arise centrally or peripherally in the lung, and growth as a **bronchial polyp-like mass** is a classic description.

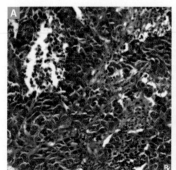
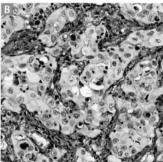
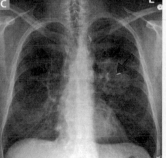
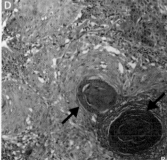

FIGURE 10-50. **Lung cancer.** A Small dark blue cells in small cell carcinoma. B Glandular pattern in adenocarcinoma. C Squamous cell carcinoma showing hilar mass on chest radiograph and D keratin pearls on histology.

Bronchial NETs are generally low-grade (well-differentiated) benign tumors with an excellent prognosis. Metastasis is rare. While most symptoms are due to mass effect (eg, dyspnea, wheezing), bronchial NETs may be associated with **carcinoid syndrome** (flushing, diarrhea, wheezing) secondary to ectopic serotonin (5-HT) production. Histology shows **nests of neuroendocrine cells** that, similarly to small cell carcinoma, stain positive for **synaptophysin, chromogranin A,** and **neuron-specific enolase.**

PRESENTATION

Patients with lung cancer generally present with nonspecific complaints, such as coughing, hemoptysis, dyspnea, and wheezing. As with all malignancies, weight loss and anorexia are common. Additionally, lung neoplasms can obstruct airways, causing distal infections (eg, lobar pneumonia). Based on the location and other characteristics (discussed below), lung cancer is also associated with certain clinical syndromes:

- **Superior vena cava (SVC) syndrome:** Tumor compression of the SVC obstructs venous drainage from the head/neck (sometimes causing facial plethora) and upper extremities. This leads to swelling, cyanosis, and venous distension in the aforementioned regions. Blanching can be appreciated in these regions (Figure 10-51A). Patients present with headaches and dizziness due to increased intracranial pressure. Commonly caused by Pancoast tumors (see below) and thrombosis from indwelling catheters (Figure 10-51B). This is a medical emergency, as patients are at increased risk of aneurysm formation/rupture within the intracranial arteries.
- **Pancoast tumor (superior sulcus tumor):** Carcinoma that arises in apex of the lung (Figure 10-51C). Can involve surrounding structures, causing a variety of syndromes (discussed below). These syndromes can coexist in a variety of combinations, collectively referred to as **Pancoast syndrome.**
  - SVC syndrome: Discussed above.
  - Horner syndrome: Ipsilateral ptosis, miosis, and anhydrosis. Due to invasion of cervical sympathetic chain.
  - Sensorimotor deficits: Due to compression of brachial plexus. A commonly tested presentation is Klumpke palsy ("claw hand"), secondary to lower trunk involvement.
  - Thoracic outlet syndrome: Use-dependent ischemic arm pain. Due to compression of subclavian vessels.
  - Hoarseness: From involvement of the recurrent laryngeal nerve (branch of the vagus nerve).
- **Paraneoplastic syndromes:** Includes hypercalcemia (squamous cell carcinoma), Cushing syndrome, SIADH, and Lambert-Eaton syndrome (small cell carcinoma).
- **Recurrent lobar pneumonia:** Due to persistent blockage (either internal obstruction of external compression) of a bronchus segment.
- **Effusions (pleural or pericardial):** Malignancy should always be considered in these cases.

In the event of metastasis, primary lung cancer most commonly spreads to the adrenals, brain, bone, and liver. In many cases, lung cancer is asymptomatic and incidentally detected as a solitary well-defined lung nodule ("coin lesion") on imaging.

Of note, metastasis to the lung (secondary lung cancer) is more common than primary lung cancer, as the lung's extensive vasculature renders it vulnerable to hematogenous seeding from distant sites. Multiple tumors on imaging should raise suspicion for metastatic disease. Metastasis to the lung is most commonly from primary breast cancer. Colon cancer, prostate cancer, and renal cell carcinoma are also frequent primary neoplasm sites.

MNEMONIC

SPHERE of complications (of lung cancer):
Superior vena cava syndrome
Pancoast tumor
Horner syndrome, **H**oarseness
Endocrine (paraneoplastic)
Recurrent pneumonia
Effusions (pleural or pericardial)

CLINICAL CORRELATION

The recurrent laryngeal nerve provides motor innervation to all of the laryngeal muscles except for the cricothyroid muscle.

KEY FACT

Bronchial hamartoma is the most common benign lung tumor. They contain islands of mature hyaline cartilage (hence the term, "hamartoma") and typically present as a well-defined coin lesion with **"popcorn" calcification** on chest x-ray. Of note, not all coin lesions are hamartomas.

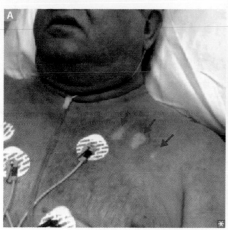
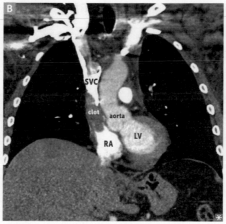
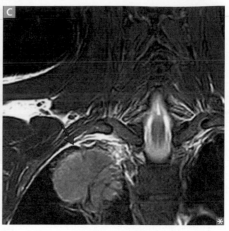

FIGURE 10-51. **Superior vena cava and Pancoast tumor.** **A** Blanching after fingertip pressure seen in superior vena cava (SVC) syndrome. **B** Coronal contrast-enhanced CT of chest showing low-density clot at junction of SVC and right atrium (RA). **C** Pancoast tumor: Chest MRI shows mass (arrow) at right lung apex. LV, left ventricle.

DIAGNOSIS

- **Chest film:** Nodule or mass within the lung.
  - **Centrally located:** Squamous and small cell.
  - **Peripherally located:** Adenocarcinoma and large cell. Involvement of the hilar lymph nodes or pleura can also be seen.
  - An exception to this is the bronchioloalveolar subtype of adenocarcinoma, which often has a more diffuse radiographic appearance, termed ground-glass opacity, similar to pneumonia.
- **CT or positron emission tomography (PET) scans:** To determine location, lymph node involvement, or metastasis for staging.
- **Cytologic examination** of sputum or washings from bronchoscopy, or tissue pathology from a **lung biopsy.**
- **PFT:** To assess whether a patient has the residual capacity to survive surgical resection of a tumor.
- **Pathology:** Multiple tumors arising at once should raise suspicion for metastatic disease from a primary tumor outside the lungs, as the lung's extensive vasculature makes it a nidus for hematogenous seeding.

TREATMENT

- **Small-cell carcinoma:** Metastases occur very early in the disease course, so surgery is not an option, only chemotherapy and/or radiation.
- **NSCLC:** Surgical resection if there is no distant spread. If metastases are present, then chemotherapy and/or radiation.

PROGNOSIS

Overall 5-year survival is about 14%. Squamous cell carcinoma has the best prognosis, and small-cell carcinoma has the worst. Early-stage disease, while rarely found, has a much better prognosis than late-stage disease.

Mesothelioma

Mesothelioma is a malignancy of the pleura, strongly associated with **asbestosis.** Classically presents with pleural thickening and **recurrent pleural effusions** (often hemorrhagic) on imaging. Electron microscopy is the gold standard for diagnosis and shows tumor cells with numerous **long, slender microvilli** and abundant tonofilaments. **Psammoma bodies** are seen on histology.

MNEMONIC

Squamous and **S**mall cell carcinomas are **S**entral (central) and strongly associated with **S**moking.

KEY FACT

Sites for metastasis of primary lung cancers (ranked by frequency):
1. Hilar lymph nodes
2. Adrenal glands
3. Liver
4. Brain
5. Bone (osteolytic)

KEY FACT

Asbestosis increases the risk for both mesothelioma and bronchogenic carcinoma. While this risk is amplified more in mesothelioma than in bronchogenic carcinoma, the latter is still more common in people with asbestos exposure.

QUESTION

A 40-year-old woman complains of progressive weakness in her right arm over 1 month. She has a 20 pack-year smoking history. Physical exam shows ptosis and miosis on the right side. What is the most likely cause?

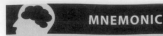
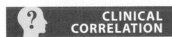

Malignancies of the Upper Respiratory Tract

Benign Laryngeal Tumors

The most common clinical presentation is hoarseness.

- **Vocal cord nodules:** Smooth hemispheric protrusions located on the true vocal cords. These occur chiefly in heavy smokers and singers.
- **Laryngeal papilloma:** A benign neoplasm on the true vocal cords that forms a soft, raspberry-like excrescence. Rarely more than 1 cm in diameter.
- **Juvenile laryngeal papillomas:** Usually singular in adults but multiple in children. Associated with human papillomavirus types 6 and 11.

Laryngeal Carcinoma

Accounts for 2% of all cancers. Presents in patients aged > 40 years, more often in men than in women. Associated with smoking, alcohol consumption, and asbestos exposure. Manifests as persistent hoarseness.

- **Glottic tumors:** On the true vocal cords, usually keratinizing.
- **Supraglottic tumors:** Above the vocal cords; one-third metastasize.
- **Subglottic tumors:** Below the vocal cords.

Nasopharyngeal Carcinoma

Strong link to Epstein-Barr virus (EBV) infection. EBV infects the host by replicating in the nasopharyngeal epithelium and then infecting nearby tonsillar B lymphocytes. High frequency in the Chinese population.

PULMONARY INFECTIONS

Pneumonia

Pneumonia is infection of the lung parenchyma. It is classified as either **community acquired** or **nosocomial** (hospital acquired). This distinction is important because individuals in the hospital setting undergo various interventions (eg, mechanical ventilation, urinary catheterization), which may predispose them to a different set of microorganisms than in the community. Specifically, *Pseudomonas aeruginosa* causes pneumonia almost exclusively in the healthcare setting.

Community-acquired pneumonia can be further classified according to presentation (typical or atypical) as well as the infiltration pattern seen on chest x-ray (lobar, patchy, or interstitial). These classifications are outlined in Figure 10-52 and elaborated on in the following discussions.

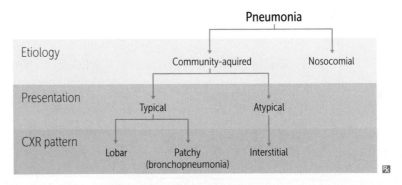

FIGURE 10-52. **Pneumonia classifications based on etiology, presentation, and pattern on chest x-ray (CXR).**

Aspiration pneumonia is another type of pneumonia that develops when oral flora (including anaerobes) are aspirated into the lung. Risk factors for developing aspiration pneumonia include decreased consciousness (eg, in the elderly and alcoholics, and in seizures) and neuromuscular diseases. Aspiration pneumonia can be acquired in the community or in a hospital setting.

The most common causes of pneumonia vary with the patient's age and are associated with specific risk factors. These organisms are listed in Tables 10-17 and 10-18, respectively.

PRESENTATION

- Community-acquired pneumonia:
  - **Typical pneumonia:** Acute onset of fever, dyspnea, and productive cough with purulent sputum. Sputum can also be blood-tinged or "rusty" in appearance due to rupture of pulmonary microvasculature. Pleuritic chest pain can also be present due to inflammation adjacent to the pleura. In some cases, elderly patients can present with epigastric pain rather than chest pain.
  - **Atypical pneumonia:** More indolent course and usually presents with dry cough.
- Nosocomial pneumonia and aspiration pneumonia have a similar presentation to typical pneumonia. Look for additional risk factors, such as an extended hospital stay or decreased consciousness.

DIAGNOSIS

- **Physical exam:**
  - Tachycardia, tachypnea, fever.
  - Crackles over the affected area on auscultation.
  - If affected airways are patent, **bronchial breath** sounds (louder, especially during exhalation) can be heard on auscultation. If the airways are completely blocked from consolidation, breath sounds will be decreased in affected areas.
  - **Dullness** to percussion, **increased fremitus,** and **egophony** suggest frank consolidation or associated effusion.
- **Chest x-ray:** Gold standard. Allows classification of pneumonia as lobar, patchy (bronchopneumonia), or interstitial (atypical).
  - **Lobar pneumonia:** Consolidation involves the entire lobe from intra-alveolar exudates. Can involve one or more lobes (Figure 10-53A,B). Most common organism is *Streptococcus pneumoniae.* Also *Legionella* and *Klebsiella.*
  - **Bronchopneumonia:** Patchy consolidation distributed around bronchioles and adjacent alveoli (Figure 10-53C). Often multifocal and bilateral (Figure 10-53D). Most common organisms are *S pneumoniae, Staphylococcus aureus, Haemophilus influenzae,* and *Klebsiella.*

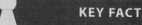

KEY FACT

Mycoplasma, Chlamydia, and *Legionella* are commonly referred to as atypical organisms because they cause atypical pneumonia and do not appear on Gram stain. Their special staining and culture requirements are as follows:
- **Mycoplasma**—Eaton agar
- **Chlamydia**—Giemsa stain
- **Legionella**—Charcoal yeast extract agar (buffered with cysteine and iron)

FLASH BACK

Fremitus refers to the vibrations transmitted through the body whenever the patient vocalizes. With increased fremitus, transmission of the patient's voice will be louder (vocal fremitus) and vibrations will be stronger (tactile fremitus) on lung auscultation and palpation, respectively.

FLASH BACK

Egophony refers to modified voice transmission through the body during lung auscultation. It is classically detected by having the patient produce and hold an "E" sound. In cases of egophony, transmission will be such that the examiner hears an "A" sound through the stethoscope.

TABLE 10-17. **Most Common Causes of Pneumonia by Age**

NEONATES (< 4 WK)	CHILDREN (4 WK–18 YR)	ADULTS (18–40 YR)	ADULTS (40–65 YR)	ELDERLY (> 65 YR)
Group B streptococci	Viruses (RSV)	*Mycoplasma*	*S pneumoniae*	*S pneumoniae*
Escherichia coli	*Mycoplasma*	*C pneumoniae*	*Haemophilus influenzae*	Influenza virus
	Chlamydia trachomatis (infants–3 yr)	*Streptococcus pneumoniae*	Anaerobes	Anaerobes
	Chlamydophila pneumoniae (school-aged children)		Viruses	*H influenzae*
	S pneumoniae		*Mycoplasma*	Gram-negative rods

TABLE 10-18.   Populations Predisposed to Pneumonia with Associated Organisms

POPULATION	ORGANISMS
Alcoholism, IV drug use	*Streptococcus pneumoniae, Klebsiella, Staphylococcus aureus*
Aspiration	Anaerobes (eg, *Peptostreptococcus, Fusobacterium, Prevotella, Bacteroides*)
Cystic fibrosis	*Pseudomonas, S aureus, S pneumoniae*
Immunocompromised	*S aureus,* enteric gram-negative rods, fungi, viruses, *Pneumocystis jirovecii* (with HIV)
Nosocomial	*S aureus, Pseudomonas, Escherichia coli,* other enteric gram-negative rods
Postviral	*S aureus, Haemophilus influenzae, S pneumoniae*

- **Interstitial (atypical) pneumonia:** Diffuse patchy inflammation localized to the interstitial areas at alveolar walls (Figure 10-53E). Sometimes very subtle on x-ray. Most common organisms are *Mycoplasma, Legionella, Chlamydia,* and viruses (influenza, respiratory syncytial virus [RSV], adenovirus).
- **Arterial blood gas testing:** Reduced Pao_2 with normal or reduced $Paco_2$ due to tachypnea.
- **Sputum Gram stain and culture:** Depends on the infecting organism. Of note, the organisms causing atypical pneumonia do not show up on Gram stain. Hence, they are commonly referred to as "atypical" organisms. The most common organisms associated with pneumonia, along with their distinguishing features and specific treatment options, are outlined in Tables 10-19 and 10-20.

TREATMENT

Antimicrobial therapy is the mainstay for bacterial and fungal pneumonia.

- Community-acquired pneumonia:
  - In general, patients without comorbidities (eg, diabetes, COPD, heart failure, renal failure, liver failure) should be treated with macrolides (eg, azithromycin, clarithromycin) or doxycycline.
  - The elderly and patients who have comorbidities or require hospitalization should be treated with a fluoroquinolone.
- Nosocomial pneumonia:
  - Treatment should be tailored toward gram-negative rods. This includes cephalosporins (specifically, ceftazidime or cefepime for *Pseudomonas* coverage), carbapenems, or piperacillin/tazobactam.
- Fungal infections:
  - If pneumonia is due to endemic mycoses, treat with itraconazole or fluconazole. Amphotericin B and newer generation -azoles are used in cases of disseminated infection.

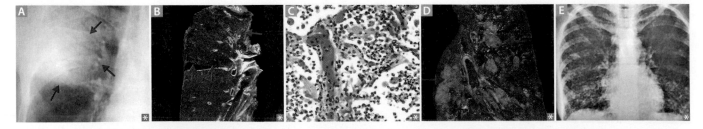

FIGURE 10-53.   Pneumonia. A Lobar pneumonia chest x-ray and B gross specimen. C Bronchopneumonia histology showing neutrophils in alveolar spaces and D gross specimen showing multifocal peribronchiolar involvement. E Interstitial pneumonia chest x-ray showing coarse bilateral reticular opacities, worse on the right.

TABLE 10-19. **Bacterial Causes of Pneumonia**

ORGANISM	CHARACTERISTICS	TREATMENT
Gram-Positive Bacteria		
Streptococcus pneumoniae	Gram-positive cocci (chains). Most common cause of community-acquired pneumonia.	Penicillins First- and second-generation cephalosporins Macrolides (if penicillin allergic) Quinolones
Staphylococcus aureus	Gram-positive cocci (clusters). Usually causes bronchopneumonia.	MSSA: First or second-generation cephalosporins Penicillinase-resistant penicillins MRSA: Vancomycin, ceftaroline, linezolid, tigecycline
Gram-Negative Bacteria		
Haemophilus influenzae	Gram-negative coccobacilli. Requires chocolate agar with hematin (factor X) and NAD+ (factor V) for culture.	Amoxicillin +/– clavulanate Second- or third-generation cephalosporins
Klebsiella pneumoniae	Gram-negative rod. Associated with aspiration pneumonia in diabetics, alcoholics, and IV drug users. Red "currant-jelly" sputum. Large mucoid colonies with abundant polysaccharide capsules.	Aminoglycosides First-, second-, or third-generation cephalosporins
Pseudomonas aeruginosa	Gram-negative rod. Non-lactose fermenting, oxidase (+). Produces pyocyanin (blue-green pigment) and has grape-like odor.	Extended-spectrum β-lactams Carbapenems Aztreonam Ciprofloxacin Aminoglycosides Colistin, polymyxin B (multidrug-resistant strains)
Legionella pneumophila	Gram-negative rod that stains poorly; requires silver stain. Grows on charcoal yeast extract culture with iron and cysteine. Aerosol transmission from environmental water sources (eg, air conditioning systems, hot water tanks, cruise ships). Labs show hyponatremia.	Macrolides Quinolones
Moraxella catarrhalis	Gram-negative diplococcus. Typically associated with otitis media (children) and COPD exacerbations (elderly), but can cause pneumonia in the latter population.	Second- or third-generation cephalosporins Macrolides Quinolones
Other Bacteria (eg, Anaerobes, Intracellular)		
Anaerobes	Part of normal oral flora. Associated with aspiration pneumonia.	Clindamycin
Mycoplasma pneumoniae	No cell wall. Not seen on Gram stain. Cultured on Eaton agar. Classic cause of atypical ("walking") pneumonia. Interstitial pattern on CXR looks worse than patient does. Outbreaks are frequently seen among military recruits and in prisons. Associated with cold-agglutinin (IgM) autoimmune hemolytic anemia.	Macrolides Doxycycline Fluoroquinolone
Chlamydia	Obligate intracellular organisms. Cell wall lacks muramic acid. Does not show up on Gram stain. Giemsa or fluorescent antibody-stained smear shows cytoplasmic inclusions. *C pneumoniae* and *C psittaci* cause atypical pneumonia.	Macrolides Doxycycline
Coxiella burnetii	Rickettsial organism. Obligate intracellular. Causes Q fever, which presents as pneumonia. Transmitted by spore inhalation from cattle/sheep amniotic fluid.	Doxycycline

COPD, chronic obstructive pulmonary disease; CXR, chest x-ray; MRSA, methicillin-resistant *S aureus;* MSSA, methicillin-sensitive *S aureus;* NAD+, oxidized nicotinamide adenine dinucleotide.

TABLE 10-20. Fungal and Viral Causes of Pneumonia

ORGANISM	CHARACTERISTICS	TREATMENT
Pneumocystis jirovecii (PCP)	Causes interstitial pneumonia in immunosuppressed patients (especially AIDS). Diagnosed by lung biopsy or lavage. Disc-shaped yeast seen with methenamine silver stain of lung tissue.	Treatment: TMP-SMX, pentamidine Prophylaxis: TMP-SMX, pentamidine, dapsone, atovaquone
Endemic mycoses	**Histoplasmosis:** Mississippi and Ohio River valleys. Found in bird/bat droppings. Macrophages filled with *Histoplasma*. **Blastomycosis:** States east of Mississippi River and Central America. Broad-based budding. **Coccidiomycosis:** Southwestern United States, California. Spherules filled with endospores. **Paracoccidioidomycosis:** Latin America. Budding yeast with "captain's wheel" formation.	Azoles Amphotericin B (for disseminated infections)
Cryptococcus neoformans	Opportunistic infection (classically HIV patients). Found in soil and pigeon droppings. Acquired through inhalation. Cryptococcosis presents like pneumonia. Can disseminate hematogenously to meninges, causing cryptococcal meningitis. Heavily encapsulated yeast. Culture on Sabouraud agar; stains with India ink and mucicarmine. Definitively diagnosed with latex agglutinin test (detects polysaccharide capsular antigen).	Cryptococcal meningitis: Amphotericin B + flucytosine Non-CNS cryptococcosis: Fluconazole
Viruses	Most commonly influenza virus, RSV, adenovirus. Causes atypical pneumonia.	Paracoccidioidomycosis

CNS, central nervous system; RSV, respiratory syncytial virus; TMP-SMX, trimethoprim-sulfamethoxazole.

- All HIV patients with a CD4+ count lower than 200 cells/mm³ should receive prophylaxis against *Pneumocystis jirovecii* (PCP). Therapy can include trimethoprim-sulfamethoxazole (TMP-SMX; most common, except with sulfa allergy), pentamidine, dapsone, or atovaquone. Existing PCP infections can be treated with TMP-SMX or pentamidine.
- Viral pneumonias are usually self-limited, requiring only supportive care, although the use of certain antiviral agents (eg, oseltamivir, zanamavir) has been shown to decrease the duration of influenza infections by approximately 24 hours.
- Refer to Table 10-19 and Table 10-20 for organism-specific treatments.

PROGNOSIS

In most cases, appropriate treatment results in complete recovery without long-term sequelae, but morbidity and mortality increase with age. Complications include:

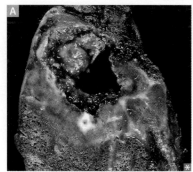

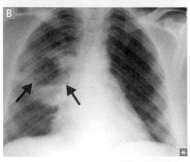

FIGURE 10-54. Lung abscess. **A** Gross specimen. **B** Cavitation with air-fluid levels (arrows) visible on x-ray of the chest.

- **Lung abscess:** Localized pus collection within the lung parenchyma (Figure 10-54A). Common complication of aspiration pneumonia or bronchial obstruction (eg, tumor). Infecting organisms include anaerobic oral flora (eg, *Bacteroides*, *Fusobacterium*, *Peptostreptococcus*) or *S aureus*. Patients typically present with symptoms of pneumonia unresponsive to antibiotics. Chest imaging shows cavitations with air-fluid levels, often in the right lung in the case of aspiration (Figure 10-54B). Treat with clindamycin.
- **Empyema:** Pus in the pleural space. Often caused by anaerobes and staphylococci. Requires drainage.

Tuberculosis

Approximately one-third of the world's population has been infected with TB, which results in 2–3 million deaths each year. The burden of disease is greatest in developing countries.

TB is primarily caused by *Mycobacterium tuberculosis*, an aerobic, rod-shaped, acid-fast bacterium (colloquially termed "red snappers" due to their appearance on Ziehl-Neelsen acid-fast stain), which is transmitted by airborne droplets from infected patients. The disease is so named because of the immune system's attempt to quarantine mycobacteria within dense granulomas ("tubercles") consisting of a core of macrophages surrounded by supporting T lymphocytes. There are three forms of TB: primary, secondary, and miliary.

- **Primary TB:** At initial infection, a **Ghon complex** develops, consisting of a peripheral parenchymal lesion called a **Ghon focus** and granulomas in involved hilar lymph nodes. The Ghon focus develops into a granuloma and eventually undergoes caseating necrosis at its core. Over time, the Ghon complex may calcify and heal into a **Ranke complex.**
- **Secondary (reactivation) TB:** Results from reactivation of a prior site of infection, where the bacteria became dormant but were never cleared. Lesions are localized to the lung apices (region of greatest aeration) with hilar lymph node involvement. Granulomatous lesions form and rupture, resulting in cavitary lesions. Scarring and calcification may be seen.
- **Miliary TB:** Disseminated disease caused by hematogenous spread of bacteria. It may follow from primary or secondary TB. The granuloma-filled lung takes the appearance of being filled with millet seeds, hence the name. Prognosis is very poor without treatment.

PRESENTATION

Pulmonary symptoms include chronic productive cough and hemoptysis. Respiratory function is generally well-preserved, perhaps because of localization of the destructive disease to the Ghon complex in primary TB and to the apices in secondary TB. Systemic symptoms include weight loss, fever, and night sweats.

DIAGNOSIS

- **Physical exam:**
  - **Primary TB:** Fever, chest pain. Often fairly normal physical exam.
  - **Secondary TB:** Cough (evolving into hemoptysis), weight loss, wasting, night sweats.
  - Crackles over the affected area on auscultation.
- **Tuberculin skin test (PPD or Mantoux test):** Acts through a type IV hypersensitivity reaction. A small amount of purified protein derivative (PPD) from *M tuberculosis* is injected subcutaneously. Induration at the site after 48–72 hours indicates prior exposure to TB. This does not differentiate between active and prior infections, and false-positives occur in individuals with prior vaccination with the variably effective BCG (bacillus Calmette-Guérin) vaccine. In contrast, the **interferon-gamma release assay** (IGRA; also known as **QuantiFERON GOLD**) is not affected by the BCG vaccine and can be used as an alternative to the PPD test in individuals who have received BCG vaccination.
- **Chest film:**
  - **Primary TB:** Nonspecific, often lower lobe infiltrate, hilar lymph node enlargement, and pleural effusion.
  - **Secondary TB:** Lesions located in the apices or superior segment of a lower lobe. Infiltrates, cavities, nodules, scarring, and/or contraction may be seen (Figure 10-55).
- Culture of the organism from sputum is needed for a definitive diagnosis. **Acid-fast staining** is useful for quicker results.

TREATMENT

Six months of treatment with isoniazid (INH), pyridoxine (vitamin B$_6$), and rifampin, supplemented during the first 2 months with pyrazinamide and ethambutol. A current global challenge is the rise of multidrug-resistant (MDR) and, more recently, extensively drug-resistant (XDR) tuberculosis. MDR-TB is resistant to at least rifampin and isonia-

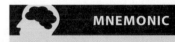

MNEMONIC

The **4 R's** of rifampin:
- **R**amps up cytochrome P450 metabolism
- Causes **R**ed or orange urine
- Leads to rapid **R**esistance when used alone
- Acts by inhibiting **R**NA polymerase

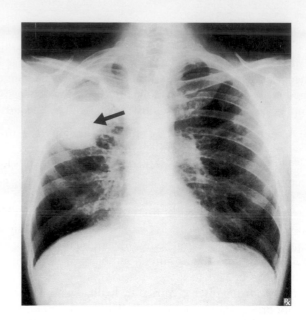

FIGURE 10-55. **Pulmonary tuberculosis.** Plain radiograph shows scarring with cavitation in the right upper lobe (arrow) and ill-defined infiltrates in the lower lobes.

zid; XDR-TB is additionally resistant to several second-line therapies. The treatment of drug-resistant TB depends heavily on culture sensitivities.

Latent tuberculosis infection (LTBI) treatment for individuals with a positive PPD but no active disease generally consists of 9 months of INH plus pyridoxine. Note that this is not an appropriate regimen for active TB.

PROGNOSIS

Most patients with primary TB are asymptomatic. Lifetime risk of reactivation is about 10% in immunocompetent patients. This is elevated in patients with AIDS or other immunosuppressive states. Reactivation TB can be complicated by miliary TB, in which distal organs are seeded with innumerable small lesions. Extrapulmonary TB includes tuberculous meningitis, Potts disease of the spine, psoas abscesses, paravertebral abscesses, tuberculous cervical lymphadenitis (scrofula), pericarditis, and kidney and GI involvement.

Upper Respiratory Tract Infections

Patients typically present with fever and sore throat. The age of the patient is also helpful in diagnosis. Physical exam may show a reddened oropharynx.

- **Pharyngitis:** Inflammation of the pharynx; manifests as a sore throat. Viral etiology is more likely than bacterial, but individuals with pharyngitis should be tested for *Streptococcus pyogenes* ("strep throat") because timely treatment with penicillin V is important for the prevention of serious sequelae such as rheumatic fever, although treatment does not prevent poststreptococcal (acute proliferative) glomerulonephritis.
- **Epiglottitis:** Syndrome of young children with an infection of the epiglottis (most frequently caused by *H influenzae*) causing pain and airway obstruction, often manifesting with uncontrollable drooling. The incidence of epiglottitis has fallen dramatically with the introduction of the *H influenzae* type b (Hib) vaccine.
- **Croup (laryngotracheobronchitis):** Croup is a common illness in children caused most often by the parainfluenza virus, influenza viruses, or respiratory syncytial virus (RSV). The typical presentation is a febrile child with barking cough, stridor, and hoarseness.

PLEURAL EFFUSION

Pleural effusion is excess fluid accumulation between the pleural layers (eg, parietal, visceral). Patients develop **dyspnea** as the accumulated fluid restricts inspiratory lung expansion. While there are several causes, workup begins with classifying the effusion as transudate, exudate, or lymphatic (discussed below).

Physical exam shows **dullness** to percussion over affected region (lung base if patient is sitting up). Chest imaging shows fluid within the chest cavity (Figure 10-56). **Thoracentesis** is both diagnostic and therapeutic. Of note, smaller effusions are often asymptomatic and self-resolving.

Transudate

Due to (1) **increased hydrostatic pressure** (ie, excess fluid backup) and/or (2) **decreased oncotic pressure** within the pulmonary vasculature. Because vascular permeability is usually unaffected, most proteins within the blood are too large to pass through the capillary membranes. Thus, transudate is **characterized by decreased protein content** within the accumulated fluid. Congestive heart failure (HF) is a common cause of increased hydrostatic pressure. Liver cirrhosis and nephrotic syndrome are common causes of decreased oncotic pressure.

Exudate

Due to **increased vascular permeability**, which is commonly associated with inflammatory processes (eg, pneumonia, malignancy), collagen vascular diseases, and trauma. Proteins are able to traverse the capillary membranes into the pleural cavity. Thus, an exudate is characterized by **increased protein content**, which may give the fluid a **cloudy** appearance.

Lymphatic

Also known as chylothorax. Leakage of lymphatic fluid (chyle) into the pleural space. Due to disruption of lymphatic flow through the thoracic duct, usually by trauma or malignancy. Lymphatic effusions are characterized by **increased triglycerides**, which gives the fluid a **milky** appearance.

PNEUMOTHORAX

Pneumothorax is the accumulation of air within the pleural space (Figure 10-57), which restricts inspiratory pulmonary expansion. Generally, pneumothoraces present with **dyspnea and unilateral chest pain.** Physical exam shows decreased or absent tactile fremitus, **hyperresonance,** and diminished breath sounds, all on the affected side. Classifications are described below.

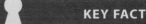

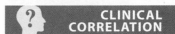

KEY FACT

Pleural effusion: Fluid accumulation in the pleural space.
Pulmonary edema: Fluid accumulation in the alveolar spaces.

CLINICAL CORRELATION

Thoracentesis is a procedure in which a needle or catheter is inserted through the chest wall to drain fluid within the pleural space.

KEY FACT

The thoracic duct is the largest lymphatic vessel in the body, draining lymph from the entire lower body as well as the left upper body (right upper body is drained by the right lymphatic duct). The thoracic duct ascends the posterior mediastinum and empties into the junction of the left subclavian and internal jugular veins.

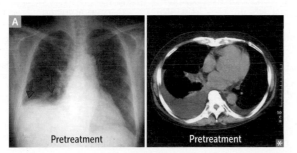
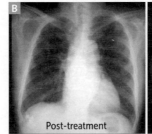
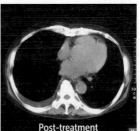

FIGURE 10-56. **Pleural effusion.** X-ray and CT findings A before and B after treatment.

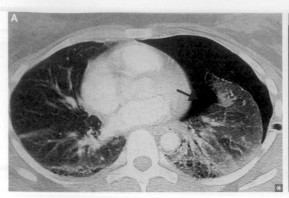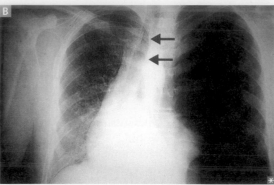

FIGURE 10-57. **Pneumothorax.** **A** CT showing collapsed left lung (arrow). **B** Chest x-ray showing left-sided tension pneumothorax; note the hyperlucent left lung field with low left hemidiaphragm (below the field of view) and rightward mediastinal/tracheal shift (arrows).

Primary Spontaneous Pneumothorax

Due to rupture of apical blebs or cysts within the lung (indicated by the term "spontaneous"). Patients typically have no known history of lung disease. Occurs most frequently in tall, thin, young males.

Secondary Spontaneous Pneumothorax

Also due to rupture of apical blebs or cysts. Develops secondary to lung disease (eg, bullae in emphysema, infections) or mechanical ventilation with excess pressures (causing barotrauma).

Traumatic Pneumothorax

Caused by blunt (eg, rib fracture) or penetrating (eg, gunshot) trauma.

Tension Pneumothorax

Can develop from any of the etiologies above. Air enters pleural space with each inspiration but cannot exit. The amount of air trapped in the pleural space increases rapidly, placing the patient at high risk for respiratory failure and circulatory shock. This is a medical emergency. High air pressure "pushes" the mediastinal contents to the contralateral side, and **contralateral tracheal deviation** is detectable on physical exam and CXR.

DIAGNOSIS

Physical examination findings for pneumothorax, as well as atelectasis, pleural effusion, and consolidation can be found in Table 10-21.

TABLE 10-21. **Lung Physical Exam Findings in Atelectasis, Pleural Effusion, Pneumothorax, and Consolidation**

ABNORMALITY	BREATH SOUNDS	PERCUSSION	FREMITUS	TRACHEAL DEVIATION
Atelectasis (bronchial obstruction)	↓	Dull	↓	Ipsilateral
Pleural effusion	↓	Dull	↓	Midline or contralateral (if large)
Simple pneumothorax[a]	↓	Hyperresonant	↓	Midline
Tension pneumothorax	↓	Hyperresonant	↓	Contralateral
Consolidation (lobar pneumonia, pulmonary edema)	Bronchial breath sounds; late inspiratory crackles	Dull	↑	Midline

[a]Simple pneumothorax = nonexpanding (in contrast to tension pneumothorax).

TREATMENT

- Supplemental oxygen to increase the rate of resorption of intrapleural air. In cases of a small asymptomatic pneumothorax, this may be sufficient for spontaneous recovery to occur.
- In larger and/or symptomatic pneumothoraces, air should be evacuated from the intrapleural space via **thoracentesis** (needle aspiration) or chest tube placement **(tube thoracostomy)** with a water seal, which acts as a one-way valve.
- In cases of recurrent pneumothorax, the pleurae may be sealed together through **pleurodesis,** in which chemical or mechanical irritation is employed in order to encourage fibrous scar tissue formation, sealing the visceral and parietal pleurae together. This effectively glues the lung to the chest wall.

ALLERGY

PRESENTATION

The term *allergy* is typically used to refer to type I hypersensitivity, mediated by IgE cross-linking after exposure to an allergen, leading to mast cell degranulation and histamine-mediated vascular permeability. Allergies manifest in a myriad of ways, but many of the symptoms affect the respiratory system, in particular, **allergic rhinitis** ("hay fever"—congestion, sneezing, itching), extrinsic **asthma,** and **anaphylaxis.** Anaphylaxis is the most severe allergy syndrome, characterized by multiorgan involvement including urticaria, edema, airway obstruction, low blood pressure, and GI symptoms. Any airway obstruction must be addressed immediately, usually through epinephrine administration.

DIAGNOSIS

The symptoms of allergies are classic and generally sufficient to establish a diagnosis. However, specific testing for allergen sensitivities may be instructive in certain cases; this is accomplished through either a **radioallergosorbent test (RAST)** of the blood for ingestion/inhalation allergies or a skin test for contact allergies.

TREATMENT

In many cases, the main "treatment" of allergies is allergen avoidance, especially in the case of hypersensitivities to foods, animals, or materials. If this is not possible, several drug classes may be used, which are listed below and discussed further in the Pharmacology section at the end of this chapter.

- H_1 **histamine blockers** (first and second generation) to treat inflammation.
- **α-Adrenergic agonists** (pseudoephedrine, phenylephrine, xylometazoline, oxymetazoline) for nasal decongestion.
- **Epinephrine** for anaphylactic shock.

Another method occasionally employed to treat allergies is **immunotherapy (desensitization),** in which successively escalating doses of allergen are injected with the goal of inducing tolerance. This is particularly useful for unpredictable and difficult-to-avoid allergens such as bee venom.

PROGNOSIS

Most cases of allergy are primarily a lifelong nuisance with seasonal or environmental variation. However, a severe allergic reaction may result in anaphylaxis, which has a poor prognosis unless immediately managed.

HYPERSENSITIVITY PNEUMONITIS

PRESENTATION

Results from inhalation of biological or chemical dust such as aerosolized mold or droppings, leading to a lymphocyte-mediated inflammatory response in the alveoli. Distinguished from asthma in that this is an alveolar disease rather than one of bronchi; additionally, unlike asthma and allergy, this is not a type I hypersensitivity reaction. Symptoms of acute disease include chest tightness, cough, wheezing, fever, and dyspnea, resolving hours after discontinuation of exposure. Symptoms of chronic disease include dyspnea, fatigue, cough, and weight loss.

DIAGNOSIS

- Probable diagnosis made with positive history of exposure, consistent CT scan (reticular, nodular, or ground glass opacities), bronchoalveolar lavage showing increased lymphocytes.
- Definitive diagnosis can be made with lung biopsy (findings include loosely organized granulomas) in conjunction with a consistent history.
- Differential diagnosis includes pneumoconiosis, IPF, COPD, and asthma.

TREATMENT

Avoid further exposure to offending agents. Glucocorticoids may help resolve symptoms.

PROGNOSIS

Usually complete or near complete recovery of lung function following cessation of antigen exposure.

Pharmacology

HISTAMINE BLOCKERS

First-Generation Histamine Blockers

DRUG NAMES

Diphenhydramine, dimenhydrinate, chlorpheniramine.

MECHANISM

Reversibly inhibit H_1 histamine receptors, which are involved in the inflammatory process. Major effects of H_1 receptor stimulation include:

- Increased nasal and bronchial mucus production
- Contraction of bronchioles
- Increased vascular permeability
- Pruritus
- Pain

USES

- **Allergies:** Due to anti-inflammatory effects (see above).
- **Motion sickness:** H_1 blockers also competitively inhibit muscarinic receptors, which contribute to the signs and symptoms associated with motion sickness.
- **Sleep aid:** H_1 blockers are lipophilic, which allows them to cross the blood-brain barrier (BBB) and act on the CNS.

KEY FACT

1st generation H_1 blocker names usually contain *-en/-ine* or *-en/-ate*.

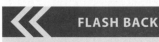

FLASH BACK

H_1 receptors mediate inflammation, whereas H_2 receptors mediate gastric acid secretion.

Side Effects

- **Sedation:** Due to CNS effects (see above).
- **Muscarinic antagonism:** Blurry vision, dry mouth, urinary retention. Can also cause confusion and hallucinations in the elderly.
- **α-Adrenergic antagonism:** Postural hypotension.

Second-Generation Histamine Blockers

Drug Names

Loratadine, fexofenadine, desloratadine, cetirizine.

Mechanism

- Reversibly inhibit H_1 receptors.
- Unlike first-generation H_1 blockers, second-generation H_1 blockers do not readily cross the BBB and are therefore far less sedating. They also do not act on muscarinic or α-adrenergic receptors.

Uses

Allergies.

Side Effects

Generally well tolerated.

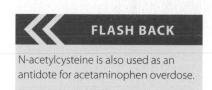

KEY FACT

Second-generation H_1 blocker names usually end in -adine.

MUCOACTIVE AGENTS

Subtypes, based on mechanism, include expectorants and mucolytics.

Drug Names

Guaifenesin, N-acetylcysteine, dornase alfa (DNAse).

Mechanism

- **Expectorants (guaifenesin):** Increase the volume of watery airway secretions. This serves to thin out respiratory secretions, making them easier to cough up.
- **Mucolytics:** Loosen mucus plugs. **N-acetylcysteine** acts by cleaving disulfide bonds within the mucus glycoproteins. **Dornase alfa (DNAse)** clears leukocytic debris through hydrolysis of DNA polymers.

Uses

- Increases clearance of respiratory secretions (eg, common cold, pneumonia, COPD).
- N-acetylcysteine and DNAse are used in cystic fibrosis (CF) patients.

Side Effects

Generally well tolerated.

FLASH BACK

N-acetylcysteine is also used as an antidote for acetaminophen overdose.

DEXTROMETHORPHAN

Mechanism

Synthetic codeine analog. Antagonizes N-methyl-D-aspartate (NMDA) glutamate receptors.

USES

Antitussive agent (suppresses cough).

SIDE EFFECTS

Mild opioid effects when used in excess (euphoria, respiratory depression, miosis, constipation). Has mild abuse potential. **Naloxone** can be given for overdose.

α-ADRENERGIC AGONISTS

DRUG NAMES

Pseudoephedrine, phenylephrine, xylometazoline, oxymetazoline.

MECHANISM

α-Adrenergic agonist.

USES

- Reduce hyperemia, edema, and nasal congestion.
- Pseudoephedrine is also illicitly used to make methamphetamine.

SIDE EFFECTS

- Hypertension.
- Pseudoephedrine can also cause CNS stimulation/anxiety.
- Rapid tolerance formation (**tachyphylaxis**).

PULMONARY HYPERTENSION DRUGS

DRUG NAMES

Bosentan, sildenafil, epoprostenol, iloprost.

MECHANISMS

- **Bosentan:** Competitively inhibits endothelin-1 receptors, thereby preventing pulmonary vasoconstriction and decreasing pulmonary vascular resistance.
- **Sildenafil:** Inhibits cGMP phosphodiesterase-5 (PDE-5), which normally breaks down nitric oxide. This prolongs the effects of nitric oxide, resulting in arterial vasodilation.
- **Epoprostenol, iloprost:** Prostacyclins (PGI_2). Have direct vasodilatory effects on pulmonary and systemic arterial vasculature. Also inhibit platelet aggregation.

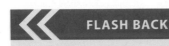

FLASH BACK

Sildenafil is also used to treat erectile dysfunction.

USES

Pulmonary hypertension.

SIDE EFFECTS

- **Bosentan:** Hepatotoxic (monitor LFTs).
- **Sildenafil:** Headaches, hypotension.
- **Epoprostenol, iloprost:** Flushing, jaw pain.

ASTHMA DRUGS

Bronchoconstriction in asthma is mediated by (1) inflammatory processes and (2) parasympathetic tone. Therapy is directed at these two pathways, outlined in Figure 10-58.

β₂-Agonists

DRUG NAMES

Albuterol, salmeterol, formoterol.

MECHANISM

Facilitate conversion of adenylate cyclase (AC) to cAMP (Figure 10-59B), which relaxes bronchial smooth muscle.

USES

- **Albuterol:** Short-acting agent used during acute exacerbations.
- **Salmeterol, formoterol:** Long-acting agents used for long-term therapy.

SIDE EFFECTS

Associated with tremors and arrhythmias.

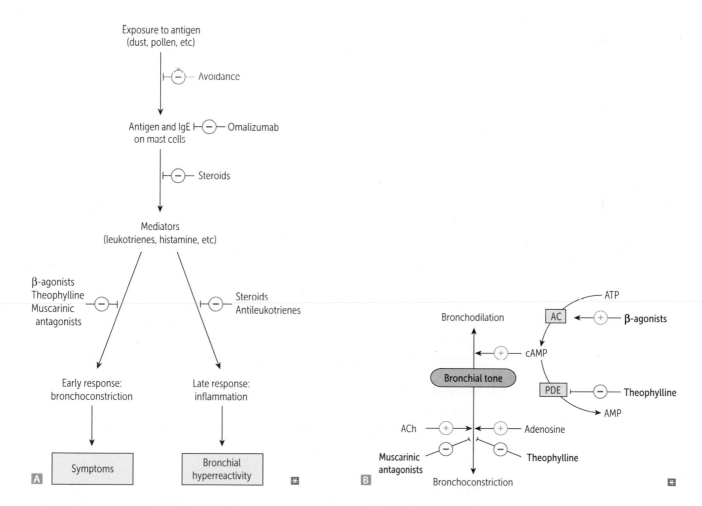

FIGURE 10-58. **Pharmacologic targets in asthma.** A Inflammatory pathway. B Parasympathetic pathway. AC, adenylyl cyclase; ACh, acetylcholine; PDE, phosphodiesterase.

Corticosteroids

DRUG NAMES

Beclomethasone, fluticasone, flunisolide.

MECHANISM

Inhibit the synthesis of virtually all cytokines. Inactivate NF-κB, which is the transcription factor that induces the production of TNF-α and other inflammatory agents.

USES

First-line therapy for **chronic asthma.**

SIDE EFFECTS

Oral candidiasis (thrush): Prevented by rinsing mouth following administration.

Muscarinic Antagonists

DRUG NAMES

Ipratropium, tiotropium.

MECHANISM

Competitively inhibit muscarinic receptors (M_3), preventing bronchoconstriction. Tiotropium is long acting.

USES

- COPD.
- Asthma.

Antileukotrienes

DRUG NAMES

Zileuton, montelukast, zafirlukast.

MECHANISM

- **Zileuton:** 5-lipoxygenase pathway inhibitor. Blocks the conversion of arachidonic acid to leukotrienes.
- **Montelukast, zafirlukast:** Competitively inhibit leukotriene receptors (CysLT1).

USES

- Considered when asthma is refractory to long-acting β_2-agonists and inhaled corticosteroids.
- Montelukast and zafirlukast are especially good for aspirin-induced asthma, in which bronchospasms result from increased leukotriene production.

SIDE EFFECTS

Zileuton is associated with hepatotoxicity.

Omalizumab

MECHANISM

Monoclonal anti-IgE antibody. Binds unbound serum IgE at the Fc region (FcεRI).

USES

Considered when asthma is refractory to long-acting β_2-agonists and inhaled corticosteroids.

SIDE EFFECTS

Generally well tolerated, but very expensive.

Methylxanthines

DRUG NAME

Theophylline.

MECHANISM

- Inhibits phosphodiesterase, which normally hydrolyzes cAMP (Figure 10-59B). This increases cAMP levels, resulting in bronchodilation.
- Also blocks the actions of adenosine (Figure 10-59B), thereby preventing bronchoconstriction.

USES

Has limited usage due to narrow therapeutic index.

SIDE EFFECTS

- Neurotoxicity (eg, seizures).
- Cardiotoxicity (eg, tachycardia, arrhythmias).
- Metabolized by cytochrome P-450.

Magnesium Sulfate

MECHANISM

Inhibits calcium influx into airway smooth muscle cells, thereby decreasing airway tone.

USES

Shown to be helpful, specifically in severe asthma exacerbations.

Methacholine

MECHANISM

Muscarinic receptor (M_3) agonist. Causes bronchoconstriction.

USES

Used in bronchial provocation to help diagnose asthma. Of note, the methacholine challenge test has high sensitivity but low specificity. Therefore, it is useful for ruling out asthma, but a positive result is not diagnostic.

NOTES

Image Acknowledgments

In this edition, in collaboration with MedIQ Learning, LLC, and a variety of other partners, we are pleased to include the following clinical images and diagrams for the benefit of integrative student learning.

Rx Portions of this book identified with the symbol Rx are copyright © USMLE-Rx.com (MedIQ Learning, LLC).

RU Portions of this book identified with the symbol RU are copyright © Dr. Richard Usatine and are provided under license through MedIQ Learning, LLC.

✳ Portions of this book identified with the symbol ✳ are listed below by Figure number.

This symbol ⊚ refers to material that is available in the public domain.

This symbol ⊚ refers to the Creative Commons Attribution license, full text at: http://creativecommons.org/licenses/by/4.0/legalcode.

This symbol ⊚ refers to the Creative Commons Attribution-Share Alike license, full text at: http://creativecommons.org/licenses/by-sa/4.0/legalcode.

Cardiovascular

Figure 1-5 **Tetralogy of Fallot: Image B. X-ray showing boot-shaped heart.** This image is a derivative work, adapted from the following source, available under ⊚: Rashid AKM: Heart diseases in Down syndrome. In: Dey S, ed: *Down syndrome*. doi 10.5772/46009. The image may have been modified by cropping, labeling, and/or captions. All rights to this adaptation by MedIQ Learning, LLC are reserved.

Figure 1-10 **Anatomic relationships of the heart: Image A. Axial CT of the heart.** This image is a derivative work, adapted from the following source, available under ⊚: Reproduced with permission from Guimarães MD, Almeida MFA, Brelinger A, et al. Diffuse bronchiolitis pattern on a computed tomography scan as a presentation of pulmonary tumor thrombotic microangiopathy: a case report. *J Med Case Rep.* 2011;5:575. doi:10.1186/1752-1947-5-575. The image may have been modified by cropping, labeling, and/or captions. All rights to this adaptation by MedIQ Learning, LLC are reserved.

Figure 1-14 **ECG finding in myocardial infarction.** This image is a derivative work, adapted from the following source, available under ⊚: Gan F, Hu D, Dai T. Acute multivessel coronary artery occlusion: a case report. *BMC Res Notes.* 2012;5:523. doi:10.1186/1756-0500-5-523.

Figure 1-17 **Fast response and slow response cardiac action potentials.** Reproduced, with permission, from Le T, et al. *First Aid for the USMLE Step 1.* New York, NY: McGraw-Hill Education, 2016.

Figure 1-24 **Frank-Starling curve.** Reproduced, with permission, from Le T, et al. *First Aid for the USMLE Step 1.* New York, NY: McGraw-Hill Education, 2016.

Figure 1-35 **Control of mean arterial pressure.** Reproduced, with permission, from Le T, et al. *First Aid for the USMLE Step 1.* New York, NY: McGraw-Hill Education, 2006.

Figure 1-37 **Waveforms.** Reproduced, with permission, from Le T, et al. *First Aid for the USMLE Step 1.* New York, NY: McGraw-Hill Education, 2015.

Figure 1-47 **Fibromuscular dysplasia.** This image is a derivative work, adapted from the following source, available under ⊚: Plouin PF, Perdu J, LaBatide-Alanore A, et al. Fibromuscular dysplasia. *Orphanet J Rare Dis.* 2007;7:28. doi 10.1186/1750-1172-2-28. The image may have been modified by cropping, labeling, and/or captions. All rights to this adaptation by MedIQ Learning, LLC are reserved.

Figure 1-48 **Features of arteriosclerosis: Image A. Hyaline arteriolosclerosis.** This image is a derivative work, adapted from the following source, available under ⊚. Courtesy of Dr. Michael Bonert. The image may have been modified by cropping, labeling, and/or captions. MedIQ Learning, LLC makes this image available under ⊚.

Figure 1-48 **Features of arteriosclerosis: Image B. Segmental glomerulosclerosis.** This image is a derivative work, adapted from the following source, available under ⊚: Tsuji K, Uchida HA, Ono T, et al. A case of focal segmental glomerulosclerosis in an adult patient with hypogammaglobulinemia superimposed on membranoproliferative glomerulonephritis in childhood. *BMC Nephrology.* 2012;13:46. doi:10.1186/1471-2369-13-46. The image may have been modified by cropping, labeling, and/or captions. All rights to this adaptation by MedIQ Learning, LLC are reserved.

Figure 1-48 **Features of arteriosclerosis: Image C. Mönckeberg arteriosclerosis.** This image is a derivative work, adapted from the following source, available under ⊚: Couri CEB, da Silva GA, Martinez JAB, Pereira F de A, de Paula FJA. Mönckeberg's sclerosis – is the artery the only target of calcification? *BMC Cardiovasc Disord.* 2005;5:34. doi:10.1186/1471-2261-5-34. The image may have been modified by cropping, labeling, and/or captions. All rights to this adaptation by MedIQ Learning, LLC are reserved.

Figure 1-51 **Classic signs of endocarditis: Image A. Janeway lesions.** This image is a derivative work, adapted from the following source, available under ⊚: Courtesy of DeNonneko.

Figure 1-51 **Classic signs of endocarditis: Image C. Osler nodes.** This image is a derivative work, adapted from the following source, available under [cc]: Yang M-L, Chen Y-H, Chen T-C, Lin W-R, et al. Case report: Infective endocarditis caused by Brevundimonas vesicularis. *BMC Infect Dis.* 2006;6:179. doi:10.1186/1471-2334-6-179. The image may have been modified by cropping, labeling, and/or captions. All rights to this adaptation by MedIQ Learning, LLC are reserved.

Figure 1-52 **Aschoff body in fibrous tissue next to myocardial vessel.** Courtesy of Dr. Daniel Wasdahl.

Figure 1-53 **Cardiomyopathies: Image A. Dilated cardiomyopathy.** This image is a derivative work, adapted from the following source, available under [cc]: Gho JMIH, van Es R, Stathonikos N, et al. High resolution systematic digital histological quantification of cardiac fibrosis and adipose tissue in phospholamban p.Arg14del mutation associated cardiomyopathy. *PLoS One.* 2014;9:e94820. doi 10.1371/journal.pone.0094820. The image may have been modified by cropping, labeling, and/or captions. All rights to this adaptation by MedIQ Learning, LLC are reserved.

Figure 1-53 **Cardiomyopathies: Image B. Hypertrophic cardiomyopathy.** Reproduced, with permission, from Le T, et al. *First Aid for the USMLE Step 1.* New York, NY: McGraw-Hill Education, 2016.

Figure 1-56 **Pitting edema.** This image is a derivative work, adapted from the following source, available under [cc]: Ong HS, Sze CW-C, Koh TW, et al. How 40 kilograms of fluid retention can be overlooked: two case reports. *Cases J.* 2009;2:33. doi:10.1186/1757-1626-2-33. The image may have been modified by cropping, labeling, and/or captions. All rights to this adaptation by MedIQ Learning, LLC are reserved.

Figure 1-59 **Aortic dissection: Image A.** This image is a derivative work, adapted from the following source, available under [cc]: Apostolakis EE, Baikoussis NG, Katsanos K, et al. Postoperative peri-axillary seroma following axillary artery cannulation for surgical treatment of acute type A aortic dissection: case report. *J Cardiothor Surg.* 2010;5:43. doi 0.1186/1749-8090-5-43. The image may have been modified by cropping, labeling, and/or captions. All rights to this adaptation by MedIQ Learning, LLC are reserved.

Figure 1-59 **Aortic dissection: Image B.** This image is a derivative work, adapted from the following source, available under [cc]: Apostolakis EE, Baikoussis NG, Katsanos K, et al. Postoperative peri-axillary seroma following axillary artery cannulation for surgical treatment of acute type A aortic dissection: case report. *J Cardiothor Surg.* 2010;5:43. doi 0.1186/1749-8090-5-43. The image may have been modified by cropping, labeling, and/or captions. All rights to this adaptation by MedIQ Learning, LLC are reserved.

Figure 1-69 **Cardiac myxoma.** This image is a derivative work, adapted from the following source, available under [cc]: Manduz S, Katrancioglu N, Karahan O, et al. Diagnosis and follow up of patients with primary cardiac tumours: a single-centre experience of myxomas. *Cardiovasc J Afr.* 2011;22(6):310-312. doi:10.5830/CVJA-2010-073. The image may have been modified by cropping, labeling, and/or captions. All rights to this adaptation by MedIQ Learning, LLC are reserved.

Figure 1-70 **Superior vena cava syndrome.** This image is a derivative work, adapted from the following source, available under [cc]: Courtesy of Dr. Herbert L. Fred and Hendrik A. van Dijk. Images of Memorable Cases: Case 11. OpenStax College Website. http://cnx.org/contents/rw1ZTFqr@3/Images-of-Memorable-Cases-Case. Accessed February 24, 2016.

Figure 1-71 **Pulmonary thromboembolism.** This image is a derivative work, adapted from the following source, available under [cc]: Kalava A, Kalstein A, Koyfman S, et al. Pulseless electrical activity during electroconvulsive therapy: a case report. *BMC Anesthesiol.* 2012;12:8. doi:10.1186/1471-2253-12-8. The image may have been modified by cropping, labeling, and/or captions. All rights to this adaptation by MedIQ Learning, LLC are reserved.

Figure 1-72 **ECG findings in acute pericarditis.** This image is a derivative work, adapted from the following source, available under [cc]: Omar HR, Fathy A, Rashad R, et al. Acute perimyocarditis mimicking transmural myocardial infarction. *Int Arch Med.* 2009;2:37. doi:10.1186/1755-7682-2-37.

Figure 1-73 **ECG finding in ST elevation myocardial infarction.** This image is a derivative work, adapted from the following source, available under [cc]: Gomes R, Andrade MJ, Santos M, et al. "Mushroom cloud": a giant left ventricular pseudoaneurysm after a myocardial infarction due to myocardial bridging – a case report. *Cardiovasc Ultrasound.* 2009;7:36. doi:10.1186/1476-7120-7-36.

Figure 1-75 **Cardiomegaly.** This image is a derivative work, adapted from the following source, available under [cc]: Haghighi A, Haack TB, Atiq M, et al. Sengers syndrome: six novel AGK mutations in seven new families and review of the phenotypic and mutational spectrum of 29 patients. *Orphanet J Rare Dis.* 2014;9:119. doi:10.1186/s13023-014-0119-3. The image may have been modified by cropping, labeling, and/or captions. All rights to this adaptation by MedIQ Learning, LLC are reserved.

Figure 1-76 **Pulmonary edema.** This image is a derivative work, adapted from the following source, available under [cc]: Hammon M, Dankerl P, Voit-Höhne HL, et al. Improving diagnostic accuracy in assessing pulmonary edema on bedside chest radiographs using a standardized scoring approach. *BMC Anesthesiol.* 2014;14:94. doi:10.1186/1471-2253-14-94. The image may have been modified by cropping, labeling, and/or captions. All rights to this adaptation by MedIQ Learning, LLC are reserved.

Figure 1-79 **Ion physiology at the distal convoluted tubule.** Reproduced, with permission, from Le T, et al. *First Aid for the USMLE Step 1.* New York, NY: McGraw-Hill Education, 2017.

Figure 1-80 **Ion physiology at the loop of Henle.** Reproduced, with permission, from Le T, et al. *First Aid for the USMLE Step 1.* New York, NY: McGraw-Hill Education, 2017.

Figure 1-81 **Ion physiology at the collecting tubule and collecting duct.** Reproduced, with permission, from Le T, et al. *First Aid for the USMLE Step 1.* New York, NY: McGraw-Hill Education, 2017.

Figure 1-82 **Ion physiology at the proximal convoluted tubule.** Reproduced, with permission, from Le T, et al. *First Aid for the USMLE Step 1.* New York, NY: McGraw-Hill Education, 2017.

Endocrine

Figure 2-3 **Pituitary gland: Image B. MRI showing pituitary microadenoma.** This image is a derivative work, adapted from the following source, available under ⓒ⊚: Faizah M, Zuhanis A, Rahmah R, et al. Precocious puberty in children: a review of imaging findings. *Biomed Imaging and Interv J.* 2012;8(1):e6. doi:10.2349/biij.8.1.e6. The image may have been modified by cropping, labeling, and/or captions. All rights to this adaptation by MedIQ Learning, LLC are reserved.

Figure 2-11 **Thyroglossal duct.** Reproduced, with permission, from Le T, et al. *First Aid for the USMLE Step 1.* New York, NY: McGraw-Hill Education, 2017.

Figure 2-12 **Thyroid follicular cells.** This image is a derivative work, adapted from the following source, available under ⓒ⊚: Terada T. Brain metastasis from thyroid adenomatous nodules or an encapsulated thyroid follicular tumor without capsular and vascular invasion: a case report. *Cases J.* 2009;2:7180. doi:10.4076/1757-1626-2-7180. The image may have been modified by cropping, labeling, and/or captions. All rights to this adaptation by MedIQ Learning, LLC are reserved.

Figure 2-24 **Osteitis fibrosis cystica.** This image is a derivative work, adapted from the following source, available under ⓒ⊚: Khaoula BA, Kaouther BA, Ines C, et al. An unusual presentation of primary hyperparathyroidism: pathological fracture. *Case Rep Orthop.* 2011;2011:521578. doi 10.1155/2011/521578. The image may have been modified by cropping, labeling, and/or captions. All rights to this adaptation by MedIQ Learning, LLC are reserved.

Figure 2-33 **Islets of Langerhans.** Reproduced, with permission, from Le T, et al. *First Aid for the USMLE Step 1.* New York, NY: McGraw-Hill Education, 2016.

Figure 2-35 **Diabetic retinopathy.** This image is a derivative work, adapted from the following source, available under ⓒ⊚: Stefanini FR, Badaro E, Falabella P, et al. Anti-VEGF for the management of diabetic macular edema. *J Immunol Res.* 2014;2014:632307. doi 10.1155/2014/632307. The image may have been modified by cropping, labeling, and/or captions. All rights to this adaptation by MedIQ Learning, LLC are reserved.

Table 2-15 **Types of thyroid cancer: Image A. Papillary carcinoma.** Courtesy of Dr. Kristine Krafts.

Gastrointestinal

Figure 3-3 **Omphalocele and gastroschisis: Image B. Gastroschisis.** This image is a derivative work, adapted from the following source, available under ⓒ⊚: Mirza B, Sheikh A. An Unusual Case of Gastroschisis. *APSP J Case Rep.* 2010;1(1):2.

Figure 3-6 **Double bubble sign.** Courtesy Dr. Evelyn Anthony.

Figure 3-7 **Pancreas divisum.** Modified, with permission, from Le T, et al. *First Aid for the USMLEx Step 1.* New York: McGraw-Hill, 2010, page 133.

Figure 3-24 **Acid secretion by parietal cells.** Reproduced, with permission, from Le T, et al. *First Aid for the USMLE Step 1.* New York, NY: McGraw-Hill Education, 2015.

Figure 3-27 **Detailed structure of the liver lobule.** Reproduced, with permission, from Le T, et al. *First Aid for the USMLE Step 1.* New York, NY: McGraw-Hill Education, 2016.

Figure 3-31 **Oral candidiasis.** ⓒ⊚ Courtesy of the US Department of Health and Human Services and Dr. Sol Silverman, Jr. The image may have been modified by cropping, labeling, and/or captions. All rights to this adaptation by MedIQ Learning, LLC are reserved.

Figure 3-34 **Large pharyngoesophageal diverticulum: Image A. Barium swallow showing two esophageal diverticula.** This image is a derivative work, adapted from the following source, available under ⓒ⊚: Elbalal M, Mohamed AB, Hamdoun A, Yassin K, et al. Zenker's diverticulum: a case report and literature review. *Pan Afr Med J.* 2014;17:267. doi:10.11604/pamj.2014.17.267.4173. The image may have been modified by cropping, labeling, and/or captions. All rights to this adaptation by MedIQ Learning, LLC are reserved.

Figure 3-34 **Large pharyngoesophageal diverticulum: Image B. Compression of esophagus.** This image is a derivative work, adapted from the following source, available under ⓒ⊚: Elbalal M, Mohamed AB, Hamdoun A, Yassin K, et al. Zenker's diverticulum: a case report and literature review. *Pan Afr Med J.* 2014;17:267. doi:10.11604/pamj.2014.17.267.4173.

Figure 3-35 **Bird-beak esophagus typical of achalasia.** This image is a derivative work, adapted from the following source, available under ⓒ⊚: Patel DA, Kim HP, Zifodya JS, Vaezi MF. Idiopathic (primary) achalasia: a review. *Orphanet J Rare Dis.* 2015;10:89. doi:10.1186/s13023-015-0302-1. The image may have been modified by cropping, labeling, and/or captions. All rights to this adaptation by MedIQ Learning, LLC are reserved.

Figure 3-38 **Changes seen with Barrett esophagus.** Reproduced, with permission, from Le T, et al. *First Aid for the USMLE Step 1.* New York, NY: McGraw-Hill Education, 2016.

Figure 3-66 **Hepatocellular carcinoma.** This image is a derivative work, adapted from the following source, available under [cc]: Dahm HH. Immunohistochemical evaluation of a sarcomatoid hepatocellular carcinoma with osteoclastlike giant cells. *Diagn Pathol.* 2015;10:40. doi:10.1186/s13000-015-0274-4.

Figure 3-67 **Methods of bile duct imaging: Image A. ERCP.** This image is a derivative work, adapted from the following source, available under [cc]: Helmy AA, Hamad MA, Aly AM, et al. Novel technique for biliary reconstruction using an isolated gastric tube with a vascularized pedicle: a live animal experimental study and the first clinical case. *Ann Surg Innov Res.* 2011;5:8. doi:10.1186/1750-1164-5-8. The image may have been modified by cropping, labeling, and/or captions. All rights to this adaptation by MedIQ Learning, LLC are reserved.

Figure 3-67 **Methods of bile duct imaging: Images B, C. MRCP datasets.** This image is a derivative work, adapted from the following source, available under [cc]: Ringe KI, Hartung D, von Falck C, Wacker F, et al. 3D-MRCP for evaluation of intra- and extrahepatic bile ducts: comparison of different acquisition and reconstruction planes. *BMC Med Imaging.* 2014;14:16. doi:10.1186/1471-2342-14-16. The image may have been modified by cropping, labeling, and/or captions. All rights to this adaptation by MedIQ Learning, LLC are reserved.

Figure 3-67 **Methods of bile duct imaging: Image D. Helical CT.** This image is a derivative work, adapted from the following source, available under [cc]: Chatzoulis G, Kaltsas A, Danilidis L, Dimitriou J, et al. Mirizzi syndrome type IV associated with cholecystocolic fistula: a very rare condition: report of a case. *BMC Surg.* 2007;7:6. doi:10.1186/1471-2482-7-6. The image may have been modified by cropping, labeling, and/or captions. All rights to this adaptation by MedIQ Learning, LLC are reserved.

Figure 3-70 **Chronic pancreatitis and pancreatic calculi.** This image is a derivative work, adapted from the following source, available under [cc]: Ahmed Ali U, Issa Y, Bruno MJ, et al. Early surgery versus optimal current step-up practice for chronic pancreatitis (ESCAPE): design and rationale of a randomized trial. *BMC Gastroenterol.* 2013;13:49. doi:10.1186/1471-230X-13-49. The image may have been modified by cropping, labeling, and/or captions. All rights to this adaptation by MedIQ Learning, LLC are reserved.

Figure 3-71 **Pancreatic cancer.** This image is a derivative work, adapted from the following source, available under [cc]: Ji J-S, Han C-W, Jang J-W, et al. Helical tomotherapy with concurrent capecitabine for the treatment of inoperable pancreatic cancer. *Radiat Oncol.* 2010;5:60. doi:10.1186/1748-717X-5-60. The image may have been modified by cropping, labeling, and/or captions. All rights to this adaptation by MedIQ Learning, LLC are reserved.

Hematology and Oncology

Figure 4-4 **Normal blood cells and stomatocytes: Image A.** This image is a derivative work, adapted from the following source, available under [cc]: Antwi-Baffour S, Asare RO, Adjei JK, Kyeremeh R, et al. Prevalence of hemoglobin S trait among blood donors: a cross-sectional study. *BMC Res Notes.* 2015;8:583. doi:10.1186/s13104-015-1583-0. The image may have been modified by cropping, labeling, and/or captions. All rights to this adaptation by MedIQ Learning, LLC are reserved.

Figure 4-4 **Supravital stain showing increased reticulocytes: Image B.** This image is a derivative work, adapted from the following source, available under [cc]: Huq S, Pietroni MAC, Rahman H, Alam MT. Hereditary Spherocytosis. *J Health Popul Nutr.* 2010;28(1):107-109. The image may have been modified by cropping, labeling, and/or captions. All rights to this adaptation by MedIQ Learning, LLC are reserved.

Figure 4-5 **Active macrophage.** [cc] Courtesy of the US Department of Health and Human Services and Dr. D.T. McClenan. The image may have been modified by cropping, labeling, and/or captions. All rights to this adaptation by MedIQ Learning, LLC are reserved.

Figure 4-6 **Categorization of anemias.** Reproduced, with permission, from Le T, et al. *First Aid for the USMLE Step 1.* New York, NY: McGraw Hill Education, 2016.

Figure 4-7 **Iron deficiency anemia: Image B. Microcytosis and hypochromia in anemia.** Reproduced, with permission, from Le T, et al. *First Aid for the USMLE Step 1.* New York, NY: McGraw-Hill Education, 2016.

Figure 4-8 **β-thalassemia major.** Courtesy of Dr. Kristine Krafts.

Figure 4-9 **Lead lines on metaphyses of long bone.** Reproduced, with permission, from Dr. Frank Gaillard and www.radiopaedia.org.

Figure 4-10 **Refractory anemia with ring sideroblasts.** [cc] Courtesy of the International Agency for Research on Cancer of the World Health Organization. The image may have been modified by cropping, labeling, and/or captions. All rights to this adaptation by MedIQ Learning, LLC are reserved.

Figure 4-12 **Hypersegmented neutrophil.** Courtesy of Dr. Kristine Krafts.

Figure 4-16 **Raynaud phenomenon.** This image is a derivative work, adapted from the following source, available under [cc]: Courtesy of Michelle Tribe. The image may have been modified by cropping, labeling, and/or captions. All rights to this adaptation by MedIQ Learning, LLC are reserved.

Figure 4-19 **Splenic infarction.** This image is a derivative work, adapted from the following source, available under [cc]: Courtesy of Mike Haggar.

Figure 4-20 **Schistocytes.** [cc] Courtesy of Professor Osaro Erhabor. The image may have been modified by cropping, labeling, and/or captions. All rights to this adaptation by MedIQ Learning, LLC are reserved.

Figure 4-25   **Petechiae on lower extremity.** This image is a derivative work, adapted from the following source, available under ⓒ⓪⌗: Cheungpasitporn W, Jirajariyavej T, Howarth CB, Rosen RM. Henoch-Schönlein purpura in an older man presenting as rectal bleeding and IgA mesangioproliferative glomerulonephritis: a case report. *J Med Case Reports.* 2011;5:364. doi:10.1186/1752-1947-5-364.

Figure 4-26   **Lymph node: Image A. Normal lymph node.** This image is a derivative work, adapted from the following source, available under ⓒ⓪⌗: Courtesy of Dr. Ed Uthman.

Figure 4-26   **Lymph node: Image B. Reactive lymph node.** This image is a derivative work, adapted from the following source, available under ⓒ⓪⌗: Vlachos K, Archontovasilis F, Falidas E, Mathioulakis S, et al. Sclerosing Mesenteritis: Diverse clinical presentations and dissimilar treatment options. A case series and review of the literature. *Int Arch Med.* 2011;4:17. doi:10.1186/1755-7682-4-17.

Figure 4-27   **Reed-Sternberg cells.** ⓒ⓪⌗ Courtesy of the US Department of Health and Human Services. The image may have been modified by cropping, labeling, and/or captions. All rights to this adaptation by MedIQ Learning, LLC are reserved.

Figure 4-28   **Hodgkin lymphoma: Image B. Mixed cellularity.** This image is a derivative work, adapted from the following source, available under ⓒ⓪⌗: Abd El All HS. Bob-1 is expressed in classic Hodgkin lymphoma. *Diagn Pathol.* 2007;2:10. doi:10.1186/1746-1596-2-10.

Figure 4-30   **Acute lymphoblastic leukemia.** This image is a derivative work, adapted from the following source, available under ⓒ⓪⌗: Bhatti FA, Hussain I, Ali MZ. Adult B lymphoblastic leukaemia/lymphoma with hypodiploidy (-9) and a novel chromosomal translocation t(7;12) (q22;p13) presenting with severe eosinophilia – case report and review of literature. *J Hematol Oncol.* 2009;2:26. doi:10.1186/1756-8722-2-26.

Figure 4-36   **Rouleaux formation.** Courtesy of Dr. Kristine Krafts.

Figure 4-38   **Birbeck granules.** ⓒ⓪⌗ Courtesy of Dr. Yale Rosen. The image may have been modified by cropping, labeling, and/or captions. All rights to this adaptation by MedIQ Learning, LLC are reserved.

Figure 4-39   **Myeloid dysplasia.** This image is a derivative work, adapted from the following source, available under ⓒ⓪⌗: Akpınar TS, Hançer VS, Nalçacı M, et al. MPL W515L/K mutations in chronic myeloproliferative neoplasms. *Turk J Haematol.* 2013;30(1):8-12. doi:10.4274/tjh.65807.

Figure 4-40   **Bone marrow fibrosis in myelofibrosis.** This image is a derivative work, adapted from the following source, available under ⓒ⓪⌗: Courtesy of Dr. Ed Uthman. The image may have been modified by cropping, labeling, and/or captions. All rights to this adaptation by MedIQ Learning, LLC are reserved.

Figure 4-45   **Common chemotoxicities.** Reproduced, with permission, from Le T, et al. *First Aid for the USMLE Step 1.* New York, NY: McGraw-Hill Education, 2016.

Figure 4-46   **Factors influencing platelet activation.** Reproduced, with permission, from Le T, et al. *First Aid for the USMLE Step 1.* New York, NY: McGraw-Hill Education, 2016.

Table 4-2   **Leukocytes: Image D. Eosinophil.** This image is a derivative work, adapted from the following source, available under ⓒ⓪⌗: Courtesy of Dr. Ed Uthman. The image may have been modified by cropping, labeling, and/or captions. All rights to this adaptation by MedIQ Learning, LLC are reserved.

Table 4-2   **Leukocytes: Image E. Basophil.** Courtesy of Dr. Kristine Krafts.

Table 4-2   **Leukocytes: Image F. Mast cell.** ⓒ⓪⌗ Courtesy of the US Department of Health and Human Services and Dr. Ayman Qasrawi. The image may have been modified by cropping, labeling, and/or captions. All rights to this adaptation by MedIQ Learning, LLC are reserved.

Table 4-2   **Leukocytes: Image G. Macrophage.** This image is a derivative work, adapted from the following source, available under ⓒ⓪⌗: De Tommasi AS, Otranto D, Furlanello T, et al. Evaluation of blood and bone marrow in selected canine vector-borne diseases. *Parasit Vectors.* 2014;7:534. doi 10.1186/s13071-014-0534-2. The image may have been modified by cropping, labeling, and/or captions. All rights to this adaptation by MedIQ Learning, LLC are reserved.

Table 4-2   **Leukocytes: Image H. Dendritic cell.** This image is a derivative work, adapted from the following source, available under ⓒ⓪⌗: Cheng J-H, Lee S-Y, Lien Y-Y, et al. Immunomodulating activity of *Nymphaea rubra* roxb. extracts: activation of rat dendritic cells and improvement of the TH1 immune response. *Int J Mol Sci.* 2012;13:10722-10735. doi 10.3390/ijms130910722. The image may have been modified by cropping, labeling, and/or captions. All rights to this adaptation by MedIQ Learning, LLC are reserved.

Table 4-3   **Red blood cell forms: Image A. Acanthocyte.** Courtesy of Dr. Kristine Krafts.

Table 4-3   **Red blood cell forms: Image B. Basophilic stippling.** Courtesy of Dr. Herbert L. Fred and Hendrik A. van Dijk. Images of Memorable Cases: Case 81. OpenStax College Website. http://cnx.org/contents/3196bf3e-1e1e-4c4d-a1acd4fc9ab65443@4@4. Published December 3, 2008. Accessed February 24, 2016.

Table 4-3   **Red blood cell forms: Image D. Degmacyte ("bite cell").** Courtesy of Dr. Kristine Krafts.

Table 4-3   **Red blood cell forms: Image G. Howell-Jolly bodies.** This image is a derivative work, adapted from the following source, available under ⓒ⓪⌗: Serio B, Pezzullo L, Giudice V, et al. OPSI threat in hematological patients. *Transl Med UniSa* 2013 May-Aug;6:2-10. The image may have been modified by cropping, labeling, and/or captions. All rights to this adaptation by MedIQ Learning, LLC are reserved.

Table 4-3   **Red blood cell forms: Image I. Ringed sideroblast.** This image is a derivative work, adapted from the following source, available under 🅭🅯. Courtesy of Paulo Henrique Orlandi Mourão. Patologista Clinico da Hospital das Clinicas UFMG e Patologista Clínico do Fundação Centro de Hematologia e Hemoterapia de Minas Gerais. The image may have been modified by cropping, labeling, and/or captions. MedIQ Learning, LLC makes this image available under 🅭🅯.

Table 4-3   **Red blood cell forms: Image K. Sickle cell.** 🅭🅯 Courtesy of the US Department of Health and Human Services and the Sickle Cell Foundation of Georgia, Jackie George, and Beverly Sinclair. The image may have been modified by cropping, labeling, and/or captions. All rights to this adaptation by MedIQ Learning, LLC are reserved.

Table 4-3   **Red blood cell forms: Image L. Spherocyte.** Courtesy of Dr. Kristine Krafts.

Table 4-11   **Histologic types of non-Hodgkin lymphoma and their characteristics: Image A. Small lymphocytic lymphoma.** This image is a derivative work, adapted from the following source, available under 🅭🅯: Tsou Y-A, Cheng Y-K, Lin C-D, Chang W-C, et al. Small B cell lymphocytic lymphoma presenting as obstructive sleep apnea. *World J Surg Oncol.* 2004;2:26. doi:10.1186/1477-7819-2-26. The image may have been modified by cropping, labeling, and/or captions. All rights to this adaptation by MedIQ Learning, LLC are reserved.

Table 4-11   **Histologic types of non-Hodgkin lymphoma and their characteristics: Image B. Follicular lymphoma.** This image is a derivative work, adapted from the following source, available under 🅭🅯: Alhaj Moustafa M, Seningen JL, Jouni H. Hypercalcemia, renal failure, and skull lytic lesions: follicular lymphoma masquerading as multiple myeloma. *J Investig Med High Impact Case Rep.* 2013;1(2):2324709613486356. doi:10.1177/2324709613486356. The image may have been modified by cropping, labeling, and/or captions. All rights to this adaptation by MedIQ Learning, LLC are reserved.

Table 4-11   **Histologic types of non-Hodgkin lymphoma and their characteristics: Image D. Mantle cell lymphoma.** This image is a derivative work, adapted from the following source, available under 🅭🅯: Agarwal A, Sadiq MA, Rhoades WR, et al. Combined systemic and ocular chemotherapy for anterior segment metastasis of systemic mantle cell lymphoma. *J Ophthalmic Inflamm Infect.* 2015;5:30. doi:10.1186/s12348-015-0060-1. The image may have been modified by cropping, labeling, and/or captions. All rights to this adaptation by MedIQ Learning, LLC are reserved.

Table 4-11   **Histologic types of non-Hodgkin lymphoma and their characteristics: Image E. Lymphoblastic lymphoma.** This image is a derivative work, adapted from the following source, available under 🅭🅯: Zhou D-M, Chen G, Zheng X-W, Zhu W-F, Chen B-Z. Clinicopathologic features of 112 cases with mantle cell lymphoma. *Cancer Biol Med.* 2015;12(1):46-52. doi:10.7497/j.issn.2095-3941.2015.0007. doi:10.1177/2324709613486356

Table 4-11   **Histologic types of non-Hodgkin lymphoma and their characteristics: Image G. Burkitt lymphoma, jaw involvement.** This image is a derivative work, adapted from the following source, available under 🅭🅯: Chaudhary S, Bansal C, Ranga U, et al. Erythrodermic mycosis fungoides with hypereosinophilic syndrome: a rare presentation. *Ecancermedicalscience.* 2013;7:337. doi:10.3332/ecancer.2013.337. The image may have been modified by cropping, labeling, and/or captions. All rights to this adaptation by MedIQ Learning, LLC are reserved.

Musculoskeletal, Skin, and Connective Tissue

Figure 5-3   **Marfan syndrome.** This image is a derivative work, adapted from the following source, available under 🅭🅯: Davari MH, Kazemi T. Marfan syndrome in an Iranian family: a case series. *Iran J Med Sci.* 2014;39(4):391-394. The image may have been modified by cropping, labeling, and/or captions. All rights to this adaptation by MedIQ Learning, LLC are reserved.

Figure 5-6   **Hemivertebra.** This image is a derivative work, adapted from the following source, available under 🅭🅯: Day G, Frawley K, Phillips G, et al. The vertebral body growth plate in scoliosis: a primary disturbance of growth? *Scoliosis.* 2008;3:3. doi:10.1186/1748-7161-3-3. The image may have been modified by cropping, labeling, and/or captions. All rights to this adaptation by MedIQ Learning, LLC are reserved.

Figure 5-9   **Prune belly syndrome: Image A. Wrinkled abdomen characteristic of prune belly syndrome secondary to absent abdominal musculature.** This image is a derivative work, adapted from the following source, available under 🅭🅯: Ome M, Wangnapi R, Hamura N, et al. A case of ultrasound-guided prenatal diagnosis of prune belly syndrome in Papua New Guinea – implications for management. *BMC Pediatr.* 2013;13:70. doi:10.1186/1471-2431-13-70. The image may have been modified by cropping, labeling, and/or captions. All rights to this adaptation by MedIQ Learning, LLC are reserved.

Figure 5-9   **Prune belly syndrome: Image B. Undersized, underdeveloped scrotum with absent testes.** This image is a derivative work, adapted from the following source, available under 🅭🅯: Ome M, Wangnapi R, Hamura N, et al. A case of ultrasound-guided prenatal diagnosis of prune belly syndrome in Papua New Guinea – implications for management. *BMC Pediatr.* 2013;13:70. doi:10.1186/1471-2431-13-70. The image may have been modified by cropping, labeling, and/or captions. All rights to this adaptation by MedIQ Learning, LLC are reserved.

Figure 5-10   **Poland syndrome: Image A. Absence of right breast and right pectoralis major muscles.** This image is a derivative work, adapted from the following source, available under 🅭🅯: Lizarraga KJ, De Salles AA. Multiple cavernous malformations presenting in a patient with Poland syndrome: a case report. *J Med Case Reports.* 2011;5:469. doi:10.1186/1752-1947-5-469. The image may have been modified by cropping, labeling, and/or captions. All rights to this adaptation by MedIQ Learning, LLC are reserved.

Figure 5-44 **Ankylosing spondylitis.** This image is a derivative work, adapted from the following source, available under [cc]: Manoj E, Ragunathan M. Disease flare of ankylosing spondylitis presenting as reactive arthritis with seropositivity: a case report. *J Med Case Reports.* 2012;6:60. doi:10.1186/1752-1947-6-60.

Figure 5-47 **Pathology and imaging of sarcoidosis: Image A. Histological sample.** Reproduced, with permission, from Le T, et al. *First Aid for the USMLE Step 1.* New York, NY: McGraw-Hill Education, 2016.

Figure 5-47 **Pathology and imaging of sarcoidosis: Image B. Typical findings on chest x-ray.** This image is a derivative work, adapted from the following source, available under [cc]: Lønborg J, Ward M, Gill A, et al. Utility of cardiac magnetic resonance in assessing right-sided heart failure in sarcoidosis. *BMC Med Imaging.* 2013;13:2. doi 10.1186/1471-2342-13-2. The image may have been modified by cropping, labeling, and/or captions. All rights to this adaptation by MedIQ Learning, LLC are reserved.

Figure 5-47 **Pathology and imaging of sarcoidosis: Image C. CT of patient with sarcoidosis.** This image is a derivative work, adapted from the following source, available under [cc]: Lønborg J, Ward M, Gill A, et al. Utility of cardiac magnetic resonance in assessing right-sided heart failure in sarcoidosis. *BMC Med Imaging.* 2013;13:2. doi 10.1186/1471-2342-13-2. The image may have been modified by cropping, labeling, and/or captions. All rights to this adaptation by MedIQ Learning, LLC are reserved.

Figure 5-48 **Cutaneous manifestations of sarcoidosis: Image A. Skin rash on a 12-year-old girl with sarcoidosis.** This image is a derivative work, adapted from the following source, available under [cc]: Shetty AK, Gedalia A. Childhood sarcoidosis: a rare but fascinating disorder. *Pediatr Rheumatol Online J.* 2008;6:16. doi:10.1186/1546-0096-6-16. The image may have been modified by cropping, labeling, and/or captions. All rights to this adaptation by MedIQ Learning, LLC are reserved.

Figure 5-48 **Cutaneous manifestations of sarcoidosis: Image B. Scaly annular violaceous plaque.** This image is a derivative work, adapted from the following source, available under [cc]: Beutler BD, Cohen PR. Sarcoidosis in melanoma patients: case report and literature review. Lee C-CR, ed. *Cancers (Basel).* 2015;7(2):1005-1021. doi:10.3390/cancers7020821. The image may have been modified by cropping, labeling, and/or captions. All rights to this adaptation by MedIQ Learning, LLC are reserved.

Figure 5-51 **Rashes of dermatomyositis: Image C. Gottron papules.** Courtesy of Dr. Christopher Crosby.

Figure 5-52 **Common skin lesions: Image C. Atopic dermatitis.** This image is a derivative work, adapted from the following source, available under [cc]: Salava A, Lauerma A. Role of the skin microbiome in atopic dermatitis. *Clin Transl Allergy.* 2014;4:33. doi:10.1186/2045-7022-4-33. The image may have been modified by cropping, labeling, and/or captions. All rights to this adaptation by MedIQ Learning, LLC are reserved.

Figure 5-52 **Common skin lesions: Image F. Rosacea.** This image is a derivative work, adapted from the following source, available under [cc]: Sand M, Sand D, Thrandorf C, et al. Cutaneous lesions of the nose. *Head Face Med.* 2010;6:7. doi:10.1186/1746-160X-6-7. The image may have been modified by cropping, labeling, and/or captions. All rights to this adaptation by MedIQ Learning, LLC are reserved.

Figure 5-52 **Common skin lesions: Image G. Seborrheic keratosis.** This image is a derivative work, adapted from the following source, available under [cc]: Kluger N, Guillot B. Sign of Leser-Trélat with an adenocarcinoma of the prostate: a case report. *Cases J.* 2009;2:8868. doi:10.4076/1757-1626-2-8868. The image may have been modified by cropping, labeling, and/or captions. All rights to this adaptation by MedIQ Learning, LLC are reserved.

Figure 5-52 **Common skin lesions: Image H. Urticaria.** This image is a derivative work, adapted from the following source, available under [cc]: Sussman G, Hébert J, Gulliver W, et al. Insights and advances in chronic urticaria: a Canadian perspective. *Allergy Asthma Clin Immunol.* 2015;11(1):7. doi:10.1186/s13223-015-0072-2. The image may have been modified by cropping, labeling, and/or captions. All rights to this adaptation by MedIQ Learning, LLC are reserved.

Figure 5-54 **Infectious skin lesions: Image C. Necrotizing fasciitis.** This image is a derivative work, adapted from the following source, available under [cc]: Smuszkiewicz P, Trojanowska I, Tomczak H. Late diagnosed necrotizing fasciitis as a cause of multiorgan dysfunction syndrome: a case report. *Cases J.* 2008;1:125. doi:10.1186/1757-1626-1-125. The image may have been modified by cropping, labeling, and/or captions. All rights to this adaptation by MedIQ Learning, LLC are reserved.

Figure 5-54 **Infectious skin lesions: Image D. Staphylococcal scalded skin syndrome.** This image is a derivative work, adapted from the following source, available under [cc]: Duijsters CE, Halbertsma FJ, Kornelisse RF, et al. Recurring staphylococcal scalded skin syndrome in a very low birth weight infant: a case report. *J Med Case Reports.* 2009;3:7313. doi:10.4076/1752-1947-3-7313.

Figure 5-54 **Infectious skin lesions: Image E. Verrucae.** Courtesy of Dr. Christopher Crosby.

Figure 5-55 **Skin conditions with blisters: Image B. Dermatitis herpetiformis.** [cc] Courtesy of the US Department of Health and Human Services. The image may have been modified by cropping, labeling, and/or captions. All rights to this adaptation by MedIQ Learning, LLC are reserved.

Figure 5-55 **Skin conditions with blisters: Image D. Stevens-Johnson syndrome.** [cc] Courtesy of the US Department of Health and Human Services and Dr. Allen W. Mathies. The image may have been modified by cropping, labeling, and/or captions. All rights to this adaptation by MedIQ Learning, LLC are reserved.

Figure 5-55 **Skin conditions with blisters: Image E. Epidermal necrolysis.** [PUBLIC DOMAIN] Courtesy of the US Department of Health and Human Services and Dr. Arthur E. Kaye. The image may have been modified by cropping, labeling, and/or captions. All rights to this adaptation by MedIQ Learning, LLC are reserved.

Figure 5-55 **Skin conditions with blisters: Image F. Pemphigus vulgaris.** This image is a derivative work, adapted from the following source, available under [CC]: Pacheco-Tovar D, López-Luna A, Herrera-Esparza R, et al. The Caspase pathway as a possible therapeutic target in experimental pemphigus. *Autoimmune Dis.* 2011;2011:563091. doi:10.4061/2011/563091.

Figure 5-56 **Miscellaneous skin conditions: Image A. Acanthosis nigricans.** This image is a derivative work, adapted from the following source, available under [CC]: Kubicka-Wołkowska J, Dębska-Szmich S, Lisik-Habib M, et al. Malignant acanthosis nigricans associated with prostate cancer: a case report. *BMC Urol.* 2014;14:88. doi:10.1186/1471-2490-14-88. The image may have been modified by cropping, labeling, and/or captions. All rights to this adaptation by MedIQ Learning, LLC are reserved.

Figure 5-56 **Miscellaneous skin conditions: Image B. Lichen planus.** [PUBLIC DOMAIN] Courtesy of the US Department of Health and Human Services and Dr. Wallace N. McLeod and Bob Craig. The image may have been modified by cropping, labeling, and/or captions. All rights to this adaptation by MedIQ Learning, LLC are reserved.

Figure 5-56 **Miscellaneous skin conditions: Image C. Pityriasis rosea.** [PUBLIC DOMAIN] Courtesy of the US Department of Health and Human Services. The image may have been modified by cropping, labeling, and/or captions. All rights to this adaptation by MedIQ Learning, LLC are reserved.

Figure 5-57 **Skin cancer lesions: Image E. Superficial spreading melanoma.** [PUBLIC DOMAIN] Courtesy of the US Department of Health and Human Services. The image may have been modified by cropping, labeling, and/or captions. All rights to this adaptation by MedIQ Learning, LLC are reserved.

Figure 5-57 **Skin cancer lesions: Image F. Nodular melanoma.** [PUBLIC DOMAIN] Courtesy of the US Department of Health and Human Services and Drs. Carl Washington and Mona Saraiya. The image may have been modified by cropping, labeling, and/or captions. All rights to this adaptation by MedIQ Learning, LLC are reserved.

Figure 5-57 **Skin cancer lesions: Image G. Lentigo maligna melanoma.** [PUBLIC DOMAIN] Courtesy of the US Department of Health and Human Services and Drs. Carl Washington and Mona Saraiya. The image may have been modified by cropping, labeling, and/or captions. All rights to this adaptation by MedIQ Learning, LLC are reserved.

Figure 5-57 **Skin cancer lesions: Image H. Acral lentiginous melanoma.** [PUBLIC DOMAIN] Courtesy of the US Department of Health and Human Services and Drs. Carl Washington and Mona Saraiya. The image may have been modified by cropping, labeling, and/or captions. All rights to this adaptation by MedIQ Learning, LLC are reserved.

Figure 5-59 **Buerger disease.** This image is a derivative work, adapted from the following source, available under [CC]: Afsharfard A, Mozaffar M, Malekpour F, Beigiboroojeni A, et al. The wound healing effects of iloprost in patients with buerger's disease: claudication and prevention of major amputations. *Iran Red Crescent Med.* 2011;13(6):420-423. The image may have been modified by cropping, labeling, and/or captions. All rights to this adaptation by MedIQ Learning, LLC are reserved.

Figure 5-60 **Kawasaki disease.** This image is a derivative work, adapted from the following source, available under [CC]: Alavi S, Fahimzad A, Jadali F, et al. Concurrent adrenal neuroblastoma and kawasaki disease: a report of a rare case. *Case Rep Pediatr.* 2013;2013:931703. doi:10.1155/2013/931703. The image may have been modified by cropping, labeling, and/or captions. All rights to this adaptation by MedIQ Learning, LLC are reserved.

Figure 5-61 **Pharmacologic interventions in gout.** Reproduced, with permission, from Le T, et al. *First Aid for the USMLE Step 1.* New York, NY: McGraw-Hill Education, 2016.

Neurology and Special Senses

Figure 6-2 **Neurulation.** Reproduced, with permission, from Le T, et al. *First Aid for the USMLE Step 1.* New York, NY: McGraw-Hill Education, 2016.

Figure 6-6 **Arnold-Chiari syndrome type I.** This image is a derivative work, adapted from the following source, available under [CC]: Marzuillo P, Grandone A, Coppola R, et al. Novel cAMP binding protein-BP (CREBBP) mutation in a girl with Rubinstein-Taybi syndrome, GH deficiency, Arnold Chiari malformation and pituitary hypoplasia. *BMC Med Genet.* 2013;14:28. doi:10.1186/1471-2350-14-28. The image may have been modified by cropping, labeling, and/or captions. All rights to this adaptation by MedIQ Learning, LLC are reserved.

Figure 6-8 **Holoprosencephaly.** This image is a derivative work, adapted from the following source, available under [CC]: Gupta AO, Leblanc P, Janumpally KC, et al. A preterm infant with semilobar holoprosencephaly and hydrocephalus: a case report. *Cases J.* 2010;3:35. doi:10.1186/1757-1626-3-35.

Figure 6-9 **Lumbar puncture.** Reproduced, with permission, from Bhushan V, Le T, Chandwani R, et al. *First Aid for the USMLE Step 1.* New York, NY: McGraw-Hill, 2006.

Figure 6-11 **Ventricular system. Sagittal view.** Reproduced, with permission, from Le T, et al. *First Aid for the USMLE Step 1.* New York, NY: McGraw-Hill Education, 2016.

Figure 6-40 **Brown-Séquard syndrome.** Reproduced, with permission, from Le T, et al. *First Aid for the USMLE Step 1.* New York, NY: McGraw-Hill Education, 2017.

Figure 6-54 **Chiari malformation.** This image is a derivative work, adapted from the following source, available under [cc 0]: Berthet S, Crevier L, Deslandres C. Abnormal movements associated with oropharyngeal dysfunction in a child with Chiari I malformation. *BMC Pediatrics.* 2014;14:1174. doi:10.1186/s12887-014-0294-3. The image may have been modified by cropping, labeling, and/or captions. All rights to this adaptation by MedIQ Learning, LLC are reserved.

Figure 6-58 **CT scans of intracranial hemorrhages: Image A. Epidural hematoma.** Courtesy of Dr. Vanja Douglas.

Figure 6-58 **CT scans of intracranial hemorrhages: Image E. Intraparenchymal hemorrhage.** This image is a derivative work, adapted from the following source, available under [cc 0]: Khanna A, Venteicher AS, Walcott BP, et al. Glioblastoma mimicking an arteriovenous malformation. *Front Neurol.* 2013;4:144. doi:10.3389/fneur.2013.00144. The image may have been modified by cropping, labeling, and/or captions. All rights to this adaptation by MedIQ Learning, LLC are reserved.

Figure 6-58 **CT scans of intracranial hemorrhages: Image F. Intraparenchymal hemorrhage.** This image is a derivative work, adapted from the following source, available under [cc 0]: Raval M, Singhal M, Guerrero D, Alonto A. Powassan virus infection: case series and literature review from a single institution. *BMC Res Notes.* 2012;5:594. doi:10.1186/1756-0500-5-594. The image may have been modified by cropping, labeling, and/or captions. All rights to this adaptation by MedIQ Learning, LLC are reserved.

Figure 6-59 **Multiple sclerosis.** This image is a derivative work, adapted from the following source, available under [cc 0]: Buzzard KA, Broadley SA, Butzkueven H. What do effective treatments for multiple sclerosis tell us about the molecular mechanisms involved in pathogenesis? *Int J Mol Sci.* 2012;13:12665-12709. doi 10.3390/ijms131012665. The image may have been modified by cropping, labeling, and/or captions. All rights to this adaptation by MedIQ Learning, LLC are reserved.

Renal

Figure 8-7 **Glomerulus: Image B. Normal glomerulus.** Reproduced, with permission, from Le T, et al. *First Aid for the USMLE Step 1.* New York, NY: McGraw-Hill Education, 2016.

Figure 8-8 **Components of the renal corpuscle.** [cc] Courtesy of the US Department of Health and Human Services and Uniformed Services University of the Health Sciences. The image may have been modified by cropping, labeling, and/or captions. All rights to this adaptation by MedIQ Learning, LLC are reserved.

Figure 8-9 **Histology of the bladder.** [cc] Courtesy of the US Department of Health and Human Services and Uniformed Services University of the Health Sciences. The image may have been modified by cropping, labeling, and/or captions. All rights to this adaptation by MedIQ Learning, LLC are reserved.

Figure 8-11 **Fluid compartments.** Reproduced, with permission, from Le T, et al. *First Aid for the USMLE Step 1.* New York, NY: McGraw-Hill Education, 2011.

Figure 8-13 **Electron photomicrograph of the glomerular filtration barrier.** [cc] Courtesy of the US Department of Health and Human Services and Dr. Ruth Bulger, Uniformed Services University of the Health Sciences. The image may have been modified by cropping, labeling, and/or captions. All rights to this adaptation by MedIQ Learning, LLC are reserved.

Figure 8-17 **Early proximal convoluted tubule.** Reproduced, with permission, from Le T, et al. *First Aid for the USMLE Step 1.* New York, NY: McGraw-Hill Education, 2017.

Figure 8-18 **Thick ascending limb of Henle.** Reproduced, with permission, from Le T, et al. *First Aid for the USMLE Step 1.* New York, NY: McGraw-Hill Education, 2017.

Figure 8-19 **Early distal convoluted tubule.** Reproduced, with permission, from Le T, et al. *First Aid for the USMLE Step 1.* New York, NY: McGraw-Hill Education, 2017.

Figure 8-20 **Collecting tubules reabsorb Na$^+$ in exchange for secreting K$^+$ or H$^+$.** Reproduced, with permission, from Le T, et al. *First Aid for the USMLE Step 1.* New York, NY: McGraw-Hill Education, 2017.

Figure 8-26 **Histology of minimal change disease.** [cc] Courtesy of the US Department of Health and Human Services. The image may have been modified by cropping, labeling, and/or captions. All rights to this adaptation by MedIQ Learning, LLC are reserved.

Figure 8-27 **Histology of focal sclerosing glomerulosclerosis.** This image is a derivative work, adapted from the following source, available under [cc]. Courtesy of Dr. Michael Bonert. The image may have been modified by cropping, labeling, and/or captions. MedIQ Learning, LLC makes this image available under [cc].

Figure 8-28 **Histologic image of membranous glomerulopathy.** [cc] Courtesy of the US Department of Health and Human Services and Uniformed Services University of the Health Sciences. The image may have been modified by cropping, labeling, and/or captions. All rights to this adaptation by MedIQ Learning, LLC are reserved.

Figure 8-29 **Diabetic nephropathy.** This image is a derivative work, adapted from the following source, available under [cc 0]: Satirapoj B, Tassanasorn S, Charoenpitakchai M, et al. Periostin as a tissue and urinary biomarker of renal injury in type 2 diabetes mellitus. Sen U, ed. *PLoS One.* 2015;10(4):e0124055. doi:10.1371/journal.pone.0124055. The image may have been modified by cropping, labeling, and/or captions. All rights to this adaptation by MedIQ Learning, LLC are reserved.

Figure 8-31 **Light microscopy of acute proliferative glomerulonephritis.** [cc] Courtesy of the US Department of Health and Human Services and Uniformed Services University of the Health Sciences. The image may have been modified by cropping, labeling, and/or captions. All rights to this adaptation by MedIQ Learning, LLC are reserved.

Figure 8-33 **Light micrograph with immunofluorescence staining of Goodpasture syndrome.** This image is a derivative work, adapted from the following source, available under 🅮 🅮 : Patel D, Nivera N, Tunkel AR. Antiglomerular basement membrane disease superimposed on membranous nephropathy: a case report and review of the literature. *J Med Case Rep.* 2010;4:237. doi:10.1186/1752-1947-4-237.

Figure 8-34 **Light microscopy of IgA nephropathy.** 🅮 Courtesy of the US Department of Health and Human Services and Uniformed Services University of the Health Sciences. The image may have been modified by cropping, labeling, and/or captions. All rights to this adaptation by MedIQ Learning, LLC are reserved.

Figure 8-35 **Immunofluorescence of IgA nephropathy.** 🅮 Courtesy of the US Department of Health and Human Services and Uniformed Services University of the Health Sciences. The image may have been modified by cropping, labeling, and/or captions. All rights to this adaptation by MedIQ Learning, LLC are reserved.

Figure 8-39 **Kidney with acute tubular necrosis.** 🅮 Courtesy of the US Department of Health and Human Services. The image may have been modified by cropping, labeling, and/or captions. All rights to this adaptation by MedIQ Learning, LLC are reserved.

Reproductive

Figure 9-13 **Female reproductive anatomy.** Reproduced, with permission, from Le T, et al. *First Aid for the USMLE Step 1.* New York, NY: McGraw-Hill Education, 2016.

Figure 9-16 **Male and female genital homologs.** Reproduced, with permission, from Le T, et al. *First Aid for the USMLE Step 1.* New York, NY: McGraw-Hill Education, 2011.

Figure 9-18 **Anatomic borders formed by the inguinal ligament.** Reproduced, with permission, from Le T, et al. *First Aid for the USMLE Step 1.* New York, NY: McGraw-Hill Education, 2011.

Figure 9-30 **Hormonal regulation of spermatogenesis.** Reproduced, with permission, from Le T, et al. *First Aid for the USMLE Step 1.* New York, NY: McGraw-Hill Education, 2011.

Figure 9-42 **Hydatidiform mole: Image A. Complete hydatidiform mole.** Reproduced, with permission, from Le T, et al. *First Aid for the USMLE Step 1.* New York, NY: McGraw-Hill Education, 2017.

Figure 9-44 **Spectrum of squamous intraepithelial lesion and cervical dysplasia.** This image is a derivative work, adapted from the following source, available under 🅮 🅮 : Courtesy of Dr. Ed Uthman. The image may have been modified by cropping, labeling, and/or captions. All rights to this adaptation by MedIQ Learning, LLC are reserved.

Figure 9-47 **Mature cystic teratoma of the ovary.** This image is a derivative work, adapted from the following source, available under 🅮 🅮 : Perazzi A, Berlanda M, Bucci M, et al. Multiple dermoid sinuses of type Vb and IIIb on the head of a Saint Bernard dog. *Acta Vet Scand.* 2013;55(1):62. doi:10.1186/1751-0147-55-62. The image may have been modified by cropping, labeling, and/or captions. All rights to this adaptation by MedIQ Learning, LLC are reserved.

Figure 9-49 **Submucosal leiomyoma.** Courtesy of Dr. Paban Sharma, Patan Hospital, Kathmandu, Nepal.

Figure 9-50 **Paget disease of the nipple.** This image is a derivative work, adapted from the following source, available under 🅮 🅮 : Muttarak M, Siriya B, Kongmebhol P, et al. Paget's disease of the breast: clinical, imaging and pathologic findings: a review of 16 patients. *Biomed Imaging Interv J.* 2011;7:e16. doi 10.2349/biij.7.2.e16. The image may have been modified by cropping, labeling, and/or captions. All rights to this adaptation by MedIQ Learning, LLC are reserved.

Figure 9-52 **Squamous cell carcinoma of the penis.** This image is a derivative work, adapted from the following source, available under 🅮 🅮 : Rouscoff Y, Falk AT, Durand M, et al. High-dose rate brachytherapy in localized penile cancer: short-term clinical outcome analysis. *Radiat Oncol.* 2014;9:142. doi:10.1186/1748-717X-9-142. The image may have been modified by cropping, labeling, and/or captions. All rights to this adaptation by MedIQ Learning, LLC are reserved.

Figure 9-54 **Hydrocele and transillumination: Image A. Hydrocele.** Courtesy of Dr. Michael J. Nowicki.

Figure 9-54 **Hydrocele and transillumination: Image B. Transillumination.** Courtesy of Dr. Michael J. Nowicki.

Figure 9-55 **Histologic specimen showing lymphocyte infiltration of the parenchyma.** Courtesy of Dr. Mark Ball.

Figure 9-56 **Transverse section of prostate showing location of BPH and prostatic carcinoma.** Reproduced, with permission, from Le T, et al. *First Aid for the USMLE Step 1.* New York, NY: McGraw-Hill Education, 2017.

Table 9-17 **Types of endometrial hyperplasia, cytologic features, and progression to endometrial carcinoma: Image A. Simple endometrial hyperplasia without nuclear atypia.** This image is a derivative work, adapted from the following source, available under 🅮 🅮 . Courtesy of Dr. Michael Bonert. The image may have been modified by cropping, labeling, and/or captions. MedIQ Learning, LLC makes this image available under 🅮 🅮 .

Table 9-17 **Types of endometrial hyperplasia, cytologic features, and progression to endometrial carcinoma: Image B. Complex hyperplasia without atypia.** This image is a derivative work, adapted from the following source, available under 🅮 🅮 : Izadi-Mood N, Yarmohammadi M, Ahmadi SA, et al. Reproducibility determination of WHO classification of endometrial hyperplasia/well differentiated adenocarcinoma and comparison with computerized morphometric data in curettage specimens in Iran. *Diang Path.* 2009;4:10. doi:10.1186/1746-1596-4-10.

Table 9-17 Types of endometrial hyperplasia, cytologic features, and progression to endometrial carcinoma: Image C. Simple hyperplasia with atypia. This image is a derivative work, adapted from the following source, available under [cc]: Izadi-Mood N, Yarmohammadi M, Ahmadi SA, et al. Reproducibility determination of WHO classification of endometrial hyperplasia/well differentiated adenocarcinoma and comparison with computerized morphometric data in curettage specimens in Iran. *Diang Path.* 2009;4:10. doi:10.1186/1746-1596-4-10.

Table 9-17 Types of endometrial hyperplasia, cytologic features, and progression to endometrial carcinoma: Image D. Complex hyperplasia with atypia. This image is a derivative work, adapted from the following source, available under [cc]: Izadi-Mood N, Yarmohammadi M, Ahmadi SA, et al. Reproducibility determination of WHO classification of endometrial hyperplasia/well differentiated adenocarcinoma and comparison with computerized morphometric data in curettage specimens in Iran. *Diang Path.* 2009;4:10. doi:10.1186/1746-1596-4-10.

Respiratory

Figure 10-9 Indications of surfactant deficiency in a premature infant: Image A. Photomicrograph showing collapsed alveoli surrounding dilated alveolar ducts lined by smooth homogeneous hyaline membranes. [cc] Courtesy of the US Department of Health and Human Services Courtesy of the Armed Forces Institute of Pathology.

Figure 10-9 Indications of surfactant deficiency in a premature infant: Image B. X-ray of the chest showing NRDS. This image is a derivative work, adapted from the following source, available under [cc]: YIN X, MENG F, QU W, et al. Clinical, radiological and genetic analysis of a male infant with neonatal respiratory distress syndrome. *Exp Ther Med.* 2013;5(4):1157-1160. doi:10.3892/etm.2013.970. The image may have been modified by cropping, labeling, and/or captions. All rights to this adaptation by MedIQ Learning, LLC are reserved.

Figure 10-12 Chest radiographs: Image A. Normal chest radiograph. This image is a derivative work, adapted from the following source, available under [cc]: Courtesy of Dr. Yale Rosen. The image may have been modified by cropping, labeling, and/or captions. All rights to this adaptation by MedIQ Learning, LLC are reserved.

Figure 10-12 Chest radiographs: Image B. Plain chest radiograph shows pleural effusion. This image is a derivative work, adapted from the following source, available under [cc]: Kashizaki F, Hatamochi A, Kamiya K, et al. Vascular-type Ehlers-Danlos syndrome caused by a hitherto unknown genetic mutation: a case report. *J Med Case Rep.* 2013;7:35. doi:10.1186/1752-1947-7-35. The image may have been modified by cropping, labeling, and/or captions. All rights to this adaptation by MedIQ Learning, LLC are reserved.

Figure 10-13 The diaphragm and penetrating structures. Reproduced, with permission, from Le T, et al. *First Aid for the USMLE Step 1.* New York, NY: McGraw-Hill Education, 2016.

Figure 10-17 Type II pneumocytes: Image A. Electron micrograph of type II pneumocytes. This image is a derivative work, adapted from the following source, available under [cc]: Chan M, Cheung C, Chui W, et al. Proinflammatory cytokine responses induced by influenza A (H5N1) viruses in primary human alveolar and bronchial epithelial cells. *Respir Res.* 2005;6(1):135. doi:10.1186/1465-9921-6-135.

Figure 10-17 Type II pneumocytes: Image B. Lamellar bodies. This image is a derivative work, adapted from the following source, available under [cc]: Chan M, Cheung C, Chui W, et al. Proinflammatory cytokine responses induced by influenza A (H5N1) viruses in primary human alveolar and bronchial epithelial cells. *Respir Res.* 2005;6(1):135. doi:10.1186/1465-9921-6-135.

Figure 10-32 Rhinosinusitis. This image is a derivative work, adapted from the following source, available under [cc]: Strek P, Zagolski O, Sktadzien J. Fatty tissue within the maxillary sinus: a rare finding. *Head Face Med.* 2006;2:28. doi 10.1186/1746-160X-2-28. The image may have been modified by cropping, labeling, and/or captions. All rights to this adaptation by MedIQ Learning, LLC are reserved.

Figure 10-35 Lateral chest film of patient with emphysema. [cc] Courtesy of Dr. James Heilman. The image may have been modified by cropping, labeling, and/or captions. All rights to this adaptation by MedIQ Learning, LLC are reserved.

Figure 10-36 Centriacinar emphysema: Image A. Gross specimen. [cc] Courtesy of the US Department of Health and Human Services and Dr. Edwin P. Ewing, Jr. The image may have been modified by cropping, labeling, and/or captions. All rights to this adaptation by MedIQ Learning, LLC are reserved.

Figure 10-36 Centriacinar emphysema: Image B. Computed tomography cross-section. This image is a derivative work, adapted from the following source, available under [cc]: Oikonomou A, Prassopoulo P. Mimics in chest disease: interstitial opacities. *Insights Imaging.* 2013;4:9-27. doi 10.1007/s13244-012-0207-7. The image may have been modified by cropping, labeling, and/or captions. All rights to this adaptation by MedIQ Learning, LLC are reserved.

Figure 10-37 Curschmann spirals. [cc] Courtesy of Dr. James Heilman. The image may have been modified by cropping, labeling, and/or captions. All rights to this adaptation by MedIQ Learning, LLC are reserved.

Figure 10-38 Mucus plug. [cc] Courtesy of Dr. Yale Rosen. The image may have been modified by cropping, labeling, and/or captions. All rights to this adaptation by MedIQ Learning, LLC are reserved.

Figure 10-39 Bronchiectasis: Image B. Permanently dilated airways. Reproduced, with permission, from Le T, et al. *First Aid for the USMLE Step 1.* New York, NY: McGraw-Hill Education, 2016.

Figure 10-54 **Lung abscess: Image A. Gross specimen.** ⊚▦ Courtesy of Dr. Yale Rosen. The image may have been modified by cropping, labeling, and/or captions. All rights to this adaptation by MedIQ Learning, LLC are reserved.

Figure 10-54 **Lung abscess: Image B. Cavitation with air-fluid levels visible on x-ray of the chest.** ⊚▦ Courtesy of Dr. Yale Rosen. The image may have been modified by cropping, labeling, and/or captions. All rights to this adaptation by MedIQ Learning, LLC are reserved.

Figure 10-56 **Pleural effusion: Image A. Before treatment.** This image is a derivative work, adapted from the following source, available under ⊚▣: Toshikazu A, Takeoka H, Nishioka K, et al. Successful management of refractory pleural effusion due to systemic immunoglobulin light chain amyloidosis by vincristine adriamycin dexamethasone chemotherapy: a case report. *Med Case Rep.* 2010;4:322. doi 10.1186/1752-1947-4-322. The image may have been modified by cropping, labeling, and/or captions. All rights to this adaptation by MedIQ Learning, LLC are reserved.

Figure 10-56 **Pleural effusion: Image B. After treatment.** This image is a derivative work, adapted from the following source, available under ⊚▣: Toshikazu A, Takeoka H, Nishioka K, et al. Successful management of refractory pleural effusion due to systemic immunoglobulin light chain amyloidosis by vincristine adriamycin dexamethasone chemotherapy: a case report. *Med Case Rep.* 2010;4:322. doi 10.1186/1752-1947-4-322. The image may have been modified by cropping, labeling, and/or captions. All rights to this adaptation by MedIQ Learning, LLC are reserved.

Figure 10-57 **Pneumothorax: Image A. CT showing collapsed left lung.** Reproduced, with permission, from Le T, et al. *First Aid for the USMLE Step 1.* New York, NY: McGraw-Hill Education, 2016.

Figure 10-57 **Pneumothorax: Image B. Chest x-ray showing left-sided tension pneumothorax.** Reproduced, with permission, from Le T, et al. *First Aid for the USMLE Step 1.* New York, NY: McGraw-Hill Education, 2016.

Figure 10-58 **Pharmacologic targets in asthma: Image A. Inflammatory pathway.** Reproduced, with permission, from Le T, et al. *First Aid for the USMLE Step 1.* New York, NY: McGraw-Hill Education, 2016.

Figure 10-58 **Pharmacologic targets in asthma: Image B. Parasympathetic pathway.** Reproduced, with permission, from Le T, et al. *First Aid for the USMLE Step 1.* New York, NY: McGraw-Hill Education, 2016.

Table 10-15 **Common inorganic pneumoconioses: Image A. Asbestosis.** ⊚▦ Courtesy of Dr. Yale Rosen. The image may have been modified by cropping, labeling, and/or captions. All rights to this adaptation by MedIQ Learning, LLC are reserved.

Table 10-15 **Common inorganic pneumoconioses: Image B. CT scan of the thorax demonstrating circumscribed calcified bilateral pleural plaques.** This image is a derivative work, adapted from the following source, available under ⊚▣: Miles SE, Sandrini A, Johnson AR, et al. Clinical consequences of asbestos-related diffuse pleural thickening: a review. *J Occup Med Toxicol.* 2008;3:20. doi 10.1186/1745-6673- 3-20. The image may have been modified by cropping, labeling, and/or captions. All rights to this adaptation by MedIQ Learning, LLC are reserved.

Table 10-15 **Common inorganic pneumoconioses: Image C. Ferruginous body.** ⊚▦ Courtesy of the US Department of Health and Human Services. The image may have been modified by cropping, labeling, and/or captions. All rights to this adaptation by MedIQ Learning, LLC are reserved.

Table 10-15 **Common inorganic pneumoconioses: Image D. Coal macule.** ⊚▦ Courtesy of the US Department of Health and Human Services. The image may have been modified by cropping, labeling, and/or captions. All rights to this adaptation by MedIQ Learning, LLC are reserved.

Table 10-15 **Common inorganic pneumoconioses: Image E. Silicotic nodule.** ⊚▦ Courtesy of the US Department of Health and Human Services. The image may have been modified by cropping, labeling, and/or captions. All rights to this adaptation by MedIQ Learning, LLC are reserved.

Index

A

A band, 21, 356, 357
a (atrial) waves, "cannon," 48
A-a gradient (alveolar-arterial O_2 gradient), 776, 777–778
AAA (abdominal aortic aneurysm), 66
AaDo$_2$ (alveolar-arterial O_2 gradient), 776, 777–778
Abciximab, 321
Abdominal aorta, 184, 185, 186
    bifurcation of, 185
        atherosclerosis at, 184
Abdominal aortic aneurysm (AAA), 66
Abdominal arterial system, 184, 185, 186
    key anastomoses of, 184, 187
Abdominal hernias, 236–238
Abdominal muscles, 674
Abdominal peritoneum, 183–184
Abdominal planes, 180–183
Abdominal quadrants, 180, 181
Abdominal regions, 180–183
Abdominal viscera, 183–184
Abdominal wall
    layers of, 181, 674
    surface anatomy of, 178–179, 181
Abducens nerve, 425, 459
    lesion of, 500, 501, 503–504
Abducens nucleus, 442
Abductor digiti minimi muscle, 349
Abductor pollicis muscle, 349
Abetalipoproteinemia, 203, 225
ABO classification, 282
ABO incompatibility, 281, 696
ABP (androgen binding protein), 682, 685
Abscess
    brain, 505
    lung, 812
Absence seizure, 489
Absolute refractory period (ARP), 19, 20
Absorption
    by small intestine, 200–203
    by stomach, 199
    vitamin B$_{12}$ deficiency due to impaired, 278
ACA (anterior cerebral artery), 422, 423, 425
    stroke involving, 478
Acalculia, 428
Acanthocyte, 273
Acantholysis, 394
Acanthosis nigricans, 394
Acarbose, 168
Accessory cuneate, 438
Accessory muscles, 334
    of respiration, 779–780
Accessory nerve, 459
    lesion of, 500
Accessory nipples, 672
Accessory pancreatic duct, 208
ACE (angiotensin-converting enzyme)
    in alveolar function, 764
    and blood pressure, 39
ACE (angiotensin-converting enzyme)
        inhibitors, 53, 659
    for heart failure, 102
    for hypertension, 99
Acetabular fractures, 341
Acetaminophen, 408–409
Acetazolamide, 95, 656–657
Acetoacetate, 162
Acetylcholine (ACh), 446, 507, 508
    effect on pacemaker action potentials of, 18

in innervation of GI tract, 189, 190
in skeletal muscle action potential, 354
Acetylcholine (ACh) receptor(s)
    and gastric secretions, 196, 197
    nicotinic, 354
Acetylcholine (ACh) receptor agonists, 509–510
Acetylcholine (ACh) receptor competitive antagonists, 509, 510
Acetylcholinesterase, 354–355
Acetyl-coenzyme A (acetyl-CoA), 508
N-Acetylcysteine, 819
ACh. See Acetylcholine (ACh)
Achalasia, 194, 195, 215–216
Achondroplasia, 325, 326
Acid(s)
    defined, 615
    nonvolatile, 616
    production of, 616
    strong, 615
    titratable, 616
    volatile, 616
    weak, 615
Acid-base disorders, mixed, 621, 773
Acid-base disturbances, 618–621, 771–773
Acid-base homeostasis, 616–618
Acid-base nomogram, 621–622
Acid-base problem solving, 622
Acidemia, 617, 621, 622
Acidophils, 112
Acidosis, 617
    anion-gap, 618, 621, 622
    dilutional, 618
    hyperchloremic, 618
    metabolic, 618–619, 620, 773
        in acid-base nomogram, 622
        clinical implications of, 621
        due to renal failure, 644
    renal tubular, 618
    respiratory, 619, 620, 771–772
        in acid-base nomogram, 622
        clinical implications of, 621
ACL (anterior cruciate ligament), 345
Acne, 389, 390
Acoustic neuroma, 444, 463, 465
Acquired immunodeficiency syndrome (AIDS), oral conditions associated with, 210
Acral lentiginous melanoma, 395, 396
Acromegaly, 120–121
Acromioclavicular joint, 344
Acrosclerosis, scleroderma, 385
Acrosome, 678, 679, 691, 692
Acrylaldehyde, 568
ACS (acute coronary syndrome), 13
    electrocardiography of, 45
ACTH. See Adrenocorticotropic hormone (ACTH)
Actin in myocardial contraction and relaxation, 22
Acting out, 538
Actinic keratosis, 395
Action potentials (APs)
    cardiac, 15, 16–20
        and cardiac pacemakers, 17–18
        conduction velocity of, 18–19
        fast-response (ventricular), 16, 17, 18
        refractory period of, 19–20
        slow-response (pacemaker), 16–17, 18
    skeletal muscle, 354
Active immunization, 710

Active transport, 596
Acute coronary syndrome (ACS), 13
    electrocardiography of, 45
Acute disseminated encephalomyelitis, 487
Acute granulocytic leukemia, 297, 302–303
Acute infective endocarditis, 58
Acute inflammatory demyelinating polyradiculopathy, 456, 466, 487–488
Acute intermittent porphyria (AIP), 288–289, 290
Acute kidney injury (AKI), 640–642
Acute lung injury, transfusion-related, 792
Acute lymphoblastic leukemia (ALL), 301–302
Acute monocytic leukemia, 303
Acute myelogenous leukemia (AML), 297, 302–303
Acute proliferative glomerulonephritis, 623, 631–632
Acute promyelocytic leukemia (APL), 302
Acute respiratory distress syndrome (ARDS), 764, 769, 792–793
Acute tubular necrosis (ATN), 641–642
Acyanotic congenital heart lesions, 6–7
Adalimumab, 404
ADAMTS13, 292
Addison disease, 152, 156–157
Adductor brevis muscle, 352
Adductor longus muscle, 102, 352
Adductor magnus muscle, 352
Adductor pollicis muscle, 349
Adenocarcinoma
    clear cell vaginal, 713
    colorectal, 234–235
    of esophagus, 219
    gastric, 222, 223
    of lung, 804–805
    pancreatic, 255
    prostatic, 680, 740–741
Adenohypophysis. See Anterior pituitary
Adenoma(s), 308
    of colon, 233
    hepatic, 248, 249
    pituitary, 115–116, 119, 436, 490, 492, 496
    pleomorphic, of salivary gland, 213
    thyroid, 134
Adenoma-carcinoma sequence, 234
Adenomatous polyps, 233
Adenomyosis, 724
Adenosine
    for arrhythmias, 104
    effect on pacemaker action potentials of, 18
Adenosine monophosphate (AMP) in muscle contraction, 359
Adenosine triphosphate (ATP) in excitation-contraction coupling, 355, 356
Adenosine triphosphate (ATP)-sensitive potassium channel, 160, 161
Adenylate cyclase mechanism, 109–110, 111
ADH. See Antidiuretic hormone (ADH)
ADHD (attention deficit/hyperactivity disorder), 579–580
Adie tonic Pupil, 461
Adjustment disorder, 551
ADPCKD (autosomal dominant polycystic kidney disease), 643–644
Adrenal androgens, 149, 153
Adrenal arteries, 147
Adrenal cortex, 147, 148–149

Adrenal gland, 147–158
  anatomy of, 147
  disorders of, 153–158
    adrenal insufficiency as, 156–157
    congenital adrenal hyperplasia as, 150, 157
    Cushing syndrome as, 152, 153–154, 155
    pheochromocytoma as, 148, 157–158
    primary hyperaldosteronism (Conn syndrome) as, 154–156
  embryology of, 147–148
  histology of, 148–149
  hormone synthesis and regulation by
    adrenal androgen, 149, 153
    glucocorticoid, 149, 150–152
    mineralocorticoid, 152–153
    steroid, 149–150
  overview of, 147
Adrenal hyperplasia, congenital, 150, 157
Adrenal insufficiency
  primary, 152, 156–157
  secondary and tertiary, 116, 152
Adrenal medulla, 147, 148
Adrenal veins, 147, 149–150
Adrenarche, adrenal androgens in, 153
Adrenocorticotropic hormone (ACTH)
  in Cushing syndrome, 153–154
  function of, 114, 116
  in glucocorticoid synthesis and regulation, 150
  in mineralocorticoid synthesis and regulation, 152
  primary hypersecretion of, 152
  regulation of secretion of, 114, 116, 147
Adrenocorticotropic hormone (ACTH)-related peptides, 117
Adrenocorticotropic hormone (ACTH) stimulation test, 156
Adrenoleukodystrophy, 488
Adult hemoglobin (Hb$\alpha_2\beta_2$), 8, 266, 267
Adult T-cell leukemia/lymphoma, 304
Adventitious breath sounds, 780
AER (apical ectodermal ridge), 331
Affect, 534
  disorders of, 536
  flat, 536, 545
  isolation of, 538
Afferent arteriole in renal tubular system, 591, 602, 603, 605, 607, 610
Afferent pupillary defect, 458
AFP. See α-fetoprotein (AFP)
Afterload, 24, 27
  and blood pressure, 37
Aging, vessel wall abnormalities due to, 295
Agoraphobia, 553
Agraphia, 428
AI (angiotensin I), 613
AICA (anterior inferior cerebellar artery), 424, 442
AICA (anterior inferior cerebellar artery) occlusion, 443
AIDS (acquired immunodeficiency syndrome), oral conditions associated with, 210
AII. See Angiotensin II (AII)
AIP (acute intermittent porphyria), 288–289, 290
Air embolism, 76, 77, 800
Air resistance, 784
Air trapping
  in bronchiectasis, 789
  in emphysema, 784
Airflow, 769
Airway(s)
  anatomy of, 754, 755
  conducting vs respiratory, 754, 755, 758–759
  in ventilation, 769–770

Airway obstruction, hypoxemia due to, 777
AKI (acute kidney injury), 640–642
ALA (δ-aminolevulinic acid), 288
Alanine aminotransferase (ALT), 256, 257
Alar plate, 413
Albinism, 391
Albright hereditary osteodystrophy, 145
Albumin, serum, 109
Albuterol, 769, 821
Alcohol, pupillary response to, 568
Alcohol use and sleep disorders, 565
Alcohol use disorder, 568–570, 572
Alcoholic hallucinosis, 570
Alcoholic hepatitis, 242–243
Aldosterone, 147, 149, 152–153
  and renal function, 612, 613–614, 615
  in renal reabsorption and secretion, 609
Aldosteronism, hypertension due to primary, 53
Alendronate, 146, 368, 402
Alexia, 428
Aliskiren, 100
Alkalemia, 617, 621, 622
Alkaline phosphatase (ALP), 257, 362
"Alkaline tide," 197
Alkalosis, 617
  contraction, 618
  metabolic, 618, 619, 620, 773
    in acid-base nomogram, 622
    clinical implications of, 621
  respiratory, 619–620, 772–773
    in acid-base nomogram, 622
    clinical implications of, 621
Alkylating agents, 310–312
ALL (acute lymphoblastic leukemia), 301–302
Allantois, 172, 584
Allergic contact dermatitis, 389, 390
Allergic rhinitis, 817
Allergy, 817
Allopurinol, 405
Allosteric regulation of muscle contraction, 358
Alogia, 545
ALP (alkaline phosphatase), 257, 362
α cells, 159
α-adrenergic agonists, 820
α_1-adrenergic receptor(s), 96, 151
  in regulation of renal blood flow and filtration, 602
α_2-adrenergic receptor(s), 96
α-adrenergic receptor antagonists, 97
α-blockers, 97
α-fetoprotein (AFP), 720
  with neural tube defects, 330, 468
  with omphalocele, 174
  screening for, 695–696
α-intercalated cells, 609, 614
Alport syndrome, 635
Alprazolam, 515, 540
ALS (amyotrophic lateral sclerosis), 457, 481
  restrictive lung disease due to, 791
ALT (alanine aminotransferase), 256, 257
Altitude, hypoxemia due to, 776, 777
Altitude sickness, 773
Altruism as defense mechanism, 537
Aluminum-containing antacids, 260, 261
Alveolar cells, 760
Alveolar dead space, 763
Alveolar duct, 756
Alveolar function, 763–764
Alveolar macrophages, 760
Alveolar oxygen tension (P$_{A}O_2$), 775–776
Alveolar period, 748, 750
Alveolar ventilation, 764–765
Alveolar-arterial O_2 gradient (A-a gradient, AaDO_2), 776, 777–778

Alveolus(i), 756, 759–760
Alzheimer disease, 482
  drugs used to treat, 527
Amaurosis fugax, 422, 503
Amelia, 331
Amiloride, 93–94, 656, 657–658
Amine hormones, 108, 109
Amino acid(s), renal reabsorption and excretion of, 605–606, 607
Amino acid metabolism, in muscle contraction, 358
δ-Aminolevulinic acid (ALA), 288
Amiodarone, 103, 104
Amitriptyline, 518, 540
AML (acute myelogenous leukemia), 297, 302–303
Amlodipine, 97–98
Ammonium (NH_4^+), renal secretion of, 617–618
Ammonium magnesium phosphate stones, 636, 637
Amnesia, 543
  dissociative, 559
Amnestic disorders, 543
Amnioblasts, 412
Amnion, 697
Amniotic fluid abnormalities, 707
Amniotic fluid embolism, 76, 77, 710, 800
Amoxapine, 518, 540
AMP (adenosine monophosphate) in muscle contraction, 359
Amphetamine(s), 541
  pupillary response to, 568
Amphetamine use disorder, 572, 573
Ampulla of ear, 462, 463
Ampulla of Vater, 208
Amygdala, 429, 431
Amylase, 257
α-Amylase
  pancreatic, 206
  salivary, 192, 193
Amyloid, common types of, 629, 630
Amyloidosis
  primary, 63
  renal, 629, 630
  vessel wall abnormalities due to, 295
Amyotrophic lateral sclerosis (ALS), 457, 481
  restrictive lung disease due to, 791
ANA(s) (antinuclear antibodies), 362
  in systemic lupus erythematosus, 380, 382
Anaerobes, pneumonia due to, 811
Anaerobic glycolysis in muscle contraction, 359
Anal delta, 339
Analgesics, clinical, 530–532
Anaphylaxis, 817
Anaplasia, 308
Anastomosis(es)
  of abdominal arterial system, 184, 187
  portal to inferior vena caval, 187, 188, 245
Anastrozole, 665, 745
Anatomic dead space, 763
Androgen(s)
  adrenal, 149, 153
  gonadal, 687, 689, 690
Androgen agonists, 741–742, 745
Androgen antagonists, 742
Androgen insensitivity, 702
Androgen-binding protein (ABP), 682, 685
Androstenedione, 149, 153, 687
Anemia, 272–287
  aplastic, 284, 287
  of chronic disease, 282–283
  classification and appearance of, 272, 273–274
  due to glucose-6-phosphate dehydrogenase deficiency, 278 279

hemolytic, 283–284, 696
  cardiac traumatic, 287
  microangiopathic, 286–287
due to hereditary spherocytosis, 279–280
immunohemolytic, 280–281
iron deficiency, 274–275
due to lead poisoning, 276–277
macrocytic, 277–278
megaloblastic, 277–278
microcytic, 272–277
normocytic, 278–287
due to paroxysmal nocturnal
    hemoglobinuria, 286
pernicious, 278, 497
physiologic, 692
due to pyruvate kinase deficiency, 286
due to renal failure, 644
due to sickle cell disease, 284–286
sideroblastic, 277
thalassemia as, 275–276
Anesthesia, stages of, 530
Anesthetics
  clinical, 530–532
  inhaled, 531
  intravenous, 531–532
Aneurysms, 56, 66–67, 68
  aortic, 66
  berry, 66, 471–472
  mycotic, 66
  syphilitic, 66
Angina
  antianginal therapy for, 100–101
  stable (effort), 85, 101
  types of, 85–86, 101
  unstable, 85, 101
  variant (Prinzmetal), 86, 101–102
Angina pectoris, 85–86
Angioedema, hereditary, 391
Angiogenic growth factors, in wound
    healing, 361
Angiosarcoma, hepatic, 250
Angiotensin I (AI), 613
Angiotensin II (AII), 99, 593
  and blood pressure, 40, 613
  in Na+ reabsorption, 608
  in regulation of renal blood flow and
    filtration, 603
  and renal function, 612, 613, 615
Angiotensin II receptor antagonists, 64,
    99–100
Angiotensin inhibitors, 98–100
Angiotensin receptor blockers (ARBs), 64, 659
  for heart failure, 102
  for hypertension, 99–100
Angiotensin-converting enzyme (ACE)
  in alveolar function, 764
  and blood pressure, 39
Angiotensin-converting enzyme (ACE)
    inhibitors, 53, 659
  for heart failure, 102
  for hypertension, 99
Angular gyrus, 426
Anion gap, 618
Anion-gap acidosis, 618, 621, 622
Anitschkow cells, 60, 61
Ankle, ligament injury of, 345–346
Ankle dorsiflexion, 341
Ankle jerk reflex, 449
Ankle joint, 345–346
Ankle plantarflexion, 341
Ankylosing spondylitis (AS), 377–379
Annular ligament, 344
Annular pancreas, 158, 178
Annulus fibrosus, 329, 338
Anopsia, 460
Anorexia nervosa, 562–564

ANP (atrial natriuretic peptide)
  in Na+ reabsorption, 608
  and renal function, 611, 612, 615
ANS (autonomic nervous system), 509
  effect on pacemaker action potentials of, 18
  and mean arterial pressure, 39
Ansoparamedian fissure, 437
Antacids, 260, 261
Antegrade ejaculation, 690
Anterior ampulla, 462
Anterior cerebral artery (ACA), 422, 423, 425
  stroke involving, 478
Anterior chamber, 502
Anterior communicating artery, 422
Anterior compartment syndrome, 495
Anterior cruciate ligament (ACL), 345
Anterior drawer sign, 345
Anterior ethmoidal artery, 783
Anterior fontanelle, 328, 329
Anterior fossa, 335
Anterior horn, 421
Anterior inferior cerebellar artery (AICA), 424,
    442
Anterior inferior cerebellar artery (AICA)
    occlusion, 443
Anterior limb, of internal capsule, 434
Anterior nuclei, 433, 435, 436
Anterior pituitary
  cell types and regulation of, 112, 114
  disease of, 119–122
  hormones of, 112–117
  structure and function of, 112
Anterior pituitary disease, 119–122
Anterior spinal artery (ASA), 424, 445
Anterior spinal artery (ASA) infarction, 110
Anterior spinal artery (ASA) occlusion, 455,
    457
Anterior superior iliac spine, 179
Anterior superior pancreaticoduodenal
    artery, 186
Anterior tibial artery, 352
Anterior tubercle, 337
Anterograde amnesia, 543
Anterograde memory loss, 430
Anterotalofibular ligament (ATFL), 345
Antiandrogens, 742, 746
Antianginal therapy, 100–101
Antiarrhythmics, 16, 103, 104
Anti-BCR-ABL agents, 317
anti-CCP (anticyclic citrullinated
    peptide), 362
Anti-CD20 antibody, 317
Anticholinergic drugs, 512
Anticoagulants, 292, 318–320
Anticonvulsants, 522–526
Anticyclic citrullinated peptide (anti-
    CCP), 362
Antidepressants, 516–520, 540–541, 549
  atypical, 516, 541
Antidiuretic hormone (ADH), 117, 118–119,
    658
  and renal function, 612, 614, 615
  syndrome of inappropriate secretion of. See
    Syndrome of inappropriate secretion
    of antidiuretic hormone (SIADH)
  and urine concentration, 609
Antidiuretic hormone (ADH) agonists, 126
Antidiuretic hormone (ADH) analog, 125
Antidiuretic hormone (ADH) antagonists,
    658–659
Anti-EGFR agents, 315–316
Anti-EGFR antibodies, 315
Antiglomerular basement membrane (anti-
    GBM) disease, 396, 399, 601, 623,
    633–634
Anti-HAV, 243

Anti-HBc, 243
Anti-HBe, 243
Anti-HBs, 243
Antihistamines, 520
Antihistone antibodies, in systemic lupus
    erythematosus, 383
Antihypertensive agents, 91–100
  angiotensin inhibitors as, 98–100
  calcium channel blockers and other
    vasodilators as, 97–98
  diuretics as, 91–95
  overview of, 91
  sympatholytics as, 95–97
Anti-La/SSB antibodies, 212
Antileukotrienes, 822
Antimetabolites, 311, 312–313
Antineutrophil cytoplasmic antibody
    (ANCA), 361
Antinuclear antibody(ies) (ANAs), 362
  in systemic lupus erythematosus, 380, 382
Antiphospholipid antibodies (aPLs), in
    systemic lupus erythematosus, 382
Antiplatelet agents, 320–321
Antiplatelet antibodies, 291
Antiport, 596
Anti proteasome, 317
Antipsychotics, 520–521
Anti-Rh factor (RhoGAM), 694, 710–711
Anti-Ro antibodies, in systemic lupus
    erythematosus, 382
Anti-Ro/SSA antibodies, 212
Antisocial personality disorder, 558, 561
Antithyroid drugs, 136–137
α1-Antitrypsin, in emphysema, 784
α1-Antitrypsin deficiency, hereditary, 701
Anti-VEGF agents, 316
Anti-VEGF antibodies, 316
Antrum
  ovarian, 687
  of stomach, 196
Anuria, 640
Anxiety, 550
  separation, 580
  and sleep disorders, 565
Anxiety disorders, 550–554
  adjustment disorder as, 551
  generalized anxiety disorder as, 550–551
  illness, 554, 556
  obsessive-compulsive disorder as, 553–554
  panic attacks as, 552
  panic disorder as, 552
  phobias as, 535, 552–553
  posttraumatic stress disorder as, 551–552
Anxiolytic(s), 513–516, 540, 549
Anxiolytic use disorder, 570–571
Aorta, 9, 12, 15
  abdominal, 184, 185, 186
    atherosclerosis at bifurcation of, 184
  coarctation of, 6
    hypertension due to, 53, 54
  overriding, 4, 5
Aortic aneurysms, 66
Aortic arch, 10
Aortic bodies in control of respiration, 779
Aortic dissection, 67, 68
Aortic pressure in diastole and systole, 31
Aortic regurgitation (AR), 5, 37, 71, 72
Aortic stenosis (AS), 10, 69–70
  congenital, 6
Aortic valve, 10, 11
  bicuspid, 5, 6
Aorticopulmonary (AP) septum, 4
AP(s). See Action potentials (APs)
APC gene, 234
Apex, cardiac, 10
Aphasia, 430–431, 479–480

Aphasia square, 430–431
Aphthous ulcers, 211
Apical ectodermal ridge (AER), 331
Apixaban, 319–320
APL (acute promyelocytic leukemia), 302
aPL(s) (antiphospholipid antibodies), in
        systemic lupus erythematosus, 382
Aplastic anemia, 285, 287
Aplastic thyroid carcinoma, 135
Apnea, sleep, 567, 769, 803
Apneustic center, 779
Appendicitis, 191, 236
Appendicular skeleton, 335
Appendix epididymis, 667
Appendix testis, 667
"Apple-peel" atresia, 177
Apraxia, 429
Aquaporins, 609, 614
AR (aortic regurgitation), 5, 37, 71, 72
Arachidonic acid, mediators derived from, 408
Arachnoid, 419, 425, 469
Arachnoid granulation, 469
ARBs (angiotensin receptor blockers), 64, 659
    for heart failure, 102
    for hypertension, 99–100
Arcuate artery, 588
Arcuate fasciculus aphasia, 480
Arcuate line, 179, 674, 675
Arcuate nucleus, 435, 436
ARDS (acute respiratory distress syndrome),
        764, 769, 792–793
Areola, 680, 681
Argyll Robertson pupil, 461, 501, 502
Aripiprazole, 521, 540
Arm muscles, 349
Arnold-Chiari malformation, 414–417
Aromatase, 687
Aromatase inhibitors, 665, 745
ARP (absolute refractory period), 19, 20
ARPCKD (autosomal recessive polycystic
        kidney disease), 644, 645
Arrhythmias, 46–52
    antiarrhythmics for, 16, 103, 104
    brady-, 46–49
    defined, 46
    tachy-, 46, 49–52
Arterial blood gas testing
    for asthma, 788
    for chronic bronchitis, 786
    for emphysema, 785
    for pulmonary embolism, 800
Arterial emboli, 77
Arterial pressure
    during cardiac cycle, 36, 37
    determinants of, 35–37
    regulation of, 37–40, 41
Arteriolar diameter and blood pressure, 37
Arterioles, 33, 34
Arteriolosclerosis, 54–55
Arteriosclerosis, 54–57
    categories of, 54–57
    complications of, 56–57
    defined, 54
    histopathology of, 56, 57
    Mönckeberg, 55
    pathogenesis of, 56
Arteriovenous fistula, 67
Arteritis
    Takayasu, 82, 398–399, 403
    temporal (giant cell), 81, 396–397, 403
Artery, 33
Arthritis
    osteo-, 327, 372–374
    psoriatic, 379–380
    reactive, 379
    rheumatoid, 373, 374–375

Articular capsule, 343
Articular cartilage, 325, 343
    loss of, 372
Articular processes, 337
Aryepiglottic muscles, 348
Arylcyclohexylamine, 532
AS (ankylosing spondylitis), 377–379
AS (aortic stenosis), 10, 69–70
ASA (anterior spinal artery), 424, 445
ASA (anterior spinal artery) infarction, 448
ASA (anterior spinal artery) occlusion, 455, 457
Asbestosis, 794, 795, 796, 807
Ascending tracts, 449
Aschoff bodies, 60, 61
Aschoff cells, 60, 61
Ascites, 183, 246
ASCUS (atypical squamous cells of
        undetermined significance), 714
ASD (atrial septal defect), 3, 5, 7
ASD (autism spectrum disorder), 577
Aseptic meningitis, 419, 420
Ash-leaf spots, 493
Asparate aminotransferase (AST), 255–256, 257
Asperger disorder, 578
Aspiration of foreign body, 779
Aspiration pneumonia, 751, 808, 809
Aspiration pneumonitis, 751
Aspirin, 320–321, 407
    defects in platelet aggregation due to, 293
    Reye syndrome due to, 244
Association visual cortex, 429
AST (aspartate aminotransferase), 255–256,
        257
Asthma, 787–788
    allergy and, 817
    characteristics of, 787
    defined, 787
    diagnosis of, 788, 789
    differential diagnosis of, 787
    exacerbations of, 788
    extrinsic, 787, 817
    intrinsic, 787
    lung volumes and capacities in, 761
    pathogenesis of, 787
    presentation of, 788
    prevalence of, 787
    prognosis for, 788
    risk factors for, 787
    treatment of, 788, 821–823
Astrocytes, 465, 490
Astrocytomas, 490
    pilocytic, 490, 492
    subependymal giant-cell, 496
Ataxia, Friedreich, 485
Ataxia-telangiectasia (AT), 493
Atelectasis, 764, 816
Atenolol, 96–97, 101
ATFL (anterotalofibular ligament), 345
Atherosclerosis, 55–57
    at bifurcation of abdominal aorta, 184
Atherosclerotic aneurysms, 66
Atherosclerotic risk factors, modifiable, 87
Athetosis, 479
Atlantoaxial dislocation, 340
Atlantoaxial joint, 344
Atlanto-occipital joint, 344
Atlas, 329
ATN (acute tubular necrosis), 641–642
Atonic seizure, 489
Atopic dermatitis, 389, 390
Atorvastatin, 105
ATP (adenosine triphosphate) in excitation-
        contraction coupling, 355, 356
ATP (adenosine triphosphate)-sensitive
        potassium channel, 160, 161
ATP7B gene, 248

Atracurium, 510
Atrial depolarization, 41
Atrial fibrillation, 30, 50, 52
Atrial flutter, 49–50
Atrial gallop, 32
"Atrial kick," 30
Atrial natriuretic peptide (ANP)
    in Na^+ reabsorption, 608
    and renal function, 611, 612, 615
Atrial pressure and mean arterial pressure, 38
Atrial repolarization, 41
Atrial septal defect (ASD), 3, 5, 7
Atrial septum, development of, 3
Atrial systole, 30
Atrial tachyarrhythmias, 49–50
Atrial (a) waves, "cannon," 48
Atrioventricular (AV) block
    complete, 14
    first-degree, 47
    second-degree, 47–48
    third-degree (complete), 48–49
Atrioventricular (AV) canal, 2
Atrioventricular (AV) canal septum, formation
        of, 2–3
Atrioventricular (AV) dissociation, 48
Atrioventricular nodal re-entrant tachycardia
        (AVNRT), 49
Atrioventricular (AV) node, 13, 14, 15, 17
    bradyarrhythmias of, 47–49
    tachyarrhythmias of, 49
Atrium(ia), cardiac, 9, 10
    primitive, 2
Atropine, 199, 512
Attention, 428–429
Attention deficit/hyperactivity disorder
        (ADHD), 579–580
Attention span, short, 535
Atypical antidepressants, 516, 541
Atypical squamous cells of undetermined
        significance (ASCUS), 714
Auditory cortex, primary, 429
Auditory hallucinations, 534
Auditory pathway, 429, 461–463
Auditory radiations, 462
Auditory system, 461
Auer rods, 303
Auerbach plexus, 190, 191, 195
Auscultation
    cardiac, 10, 11
    pulmonary, 780
Auspitz sign, 390
Autism spectrum disorder (ASD), 577
Autocrine secretion, 108
Autoimmune diseases during pregnancy, 694
Autoimmune gastritis, 220
Automaticity, 13, 17
Autonomic drugs, 508–512
    anticholinergic (muscarinic) drugs as, 512
    cholinesterase inhibitors as, 511
    cholinomimetic agents as, 511
    neuromuscular junction blocking agents as,
        509–510
Autonomic nervous system (ANS), 509
    effect on pacemaker action potentials of, 18
    and mean arterial pressure, 39
Autoregulation, 40
    of renal blood flow and filtration, 603
Autosomal dominant polycystic kidney disease
        (ADPCKD), 643–644
Autosomal recessive polycystic kidney disease
        (ARPCKD), 644, 645
AV. See Atrioventricular (AV)
AVNRT (atrioventricular nodal re-entrant
        tachycardia), 49
Avoidant personality disorder, 553, 560, 562
Axial skeleton, 335

Axillary artery and vein, 682
Axillary lymph nodes, 680
Axillary nerve, 351
Axillary nerve injury, 350, 495
Axis, 329
Axon(s), 354, 464, 465
Axoneme, 678
Azotemia, 640
   in nephritic syndrome, 630
Azygos vein, 755
Azygos venous system, 185

B

B lymphocyte (B-cell), 268, 269, 270
Babinski sign, 451
BAC (bronchoalveolar adenocarcinoma), 804–805
Bachmann bundle, 15
Bacterial embolism, 800
Bacterial endocarditis, 58–59, 61–62
Bacterial infection of CNS, 505
Bacterial meningitis, 419, 420
Bacterial overgrowth syndrome, 225
   vitamin B_{12} deficiency due to, 278
Bacterial vaginosis, 732, 733
Bacteriuria, asymptomatic, 638
Baker cyst, 353, 374
Balance, 445
Balanitis, 733
Balanoposthitis, 733
Balint syndrome, 429
Ball and socket joints, 343
"Bamboo" spine, 378
Barbiturate(s), 513, 514, 531–532, 540
Barbiturate use disorder, 570, 572
Barlow maneuver, 333–334
Baroreceptor(s), 614
Baroreceptor reflex and mean arterial pressure, 37, 38, 39
"Barrel chest," 780, 785
Barrett esophagus, 195, 217–219
Bartholin glands, 671
Bartter syndrome, 645
Basal cell carcinoma (BCC), 395
Basal electrical rhythm, 196
Basal ganglia, 431–432
   degenerative diseases due to lesions of, 484–485
Basal plate, 413
Base(s)
   defined, 615
   strong, 615
   weak, 615
Basilar artery, 442
Basilar membrane, 462
Basilar skull fracture, 339
Basket cell, 439
Basophil(s), 112, 268, 270, 271
Basophilic stippling, 273
Battle sign, 339
BBB (blood-brain barrier), 420
BBB (bundle branch block), 44–45
BCC (basal cell carcinoma), 395
B-cell (B lymphocyte), 268, 269, 270
BCR-ABL, molecular therapy targeting, 317
Beck triad, 79
Becker muscular dystrophy, 388
Beckwith-Wiedemann syndrome, 174, 649
Beclomethasone, 822
Behavioral disorders, 536
Bell palsy, 457, 458
La belle indifference, 555
The bends, 77
Benedikt syndrome, 441
Benign prostatic hyperplasia (BPH), 590, 680, 738–739

Benign tumors, 308–309
Benzodiazepine(s) (BZDs), 513, 515, 532, 540
   and sleep disorders, 565
Benzodiazepine (BZD) use disorder, 570, 572
Benztropine, 512
Bereavement, 550
Berger disease, 634–635
Beriberi, 62
Bernard-Soulier disease, 293
Berry aneurysms, 66, 471–472
Berylliosis, 794, 795, 796
β cells, 159
   insulin secretion by, 160, 161
β-adrenergic receptor(s), in salivary secretion, 193
β_1-adrenergic receptor(s), 96–97
β_2-adrenergic receptor(s), 96–97
β-adrenergic receptor agonists, 102–103
β_1-adrenergic receptor agonists, 613
β_2-adrenergic receptor agonists, 821
β-adrenergic receptor antagonists. See β-blockers
β_1-adrenergic receptor antagonists, 613
β-blockers
   for angina pectoris, 86, 100, 101
   for arrhythmias, 104
   effect on pacemaker action potentials of, 18
   for heart failure, 102
   for hypertension, 96–97
β-intercalated cells, 609
Bethanechol, 511
Betz cells, 425, 450
Bevacizumab, 316
Bicarbonate (HCO_3^-)
   carbon dioxide transport by, 771
   gastric secretion of, 197, 198
   renal reabsorption of, 609
   renal regulation of, 617–618
   small intestinal secretion of, 202
Biceps brachii muscle, 349
Biceps femoris muscle, 352
Biceps jerk reflex, 449
Bicornuate uterus, 673
Bicuspid aortic valves, 5, 6
Bile, 209–210
Bile acid(s), 209
Bile acid resins, 105
Bile acid sequestrants, 209
Bile canaliculus, 207
Bile ductule, 207
Bi-level positive airway pressure (BiPAP), 803
Biliary atresia, extrahepatic, 177
Biliary cirrhosis, primary, 246–247
Bilirubin, 208–209, 256
Biliverdin, 208
Binge eating/purging, 562–563
Binge-eating disorder, 564–565
Binswanger leukoencephalopathy, 479
BiPAP (bi-level positive airway pressure), 803
Bipolar disorder, 546, 547, 548–550
   and sleep disorders, 565
Birbeck granules, 306
Bird-beak esophagus, 216
Bismuth, 260
Bisphosphonates, 146, 368, 402
"Bite cell," 273
Bitemporal hemianopsia, 120, 121–122, 422, 460
Bladder
   anatomy of, 589
   exstrophy of, 669
   histology of, 594
Blastomycosis, pneumonia due to, 812
Bleeding, GI, 274

Bleeding disorders, 290–295
   due to clotting factor deficiencies, 293–294
   disseminated intravascular coagulation as, 291, 292, 294
   laboratory findings in, 290, 291
   due to liver disease, 291, 294
   due to platelet disorders, 290–293
   due to vessel wall abnormalities, 291, 295
Bleeding time, 291
Blisters, conditions with, 392–394
Blood
   anatomy of, 267–272
   composition of, 32, 33
Blood bicarbonate buffer, 617
Blood cells, 267–272
   formation of, 266, 268
Blood clot, 76
Blood flow, 34
   laminar vs turbulent, 34, 67
   velocity of, 33, 34
Blood gas(es), 770–779
   carbon dioxide transport in, 771, 772
   control of respiration in, 778–779
   hypercapnia in, 778
   hypoxemia in, 775–778
   oxygen transport in, 770–771
   pulmonary circulation in, 773–775
   respiratory acid-base disturbances in, 771–773
Blood gas testing
   for asthma, 788
   for chronic bronchitis, 786
   for emphysema, 785
   for pulmonary embolism, 800
Blood groups, 282
Blood loss, 288
Blood pressure (BP)
   determinants of, 35–37
   regulation of, 37–40, 41, 444
Blood volume
   and cardiac and vascular function curves, 28, 29
   and mean arterial pressure, 38
Blood-brain barrier (BBB), 420
Blood-testis barrier, 682
"Blue bloater," 786
BMD (bone mineral density), 367
BNP (brain natriuretic peptide), 611
Body dysmorphic disorder, 554, 556
Body fluid(s)
   composition of, 596
   intercompartmental water dynamics between, 598, 599, 600
   volume of
      estimating, 597
      measuring, 597–598
Body plethysmography, 763
Boerhaave syndrome, 215
Bohr effect, 770
Bohr equation, 763
Bombesin, 196, 197–199, 204
Bone(s)
   compact, 325, 335
   major, 335–338
   Paget disease of, 327, 369–370
   during pregnancy, 694
   spongy, 325, 335
   von Recklinghausen disease of, 144, 326, 370
Bone cells, 324, 325
Bone cysts, 372
Bone development, 324–325
   congenital malformations involving, 326–328
Bone metabolism, 324
Bone mineral density (BMD), 367

Bone remodeling, 143, 367
Bone tumors, 362–367
    benign, 363–364
    classification of, 362
    common, 364
    diagnosis of, 362
    malignant, 364–367
    presentation of, 362
    primary, 362, 363–367
    prognosis for, 363
    secondary, 362
    treatment of, 363
Bone turnover, hypercalcemia due to
        increased, 144
Bony labyrinth, 462, 463
Bony metastases, 362
Borderline personality disorder, 558, 561
Bortezomib, 317
Bosentan, 775, 820
Bouchard nodes, 373
Boutonnière deformity, 374
Bowen disease, 734
Bowenoid papulosis, 734
Bowman capsule
    histology of, 590, 591–592
    physiology of, 607
Bowman space, 592
Boyle's law, 761
BP (blood pressure)
    determinants of, 35–37
    regulation of, 37–40, 41, 444
BPH (benign prostatic hyperplasia), 590, 680,
        738–739
Brachial plexus
    anatomy of, 351
    lesions of, 496
Brachialis muscle, 349
Brachioradialis muscle, 349
Brachydactyly, 332
Bradyarrhythmias, 46–49
Bradycardia, 42
    sinus, 42, 46–47
Bradycardia-tachycardia syndrome, 47
Bradykinin, 603, 611
Brain, 412–446
    blood supply to, 422–423
    brain stem of, 440–445
    Brodmann areas of, 425, 427
    cerebellum of, 437–440
    cerebral cortex of, 425–431
    congenital malformations of, 414–418
    deep structures of, 431–436
        basal ganglia as, 431–432
        hypothalamus as, 435–436
        internal capsule as, 434–435
        thalamus as, 432–434
    development of, 414
    dural veins and sinuses of, 424–425
    meninges of, 419–420
    neurotransmitters in, 445
    primary neoplasms of, 490–492
    ring-enhancing lesions of, 58
    ventricles of, 420
    ventricular system of, 420–422
Brain abscess, 505
Brain natriuretic peptide (BNP), 611
Brain stem, 440–445
    lesions of, 501
    medulla of, 444–445
    midbrain of, 440, 441
    pons of, 440–444
    vascular lesions of, 478
Brain vesicles, 414, 416
Branchial arches, 138
Branchial clefts, 137, 348
Branchial cysts, 137

Branchial membranes, 137
Branchial pouches, 137–138, 139, 140
BRCA mutation, 717
Breast(s)
    anatomy of, 679–680, 681, 682
    development of, 672, 685
    disorders of, 727–731
        benign, 727–728
        malignant, 727, 728–731
    Paget disease of, 729, 730
Breast budding, 672, 685
Breast cancer, 727, 728–731
    in situ, 680, 729
    invasive, 729–731
        ductal, 729–731
        lobular, 731
    obesity and, 687
    Paget disease of breast as, 729, 730
    presentation of, 728–729
    treatment for, 729
Breast milk, 698
Breast-feeding, 698
Breath sounds, 780
Breathing during respiratory cycle, 766–769
Breathing motion, paradoxical, 758
Brenner tumor, 718
Brevicollis, 330
Bridging veins, 419, 424
Brief psychotic disorder, 546
Broad ligament, 671, 672, 680
Broca aphasia, 430, 431, 480
Broca area, 427
Brodmann areas, 425, 427
Bromocriptine, 125, 528–529
Bronchial arteries, 754, 756
Bronchial hamartoma, 348, 806
Bronchial neuroendocrine tumors, 805–806
Bronchial veins, 755
Bronchiectasis, 788–790
Bronchioles
    anatomy of, 756
    congenital cysts of, 753
    development of, 749
    terminal, 756
Bronchitis, chronic, 786–787
Bronchoalveolar adenocarcinoma (BAC),
        804–805
Bronchoconstriction, 787
Bronchogenic carcinoma, 807
Bronchopneumonia, 809, 810
Bronchopulmonary lymph node, 756
Bronchopulmonary segments, 754, 756
Bronchus(i)
    anatomy of, 754, 756
    development of, 749
    respiratory, 756
Brown-Séquard syndrome, 453, 454, 455,
        494–496
Brudzinski sign, 420
Brunner glands, 202
Brush border, 200, 202, 203
Buccopharyngeal membrane, 412
Buck fascia, 674, 676
Budd-Chiari syndrome, 245
Buerger disease, 83, 398, 403, 634
Buffer(s), 615–616, 617
Buffer systems, 616–617
Bulbourethral gland, 676
Bulbus cordis, 2
Bulimia nervosa, 563, 564
Bulla, 389
Bullous pemphigoid, 393
Bumetanide, 93, 94, 656, 657
Bundle branch(es), 14, 15
Bundle branch block (BBB), 44–45
Bundle of His, 14, 15

Bundle of Kent, 49
Buprenorphine, 515–516, 574
Bupropion, 519, 541
Burkitt lymphoma, 297, 301
Bursitis
    pes anserine, 353
    prepatellar, 353
Burton lines, 277
Buserelin, 741
Buspirone, 516, 540
Busulfan, 311–312
BZD(s) (benzodiazepines), 513, 515, 532, 540
    and sleep disorders, 565
BZD (benzodiazepine) use disorder, 570, 572

C

C. See Compliance (C)
C (parafollicular) cells, 126, 127
C3 nephritic factor (C3NeF), 627
C5 root, damage to, 350
C6 root, damage to, 350
C8 root, damage to, 350
Ca^{2+}. See Calcium (Ca^{2+})
CA-125, 717
Cabergoline, 125
CABG (coronary artery bypass graft), 86
Cachexia, cancer, 310
Café-au-lait macules, 493
Caffeine and sleep disorders, 565
Caffeine use disorder, 572
CAH (congenital adrenal hyperplasia), 150,
        157
CAIS (complete androgen insensitivity), 702
Calcaneofibular ligament, 345
Calcarine fissure, 426
Calcitonin, 137, 143
    for bone disorders, 402–403
    in bone metabolism, 324
    for osteoporosis, 368
    pharmacologic use of, 146
    synthesis of, 126
Calcitriol, 142, 143, 146
Calcium (Ca^{2+})
    distribution of total body, 139, 151
    intracellular and extracellular
        concentrations of, 15–16
    renal reabsorption of, 612
        during pregnancy, 694
    serum, 362
    small intestinal absorption of, 202
Calcium (Ca^{2+}) channel(s), 466
    in excitation-contraction coupling, 20–21
    voltage-gated, 16–17
        in myocardial contraction and
            relaxation, 22
Calcium (Ca^{2+}) channel blockers
    for angina pectoris, 86, 100, 101
    for arrhythmias, 104
    for hypertension, 97–98
Calcium (Ca^{2+}) deficiency, 369
Calcium (Ca^{2+}) disorders, 144–146
Calcium drugs, 146
Calcium gluconate for hyperkalemia, 18
Calcium (Ca^{2+}) homeostasis, 139–143
Calcium (Ca^{2+})-induced calcium (Ca^{2+})
        release, 467
    in excitation-contraction coupling, 20–21
    in myocardial contraction and relaxation, 22
Calcium (Ca^{2+}) influx
    in excitation-contraction coupling, 20–21
    in myocardial contraction and relaxation, 22
Calcium oxalate stones, 636, 637
Calcium phosphate stones, 636, 637
Calcium pyrophosphate dihydrate deposition
        disease (CPPD), 376–377
Calcium (Ca^{2+}) sequestration, 145–146

Calcium-containing antacids, 260, 261
Calciuria, idiopathic, 613
Calmodulin in excitation-contraction coupling, 358
Caloric nystagmus, 442–444
cAMP (cyclic adenosine monophosphate), 110
    in insulin secretion, 160
    urinary, 612
Camper fascia, 674
Canagliflozin, 169
Canalicular period, 748, 750
c-ANCA (cytoplasmic antineutrophil cytoplasmic antibody), 82, 361
Cancer cachexia, 310
Cancer immunotherapy, 317
Candesartan, 659
Candida albicans, 732
Candidiasis
    oral, 210, 211
    vaginal, 732
Cannabis use disorder, 576
"Cannon" a (atrial) waves, 48
Capacitance, 34
Capacitated sperm, 691
Capillaries, 33
Capillary fluid exchange, 35
Capillary hydrostatic pressure, 35
Capillary oncotic pressure, 35
Capitate, 339
Caplan syndrome, 795
Captopril, 99, 102, 659
"Caput medusae" sign, 8
Carbachol, 511
Carbamazepine, 525
Carbidopa, 529
Carbohydrate(s), small intestinal absorption of, 202
Carbohydrate metabolism in muscle contraction, 358
Carbon dioxide (CO_2) transport, 771, 772
Carbon monoxide (CO) poisoning, 771
Carbonic acid, 609
Carbonic anhydrase, 197, 771
Carbonic anhydrase inhibitors, 95, 655, 656–657
Carboplatin, 311
Carboxypeptidase, 206
Carcinoembryonic antigen (CEA), 235
Carcinoid syndrome, 59–60, 235, 806
Carcinoid tumors, 59–60, 235
    bronchial, 805–806
Carcinoma, 309
Carcinoma in situ
    cervical, 713–714
    ductal, 680, 729
    lobular, 680, 729
Carcinomatous meningitis, 420
Cardia of stomach, 196
Cardiac action potentials, 15, 16–20
    and cardiac pacemakers, 17–18
    conduction velocity of, 18–19
    fast-response (ventricular), 16, 17, 18
    refractory period of, 19–20
    slow-response (pacemaker), 16–17, 18
Cardiac catheterization, 90
Cardiac conduction system, 13–14, 15
Cardiac cycle, 29–32
    arterial pressure during, 36, 37
    heart sounds in, 31–32
    pressure tracings during, 30–31
    Wiggers diagram of, 29–30
Cardiac defect associations, congenital, 7
Cardiac electrophysiology, 14–20
    anatomy of conduction system in, 14–15
    cardiac action potentials in, 15, 16–20
    cardiac pacemakers in, 17–18

conduction velocity in, 18–19
    refractory period in, 19–20
    resting membrane potential in, 15–16
Cardiac function curves, 27–29
Cardiac glycosides, 102, 103
Cardiac murmurs. *See* Heart murmurs
Cardiac muscle
    anatomy of, 347
    contraction of, 20–23
    development of, 333
Cardiac myocytes, 14–15, 17–18
    characteristics of, 20
    contraction of, 20–23
Cardiac myxoma, 73
Cardiac output (CO), 23–26
    afterload in, 24
    contractility (inotropy) in, 25
    defined, 23
    determinants of, 24–26
    ejection fraction and, 23
    Fick's, 23
    Frank-Starling relationship in, 25–26
    length-tension relationship in, 25
    and mean arterial pressure, 35, 37
    normal resting, 23
    during pregnancy, 693
    preload in, 25, 28
    and pulmonary vascular resistance, 774
    stroke volume and, 23, 24
    and venous return, 28
Cardiac pacemakers, 17–18
Cardiac rhabdomyoma, 73
Cardiac tamponade, 11, 79–80
Cardiac traumatic hemolytic anemia, 287
Cardiac tumors, 73
Cardinal ligament, 671, 672
Cardinal veins, 2
Cardiogenic shock, 78
Cardiomegaly, 9, 90
Cardiomyopathy, 61–63
    defined, 61
    dilated, 61–62, 63
    hypertrophic, 62–63, 71
        obstructive, 10, 11
    nonischemic, 62
    restrictive, 62, 63
Cardiovascular (CV) disorders, 52–89
    aneurysms as, 66–67
    arteriosclerosis as, 54–57
    cardiac tumors as, 73
    cardiomyopathies as, 61–63
    chronic ischemic heart disease as, 89
    congestive heart failure as, 63–65
    coronary steal phenomenon as, 86
    emboli as, 76–77
    endocarditis as, 58–60
    heart murmurs as, 67–73
    hypertension as, 52–54
    ischemic heart disease as, 85–86
    myocardial infarction as, 87–89
    myocarditis as, 57
    pericardial disease as, 78–81
    peripheral vascular disease as, 81–85
    rheumatic fever as, 60–61
    shock as, 77–78
    venous disease as, 73–75
Cardiovascular (CV) system, 1–106
    anatomy of, 9–14
        conduction system in, 13–14
        coronary artery in, 12–13
        heart valves and sites of auscultation in, 10, 11
        layers of heart in, 10–12
        relationship of heart and great vessels in, 10
        surfaces and borders of heart in, 9–10

disorders of. *See* Cardiovascular (CV) disorders
    embryology of, 2–9
        congenital cardiac defect associations in, 7
        congenital heart lesions in, 4–7
        development of heart in, 2–4
        fetal circulation in, 8–9, 696–698
        fetal erythropoiesis in, 8
        fetal-postnatal derivatives in, 8
    imaging/diagnostic tests of, 90–91
    pharmacology of, 91–105
        antianginal therapy in, 100–101
        antiarrhythmics in, 16, 103, 104
        antihypertensive agents in, 91–100
        drugs used in heart failure in, 101–103
        lipid-lowering agents in, 103, 105
    physiology of, 14–52
        arrhythmias in, 46–52
        cardiac and vascular function curves in, 27–29
        cardiac cycle in, 29–32
        cardiac electrophysiology in, 14–20
        cardiac muscle and contraction in, 20–23
        cardiac output in, 23–26
        electrocardiography in, 40–45
        hemodynamics and peripheral vascular circulation in, 32–35, 36
        measurement and regulation of arterial pressure in, 35–40
        pressure-volume loops in, 26–27
    during pregnancy, 693, 695
Cardioversion, 52
Carmustine, 311
Carotid bodies in control of respiration, 779
Carpal bones, 338, 339
Carpal tunnel injury, 350
Carrier-mediated diffusion, 595
Cartilaginous joints, 343–344
Carvedilol, 96–97, 102
Casts, urinary, 623
Catalase, 57
Cataracts, 502
Catatonia, 536
Catatonic features, major depressive disorder with, 548
Catecholamines, effect on pacemaker action potentials of, 18
Catechol-O-methyltransferase (COMT) inhibitors, 530
Cauda equina, 447
Cauda equina syndrome, 448, 456
Caudal artery, 158
Caudate nucleus, 431, 432, 434
Cavernous artery, 677
Cavernous hemangioma, 250
Cavernous sinus, 424, 425
Cavernous sinus syndrome, 425, 501
CBG (corticosteroid-binding globulin), 109
CBT (cognitive behavioral therapy), 539
CCK (cholecystokinin), 196, 204, 209
CCMS (countercurrent multiplier system), 609–610
CD (Crohn disease), 230
CD20 antibody, molecular therapy targeting, 317
CDH (congenital diaphragmatic hernia), 333, 752, 753
CEA (carcinoembryonic antigen), 235
Cecum, 173
Celecoxib, 407
Celiac artery, anastomoses with, 187
Celiac disease, 200, 224
Celiac ganglia, 189
Celiac sprue, 224, 225
Celiac trunk, 147, 158, 172, 184, 185, 186

Cell body, 464
Cell cycle–independent chemotherapy drugs, 311
Cellular casts, 623
Cellulitis, 391, 392
Celomic metaplasia, 723
Central artery of the retina, 422
Central diabetes insipidus, 122, 123, 125–126, 435
Central lobule, 437
Central nervous system (CNS) lymphoma, primary, 496
Central nervous system (CNS) neurotransmitters, 507–508
Central pontine myelinolysis (CPM), 124, 444, 488, 497, 651
Central retinal artery, 459, 460, 502
Central retinal vein, 459, 460, 502
Central sleep apnea (CSA), 567, 803
Central sulcus, 418, 425, 426
Central venous pressure (CVP) and mean arterial pressure, 35
Centrally acting sympatholytics, 97
Cephalic phase of gastric secretion, 197
Cerebellar glomeruli, 437
Cerebellar lesions, degenerative diseases due to, 481, 484
Cerebellar peduncles, 437
Cerebellar tonsil(s), 437
herniation of, 414–416, 504, 505
Cerebellopontine angle, 461
Cerebellum, 437–440
anatomy of, 437–438, 439
dysfunction and syndromes of, 439–440
layers of, 437, 439
major pathways of, 438
neurons and fibers of, 439
regional anatomy of, 437
Cerebral aqueduct (of Sylvius), 420, 421, 440, 469
congenital stenosis of, 470
Cerebral contusion, 489–490
Cerebral cortex, 425–431
in control of respiration, 779
degenerative diseases due to lesions of, 482–483
frontal lobe of, 425–427
occipital lobe of, 429
organization of, 425
parietal lobe of, 427–429
temporal lobe of, 429–431
Cerebral edema, 488
Cerebral herniation, 503–505
Cerebrospinal fluid (CSF), 420, 468, 469
in meningitis, 420
Cerebrovascular disorders, 473–478
embolic stroke (hemorrhagic infarction) as, 474–475
intracranial hemorrhage as, 475–476, 477
lacunar infarcts as, 476–478
stroke presentation by location of occlusion in, 478
thrombotic stroke (pale infarction) as, 473–474
Certolizumab, 404
Ceruloplasmin, 258
Cervical carcinoma
in situ, 713–714
invasive, 714–715
Cervical dysplasia, 713–714
Cervical dystonia, 348
Cervical intraepithelial neoplasia (CIN), 713–714
Cervical pathology, 713–715
Cervical vertebrae, 337
Cervicitis, acute, 715

Cervix, 672, 680
Cetirizine, 819
Cetrorelix, 741
Cetuximab, 315
Cevimeline, 511
CFU-GEMM (colony-forming unit–granulocyte, erythrocyte, monocyte/macrophage, megakaryocyte), 268
CFU-GM (colony-forming unit–granulocyte, macrophage), 268
cGMP (cyclic guanosine monophosphate), 110
Chagas disease, 57, 62
achalasia due to, 215
Chancroid, 731
Chandelier sign, 722
Charcot triad, 252, 442, 456
Charcot-Bouchard microaneurysms, 435
Charcot-Leyden crystals, 788
Charcot-Marie-Tooth disease, 499
Chauffer fracture, 342
Chediak-Higashi syndrome, 279
Chemoreceptor(s) in control of respiration, 779
Chemoreceptor trigger zone, 444
Chemotherapy drugs, 310–318
alkylating agents as, 310–312
antimetabolites as, 311, 312–313
cell cycle–independent, 311
classes of, 310, 311
common side effects of, 318
drugs that target tubulin as, 314
hormonal agents as, 315
microtubule inhibitors as, 311
native cytokines as, 318
targeted molecular therapeutics as, 315–317
targets of, 312
topoisomerase inhibitors as, 311, 313–314
Chest wall
outward recoil of, 767
palpation of, 781
Chewing reflex, 192
Cheyne-Stokes respirations, 803
CHF. See Congestive heart failure (CHF)
Chiari malformation, 414–417, 470, 471
Chief cells, 138–139, 140, 196
Child abuse, 581
Childhood psychiatric disorders, 577–581
attention deficit/hyperactivity disorder as, 579–580
child abuse as, 581
disruptive behavior disorders as, 578–579
intellectual disability as, 581
pervasive developmental disorders as, 577–578
selective mutism as, 581
separation anxiety disorder as, 580
Tourette disorder as, 580
Chlamydia, pneumonia due to, 811
Chlamydia trachomatis, 731
Chlordiazepoxide, 515, 540
Chloride (Cl-), small intestinal secretion of, 202
Chlorpheniramine, 818–819
Chlorpromazine, 520–521, 540
Chocolate cysts, 723
Cholangiocarcinoma, 250, 252
Cholangiopancreatography
endoscopic retrograde, 178, 251, 252
magnetic resonance, 178, 251, 252
Cholangitis, 252
primary sclerosing, 253
Cholecalciferol, 142, 143
Cholecystitis, 252
Cholecystokinin (CCK), 196, 204, 209
Choledocholithiasis, 252

Cholelithiasis, 208, 210, 250–252
Cholera toxin, 203
Cholescintigraphy, 252
Cholesterol
in bile synthesis, 209
during pregnancy, 694
in steroid hormone synthesis, 149
Cholesterol absorption inhibitors, 105
Cholesterol desmolase in steroid hormone synthesis, 149
Cholesterol embolism, 76
Cholesterol ester hydrolase, 206
Cholesterol stones, 250, 251
Cholestyramine, 105
Choline acetyltransferase, 507, 508
Cholinesterase inhibitors, 511
Cholinomimetic agents, 511
Chondroma, 308
Chondrosarcoma, 363, 364–365
Chordoma, 329
Chorea, 478, 479
Choriocarcinoma, 695
ovarian, 712, 719, 720
testicular, 737, 738
Chorionic plate, 697
Chorionicity, 698
Choroid, 502
Choroid plexus, 420, 469
Christmas disease, 293
Chromatid, 682, 683
Chromatolysis, 465
Chromophobe(s), 112
Chromophobe renal carcinomas, 647
Chronic bronchitis, 786–787
Chronic disease, anemia of, 282–283
Chronic eosinophilic pneumonia, 798
Chronic granulocytic leukemia, 297, 303–304
Chronic granulomatous disease, 279
Chronic ischemic heart disease (CIHD), 89
Chronic kidney disease (CKD), 640, 642–643
Chronic kidney injury (CKI), 640, 642–643
Chronic lymphocytic leukemia (CLL), 300, 302
Chronic myelogenous leukemia (CML), 297, 303–304
Chronic obstructive pulmonary disease (COPD), 783, 786. See also Chronic bronchitis; Emphysema
Chronic renal failure, 640, 642–643
Churg-Strauss syndrome, 84, 400–401, 403
Chvostek sign, 145
Chylomicrons, 203
Chylothorax, 815
Chyme, 196–197, 200
Chymotrypsin, 206
Chymotrypsinogen, 206
Cigarette smoking
and emphysema, 784
and lung cancer, 804
Ciguatoxin, 513
CIHD (chronic ischemic heart disease), 89
Cilia of respiratory epithelium, 759
Ciliary body, 502
Ciliary dyskinesia, primary, 2, 760, 789
Ciliary ganglion, 462
Cilostazol, 321
Cimetidine, 199, 258–259
CIN (cervical intraepithelial neoplasia), 713–714
Cingulate gyrus, 426
Cingulate herniation, 504, 505
Circadian rhythm sleep disorder, 566
Circle of Willis, 422–424
Circulation
co-dominant, 13
enterohepatic, 207

fetal, 8–9, 696–698
left-dominant, 13
peripheral vascular, 32–35, 36
pulmonary, 773–775
right-dominant, 13
Circumferential thought, 535
Cirrhosis, 244–246
primary biliary, 246–247
Cis deletion, 276
Cisplatin, 311
Citalopram, 517, 540
CJD (Creutzfeldt-Jakob disease), 483
CK (creatine kinase), 361
CKD (chronic kidney disease), 640, 642–643
CKI (chronic kidney injury), 640, 642–643
CK-MB (creatine kinase MB isoenzyme), 88, 361
Cl⁻ (chloride), small intestinal secretion of, 202
Clang associations, 535
Clara cells, 759
Clarke nucleus, 438
Claustrum, 431
Clavicle, fracture of, 341
Clear cell adenocarcinoma, vaginal, 713
Clear cell carcinoma
of endometrium, 725
renal, 647
Clearance ratio, 599
Cleft foot, 331
Cleft hand, 331
Climbing fibers, 439
Clinodactyly, 331
Clitoris, development of, 671, 673
CLL (chronic lymphocyte leukemia), 300, 302
Cloacal membrane, 412
Clodronate, 402
Clofibrate, 105
Clomiphene, 745
Clomipramine, 518, 540
Clonazepam, 540
Clonidine, 97
Clopidogrel, 321
Clostridium difficile, pseudomembranous colitis due to, 231
Clostridium tetani, 357
Clotting factor deficiencies, 293–294
Clozapine, 521, 540
CLP (common lymphoid progenitor), 268
Clubfoot, congenital, 331
Clue cells, 733
CML (chronic myelogenous leukemia), 297, 303–304
CMP (common myeloid progenitor), 268
CNS (central nervous system) lymphoma, primary, 496
CNS (central nervous system) neurotransmitters, 507–508
CO (cardiac output). *See* Cardiac output (CO)
CO (carbon monoxide) poisoning, 771
CO₂ (carbon dioxide) transport, 771, 772
Coagulation, disseminated intravascular, 291, 292, 294
Coagulation cascade, 292
Coagulation factor inhibitors, 294
Coal worker's pneumoconiosis (CWP), 794, 795, 796
Coarctation of the aorta, 6
hypertension due to, 53, 54
Cobalamin, small intestinal absorption of, 203
Cocaine, pupillary response to, 568
Cocaine use disorder, 572, 573
Coccidioidomycosis, pneumonia due to, 812
Coccyx, 329, 337
Cochlear duct, 462

Cochlear nerve, 461, 462
Cochlear nuclei, 462
Cocked state, 356
Codeine, 515–516
Codman triangle, 366
Co-dominant circulation, 13
Cognitive behavioral therapy (CBT), 539
Cognitive disorders, 539–543
amnestic, 543
delirium as, 539–542
dementia as, 542–543
Colchicine, 404–405
Cold agglutinin immune hemolytic anemia, 280, 281
Cold caloric testing, 442–443
Colestipol, 105
Colic arteries, 186
Colipase, 206
Colitis
defined, 229
infectious, 231–232
pseudomembranous, 231
ulcerative, 230
Collagen synthesis, 328
Collecting ducts
histology of, 593
physiology of, 609, 610
Collecting system
development of, 584
duplex, 586
Collecting tubules
histology of, 590, 591, 593
physiology of, 607–610
Colles fascia, 674, 676, 681
Colles fracture, 342, 344, 367
Colloid, 127
Colloid carcinoma of breast, 730
Colon
in bilirubin production, 209
congenital mega-, 172, 229
development of, 173
diverticular disease of, 226–228
Hirschsprung disease of, 229
inflammatory diseases of, 229–232
Crohn disease and ulcerative colitis as, 230
infectious colitis as, 231–232
pseudomembranous colitis as, 231
intussusception of, 228
malabsorption syndromes of, 224–225
omphalocele of, 229
physiology of, 204–205
sigmoid, 184
tumors of, 232–235
adenomatous polyps as, 233
benign polyps as, 232–233
carcinoid tumors as, 235
colorectal cancer as, 234–235
polyposis syndromes as, 233–234
Colon cancer, hereditary nonpolyposis, 233, 234
Colony-forming unit–granulocyte erythrocyte, monocyte/macrophage, megakaryocyte (CFU-GEMM), 268
macrophage (CFU-GM), 268
Colorectal cancer, 234–235
Coma, myxedema, 133
Combined motor and sensory lesions, 455–456
Combined upper and lower motor neuron lesions, 455, 457
Comminuted fractures, 340
Common bile duct, 208
Common carotid artery, 682
Common fibular nerve damage, 353
Common hepatic artery, 158, 186
Common hepatic duct, 208

Common iliac arteries, 184, 185, 589
Common iliac vein, 187
Common lymphoid progenitor (CLP), 268
Common myeloid progenitor (CMP), 268
Common peroneal nerve, 352
damage to, 353, 495
Compact bone, 325, 335
Compartment syndrome, 343, 345–346
anterior, 495
Compensation states, 618, 621
Complete androgen insensitivity (CAIS), 702
Complete atrioventricular (AV) block, 14, 48–49
Complete block, 44
Complete mole, 711–712
Complex seizure, 489
Compliance (C), 34
lung, 766, 784
of lung–chest wall system, 766, 767
venodilators and, 29
Compliance curve, 26
Compression fracture, vertebral, 367
Compulsions, 536, 554
COMT (catechol-O-methyltransferase) inhibitors, 530
Concentration, 595
Concrete thinking, 535
Conduct disorder, 578–579
Conducting airways, 754, 755, 758–759
Conducting cells, 14–15
Conduction aphasia, 431
Conduction blocks, 14, 47–49
Conduction deafness, 463
Conduction system of heart, 13–14, 15
Conduction velocity, 18–19
Condyloid joints, 343
Condylomata acuminata, 712–713, 732
Cones, 459
Confluence of the sinuses, 424
Congenital adrenal hyperplasia (CAH), 150, 157
Congenital diaphragmatic hernia (CDH), 333, 752, 753
Congenital heart lesions, 4–7
acyanotic, 6–7
cyanotic, 4–5
Congenital hip dislocation, 332
Congenital malformations
of gastrointestinal tract, 174–178
duodenal atresia as, 176–177
esophageal atresia with tracheoesophageal fistula as, 176
extrahepatic biliary atresia as, 177
gastroschisis as, 174–175
intestinal malrotation and volvulus as, 175–176
omphalocele as, 174
pancreas divisum as, 177–178
post-duodenal atresia as, 177
pyloric stenosis as, 177
of reproductive system
early, 662, 666
female, 673
male, 669, 734–735
of respiratory system, 751–753
skeletal
involving osteogenesis, 326–328
of limbs, 331–332
of ribs, 331
of skull, 328–329
of vertebral column, 329–330
Congenital megacolon, 172, 229
Congestive heart failure (CHF), 63–65
classification of, 102
defined, 63
left-sided, 63–65

Congestive heart failure (continued)
  pathophysiology of, 65
  portal hypertension with, 245
  due to renal failure, 643
  right-sided, 65
Conivaptan, 126
Conjoined tendon, 182
Conjugate gaze, 503, 504
Conn syndrome, 154–156
  hypertension due to, 53
Connective tissue disorders, 377–389
  aneurysms due to, 66
  drugs used to treat, 406
  laboratory values pertinent to, 361–362
  mixed, 385–386
  muscular dystrophy as, 388–389
  polymyositis and dermatomyositis as,
    387–388
  sarcoidosis as, 383–384
  scleroderma/systemic sclerosis as, 385
  seronegative spondyloarthropathies as,
    377–380
  Sjögren syndrome as, 386–387
  systemic lupus erythematosus as, 380–383
Consciousness, 444
Consolidation, 816
Constipation
  opioid-induced, 576
  during pregnancy, 693
Continuous positive airway pressure (CPAP),
    769, 803
Contractile cells, 14–15
Contractility
  autonomic effects on, 39
  and blood pressure, 37
  factors affecting, 23, 24
  Frank-Starling relationship and, 25–26
  length-tension relationship and, 25
  and pressure-volume loop, 27
Contralateral neglect, 428
Contrast nephropathy, 642
Contrecoup fracture, 340
Contrecoup injuries, 489
Conus medullaris, 447
Conus medullaris syndrome, 448, 456
Conversion disorder, 537, 554, 555–556
Coombs test, 280
Cooper ligaments, 680, 681
COPD (chronic obstructive pulmonary
    disease), 783, 786. See also Chronic
    bronchitis; Emphysema
Coporphobilinogen, 288
Copper in wound healing, 361
Cor pulmonale, 787
Coracobrachialis muscle, 349
Cornea, 502
Corona radiata, 684, 687, 691, 692
Coronal suture, 328, 329, 335, 336
Coronary angioplasty, percutaneous
    transluminal, 86
Coronary artery, 12–13, 14
Coronary artery bypass graft (CABG), 86
Coronary artery vasospasm, 86
Coronary perfusion pressure, 69
Coronary sinus, 12
Coronary steal phenomenon, 86
Coronary syndrome, acute, 13
  electrocardiography of, 45
Coronary thrombus, 13
Coronoid process, 336
Corpus albicans, 687, 688
Corpus callosum, 426, 431
Corpus cavernosum, 676, 677
Corpus luteum, 686, 687, 688
Corpus luteum cysts, 717
Corpus spongiosum, 676, 677

Corrected reticulocyte count (CRC), 288
Cortex, 418
Cortical nephrons, 593
Corticobulbar tract, 442
Corticopontine tract, 438, 440
Corticospinal tracts, 440, 442, 449, 450–451
Corticosteroid(s)
  for asthma, 822
  for connective tissue disorders, 406
  synthetic (exogenous), 151
  for systemic lupus erythematosus, 155–156
Corticosteroid-binding globulin (CBG), 109
Corticotropin-releasing hormone (CRH), 113,
    147, 150
Corticotropin-releasing hormone (CRH)
    stimulation test, 154
Cortisol, 147, 150, 151–152
Costodiaphragmatic recess, 755
Costophrenic angle, 755
Cotransport, 596
Countercurrent exchanger, 610
Countercurrent multiplier system (CCMS),
    609–610
Countertransference, 536–537
Countertransport, 596
Count-off method to measure heart rate on
    ECG, 42
Coup injuries, 489
Coupling in thyroid hormone synthesis, 129
Cowden syndrome, 233
Cowper gland, 676
Coxa valga, 343, 344
Coxa vara, 343, 344
Coxiella burnetii, pneumonia due to, 811
CPAP (continuous positive airway pressure),
    769, 803
C-peptide, 159
CPM (central pontine myelinolysis), 124, 444,
    488, 497, 651
CPPD (calcium pyrophosphate dihydrate
    deposition disease), 376–377
Crackles, 780, 809
Cranial nerve(s), 457–459
Cranial nerve lesions, 457, 458, 460
Cranial nerve palsy, 499–503
Craniopharyngioma, 436, 490, 491, 496
Craniosynostoses, 328
CRC (corrected reticulocyte count), 288
C-reactive protein (CRP), 56, 361
Creatine kinase (CK), 361
Creatine kinase MB isoenzyme (CK-MB),
    88, 361
Creatinine, 601–602
Creatinine clearance, 602
Cremasteric muscle and fascia, 182, 677, 678
Cremasteric reflex, 677
Crepitus, 781
Crescent formation in rapidly progressive
    glomerulonephritis, 632, 633
CREST syndrome, 385
Cretinism, 133, 327, 694
Creutzfeldt-Jakob disease (CJD), 483
CRH (corticotropin-releasing hormone), 113,
    147, 150
CRH (corticotropin-releasing hormone)
    stimulation test, 154
Cribriform plate, 459
  foramina of, 336
Cricoarytenoid joints, 348
Cricoarytenoid muscles, 348
Cricoid cartilage, 749
Cricothyroid muscles, 348
Crigler-Najjar syndrome, 238, 241–242
Crohn disease (CD), 230
Cross-bridges, 356
Croup, 814

CRP (C-reactive protein), 56, 361
Crush injury, 652
Cryoglobulinemic vasculitis, 85
Cryptococcus neoformans, 812
Cryptorchidism, 669, 734–735, 737
Cryptosporidia, 232
Cryptosporidiosis, 232
Crypts of Lieberkühn, 200, 201, 202
CSA (central sleep apnea), 567, 803
CSF (cerebrospinal fluid), 420, 468, 469
  in meningitis, 420
Culmen, 437
Cuneate fasciculus, 449, 451, 452
Cuneus, 426
Curling ulcers, 220
Curschmann spirals, 788
Cushing disease, 152, 154
Cushing reflex, 489
Cushing response, 489
Cushing syndrome, 152, 153–154, 155
  hypertension due to, 53
  paraneoplastic, 310
  vessel wall abnormalities due to, 295
Cushing triad, 489
Cushing ulcers, 220
Cutaneous innervation, 447
Cutaneous T-cell lymphomas, 299, 301
CV. See Cardiovascular (CV)
CVP (central venous pressure) and mean
    arterial pressure, 35
CWP (coal worker's pneumoconiosis), 794,
    795, 796
Cyanosis, 4, 5, 7
Cyanotic congenital heart lesions, 4–5
Cyclic adenosine monophosphate
    (cAMP), 110
  in insulin secretion, 160
  urinary, 612
Cyclic guanosine monophosphate
    (cGMP), 110
Cyclooxygenase-2 inhibitors, 407
Cyclophosphamide, 84, 310–311, 406
Cyclothymic disorder, 550
Cyst(s)
  Baker, 353, 374
  bone, 372
  chocolate, 723
  congenital bronchiolar, 753
  dermoid, 720
  follicular, 717
Cystadenocarcinoma
  mucinous, 718
  serous, 718
Cystadenoma, 309
  mucinous, 718
  serous, 718
Cystic duct, 208
Cystic fibrosis, 205, 789
Cystic kidney disease, 643–645
Cystic teratoma, 720
Cystine stones, 636, 637
Cytarabine, 313
Cytokines
  in bone metabolism, 325
  in cancer treatment, 318
  immune, 788
Cytoplasmic antineutrophil cytoplasmic
    antibody (c-ANCA), 82, 361
Cytotrophoblasts, 696, 697

D

D cells, 196, 204
Dacrocytes, 273, 307
Dactylitis in psoriatic arthritis, 380
Danazol, 745
Dandy-Walker malformation/syndrome, 417,
    470

Dantrolene, 467, 531
Dapagliflozin, 169
Darrow-Yannet diagram, 599
Dasatinib, 317
DCIS (ductal carcinoma in situ), 680, 729
DCN (diffuse cortical necrosis), 639–640
DCT (distal convoluted tubule)
    histology of, 590, 591, 593
    physiology of, 608–609, 610
DDH (developmental dysplasia of the hip),
        333–334
D-dimer level, 800
DDP-4 (dipeptidyl peptidase 4) inhibitors, 169
de Quervain thyroiditis, 132, 133
Dead space
    alveolar, 763
    anatomic, 763
    physiologic (total), 763, 777
Deafness, 463
Decidua basalis, 697
Declive, 437
Deep cerebellar nuclei, 438
Deep inguinal ring, 182
Deep peroneal nerve, 352
Deep tendon reflexes, 447–448, 449
Deep venous thrombosis (DVT), 74–75,
        798–799
Defense mechanisms, 537–538
Defibrillation, 52
Degenerative diseases, 480–485
    Alzheimer disease as, 482
    amyotrophic lateral sclerosis as, 481
    due to basal ganglia lesions, 484–485
    due to cerebellar lesions, 481, 484
    due to cerebral cortex lesions, 482–483
    dementia with Lewy bodies as, 483
    Friedreich ataxia as, 485
    frontotemporal dementia (Pick disease)
        as, 482
    Huntington disease as, 484
    due to motor neuron lesions, 481
    multi-infarct (vascular) dementia as, 479,
        483
    olivopontocerebellar atrophy as, 485
    Parkinson disease as, 484
    poliomyelitis as, 481
    prion diseases as, 483
    progressive supranuclear palsy as, 480–481
    due to spinocerebellar lesions, 485
    treatments for, 527–530
    Werdnig-Hoffman disease (infantile spinal
        muscular atrophy) as, 481
    Wilson disease (hepatolenticular
        degeneration) as, 481, 485
Deglutition, 194–195
Degmacyte, 273
Dehydroepiandrosterone (DHEA), 153, 689
Dehydroepiandrosterone sulfate (DHEA-S),
        147, 149, 153
Deiodinase, 129
Deiodination, 130
Dejerine-Roussy syndrome, 434
Delirium, 539–542
Delirium tremens (DTs), 570
Delta wave, 49
Delta-delta analysis, 621
δ cells, 159
Deltoid paralysis, 496
Delusions, 535, 543, 545
Demeclocycline, 126, 656
Dementia, 542–543
Dementia with Lewy bodies (DLB), 483
Demyelinating diseases, 481–488
    acute disseminated (postinfectious)
        encephalomyelitis as, 487
    acute inflammatory demyelinating
        polyradiculopathy as, 487–488

multiple sclerosis as, 481–484, 486
osmotic demyelination syndrome (central
        pontine myelinolysis) as, 488
progressive multifocal leukoencephalopathy
        as, 486
Dendrites, 461, 465
Dendritic cells, 271, 272
Denial, 538
Denosumab, 368
Dens, 329
Dentate nucleus, 438
Dentatorubrothalamic tract, 438
Denys-Drash syndrome, 649
11-Deoxycortisol, 151
Deoxyribonuclease, 206
Dependent personality disorder, 562
Depersonalization/derealization disorder, 559
Depolarization, 41, 42
Depolarizing agents, 509–510
Depressant use disorder, 568–571
Depressed fractures, 340
Depression
    postpartum, 548
    and sleep disorders, 565
Depressive disorder
    major, 546, 547–548, 549, 550
    persistent, 548
Derangement states, 618
Derealization disorder, 559
Dermatitis
    allergic contact, 389, 390
    atopic, 389, 390
    herpetiformis, 224, 393
    lupus, 380, 381
Dermatologic disorders. See Skin disorders
Dermatomes of hand, 351
Dermatomyositis (DM), 387–388
Dermoid cyst, 720
DES (diethylstilbestrol), 744
Descending colon, 173
Descending nucleus, 445
Descending sympathetic tract, 445
Descending tracts, 445, 449
Desensitization, 817
Desflurane, 531
Desipramine, 518, 540
Desloratadine, 819
Desmoplasia, 308
Desmopressin, 125, 658
Detrusor muscle, 589
Detumescence, 690, 691
Developmental dysplasia of the hip (DDH),
        333–334
DEXA (dual-energy X-ray absorptiometry)
        scans, 367–368
Dexamethasone suppression test (DST), 154,
        155
Dexlansoprazole, 259–260
α-Dextrinase, small intestinal secretion of, 202
Dextroamphetamine, 541
Dextrocardia, 2
Dextromethorphan, 515–516, 819–820
DHEA (dehydroepiandrosterone), 153, 689
DHEA-S (dehydroepiandrosterone sulfate),
        147, 149, 153
DHT (dihydrotestosterone) in sexual
        differentiation, 662
Diabetes, gestational, 694
Diabetes insipidus (DI), 122–123, 125–126
    central, 122, 123, 125–126, 435
    nephrogenic, 122, 123
Diabetes mellitus (DM), 162–164
    complications of, 163
    diagnosis of, 163
    during pregnancy, 159
    presentation of, 163

treatment of, 163, 166–169
    type 1, 159, 162, 166–167
    type 2, 162, 167–169
Diabetic ketoacidosis (DKA), 163–164
Diabetic mother, cardiac defects in offspring
        of, 7
Diabetic nephropathy, 163, 628, 629
Diabetic neuropathy, 163, 499
Diabetic polyradiculopathy, 497
Diabetic retinopathy, 163
Diagonal conjugate, 339
Dialysis, 640, 641
Diaphragm
    anatomy of, 754, 756–757
    development of, 333, 750, 751
    in inspiration, 765
    structures passing through, 353
Diaphragmatic hernia, congenital, 333, 752,
        753
Diarrhea, causes of, 231
Diastole, 27, 30
    pressure changes during, 30–31
    ventricular, 26, 27, 30
Diastolic pressure, 36–37
Diazepam, 515, 540
DIC (disseminated intravascular coagulation),
        291, 292, 294
Dictyate, 684
Dictyotene, 684
Diencephalon, 426
    development of, 111, 116
Diethylstilbestrol (DES), 744
Diffuse cortical necrosis (DCN), 639–640
Diffuse large-cell lymphoma, 300
Diffuse membranous glomerulopathy,
        626–627
Diffuse proliferative nephritis, 630
Diffusion
    carrier-mediated, 595
    simple, 595
Diffusion capacity of lung for carbon dioxide
        ($D_{L}CO$), 776–777
Diffusion impairment, hypoxemia due to
        decreased, 776
Diffusion-limited gas, 776
Digastric muscle, 348
DiGeorge syndrome, 4, 137, 145, 654
Digestive system. See Gastrointestinal (GI)
        system
Digital rectal exam (DRE), 739
Digitalis and contractility, 24
Digoxin, 102, 103
Dihydrogen phosphate ($H_2PO_4^-$), renal
        secretion of, 617
Dihydropyridines, 97
Dihydropyridine receptor, 355
Dihydrotestosterone (DHT) in sexual
        differentiation, 662
1,25-Dihydroxycholecalciferol [1,25-$(OH)_2$
        vitamin D], 142, 143, 611
Diiodotyrosine (DIT), 128
Dilated cardiomyopathy, 61–62, 63
Dilator pupillae muscle, 332
Diltiazem, 97–98, 101, 104
Dilution tests, 762–763
Dimenhydrinate, 818–819
"Dinner fork" deformity, 342, 344
Dipalmitoylphosphatidylcholine (DPPC), 764
Dipeptidyl peptidase 4 (DDP-4) inhibitors, 169
Diphenhydramine, 818–819
Diphenoxylate, 515–516
Diploid, 682, 683
Dipyridamole, 321
Direct Coombs test, 280
Direct factor Xa inhibitors, 319–320
Disaccharidase deficiency, 225

Disease-modifying antirheumatic drugs (DMARDs), 375
Dislocations
  atlantoaxial, 340
  radial head, 350
  of shoulder, 342, 350
  of vertebrae, 340
Disopyramide, 104
Disordered thinking, 543
Displacement, 538
Disruptive behavior disorders, 578–579
Disseminated intravascular coagulation (DIC), 291, 292, 294
Dissociation, 538
Dissociative amnesia, 559
Dissociative disorders, 558, 559
Dissociative fugue, 559
Dissociative identity disorder, 559
Distal convoluted tubule (DCT)
  histology of, 590, 591, 593
  physiology of, 608–609, 610
Distal radius, fracture of, 342, 344
Distributive shock, 78
DIT (diiodotyrosine), 128
Diuretics, 91–95, 655–658
  carbonic anhydrase inhibitors as, 95, 655, 656–657
  electrolyte changes associated with, 93–94
  for heart failure, 102
  loop, 93, 94, 608, 655, 656, 657
  osmotic, 94–95, 655, 656
  potassium-sparing, 93–94, 614, 655, 656, 657–658
  thiazide, 655, 657
    as antihypertensive agents, 92, 94
    electrolyte changes with, 656
    hypercalcemia due to, 144
    for idiopathic calciuria, 613
    renal mechanism of, 608
    side effects of, 609
Diverticular disease, intestinal, 226–228
Diverticulitis, 227–228
Diverticulosis, 226–227
Diverticulum(a)
  epiphrenic, 214
  esophageal, 214
  intestinal, 226–228
  Meckel, 172, 226
  midesophageal, 214
  pharyngoesophageal (Zenker), 214
Dizygotic twins, 697, 698, 699
DKA (diabetic ketoacidosis), 163–164
DLB (dementia with Lewy bodies), 483
DLCO (diffusion capacity of lung for carbon dioxide), 776–777
DM (dermatomyositis), 387–388
DM (diabetes mellitus). See Diabetes mellitus (DM)
DMARDs (disease-modifying antirheumatic drugs), 375
DNase (dornase alfa), 819
Dobutamine, 102–103
Docetaxel, 314
Donepezil, 527
Donovanosis, 732
Dopamine, 113, 446, 507, 508
  in regulation of renal blood flow and filtration, 603
Dopamine agonists, 125
Dornase alfa (DNase), 819
Dorsal acoustic stria, 462
Dorsal cochlear nucleus, 442, 462
Dorsal column lesions, 455
Dorsal column–medial lemniscus pathway, 451, 452
Dorsal interossei muscle, 351
Dorsal primary ramus, 332

Dorsal respiratory group, 778–779
Dorsal root ganglion cell, 452
Dorsal spinocerebellar tract, 445, 449
Dorsalis pedis (DP) artery, 352
Dorsomedial nucleus, 435, 436
Double uterus, 673
Double Y males, 701
"Double-bubble" sign, 176, 177
Double-tract sign, 177
Down syndrome
  cardiac defects in, 7
  duodenal atresia in, 176
  limb defects in, 331
Downregulation, 111
Doxacurium, 510
Doxazosin, 97
Doxepin, 518, 540
DP (dorsalis pedis) artery, 352
DPPC (dipalmitoylphosphatidylcholine), 764
DRE (digital rectal exam), 739
Dressler syndrome, 80
Drug-induced hypertension, 53
Drug-induced lupus, 383
DST (dexamethasone suppression test), 154, 155
DTs (delirium tremens), 570
Dual-energy X-ray absorptiometry (DEXA) scans, 367–368
Dubin-Johnson syndrome, 238, 240
Duchenne muscular dystrophy, 388
Ductal carcinoma in situ (DCIS), 680, 729
Ductus arteriosus, 9, 173, 698
  closure of, 696
  patent, 5, 6, 7, 8, 73, 697
Ductus deferens, 668
Ductus venosus, 8, 9, 173, 698
Duloxetine, 518–519, 540
Duodenal atresia, 176–177
Duodenal ulcers, 221–222
Duodenoduodenostomy, 177
Duodenojejunostomy, 177
Duodenum
  anatomy and histologic characteristics of, 199
  development of, 173
Duplex collecting system, 586
Dura mater, 419, 425, 469
Dural veins, 424–425
Dural venous sinuses, 424–425
DVT (deep venous thrombosis), 74–75, 798–799
Dwarfism, 325, 327
Dynamic hyperinflation in emphysema, 784
Dyneins, 2, 464
Dysgerminoma, 719
Dyskinesias, 478–479
Dyslexia, 428
Dysplasia, 308
Dyspnea, 779
Dyssomnias, 565, 566–567
Dyssynergia, 439
Dysthymic disorder, 548
Dystocia, 338
Dystrophin, 388

E

EA (esophageal atresia), 176, 213–214, 751–752
Eating disorders, 562–565
Eburnation, 372
EBV (Epstein-Barr virus), 310, 808
ECF. See Extracellular fluid (ECF)
ECG. See Electrocardiography (ECG)
Echocardiography, 90
ECL (enterochromaffin-like) cells, 196, 204
Eclampsia, 708
ECT (electroconvulsive therapy), 539, 549

Ectopia lentis, 328
Ectopic pregnancy, 691, 707
Ectopic rhythms, 51
ECV (extracellular circulating volume), 37
Eczema, 389, 390
Edema, 35, 36
  cerebral, 488
  exudative vs transudative, 35, 36
  in nephrotic syndrome, 624–625
  pitting, 65
  pulmonary, 90, 761, 792, 815, 816
Edinger-Westphal nucleus, 462
Edrophonium, 511
EDV (end-diastolic volume), 26
Edwards syndrome, 331
EF (ejection fraction), 23, 25
  heart failure with preserved, 64
  heart failure with reduced, 63–64
Effective refractory period (ERP), 19, 20
Effective renal plasma flow (ERPF), 604
Efferent arteriole in renal tubular system, 591, 602, 603, 605, 607, 610
Efferent ductules, 666, 667
EGFR (epidermal growth factor receptor), molecular therapy targeting, 315–316
Ego-dystonic response, 553
Egophony, 780, 809
Ehlers-Danlos syndrome, vessel wall abnormalities due to, 295
Eisenmenger syndrome, 7, 70, 778
Ejaculation, 690, 691
Ejaculatory duct, 667, 668, 676
Ejection fraction (EF), 23, 25
  heart failure with preserved, 64
  heart failure with reduced, 63–64
E_K (equilibrium potential), 15–16
E_K (Nernst potential), 15–16
Elastase, 206
  in emphysema, 784
Elastic recoil in emphysema, 784
Elbow
  golfer's, 349
  pulled (nursemaid's), 344
  tennis, 349
Elbow joints, 344
Electrical alternans, 79
Electrical axes of heart, 41
Electrocardiography (ECG), 40–45
  of acute coronary syndrome, 45
  golden rules of, 41–42
  heart rate in, 42–43
  heart rhythm in, 42
  interpretation of, 42–45
  intervals in, 42, 43
  leads in, 41
  mean QRS axis in, 43–44
  of myocardial infarction, 87, 88
  P-wave abnormalities in, 44
  QRS abnormalities in, 44–45
  waveforms in, 41–42
Electroconvulsive therapy (ECT), 539, 549
Electrolyte abnormalities, 650–654
  hypercalcemia as, 650, 653–654
  hyperkalemia as, 650, 651–652
  hypernatremia as, 650
  hypocalcemia as, 650, 653, 654
  hypokalemia as, 650, 652, 653
  hypomagnesemia as, 650, 654
  hyponatremia as, 650, 651
Elliptocyte, 273
Embolic stroke, 474–475
Emboliform nucleus, 438
Embolus(i) and embolism, 76–77
  amniotic fluid, 76, 77, 710, 800
  arterial, 77
  bacterial, 800

cholesterol, 76
defined, 76
fat, 76, 77, 800
gas (air), 76, 77, 800
paradoxical, 77
pulmonary, 75, 76–77, 799–801
hypoxemia due to, 777–778
saddle, 76–77
septic, 76
from endocarditis, 58, 59
thrombo-, 76, 800
tumor cell, 800
types of, 76
Embryonal carcinoma
ovarian, 719, 720
testicular, 738
Embryonal rhabdomyosarcoma variant, 713
Emesis, 195, 197
metabolic alkalosis due to, 619
Emotion, 430, 433
Emphysema, 784–786
causes of, 784, 785
centriacinar (centrilobular), 785, 786
vs chronic bronchitis, 786
defined, 784
diagnosis of, 785
diffusion impairment in, 776
lung compliance in, 766, 784
lung volumes and capacities in, 761
mechanics of breathing with, 768
panacinar (panlobar), 785
pathophysiology of, 784
presentation of, 785
prognosis for, 786
treatment of, 785
Empty sella syndrome (ESS), 112
Enalapril, 99, 659
Encephalitis, HIV, 165
Encephalomyelitis, acute disseminated
(postinfectious), 487
Encephalopathy(ies)
hepatic, 246
spongiform, 483
Enchondroma, 363, 364
Enchondromatosis, 363
End-diastolic volume (EDV), 26
Endemic mycoses, pneumonia due to, 812
Endocardial cushion(s), 2–3
Endocardial cushion defects, 3
Endocarditis, 58–60
in carcinoid syndrome, 59–60
defined, 58
infective (bacterial), 58–59, 61–62
Libman-Sacks, 59, 382
marantic (nonbacterial), 59
due to rheumatic fever, 60–61
right-sided, 58
septic emboli from, 58, 59
Endocardium, 11, 12
Endochondral ossification, 326–327
Endocrine disorders
of adrenal gland, 153–158
of pancreas
diabetes mellitus as, 162–164
insulinoma as, 164
islet cell tumors as, 165–166
of parathyroid gland, 144–146
pituitary disease as
anterior, 119–122
posterior, 122–124
of thyroid, 131–135, 136
Endocrine secretion, 108
Endocrine system, 107–170
adrenal gland in, 147–158
anatomy of, 147
disorders of, 153–158

embryology of, 147–148
histology of, 148–149
hormone synthesis and regulation by,
149–153
hypothalamus and pituitary in, 108–126
anterior pituitary disease of, 119–122
hormone basics of, 108–111
hypothalamic-pituitary axis for, 112–119
pharmacology of, 124–126
posterior pituitary disease of, 122–124
pancreas in, 158–169
anatomy of, 158
in diabetes mellitus, 162–164
embryology of, 159
vs exocrine, 108
and glucagon, 161–162
histology of, 159
and insulin, 159–161
insulinoma of, 164
islet cell tumors of, 165–166
pharmacology of, 166–169
and somatostatin, 162
parathyroid gland in, 137–146
anatomy of, 137, 138
in calcium and phosphate homeostasis,
139–146
disorders of, 144–146
embryology of, 137–138, 139, 140
histology of, 138–139
overview of, 137
pharmacology of, 146
during pregnancy, 694
thyroid in, 126–137
anatomy of, 126, 127
disorders of, 131–135, 136
embryology of, 127
histology of, 127, 128
overview of, 126
pharmacology of, 135–137
Endodermal sinus tumor, 719, 720
Endolymph, 463
Endolymphatic cavity, 462
Endometrial artery, 696, 697
Endometrial carcinoma, 725–726
Endometrial hyperplasia, 724–725
Endometrial vein, 696, 697
Endometrioid carcinoma, 718, 725
Endometrioma, 723
Endometriosis, 722–724
Endometritis, 722
Endometrium, 589, 672, 680
Endoneurium, 468
Endopelvic fascia, 681
Endoscopic retrograde
cholangiopancreatography (ERCP),
178, 251, 252
Endplate, 467
Entacapone, 530
Entamoeba histolytica, 232
Enteric nervous system, 190, 191
Enterochromaffin-like (ECL) cells, 196, 204
Enterocytes, 200, 202, 203
Enteroendocrine cells, 200
Enterohepatic circulation, 207
Enterokinase, 205
Enteropathy, gluten-sensitive, 224, 225
Enteropeptidase, 205
Enzyme markers of GI pathology, 255–258
alanine aminotransferase as, 256, 257
alkaline phosphatase as, 257
amylase as, 257
aspartate aminotransferase as, 255–256, 257
ceruloplasmin as, 258
γ-glutamyl transferase as, 256–257
lipase as, 258
prothrombin time as, 258

Eosinopenia, 296
Eosinophil(s), 268, 270, 271
Eosinophilia, 269
Eosinophilic granuloma, 306
Eosinophilic pneumonia, chronic, 798
Epaxial division, 332
Epaxial myotomes, 333
Ependymal cells, 465
Ependymoma, 490, 492, 494
Epi (epinephrine), 151, 507, 508
in regulation of renal blood flow and
filtration, 602
Epiblast, 266, 412
Epicardium, 11, 12
Epicondylitis, 349
Epidermal growth factor receptor (EGFR),
molecular therapy targeting,
315–316
Epidermis, 361
Epididymis, 667, 668, 676, 678
Epididymitis, 735
Epidural hematoma, 335, 337–338, 419
Epidural hemorrhage, 419, 475
Epidural space, 419
Epigastric region, 180, 181
Epiglottis, 749, 814
Epinephrine (Epi), 151, 507, 508
in regulation of renal blood flow and
filtration, 602
Epineurium, 468
Epiphrenic diverticula, 214
Epiphyseal plate, 325
Epiploic foramen, 184
Epispadias, 669
Epistaxis, 783
during pregnancy, 693
Epithelial cell casts, 623
Epithelial cell tumors, ovarian, 717–718
Epithelial tumors, 308
Eplerenone, 93–94, 656, 657–658
EPO (erythropoietin), 611
impaired responsiveness to, 282
EPO (erythropoietin) receptors, 611
Epoprostenol, 820
Epothilone, 314
Epstein-Barr virus (EBV), 310, 808
EPT (estrogen-progesterone therapy), 700
Eptifibatide, 321
Equilibrium potential (E_K), 15–16
Equivalent, 595
Erb palsy, 350, 496
ERBB2 protooncogene, 729
ERCP (endoscopic retrograde
cholangiopancreatography), 178,
251, 252
Erection, 689, 690, 691
Erector pili muscles, 347
Ergocalciferol, 142
Ergometrine, 744
Erlotinib, 315–316
ERP (effective refractory period), 19, 20
ERPF (effective renal plasma flow), 604
ERV (expiratory reserve volume), 761, 762
Erythema marginatum, 60
Erythema multiforme, 393
Erythema nodosum, 384
Erythroblastosis fetalis, 281, 710–711
Erythrocyte(s)
fetal, 8
formation of, 267–268, 269
forms of, 273–274
and oxidative stress, 278–279
Erythrocyte sedimentation rate (ESR), 361
Erythrocythemia, 306, 307
Erythroplasia of Queyrat, 734
Erythropoiesis, fetal, 8

Erythropoietin (EPO), 611
  impaired responsiveness to, 282
Erythropoietin (EPO) receptors, 611
Escape rhythms, 51
Escitalopram, 517, 540
Esmolol, 96–97, 104
Esomeprazole, 259–260
Esophageal atresia (EA), 176, 213–214,
    751–752
Esophageal cancer, 219
Esophageal closure, 751
Esophageal disorder(s), 213–219
  achalasia as, 215–216
  Barrett esophagus as, 217–219
  Boerhaave syndrome as, 215
  esophageal atresia and tracheoesophageal
      fistula as, 213–214
  esophageal cancer as, 219
  esophageal diverticula as, 214
  esophageal varices as, 215
  esophageal web as, 215
  gastroesophageal reflux disease as, 216–217
  hiatal hernia as, 216
  Mallory-Weiss tear as, 215
  motility, 194
Esophageal diverticula, 214
Esophageal phase of swallowing, 194
Esophageal varices, 215
Esophageal web, 215
Esophagus
  anatomy and physiology of, 195
  Barrett, 195, 217–219
  bird-beak, 216
  during swallowing, 194
ESR (erythrocyte sedimentation rate), 361
ESS (empty sella syndrome), 112
Essential thrombocythemia, 306, 307–308
Estradiol, 687, 689
Estriol, unconjugated, 330
Estrogen(s), 687, 689, 690
  in bone metabolism, 324, 325
  in bone remodeling, 367
  insulin and, 687
  in menstrual cycle, 688
Estrogen agonists, 744
Estrogen hormone replacement therapy, 700
Estrogen receptor(s), in breast cancer, 729
Estrogen receptor antagonists, 729
Estrogen-progesterone therapy (EPT), 700
Estrone, 687, 689
Eszopiclone, 540
Etanercept, 404
Ethacrynic acid, 93, 94, 656, 657
Ethinyl estradiol, 744
Ethmoid bone, 335
Ethmoid sinus, 782
Ethosuximide, 524
Etidronate, 402
Etoposide, 313–314
Ewing sarcoma, 297, 363, 364, 365–366
EWS-FLI1 fusion gene, 365
Excitation-contraction coupling, 20–21
  of skeletal muscle, 355–357
  of smooth muscle, 358
Excoriation, 389
Executive functions, 427
Exemestane, 665, 745
Exenatide, 168–169
Exercise, metabolic needs of skeletal muscle
    during, 358–359
Exercise stress testing, 90
Exocrine secretion, 108
Expectorants, 819
Expiration, 766
  mechanics of breathing during, 766, 768
Expiratory muscles, 758, 766

Expiratory reserve volume (ERV), 761, 762
Exstrophy of bladder, 669
Extensor digitorum longus muscle, 352
Extensor hallucis longus muscle, 352
Extensor muscles
  of arm, 349
  of knee, 351
External acoustic meatus, 462
External genitalia
  development of
    early, 664, 665
    female, 671–672, 673
    male, 666–669
  differentiation of, 665
External iliac artery, 184, 185, 589
  anastomoses with, 187
External iliac vein, 187
External intercostal muscles, 765
External oblique fascia, 182
External oblique muscle, 179, 182
External occipital protuberance, 336
External spermatic fascia, 182
Extracellular circulating volume (ECV), 37
Extracellular fluid (ECF)
  composition of, 596–597
  intercompartmental water dynamics
      between intracellular and, 598, 599,
      600
  osmolarity of, 598
  pathophysiology of, 598
  volume of
    estimating, 597
    measuring, 597–598
Extraglomerular mesangial cells, 592, 594
Extrahepatic biliary atresia, 177
Extranodal marginal zone lymphoma, 189, 299
Extraocular muscles, 458
Extraperitoneal tissue, 182
Extrapyramidal diseases, 478
Extrinsic innervation of GI tract, 189–190
Extrinsic laryngeal muscles, 348
Exudate, 755, 815
Exudative edema, 35, 36
Exudative effusion, 755, 815
Eye, structure of, 502
Eye movement(s), 427, 458
  defects in, 500–501
Ezetimibe, 105

F

F cells, 204
Facet joints, 344
Facial bones, 335
Facial nerve, 459
  lesions of, 457, 458, 500, 502
Facial nerve palsy, 457, 458
Facilitated diffusion, 595
Factitious disorders, 557–558
Factor Xa inhibitors, direct, 319–320
Falciform ligament, 206
Fallopian tubes, 670, 672, 679, 680, 686, 691
False pelvis, 338, 339
Familial adenomatous polyposis (FAP), 233
Familial hypocalciuric hypercalcemia
    (FHH), 144
Famotidine, 258–259
Fanconi syndrome, 644, 645
Fasciculations, 453
Fasciitis, necrotizing, 392
Fast-conducting pain fibers, 453
Fastigial nucleus, 438
Fast-response action potentials, 16, 17, 18
Fat embolism, 76, 77, 800
Fat necrosis, 728
Fatty acid metabolism in muscle
    contraction, 358

Fatty casts, 623
Fatty streaks, 56
Fe^{2+} (iron)
  serum, 275
  small intestinal absorption of, 203
Fe^{2+} (ferrous) iron, 770
Fe^{3+} (ferric) iron, 770
Fear, 430
Febuxostat, 405
Fecalith, 227
Feedback, 111
Female pseudohermaphroditism, 666
Female reproductive disorders, 703–733
  of breast, 727–731
  cervical, 713–715
  congenital malformations as, 673
  ovarian, 715–721
  of pregnancy, 703–712
  uterine, 721–727
  vaginal, 712–713
Female reproductive system
  anatomy of, 679–681
  development of, 669–673
  drugs that modulate, 744–746
  fertilization in, 691–692
  gonadal steroids in, 687, 689, 690
  homologs in male and, 674, 675
  menopause in, 698–700
  menstrual cycle and ovulation in, 686–687,
      688
  oogenesis in, 684–686
  pregnancy in, 692–698
  sexual response in, 689–691
Femoral artery, 182, 351, 352
Femoral hernia, 181, 182, 236, 237, 674
Femoral neck fracture, 342
Femoral nerve, 182, 352
  damage to, 353, 495
Femoral ring, 676
Femoral triangle, 182, 183, 676
  trauma in, 353
Femoral vein, 182, 676
Fenestrated capillary endothelium, 600, 601
Fenofibrate, 105
Fenoldopam, 98
Fentanyl, 515–516, 532
Ferric (Fe^{3+}) iron, 770
Ferritin, 275
Ferrous (Fe^{2+}) iron, 770
Fertilization, 684, 686, 687, 691–692
Fetal alcohol syndrome, 418
Fetal circulation, 8–9, 696–698
Fetal D antigen, 281
Fetal erythrocytes, 8
Fetal erythropoiesis, 8
Fetal hemoglobin (HbF, $Hb\alpha_2\gamma_2$), 8, 266, 267,
    285, 696, 770
Fetal shunts, 696, 698
Fetal-postnatal derivatives, cardiac, 8
FEV_1 (forced expiratory volume in
    1 second), 761
  during pregnancy, 693
FEV_1/FVC (forced expiratory volume in
    1 second/forced vital capacity) ratio,
    761, 783
Fexofenadine, 819
FF (filtration fraction), 604
  changes in, 604–605
FFI (fatal familial insomnia), 483
FGF (fibroblast growth factor), 331
  in wound healing, 361
FHH (familial hypocalciuric
    hypercalcemia), 144
Fibrates, 105
Fibrillation(s), 453
  atrial, 30, 50, 52
  ventricular, 51–52

Fibrinogen, 291
Fibrinous pericarditis, 60
Fibroadenoma, 727, 728
Fibroblast growth factor (FGF), 331
  in wound healing, 361
Fibrocartilage, 344
Fibrocystic changes, 727
Fibroid, 726
Fibroma, 308
  sex cord stromal, 720
Fibromuscular dysplasia, hypertension due to,
  53–54, 55
Fibrotic lung disease. See Idiopathic
  pulmonary fibrosis (IPF)
Fibrous capsule, 343
Fibrous dysplasia, 371
Fibrous joints, 344
Fibrous pericardium, 11, 12
Fibrous plaques, 56, 57
Fibular collateral ligament, 345
Fick's cardiac output, 23
Fifth intercostal space, 10
Fifth metatarsal fracture, 342
Filtration fraction (FF), 604
  changes in, 604–605
Fimbriae, 679, 680, 686
Finasteride, 739, 743
Finger agnosia, 428
First-degree AV block, 47
First-order neurons, 451, 453
"First-pass metabolism," 207
Fissure of Rolando, 426
Fistula, tracheoesophageal, 176, 213–214,
  751–752
Fitz-Hugh-Curtis syndrome, 722
Fixation, 538
Flail chest, 758
Flat affect, 536, 545
Flecainide, 104
Flexor carpi ulnaris muscle, 349
Flexor digiti minimi muscle, 349
Flexor digitorum longus muscle, 352
Flexor digitorum profundus muscle, 349
Flexor hallucis longus muscle, 352
Flexor muscles
  of arm, 349
  of hip, 351
  of toes, 352
Flexor pollicis brevis muscle, 349
Flight of ideas, 535
Flocculonodular lobe, 437
Flow, 769
Fluid compartment(s)
  composition of, 596–597
  intercompartmental water dynamics
    between, 598, 599, 600
  volume of
    estimating, 596
    measuring, 596–597
Fluid overload in pregnancy, 692
Flunisolide, 822
5-Fluorouracil (5-FU), 313
Fluoxetine, 517, 540
Fluphenazine, 540
Flutamide, 742
Fluticasone, 822
Fluvoxamine, 517
Focal nodular hyperplasia (FNH), 249
Focal segmental glomerulosclerosis (FSGS),
  626, 627–628
Folate, small intestinal absorption of, 203
Folic acid, during pregnancy, 330
Folic acid deficiency, 277–278
Folium vermis, 437
Follicle-stimulating hormone (FSH), 683, 685
  with age, 687, 689

in menstrual cycle, 686–687, 688
  in spermatogenesis, 683, 685
Follicular cysts, 717
Follicular development, 685, 687
Follicular lymphoma, 297, 300
Follicular phase, 686, 688
Follicular thyroid carcinoma, 135
Fontanelles, 328, 329
Footdrop, 353
Foramen(ina), 335, 336
Foramen cecum, 127, 140, 749
Foramen lacerum, 336
Foramen magnum, 336
Foramen of Luschka, 420, 421, 469
Foramen of Magendie, 420, 421, 469
Foramen of Monro, 420, 421
Foramen ovale, 3, 8, 9, 336, 698
  patent, 2
  structures passing through, 336
Foramen primum, 3
Foramen rotundum, 336
Foramen secundum, 3
Foramen spinosum, 336
Forced expiratory volume in 1 second
  (FEV$_1$), 761
  during pregnancy, 693
Forced expiratory volume in 1 second/forced
  vital capacity (FEV$_1$/FVC) ratio,
  761, 783
Forced vital capacity (FVC), 761
  during pregnancy, 693
Forearm jerk reflex, 449
Forearm muscles, 349
Forebrain, development of, 414, 416
Foregut, 177
Foreign body aspiration, 779
Foreskin, 668, 676
Formication, 572
Formoterol, 821
Fornix, 426
Forteo (recombinant parathyroid
  hormone), 404
Fossa ovalis, 9
Fourth ventricle, 420, 421, 469
Fovea, 502
Fracture(s)
  comminuted, 340
  contrecoup, 340
  depressed, 340
  hip, 367
  of lower limb, 342
  of pelvis, 341
  of skull, 339–340
  of upper limb, 341–342, 350
  of vertebrae, 340
  vertebral compression, 367
Frank-Starling relationship, 25–26
Fraternal twins, 697, 698, 699
FRC (functional residual capacity), 761, 762
Free water, 606
Fremitus, 809
Friedreich ataxia, 485
Frontal bone, 329, 335, 336
Frontal eye fields, 427
Frontal lobe, 425–427
Frontal sinus, 782
Frontal suture, 328, 329
Frontotemporal dementia, 482
FSGS (focal segmental glomerulosclerosis),
  626, 627–628
FSH. See Follicle-stimulating hormone (FSH)
5-FU (5-fluorouracil), 313
Fugue, dissociative, 559
Functional residual capacity (FRC), 761,
  762
Fundus of stomach, 196

Fungal infection of CNS, 505
Fungal meningitis, 419, 420
Furosemide, 93, 94, 102, 656, 657
Fusiform gyrus, 426
FVC (forced vital capacity), 761
  during pregnancy, 693

G

G cells, 196, 197–199, 204
G protein-coupled receptor (GPCR), 110, 111
GABA (γ-aminobutyric acid), 446, 508
GABA (γ-aminobutyric acid) receptor, in
  alcohol use disorder, 568, 569
Gabapentin, 526
GABHS (group A β-hemolytic streptococci)
  glomerulonephritis due to, 631–632
  rheumatic fever due to, 60, 631
GAD (generalized anxiety disorder), 550–551
Gain, primary vs secondary, 537
Galantamine, 527
Gallbladder
  anatomy and physiology of, 207–208
  in bilirubin production, 208
  porcelain, 251
Gallbladder carcinoma, 252
Gallbladder disease, 250–253
  cholecystitis as, 252
  cholelithiasis as, 250–252
  gallbladder carcinoma/cholangiocarcinoma
    as, 252
  primary sclerosing cholangitis as, 253
Gallstones, 208, 210, 250–252
  during pregnancy, 693
GALT (gut-associated lymphoid tissue), 189
Gametogenesis, 681–686, 687
γ-aminobutyric acid (GABA), 446, 508
γ-aminobutyric acid (GABA) receptor, in
  alcohol use disorder, 568, 569
Ganglion cells, 459
Ganirelix, 741
Gap junctions, 21, 358
Gardner syndrome, 233
Gardnerella vaginalis, 732
Gas embolism, 76, 77, 800
Gas exchange, 763–764
Gastric acid, 196, 197–199
Gastric adenocarcinoma, 222, 223
Gastric arteries, 186
Gastric cancer, 222–224
Gastric disorders, 219–223
  gastric cancer as, 222–224
  gastritis as, 219–221
  Ménétrier disease as, 221
  peptic ulcer disease as, 221–222
  Zollinger-Ellison syndrome as, 222
Gastric epiploic arteries, 186
Gastric inhibitory peptide (GIP), 196, 199, 204
Gastric lymphoma, 223
Gastric phase of gastric secretion, 197
Gastric secretions
  general regulation of, 197, 198
  of hydrochloric acid, 196, 197–199
  types of, 197, 198
Gastric ulcers, 221
Gastrin, 196, 197, 198, 199, 204
Gastrinoma, 165
Gastrin-releasing peptide (GRP), 196, 197–
  199, 204
Gastritis, 219–221
  acute, 220
  autoimmune, 220
  chronic (atrophic), 220–221
  hemorrhagic, 220
Gastrocnemius muscle, 352
Gastrocolic reflex, 205
Gastroduodenal artery, 198, 186

Gastroesophageal reflux disease (GERD), 195, 216–217
  and Barrett esophagus, 218–219
  during pregnancy, 693
Gastrointestinal (GI) bleeding, 274
Gastrointestinal (GI) disorders, 210–258
  abdominal hernias as, 236–238
  appendicitis as, 236
  congenital malformations as, 174–178
    duodenal atresia as, 176–177
    esophageal atresia with tracheoesophageal fistula as, 176
    extrahepatic biliary atresia as, 177
    gastroschisis as, 174–175
    intestinal malrotation and volvulus as, 175–176
    omphalocele as, 174
    pancreas divisum as, 177–178
    post-duodenal atresia as, 177
    pyloric stenosis as, 177
  enzyme markers of, 255–258
    alanine aminotransferase as, 256, 257
    alkaline phosphatase as, 257
    amylase as, 257
    aspartate aminotransferase as, 255–256, 257
    ceruloplasmin as, 258
    γ-glutamyl transferase as, 256–257
    lipase as, 258
    prothrombin time as, 258
  of esophagus, 213–219
    achalasia as, 215–216
    Barrett esophagus as, 217–219
    Boerhaave syndrome as, 215
    esophageal atresia and tracheoesophageal fistula as, 213–214
    esophageal cancer as, 219
    esophageal diverticula as, 214
    esophageal varices as, 215
    esophageal web as, 215
    gastroesophageal reflux disease as, 216–217
    hiatal hernia as, 216
    Mallory-Weiss tear as, 215
  of exocrine pancreas, 253–255
    acute pancreatitis as, 253
    chronic pancreatitis as, 254
    pancreatic adenocarcinoma as, 255
  gallbladder disease as, 250–253
    cholecystitis as, 252
    cholelithiasis as, 250–252
    gallbladder carcinoma/cholangiocarcinoma as, 252
    primary sclerosing cholangitis as, 253
  liver disease as, 238–250
    alcoholic hepatitis as, 242–243
    cirrhosis and portal hypertension as, 244–246
    hepatic tumors as, 248–250
    hereditary hyperbilirubinemias as, 240–242
    due to inborn errors of metabolism, 247–248
    infectious hepatitis as, 242, 243
    jaundice as, 238–240
    primary biliary cirrhosis as, 246–247
    Reye syndrome as, 244
  of oral cavity, 210–212
    of mouth and jaw, 210–211
    of salivary glands, 211–213
  pharmacology for, 258–263
    antacids in, 260, 261
    bismuth and sucralfate in, 260
    H_2 blockers in, 258–259
    infliximab in, 260–261
    metoclopramide in, 262

octreotide in, 260
ondansetron in, 262
orlistat in, 262–263
osmotic laxatives in, 261
proton pump inhibitors in, 259–260
sulfasalazine in, 262
  of small and large intestine, 224–235
    diverticular disease as, 226–228
    Hirschsprung disease (congenital megacolon) as, 229
    inflammatory diseases of colon as, 229–232
    intussusception as, 228
    malabsorption syndromes as, 224–225
    omphalocele as, 229
    tumors of colon as, 232–235
  of stomach, 219–223
    gastric cancer as, 222–224
    gastritis as, 219–221
    Ménétrier disease as, 221
    peptic ulcer disease as, 221–222
    Zollinger-Ellison syndrome as, 222
Gastrointestinal (GI) system, 171–264
  anatomy of, 178–192
    abdominal planes and regions in, 180–183
    abdominal wall in, 178–179, 181
    arterial supply in, 184–187
    lymphatic drainage in, 188–189
    nerve supply in, 189–192
    peritoneum and abdominal viscera in, 183–184
    venous drainage in, 185–188
  disorders of. See Gastrointestinal (GI) disorders
  embryology of, 172–178
  physiology of, 193–210
    colon in, 204–205
    esophagus in, 195
    exocrine pancreas in, 205–206
    hypothalamus in, 192
    liver and gallbladder in, 206–210
    mouth in, 192–195
    small intestine in, 199–204
    stomach in, 195–199
  during pregnancy, 693–694, 695
Gastroschisis, 174–175
Gastrulation, 412
Gaze deviation, 427
GBM (glomerular basement membrane), 601
  in nephrotic syndrome, 623
GBS (Guillain-Barré syndrome), 456, 466, 487–488
  restrictive lung disease due to, 791
GCA (giant-cell arteritis), 81, 396–397, 403
Gefitinib, 315–316
Gemelli inferior muscle, 351
Gemelli superior muscle, 351
Gemfibrozil, 105
Gender, 662
General anesthetics, 530–532
Generalized anxiety disorder (GAD), 550–551
Generalized seizures, 488, 489
Genetic sex, 662
Geniculocalcarine tract, 460
  lesion of, 461
Genioglossus muscle, 347
Geniohyoid muscle, 348
Genital ducts
  development of, 663, 664
  differentiation of, 665
Genital herpes, 732
Genital infections, 731–733
Genital tubercle, 664, 665, 669, 673
Genital warts, 712–713
Genitofemoral nerve, 677

Genotypic sex, 662
Genu of internal capsule, 434, 435
GERD (gastroesophageal reflux disease), 195, 216–217
  and Barrett esophagus, 218–219
  during pregnancy, 693
Germ cell tumors, 674
  ovarian, 718–720
  testicular, 737–738
Gerstmann syndrome, 428
Gestational diabetes, 694
Gestational hypertension, 708
Gestational neoplasms, 711–712
GFAP (glial fibrillary acidic protein), 465
GFR (glomerular filtration rate), 593, 601–602, 640
  measurement of, 604–605
  regulation of, 602–603
GH. See Growth hormone (GH)
Ghon complex, 813
Ghon focus, 813
GHRH (growth hormone-releasing hormone), 113
GI. See Gastrointestinal (GI)
Giant-cell arteritis (GCA), 81, 396–397, 403
Giant-cell tumor, 363, 364, 365
Gigantism, 120–121, 327
Gilbert syndrome, 238, 241
GIP (gastric inhibitory peptide), 196, 199, 204
Gitelman syndrome, 646
Glans penis, 668, 669, 676, 677
Glanzmann thrombasthenia, 293
Glaucoma, 503
Glenohumeral joint, 344
Glial fibrillary acidic protein (GFAP), 465
Glioblastoma multiforme, 490, 491
Glipizide, 167
-gliptins, 169
Global aphasia, 431, 480
Globoid cell leukodystrophy, 487
Globose nucleus, 438
Globus pallidus, 431, 432, 434
Glomerular basement membrane (GBM), 601
  in nephrotic syndrome, 623
Glomerular capillaries, 591
Glomerular capsule, 590, 591–592
Glomerular filtrate, 601
Glomerular filtration barrier, 600–601
Glomerular filtration rate (GFR), 593, 601–602, 640
  measurement of, 604–605
  regulation of, 602–603
Glomerular markers, 599
Glomerulonephritis
  acute proliferative (poststreptococcal, infectious), 623, 631–632
  membranoproliferative, 627–628
  rapidly progressive, 623, 632–633
Glomerulopathy(ies)
  diffuse membranous, 626–627
  membranous, 623
  with nephritic syndrome, 623, 624, 630–636
    acute proliferative (poststreptococcal, infectious) glomerulonephritis as, 623, 631–632
    antiglomerular basement membrane disease (Goodpasture) syndrome as, 601, 623, 633–634
    granulomatosis with polyangiitis as, 635–636
    hereditary nephritis (Alport syndrome) as, 635
    IgA nephropathy (Berger disease) as, 631, 634–635
    rapidly progressive glomerulonephritis as, 623, 632–633

with nephrotic syndrome, 623–628
diffuse membranous glomerulopathy as, 626–627
focal segmental glomerulosclerosis as, 626, 627–628
glomerular basement membrane in, 601
membranoproliferative glomerulonephritis as, 627–628
minimal change disease as, 625–626
proteinuria in, 592, 624
nomenclature for, 624
Glomerulosclerosis, focal segmental, 626, 627–628
Glomerulus
histology of, 590, 591
physiology of, 607, 610
Glossopharyngeal nerve, 459
"-glossus," muscles ending in, 347
GLP-1 (glucagon-like peptide-1), 204
GLP-1 (glucagon-like peptide-1) analogs, 168–169
Glucagon, 151, 161–162
Glucagon-like peptide-1 (GLP-1), 204
Glucagon-like peptide-1 (GLP-1) analogs, 168–169
Glucagonoma, 165–166
Glucocorticoids, 149, 150–152, 687
endogenous, 151
synthesis and regulation of, 150
Gluconeogenesis, 151
Glucose, renal reabsorption and excretion of, 605, 607
Glucose metabolism in muscle contraction, 358
Glucose titration curve, 606
Glucose transporter-2 (GLUT2), 160, 161
Glucose transporter-4 (GLUT4), 160, 161
in muscle contraction, 360
Glucose uptake, insulin-independent, 160
Glucose-6-phosphate dehydrogenase (G6PD) deficiency, 278–279
Glucosuria, 165–166, 605
GLUT2 (glucose transporter-2), 160, 161
GLUT4 (glucose transporter-4), 160, 161
in muscle contraction, 360
Glutamate, 508
γ-glutamyl transferase, 256–257
Gluteal muscles, 351
Gluten-sensitive enteropathy, 224, 225
Gluteus maximus muscle, 351
Gluteus medius muscle, 351
Gluteus minimus muscle, 351
Glyburide, 167
Glycine, 508
Glycogen metabolism in muscle contraction, 358
Glycogen phosphorylase in muscle contraction, 359
Glycogen synthase in muscle contraction, 359
Glycogenolysis in muscle contraction, 360
Glycolysis in muscle contraction, 359
Glycoprotein(s), 117
Glycoprotein IIb/IIIa inhibitors, 321
Glycopyrrolate, 512
Glycosylated hemoglobin A_{1c} (HbA_{1c}), 163
Glycosylphosphatidylinositol (GPI), 286
GnRH. See Gonadotropin-releasing hormone (GnRH)
Goblet cells, 200, 202, 759
Goiter, 125–126
toxic multinodular, 132
Golfer's elbow, 349
Golgi cell, 439
Golgi tendon organs, 453, 468
Golimumab, 404

Gonad(s)
development of, 662, 663
differentiation of, 665
lymphatic drainage of, 675
venous drainage of, 675
Gonadal agenesis, 666
Gonadal arteries, 184
Gonadal differentiation, male, 666–667
Gonadal ridge, 662, 663
Gonadal sex, 662
Gonadal steroids, 687, 689, 690
Gonadal veins, 588
Gonadotropin(s)
with age, 687, 689
in menstrual cycle, 686–687, 688
in spermatogenesis, 683, 685
Gonadotropin axis, drugs that modulate, 741
Gonadotropin-releasing hormone (GnRH), 113
Gonadotropin-releasing hormone (GnRH) agonist, 124
Gonadotropin-releasing hormone (GnRH) mixed agonists/antagonists, 741, 742
Gonadotropin-releasing hormone (GnRH) pure antagonists, 741
Gonorrhea, 731
Goodpasture syndrome
granulomatosis with polyangiitis vs, 399
renal disorder in, 601, 623, 633–634
respiratory disorder in, 797
vasculitis in, 396
Goserelin, 315, 741
Gottron papules, 387
Gout, 375–376, 377
drugs used to treat, 404–406
GPA (granulomatosis with polyangiitis), 83–84, 399–400, 403, 635–636, 797–798
GPCR (G protein-coupled receptor), 110, 111
G6PD (glucose-6-phosphate dehydrogenase) deficiency, 278–279
GPI (glycosylphosphatidylinositol), 286
Graafian follicles, 684
Gracile fasciculus, 449, 451, 452
Gracilis muscle, 352
Grading of tumors, 309
Gram-negative bacteria, pneumonia due to, 811
Gram-positive bacteria, pneumonia due to, 811
Grand mal seizure, 489
Granular casts, 623
Granular cells, 593
Granular neuron, 438
Granule cells, 439
Granule layer of cerebellum, 437
Granuloma(s)
eosinophilic, 306
noncaseating, 383
Granuloma inguinale, 732
Granulomatosis, Wegener, 83–84, 399–400, 403, 635–636, 797–798
Granulomatosis with polyangiitis (GPA, GWP), 83–84, 399–400, 403, 635–636, 797–798
Granulomatous disease, chronic, 279
Granulosa cell(s), 686, 687, 688
Granulosa cell tumor, 721
Graves disease, 132
Gray communicating rami, 449
Gray matter, 449
Great cerebral vein of Galen, 424
Great saphenous vein, 352
Great vessels
relationship of heart and, 10
transposition of, 4, 5
Greater palatine artery, 703

Greater pelvis, 338, 339
Greater sac, 184
Greater sciatic foramen, 339
Greater tuberosity fracture, 341
Grief reaction, 550
Group A β-hemolytic streptococci (GABHS)
glomerulonephritis due to, 631–632
rheumatic fever due to, 60, 631
Growth factors in bone remodeling, 367
Growth hormone (GH), 114, 115, 116, 151
Growth hormone (GH) analog, 125
Growth hormone (GH) excess, 120–121
Growth hormone-inhibitory hormone, 113
Growth hormone-releasing hormone (GHRH), 113
GRP (gastrin-releasing peptide), 196, 197–199, 204
Guaifenesin, 819
Gubernaculum
development of, 664, 665
in male reproductive system development, 667, 668, 677
Guillain-Barré syndrome (GBS), 456, 465, 487–488
restrictive lung disease due to, 791
Gustatory pathway, 464
Gustatory system, 464
Gut-associated lymphoid tissue (GALT), 189
Guyon canal syndrome, 350
GWP (granulomatosis with polyangiitis), 83–84, 399–400, 403, 635–636, 797–798
Gynecomastia, 728
Gyrus(i), 418, 426

H

H^+ (hydrogen), renal regulation of, 617–618
H band, 21, 356, 357
H_1 blockers, 818–819
H_1 receptors, 818
H_2 receptor(s), 199
H_2 receptor antagonists (H_2 blockers), 199, 258–259
$H_2PO_4^-$ (dihydrogen phosphate), renal secretion of, 617
Haemophilus ducreyi, 731, 732
Haemophilus influenzae, 811
Hair cells, 461, 462, 463
Hairy cell leukemia, 304
Hairy leukoplakia, 210, 211
Haldane effect, 771, 772
Hallucinations, 534, 536, 543–544, 545
Hallucinogen use disorder, 575
Hallucinosis, alcoholic, 570
Haloperidol, 540
Halothane, 531
Hamartoma, 309
bronchial, 348, 806
Hamate, 339
fracture of hook of, 350
Hampton hump, 800
Hamstring muscles, 352
Hand
dermatomes of, 351
intrinsic muscles of, 351
Hand-Schüller-Christian disease, 305
Haploid, 682, 683
Haptoglobin, 279
Hartnup disease, 200, 605–606
Hashimoto thyroiditis, 133
Haustrations, 205
Hay AV block, 47–48
"Hay fever," 817
Hb. See Hemoglobin (Hb)
HbA_{1c} (glycosylated hemoglobin A_{1c}), 163
HBcAg, 243
HBeAg, 243

HbF (fetal hemoglobin), 8, 266, 267, 285, 696, 770
HbH (hemoglobin H) disease, 276
HbS (hemoglobin S), 284
HBsAg, 243
Hbα$_2$β$_2$ (adult hemoglobin), 8, 266, 267
Hbα$_2$γ$_2$ (fetal hemoglobin), 8, 266, 267, 285, 696, 770
HCAs (heterocyclic agents), 516, 519–520
HCC (hepatocellular carcinoma), 249–250
hCG (β-human chorionic gonadotropin), 117, 330
hCG (human chorionic gonadotropin), 686, 687, 695, 712, 720
HCl (hydrochloric acid), 196, 197–199
HCM (hypertrophic cardiomyopathy), 62–63, 71
HCO$_3$⁻. *See* Bicarbonate (HCO$_3$⁻)
HCTZ (hydrochlorothiazide), 92, 94, 656, 657
HD (Hirschsprung disease), 172, 229
Head muscles
  anatomy of, 347–348
  development of, 332
Head trauma, 489
Headache syndromes, 505–507
Hearing, 429
Hearing defects, 463
Heart. *See also* Cardiovascular (CV) system
  conduction system of, 13–14
  congenital lesions of, 4–7
  development of, 2–4, 5
  electrical axes of, 41
  electrocardiography of, 40–45
  electrophysiology in, 14–20
  imaging/diagnostic tests of, 90–91
  layers of, 10–12
  relationships of great vessels and, 10
  surfaces and borders of, 9–10
Heart disease
  ischemic, 85–86
  rheumatic
    acute, 60–61
    chronic, 61
Heart failure
  congestive, 63–65
  drugs used in, 101–103
  left-sided, 63–65
  with preserved ejection fraction, 64
  with reduced ejection fraction, 63–64
  right-sided, 65
Heart murmurs, 67–73
  classification of, 68, 69
  continuous (due to patent ductus arteriosus), 68, 73
  diastolic, 68, 71–72
    due to aortic valve regurgitation, 71, 72
    due to mitral stenosis, 72, 73
    due to pulmonic regurgitation, 72
  mechanism of, 67–68
  systolic, 68–71
    due to aortic stenosis, 69–70
    crescendo-decrescendo, 10
    grading of, 71
    holosystolic blowing, 10, 69
    due to mitral regurgitation, 68–69, 71
    due to mitral valve prolapse, 69–70, 71
    due to pulmonic stenosis, 70
    due to tricuspid regurgitation, 69
    due to ventricular septal defect, 70
Heart rate (HR)
  autonomic effects on, 39
  and blood pressure, 37
  and cardiac output, 24
  and contractility, 24
  normal, 42
  during pregnancy, 693

Heart sounds, 31–32
Heart tube, 2
Heart valves, 10–11
  in endocarditis, 58
Heart-hand syndrome, 332
Heavy alkaline mucus, small intestinal secretion of, 202
Heberden nodes, 373
Heinz body, 273, 278
Helicobacter pylori, 220, 260
Heliotrope rash, 387
HELLP syndrome, 709
Hemangioblastoma, 490, 491
Hemangioma, 250
Hematocele, 736
Hematocrit, 33, 269
Hematologic disorders, 272–308
  anemia as, 272–287
    classification and appearance of, 272, 273–274
    macrocytic, 277–278
    microcytic, 272–277
    normocytic, 278–287
  blood loss as, 288
  heme pathology as, 288–290
  hemorrhagic, 290–295
    due to clotting factor deficiencies, 293–294
    disseminated intravascular coagulation as, 291, 292, 294
    laboratory findings in, 290, 291
    due to liver disease, 294
    due to platelet disorders, 290–293
    due to vessel wall abnormalities, 295
  myeloproliferative syndromes as, 306–308
  pharmacology for, 318–322
    anticoagulants in, 318–320
    antiplatelet agents in, 320–321
    thrombolytics in, 322
  white cell disorders as, 295–306
    Langerhans cell histiocytosis as, 305–306
    leukemias as, 301–304
    leukopenia as, 295–296
    lymphomas as, 297–301
    plasma cell disorders as, 304–305
    reactive proliferation as, 296–297
Hematologic system
  anatomy of, 267–272
  disorders of. *See* Hematologic disorders
  embryology of, 266–267
  during pregnancy, 695
Hematoma
  epidural, 335, 337–338, 419
  subdural, 419
Hematopoiesis, 266, 268
Hematopoietic progenitor cell (HPC), 268
Hematuria in nephritic syndrome, 630
Heme, 274
  metabolism of, 208–209
  pathology of, 288–290
  production of, 288, 289
Heme moiety, 770
Hemianopsia
  bitemporal, 120, 121–122, 422, 460
  homonymous, 460
  with macular sparing, 460
Hemiazygos vein, 755
Hemiballismus, 432, 479
Hemiblock, 44–45
Hemiparesis, spastic, 451
Hemiplegia, alternating, 440, 441
Hemisection of spinal cord, 453, 454, 455
Hemivertebra, 330
Hemochromatosis, 247–248
Hemodynamic(s), 32–35, 36
Hemodynamic parameters, 33–34

Hemoglobin (Hb), 8
  adult, 8, 266, 267
  electrophoresis of, 284
  fetal, 8, 266, 267, 284, 285, 696, 770
  mean cell, 269
  oxygen transport by, 770
  pathologic forms of, 267
  types of, 266–267
Hemoglobin A$_{1c}$, glycosylated, 163
Hemoglobin Bart, 276
Hemoglobin dissociation curve, 770–771
Hemoglobin H (HbH) disease, 276
Hemoglobin S (HbS), 284
Hemoglobinuria, paroxysmal nocturnal, 286
Hemolytic anemias, 283–284, 696
  cardiac traumatic, 287
  microangiopathic, 286–287
Hemolytic symptoms of sickle cell disease, 285
Hemolytic uremic syndrome (HUS), 292
Hemoperitoneum, 183
Hemophilia, 291, 293
Hemorrhage
  epidural, 419, 475, 477
  intracerebral/parenchymal, 419
  intracranial, 475–476, 477
  intraparenchymal, 476, 477
  subarachnoid, 419, 471–472, 476, 477–478
  subdural, 419, 475, 477
Hemorrhagic disorders, 290–295
  due to clotting factor deficiencies, 293–294
  disseminated intravascular coagulation as, 291, 292, 294
  laboratory findings in, 290, 291
  due to liver disease, 294
  due to platelet disorders, 290–293
  due to vessel wall abnormalities, 295
Hemorrhagic infarction, 474–475
Hemosiderosis, 248
Hemostasis, 290
Henderson-Hasselbalch equation, 616, 617
Henoch-Schönlein purpura (HSP), 84–85, 401–402, 403
  IgA nephropathy due to, 634, 635
  vessel wall abnormalities due to, 295
Heparin, 319
Heparin-induced thrombocytopenia (HIT), 290
Hepatic adenoma, 248, 249
Hepatic artery proper, 158, 186
Hepatic encephalopathy, 246
Hepatic flexure, 173
Hepatic tumors, 248–250
Hepatic veins, 187
Hepatitis
  alcoholic, 242–243
  infectious, 242, 243
Hepatitis A, 242
Hepatitis B, 242, 310
Hepatitis C, 242
Hepatitis D, 242
Hepatitis E, 242
Hepatobiliary iminodiacetic acid (HIDA) scan, 252
Hepatoblastoma, 250
Hepatocellular carcinoma (HCC), 249–250
Hepatocytes, 206, 207
Hepatoduodenal ligament, 184
Hepatolenticular degeneration, 248, 481, 485
Hepatorenal syndrome, 246
Hepcidin, 282
HER2/neu antagonists, 746
HER2/neu receptor, molecular therapy targeting, 316
Herald patch, 394
Hereditary angioedema, 391
Hereditary hemorrhagic telangiectasia, 295

Hereditary motor and sensory neuropathy, 499
Hereditary nephritis, 635
Hereditary nonpolyposis colon cancer (HNPCC), 233, 234
Hereditary spherocytosis (HS), 279–280
Hermaphroditism, true, 666, 702
Hernia(s)
  abdominal, 236–238
  congenital diaphragmatic, 333, 752, 753
  femoral, 181, 182, 236, 237, 674
  hiatal, 196, 216, 757
  incisional, 236
  inguinal, 237, 669
    direct, 181, 182, 236, 237, 666, 674
    indirect, 181, 182, 236, 237, 666
  irreducible (incarcerated), 237
  paraesophageal, 216
  reducible, 237
  sliding, 216
  strangulated, 237
  umbilical, 236, 237
Herniated disk, 340–341, 456
Herniation
  of cerebellar tonsils, 414–416
  cerebral, 503–505
  intervertebral disk, 340–341, 456
  of nucleus pulposus, 340–341, 412
Heroin use disorder, 573–574
Herpes simplex virus 1 (HSV-1)
  genital herpes due to, 732
  herpetic stomatitis due to, 210, 211
Herpes simplex virus 2 (HSV-2), genital herpes due to, 732
Herpetic stomatitis, 210, 211
Heterocyclic agents (HCAs), 516, 519–520
HGSIL (high-grade squamous intraepithelial lesion), 714
5-HIAA (5 hydroxyindoleacetic acid) in carcinoid syndrome, 60
Hiatal hernia, 196, 216, 757
HIDA (hepatobiliary iminodiacetic acid) scan, 252
High altitude, hypoxemia due to, 776, 777
High-grade squamous intraepithelial lesion (HGSIL), 714
Hindbrain, 414, 416
Hindgut, 172
Hinge joints, 343
Hip, developmental dysplasia of, 333–334
Hip dislocation, congenital, 332
Hip flexion, 341
Hip fracture, 367
Hip joint, 344
Hippocampus, 429–430
Hirschsprung disease (HD), 172, 229
Histamine
  in alveolar function, 764
  as CNS neurotransmitter, 508
  gastric secretion of, 196, 199, 204
Histamine blockers, 818–819
Histiocytosis, Langerhans cell, 305–306
Histoplasmosis, pneumonia due to, 812
Histrionic personality disorder, 561
HIT (heparin-induced thrombocytopenia), 290
HIV (human immunodeficiency virus), oral conditions associated with, 210
HIV (human immunodeficiency virus) encephalitis, 465
Hives, 390–391
HLA-B27 gene, 377
HM (hydatidiform mole), 695, 711–712
HMG-CoA (3-hydroxy-3-methylglutaryl-coenzyme A) reductase inhibitors, 105

HNPCC (hereditary nonpolyposis colon cancer), 233, 234
HOCM (hypertrophic obstructive cardiomyopathy), 10, 11
Hodgkin lymphoma, 297–298, 299
Holoprosencephaly, 418
Holt-Oran syndrome, 332
Homeobox-containing (Hox) genes, 331
Homicidal thoughts, 535
Homonymous hemianopsia, 460
Horizontal fissure, 437
Hormonal agents for cancer, 315
Hormone(s)
  amine, 108, 109
  basics of, 108–111
  peptide/protein, 108–109
    in second-messenger pathways, 109–111
  regulatory control of, 111
  site of action of, 108
  steroid (lipid-soluble), 108, 109
    plasma transport of, 109
  types by mechanism of action of, 108–109
Hormone replacement therapy (HRT), estrogen, 700
Horner syndrome, 444, 445, 451, 461
Horseshoe kidney, 585–586
Housemaid's knee, 353
Howell-Jolly bodies, 273
Hox (homeobox-containing) genes, 331
HPC (hematopoietic progenitor cell), 268
HPV (human papillomavirus), 310, 712, 713, 714–715, 732
HR. See Heart rate (HR)
HRT (hormone replacement therapy), estrogen, 700
HS (hereditary spherocytosis), 279–280
HSV-1 (herpes simplex virus 1)
  genital herpes due to, 732
  herpetic stomatitis due to, 210, 211
HSV-2 (herpes simplex virus 2), genital herpes due to, 732
HTLV-1 (human T-cell leukemia virus type 1), 304, 310
Human chorionic gonadotropin (hCG), 686, 687, 695, 712, 720
β-Human chorionic gonadotropin (hCG), 117, 330
Human herpesvirus-8, 310
Human immunodeficiency virus (HIV), oral conditions associated with, 210
Human immunodeficiency virus (HIV) encephalitis, 465
Human papillomavirus (HPV), 310, 712, 713, 714–715, 732
Human placental lactogen, 694
Human T-cell leukemia virus type 1 (HTLV-1), 304, 310
Humerus, fractures of, 342, 350
Humor as defense mechanism, 537
Huntington disease, 432, 484, 487–488
HUS (hemolytic uremic syndrome), 292
Hyaline arteriolosclerosis, 54, 55
Hyaline cartilage, 343–344
Hyaline casts, 623
Hyaline membranes, 793
Hydatidiform mole (HM), 695, 711–712
Hydralazine, 98
Hydrocele, 183, 666, 735–736
Hydrocephalus, 417–418, 421–422
  communicating, 421–422, 469, 470–473
  ex vacuo, 422, 473
  mimics of, 473
  noncommunicating, 421, 469–470
  normal-pressure, 422, 472–473
  due to ventricular system malformations, 468–469

Hydrochloric acid (HCl), 196, 197–199
Hydrochlorothiazide (HCTZ), 92, 94, 656, 657
Hydrocodone, 515–516
Hydrogen (H+), renal regulation of, 617–618
Hydromorphone, 515–516
Hydronephrosis, 585
Hydrops fetalis, 276, 281
3-hydroxy-3-methylglutaryl-coenzyme A (HMG-CoA) reductase inhibitors, 105
β-Hydroxybutyrate, 162
25-Hydroxycholecalciferol, 142, 143
5-Hydroxyindoleacetic acid (5-HIAA) in carcinoid syndrome, 60
1α-Hydroxylase, 142, 143, 612
11β-Hydroxylase
  deficiency of, 153, 157
  in steroid hormone synthesis, 149
17α-Hydroxylase
  deficiency of, 150, 157
  in steroid hormone synthesis, 150
21-Hydroxylase
  deficiency of, 150, 157
  in steroid hormone synthesis, 149
3β-Hydroxysteroid dehydrogenase, in steroid hormone synthesis, 149
11β-Hydroxysteroid dehydrogenase, 152
5-Hydroxytryptamine, 508, 509
Hydroxyurea, 284
Hymen, 673
Hyoscyamine, 512
Hypaxial division, 332
Hyperactivity, 536
Hyperaldosteronism
  metabolic alkalosis due to, 619
  primary, 154–156
Hyperalimentation, metabolic acidosis due to, 618
Hyperbilirubinemia, 238–242
Hypercalcemia, 650, 653–654
  causes of, 796
  familial hypocalciuric, 144
  due to increased bone turnover, 144
  malignancy-induced, 144, 145, 310, 362, 805
  metabolic alkalosis due to, 619
  due to milk-alkali syndrome, 144
  presentation of, 144, 805
  due to thiazide diuretics, 144
  due to vitamin D toxicity, 144
Hypercapnia, 778
Hyperchloremic acidosis, 618
Hypercoagulability, 799
  in nephrotic syndrome, 625
Hypercortisolism, primary, 152
Hyperextension of neck, 341
Hyperflexion of neck, 340
Hyperglycemia during pregnancy, 694
Hyperinflated lungs, 780, 785
Hyperinflation, dynamic, in emphysema, 784
Hyperinsulinemia during pregnancy, 694
Hyperkalemia, 650, 651–652
  calcium gluconate for, 18
  due to renal failure, 644
Hyperlipidemia in nephrotic syndrome, 625
Hypernatremia, 650
Hyperosmolar urine, 606
Hyperosmotic disturbances, 598
Hyperosmotic urine, 614
Hyperparathyroidism, 144, 145, 327
Hyperplasia, 308
Hyperplastic arteriolosclerosis, 55
Hyperplastic polyps, 232, 233
Hyperpolarization, 17

Hypersegmented neutrophils, 268, 278
Hypersensitivity
    type I, 817
    type II, 623
    type III, 623
Hypersensitivity pneumonitis, 818
Hypersomnia, primary, 566
Hypertension, 52–54
    defined, 52
    epidemiology of, 52
    gestational, 708
    long-term consequences of, 52–53
    malignant, 54, 55
    in nephritic syndrome, 630
    persistent, 53–54
    portal, 188, 244–246
    in pregnancy, 708–709
    primary (essential), 52, 53
    pulmonary, 801–802, 820
    due to renal failure, 644
    risk factors for, 52
    secondary, 53–54, 59–60
    stages of, 52
Hypertensive emergency, 54
Hypertensive urgency, 54
Hyperthermia, malignant, 467, 531
Hyperthyroidism, 128, 131–132, 134
    hypertension due to, 53, 54
Hypertrophic cardiomyopathy (HCM), 62–63, 71
Hypertrophic obstructive cardiomyopathy (HOCM), 10, 11
Hypertrophic osteoarthropathy, paraneoplastic, 310, 804
Hypertrophic scar, 328
Hyperventilation during pregnancy, 693
Hyperviscosity syndrome, 305
Hypnotic(s), 513–516
    nonbenzodiazepine, 540
Hypnotic use disorder, 570–571
Hypoactivity, 536
Hypoalbuminemia, 145
    in nephrotic syndrome, 624
Hypoblast, 412
Hypocalcemia, 145–146, 650, 653, 654
Hypocalciuric action, 612
Hypochondriac regions, 180, 181
Hypogastric region, 180, 181
Hypoglossal canal, 336
Hypoglossal nerve, 347, 459
Hypoglossus muscle, 347
Hypoglycemia, 164
    factitious, 164
    during pregnancy, 694
Hypoglycemic drugs, oral, 167–169
Hypokalemia, 650, 652, 653
    metabolic alkalosis due to, 619
Hypomagnesemia, 145, 650, 654
Hypomania, 546, 547, 548–550
Hyponatremia, 124, 650, 651
Hypo-osmotic volume expansion, 598
Hypoparathyroidism
    primary, 145
    pseudo-, 145
Hypophyseal portal veins, 113
Hypophyseal veins, 113
Hypophysis. See Pituitary
Hypopituitarism, 121–122
    postpartum, 121, 133, 709–710
Hyposmotic urine, 614
Hypospadias, 669
Hypothalamic nuclei, 435, 436
Hypothalamic-pituitary axis, 112–119
    anterior pituitary in
        cell types and regulation of, 112, 114
        hormones of, 112–117
        structure and function of, 112

hypothalamus in
    hormones of, 113
    structure and function of, 112
    pituitary in, 112, 113
    posterior pituitary in
        hormones of, 117–119
        structure and function of, 112, 113
Hypothalamic-pituitary-thyroid axis, 130, 131
Hypothalamospinal tract, 449, 451
Hypothalamus, 108–126, 435–436
    diseases of, 435–436
    in GI system, 192
    hormones of, 113
    in hypothalamic-pituitary axis, 112–119
    pharmacology of, 124–126
    structure and function of, 112
Hypothenar muscles, 349
Hypothyroidism, 133, 134
    during pregnancy, 694
Hypoventilation, hypoxemia due to, 776
Hypovolemic shock, 78
Hypoxemia, 775–778
    defined, 775
    etiology of, 776–778
    vs hypoxia, 775
    $P_{A}O_2$ and, 775–776
Hypoxia, 775
Hysteresis curve, 766
Hysterosalpingogram, 673

I

I band, 21, 356, 357
I cells, 196, 204
Ibandronate, 368, 402
IBD (inflammatory bowel disease), 230
Ibuprofen, 407
IC (inspiratory capacity), 761, 762
ICC (interstitial cells of Cajal), 196
ICF. See Intracellular fluid (ICF)
ICP (inferior cerebellar peduncle), 437, 438
ICP (intracranial pressure), increased, 468–469, 488
ID (intellectual disability), 581
Idea of reference, 536
Ideal gas law, 761
Identical twins, 697, 698, 699
Identification, 538
Idiopathic pulmonary fibrosis (IPF), 796–797
    diagnosis of, 797
    diffusion impairment in, 776
    lung compliance in, 766
    lung volumes and capacities in, 762
    mechanics of breathing in, 768
    pathogenesis of, 796
    presentation of, 797
    prognosis for, 797
    treatment of, 797
Idiopathic thrombocytopenic purpura (ITP), 85, 291–292
IF (intrinsic factor), 196, 198
IF (intrinsic factor) deficiency, 278
Ifosfamide, 310–311
IgA (immunoglobulin A) nephropathy, 634–635
IGF-1 (insulin-like growth factor-1), 114
IgG (immunoglobulin G), maternal, 694
IGRA (interferon-gamma release assay), 813
IHD (ischemic heart disease), 85–86
    chronic, 89
IL. See Interleukin (IL)
Ileal artery, 186
Ileocecal valve, 199
Ileocolic artery, 186
Ileum, 199
Iliac crest, 338
Iliac regions, 180, 181

Iliacus muscle, 587, 588
Ilioinguinal nerve, 179, 677
Iliopsoas muscle, 352, 588
Ilium, 338
Illness anxiety disorder, 554, 556
Illusion, 536
Iloprost, 820
IMA (inferior mesenteric artery), 172, 184, 185, 186
    anastomoses with, 187
Imatinib, 317
Imipramine, 518, 540
IML (intermediolateral) cell column, 449
Immotile cilia syndrome, 2, 760, 789
Immune cytokines, 788
Immune system during pregnancy, 694
Immune-mediated thrombocytopenia, 291
Immunization, passive vs active, 710
Immunoglobulin A (IgA) nephropathy, 634–635
Immunoglobulin G (IgG), maternal, 694
Immunohemolytic anemias, 280–281
Immunotherapy
    for allergy, 817
    cancer, 317
Impetigo, 392
Implantation, 687
Inamrinone, 102
Inborn errors of metabolism, liver disease due to, 247–248
Incisional hernia, 236
Incomplete block, 44
Incus, 462
Indifferent stage, 662
Indirect Coombs test, 280
Indomethacin, 407
Induction theory of endometriosis, 723
Infant respiratory distress syndrome, 764, 793–794
Infantile spinal muscular atrophy, 457, 481
Infections
    CNS, 503, 505
    metabolic acidosis due to, 619
    pulmonary, 808–814
        pneumonia as, 808–812
        tuberculosis as, 774, 812–814
        upper respiratory tract, 814
    sexually transmitted and other genital, 731–733
    skin, 391–392
    urinary tract, 638–639
    vessel wall abnormalities due to, 295
Infectious colitis, 231–232
Infectious glomerulonephritis, 623, 631–632
Infectious hepatitis, 242, 243
Infective endocarditis, 58–59, 61–62
Inferior adrenal arteries, 147
Inferior cerebellar peduncle (ICP), 437, 438
Inferior colliculus, 462, 463
Inferior epigastric artery, 179, 182, 674, 676
Inferior epigastric vein, 182, 674, 676
Inferior frontal gyrus, 426
Inferior gluteal nerve injury, 353
Inferior hypophyseal artery, 113, 117
Inferior mesenteric artery (IMA), 172, 184, 185, 186
    anastomoses with, 187
Inferior mesenteric ganglia, 189
Inferior nasal conchae, 335
Inferior oblique muscle, 458
Inferior olivary nucleus, 438, 445
Inferior pancreaticoduodenal artery, 158, 186
Inferior phrenic artery, 184
Inferior phrenic vein, 187
Inferior rectus muscle, 458
Inferior sagittal sinus, 424

Inferior temporal gyrus, 426
Inferior thyroid artery, 126
Inferior thyroid vein, 126, 127
Inferior vena cava (IVC), 9, 185, 187
Inferior vena cava (IVC) syndrome, 75
Inflammatory bowel disease (IBD), 230
Inflammatory ductal carcinoma, 730–731
Infliximab, 260–261, 404
Infrahyoid muscles, 348
Infraspinatus muscle, 349
Infundibulopelvic ligament, 672
Inguinal canal, 181–183
Inguinal groove, 179
Inguinal hernia, 237, 669
    direct, 181, 182, 236, 237, 666, 674
    indirect, 181, 182, 236, 237, 666
Inguinal ligament, 179, 182, 674, 675, 676
Inguinal triangle, 182, 183, 237, 674, 676
Inhibin, 683, 685
Inner hair cells, 462
Inositol triphosphate (IP$_3$) mechanism, 110
Inotropic agents, positive vs negative, 26
Inotropic effect, positive vs negative, 24
Inotropy
    and cardiac and vascular function curves,
        28, 29
    intracellular calcium and, 22
    length-tension relationship and, 25
INR (international normalized ratio), 320
Insomnia
    fatal familial, 483
    primary, 566
Inspection in pulmonary physical examination,
    779–780
Inspiration, 765
    mechanics of breathing during, 766, 768
Inspiratory capacity (IC), 761, 762
Inspiratory muscles, 758, 765
Inspiratory reserve volume (IRV), 761, 762
Inspired O_2, hypoxemia due to decreased,
    776, 777
Insulin, 159–161
    action of, 160–161
    biosynthesis of, 159
    and estrogen, 687
    intermediate-acting, 167
    long-acting, 167
    rapid-acting, 167
    secretion of, 160, 161
    short-acting, 167
    for type 1 diabetes, 166–167
    types of, 167
Insulin aspart, 167
Insulin detemir, 167
Insulin glargine, 167
Insulin glulisine, 167
Insulin lispro, 167
Insulin receptor activation, 160
Insulin regulation of muscle contraction, 358
Insulin resistance during pregnancy, 694
Insulin-independent glucose uptake, 160
Insulin-like growth factor-1 (IGF-1), 114
Insulinoma, 165
Intellectual disability (ID), 581
Intellectualization, 538
Intercalated disks, 21
Intercellular communication, 466–468
Intercostal artery, 757
Intercostal nerve, 757
Intercostal vein, 757
Intercostobrachial nerve, 351
Interferon-alpha in cancer treatment, 318
Interferon-gamma release assay (IGRA,
        QuantiFERON GOLD), 813
Interleukin-1 (IL-1)
    in bone metabolism, 325
    in bony metastases, 362

Interleukin-2 (IL-2) in cancer treatment, 318
Interleukin-4 (IL-4), 788
Interleukin-5 (IL-5), 788
Interleukin-6 (IL-6) in bone metabolism, 325
Interlobar artery, 588
Interlobular artery, 588
Intermediate acoustic stria, 462
Intermediolateral (IML) cell column, 449
Internal acoustic meatus, 336
Internal anal sphincter, 205
Internal arcuate fibers, 452
Internal capsule, 431, 434–435
Internal carotid artery, 425
Internal genitalia, development of
    female, 670–671
    male, 668
Internal iliac artery, 9, 184, 185, 589
    anastomoses with, 187
Internal iliac vein, 187
Internal jugular vein, 424, 682
Internal laryngeal nerve, 348
Internal medullary lamina, 433
Internal oblique fascia, 182
Internal oblique muscle, 179, 182
Internal spermatic fascia, 182
Internal thoracic artery, 682
    anastomoses with, 187
Internal thoracic vein, 682
International normalized ratio (INR), 320
Internuclear ophthalmoplegia, 442, 486, 503
Interossei muscles, 351
Interosseous ligaments, 344
Interscalene triangle, 331
Interstitial cells of Cajal (ICC), 196
Interstitial fluid
    composition of, 596
    measuring volume of, 598
Interstitial hydrostatic pressure, 35
Interstitial lung diseases, 792–798
    acute respiratory distress syndrome as, 764,
        769, 792–793
    chronic eosinophilic pneumonia as, 798
    Goodpasture syndrome as, 797
    granulomatosis with polyangiitis as, 797–798
    idiopathic pulmonary fibrosis as, 762, 766,
        768, 776, 796–797
    neonatal (infant) respiratory distress
        syndrome as, 764, 793–794
    pneumoconiosis as, 794–795
    sarcoidosis as, 795–796
Interstitial oncotic pressure, 35
Intertubercular plane, 181
Intervals on electrocardiogram, 42, 43
Interventricular septum, 3–4
Intervertebral disk, 338
    herniation of, 340–341, 456
Intestinal arteries, 186
Intestinal crypts, 200, 201, 202
Intestinal lipase, small intestinal secretion
    of, 202
Intestinal lymphangiectasia, 225
Intestinal malrotation, 175–176
Intestinal phase of gastric secretion, 197
Intestinal villi, 191, 199, 200, 201
Intra-alveolar pressure, 767, 768–769
Intrabiventral fissure, 437
Intracellular fluid (ICF)
    composition of, 596–597
    intercompartmental water dynamics
        between extracellular and, 598, 599,
        600
    osmolarity of, 598
    volume of
        estimating, 597
        measuring, 597–598
Intracellular receptor, 110

Intracerebral hemorrhage, 419
Intracranial hemorrhage, 475–476, 477
Intracranial pressure (ICP), increased, 468–
    469, 488
Intraculminate fissure, 437
Intraductal papilloma, 728
Intraglomerular mesangial cells, 592, 593
Intramembranous ossification, 326
Intraparenchymal hemorrhage, 476, 477
Intraparietal sulcus, 426
Intrapleural pressure, 767, 768–769
Intraventricular septum (IVS), 4
Intrinsic factor (IF), 196, 198
Intrinsic factor (IF) deficiency, 278
Intrinsic innervation of GI tract, 190, 191
Intrinsic laryngeal muscles, 348
Intrinsic tyrosine kinase, 110
Intussusception, 228
Inulin, 599, 601
Invasive ductal carcinoma, 729–731
Invasive lobular carcinoma, 731
Inward recoil of lungs, 767
Iodide, 137
Iodide extraction in thyroid hormone
        synthesis, 128
Iodide trapping, 128
Iodine, 137
Iodine deficiency, 133
Ion channels, 466
IP$_3$ (inositol triphosphate) mechanism, 110
IPF. See Idiopathic pulmonary fibrosis (IPF)
Ipratropium, 512, 769, 822
Irbesartan, 659
Iris, 502
Iron (Fe^{2+})
    serum, 275
    small intestinal absorption of, 203
Iron deficiency anemia, 274–275
Iron poisoning, metabolic acidosis due to, 619
Irritant receptors, 779
IRV (inspiratory reserve volume), 761, 762
Ischemic heart disease (IHD), 85–86
    chronic, 89
Ischial spine, 352
Ischial tuberosity, 338, 339
Ischium, 338
Islet cell tumors, 165–166
Islets of Langerhans, 159
Isocarboxazid, 517–518, 541
Isoflurane, 531
Isolation of affect, 538
Isomaltase, small intestinal secretion of, 202
Isoniazid, 814
Iso-osmotic volume contraction, 598
Isosorbide dinitrate, 101
Isosorbide mononitrate, 101
Isovolumetric contraction, 27, 29, 30
Isovolumetric relaxation, 27, 29, 30
ITP (idiopathic thrombocytopenic purpura),
    85, 291–292
IVC (inferior vena cava), 9, 185, 187
IVC (inferior vena cava) syndrome, 75
IVS (intraventricular septum), 4
Ixabepilone, 314

J

J (juxtacapillary) receptors, 779
Janeway lesions, 58, 59
Janus kinase (JAK) inhibitors, 110
Janus kinase/signal transducer and activator
        (JAK/STAT) mechanism, 110–111
Jaundice, 209, 238–242
Jaw disorders, 210–211
JC virus, 486
Jejunal artery, 186

Jejunum
anatomy and histologic characteristics of, 199
development of, 173
JG (juxtaglomerular) apparatus
histology of, 593
and mean arterial pressure, 37, 38
JG (juxtaglomerular) cells, histology of, 591, 593
Jod-Basedow effect, 130
Joint(s), types of, 343–344
Joint capsule receptors, 468
Joint disorders
gout as, 375–376
drugs used to treat, 404–406
due to injuries, 344–346
osteoarthritis as, 372–374
pseudogout as, 376–377
rheumatoid arthritis as, 374–375
Joint receptors, 779
Jones criteria for rheumatic fever, 60
Jones fracture, 342
Jugular foramen, 336, 424
Jugular venous distention (JVD), 31
Jugular venous pulses (JVPs) in diastole and systole, 31
Junctional escape rhythm, 49
Junctional zone, 355
Juvenile polyps, 232, 233
Juxtacapillary (J) receptors, 779
Juxtaglomerular (JG) apparatus
histology of, 593
and mean arterial pressure, 37, 38
Juxtaglomerular (JG) cells
histology of, 591, 593
and mean arterial pressure, 39
Juxtamedullary nephrons, 593
JVD (jugular venous distention), 31
JVPs (jugular venous pulses) in diastole and systole, 31

K

K⁺. *See* Potassium (K⁺)
K cells, 204
Kallikrein in alveolar function, 764
Kallmann syndrome, 464, 703
Kartagener syndrome, 2, 760, 789
Karyotype, 662
Kawasaki disease (KD), 82–83, 401, 403
Kayser-Fleischer rings, 248
Keloid, 328
Keratoacanthoma, 395
Keratoconjunctivitis sicca, 211–212
Keratosis
actinic, 395
seborrheic, 390
Kernicterus, 281
Kernig sign, 420
Ketamine, 532
Ketoacidosis, diabetic, 163–164
Ketoconazole, 746
Ketone bodies, 162
Ketorolac, 407
Kidney(s)
in acid-base homeostasis, 617–618
anatomy of, 587–588, 589
in bilirubin production, 209
development of, 584–587
endocrine functions of, 611
hormones acting on, 611–615
horseshoe, 585–586
multicystic dysplastic, 586
Kidney disease
chronic, 640, 642–643
cystic, 643–645
Kidney injury
acute, 640–642

chronic, 640, 642–643
postrenal, 641
prerenal, 641
renal, 641
Kidney stones, 636–637
Kiesselbach plexus, 783
Kimmelstiel-Wilson lesions, 628, 629–630
Kinesins, 464
Kinetic labyrinth, 463
Kinocilium, 463
Klebsiella granulomatis, 732
Klebsiella pneumoniae, 811
Klinefelter syndrome, 700
Klippel-Feil syndrome, 330
Klumpke palsy, 331, 350, 498–499
Klüver-Bucy syndrome, 430
Knee
common pathology of, 353
housemaid's, 353
Knee extension, 341
Knee jerk reflex, 449
Knee joint, 345
Koilocytes, 712
Koilocytic change, 712–713
Krabbe disease, 487
K-RAS gene, 234
Krukenberg tumor, 223–224, 721
Kulchitsky cells, 804
Kupffer cells, 207, 249
Kuru, 483
Kussmaul sign, 80–81
Kyphoscoliosis, restrictive lung disease due to, 791
Kyphosis, 337

L

L cells, 204
LA (left atrium), 9, 10
Labia majora, 671, 673, 680
Labia minora, 671, 673, 680
Labioscrotal folds, 664, 665
Labioscrotal swelling, 669, 673
Labor modulators, 744
Labyrinth, 462, 463
Lachman test, 345
Lacrimal bones, 335
Lactase
deficiency of, 224
small intestinal secretion of, 202
Lacteal, 201, 203
Lactose intolerance, 224
Lactulose, 261
Lacunar infarcts, 476–478, 479
nonembolic, 435
LAD (left anterior descending) artery, 12, 13
infarction of, 78
Ladd bands, 175
Lambdoid suture, 328, 329, 335, 336
Lambert-Eaton myasthenic syndrome (LEMS), 467, 468, 804
Lamina, 336, 337
Laminar flow, 34, 67
Lamotrigine, 525–526, 541
Langerhans cell(s), 305
Langerhans cell histiocytosis, 305–306
Language comprehension, 430
Language production, 427
Lansoprazole, 259–260
LAP (left atrial pressure), 31
Laplace's law, 764
Large cell carcinoma (LCC) of lung, 805
Large intestine. *See* Colon
Large-vessel vasculitis, 81–82, 403
Larson syndrome, 325
Laryngeal atresia, 752
Laryngeal carcinoma, 808

Laryngeal muscles, 348
Laryngeal tumors, benign, 808
Laryngomalacia, 752
Laryngopharynx, 749
Laryngotracheal diverticulum, 750
Laryngotracheal tube, 749
Laryngotracheobronchitis, 814
Larynx, 348
development of, 748–749
Latch-bridges, 358
Lateral ankle ligaments, torn, 345
Lateral cerebral fissure, 425, 426
Lateral collateral ligament, 345
Lateral corticospinal tract, 449, 450–451
Lateral cricoarytenoid muscles, 348
Lateral dorsal nucleus, 433
Lateral epicondyle of humerus, fracture of, 350
Lateral epicondylitis, 349
Lateral funiculus, 453
Lateral geniculate nucleus, 433, 462
Lateral hemisphere, 437
Lateral horn, 449
Lateral hypothalamic area (LHA), 192
Lateral inferior pontine syndrome, 442, 443
Lateral lemniscus, 461, 462
Lateral malleolus, 353
Lateral mammary vessels, 682
Lateral medullary syndrome, 445, 478
Lateral meniscus, 345
Lateral nucleus, 435, 436
Lateral pontine syndrome, 478
Lateral rectus muscle, 458
Lateral spinothalamic tract, 440, 449, 453, 454
Lateral striate arteries, 435
Lateral thoracic artery, 682
Lateral ventral nucleus, 433
Lateral ventricles, 420, 421, 431, 434, 469
Law of Laplace, 66
Laxative(s), osmotic, 261
Laxative abuse, metabolic alkalosis due to, 619
LCA (left coronary artery), 12, 13
LCC (large cell carcinoma) of lung, 805
LCIS (lobular carcinoma in situ), 680, 729
LCX (left circumflex coronary artery), 12, 13
L-dopa (levodopa), 529
Lead(s), electrocardiogram, 41
Lead lines, 277
Lead poisoning, 276–277
Lecithin–sphingomyelin ratio, 764
Left anterior descending (LAD) artery, 12, 13
infarction of, 78
Left anterior fascicle, 14, 15
Left atrial pressure (LAP), 31
Left atrium (LA), 9, 10
Left axis deviation, 44
Left bundle branch, 14, 15
Left bundle branch block, 44–45
Left circumflex coronary artery (LCX), 12, 13
Left colic artery, 186
Left coronary artery (LCA), 12, 13
Left gastric artery, 186
Left hepatic artery, 186
Left hypochondriac region, 180, 181
Left iliac region, 180, 181
Left lower quadrant (LLQ), 181
Left lumbar region, 180, 181
Left (obtuse) marginal artery, 12
Left posterior fascicle, 14, 15
Left upper quadrant (LUQ), 181
Left ventricle (LV), 10
Left ventricular (LV) afterload, 24
Left ventricular end-diastolic pressure (LVEDP), preload and, 25
Left ventricular end-diastolic volume (LVEDV), preload and, 25
Left ventricular (LV) hypertrophy, 44, 45

Left ventricular (LV) pressure in diastole and systole, 30
Left-dominant circulation, 13
Left-sided heart failure, 63–65
Left-to-right shunts, 7
  hypoxemia due to, 778
Leg muscles, 351–352
Legg-Calvé-Perthes disease, 343
Legionella pneumophila, 811
Leiomyoma, 726
Leiomyosarcoma, 726–727
LEMS (Lambert-Eaton myasthenic syndrome), 467, 468, 804
Length-tension relationship and contractility, 25
Lens, 502
  dislocation of, 504
Lentiform nucleus, 452
Lentigo maligna melanoma, 395, 396
Leptin, 192
LES (lower esophageal sphincter), 194, 195
Leser-Trélat triad, 223, 390
Lesser pelvis, 338, 339
Lesser sac, 184
Lesser sciatic foramen, 339
Letterer-Siwe disease, 305
Leukemia, 301–304
  acute
    lymphoblastic, 301–302
    monocytic, 303
    myelogenous (acute granulocytic), 297, 302–303
    promyelocytic, 302
  chronic
    lymphocytic, 300, 302
    myelogenous (chronic granulocytic), 297, 303–304
  classification of, 301
  defined, 301
  epidemiology of, 301
  hairy cell, 304
Leukemia/lymphoma, adult T-cell, 304
Leukocyte(s), 268–271
Leukocyte adhesion deficiency, 269
Leukocyte disorders, 295–306
  Langerhans cell histiocytosis as, 305–306
  leukemias as, 301–304
  leukopenia as, 295–296
  lymphomas as, 297–301
  plasma cell disorders as, 304–305
  reactive proliferation as, 296–297
Leukocytosis, 267, 296–297
Leukodystrophy
  globoid cell, 487
  metachromatic, 487
Leukoencephalopathy
  Binswanger, 479
  progressive multifocal, 486, 487
Leukoerythroblastosis, 307
Leukopenia, 295–296
Leukoplakia, 210, 211
Leuprolide, 124, 315, 741
Levator veli palatini, 347
Levodopa (L-dopa), 529
Levothyroxine (T$_4$), 135, 136, 137–138
Lewy bodies, dementia with, 483
Leydig cell(s), 666, 682–683, 684
Leydig cell tumor, 738
LGSIL (low-grade squamous intraepithelial lesion), 714
LH. *See* Luteinizing hormone (LH)
LHA (lateral hypothalamic area), 192
Libman-Sacks endocarditis (LSE), 59, 382
Lichen planus, 210, 211, 394
Liddle syndrome, 646
Lidocaine, 104, 464

Ligamentum arteriosum, 172
Ligamentum teres hepatis, 172
Ligamentum venosum, 172
Limb(s)
  bones of, 338
  congenital malformations of, 331–332
  development of, 331
  fractures of, 341–342
  muscular development of, 333
Limb leads, 41
Linagliptin, 169
Linea alba, 178, 179, 182, 675
Linea nigra, 694
Linea semilunaris, 178, 179
Linear skull fracture, 339
Lines of Zahn, 800, 801
Lingual gyrus, 426
Lingual lipase, 193
Lingula, 437
Lipase, 258
  intestinal, 202
  lingual, 193
  pancreatic, 206
Lipid(s), small intestinal absorption of, 202, 203
Lipid metabolism in muscle contraction, 358
Lipid-lowering agents, 103, 105
Lipid-soluble hormones, 108, 109
  plasma transport of, 109
Lipiduria in nephrotic syndrome, 625
Lipocortin, 151
Lipoid nephrosis, 625–626
Liraglutide, 168–169
Lisdexamfetamine, 605
Lisfranc fracture, 342
Lisinopril, 99, 659
Lissauer tract, 453
Lithium, 521–522, 539, 541
  hypothyroidism due to, 133
Liver
  anatomy and physiology of, 206–207
  in bilirubin production, 208
  formation of blood cells in, 266
Liver cell plates, 207
Liver disease, 238–250
  alcoholic hepatitis as, 242–243
  bleeding disorders due to, 291, 294
  cirrhosis and portal hypertension as, 244–246
  hepatic tumors as, 248–250
  hereditary hyperbilirubinemias as, 240–242
  due to inborn errors of metabolism, 247–248
  infectious hepatitis as, 242, 243
  jaundice as, 238–240
  primary biliary cirrhosis as, 246–247
  Reye syndrome as, 244
Liver lobule, 206
Liver sinusoids, 206, 207
LLQ (left lower quadrant), 181
LMN (lower motor neuron) lesions, 455, 457, 460, 494, 497, 502
Lobar pneumonia, 809, 810, 816
"Lobster-claw deformities," 331
Lobular carcinoma in situ (LCIS), 680, 729
Local anesthetics, 464
Locked-in syndrome, 444, 488
Locus ceruleus, 508
Lofgren syndrome, 384
Lomustine, 311
Long QT interval/syndrome, 42, 43
Long saphenous vein, 352
Long thoracic nerve damage, 350
Loop diuretics, 93, 94, 608, 655, 656, 657
Loop of Henle
  histology of, 590, 591, 592
  physiology of, 608–610

Loose associations, 545
Loperamide, 515–516
Loratadine, 819
Lorazepam, 515, 540
Lordosis, 337, 338
  during pregnancy, 694
Losartan, 99–100, 102, 659
Louis-Bar syndrome, 493
Lovastatin, 105
Lower esophageal sphincter (LES), 194, 195
Lower extremity nerve injury, 495
Lower limbs
  anatomic landmarks of, 353
  bones of, 338
  fractures of, 342
  muscles of
    anatomy of, 351–352
    nerve damage affecting, 352–353
  quick motor exam of, 341
Lower motor neuron (LMN) lesions, 455, 457, 460, 494, 497, 502
Low-grade squamous intraepithelial lesion (LGSIL), 714
LSD (lysergic acid diethylamide), pupillary response to, 568
LSD (lysergic acid diethylamide) use disorder, 575
LSE (Libman-Sacks endocarditis), 59, 382
Lumbar arteries, 185
Lumbar puncture, 338, 419, 420, 469
Lumbar vertebrae, 337
Lumber regions, 180, 181
Lumbrical muscles, 351
Lung(s)
  in acid-base homeostasis, 618
  anatomy of, 754–756
  blood supply of, 754–755, 756
  development of, 749, 750
  inward recoil of, 767
Lung abscess, 812
Lung buds, 749, 750
Lung cancer, 803–807
  adenocarcinoma as, 804–805
  bronchial neuroendocrine (carcinoid), 805–806
  categories of, 804
  complications of, 806
  diagnosis of, 807
  incidence of, 803
  large cell, 805
  metastatic, 806, 807
  presentation of, 806
  prognosis for, 807
  risk factors for, 804
  small cell, 804, 805
  squamous cell, 805
  treatment of, 807
Lung capacities, 761–763
Lung compliance (C), 766, 784
Lung consolidation, 816
Lung disease
  fibrotic, 762, 766, 768, 776, 796–797
  interstitial, 792–798
    acute respiratory distress syndrome as, 764, 769, 792–793
    chronic eosinophilic pneumonia as, 798
    Goodpasture syndrome as, 797
    granulomatosis with polyangiitis, 797–798
    idiopathic pulmonary fibrosis as, 762, 766, 768, 776, 796–797
    neonatal (infant) respiratory distress syndrome as, 764, 793–794
    pneumoconiosis as, 794–795
    sarcoidosis as, 795–796

Lung disease (continued)
  obstructive, 783–790
    asthma as, 761, 787–788, 789
    bronchiectasis as, 788–790
    chronic bronchitis as, 786–787
    emphysema as, 761, 766, 768, 776,
      784–786
    lung volumes and capacities in, 761, 762,
      763, 783
  restrictive, 790–798
    acute respiratory distress syndrome as,
      764, 769, 792–793
    chronic eosinophilic pneumonia as, 798
    extrapulmonary, 790–791
    Goodpasture syndrome as, 797
    granulomatosis with polyangiitis as,
      797–798
    idiopathic pulmonary fibrosis as, 762, 766,
      768, 776, 796–797
    interstitial, 792–798
    lung volumes and capacities in, 762, 763
    neonatal (infant) respiratory distress
      syndrome as, 764, 793–794
    pneumoconiosis as, 794–795
    sarcoidosis as, 795–796
Lung percussion, 780–781
Lung stretch receptors, 779
Lung volumes, 761–763
  and pulmonary resistance, 770
  and pulmonary vascular resistance, 773–774
Lung–chest wall system, compliance of, 766,
  767
Lupus, drug-induced, 383
Lupus dermatitis, 380, 381
Lupus nephritis, 381, 382, 629–630
LUQ (left upper quadrant), 181
Luteal phase, 688
Luteinizing hormone (LH), 114
  with age, 687, 689
  in menstrual cycle, 686–687, 688
  in spermatogenesis, 683, 685
LV. See Left ventricle (LV)
LVEDP (left ventricular end-diastolic
  pressure), preload and, 25
LVEDV (left ventricular end-diastolic volume),
  preload and, 25
17,20-Lyase in steroid hormone synthesis, 150
Lyme disease, 499
Lymph nodes, normal vs reactive, 296
Lymphadenopathy, 189
Lymphangiectasia, intestinal, 225
Lymphatic(s), 35
Lymphatic drainage, 187
  of GI tract, 188–189
Lymphatic duct, 203
Lymphatic effusion, 815
Lymphoblastic lymphoma, 301
Lymphocyte(s), 269, 270
Lymphocytic leukocytosis, 296–297
Lymphogranuloma venereum, 731
Lymphoma, 297–301
  adult T-cell leukemia/, 304
  Burkitt, 297, 301
  cutaneous T-cell, 299, 301
  diffuse large-cell, 300
  extranodal marginal zone, 189, 299
  follicular, 297, 300
  gastric, 223
  Hodgkin, 297–298, 299
  lymphoblastic, 301
  mantle cell, 297, 300
  mucosa-associated lymphoid tissue (MALT),
    189, 299
  non-Hodgkin, 297, 298, 300–301
  primary CNS, 496
  small lymphocytic, 300, 302

  testicular, 738
  thyroid, 134
Lymphopenia, 295, 296
Lynch syndrome, 233
Lysergic acid diethylamide (LSD), pupillary
  response to, 568
Lysergic acid diethylamide (LSD) use
  disorder, 575

M

M (microfold) cells, 200
M line, 21
Macroglobulinemia, Waldenström, 295, 305
Macro-ovalocyte, 274
Macrophages, 268, 271, 272
  alveolar, 760
Macrovascular complications of diabetes, 163
Macula densa, 591, 592, 593
Macular degeneration, 502
Macule, 389
Magnesium (Mg^{2+}), for arrhythmias, 104
Magnesium ammonium phosphate stones,
  636, 637
Magnesium citrate, 261
Magnesium hydroxide, 261
Magnesium sulfate, 823
Magnesium-containing antacids, 260, 261
Magnetic resonance
      cholangiopancreatography (MRCP),
    178, 251, 252
Magnocellular neurons, 117
Main pancreatic duct, 208
Major basic protein (MBP), 788
Major calyces, 588
Major depressive disorder (MDD), 546, 547–
  548, 549, 550
Major salivary glands, 192
Malabsorption syndromes, 224–225
Malar rash, 380, 381
Male pseudohermaphroditism, 666
Male reproductive disorders, 733–741
  congenital malformations as, 669
  penile, 733–734
  prostatic, 738–741
  testicular, 734–738
Male reproductive system
  anatomy of, 675–679
  development of, 666–669
  drugs that modulate, 741–743
  gonadal steroids in, 687, 689, 690
  homologs in female and, 674, 675
  sexual response in, 689–691
  spermatogenesis in, 682–684
Malignancy-induced hypercalcemia, 144, 145,
  310, 362
Malignant hypertension, 54, 55
Malignant hyperthermia, 467, 531
Malignant melanoma, 395–396
  oral, 211
  vaginal, 713
Malignant tumors, 308, 309–310
Malingering, 557, 558
Malleus, 462
Mallory bodies, 243
Mallory-Weiss tear, 215
Malrotation, 175–176
MALT (mucosa-associated lymphoid tissue)
    lymphoma, 189, 299
Maltase, small intestinal secretion of, 202
Mamillary body, 435, 436
Mammary glands, 672
Mammary ridge, 672
Mammary vessels, 682
Mandible, 335, 336
Mania, 546, 547, 548–550
Mannitol, 94–95, 656

Mantle cell lymphoma, 297, 300
Mantoux test, 813
MAO (monoamine oxidase) inhibitors, 516,
  517–518, 529–530, 541
MAP (mean arterial pressure)
  determinants of, 35–37
  regulation of, 35–40
MAP (mitogen-activated protein) kinase, 160
Maprotiline, 520
Marantic endocarditis, 59
Marble bone disease, 326, 368–369
Marcus Gunn pupil, 458, 502
Marfan syndrome, 326–328, 329–330
  cardiac defects in, 7, 68
Marginal artery, 12, 13
Marijuana use disorder, 576
Mast cells, 270, 271
Mastication muscles, 347
Mastitis, acute, 728
Mastoid fontanelles, 328
Mastoid process, 336
Mature follicle, 687
Maxillae, 335, 336
Maxillary nerve, 425
Maxillary sinus, 782
Maximum expiration, mechanics of breathing
  at, 768–769
Maximum inspiration, mechanics of breathing
  at, 768
MBP (major basic protein), 788
MCA (middle cerebral artery), 422, 423
  stroke involving, 478
McBurney point, 191, 236, 338
McCune-Albright syndrome, 371
MCDK (multicystic dysplastic kidney), 586
MCHC (mean corpuscular hemoglobin
  concentration), 269
MCP (middle cerebellar peduncle), 437, 438,
  442
MCTD (mixed connective tissue disease),
  384–385
MCV (mean corpuscular volume), 269
MDD (major depressive disorder), 546, 547–
  548, 549, 550
Mean arterial pressure (MAP)
  determinants of, 35–37
  regulation of, 35–40
Mean cell hemoglobin, 269
Mean corpuscular hemoglobin concentration
  (MCHC), 269
Mean corpuscular volume (MCV), 269
Mean systemic pressure, 23
  and cardiac and vascular function curves,
  28, 29
Mechanical ventilation, 769
Meckel diverticulum, 172, 226
Meckel scan, 226
Medial antebrachial cutaneous nerve, 351
Medial brachial cutaneous nerve, 351
Medial collateral ligament, 345
Medial dorsal nuclei, 433
Medial epicondyle fracture
  of arm, 342
  of humerus, 350
Medial epicondylitis, 349
Medial geniculate nucleus (MGN), 433, 462,
  463
Medial inferior pontine syndrome, 442
Medial lemniscus, 442, 445
Medial longitudinal fasciculus (MLF), 442,
  445
  lesion of, 503
Medial longitudinal fasciculus (MLF)
    syndrome, 442, 486, 503
Medial malleolus, 352
Medial mammary vessels, 682

Medial medullary syndrome, 445
Medial meniscus, 345
Medial nuclei, 433
Medial occipitotemporal gyrus, 426
Medial rectus muscle, 458
Medial sacral artery, 185
Medial umbilical ligaments, 172, 182
Median nerve, 338, 349, 351
    damage to, 350, 495
Median sacral vein, 187
Median umbilical ligament, 172, 182
Medium-vessel vasculitis, 82–83, 403
Medroxyprogesterone, 744
Medulla, 437, 444–445
    in control of respiration, 779
Medullary carcinoma of breast, 730
Medullary cavity, 325, 335
Medullary pyramids, 588
Medullary respiratory center, 778–779
Medullary thyroid carcinoma, 135
Medulloblastoma, 490, 492
Megacolon, congenital, 172, 229
Megakaryocytes, 268, 307, 308
Megaloblastic anemia, 277–278
Meigs syndrome, 720, 721
Meiosis, 683
Meissner corpuscles, 452, 453, 468
Meissner nerve plexus, 190, 195
Melancholia, 547, 548
Melanocytic nevus, 390
Melanoma, 395–396
    oral, 211
    vaginal, 713
Melasma, 391

Membrane conductance, 15–16
Membrane potential (Vm), 15–16
Membranoproliferative glomerulonephritis
    (MPGN), 627–628
Membranous glomerulopathy, 623
    diffuse, 626–627
Membranous labyrinth, 463
Membranous urethra, 589
Memory, 429–430, 433
Memory loss, 430
MEN (multiple endocrine neoplasia), 135, 136
Menarche, 686
Ménétrier disease, 221
Meninges
    anatomy of, 419
    pathology of, 419–420
Meningioma, 420, 490, 491, 494
    olfactory groove, 463
Meningismal signs, 420
Meningismus, 470
Meningitis
    bacterial, 419, 420
    carcinomatous, 420
    causes of, 419, 503, 505
    communicating hydrocephalus due to,
        470–471
    CSF characteristics of, 420
    defined, 419, 503
    fungal, 419, 420
    signs of, 420
    viral (aseptic), 419, 420
Meningocele, 330, 414
Meningoencephalocele, 330, 414
Meningohydroencephalocele, 330, 414
Meningomyelocele, 414, 470
Menopause, 698–700
    adrenal androgens in, 153
Menstrual cycle, 686–687, 688
Menstruation, 687, 688
    retrograde, 723
Mental foramen, 336

Mental retardation, 581
Meperidine, 515–516
6-Mercaptopurine (6-MP), 313
Merkel corpuscles, 453, 468
Meromelia, 331
Mesencephalon, 414, 416
Mesenchymal tumors, 308
Mesenteric artery, 201
Mesenteric vein, 201
Mesentery, 184
Mesonephric duct, 585
    derivatives of
        female, 669, 670, 674
        male, 668, 674
    development of, 663, 664
Mesonephros, 584, 585
Mesothelioma, 807
Mestranol, 744
Metabolic acidosis, 618–619, 620, 773
    in acid-base nomogram, 622
    clinical implications of, 621
    due to renal failure, 644
Metabolic alkalosis, 618, 619, 620, 773
    in acid-base nomogram, 622
    clinical implications of, 621
Metabolic syndrome, 54
Metachromatic leukodystrophy, 487
Metanephric mesenchyme, 585
Metanephros, 584, 585
Metaplasia, 308
Metastasis(es), bony, 362
Metastatic lung cancer, 806, 807
Metastatic tumors
    of liver, 250
    ovarian, 721
Metencephalon, 414, 416
Metformin, 168
Methacholine, 511, 823
Methacholine challenge test, 788
Methadone, 515–516, 574
Methamphetamine, 541
Methemoglobin, 770
Methemoglobinemia, 770
Methimazole, 128, 136–137
Methotrexate, 312
Methylated B_{12}, 497
Methylcobalamin, 497
Methyldopa, 97
Methylnaltrexone, 576
Methylphenidate, 541
Methyltestosterone, 741–742
Methylxanthines, 823
Metoclopramide, 262
Metolazone, 92, 94, 656, 657
Metoprolol, 96–97, 101, 102, 104
Metyrapone stimulation test, 157
Meyer loop, 460
Mg^{2+}. See Magnesium (Mg^{2+})
MGN (medial geniculate nucleus), 433, 462,
    463
MI. See Myocardial infarction (MI)
Micelles, 203
Microaneurysms, 67
Microangiopathic hemolytic anemia, 286–287
Microangiopathies, thrombotic, 292
Microcephaly, 328, 418
Microfold (M) cells, 200
Microglia, 465
    HIV-infected, 466
Microscopic polyangiitis, 84, 403
Microscopic polyarteritis, 400
Microtubule inhibitors, 311
Microvascular complications of diabetes, 163
Microvilli, 199
Micturition, 594
Midaxillary line, 757

Midazolam, 515, 532, 540
Midbrain, 437, 440, 441
    development of, 414, 416
Midclavicular lines, 181, 757
Middle adrenal arteries, 147
Middle cerebellar peduncle (MCP), 437, 438,
    442
Middle cerebral artery (MCA), 422, 423
    stroke involving, 478
Middle colic artery, 186
Middle cranial fossa, 459
Middle fossa, 335
Middle frontal gyrus, 426
Middle suprarenal artery, 184, 185
Middle temporal gyrus, 426
Middle temporal sulcus, 426
Middle thyroid vein, 126, 127
Midgut, 172, 173
Midgut volvulus, 175, 176
Midhumerus fracture, 350
Midpelvis, 339
Midsternal line, 757
MIF (Müllerian-inhibiting factor) in sexual
    differentiation, 662
Mifepristone, 746
Migraines, 505–506
Migrating motor complex (MMC), 196, 200,
    205
Migratory thrombophlebitis, 75, 255
Migratory venous thrombosis,
    paraneoplastic, 310
Miliary tuberculosis, 813
Milk "letdown" reflex, 698
    hypercalcemia due to, 144
    metabolic alkalosis due to, 619
Milrinone, 102
Mineralocorticoid(s), 152–153, 687
Mineralocorticoid escape, 614
Mineralocorticoid receptors (MRs), 613
Minimal change disease, 625–626
Minor calyces, 588
Minor salivary glands, 192
Minoxidil, 98, 743
Minute ventilation (MV), 764
    during pregnancy, 693
Mirtazapine, 519–520, 541
MIT (monoiodotyrosine), 128
Mitochondrially inherited disorders, 678
Mitogen-activated protein (MAP) kinase, 160
Mitosis, 683
Mitral regurgitation (MR), 10, 68–69, 71
Mitral stenosis (MS), 72, 73
    due to rheumatic heart disease, 61, 72
Mitral valve (MV), 10, 11
Mitral valve (MV) insufficiency, 7
Mitral valve prolapse (MVP), 63, 68, 70–71
Mivacurium, 510
Mixed acid-base disorders, 621, 773
Mixed connective tissue disease (MCTD),
    384–385
Mixed stones, 250, 251
Mixed transcortical aphasia, 431
Mixing studies, 291
MLCK (myosin light-chain kinase), 358
MLF (medial longitudinal fasciculus), 442,
    445
    lesion of, 503
MLF (medial longitudinal fasciculus)
    syndrome, 442, 486, 503
MMC (migrating motor complex), 196, 200,
    205
Mobitz Type I AV block, 47–48
Mobitz Type II AV block, 47–48
Molecular layer of cerebellum, 437
Mönckeberg arteriosclerosis, 55

Monoamine oxidase (MAO) inhibitors, 516, 517–518, 529–530, 541
Monoclonal gammopathy of uncertain significance, 305
Monocular input, 461
Monocyte, 268, 269–271
Monoiodotyrosine (MIT), 128
Monosodium urate (MSU) crystal deposition, 375–376
Monozygotic twins, 697, 698, 699
Montelukast, 822
Mood, 534, 546
Mood disorders, 546–550
  bipolar, 546, 547, 548–550
  major depressive, 546, 547–548, 549, 550
Mood stabilizers, 521–522, 541
Moraxella catarrhalis, 811
Morphine, 515–516, 532
Mosaicism, 702
Mossy fibers, 439
Motilin, 204
Motivators, psychological, 537
Motor activity disorders, 536
Motor cortex, 428
  primary, 426, 427
Motor endplates, 354
Motor homunculus, 428
Motor neuron lesions, degenerative diseases due to, 481
Motor pathway(s), 449
  lesions of, 455
Motor relay station, 434
Motor speech area, 427
Motor unit, 354
Mouth
  anatomy and physiology of, 192–195
  disorders of, 210–211
Movement, 426–427
  stereotyped, 536
6-MP (6-mercaptopurine), 313
MPGN (membranoproliferative glomerulonephritis), 627–628
MR (mitral regurgitation), 10, 68–69, 71
MR(s) (mineralocorticoid receptors), 613
MRCP (magnetic resonance cholangiopancreatography), 178, 251, 252
MS (mitral stenosis), 72, 73
  due to rheumatic heart disease, 61, 72
MS (multiple sclerosis), 442, 456, 457, 481–484, 486
MSU (monosodium urate) crystal deposition, 375–376
Mucin, 192
Mucinous carcinoma of breast, 730
Mucinous cystadenocarcinoma, 718
Mucinous cystadenoma, 718
Mucinous tumors, ovarian, 718
Mucoactive agents, 819
Mucoepidermoid carcinoma of salivary gland, 213
Mucolytics, 819
Mucosa, 201
Mucosa-associated lymphoid tissue (MALT) lymphoma, 189, 299
Mucous salivary secretions, 192
Mucus
  gastric secretion of, 196, 197
  small intestinal secretion of, 202
Mucus plug in asthma, 788, 789
Mucus-secreting cells of stomach, 196
Müllerian agenesis, 703
Müllerian duct
  derivatives of
    female, 669, 670, 674
    male, 668, 674
  development of, 663, 664

Müllerian-inhibiting factor (MIF) in sexual differentiation, 662
Multicystic dysplastic kidney (MCDK), 586
Multifunctional signals, 108
Multi-infarct dementia, 479, 483
Multinucleated giant cells, 383
Multiple endocrine neoplasia (MEN), 135, 136
Multiple myeloma, 304–305, 632
Multiple personality disorder, 559
Multiple sclerosis (MS), 442, 456, 457, 481–484, 486
Mumps, 212
Munchausen syndrome, 557, 558
Munchausen syndrome by proxy, 557, 558
Mural thrombus, 50
Murmurs. *See* Heart murmurs
Murphy sign, 252
Muscarinic antagonists, 822
Muscarinic drugs, 512
Muscarinic receptor blockade, 521
Muscarinic receptors
  in gastric secretion, 196, 197
  in salivary secretion, 193
Muscle(s)
  accessory, 334
  cardiac, 347
  of head and neck, 347–348
  important, 347–354
  of lower limb, 351–353
  skeletal
    anatomy of, 346, 355
    development of, 332–333
    physiology of, 354–357
  smooth
    anatomy of, 346–347
    development of, 333
    locations of, 358
    physiology of, 357–358
  types of, 346–347
  of upper limb, 348–351
Muscle contraction
  energy sources for, 358–360
  skeletal, 355–357
  smooth, 358
Muscle receptors, 779
Muscle spindles, 453, 468
Muscle stretch reflexes, 447–448, 449
Muscular disorders
  congenital malformations as, 332–334
  important laboratory values for, 361–362
  due to inflammation, 353
  due to injury
    of lower limb, 352–353
    of upper limb, 349, 350
  muscular dystrophy as, 388–389
Muscular dystrophy, 388–389
Muscular system
  anatomy of, 346–353
    head and neck muscles in, 347–348
    lower limb muscles in, 351–353
    types of muscle in, 346–347
    upper limb muscles in, 348–351
  development of, 332–334
  disorders of. *See* Muscular disorders
  physiology of, 354–360
Muscularis externa, 201
Muscularis mucosae, 191, 201
Musculocutaneous nerve, 351
  damage to, 350, 495
Musculoskeletal disorders, 362–389
  bone tumors as, 362–367
  fibrous dysplasia as, 371
  gout as, 375–376
  laboratory values pertinent to, 361–362
  osteitis fibrosa cystica as, 370

  osteoarthritis as, 372–374
  osteomalacia/rickets as, 369
  osteomyelitis as, 371–372
  osteopetrosis (marble bone disease) as, 368–369
  osteoporosis as, 367–368
  Paget disease of bone as, 369–370
  pharmacology for, 402–409
  pseudogout as, 376–377
  rheumatoid arthritis as, 374–375
Musculoskeletal system, 323–410
  anatomy of, 335–353
  disorders of. *See* Musculoskeletal disorders
  embryology of, 324–334
  important laboratory values for, 361–362
  pharmacology for, 402–409
  physiology of, 354–362
Mutism, selective, 581
MV (minute ventilation), 764
  during pregnancy, 693
MV (mitral valve), 10, 11
MV (mitral valve) insufficiency, 7
MVP (mitral valve prolapse), 63, 68, 70–71
Myasthenia gravis, 194, 467, 468
  paraneoplastic, 310
  restrictive lung disease due to, 791
MYC gene, 309
Mycobacterium tuberculosis, 813
Mycoplasma pneumoniae, 811
Mycosis fungoides, 299
Mycotic aneurysms, 66
Myelencephalon, 414, 416
Myelin, 464
Myelin sheath, 354, 465
Myelination, 464
Myelinolysis, central pontine, 124, 444, 488, 497, 651
Myelofibrosis, 306, 307
Myeloid dysplasia, 307
Myeloid metaplasia, 307
Myeloma, multiple, 304–305, 632
Myeloma cast nephropathy, 632
Myeloperoxidase deficiency disease, 279
Myelophthisis, 362
Myeloproliferative syndromes, 306–308
Myenteric plexus, 190, 191, 195
Mylohyoid muscle, 348
Myoblasts, 332
Myocardial contraction, 21–23
Myocardial infarction (MI), 87–89
  cardiac enzymes in, 87–88, 89
  diagnosis of, 87–88, 89
  ECG of, 87, 88
  etiology of, 87
  gross and microscopic changes to heart in, 87
  non-ST-elevation, 13, 87, 89
  presentation of, 87, 88
  prognosis for, 88–89
  ST-elevation, 13, 14, 87, 88, 89
  treatment of, 89
Myocardial relaxation, 21–23
Myocarditis, 57
  due to rheumatic fever, 60
Myocardium, 11, 12, 347
Myoclonic seizure, 489
Myoclonus
  nocturnal, 568
  physiologic, 488
Myocytes
  cardiac, 14–15, 17–18
    characteristics of, 20
    contraction of, 20–23
  skeletal, 20, 354
Myofibrils, 21, 332
  and excitation-contraction coupling, 355, 356

Myofilaments, 21, 332
Myogenic feedback, in autoregulation of renal
    blood flow and filtration, 603
Myometrium, 589, 671, 672, 680
Myosin, in myocardial contraction and
    relaxation, 22
Myosin light chains, 356
Myosin light-chain kinase (MLCK), 358
Myosin light-chain phosphatase, 358
Myotatic reflexes, 447–448, 449
Myotomes, 332–333
Myotubes, 332
Myxedema coma, 133
Myxoma, cardiac, 73

N

Na+. *See* Sodium (Na+)
Nafarelin, 741
Na+-K+-2Cl– (sodium-potassium-chloride)
    symporter, 608
Na+/K+-ATPase (sodium/potassium–adenosine
    triphosphatase) pump, 607
Naloxegol, 576
Naloxone, 576
Naltrexone, 576
Naproxen, 407
Narcissistic personality disorder, 561
Narcolepsy, 566
Nasal bones, 335
Nasal cavity, 754, 782
Nasal congestion during pregnancy, 693
Nasopharyngeal carcinoma, 808
Nasopharynx, disorders of, 781–783
Native pacemakers, 13, 17–18
    intrinsic factor, 333
Natural killer (NK) cells, 260, 269, 270
NBTE (nonbacterial thrombotic
    endocarditis), 59
NE (norepinephrine), 446, 507, 508
    in regulation of renal blood flow and
        filtration, 602
Near reflex and accommodation pathway, 461
Neck
    hyperextension of, 341
    hyperflexion of, 340
    wry, 348
Neck muscles
    anatomy of, 347–348
    development of, 332
Necrotizing fasciitis, 392
Nefazodone, 519–520
Negative feedback, 111
Negative inotropic agents, 26
Negative inotropic effect, 24
Negative inotropy and cardiac and vascular
    function curves, 28, 29
Negative pressure, 767
Negative symptoms of schizophrenia, 544,
    545
Neisseria gonorrhoeae, 731
Neonatal respiratory distress syndrome
    (NRDS), 764, 793–794
Neoplasia, 308
Neostigmine, 511
Nephritic syndrome, 623, 624, 630–636
    acute proliferative (poststreptococcal,
        infectious) glomerulonephritis as,
        623, 631–632
    antiglomerular basement membrane disease
        (Goodpasture) syndrome as, 601,
        623, 633–634
    granulomatosis with polyangiitis as, 635–636
    hereditary nephritis (Alport syndrome)
        as, 635
    IgA nephropathy (Berger disease) as,
        634–635

rapidly progressive glomerulonephritis as,
    623, 632–633
Nephritis
    diffuse proliferative, 630
    hereditary, 635
    lupus, 381, 382, 629–630
Nephroblastoma, 648–649
Nephrogenic diabetes insipidus, 122, 123
Nephrogenic rests, 648
Nephron(s)
    cortical vs juxtamedullary, 593
    development of, 584
    histology of, 590–593
    physiology of, 607–610
Nephron unit, 607
Nephropathy(ies)
    associated with systemic disorders, 628–630
    contrast, 642
    diabetic, 163, 628, 629
    myeloma cast, 632
Nephrosclerosis, benign vs malignant, 55
Nephrosis, lipoid, 625–626
Nephrotic syndrome, 623–628
    diffuse membranous glomerulopathy as,
        626–627
    focal segmental glomerulosclerosis as, 626,
        627–628
    glomerular basement membrane in, 601
    membranoproliferative glomerulonephritis
        as, 627–628
    minimal change disease as, 625–626
    proteinuria in, 592, 624
Nephrotoxic drugs, 660
Nernst potential (E_x), 15–16
Nerve roots, 447
Nerve supply of GI tract, 189–192
Nervous system, 411–532
    brain in, 412–446
        blood supply to, 422–423
        brain stem of, 440–445
        cerebellum of, 437–440
        cerebral cortex of, 425–431
        congenital malformations of, 414–418
        deep structures of, 431–436
        development of, 414
        dural veins and sinuses of, 424–425
        meninges of, 419–420
        neurotransmitters in, 445
        ventricles of, 420
        ventricular system of, 420–422
    cells of, 464–466
    cranial nerves in, 457–459
    development of, 412, 413
        and neural tube defects, 412–414, 415,
            468
    disorders of. *See* Neurologic disorders
    intercellular communication in, 466–468
    pharmacology of, 507–532
        antidepressants in, 516–520
        anxiolytics and hypnotics in, 513–516
        autonomic drugs in, 508–512
        clinical anesthetics and analgesics in,
            530–532
        CNS neurotransmitters in, 507–508
        mood stabilizers and anticonvulsants in,
            521–526
        neuroleptics in, 520–521
        seafood toxins in, 512–513
        treatments for neurodegenerative disease
            in, 527–530
    sensory systems and pathways in, 459–464
        auditory, 461–463
        gustatory, 464
        olfactory, 463–464
        vestibular, 463
        visual, 459–461

spinal cord in, 446–457
    blood supply to, 446
    cross-section of, 449
    function of, 446
    hemisection of, 453, 454
    lesions of, 455–457
    levels of, 446–447
    myotatic reflex of, 447–448
    tracts of, 449, 453, 454
    unique structures of, 447, 448
NET(s) (neuroendocrine tumors), bronchial,
    805–806
Net filtration pressure, 35
Net fluid flow, 35
Neural crest cells, 413
Neural crest derivatives, 413, 415
Neural fold, 413
Neural groove, 412
Neural plate, 412, 413
Neural tube, 329, 412, 413, 468
Neural tube defects, 330, 412–414, 415, 468
Neuralgia, trigeminal, 501, 506–507
Neuroblastoma, 149, 649–650
Neurocutaneous disorders, 492, 493–494
Neurocysticercosis, 488
Neurodegenerative diseases. *See* Degenerative
    diseases
Neuroendocrine cell nuclei, 113
Neuroendocrine tumors (NETs), bronchial,
    805–806
Neurofibroma, 491
Neurofibromatosis type 1 (NF1), 493
Neurofibromatosis type 2 (NF2), 444, 463, 493
Neurohypophysis. *See* Posterior pituitary
Neuroleptic(s), 520–521
Neuroleptic malignant syndrome, 167
Neurologic disorders, 468–507
    aphasias as, 479–480
    cerebral contusion as, 489–490
    cerebral edema as, 488
    cerebrovascular, 473–478
        embolic stroke (hemorrhagic infarction)
            as, 474–475
        intracranial hemorrhage as, 475–476, 477
        lacunar infarcts as, 476–478
        stroke presentation by location of
            occlusion in, 478
        thrombotic stroke (pale infarction) as,
            473–474
    CNS infections as, 503, 505
    congenital malformations of brain as, 414
    cranial nerve palsies as, 457–459, 499–503
        defects in eye movement due to, 500–501
        due to facial lesions, 502
        internuclear ophthalmoplegia (medial
            longitudinal fasciculus syndrome) as,
            503, 504
        uveitis due to, 502
        visual field defects due to, 502
    degenerative, 480–485
        Alzheimer disease as, 482
        amyotrophic lateral sclerosis as, 481
        due to basal ganglia lesions, 484–485
        due to cerebellar lesions, 481, 484
        due to cerebral cortex lesions, 482–483
        dementia with Lewy bodies as, 483
        Friedreich ataxia as, 485
        frontotemporal dementia (Pick disease)
            as, 482
        Huntington disease as, 484
        due to motor neuron lesions, 481
        multi-infarct (vascular) dementia as, 479,
            483
        olivopontocerebellar atrophy as, 485
        Parkinson disease as, 484

Neurologic disorders (continued)
  degenerative (continued)
    poliomyelitis as, 481
    prion diseases as, 483
    progressive supranuclear palsy as, 480–481
    due to spinocerebellar lesions, 485
    treatments for, 527–530
    Werdnig-Hoffman disease (infantile spinal muscular atrophy) as, 481
    Wilson disease (hepatolenticular degeneration) as, 481, 485
  demyelinating, 481–488
    acute disseminated (postinfectious) encephalomyelitis as, 487
    acute inflammatory demyelinating polyradiculopathy as, 487–488
    multiple sclerosis as, 481–484, 486
    osmotic demyelination syndrome (central pontine myelinolysis) as, 488
    progressive multifocal leukoencephalopathy as, 486
  dyskinesias as, 478–479
  headache syndromes as, 505–507
  herniation syndromes as, 503–505
  hydrocephalus as, 417–418, 421–422
    communicating, 421–422, 470–473
    ex vacuo, 422
    mimics of, 473
    noncommunicating, 421, 469–470
    normal-pressure, 422
  due to lower extremity nerve injury, 495
  of meninges, 419–420
  neural tube defects as, 412–414, 415, 468
  neurocutaneous, 492–494
  of peripheral nervous system, 502
    Guillain-Barré syndrome as, 456
    hereditary motor and sensory neuropathy (Charcot-Marie-Tooth disease) as, 502
  primary brain neoplasms as, 490–492
  seizures as, 488, 489
  spinal cord lesions as, 455–457, 494–499
    Brown-Séquard syndrome as, 453, 454, 494–496
    combined motor and sensory, 455–456
    intervertebral disk herniation as, 456
    of motor pathway, 455, 494, 496
    patterns of, 457
    poliomyelitis as, 496
    of sensory pathway, 455
    subacute combined degeneration (vitamin B_{12}) deficiency as, 497–498
    syringomyelia as, 498
    tabes dorsalis (tertiary syphilis) as, 497
    terminal cord syndromes as, 456
    thoracic outlet syndrome (Klumpke palsy) as, 498–499
  due to upper extremity nerve injury, 495
  ventricular system malformations as, 468–469, 470
Neuroma, acoustic, 444, 463, 465
Neuromuscular blockade, 354
Neuromuscular junction (NMJ), 354, 467
  diseases of, 467, 468
Neuromuscular junction (NMJ)-blocking agents, 509–510
Neuron(s), 464–465
  bipolar, 464
  first-order, 451, 453
  multipolar, 464
  pseudounipolar, 464
  red, 473
  second-order, 452, 453
  third-order, 452, 453
  unipolar, 464

Neuropathy
  diabetic, 163, 499
  hereditary motor and sensory, 499
Neuropeptides in innervation of GI tract, 190
Neurotransmitters, 446
  CNS, 507–508
Neurulation, 412, 413
Neutropenia, 295, 296
Neutrophil(s), 268–269, 270
  hypersegmented, 268, 278
Neutrophilic leukopenia, 296
Nevus, melanocytic, 390
NF1 (neurofibromatosis type 1), 493
NF2 (neurofibromatosis type 2), 444, 463, 493
NH_4^+ (ammonium), renal secretion of, 617–618
NHL (non-Hodgkin lymphoma), 297, 298, 300–301
Niacin, 105
Nicotine use disorder, 572
Nicotinic ACh receptors, 354
Nicotinic acid, 105
Nifedipine, 97–98, 101
Nightmares, 567
Nikolsky sign, 394
Nilotinib, 317
Nipples
  accessory, 672
  anatomy of, 680, 681
  Paget disease of, 729, 730
Nissl bodies, 464, 465
Nitrates, 86, 100, 101
Nitric oxide releasers, 98
Nitroglycerin, 101, 102
Nitroprusside, 98, 102
Nitrosoureas, 311
Nivolumab, 317
Nizatidine, 258–259
NK (natural killer) cells, 268, 269, 270
NMJ (neuromuscular junction), 354, 465, 467
  diseases of, 467, 468
NMJ (neuromuscular junction)-blocking agents, 509–510
Nociceptors, 779
Nocturnal myoclonus, 568
Node of Ranvier, 354, 465
Node of Virchow, 223
Nodular melanoma, 395, 396
Nodule, 389
Nodulus, 437
Nonbacterial endocarditis, 59
Nonbacterial thrombotic endocarditis (NBTE), 59
Noncaseating granulomas, 383
Nondepolarizing agents, 509, 510
Nongonococcal urethritis, 731
Non-Hodgkin lymphoma (NHL), 297, 298, 300–301
Nonionic diffusion, 595
Non-ST-elevation myocardial infarction (NSTEMI), 13, 87, 89
Nonsteroidal anti-inflammatory drugs (NSAIDs), 407, 408
Norepinephrine (NE), 446, 507, 508
  in regulation of renal blood flow and filtration, 602
Norethindrone, 744
Nortriptyline, 518, 540
Nose bleed, 783
  during pregnancy, 693
Notochord, 329, 412, 413
NPH insulin, 167
NRDS (neonatal respiratory distress syndrome), 764, 793–794
NSAIDs (nonsteroidal anti-inflammatory drugs), 407, 408

NSTEMI (non-ST-elevation myocardial infarction), 13, 87, 89
Nuclear imaging of cardiovascular system, 90
Nuclei, 418
Nucleus ambiguus, 445
Nucleus basalis of Meynert, 507
Nucleus cuneatus, 452
Nucleus gracilis, 452
Nucleus pulposus, 338, 457
  herniation of, 340–341, 412
Nursemaid's elbow, 344
Nystagmus, caloric, 442–444

O

O_2. See Oxygen (O_2)
OA (osteoarthritis), 327, 372–374
Oat cell carcinoma, 804, 805
Obesity
  and breast cancer, 687
  restrictive lung disease due to, 791
Obesity hypoventilation syndrome (OHS), 803
Oblique cricoarytenoid muscles, 348
Obsessions, 535, 553
Obsessive-compulsive disorder (OCD), 553–554
Obsessive-compulsive personality disorder (OCPD), 562
Obstetric conjugate, 339
Obstructive lung disease, 783–790
  asthma as, 761, 787–788, 789
  bronchiectasis as, 788–790
  chronic bronchitis as, 786–787
  emphysema as, 761, 766, 768, 776, 784–786
  lung volumes and capacities in, 761, 762, 763, 783
Obstructive shock, 78
Obstructive sleep apnea (OSA), 567, 769, 803
Obturator artery, 352
Obturator externus muscle, 352
Obturator internus muscle, 351
Obturator nerve, 352
  injury to, 353, 495
Occipital bone, 329, 335
Occipital horn, 421
Occipital lobe, 429
Occipital myotomes, 332
Occipital sinus, 424
OCD (obsessive-compulsive disorder), 553–554
OCP (oral contraceptive pill), 746
  hypertension due to, 59–60
OCPD (obsessive-compulsive personality disorder), 562
Octreotide, 125, 162, 260
  for carcinoid syndrome, 60
Oculomotor nerve, 425, 459, 462
Oculomotor nucleus, 440
Oculomotor paralysis, 500–501
Odontoid process, 329
ODS (osmotic demyelination syndrome), 124, 444, 488
OHS (obesity hypoventilation syndrome), 803
Olanzapine, 521, 540
Olfactory cells, 761
Olfactory groove meningioma, 463
Olfactory hallucinations, 534
Olfactory nerve, 459, 463
Olfactory pathways, 464
Olfactory system, 463
Oligodendrocytes, 464, 465
Oligodendroglia, 465
Oligodendroglioma, 490, 491
Oligohydramnios, 707, 752
Oliguria, 640
  in nephritic syndrome, 630
Olivocerebellar tract, 438
Olivopontocerebellar atrophy, 485
Ollier disease, 363

Omalizumab, 822–823
Omental bursa, 184
Omental foramen, 184
Omeprazole, 199, 259–260
Omohyoid muscle, 348
Omphalocele, 174, 229
Omphalomesenteric duct, 226
Oncogenes, 309
Oncogenic viruses, 309–310
Oncologic disorders
    myeloproliferative syndromes as, 306–308
    pharmacology for, 310–317
        alkylating agents in, 310–312
        antimetabolites in, 312–313
        drugs that target tubulin in, 314
        hormonal agents in, 315
        native cytokines in, 318
        targeted molecular therapeutics in, 315–317
        topoisomerase inhibitors in, 313–314
    solid tumors as, 308–310
    white cell disorders as, 295–306
        Langerhans cell histiocytosis as, 305–306
        leukemias as, 301–304
        leukopenia as, 295–296
        lymphomas as, 297–301
        plasma cell disorders as, 304–305
        reactive proliferation as, 296–297
Ondansetron, 262
Oocyte, 684, 685, 686, 687
Oogenesis, 684–686, 687
Oogonia, 669–670
Ootid, 685
Ophthalmic artery, 422
Ophthalmoplegia, internuclear, 442, 486, 503
Opiate(s), endogenous, 574
Opiate overdose, 575
Opiate use disorder, 573–574
Opioid(s), 406–407, 515–516, 532
    pupillary response to, 568
Opioid-induced constipation, 576
Opponens digiti minimi muscle, 349
Opponens pollicis muscle, 349
Oppositional defiant disorder, 579
Optic canal, 336
Optic chiasm, 117, 425, 460, 462
    compression of, 120, 121–122
    lesion of, 461
Optic disc, 502
Optic nerve, 459, 460, 502
    lesion of, 461
Optic neuritis, 504
Optic tract, 460
    lesion of, 461
Oral candidiasis, 210, 211
Oral cavity
    anatomy and physiology of, 192–195
    disorders of, 210–213
Oral contraceptive pill (OCP), 746
    hypertension due to, 59–60
Oral hypoglycemic drugs, 167–169
Oral stage of swallowing, 194
Orchiectomy, inguinal-approach, 736
Orchitis, 735
Organ of Corti, 461, 462
Organification in thyroid hormone synthesis, 128
Organophosphate poisoning, 511
Orgasm, 690, 691
Orlistat, 262–263
Oropharynx, 749
Orotic aciduria, 277
Orthopnea, 64
Ortolani maneuver, 333–334
OSA (obstructive sleep apnea), 567, 769, 803
Osler nodes, 58, 59

Osler-Weber-Rendu syndrome, vessel wall abnormalities due to, 295
Osmolality, 598
Osmolarity, 595, 598
    urine, 606–607
Osmole, 595
Osmoreceptors, 614
Osmoregulation in pregnancy, 692
Osmosis, 595
Osmotic damage due to diabetes, 163
Osmotic demyelination syndrome (ODS), 124, 444, 488
Osmotic diuretics, 94–95, 655, 656
Osmotic laxatives, 261
Osmotic pressure, 596
Ossicles, 462
Ossification
    intramembranous vs endochondral, 326–327
    primary vs secondary centers of, 324, 325
Osteitis deformans, 327, 369–370
Osteitis fibrosa cystica, 144, 326, 370
Osteoarthritis (OA), 327, 372–374
Osteoarthropathy, paraneoplastic hypertrophic, 310, 804
Osteoblast(s), 324, 325
Osteoblastic lesions, 362
Osteoblastoma, 364
Osteochondroma, 363, 364
Osteochondroprogenitors, 324
Osteoclasts, 324, 325
Osteocytes, 324, 325
Osteodystrophy
    Albright hereditary, 145
    renal, 146, 644
Osteogenesis, 324–325
    congenital malformations involving, 326–328
Osteogenesis imperfecta, 326, 339–340
Osteogenic sarcoma, 363, 364, 366–367
Osteoid osteoma, 363, 364
Osteolytic lesions, 362
Osteoma, 364
    osteoid, 363, 364
Osteomalacia, 143, 326, 360, 369
Osteomyelitis, 371–372
Osteonecrosis, 327
Osteopetrosis, 326, 368–369
Osteophytes, 372, 373
Osteoporosis, 326, 367–368
    postmenopausal, 146
Osteosarcoma, 363, 364, 366–367
Ostium primum, 3
Ostium secundum, 3
Outer hair cells, 462
Outward recoil of chest wall, 767
Ovarian artery, 589, 672, 680
Ovarian cycle, 686–687, 688
Ovarian failure, premature, 715
Ovarian follicle, 685
Ovarian hypoplasia, 673
Ovarian insufficiency, primary, 715
Ovarian neoplasms, 717–721
    epithelial cell, 717–718
    germ cell, 718–720
    metastatic, 721
    sex cord stromal, 720–721
Ovarian round ligament, 671, 672, 680
Ovarian veins, 187
Ovary(ies)
    anatomy of, 680
    development of, 669–670
    disorders of, 715–721
        follicular cysts as, 717
        ovarian neoplasms as, 717–721
        polycystic ovarian syndrome as, 716–717
        primary ovarian insufficiency as, 715

Overabundance of thoughts, 535
Overriding aorta, 4, 5
Oviduct, 670, 672, 679, 680, 686, 691
Ovotesticular disorder of sex development, 666, 702
Ovulation, 685, 686–687, 688, 691
Ovum(a), 679, 684, 685, 691, 692
Oxaliplatin, 311
Oxazepam, 515, 540
Oxidative stress, red blood cells and, 278–279
Oxybutynin, 512
Oxycodone, 515–516
Oxygen (O_2) capacity, 770
Oxygen (O_2) consumption and cardiac output, 23
Oxygen (O_2) content, 770
Oxygen dissociation curve, 266, 267
Oxygen (O_2) saturation (SpO_2), 770
Oxygen (O_2) tension, 775
Oxygen transport, 770–771
Oxygen-hemoglobin dissociation curve, 770–771
Oxymetazoline, 820
Oxymorphone, 515–516
Oxyphil cells, 138–139
Oxytocin, 117, 118, 698, 744

P

P wave, 41, 42
    abnormalities of, 44
p53 gene, 234
PA (pulmonary artery), 9, 12, 754, 756
PA (pulmonary artery) catheter, 31
Pacemaker(s)
    cardiac, 17–18
    native, 13, 17–18
Pacemaker action potentials, 16–17, 18
Pacinian corpuscles, 452, 453, 468
Paclitaxel, 314
Paget disease
    of bone, 327, 369–370
    of breast, 729, 730
PAH (*para*-aminohippuric acid), 604, 606
PAH (pulmonary arterial hypertension), 801–802
Pain
    drugs used to treat, 406–409
    referred, 191–192
    visceral vs parietal, 191
Pain fibers, fast- vs slow-conducting, 453
PAIS (partial androgen insensitivity), 702
"Palat-," muscles including, 347
Palatine bones, 335
Palatoglossus muscle, 347
Palatopharyngeal folds, 194
Palatopharyngeus muscle, 347
Pale infarcts, 87, 473–474
Palmar interossei muscle, 351
Palpation in pulmonary physical examination, 781
Pamidronate, 402
Pampiniform venous plexus, 677
PAN (polyarteritis nodosa), 82, 397–398, 403
p-ANCA (perinuclear antineutrophil cytoplasmic antibody), 82, 361
Pancoast syndrome, 806, 808
Pancoast tumor, 806, 807
Pancreas
    annular, 158, 178
    divisum, 177–178
    endocrine, 158–169
        anatomy of, 158
        in diabetes mellitus, 162–164
        embryology of, 159
        exocrine vs, 108

Pancreas (continued)
  endocrine (continued)
    and glucagon, 161–162
    histology of, 159
    and insulin, 159–161
    insulinoma of, 164
    islet cell tumors of, 165–166
    pharmacology of, 166–169
    and somatostatin, 162
  exocrine
    anatomy and physiology of, 205–206
    diseases of, 253–255
    endocrine vs, 108
  rupture of, 158
Pancreatic adenocarcinoma, 255
Pancreatic arteries, 158
Pancreatic calculi, 254
Pancreatic enzymes, 205–206
Pancreatic fistulas, metabolic acidosis due
    to, 619
Pancreatic insufficiency, 205, 225, 254
  vitamin B_{12} deficiency due to, 278
Pancreatic lipase, 206
Pancreatic polypeptide, 204
Pancreaticoduodenal arteries, 158
Pancreaticoduodenectomy, 255
Pancreatitis
  acute, 253
  chronic, 254
Pancuronium, 510
Panencephalitis, subacute sclerosing, 487
Paneth cells, 200
Panhypopituitarism, 121–122
Panic attacks, 552
Panic disorder (PD), 552
Panitumumab, 315
Pannus, 374
Pantoprazole, 259–260
PaO_2 (alveolar oxygen tension), 775–776
Papez circuit, 430
Papillary carcinoma of breast, 730
Papillary renal cell carcinoma, 647
Papillary serous cell carcinoma of
    endometrium, 725
Papillary thyroid carcinoma, 135
Papilledema, 460
Papilloma, 309
  intraductal, 728
Papule, 389
para-aminohippuric acid (PAH), 604, 606
Paracellular transport, 595
Paracentral lobule, 426
Paracoccidioidomycosis, 812
Paracrine secretion, 108
Paradoxical breathing motion, 758
Paradoxical emboli, 77
Paraesophageal hernia, 216
Parafollicular (C) cells, 126, 127
Parahippocampal gyrus, 426
Parallel fibers, 439
Paramedian branch, 442
Paramesonephric duct
  derivatives of
    female, 669, 670, 674
    male, 668, 674
  development of, 663, 664
Paranasal sinuses, 781–783
Paraneoplastic syndrome(s), 310
  endocarditis as, 59
Paranoid personality disorder, 560
Parasitic infection of CNS, 505
Parasomnias, 565, 566, 567
Parasternal line, 757
Parasternal pericardiocentesis, 91
Parasympathetic innervation of GI tract, 189,
    190

Parasympathetic stimulation
  and contractility, 24
  and pulmonary resistance, 769
Parathyroid gland, 137–146
  anatomy of, 137, 138
  in calcium and phosphate homeostasis,
      139–143
    disorders of, 144–146
    pharmacology of, 146
  embryology of, 137–138, 139, 140
  histology of, 138–139
  overview of, 137
Parathyroid hormone (PTH), 137
  in bone metabolism, 324, 325
  in bone remodeling, 367
  in calcium and phosphate homeostasis,
      140–141
  in calcium and phosphate metabolism, 611
  in calcium disorders, 144–146
  mechanisms of action of, 141, 142
  in musculoskeletal and connective tissue
      disorders, 362
  in phosphate reabsorption, 608
  recombinant, 404
  regulation of, 141
  and renal function, 612, 615
  synthesis of, 140–141
Parathyroid hormone–related peptide
    (PTHrP), 362, 367
Parathyroid hyperplasia, 145
Parathyroid tissue, ectopic, 138
"Paraumbilical" veins, 8
Paraventricular nucleus, 117, 435, 436
Paravermis, 437
Parenchymal hemorrhage, 419
Parietal bones, 329, 335, 336
Parietal cells, 196
  acid secretion by, 197
Parietal lobe, 427–429
Parietal pain, 191
Parietal peritoneum, 182, 183, 191
Parietal pleura, 750, 755, 756
Parieto-occipital fissure, 426
Parinaud syndrome, 441, 491
Parkinson disease (PD), 432, 484
  drugs used to treat, 528–530
Parotid gland, 192
Paroxetine, 517, 540
Paroxysmal nocturnal dyspnea (PND), 64
Paroxysmal nocturnal hemoglobinuria, 286
Paroxysmal supraventricular tachycardia, 49
Pars interarticularis defect or fracture, 341
Partial androgen insensitivity (PAIS), 702
Partial mole, 711–712
Partial pressure of carbon dioxide (Pco_2) and
    arterial pressure, 38
Partial pressure of oxygen (Po_2) and arterial
    pressure, 38
Partial seizures, 489
Passive aggression, 538
Passive aggressive personality disorder, 558
Passive immunization, 710
Passive transport, 595–596
Patau syndrome, 331, 418
Patch, 389
Patent ductus arteriosus (PDA), 5, 6, 7, 8, 73,
    697
Patent foramen ovale (PFO), 2
Patent process vaginalis, 666
Patent urachus, 584
PAW (pulmonary artery wedge), 31
PBC (primary biliary cirrhosis), 246–247
PCA (posterior cerebral artery), 423, 424, 441
  stroke involving, 478
Pco_2 (partial pressure of carbon dioxide) and
    arterial pressure, 38

PCOS (polycystic ovarian syndrome), 716–717
PCP (Pneumocystis jirovecii) pneumonia, 812
PCP (phencyclidine) use disorder, 575
PCT (proximal convoluted tubule)
  histology of, 590, 591, 592
  physiology of, 607–608, 610
PCV (polycythemia vera), 306–307
PCWP (pulmonary capillary wedge
    pressure), 31
PD (panic disorder), 552
PD (Parkinson disease), 432, 484
  drugs used to treat, 528–530
PD-1, monoclonal antibody targeting, 317
PDA (patent ductus arteriosus), 5, 6, 7, 8, 73,
    697
PDA (posterior descending/interventricular
    artery), 12, 13
PDE-5 (phosphodiesterase-5), 691
PDE-5 (phosphodiesterase-5) inhibitors, 102,
    743
PE (pulmonary embolism), 75, 76, 799–801
  hypoxemia due to, 777–778
Pectineus muscle, 352
Pectoral girdle, 338
Pectoralis major muscle, 681
Pectoralis minor muscle, 681
Pedicle, 337
Pedunculopontine nucleus, 432
PEEP (positive end-expiratory pressure), 769
Pellagra due to carcinoid syndrome, 59
Pelvic brim, 339
Pelvic fasciae, 674, 676, 679, 681
Pelvic girdle, 338
Pelvic inflammatory disease (PID), 721–722
Pelvic inlet, 338, 339
Pelvic nerves, 189, 190
Pelvic outlet, 338, 339
Pelvic peritoneum, 183–184
Pelvis
  bones of, 338, 339
  fractures of, 341
Pemetrexed, 312–313
Pemphigoid, bullous, 393
Pemphigus vulgaris, 393, 394
Pencil-in-cup deformity in psoriatic
    arthritis, 380
Penile squamous cell carcinoma, 734
Penile urethra, 590
Penis
  anatomy of, 677
  development of, 668, 669
  disorders of, 733–734
Pentobarbital, 514, 540
Pepsinogen, 196, 198
Peptic ulcer disease, 221–222
Peptidases, small intestinal secretion of, 202
Peptide hormones, 108–109
  in second-messenger pathways, 109–111
Peptide YY, 192
Perception, disorders of, 536
Percussion in pulmonary physical examination,
    780–781
Percutaneous transluminal coronary
    angioplasty, 86
Perfusion pressure, 40
Perfusion-limited gas, 776
Pergolide, 528–529
Pericardial cavity, 11
Pericardial disease, 78–81
  cardiac tamponade as, 79–80
  pericardial effusion as, 78–79
  pericarditis as
    acute, 80, 81
    chronic constrictive, 80–81
Pericardial effusion, 78–79
Pericardiocentesis, 79, 80, 91

Pericarditis, 12, 89
  acute, 80, 81
  causes of, 80
  chronic constrictive, 80–81
  fibrinous, 60
  types of, 80
Pericardium, 11, 78
Perilymphatic cavity, 462
Perimacular input, 461
Perimetrium, 671
Perineal body, 339
Perineurium, 468
Perinuclear antineutrophil cytoplasmic
        antibody (p-ANCA), 82, 361
Periosteum, 325
Peripheral nerves, 447
  lesions of, 456
  organization of, 468
Peripheral neuropathy, 499
  diabetic, 163, 499
Peripheral spinal nerves, 191
Peripheral vascular circulation, 32–35, 36
Peripheral vascular disease, 81–85
  large-vessel, 81–82
  medium-vessel, 82–83
  small-vessel, 83–85
Perirenal space, 588
Peristalsis, 200, 346
  primary, 194
  secondary, 195
Peritoneal cavity, 183–184
Peritoneum, 183–184
  female, 681
  parietal, 182
Perivitelline space, 684, 692
Pernicious anemia, 278, 497
Peroneal artery, 352
Peroneal ligaments, 671
Peroneus brevis muscle, 352
Peroneus longus muscle, 352
Peroneus tertius muscle, 352
Persistent depressive disorder, 548
Personality disorders
  antisocial, 558, 561
  avoidant, 553, 560, 562
  borderline, 558, 561
  cluster A, 558, 559, 560
  cluster B, 558, 560, 561
  cluster C, 558, 560, 562
  dependent, 562
  histrionic, 561
  narcissistic, 561
  not otherwise specified (NOS), 558
  obsessive-compulsive, 562
  paranoid, 560
  passive aggressive, 558
  sadistic, 558
  sadomasochistic, 558
  schizotypal and schizoid, 544, 558, 560
Pertuzumab, 746
Pervasive developmental disorders, 577–578
Pes anserine bursitis, 353
Pes anserinus, 353
Petechiae, 292
Petit mal seizure, 489
Peutz-Jeghers syndrome, 234
Peyer patches, 189
Peyronie disease, 733
PFA (platelet function analyzer)-100 test, 291
PFO (patent foramen ovale), 2
PFT (pulmonary function testing)
  for asthma, 788
  for chronic bronchitis, 786
  for emphysema, 785
pH, physiologic, 617

Ph (Philadelphia) chromosome, 303
Pharyngeal arches, 748–749
Pharyngeal phase of swallowing, 194
Pharyngitis, 814
Pharyngoesophageal diverticulum, 214
Pharynx, 754
Phencyclidine (PCP) use disorder, 575
Phenelzine, 517–518, 541
Phenobarbital, 514, 524–525, 540
Phenotypic sex, 662
Phenylephrine, 820
Phenytoin, 525
Pheochromocytoma, 148, 157–158
  hypertension due to, 53, 54
Philadelphia (Ph) chromosome, 303
Phimosis, 734
Phobias, 535, 552–553
Phosphate, renal reabsorption of, 608, 612
Phosphate homeostasis, 139–143
Phosphatidylinositol-3-kinase, 160
Phosphaturia, 612
Phosphodiesterase-5 (PDE-5), 691
Phosphodiesterase-5 (PDE-5) inhibitors, 102,
        743
Phospholipase A$_2$, 206
Photoreceptors, 459
Phrenic arteries, 147, 184
Phrenic nerve, 353, 757
Phrenic vein, 147, 187
Phyllodes tumor, 728
Physical examination, pulmonary, 779–781
Physiologic dead space, 763, 777
Physostigmine, 511
PICA (posterior inferior cerebellar artery),
        423, 424
  stroke involving, 478
PICA (posterior inferior cerebellar artery)
        syndrome, 444, 445
Pick disease, 482
PID (pelvic inflammatory disease), 721–722
Pigment stones, 250, 251
Pigmented lesions, 391
Pilocarpine, 511
Pilocytic astrocytoma, 490, 492
Pimozide, 540
Pinealoma, 491
"Pink puffer," 785
Pioglitazone, 168
Piriformis muscle, 351
Piriformis syndrome, 351, 352
Pisiform, 339
Pitting edema, 65
Pituitary, 108–126
  anterior
    cell types and regulation of, 112, 114
    disease of, 119–122
    hormones of, 112–117
    structure and function of, 112
  in hypothalamic-pituitary axis, 112–119
  ischemic necrosis of, 121
  pharmacology of, 124–126
  posterior
    disease of, 122–124
    hormones of, 117–119
    structure and function of, 112, 113
  during pregnancy, 694
  structure and function of, 112, 113
Pituitary adenoma, 115–116, 119, 436, 490,
        492, 496
Pituitary disease
  anterior, 119–122
  posterior, 122–124
Pituitary tumors, 119, 120
Pityriasis rosea, 394
Pivot joints, 343

Placenta, 696, 697
  accreta, 705–706
  fused, 698
  increta, 706
  percreta, 706
  previa, 706–707
Placental abruption, 705, 706
Placental disorders, 705–707
Plane joints, 343
Plantar flexor muscles, 352
Plantaris muscle, 352
Plaques, 389
  fibrous, 56, 57
Plasma, 32, 33, 267, 596
  measuring volume of, 598
Plasma cell(s), 269, 270
Plasma cell disorders, 304–305
Platelet activation, factors influencing, 320
Platelet count, 291
Platelet defects
  of adhesion, 293
  of aggregation, 293
  of function, 293
  hemorrhagic, 290–293
  qualitative, 291
Platelet formation, 268
Platelet function analyzer (PFA)-100
        test, 291
Platelet plug formation, 290
Platelet-derived growth factor in wound
        healing, 361
Pleomorphic adenoma of salivary gland, 213
Pleura
  anatomy of, 755, 756, 757
  parietal, 750, 755, 756
  visceral (pulmonary), 750, 755, 756
Pleural cavities
  anatomy of, 755
  development of, 750, 751
Pleural effusions, 755, 756, 757, 815, 816
Pleural reflections, 755, 757
Pleural rub, 780
Pleurodesis, 817
Pleuroperitoneal folds, 750
Pleuroperitoneal membranes, 750, 751
Plicae circulares, 199, 200, 201
Ploidy, 682
Plummer disease, 132
Plummer-Vinson syndrome, 275
PM (polymyositis), 387–388
PMI (point of maximal impulse), 9, 10
PML (progressive multifocal
        leukoencephalopathy), 486, 487
PMNs (polymorphonuclear neutrophils), 267
PND (paroxysmal nocturnal dyspnea), 64
Pneumoconiosis, 794–795, 796
Pneumocystis jirovecii pneumonia (PCP), 812
Pneumocytes, 760
Pneumonia, 808–812
  aspiration, 751, 808, 809
  bacterial, 811
  broncho-, 809, 810
  causes of, 809, 811, 812
  chronic eosinophilic, 798
  classification of, 808
  community-acquired, 808, 810
  defined, 808
  diagnosis of, 809–810
  fungal, 810, 812
  interstitial (atypical), 809, 810
  lobar, 809, 810, 816
  nosocomial (hospital-acquired), 808, 810
  Pneumocystis jirovecii (Pneumocystic carinii),
        812
  presentation of, 809
  prognosis for, 812

Pneumonia (*continued*)
risk factors for, 809, 810
treatment of, 810–812
typical, 809
viral, 812
Pneumonitis
aspiration, 751
hypersensitivity, 818
Pneumoperitoneum, 183
Pneumotaxic center, 779
Pneumothorax, 755, 815–817
Po$_2$ (partial pressure of oxygen) and arterial
pressure, 38
Podagra, 375
Podocytes, 591, 601
Point of maximal impulse (PMI), 9, 10
Poiseuille's law, 769
Poland syndrome, 334
Polar bodies, 685, 686, 692
Poliomyelitis (polio), 457, 481, 496
restrictive lung disease due to, 791
Poliovirus, 486
Polyangiitis
granulomatosis with, 83–84, 399–400, 403,
635–636, 797–798
microscopic, 84, 403
Polyarteritis, microscopic, 400
Polyarteritis nodosa (PAN), 82, 397–398, 403
Polycystic kidney disease
autosomal dominant, 643–644
autosomal recessive (childhood), 644, 645
Polycystic ovarian syndrome (PCOS),
716–717
Polycythemia vera (PCV), 306–307
Polydactyly, 331, 332
Polydipsia, primary, 122, 123
Polyethylene glycol, 261
Polyhydramnios, 213, 707
Polymorphonuclear neutrophils (PMNs), 267
Polymyositis (PM), 387–388
Polyp, 309
Polyp(s), of colon
adenomatous, 233
benign, 232
Polyposis, familial adenomatous, 233
Polyposis syndromes, 233–234
Polyradiculopathy
acute inflammatory demyelinating, 456,
466, 487–488
diabetic, 497
Polyuria, 640
POMC (proopiomelanocortin), 116, 118
Pons, 437, 440–444
in control of respiration, 779
Pontine arteries, 424
Pontine nuclei, 442
Pontocerebellar fibers, 442
Pontocerebellar tract, 438
Pope blessing, 496
Popliteus muscle, 352
Porcelain gallbladder, 251
Porphobilinogen deaminase, 288
Porphyria, 288–290
acute intermittent, 288–289, 290
cutanea tarda, 289, 290
Portal hypertension, 188, 244–246
Portal to inferior vena caval anastomoses, 187,
188, 245
Portal triads, 206, 207
Portal vein, 9, 158, 187, 207
Portal venous system, 187–188, 207
Portosystemic anastomoses, 187, 188
Positive end-expiratory pressure (PEEP), 769
Positive feedback, 111
Positive inotropic agents, 26
Positive inotropic effect, 24

Positive inotropy and cardiac and vascular
function curves, 28, 29
Positive pressure, 767
Positive symptoms of schizophrenia, 544, 545
Postcentral gyrus, 426
Postcentral primary sensory areas, 427
Post-duodenal atresia, 177
Posterior abdominal wall, 587
Posterior ampulla, 462
Posterior cerebral artery (PCA), 423, 424, 441
stroke involving, 478
Posterior chamber, 502
Posterior communicating artery, 424
Posterior cranial fossa, 459
Posterior cricoarytenoid muscles, 348
Posterior cruciate ligament, 345
Posterior descending/interventricular artery
(PDA), 12, 13
Posterior drawer sign, 345
Posterior fontanelle, 328, 329
Posterior fossa, 335
Posterior inferior cerebellar artery (PICA),
423, 424
stroke involving, 478
Posterior inferior cerebellar artery (PICA)
syndrome, 444, 445
Posterior limb of internal capsule, 434
Posterior nucleus, 435, 436
Posterior pituitary
disease of, 122–124
hormones of, 117–119
structure and function of, 112, 113
Posterior superior pancreaticoduodenal
artery, 186
Posterior tibial artery, 352
Posterior tubercle, 337
Posterior urethral valve, 586–587
Postganglionic fibers in innervation of GI tract,
189, 190
Postinfectious encephalomyelitis, 487
Postmenopausal osteoporosis, 146
Postpartum blues, 548
Postpartum depression, 548
Postpartum psychosis, 548
Poststreptococcal glomerulonephritis, 623,
631–632
Poststreptococcal rheumatic fever, 60, 631
Postsynaptic membrane, 354, 466
Posttraumatic stress disorder (PTSD), 551–552
Potassium (K$^+$)
intracellular and extracellular
concentrations of, 15–16
renal reabsorption of, 609
Potassium (K$^+$) channel(s), 466
ATP-sensitive, 160, 161
voltage-gated, 16
Potassium (K$^+$) channel blockers, 104
Potassium-sparing diuretics, 93–94, 614, 655,
656, 657–658
Potentiation, 199
Pott disease, 371
Pott fracture, 342, 346
Potter sequence, 584–585
Potter syndrome, 752
Pouch of Rathke, 112
Poupart ligament, 179, 182, 674, 675, 676
Poverty of speech, 545
Poverty of thought, 535
Power-stroke state, 356
PPD (purified protein derivate), 813
PPIs (proton pump inhibitors), 199, 259–260
PR interval, 43
Pramipexole, 528–529
Pravastatin, 105
Prazosin, 97
Precentral gyrus, 426

Precentral sulcus, 426
Prechordal plate, 412
Precordial leads, 41
Preculminate fissure, 437
Precuneus, 426
Preeclampsia, 654, 696, 708, 709
Prefrontal cortex, 427
Pregabalin, 526
Preganglionic fibers in innervation of GI tract,
189, 190
Pregnancy, 692–698
blood system during, 695
and breast-feeding, 698
cardiovascular system during, 693, 695
digestive system during, 693–694, 695
disorders of, 703–712
amniotic fluid abnormalities as, 707
amniotic fluid embolism syndrome
as, 710
erythroblastosis fetalis as, 710–711
gestational neoplasms as, 711–712
HELLP syndrome as, 709
hypertension as, 708–709
placental, 705–707
Sheehan syndrome as, 709–710
due to teratogens, 703–705
ectopic, 691, 707
endocrine system during, 694
fetal circulation during, 696–698
folic acid during, 330
immune system during, 694
osmoregulation during, 692
placenta during, 696, 697
prenatal testing during, 695–696
respiratory system during, 693, 695
skin and bones during, 694
"triple screen" during, 330
twin, 697, 698, 699
urinary system during, 693, 695
weight during, 695
Pregnenolone in steroid hormone
synthesis, 149
Prehn sign, 735
Prehypertension, 52
Preload
and blood pressure, 37
and cardiac output, 28
defined, 25
in Frank-Starling relationship, 26
measurement of, 25
medications and, 24
and pressure-volume loop, 27
and venous return, 25, 28
Premature ovarian failure, 715
Premature ventricular contraction (PVC), 51
Premotor cortex, 426–427
Prenatal testing, 695–696
Prenotochordal cells, 412
Preoptic area, 435
Preoptic myotomes, 332
Preoptic nucleus, 436
Prepatellar bursitis, 353
Prepuce, 668, 676
Prepyramidal fissure, 437
Pressure-volume (PV) loops, 26–27
Presynaptic membrane, 466
Pretectal nucleus, 462
Prevertebral ganglion, 189
Priapism, 733
Primary active transport, 596
Primary auditory cortex, 429
Primary biliary cirrhosis (PBC), 246–247
Primary ciliary dyskinesia, 2, 760, 789
Primary CNS lymphoma, 496
Primary fissure, 437
Primary follicle, 687

Primary gain, 537
Primary motor cortex, 426, 427
Primary ovarian insufficiency, 715
Primary sclerosing cholangitis, 253
Primary sensory cortex, 428
Primary visual cortex, 427, 429
Primitive node, 412
Primitive streak, 412
Primordial follicles, 669, 670
Primordial germ cells, 662, 663, 669, 670
Principal cells, 609
Prinzmetal angina, 86, 101–102
Prion diseases, 483
PRL (prolactin), 112–114, 115, 698
Probenecid, 405–406
Procainamide, 104
Procarboxypeptidase, 206
Processus vaginalis, 183
    development of, 666
    patent, 666
Procolipase, 206
Proelastase, 206
Proerythroblasts, 611
Profunda femoral artery, 352
Progesterone, 689
    in menstrual cycle, 686, 688
Progesterone agonists, 744
Progesterone inhibitors, 746
Progesterone receptors in breast cancer, 729
Progestins, 689, 690
Progestogens, 687
Progressive multifocal leukoencephalopathy
    (PML), 486, 487
Progressive supranuclear palsy, 480–481

Prolactin (PRL), 112–114, 115, 698
Prolactin-inhibiting factor, 112
Prolactinoma, 119–120, 121–122
Prolymphocytic transformation, 300, 302
Pronator muscles of arm, 349
Pronephros, 584, 585
Proopiomelanocortin (POMC), 116, 118
Propafenone, 104
Proper hepatic artery, 158, 186
Prophospholipase, 206
Propofol, 532
Propranolol, 96–97, 101, 104
Propylthiouracil (PTU), 128, 136–137
Prosencephalon, 414, 416
Prostaglandins, 8
    in alveolar function, 764
    in regulation of renal blood flow and
        filtration, 603, 611
Prostate
    anatomy of, 589, 676, 678–679, 680
    development of, 668
    diseases of, 738–741
        benign prostatic hyperplasia as, 738–739
        prostatic adenocarcinoma as, 740–741
        prostatitis as, 739–740
Prostate-specific antigen (PSA), 740
Prostatic adenocarcinoma, 680, 740–741
Prostatic hyperplasia, benign, 590, 680,
    738–739
Prostatic urethra, 589
Prostatitis, 739–740
Protein, small intestinal absorption of, 202
Protein A, 57
Protein hormones, 108–109
    in second-messenger pathways, 109–111
Protein metabolism in muscle contraction, 358
Proteinuria, 591, 592
    in nephritic syndrome, 630
    in nephrotic syndrome, 592, 624
Prothrombin time (PT), 258, 291, 294
Proton pump inhibitors (PPIs), 199, 259–260

Protriptyline, 518
Proximal convoluted tubule (PCT)
    histology of, 590, 591, 592
    physiology of, 607–608, 610
Prune belly syndrome, 333–334
PSA (prostate-specific antigen), 740
Psammoma bodies, 491, 494, 718, 807, 808
Pseudocholinesterase, 510
Pseudoephedrine, 820
Pseudoglandular period, 748, 750
Pseudogout, 376–377
Pseudohermaphrodite, 666, 701
    female, 702
    male, 701–702
Pseudohypoparathyroidism, 145
Pseudomembranous colitis, 231
Pseudomonas aeruginosa, 811
Pseudomyxoma peritonei, 718
Pseudotumor cerebri, 422
Psoas major muscle, 587, 588
Psoas minor muscle, 587, 588
Psoriasis, 390
Psoriatic arthritis, 379–380
Psychiatric disorders, 533–582
    of affect, behavior, or motor activity, 536
    anxiety disorders as, 550–554
        adjustment disorder as, 551
        generalized anxiety disorder as, 550–551
        obsessive-compulsive disorder as, 553–554
        panic attacks as, 552
        panic disorder as, 552
        phobias as, 535, 552–553
        posttraumatic stress disorder as, 551–552
    approaches to treating, 539, 540–541

    attention deficit/hyperactivity disorder as,
        579–580
    child abuse as, 581
    disruptive behavior disorders as, 578–579
    intellectual disability as, 581
    pervasive developmental disorders as,
        577–578
    selective mutism as, 581
    separation anxiety disorder as, 580
    Tourette disorder as, 580
    classification of, 534–536
    cognitive, 539–543
        amnestic disorders as, 543
        delirium as, 539–542
        dementia as, 542–543
    and defense mechanisms, 537–538
    defined, 534
    dissociative disorders as, 558, 559
    eating disorders as, 562–565
    factitious disorders and malingering as,
        557–558
    with known biologic causes, 536, 537
    mood disorders as, 546–550
        bipolar disorder as, 546, 547, 548–550
        major depressive disorder as, 546, 547–
            548, 549, 550
    of perception, 536
    personality disorders as, 558–562
    and psychological motivators, 537
    schizophrenia and other psychotic disorders
        as, 543–546
    secondary disorders as, 536, 537
    sleep disorders as, 565–568
    somatic symptom and related disorders as,
        554–556
    substance use disorders as, 568–576
        alcohol use disorder as, 568–570
        cannabis use disorder as, 544, 576
        depressant use disorder as, 568–571
        hallucinogen (phencyclidine and lysergic
            acid diethylamide) use disorder
            as, 575

    opiate use disorder as, 573–574
    pupillary responses to, 568
    secondary vs, 536, 537
    sedative, hypnotic, and anxiolytic use
        disorder as, 570–571
    stimulant use disorder as, 571–572
    terminology for, 534
    of thought content, 535
    of thought process, 535
    transference and countertransference in
        treating, 536–537
Psychoactive medications, 539, 540–541
Psychodynamic therapy, 539
Psychological motivators, 537
Psychomotor agitation, 536
Psychomotor retardation, 536
Psychopathology, 534
Psychopharmacotherapy, 539, 540–541
Psychosis, 534, 543
    postpartum, 548
Psychosocial treatments, 539
PT (prothrombin time), 258, 291, 294
Pterion, 335, 336
PTH. *See* Parathyroid hormone (PTH)
PTHrP (parathyroid hormone–related
    peptide), 362, 367
PTSD (posttraumatic stress disorder), 551–552
PTT (partial thromboplastin time), 291, 293
PTU (propylthiouracil), 128, 136–137
Ptyalin, 192, 193
Pubic symphysis, 676, 681
Pubis, 338
Pudendal nerve, 352

Pulmonary aplasia, 753
Pulmonary arterial hypertension (PAH),
    801–802
Pulmonary artery (PA), 9, 12, 754, 756
Pulmonary artery (PA) catheter, 31
Pulmonary artery wedge (PAW), 31
Pulmonary blood flow, regulation of, 775
Pulmonary capillary wedge pressure
    (PCWP), 31
Pulmonary circulation, 773–775
Pulmonary edema, 90, 761, 792, 815, 816
    due to renal failure, 643
Pulmonary embolism (PE), 75, 76, 799–801
    hypoxemia due to, 777–778
Pulmonary fibrosis, idiopathic. *See* Idiopathic
    pulmonary fibrosis (IPF)
Pulmonary function testing (PFT)
    for asthma, 788
    for chronic bronchitis, 786
    for emphysema, 785
Pulmonary hypertension, 801–802, 820
Pulmonary hypoplasia, 752, 753
Pulmonary infections, 808–814
    pneumonia as, 808–812
    tuberculosis as, 774, 812–814
    upper respiratory tract, 814
Pulmonary physical examination, 779–781
Pulmonary pleura, 750, 755, 756
Pulmonary resistance, 769–770
Pulmonary surfactant, 760, 764
    deficiency in, 753, 754
Pulmonary system. *See* Respiratory system
Pulmonary vascular disease, 798–803
    deep venous thrombosis as, 798–799
    pulmonary embolism as, 799–801
    pulmonary hypertension as, 801–802
    sleep apnea as, 803
Pulmonary vascular resistance (PVR), 5, 762,
    773–774, 775
    in fetus, 776
Pulmonary veins, 755, 756
Pulmonary venous return, total anomalous, 5

Pulmonic stenosis, 4, 5, 70
Pulmonic valve, 10, 11
Pulse pressure, 37
Pulseless disease, 82, 398–399, 403
Pulsus paradoxus, 79, 788
Pulvinar nucleus, 433
Pupil, 502
    Adie tonic, 461
    Argyll Robertson, 461, 501, 502
    Marcus Gunn, 458, 502
Pupillary constrictor muscle, 462
Pupillary defect, afferent, 458
Pupillary dilation pathway, 461
Pupillary light reflex pathway, 461, 462
Pupillary responses to substance intoxication
        or withdrawal, 568
Purging, 562–563
Purified protein derivate (PPD), 813
Purkinje cell(s), 17, 438, 439
Purkinje cell layer of cerebellum, 437, 438
Purkinje fibers, 14, 15
Purkinje neuron, 438
Purpura
    Henoch-Schönlein, 84–85, 401–402, 403
        IgA nephropathy due to, 634, 635
        vessel wall abnormalities due to, 295
    thrombocytopenic
        idiopathic, 85, 291–292
        thrombotic, 292
Pustule, 389
Putamen, 431, 432, 434
PV (pressure-volume) loops, 26–27
PVC (premature ventricular contraction), 51
PVR (pulmonary vascular resistance), 5, 762,
        773–774, 775
    in fetus, 776
Pyelonephritis
    acute, 638–639
    chronic, 639
Pyloric sphincter, 196, 197
Pyloric stenosis, 177, 197
Pyloromyotomy, 177
Pyramidal decussation, 444, 450, 451
Pyramidal tract, 440
Pyramidalis muscle, 182
Pyramis, 437
Pyridostigmine, 511
Pyruvate kinase deficiency, 286
Pyuria, sterile, 638

Q

QRS axis, mean, 43–44
QRS complex(es), 41, 42, 43
    abnormalities of, 44–45
    narrow, 49
QT interval, 43
    long, 42, 43
Quad screen, 469, 696
Quadratus femoris muscle, 351
Quadratus lumborum muscle, 587
Quadriceps muscle, 352
QuantiFERON GOLD (interferon-gamma
        release assay), 813
Quetiapine, 521, 540
Quinidine, 104

R

r (resistance). See Resistance (r, R)
R (resistance). See Resistance (r, R)
R (respiratory quotient), 775
RA (rheumatoid arthritis), 373, 374–375
RA (right atrium), 10
RAAS (renin-angiotensin-aldosterone system),
        99, 100, 152
    and mean arterial pressure, 37–38, 39–40
    and renal function, 612–613

Rabeprazole, 259–260
Rabies, 487
"Raccoon eyes," 339
Radial groove, 338
Radial head dislocation, 350
Radial nerve, 338, 349, 351, 498
    damage to, 350, 495
Radial nerve palsy, 339–340
Radial traction in emphysema, 784
Radicular nerves, 447
Radioallergosorbent test (RAST), 817
Radiocarpal joint, 344
Radiohumeral joint, 344
Radioiodine, 137
Radioulnar joint, 344
Rales, 780
Raloxifene, 315, 368, 404, 729, 745
Ramipril, 659
Ranitidine, 258–259
Raphe nucleus, 508
Rapid ejection, 30
Rapid ventricular filling, 30
Rapid ventricular rate (RVR), atrial fibrillation
        with, 50
Rapidly progressive glomerulonephritis
        (RPGN), 623, 632–633
RAS (renin-angiotensin system), 152
RAS gene, 234
RAST (radioallergosorbent test), 817
Rate-limited transport, 596
Rate-limiting enzyme (RLE)
    in glucocorticoid synthesis, 150
    in steroid hormone synthesis, 149
Rathke pouch, 436, 491
Rationalization, 538
Raynaud disease, 83
Raynaud phenomenon, 83, 281
RB (retinoblastoma) gene, 309
RBCs. See Red blood cell(s) (RBCs)
RBF (renal blood flow), 602–603
RCA (right coronary artery), 12, 13–14
RCC (renal cell carcinoma), 647–648
RDS (respiratory distress syndrome), 753, 754
    acute, 764, 769, 792–793
    neonatal (infant), 764, 793–794
RDW (red blood cell distribution width), 269
Reabsorption, 605–607
Reaction formation, 538
Reactive arthritis (ReA), 379
Reactive proliferation of white blood cells,
        296–297
Reality testing, 534
Receptor(s), 466
Receptor up- and downregulation, 111
Receptor-associated tyrosine kinase (RTK)
        mechanism, 110
Recombinant parathyroid hormone
        (Forteo), 404
Rectosphincteric reflex, 205
Rectus abdominis muscle, 179, 182, 674, 675,
        676
Rectus sheath, 674, 675, 681
Recurrent laryngeal nerve, 348, 806
Red blood cell(s) (RBCs)
    formation of, 267–268, 269
    forms of, 273–274
    and oxidative stress, 278–279
Red blood cell (RBC) casts, 623
Red blood cell distribution width (RDW), 269
Red degeneration, 726
Red infarcts, 87
Red neurons, 473
Red nucleus, 438, 440
Reduced ejection, 30
Reduced ventricular filling, 30

5α-Reductase inhibitors, 739, 743
5α-Reductase type 2 deficiency, 666, 701–702
Reed-Sternberg cells, 297, 298
Re-entry, 50
Referred pain, 191–192
Refractory period, 19–20
Regression, 538
Regurgitant flow theory of endometriosis, 723
Reinke crystals, 721, 738
Relative refractory period (RRP), 19, 20
Relaxin, 694
Released state, 356
Renal agenesis, 584
Renal amyloidosis, 629, 630
Renal arteries, 147, 184, 588, 589
Renal artery stenosis, 53, 54
Renal blood flow (RBF), 602–603
Renal calculi, 636–637
Renal calyces, 588
    histology of, 590, 594
Renal cell carcinoma (RCC), 647–648
Renal clearance, 599–600
Renal compensation, 621, 771, 772
Renal corpuscles, 590, 591, 592
Renal cortex, 588
Renal development, 584–587
Renal disorders, 623–654
    acute and chronic kidney injury, 640–643
    congenital abnormalities as, 584–587
    cystic kidney disease as, 643–645
    diffuse cortical necrosis as, 639–640
    electrolyte abnormalities as, 650–654
    glomerulopathies as, 623, 624
    inherited renal syndromes as, 645–646
    with nephritic syndrome, 623, 624, 630–636
        acute proliferative (poststreptococcal,
            infectious) glomerulonephritis as,
            623, 631–632
        antiglomerular basement membrane
            disease (Goodpasture) syndrome as,
            601, 623, 633–634
        granulomatosis with polyangiitis as,
            635–636
        hereditary nephritis (Alport syndrome)
            as, 635
        IgA nephropathy (Berger disease) as, 631,
            634–635
        rapidly progressive glomerulonephritis as,
            623, 632–633
    nephropathies associated with systemic
        disorders as, 628–630
    with nephrotic syndrome, 623–628
        diffuse membranous glomerulopathy as,
            626–627
        focal segmental glomerulosclerosis as,
            626, 627–628
        glomerular basement membrane in, 601
        membranoproliferative
            glomerulonephritis as, 627–628
        minimal change disease as, 625–626
        proteinuria in, 592, 624
    renal papillary necrosis as, 640
    renal stones (urolithiasis) as, 636–637
    tumors of renal system as, 647–650
    urinary casts as, 623
    urinary tract infections as, 638–639
Renal ectopy, 585
Renal excretion, 605–607
Renal failure
    chronic, 640, 642–643
    consequences of, 643, 644
Renal medulla, 588
Renal osteodystrophy, 146, 612, 644
Renal output medullary potassium (ROMK)
        channels, 608, 609
Renal papillae, 588

Renal papillary necrosis, 640
Renal parenchymal disease, hypertension due
    to, 53
Renal pelvis, 588
    histology of, 590, 594
Renal plasma flow, 604
Renal pyramids, 588
Renal secretion, 605–607
Renal stones, 636–637
Renal syndromes, inherited, 645–646
Renal system, 583–660
    in acid-base homeostasis, 616–622
    anatomy of, 587–590
    disorders of. See Renal disorders
    embryology of, 584–587
    endocrine functions of, 611
    filtration fraction in, 604–605
    fluid compartments in, 596–599
    glomerular filtrate in, 601
    glomerular filtration barrier in, 600–601
    glomerular filtration rate in, 601–602
    histology of, 590–594
    hormones acting on, 611–615
    nephron physiology and tubular system in,
        607–610
    pharmacology of, 655–660
        angiotensin receptor blockers in, 659
        angiotensin-converting enzyme inhibitors
            in, 659
        antidiuretic hormone antagonists in,
            658–659
        antidiuretic hormone (vasopressin,
            desmopressin) in, 658
        diuretics in, 655–658
        nephrotoxic drugs in, 660
    during pregnancy, 693, 695
    reabsorption and secretion in, 605–607
    regulation mechanisms in, 602–603
    renal blood flow in, 602, 604
    renal clearance by, 599–600
    renal plasma flow in, 604
    transport in, 594–596
Renal transport, 594–596
Renal tubular acidosis, 618
Renal tubular system
    histology of, 590, 591, 592–593
    physiology of, 607–610
Renal tumors, 647–650
Renal vascular resistance and filtration
    fraction, 604–605
Renal veins, 147, 187, 588
Renin, 612–613
Renin-angiotensin system (RAS), 152
Renin-angiotensin-aldosterone system (RAAS),
    99, 100, 152
    and mean arterial pressure, 37–38, 39–40
    and renal function, 612–613
Renshaw cells, 450
Repaglinide, 168
Repolarization, 41, 42
Repression, 538
Reproductive disorders, 700–741
    developmental
        early, 662, 666
        female, 673
        male, 669
    female, 703–733
        of breast, 727–731
        cervical, 713–715
        developmental, 673
        ovarian, 715–721
        of pregnancy, 703–712
        uterine, 721–727
        vaginal, 712–713
    genetic
        double Y males (XYY syndrome) as, 701

female pseudohermaphrodite as, 702
        Kallmann syndrome as, 703
        Klinefelter syndrome as, 700
        male pseudohermaphrodite as, 701–702
        Müllerian agenesis as, 703
        ovotesticular disorder of sex development
            as, 702
        Turner syndrome as, 700–701
    male, 733–741
        developmental, 669
        penile, 733–734
        prostatic, 738–741
        testicular, 734–738
    sexually transmitted and other genital
        infections as, 731–733
Reproductive system, 661–746
    anatomy of, 674–681
        female, 679–681
            lower abdomen and perineum in,
                674–675
            male, 675–679
    development of, 662–673
        determination of sex in, 662
        differentiation in, 665
        disorders of, 662, 666
        early, 662–665
        female, 669–673
        male, 666–669
        male and female genital homologs in,
            674, 675
    disorders of. See Reproductive disorders
    female
        anatomy of, 679–681
        development of, 669–673
        fertilization in, 691–692
        gonadal steroids in, 687, 689, 690
        homologs in male and, 674, 675
        menopause in, 698–700
        menstrual cycle and ovulation in, 686–
            687, 688
        oogenesis in, 684–686
        pregnancy in, 692–698
        sexual response in, 689–691
    male
        anatomy of, 675–679
        development of, 666–669
        gonadal steroids in, 687, 689, 690
        homologs in female and, 674, 675
        sexual response in, 689–691
        spermatogenesis in, 682–684
    pharmacology of, 741–745
        drugs that modulate female reproductive
            system in, 744–746
        drugs that modulate gonadotropin axis
            in, 741
        drugs that modulate male reproductive
            system in, 741–743
    physiology of, 681–700
        fertilization in, 691–692
        gametogenesis in, 681–686, 687
        gonadal steroids in, 687, 689, 690
        menopause in, 698–700
        menstrual cycle and ovulation in, 686–
            687, 688
        pregnancy in, 692–698
        sexual response in, 689–691
Residual volume (RV), 761, 762
Resistance (r, R), 34
    air, 784
    pulmonary, 769–770
Respiration(s)
    Cheyne-Stokes, 803
    control of, 778–779
    forced, 758
    quiet, 758
    spontaneous, 767

Respiratory acidosis, 619, 620
    in acid-base nomogram, 622
    clinical implications of, 621
    renal compensation for, 771–772
Respiratory airways, 754, 755, 758–759
Respiratory alkalosis, 619–620, 772–773
    in acid-base nomogram, 622
    clinical implications of, 621
Respiratory bronchi, 756
Respiratory compensation, 618, 621
Respiratory cycle, mechanics of breathing
    during, 766–769
Respiratory disorders, 779–818
    allergy as, 817
    congenital malformations as, 751–753
    flail chest as, 758
    hypersensitivity pneumonitis as, 818
    infectious, 808–814
        pneumonia as, 808–812
        tuberculosis as, 774, 812–814
        upper respiratory tract, 814
    of nasopharynx, 781–783
    neoplastic, 803–808
        lung cancer as, 803–807
        mesothelioma as, 807
        of upper respiratory tract, 808
    obstructive, 783–790
        asthma as, 761, 787–788, 789
        bronchiectasis as, 788–790
        chronic bronchitis as, 786–787
        emphysema as, 761, 766, 768, 776,
            784–786
        lung volumes and capacities in, 761, 762,
            763, 783
    pathology on physical examination with,
        779–781
    pleural effusion as, 815
    pneumothorax as, 815–817
    restrictive, 790–798
        acute respiratory distress syndrome as,
            764, 769, 792–793
        chronic eosinophilic pneumonia as, 798
        extrapulmonary, 790–791
        Goodpasture syndrome as, 797
        granulomatosis with polyangiitis as,
            797–798
        idiopathic pulmonary fibrosis as, 762, 766,
            768, 776, 796–797
        interstitial, 792–798
        lung volumes and capacities in, 762, 763
        neonatal (infant) respiratory distress
            syndrome as, 764, 793–794
        pneumoconiosis as, 794–795
        sarcoidosis as, 795–796
    vascular, 798–803
        deep venous thrombosis as, 798–799
        pulmonary embolism as, 799–801
        pulmonary hypertension as, 801–802
        sleep apnea as, 803
Respiratory distress syndrome (RDS), 753, 754
    acute, 764, 769, 792–793
    neonatal (infant), 764, 793–794
Respiratory epithelium, 759
Respiratory muscles, 757–758
    accessory, 779–780
Respiratory quotient (R), 775
Respiratory rate (RR) during pregnancy, 693
Respiratory regulation, 444
Respiratory system, 747–824
    anatomy of, 753–761
        airways in, 754, 755
        diaphragm in, 756–757
        external, 757, 758
        gross, 753, 754
        lungs in, 754–756
        muscles of respiration in, 757–758

Respiratory system (continued)
  development of, 748–751
    bronchi and bronchioles in, 749
    diaphragm in, 750–751
    larynx in, 748–749
    lungs in, 750
    pleural cavities in, 750
    trachea in, 749
  disorders of. See Respiratory disorders
  histology of, 758–761
    alveoli in, 758–760
    olfactory cells in, 761
    respiratory epithelium in, 758
  pharmacology of, 818–823
    α-adrenergic agonists as, 820
    asthma drugs in, 821–823
    dextromethorphan in, 819–820
    histamine blockers in, 818–819
    mucoactive agents in, 819
    pulmonary hypertension drugs in, 820
  physiology of, 761–779
    blood gases in, 770–779
    ideal gas law and Boyle's law in, 761
    lung volumes and capacities in, 761–763
    ventilation in, 763–770
  during pregnancy, 693, 695
Respiratory tract cancers, 803–808
  lung cancer as, 803–807
  mesothelioma as, 807
  upper, 808
Rest(s)
  mechanics of breathing at, 766, 768
  nephrogenic, 648
Restiform body, 442, 445
Resting membrane potential, 15–16
Restless legs syndrome, 567, 568
Restrictive cardiomyopathy, 62, 63
Restrictive lung disease, 790–798
  acute respiratory distress syndrome as, 764,
    769, 792–793
  characteristics of, 790
  chronic eosinophilic pneumonia as, 798
  classification of, 790
  extrapulmonary, 790–791
  Goodpasture syndrome as, 797
  granulomatosis with polyangiitis as, 797–798
  idiopathic pulmonary fibrosis as, 762, 766,
    768, 776, 796–797
  interstitial, 792–798
  lung volumes and capacities in, 762, 763
  neonatal (infant) respiratory distress
    syndrome as, 764, 793–794
  pneumoconiosis as, 794–795
  sarcoidosis as, 795–796
Retching, 195
Rete testes, 666, 667, 676
Reticular formation, 444
Reticulocyte(s), 267–268
Reticulocyte count, 267–268
  corrected, 288
Reticuloendothelial system in bilirubin
    production, 208
Retina, 459–460, 502
Retinoblastoma, 492
Retinoblastoma (RB) gene, 309
Retinopathy, diabetic, 163
Retractions, 779–780
Retrograde amnesia, 543
Retrograde memory loss, 430
Retrograde menstruation, 723
Retrolenticular limb of internal capsule, 435
Retroperitoneal organs, 184, 587–590
Retropulsion, 197
Rett syndrome, 578
Reverse enterogastric reflex, 197
Reverse T$_3$ (rT$_3$), 109, 130
Reye syndrome, 244

Reynolds pentad, 252
RF (rheumatoid factor), 362, 374
Rh classification, 282
Rh factor, 281
Rh immunoglobulin (RhoGAM), 694,
    710–711
Rh incompatibility, 694, 710–711
Rhabdomyolysis, 359–360
Rhabdomyoma, cardiac, 73
Rhabdomyosarcoma, embryonal, 713
Rheumatic fever, 60–61, 631, 814
Rheumatic heart disease, 60–61
Rheumatoid arthritis (RA), 373, 374–375
Rheumatoid factor (RF), 362, 374
Rheumatoid nodules, 374
Rhinitis, allergic, 817
Rhinosinusitis, 781–783
RhoGAM (Rh immunoglobulin), 694,
    710–711
Rhombencephalon, 414, 416
Rhonchi, 780
Rib(s)
  accessory, 331
  congenital malformations of, 331
  development of, 330
  "floating," 330
  "true" vs "false," 330
"Rib notching," 6
Ribonuclease, 206
Richter syndrome, 300
Rickets, 142, 326, 360, 369
Riedel thyroiditis, 133
Rifampin, 813
Right atrium (RA), 10
Right bundle branch, 14, 15
Right bundle branch block, 44–45
Right colic artery, 186
Right coronary artery (RCA), 12, 13–14
Right hepatic artery, 186
Right hypochondriac region, 180, 181
Right iliac region, 180, 181
Right lower quadrant (RLQ), 181
Right lumbar region, 180, 181
Right (acute) marginal artery, 12
Right upper quadrant (RUQ), 181
Right ventricle (RV), 9, 10
Right ventricular (RV) afterload, 24
Right ventricular (RV) hypertrophy, 4, 5,
    44, 45
Right ventricular (RV) outflow obstruction,
    4, 5
Right-dominant circulation, 13
Right-heart catheterization, 31
Right-sided heart failure, 65
Right-to-left shunting, 4–5
  hypoxemia due to, 778
Rima glottidis, 348
Ringed sideroblast(s), 274
  refractory anemia with, 277
Ring-enhancing brain lesions, 58
Rinne test, 463
Risedronate, 368, 402
Risperidone, 521, 540
Ritodrine, 744
Rituximab, 317
Rivaroxaban, 319–320
Rivastigmine, 527
RLE (rate-limiting enzyme)
  in glucocorticoid synthesis, 150
  in steroid hormone synthesis, 149
RLQ (right lower quadrant), 181
Rocuronium, 510
Rods, 459
Romberg sign, 445, 448
ROMK (renal output medullary potassium)
    channels, 608, 609
Ropinirole, 528–529

Rosacea, 390
Rose spots, 232
Rosenthal fibers, 492
Rosiglitazone, 168
Rotator cuff muscles, 348–349
Roth spots, 58
Rotor syndrome, 238, 241
Rouleaux formation, 305
RPGN (rapidly progressive
    glomerulonephritis), 623, 632–633
RR (respiratory rate) during pregnancy, 693
RRP (relative refractory period), 19, 20
rT$_3$ (reverse T$_3$), 109, 130
RTK (receptor-associated tyrosine kinase)
    mechanism, 110
RU-486, 746
Rubella, cardiac defects due to congenital, 7
Rubrospinal tract, 449
Ruffini corpuscle, 453
RUQ (right upper quadrant), 181
Russell sign, 564
RV (residual volume), 761, 762
RV (right ventricle). See Right ventricle (RV)
RVR (rapid ventricular rate), atrial fibrillation
    with, 50
Ryanodine receptors, 22, 355

S

S cells, 196, 199, 204
S$_1$ heart sound, 31–32
S$_2$ heart sound, 31–32
S$_2$ splitting, 31–32
S$_3$ heart sound, 32, 63, 69
S$_4$ heart sound, 32
SA (sinoatrial) node, 13, 15, 17
  bradyarrhythmias of, 46–47
  tachyarrhythmias of, 49
Saccular period, 748, 750
Saccule, 462, 463
Sacral promontory, 338
Sacral vein, 187
Sacral vertebrae, 337
Sacrococcygeal teratomas, 412
Sacrotuberous ligament, 339
Sacrum, 329
Saddle embolus, 76–77
Saddle joints, 343
Sadistic personality disorder, 558
Sadomasochistic personality disorder, 558
Sagittal sulcus, 425
Sagittal suture, 328, 329, 335
SAH (subarachnoid hemorrhage), 419, 471–
    472, 476, 477–478
Salicylate, Reye syndrome due to, 244
Salicylate poisoning, 621
Saliva
  antibacterial actions of, 194
  composition of, 193–194
Salivary gland(s)
  anatomy and physiology of, 192–193
  disorders of, 211–213
Salivary gland hypertrophy, 212
Salivary gland stones, 211, 212
Salivary gland tumors, 212, 213
Salivary secretions, 192–193
Salmeterol, 744, 821
Salmonella typhi, 232
Salpinges, 670, 672, 679, 680, 686, 691
Sampson's theory of endometriosis, 723
Samter's triad, 787
Saphenous nerve, 352
Sarcoidosis, 383–384, 795–796
Sarcoma, 309
  botryoides, 713
  Ewing, 297, 363, 364, 365–366
  osteogenic, 363, 364, 366–367

Sarcomere, 21, 22, 25
    in excitation-contraction coupling, 356,
        357
Sarcoplasmic reticulum (SR), 21, 355
Sartorius muscle, 182, 352, 676
Saturday night palsy, 339–340, 350, 496
"Sausage digits" in psoriatic arthritis, 380
Saxagliptin, 169
SCA (superior cerebellar artery), 424
Scale, 389
Scalene muscles in inspiration, 765
Scaphoid, 339
    fracture of, 342
Scapula, winged, 350, 496
Scar, hypertrophic, 328
Scarpa fascia, 674, 676, 681
SCC. See Squamous cell carcinoma (SCC)
SCFE (slipped capital femoral epiphysis), 343,
        345–346
Schaumann bodies, 383
Schilling test, 220, 278
Schirmer test, 212
Schistocytes, 274, 287
Schistosomiasis, 648
Schizoaffective disorder, 546
Schizoid personality disorder, 544, 558, 560
Schizophrenia, 543–545
Schizophreniform disorder, 546
Schizotypal personality disorder, 544, 558,
        560
Schwann cells, 354, 464, 465–466
Schwannomas, 465–466, 490, 491
    vestibular, 444, 493
Sciatic nerve, 351, 352, 497
Sciatica, 340, 351, 352
SCLC (small cell lung cancer), 804, 807
Sclera, 502
Scleroderma, 194, 384
Scleroderma acrosclerosis, 385
Sclerosing cholangitis, primary, 253
SCM (sternocleidomastoid) muscle, 347–348
    in inspiration, 765
Scoliosis, 338
    restrictive lung disease due to, 791
Scombroid poisoning, 513
Scopolamine, 512
SCP (superior cerebellar peduncle), 437, 438
"Scrotal ligament," 677
Scrotal/penile raphe, 668
Scrotum, 668, 669, 676, 677, 678
Scurvy
    musculoskeletal disorders due to, 360
    vessel wall abnormalities due to, 295
Seafood toxins, 512–513
Seasonal affective disorder, 548
Seborrheic keratosis, 390
Secobarbital, 514, 540
Second intercostal space, 10
Secondary active transport, 596
Secondary fissure, 437
Secondary gain, 537
Second-degree AV block, 47–48
Second-messenger pathways, peptide
        hormones in, 109–111
Second-order neurons, 452, 453
Secretin, 196, 199, 204, 209
Secretions and pulmonary resistance, 769
Secretory vesicles, 466
Sedative use disorder, 570–571
Segmental artery, 588
Segmental nerves, 447
Seizures, 430, 488, 489
    due to alcohol withdrawal, 570
    eclamptic, 708
Selective estrogen receptor modulators
        (SERMs), 315, 368, 404, 745

Selective mutism, 581
Selective serotonin reuptake inhibitors
        (SSRIs), 516, 517, 540
Selegiline, 530, 541
Sella turcica, 112, 436
Semen, 690–691
Semicircular canals, 462
Semimembranosus muscle, 352
Seminal emission, 690
Seminal vesicle, 667, 668, 676
Seminiferous tubules, 667, 676, 677, 684
Seminoma, 737, 738
Semitendinosus muscle, 352
Sensation, 428
Sensorineural deafness, 463
Sensory corpuscles, 451, 453, 468
Sensory cortex, 428
    primary, 428
Sensory homunculus, 428
Sensory pathway(s), 449, 451–453
    lesions of, 455
Sensory receptors, 451, 453
Sensory relay station, 433
Sentinel node biopsy, 729
Separation anxiety disorder, 580
Septate uterus, 673
Septic emboli, 76
    from endocarditis, 58, 59
Septum(a)
    cardiac, 2
    primum, 3
    secundum, 3
    transversum, 750, 751
Sequestration symptoms of sickle cell
        disease, 285
SERMs (selective estrogen receptor
        modulators), 315, 368, 404, 745
Seronegative spondyloarthropathies, 377–380
Serosa, 201
Serotonin, 446, 508, 509
Serotonin-norepinephrine reuptake inhibitors
        (SNRIs), 518–519, 540
Serous cystadenocarcinoma, 718
Serous cystadenoma, 718
Serous pericardium, 11, 12
Serous salivary secretions, 192
Serous tumors, ovarian, 718
Sertoli cell(s), 666, 682, 683, 684
Sertoli cell tumor, 738
Sertoli-Leydig cell tumor, 721
Sertraline, 517, 540
Serum, 32, 33
Sevoflurane, 531
Sex, determination of, 662
Sex cord stromal tumors
    ovarian, 720–721
    testicular, 738
Sex hormone-binding globulin (SHBG), 109
Sex-determining region (SRY) gene, 662
Sexual development, 662–673
    determination of sex in, 662
    differentiation in, 665
    disorders of, 662, 666
    early, 662–665
    female, 669–673
    male, 666–669
    male and female genital homologs in, 674,
        675
    ovotesticular disorder of, 666, 702
Sexual differentiation, 662, 664, 665
Sexual response, 689–691
Sexually transmitted infections (STIs),
        731–733
Sézary syndrome, 299, 301
SGLT-2 (sodium-glucose cotransporter 2)
        inhibitors, 169

Shagreen patches, 493
SHBG (sex hormone-binding globulin), 109
Sheehan syndrome, 121, 133, 709–710
Shock, 77–78
Short gastric arteries, 186
Short gut syndrome, 175
Short portal vessel, 113
Short saphenous vein, 352
Shoulder dislocation, 342, 350
Shoulder joints, 344
Shoulder sign, 177
Shunt(s)
    fetal, 696, 698
    hypoxemia due to, 778
    left-to-right, 7
    right-to-left, 4–5
    transjugular intrahepatic portosystemic, 215
    ureteroenteric, 619
SIADH. See Syndrome of inappropriate
        secretion of antidiuretic hormone
        (SIADH)
Sialolithiasis, 211, 212
Sicca, 386
Sick sinus syndrome (SSS), 47
Sickle cell, 274, 284
Sickle cell disease, 284–286
Sickle cell trait, 283
Sickle β-thalassemia, 284
Sideroblast(s), ringed, 274
    refractory anemia with, 277
Sideroblastic anemia, 277
Sigmoid artery, 186
Sigmoid colon, 184
Sigmoid sinus, 474
Signal propagation mechanisms, 109–111
Signet ring cells, 222, 223
SIL (squamous intraepithelial lesion), 714
Sildenafil, 691, 743, 820
"Silent chest," 787
Silicosis, 794, 795, 796
Simple diffusion, 595
Simple seizure, 489
Simvastatin, 105
Sinoatrial (SA) node, 13, 15, 17
    bradyarrhythmias of, 46–47
    tachyarrhythmias of, 49
Sinovaginal bulbs, 671
Sinus bradycardia, 42, 46–47
Sinus rhythm, normal, 42
Sinus tachycardia, 42, 49
Sinus venosus (SV), 2
Sinusitis, 781–783
Sinusoids, liver, 206, 207
Sipple syndrome, 135
Sister Mary Joseph sign, 223
Sjögren syndrome, 211–212, 386–387
Skeletal disorders
    bone tumors as, 362–367
    congenital malformations as, 324–332
        of limbs, 331–332
        of osteogenesis, 326–328
        of ribs, 332
        of skull, 328–329
        of vertebral column, 329–330
    drugs used to treat, 402–404
    fibrous dysplasia as, 371
    fractures and other mechanical disorders as,
        339–343
    important laboratory values for, 361–362
    oncologic, 362–367
    osteitis fibrosa cystica as, 370
    osteomyelitis as, 371–372
    osteopetrosis (marble bone disease) as,
        368–369
    osteoporosis as, 367–368
    Paget disease of bone as, 369–370

Skeletal muscle
  anatomy of, 346, 355
  development of, 332–333
  physiology of, 354–357
Skeletal myocytes, 20, 354
Skeletal system
  anatomy of, 335–339
  development of, 324–332
    of limbs, 331
    osteogenesis in, 324–325
    of ribs, 330
    of skull, 328
    of vertebral column, 329
  disorders of. *See* Skeletal disorders
Skeleton, axial vs appendicular, 335
Skene glands, 671
Skin
  anatomy of, 360
  disorders of. *See* Skin disorders
  during pregnancy, 694
  would healing by, 360–361
Skin cancer, 395–396
Skin disorders, 389–396
  acanthosis nigricans as, 394
  acne as, 389, 390
  actinic keratosis as, 395
  albinism as, 391
  allergic contact dermatitis as, 389, 390
  atopic dermatitis (eczema) as, 390
  with blisters, 392–394
  bullous pemphigoid as, 393
  cellulitis as, 391
  common, 389–391
  dermatitis herpetiformis as, 393
  erythema multiforme as, 393
  impetigo as, 392
  infectious, 391–392
  lichen planus as, 394
  melanocytic nevus as, 390
  melasma as, 391
  necrotizing fasciitis as, 392
  pemphigus vulgaris as, 394
  pigmented, 391
  pityriasis rosea as, 394
  psoriasis as, 390
  rosacea as, 390
  seborrheic keratosis as, 390
  skin cancer as, 395–396
  staphylococcal scalded skin syndrome
    as, 392
  urticaria as, 390–391
  verrucae as, 392
  vitiligo as, 391
Skin infections, 391–392
Skin lesions, terminology for, 389
Skull
  bones of, 335, 336
  congenital malformations of, 328
  development of, 328, 329
  fractures of, 339–340
SLE. *See* Systemic lupus erythematosus (SLE)
Sleep apnea, 567, 769, 803
Sleep disorders, 565–568
Sleep terrors, 567
Sleepwalking, 567
Sliding hernia, 216
Slipped capital femoral epiphysis (SCFE),
    343, 345–346
Slipped disk, 340–341
SLL (small lymphocytic lymphoma), 300, 302
Slow-conducting pain fibers, 453
Slow-response action potentials, 16–17, 18
SMA. *See* Superior mesenteric artery (SMA)
Small cell lung cancer (SCLC), 804, 805
Small intestine
  absorption in, 200–203

anatomy and histologic characteristics of,
    199–200, 201, 202
  diverticular disease of, 226–228
  hormones and peptides of, 204
  intussusception of, 228
  malabsorption syndromes of, 224–225
  omphalocele of, 229
Small lymphocytic lymphoma (SLL), 300, 302
Small saphenous vein, 352
Small-vessel vasculitis, 83–85, 403
Smith fracture, 342
Smoking
  and emphysema, 784
  and lung cancer, 804
Smooth muscle
  anatomy of, 346–347
  development of, 333
  locations of, 358
  physiology of, 357–358
SNRIs (serotonin-norepinephrine reuptake
    inhibitors), 518–519, 540
Social judgment, 427
Social phobia, 552–553
Sodium (Na+)
  intracellular and extracellular
    concentrations of, 15–16
  renal reabsorption of, 607, 608
Sodium (Na+) channel(s), 466
  I(f) ("funny"), 17
  voltage-gated, 16
Sodium (Na+) channel blockers, 104
Sodium (Na+) channel inactivation gates, 19
Sodium (Na+) excretion in pregnancy, 692
Sodium (Na+) gradient, transmembrane, 607
Sodium (Na+) retention
  in pregnancy, 692
  due to renal failure, 644
Sodium (Na+) suppression test, 156
Sodium glucose cotransporter 2 (SGLT-2)
    inhibitors, 169
Sodium/potassium–adenosine triphosphatase
    (Na+/K+-ATPase) pump, 607
Sodium-potassium-chloride (Na+-K+-2Cl−)
    symporter, 608
Soft palate, 749
Soleus muscle, 352
  accessory, 334
Solid tumors, 308–310
Solifenacin, 512
Soma, 464
Somatic nervous system, 509
Somatic symptom disorder, 554, 555
Somatic treatments for psychiatric
    disorders, 539
Somatization disorder, 555, 557
Somatoform disorders, 557
Somatomammotropins, 117
Somatomedin, 114
Somatostatin, 113, 162, 196, 204, 209
Somatostatin analog, 125
Somatostatinoma, 165, 166
Somatotropic hormone, 114, 115, 116
Somatotropin, 114, 115, 116, 125
Somnambulism, 567
Sonic hedgehog protein, 331
Sorafenib, 316
Sorbitol, 261
Sotalol, 104
Space of Disse, 207
Spasmodic torticollis, 348
Spastic hemiparesis, 451
Spatial relationships, 428
Specific phobia, 553
Speech, poverty of, 545
Speech comprehension area, 427

Sperm cells, 677–678, 679, 691, 692
Spermatic cord, 182, 677, 678
Spermatic fascia, 678
Spermatid, 683, 684
Spermatocele, 736
Spermatocyte, 683, 684
Spermatogenesis, 682–684, 685
Spermatogonium(ia), 682, 683, 684
Spermatozoon, 683, 684
Sphenoid bone, 335
Sphenoid fontanelle, 328
Sphenoid sinus, 425, 782
Sphenopalatine artery, 783
Sphenoparietal sinus, 424
Spherocyte, 274
Spherocytosis, hereditary, 279–280
Sphincter muscle, 332, 346
Sphincter of Oddi, 208
Spina bifida, 330, 413
  occulta, 414
Spinal cord, 446–457
  blood supply to, 446
  cross-section of, 449
  function of, 446
  hemisection of, 453, 454, 455
  lesions of, 455–457, 494–499
  levels of, 446–447
  myotatic reflex of, 447–448
  tracts of, 449–453, 454
  transection of, 453
  unique structures of, 447, 448
Spinal cord tracts, 449–453, 454
Spinal muscular atrophy, infantile, 457, 481
Spinal reflex collaterals, 451
Spinal trigeminal nucleus, 452
Spine, "bamboo," 378
Spinocerebellar lesions, degenerative diseases
    due to, 485
Spinothalamic tract, 442, 445, 453, 454
Spinous process, 337
Spiral ganglion, 461, 462
Spironolactone, 93–94, 102, 656, 657–658,
    746
Splanchnic mesoderm, 332
Splanchnic nerve, 189, 190
Splay, 605
Spleen, formation of blood cells in, 266
Splenic artery, 158, 186
Splenic flexure, 184
Splenic infarction, 285
Splenic vein, 187
Splinter hemorrhages due to endocarditis,
    58, 59
Splitting, 538
SpO2 (oxygen saturation), 770
Spondylitis, ankylosing, 377–379
Spondyloarthropathies, seronegative, 377–380
Spondylolisthesis, 330, 338, 341, 377
Spondylolysis, 330, 341, 377
Spongiform encephalopathies, 483
Spongy bone, 325, 335
Sprue
  celiac, 224, 225
  tropical, 225
Squamosal sutures, 328, 335
Squamous cell carcinoma (SCC)
  of bladder, 648
  of esophagus, 219
  of lung, 805
  of mouth, 211
  penile, 734
  of skin, 395
  vaginal, 713
Squamous cell hyperplasia of mouth, 210
Squamous intraepithelial lesion (SIL), 714
SR (sarcoplasmic reticulum), 21, 355

SRY (sex-determining region) gene, 662
SSc (systemic sclerosis), 384
SSPE (subacute sclerosing panencephalitis), 487
SSRIs (selective serotonin reuptake inhibitors), 516, 517, 540
SSS (sick sinus syndrome), 47
ST segment, in acute coronary syndrome, 45
ST segment depression, 45, 87
ST segment elevation, 45, 87
  in myocarditis, 57
Staghorn kidney stone, 636, 637
Staging of tumors, 309
Stapes, 462
Staphylococcal scalded skin syndrome, 392
Staphylococcus aureus
  endocarditis due to, 58
  pneumonia due to, 811
  virulence factors of, 57
Staphylococcus epidermidis, endocarditis due to, 58
Starling equation, 35, 605
Starling forces, 35, 605
Static compliance curve, 766
Static labyrinth, 463
"Statins," 105
Status asthmaticus, 788
Status epilepticus, generalized convulsive, 488
Steatorrhea, 224, 254
Steinberg sign, 328
ST-elevation myocardial infarction (STEMI), 13, 14, 87, 88, 89
Stellate cell, 207, 439
Stenotic lesions, 6
Stereotyped movement, 536
Sternal lands, 602
Sternocleidomastoid (SCM) muscle, 347–348
  in inspiration, 765
Sternohyoid muscle, 348
Sternothyroid muscle, 348
Steroid hormones, 108, 109, 683
  adrenal, 149–150
  in bone metabolism, 324
  gonadal, 687, 689, 690
  plasma transport of, 109
Stevens-Johnson syndrome, 393
Stimulant(s), 541
Stimulant use disorder, 572–573
STIs (sexually transmitted infections), 731–733
Stomach, 195–199
  absorption by, 199
  anatomy and histology of, 195–196
  disorders of, 219–223
    gastric cancer as, 222–224
    gastritis as, 219–221
    Ménétrier disease as, 221
    peptic ulcer disease as, 221–222
    Zollinger-Ellison syndrome as, 222
  mechanical contractions of, 196–197
  secretions of
    general regulation of, 197, 198
    of hydrochloric acid, 197–199
Stomatitis, herpetic, 210, 211
Stomatocytes, 268
Straight sinus, 424
Stratum basale, 360, 361
Stratum corneum, 360, 361
Stratum granulosum, 360, 361
Stratum lucidum, 360, 361
Stratum spinosum, 360, 361
"Strep throat," 814
Streptococcal infection, evidence of, 60
Streptococcus pneumoniae, 811
Streptococcus pyogenes, 814
Streptococcus viridans, 58
Streptokinase, 322

Streptozocin, 311
Stress hormones, 151
Stress testing, 90–91
Stretch feedback in autoregulation of renal blood flow and filtration, 603
Striatum, 431, 432
Stridor, 780
String sign, 177
Stroke(s)
  embolic, 474–475
    neurologic deficits associated with common, 423
    presentation by location of occlusion of, 478
    thrombotic, 473–474
Stroke volume (SV), 23, 24, 25
  and blood pressure, 37
  during pregnancy, 693
Struma ovarii, 132, 720
Struvite stones, 636, 637
Sturge-Weber syndrome (SWS), 493
Styloglossus muscle, 347
Stylohyoid muscle, 348
Styloid process, 336
Stylopharyngeus muscle, 348
Subacute combined degeneration, 455, 457, 497–498
Subacute granulomatous thyroiditis, 132, 133
Subacute infective endocarditis, 58
Subacute sclerosing panencephalitis (SSPE), 487
Subarachnoid granulations, 421
Subarachnoid hemorrhage (SAH), 419, 471–472, 476, 477–478
Subarachnoid space, 419, 425, 469
Subchondral sclerosis, 372
Subclavian artery, 682
  anastomoses with, 187
Subclavian vein, 682
Subcostal pericardiocentesis, 91
Subcostal plane, 181
Subdural hematoma, 419
Subdural hemorrhage, 419, 475, 477
Subdural space, 419
Subendocardial infarction, 12
Subependymal giant-cell astrocytoma, 496
Subfalcine herniation, 504, 505
Sublenticular limb of internal capsule, 435
Sublimation, 537
Sublingual glands, 192
Subluxation, 373
Submandibular gland, 192
Submaxillary gland, 192
Submucosa, 201
Submucosal gland, 191
Submucosal nerve plexus, 190, 195
Subscapularis muscle, 348, 349
Substance use disorders, 568–576
  alcohol, 568–570
  cannabis, 544, 576
  depressant, 568–571
  hallucinogen (phencyclidine and lysergic acid diethylamide), 575
  opiate, 573–574
  pupillary responses to, 568
  secondary psychiatric vs, 536, 537
  sedative, hypnotic, and anxiolytic, 570–571
  stimulant, 571–572
Substance-induced psychotic disorder, 546
Substantia gelatinosa, 453
Substantia nigra, 431, 432, 440
Substantia nigra pars compacta, 507
Subthalamic nucleus, 431
Subxiphoid pericardiocentesis, 79
Succinylcholine, 509–510
Sucralfate, 260
Sucrase, small intestinal secretion of, 202

Sufentanil, 532
Suicidal thoughts, 535
Sulcus, 418
  limitans, 413
Sulfasalazine, 262
Sulfonylureas, 167
Sunitinib, 316
Superficial fibular nerve, 352
Superficial inguinal ring, 182
Superficial peroneal nerve, 352
Superficial spreading melanoma, 395, 396
Superior adrenal arteries, 147
Superior articular process, 337
Superior cerebellar artery (SCA), 424
Superior cerebellar peduncle (SCP), 437, 438
Superior cerebral veins, 424
Superior cervical ganglion, 189
Superior frontal gyrus, 426
Superior gluteal nerve damage, 353
Superior hypophyseal artery, 113
Superior labial artery, 783
Superior mesenteric artery (SMA)
  and adrenal glands, 147
  anastomoses with, 187
  and GI tract, 184, 185, 186
    development of, 172, 173
  and pancreas, 158
Superior mesenteric artery (SMA) syndrome, 184
Superior mesenteric ganglia, 189
Superior mesenteric vein, 187
Superior oblique muscle, 458
Superior olivary nucleus, 461, 462
Superior ophthalmic vein, 424
Superior orbital fissures, 336
  structures passing through, 335
Superior pancreaticoduodenal artery, 158, 186
Superior posterior fissure, 437
Superior rectal artery, 186
Superior rectus muscle, 458
Superior sagittal sinus, 421, 424, 469
Superior sulcus tumor, 806, 807
Superior temporal gyrus, 426
Superior temporal sulcus, 426
Superior thyroid artery, 126, 127
Superior thyroid vein, 126, 127
Superior vena cava (SVC), 9, 10, 12, 15
Superior vena cava (SVC) syndrome, 75, 806, 807
Supinator muscles of arm, 349
Suppression, 537
Suprachiasmatic nucleus, 435, 436
Supraclavicular fossa, 757
Supracondylar fracture, 342, 350
Suprahyoid muscles, 348
Supramarginal gyrus, 426
Supraoptic nucleus, 117, 435, 436
Suprarenal gland. *See* Adrenal gland
Suprarenal vein, 187
Supraspinatus muscle, 349
Supraventricular tachyarrhythmias, 49–50
Supraventricular tachycardia (SVT)
  hemodynamically unstable, 103
  paroxysmal, 49
Sural nerve, 352
Surface tension, 764
Surfactant, 760, 764
  deficiency of, 753, 754
Suspensory ovarian ligament, 671
Sutures, 328, 329, 335
SV (sinus venosus), 2
SV (stroke volume), 23, 24, 25
  and blood pressure, 37
  during pregnancy, 693

SVC (superior vena cava), 9, 10, 12, 15
SVC (superior vena cava) syndrome, 75, 806, 807
SVR. *See* Systemic vascular resistance (SVR)
SVT (supraventricular tachycardia)
  hemodynamically unstable, 103
  paroxysmal, 49
Swallowing, 194–195
Swallowing center, 194
Swallowing reflex, 194
Swan-Ganz catheter, 31
Swan-neck deformity, 374
SWS (Sturge-Weber syndrome), 493
Sydenham chorea, 60
Sylvan fissure, 418, 425, 426
Sympathetic innervation of GI tract, 189, 190
Sympathetic nervous system in regulation of renal blood flow and filtration, 602
Sympathetic receptors, function of, 95–96
Sympathetic stimulation
  and contractility, 24
  and pulmonary resistance, 769
Sympatholytics, 95–97
Symport, 596
Synapses, 466
Synaptic cleft, 354, 466
Synaptic vesicle, 354
Syncytiotrophoblasts, 696
Syncytium, 697
Syndactyly, 332
Syndrome of inappropriate secretion of antidiuretic hormone (SIADH), 123–124, 435, 614
  intercompartmental water dynamics in, 599
  paraneoplastic, 310
  renal clearance in, 600
Synovial fluid, 343
Synovial joints, 343
Synovial membrane, 343
Syphilis, 731
  tertiary, 457, 497
Syphilitic aneurysms, 66
Syringomyelia, 414, 456, 457, 470, 498
Systemic lupus erythematosus (SLE), 380–383
  diagnosis of, 382–383
  diagnostic criteria for, 380, 381
  epidemiology of, 380
  during pregnancy, 694
  presentation of, 380–382
  prognosis for, 383
  treatment of, 383
    corticosteroids for, 155–156
Systemic sclerosis (SSc), 384
Systemic vascular resistance (SVR), 5, 774
  and cardiac and vascular function curves, 28, 29
  and mean arterial pressure, 35, 37
  during pregnancy, 693
Systole, 27, 30
  atrial, 30
  pressure changes during, 30–31
  ventricular, 26, 27, 30
Systolic pressure, 36, 37

T

T lymphocyte (T-cell), 268, 269, 270
T tubules, 21
T wave, 41, 42
T wave inversions in myocarditis, 57
T1 root damage, 350
T_3 (triiodothyronine), 116, 126, 129–131
T_4 (levothyroxine), 135, 136, 137–138
T_4 (thyroxine), 116, 126, 129–131
Tabes dorsalis, 457, 497
Tachyarrhythmias, 46, 49–52

Tachycardia, 12, 42
  atrioventricular nodal re-entrant, 49
  sinus, 42, 49
  supraventricular
    hemodynamically unstable, 103
    paroxysmal, 49
  ventricular, 51
Tachypnea, 779
Tactile fremitus, 781
Tactile hallucinations, 534
Tadalafil, 743
Tail of Spence, 680
Takayasu arteritis, 82, 398–399, 403
Talipes equinovarus, 331
Talocrural joint, 345–346
Tamm-Horsfall mucoprotein, 623
Tamoxifen, 315, 368, 404, 729, 745
Tamsulosin, 743
Tangential thought, 535
TAO (thromboangiitis obliterans), 83, 398, 403, 634
Target cell, 274
Targeted molecular therapeutics, 315–317
Tartrate-resistant acid phosphatase (TRAP), 304
Taste buds, 464
Taxanes, 314
TB (tuberculosis), 774, 812–814
TBG (thyroid-binding globulin), 131–132, 693
TBG (thyroxine-binding globulin), 109, 129
TBW (total body water)
  composition of, 596–597
  measuring volume of, 598
TCAs (tricyclic antidepressants), 518, 540
T-cell (T lymphocyte), 268, 269, 270
T-cell leukemia/lymphoma, adult, 304
T-cell lymphomas, cutaneous, 299, 301
TDF (testis-determining factor), 662
Teardrop cells, 273, 307
Tectorial membrane, 462
Tectum, 440
  compression of, 441
TEF (tracheoesophageal fistula), 176, 213–214, 751–752
Tegmentum, 440
Tela subcutanea, 681
Telangiectasia, hereditary hemorrhagic, 295
Telencephalon, 414, 416
Temazepam, 515
Temporal arteritis, 81, 396–397, 403
Temporal bones, 335, 336
Temporal lobe, 429–431
Temporomandibular joint, 336
Teniposide, 313–314
Tennis elbow, 349
Tensilon test, 467
Tension pneumothorax, 816
Tension-type headaches, 506
Tensor fascia lata muscle, 352
Tensor veli palatini muscle, 347
Teratogens, 703–705
Teratoma(s), 309
  ovarian, 719, 720
  sacrococcygeal, 412
  testicular, 737–738
Terazosin, 97
Terbutaline, 744
Teres minor muscle, 349
Teriparatide, 404
Terminal bronchiole, 756
Terminal button of motor neuron, 354, 355
Terminal cord syndrome, 456
Terminal lines, 338
Terminal sacs, 750
Testicles. *See* Testis(es)
Testicular artery, 589, 677

Testicular neoplasms, 737–738
Testicular torsion, 677, 735
Testicular veins, 187
Testis(es)
  anatomy of, 676, 678
  descent of, 666, 667, 735
  development of, 666–667
  diseases of, 734–738
    congenital, 734–735
    infectious, 735
    neoplastic, 737–738
    structural/anatomic, 735–736
Testis-determining factor (TDF), 662
Testosterone
  adrenal synthesis of, 147
  as androgen agonist, 741–742
  gonadal, 687, 689
  in sexual differentiation, 662
  in spermatogenesis, 683, 685
Tetanospasmin, 450
Tetanus, 357
Tetanus toxin, 450
Delta-9-tetrahydrocannabinol (THC), 576
Tetralogy of Fallot, 4, 5, 778
Tetrodotoxin, 512–513
TGB (thyroglobulin), 127, 128, 131–132, 693
TGF (transforming growth factor)-α in wound healing, 361
TGF (transforming growth factor)-β, in wound healing, 361
Thalamic nuclei, 432, 433
Thalamic pain syndrome, 434
Thalamus, 431, 432–434
Thalassemia, 275–276
α-Thalassemia, 276
α-Thalassemia trait, 276
β-Thalassemia, 8, 275–276
Thalidomide, 331
THC (delta-9-tetrahydrocannabinol), 576
Theca cells, 686, 687, 688
Theca lutein cysts, 717
Thelarche, 672, 685
Thenar muscles, 349
Theophylline, 823
Thiamine deficiency, 62
Thiazide diuretics, 655, 657
  as antihypertensive agents, 92, 94
  electrolyte changes with, 656
  hypercalcemia due to, 144
  for idiopathic calciuria, 613
  renal mechanism of, 608
  side effects of, 609
Thiazolidinediones, 168
Thick ascending limb, 591, 608, 609–610
Thick filaments, 357
Thigh muscles, 351–352
Thin ascending limb, 608, 609–610
Thin descending limb, 591, 608, 609–610
Thin filaments, 357
Thinking
  concrete, 535
  disordered, 543
Thionamides, 136–137
Thiopental, 514, 531–532, 540
Thioridazine, 520–521, 540
Third spacing, 183
Third ventricle, 420, 421, 425, 469
Third-degree AV block, 48–49
Third-order neurons, 452, 453
Thoracentesis, 757, 758, 815, 817
Thoracic aortic aneurysms, 66
Thoracic duct, 35, 815
Thoracic outlet syndrome, 331, 350, 498–499
Thoracic vertebrae, 337
Thought blocking, 535, 545
Thought content disorders, 535

Thought disorder, 534
Thought process disorders, 535
Thrombasthenia, Glanzmann, 293
Thrombin time, 291
Thromboangiitis obliterans (TAO), 83, 398, 403, 634
Thrombocythemia, essential, 306, 307–308
Thrombocytopenia, 290–293
  heparin-induced, 290
  immune-mediated, 291
Thromboembolism, 76, 800
Thrombolytics, 292, 322
Thrombophlebitis, migratory, 75, 255
Thrombosis, deep venous, 74–75
Thrombotic microangiopathies, 292
Thrombotic stroke, 473–474
Thrombotic thrombocytopenic purpura (TTP), 292
Thrombus
  coronary, 13
  mural, 50
Thrush, 210, 211
Thymus, blood cell formation in, 266
Thyroarytenoid muscles, 348
Thyrocervical trunk, 127
Thyroglobulin (TGB), 127, 128, 131–132, 693
Thyroglossal duct, 127, 140
Thyroglossal duct cysts, 127, 137
Thyrohyoid muscle, 348
Thyroid, 126–137
  anatomy of, 126, 127
  disorders of, 131–135
    drugs for, 135–137
    hyperthyroidism as, 131–132, 134
    hypothyroidism as, 132–133, 134
    multiple endocrine neoplasia as, 135, 136
    thyroid neoplasms as, 134–135
  embryology of, 127
  histology of, 127, 128
  overview of, 126
  during pregnancy, 694
Thyroid adenoma, 134
Thyroid cancer, 134–135
Thyroid cartilage, 749
Thyroid diverticulum, 127
Thyroid follicular cells, 127, 128
Thyroid hormones, 116, 126
  in bone remodeling, 367
  downstream effects of, 130–131
  regulation of, 130, 131
  release of, 129
  synthesis and secretion of, 128–130
  transport and metabolism of, 129–130
Thyroid lymphoma, 134
Thyroid neoplasms, 134–135
Thyroid peroxidase, 128
Thyroid storm, 131
Thyroid tissue, ectopic, 127
Thyroid-binding globulin (TBG), 131–132, 693
Thyroidea ima artery, 127
Thyroiditis
  Hashimoto, 133
  Riedel, 133
  subacute granulomatous (de Quervain), 132, 133
Thyroid-stimulating hormone (TSH), 114, 116, 130, 131
Thyrotoxicosis, 131
Thyrotropin, 114, 116
Thyrotropin-releasing hormone (TRH), 113, 130, 131
Thyroxine (T₄), 116, 126, 129–131
Thyroxine-binding globulin (TBG), 109, 129
TIA (transient ischemic attack), 422
TIBC (total iron-binding capacity), 275

Tibial collateral ligament, 345
Tibial fractures, 342
Tibial nerve, 352
  injury to, 353, 495
Tibialis anterior muscle, 352
Tibialis posterior muscle, 352
Tibiofibular ligament, 345
Ticlopidine, 321
Tidal volume (TV, V_T), 761, 762
  during pregnancy, 693
Tiludronate, 402
Tiotropium, 512, 822
TIPS (transjugular intrahepatic portosystemic shunt) procedure, 215
Tirofiban, 321
Tissue plasminogen activator (tPA), 322
TLC (total lung capacity), 761, 762
  during pregnancy, 693
TN (trigeminal neuralgia), 501, 506–507
TNF-α (tumor necrosis factor-alpha), in bony metastases, 362
TNF-α (tumor necrosis factor-alpha) antagonists, 404
TNM staging system, 309
Toe plantarflexion, 341
Tolbutamide, 167
Tolcapone, 530
Tolterodine, 512
Tolvaptan, 126, 656–657
Tonic seizure, 489
Tonic-clonic seizure, 489
Topoisomerase inhibitors, 311, 313–314
Topotecan, 314
Torsade de pointes, 51
Torticollis
  congenital, 334, 348
  spasmodic, 348
Total anomalous pulmonary venous return, 5
Total body water (TBW)
  composition of, 596–597
  measuring volume of, 598
Total dead space, 763
Total iron-binding capacity (TIBC), 275
Total lung capacity (TLC), 761, 762
  during pregnancy, 693
Total parenteral nutrition (TPN), metabolic acidosis due to, 618
Total peripheral resistance and cardiac and vascular function curves, 28
Tourette disorder, 580
Toxic epidermal necrolysis, 393
Toxic multinodular goiter, 132
tPA (tissue plasminogen activator), 322
TPN (total parenteral nutrition), metabolic acidosis due to, 618
Trachea
  anatomy of, 754
  development of, 749
Tracheal deviation, 781
Tracheoesophageal fistula (TEF), 176, 213–214, 751–752
Tracheoesophageal septum, 749, 751
Tract of Lissauer, 453
Tractus solitarius, 445
TRALI (transfusion-related acute lung injury), 792
Trans deletion, 276
Transcellular transport, 595
Transference, 536–537
Transforming growth factor (TGF)-α in wound healing, 361
Transforming growth factor (TGF)-β, in wound healing, 361
Transfusion(s), bleeding disorders due to, 291
Transfusion-related acute lung injury (TRALI), 792

Transient ischemic attack (TIA), 422
Transitional cell carcinomas of urinary tract, 648
Transjugular intrahepatic portosystemic shunt (TIPS) procedure, 215
Transmembrane sodium (Na⁺) gradient, 607
Transmural infarction, 12
Transmural ischemia, 85
Transport maximum, 605
Transposition of the great vessels, 4, 5
Transpulmonary pressure, 767
Transtentorial herniation, 505
Transudate, 755, 815
Transudative edema, 35, 36
Transudative effusion, 755, 815
Transversalis fascia, 182
Transverse colon, 173
Transverse cricoarytenoid muscles, 348
Transverse foramen, 337
Transverse processes, 337
Transverse sinus, 424
Transverse temporal gyri of Heschl, 463
Transverse tubules (T-tubules), 354, 355
Transversus abdominis muscle, 179, 182
Tranylcypromine, 517–518, 541
TRAP (tartrate-resistant acid phosphatase), 304
Trapezium, 339
Trapezoid, 339
Trapezoid body, 461, 462
Trastuzumab, 316, 746
Trazodone, 519–520, 541
Trendelenburg sign, 353
Treponema pallidum, 731
TRH (thyrotropin-releasing hormone), 113, 130, 131
Triamterene, 93–94, 656, 657–658
Triazolam, 515, 540
Triceps brachii muscle, 349
Triceps jerk reflex, 449
Trichomonas vaginalis, 732
Trichomoniasis, 732
Tricuspid atresia, 5
Tricuspid regurgitation, 69
Tricuspid valve, 10, 11
Tricyclic antidepressants (TCAs), 518, 540
Trifluoperazine, 540
Trigeminal nerve, 452, 459
  motor lesion of, 500
Trigeminal neuralgia (TN), 501, 506–507
Triiodothyronine (T₃), 116, 126, 129–131
"Triple screen," 330
Triquetrum, 339
Trisomy 13, 331
Trisomy 18, 331
Trisomy 21, 331
Trisomy syndromes, 331
Trochlear nerve, 425, 459
  lesion of, 500, 501
Tropheryma whippelii, 224–225
Trophic hormone secreting cells, 113
Trophoblasts, 696
Tropical sprue, 225
Tropomyosin
  in excitation-contraction coupling, 356
  in myocardial contraction and relaxation, 22
Troponin, in myocardial infarction, 88
Troponin C, in myocardial contraction and relaxation, 22
Trousseau sign, 145, 255
Trousseau syndrome, paraneoplastic, 310
True pelvis, 338, 339
Truncus arteriosus, 2
  persistent, 4, 5
Trunk, muscular development of, 332–333
Trypanosoma cruzi, 57, 62
  achalasia due to, 215

Trypsin, 205, 206
Trypsinogen, 205, 206
TSC (tuberous sclerosis complex), 493
T-score, 367
TSH (thyroid-stimulating hormone), 114, 116, 130, 131
TTP (thrombotic thrombocytopenic purpura), 292
T-tubules (transverse tubules), 354, 355
Tube thoracostomy, 817
Tuber vermis, 437
Tuberculin skin test, 813
Tuberculosis (TB), 774, 812–814
Tuberous sclerosis, 73, 496
Tuberous sclerosis complex (TSC), 493
Tubular adenomas, 233
Tubular carcinoma of breast, 730
Tubulin, drugs that target, 314
Tubuloglomerular feedback, 603
Tubulovillous polyps, 233
Tumor(s)
    nomenclature for, 308
    solid, 308–310
Tumor cell embolism, 800
Tumor grading, 309
Tumor lysis syndrome, 302, 636
Tumor necrosis factor-alpha (TNF-α), in bony metastases, 362
Tumor necrosis factor-alpha (TNF-α) antagonists, 404
Tumor staging, 309
Tumor suppressor genes, 309
Tunica albuginea, 666, 667, 676, 677
Tunica dartos, 677, 678
Tunica muscularis externa, 191
Tunica serosa, 191
Tunica submucosa, 191
Tunica vaginalis, 666, 667, 678
Turbulent flow, 34, 67
Turcot syndrome, 233
Turner syndrome, 700–701
    cardiac defects in, 7
TV (tidal volume), 761, 762
    during pregnancy, 693
22q11 deletions, cardiac defects in, 7
Twinning, 697, 698, 699
Twitch, 356
Two-hit hypothesis, 309
Type C fibers, 191
Typhoid fever, 232

U

U wave, 41
UC (ulcerative colitis), 230
UDP (uridine diphosphate), 208, 209
UES (upper esophageal sphincter), 194, 195
Ulcer(s)
    aphthous, 211
    Curling, 220
    Cushing, 220
    duodenal, 221–222
    gastric, 221
    peptic, 221–222
Ulcerative colitis (UC), 230
Ulnar nerve, 338, 349, 351
    damage to, 350, 495
Ulnohumeral joint, 344
Ultimobranchial body, 140
Umbilical artery(ies), 8, 9, 173, 697
    single, 176
Umbilical hernia, 236, 237
Umbilical region, 180, 181
Umbilical vein, 8, 9, 173, 697
UMN (upper motor neuron) lesions, 455, 457, 460, 494, 497, 502
Uncal herniation, 504, 505

Uncus, 426
"Unhappy triad," 345
Unicornuate uterus, 673
Upper esophageal sphincter (UES), 194, 195
Upper extremity nerve injury, 495
Upper limbs
    bones of, 338
    fractures of, 341–342
    muscles of, 348–351
    nerve damage of, 349, 350, 351
Upper motor neuron (UMN) lesions, 455, 457, 460, 494, 497, 502
Upper respiratory tract cancers, 808
Upper respiratory tract infections, 814
Upregulation, 111
Urachal fistula, 584
Urachal remnants, 589
Urachus, 172
    patent, 584
Urea, 606, 609, 656
Ureaplasma urealyticum, 731
Uremia, 640
Uremic syndrome, 644
Ureter(s)
    anatomy of, 588–589, 679, 680
    histology of, 590, 594
Ureter bud, 585
Ureteral peristalsis, 594
Ureteral stones, 589
Ureteroenteric shunts, metabolic acidosis due to, 619
Urethra
    male, 676
    membranous, 589
    penile, 590
    prostatic, 589
Urethral orifice, 673
Urethral valve
    anatomy of, 589–590
    female, 590
    male, 589–590
    posterior, 586–587
Urethritis, nongonococcal, 731
Uric acid stones, 636, 637
Uridine diphosphate (UDP), 208, 209
Urinary casts, 623
Urinary system. *See* Renal system
Urinary tract infections (UTIs), 638–639
Urine, hyperosmolar, 606
Urine concentration, 609
Urine osmolarity, 606–607
URO (uroporphyrinogen decarboxylase), 289
Urobilinogen, 209
Urogenital delta, 339
Urogenital diaphragm, 676, 681
Urogenital folds, 664, 665, 669, 673
Urogenital sinus, 584, 585
    development of, 665, 667, 668, 669, 673
Urolithiasis, 636–637
Uroporphyrin, 289
Uroporphyrinogen decarboxylase (URO), 289
Urticaria, 390–391
Uterine artery, 589, 672, 680
Uterine canal
    abnormalities of, 673
    atresia of, 673
Uterine contractants, 744
Uterine cycle, 686–687, 688
Uterine neoplasms, 724–727
    endometrial carcinoma as, 725–726
    endometrial hyperplasia as, 724–725
    leiomyoma (fibroid) as, 726
    leiomyosarcoma as, 726–727
Uterine relaxants, 744

Uterine round ligament, 671, 672
Uterine tube, 670, 672, 679, 680, 686, 691
Uterosacral ligaments, 672
Uterus, 589, 680
    bicornuate, 673
    development of, 670, 671, 672
    disorders of, 721–727
        adenomyosis as, 724
        endometriosis as, 722–724
        endometritis as, 722
        neoplasms as, 724–727
        pelvic inflammatory disease as, 721–722
    double, 673
    septate, 673
    unicornuate, 673
UTIs (urinary tract infections), 638–639
Utricle, 462, 463
Utriculus prostaticus, 667
Uvea, 502
Uveal tract, 502
Uveitis, 502
Uvula, 437

V

V1 receptors, 614
VACTERL association, 176, 586, 752
Vagal nerves, 189
Vagina, 670, 672, 680
Vaginal diseases, 712–713
Vaginal plate, 671
Vaginal tumors, 713
Vaginismus, 712
Vaginosis, bacterial, 732, 733
Vagotomy, 199
Vagovagal reflex, 196–197
Vagus nerve, 196, 347, 459
    lesion of, 500
Valgus, 344
Valproic acid, 522–524, 541
Valsartan, 99–100, 659
Vardenafil, 743
Variant Creutzfeldt-Jakob disease (vCJD), 483
Varices, esophageal, 215
Varicocele, 185, 675, 735
Varicose veins, 73–74
Varus, 344
Vas deferens, 676, 677
Vasa efferentia, 666, 667
Vasa recta, 610
Vascular dementia, 479, 483
Vascular endothelial growth factor (VEGF)
    molecular therapy targeting, 316
    in wound healing, 361
Vascular function curves, 27–29
Vascular smooth muscle tone, autonomic effects on, 39
Vasculature, components of, 33
Vasculitis(ides), 396–402
    Churg-Strauss, 400–401, 403
    cryoglobulinemic, 85
    giant-cell (temporal) arteritis as, 396–397, 403
    Goodpasture syndrome as, 396, 399
    granulomatosis with polyangiitis (Wegener granulomatosis) as, 399–400, 403
    Henoch-Schönlein purpura as, 401–402, 403
    Kawasaki disease as, 401, 403
    large-vessel, 81–82, 403
    medium-vessel, 82–83, 403
    microscopic polyangiitis as, 403
    polyarteritis nodosa as, 397–398, 403
    small-vessel, 83–85, 403
    Takayasu arteritis ("pulseless disease") as, 398–399, 403
    thromboangiitis obliterans (Buerger disease) as, 398, 403

Vasoactive intestinal peptide (VIP), 204
Vasoconstriction, 34, 346
    and blood pressure, 37
Vasoconstrictors, 708
    in autoregulation, 40
Vasodilation, 34
    and blood pressure, 37
Vasodilators, 708
    in autoregulation, 40
    for heart failure, 102
    for hypertension, 97–98
Vasomotor center and mean arterial pressure,
    37, 38
Vaso-occlusive symptoms of sickle cell
    disease, 285
Vasopressin, 117, 118–119. *See also*
    Antidiuretic hormone (ADH)
Vasopressin analog, 125
VC (vital capacity), 761, 762
vCJD (variant Creutzfeldt-Jakob disease), 483
Vecuronium, 510
VEGF (vascular endothelial growth factor)
    molecular therapy targeting, 316
    in wound healing, 361
Veins, 33
    varicose, 73–74
Venlafaxine, 518–519, 540
Venodilators and compliance, 29
Venous disease, 73–75
    deep venous thrombosis as, 74–75
    inferior vena cava syndrome as, 75
    migratory thrombophlebitis (Trousseau
        syndrome) as, 75
    superior vena cava syndrome as, 75
    varicose veins as, 73–74
Venous return
    and cardiac output, 25, 26, 28
    preload and, 25, 28
Venous sinuses of brain, 424–425
Ventilation, 763–770
    airways in, 769–770
    alveolar, 763–765
    lung compliance in, 766
    mechanical, 769
    mechanics of breathing during respiratory
        cycle in, 766–769
    minute, 764
        during pregnancy, 693
Ventilation rate, 764–766
Ventilation/perfusion (V̇/Q̇) mismatch, 774,
    775
    hypoxemia due to, 777–778
Ventilation/perfusion (V̇/Q̇) scanning, 774
Ventral anterior nucleus, 433
Ventral cochlear nucleus, 462
Ventral corticospinal tract, 449, 451
Ventral lateral nucleus, 433
Ventral posterior nucleus, 433
Ventral posterolateral (VPL) nucleus, 433, 452
Ventral posteromedial nucleus, 433
Ventral primary ramus, 332
Ventral respiratory group, 779
Ventral spinal artery, 424
Ventral spinocerebellar tract, 445, 449
Ventral spinothalamic tract, 449
Ventral trigeminal area, 507
Ventral white commissure, 451, 453, 454
Ventricle(s)
    of brain, 420
    cardiac, 9, 10
    primitive, 9
Ventricular action potential, 16, 17, 18
Ventricular compliance, preload and, 25
Ventricular contraction, premature, 51
Ventricular depolarization, 41
Ventricular diastole, 26, 27, 30
Ventricular ejection, 27, 29, 30

Ventricular escape rhythm, 49
Ventricular fibrillation (VF), 51–52
Ventricular filling, 27, 29, 30
Ventricular gallop, 32
Ventricular hypertrophy, 44, 45
Ventricular pressure and mean arterial
    pressure, 38
Ventricular repolarization, 41
Ventricular septal defect (VSD), 4, 5, 7, 70
Ventricular system, 420–422
    malformations of, 468–469, 470
Ventricular systole, 26, 27, 30
Ventricular tachyarrhythmias, 49, 51–52
Ventricular tachycardia, 51
Ventriculomegaly, ex vacuo, 422, 473
Ventrolateral nucleus, 438
Ventromedial nucleus of the hypothalamus
    (VNH), 192, 435, 436
Venule, 33
Verapamil, 97–98, 101, 104
Vermis, 437
Verner-Morrison syndrome, 165, 166
Verrucae, 392
Vertebrae
    anatomy of, 336–338
    fractures and dislocations of, 340
    variations in number of, 329
Vertebral arch, 336
Vertebral artery, 445
Vertebral body, 336, 337
Vertebral column
    bones of, 336–338
    congenital malformations of, 329–330
    development of, 329
Vertebral compression fracture, 367
Vertebral foramen, 337
Vertebral joints, 344
Vertebrobasilar system, 424
Vertigo, 463
Vesicle, 389
Vesicoureteric reflux, 585
Vessel wall abnormalities, hemorrhagic
    disorders due to, 291, 295
Vestibular nucleus, 442, 445
Vestibular pathways, 463
Vestibular schwannoma, 444, 493
Vestibular system, 462, 463
Vestibule, 462
Vestibulocochlear nerve, 459
Vestibulospinal tract, 449
VF (ventricular fibrillation), 51–52
VHL (von Hippel–Lindau) syndrome, 491,
    494, 647
Vibrio cholerae, 203
Villous adenomas, 233
Villus(i), 191, 199, 200, 201
Vinblastine, 314
Vinca alkaloids, 314
Vincristine, 314
VIP (vasoactive intestinal peptide), 204
VIPoma, 165, 166
Viral hepatitis, 242, 243
Viral infection of CNS, 505
Viral meningitis, 419, 420
Virchow triad, 74, 798
Viridans group streptococci, 58
Visceral pain, 191
Visceral peritoneum, 183, 191, 201
Visceral pleura, 750, 755, 756
Visceral sensation, 190–192
Vision, 428, 429
Visual cortex
    association, 429
    lesion of, 461
    primary, 427, 429
Visual field defects, 460, 502

Visual hallucinations, 534
Visual pathway, 459–461, 462
    lesions of, 461
Visual radiation, 460
Visual recognition, 429
Visual system, 459
Vital capacity (VC), 761, 762
Vitamin(s), small intestinal absorption
    of, 202
Vitamin B_1 deficiency, 62
Vitamin B_3, 105
Vitamin B_{12}
    absorption of, 277, 278
    deficiency in, 277–278, 497–498
    methylated, 497
    small intestinal absorption of, 203
Vitamin C
    vessel wall abnormalities due to deficiency
        in, 295
    in wound healing, 361
Vitamin D, 137, 142–143
    in bone metabolism, 324
    in bone remodeling, 367
    deficiency in, 369
    renal formation of, 611
1,25-$(OH)_2$ Vitamin D
    (1,25-dihydroxycholecalciferol), 142,
    143, 611
Vitamin D resistance, 611
Vitamin D toxicity, hypercalcemia due to, 144
Vitamin D_2, 142
Vitamin D_3, 142
Vitamin K deficiency, 291, 294
Vitelline duct, 172
Vitelline veins, 2
Vitiligo, 391
Vitreous chamber, 502
Vm (membrane potential), 15–16
VNH (ventromedial nucleus of the
    hypothalamus), 192, 435, 436
Vocal folds, 348, 749
Vocalis muscles, 348
Volkmann ischemic contracture, 342
Voltage-gated Ca^{2+} channels, 16–17
    in myocardial contraction and relaxation, 22
Voltage-gated K^+ channels, 16
Voltage-gated Na^+ channels, 16
Volume contraction, 598, 599
Volume expansion, 598, 599
Volume overload in pregnancy, 692
Volume-versus-pressure graph, 766
Voluntary stage of swallowing, 194
Volvulus, 175–176
Vomer, 335
Vomiting, 195, 197
Vomiting center, 444
von Hippel–Lindau (VHL) syndrome, 491,
    494, 647
von Recklinghausen disease, 144, 326, 370,
    493
von Willebrand disease, 291, 293
von Willebrand factor (vWF), 292
VPL (ventral posterolateral) nucleus, 433, 452
V̇/Q̇ (ventilation/perfusion) mismatch, 774,
    775
    hypoxemia due to, 777–778
V̇/Q̇ (ventilation/perfusion) scanning, 774
VSD (ventricular septal defect), 4, 5, 7, 70
V_T (tidal volume), 761, 762
    during pregnancy, 693
Vulva, squamous cell carcinoma of, 713
vWF (von Willebrand factor), 292

W

WAGR complex, 649
Waiter tip, 350, 496

Waldenström macroglobulinemia, 295, 305
Wall stress
    and blood pressure, 37
    and cardiac output, 24
Wallenberg syndrome, 444, 445, 478
Wallerian degeneration, 465
Warfarin, 319, 320
Warm antibody hemolytic anemia, 280, 281
Wart(s), 392
    genital, 712–713
Warthin tumor, 213
Water, free, 606
Water balance, regulation of, 614
Water retention due to renal failure, 644
Waterhouse-Friderichsen syndrome, 156
Watershed zones, 184
Waveforms, electrocardiogram, 41–42
WBCs. See White blood cell(s) (WBCs)
WD. See Wolffian duct (WD)
Weber syndrome, 440, 441
Weber test, 463
Wegener granulomatosis, 83–84, 399–400,
        403, 635–636, 797–798
Weight during pregnancy, 695
Wells criteria for pulmonary embolism, 76
Wenckebach AV block, 47–48
Werdnig-Hoffmann disease, 457, 481
Werner syndrome, 135
Wernicke aphasia, 431, 479, 480
Wernicke area, 427, 429, 430
Wernicke-Korsakoff syndrome, 479
Westermark sign, 800
"Wheal-and-flare" reaction, 390–391
Wheezes, 780, 787
Whiplash, 341
Whipple disease, 224–225

Whipple operation, 255
Whipple triad, 164
White blood cell(s) (WBCs), 268–271
White blood cell (WBC) casts, 623
White blood cell (WBC) disorders, 295–306
    Langerhans cell histiocytosis as, 305–306
    leukemias as, 301–304
    leukopenia as, 295–296
    lymphomas as, 297–301
    plasma cell disorders as, 304–305
    reactive proliferation as, 296–297
White communicating rami, 449
White matter, 449
Wickham striae, 210, 394
Wiggers diagram, 29–30
Wilms tumor, 648–649
Wilson disease, 248, 481, 485
Winged scapula, 350, 496
Winslow foramen, 184
Withdrawal
    alcohol, 570
    cannabis, 576
    opiate, 574
    sedative, hypnotic, and anxiolytic, 571
    stimulant, 573
Wolff-Chaikoff effect, 130
Wolffian duct (WD), 584
    derivatives of
        female, 669, 670, 674
        male, 668, 674
    development of, 663, 664
Wolff-Parkinson-White syndrome, 49
Wound healing, 360–361
Wrist drop, 339–340, 350, 496
Wrist joint, 344
Wry neck, 348

X

X chromosome, 662
Xanthine oxidase inhibitors, 405
Xeroderma pigmentosum, 395
Xerophthalmia, 386, 502
Xerostomia, 211–212, 386
Xylometazoline, 820
XYY syndrome, 701

Y

Y chromosome, 662
Yolk sac tumor
    ovarian, 719, 720
    testicular, 737, 738

Z

Z line, 21, 356, 357
Zafirlukast, 822
Zaleplon, 540
Zenker diverticulum, 214
Zileuton, 822
Zinc in wound healing, 361
Ziprasidone, 521, 540
Zoledronate, 402
Zoledronic acid, 368
Zollinger-Ellison syndrome, 165, 222
Zolpidem, 540
Zona fasciculata, 149, 689
Zona glomerulosa, 148–149, 689
Zona pellucida, 684, 687, 691, 692
Zona reticularis, 149, 689
Zone of polarizing activity, 331
Zonular fibers, 502
Zygomatic arch, 336
Zygomatic bones, 335
Zygote, 685, 686, 691

NOTES

NOTES

NOTES

NOTES

NOTES

NOTES

NOTES

NOTES

About the Senior Editors

Tao Le, MD, MHS

Tao developed a passion for medical education as a medical student. He currently edits more than 15 titles in the *First Aid* series. In addition, he is Founder and Chief Education Officer of USMLE-Rx for exam preparation and ScholarRx for undergraduate medical education. As a medical student, he was editor-in-chief of the University of California, San Francisco (UCSF) *Synapse*, a university newspaper with a weekly circulation of 9000. Tao earned his medical degree from UCSF in 1996 and completed his residency training in internal medicine at Yale University and fellowship training at Johns Hopkins University. Tao subsequently went on to cofound Medsn, a medical education technology venture, and served as its chief medical officer. He is currently chief of adult allergy and immunology at the University of Louisville.

William L. Hwang, MD, PhD

William is currently a resident physician-scientist in the Harvard Radiation Oncology Program. He previously completed an Internal Medicine internship at Massachusetts General Hospital. In 2015, William graduated summa cum laude from the Harvard-MIT MD-PhD program and was awarded the Seidman Prize for Best Senior Thesis. He earned his PhD in Biophysics in the laboratory of Xiaowei Zhuang, elucidating the mechanism and regulation of chromatin remodeling using a combination of single-molecule biophysics and molecular biology approaches. Prior to that, William completed his undergraduate studies at Duke University with degrees in Biomedical Engineering, Electrical and Computer Engineering, and Physics on an Angier B Duke Scholarship. He then made the hop across the pond to complete a Masters in Chemistry at the University of Oxford as a Rhodes Scholar. Outside of the clinic/lab, he is passionate about educational outreach and directs a nonprofit educational organization, United InnoWorks Academy, which develops innovative STEM programs for underserved youth. In his free time, he enjoys traveling with his wife, Katie, and playing volleyball.

About the Editors

Vinayak Muralidhar, MD, MSc

Vinayak is currently an intern in internal medicine at Brigham and Women's Hospital and will be starting a residency in radiation oncology at the Harvard Radiation Oncology Program in July 2017. He earned an MD magna cum laude from the joint Harvard-MIT Health Sciences and Technology program, where he conducted basic research in cancer metabolism and clinical research in prostate cancer. His work in medical school was awarded the Soma Weiss Award for Medical Student Research and the Elizabeth D. Hay Award for Basic Science Research. Vinayak also earned an MSc with Distinction in Evidence-Based Social Intervention from the University of Oxford on a Marshall Scholarship, where he studied selective outcome reporting bias in clinical trials. He attended MIT as an undergraduate, where he earned degrees in mathematics and biology and was named by *USA Today* to the 2010 All-USA College Academic First Team.

Jared A. White, MD

This is Jared's third project with the First Aid team. He previously served as an author of *First Aid for the USMLE Step 1, 2015* and as a question writer on *USMLE-Rx Step 1 Qmax*. Jared grew up in the town of Taylorsville, Mississippi. He completed his undergraduate degree at Belhaven University in Jackson, Mississippi and attended the University of Mississippi School of Medicine. He is currently completing a residency in plastic surgery at the University of Florida, College of Medicine. Jared's greatest joy in life is his family. He and his wife, Morgan, have two children, John and Hazel.

M. Scott Moore, DO

Scott's passions in medicine are clinical pathology, osteopathy, and education. After earning an AAS degree in clinical laboratory sciences and a BA in German from Weber State University, a DO from Midwestern University's Arizona College of Osteopathic Medicine, and completing a pathology internship at the University of Arizona, he was hired as a clinical research fellow at Affiliated Dermatology in Scottsdale. He and his wife have been married since college and they just welcomed twins to their family. In his free time he is an avid runner, guitarist, his wife's sous-chef, and plays his fair share of peek-a-boo.

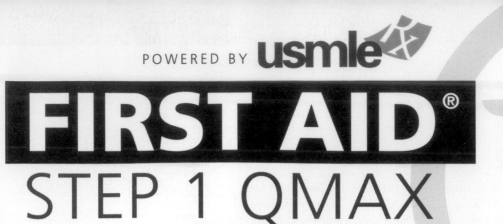
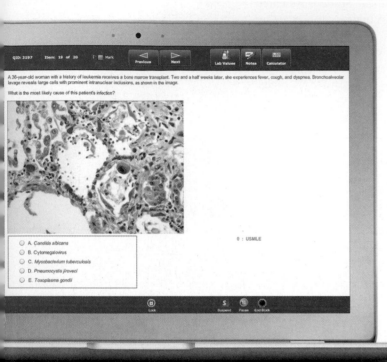
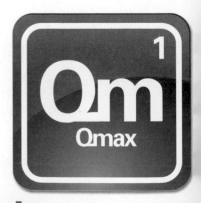